Pharmacology

For Churchill Livingstone:

Commissioning editor: Laurence Hunter
Project editor: Barbara Simmons
Project controller: Nancy Arnott
Design direction: Erik Bigland

Pharmacology

H. P. Rang MB BS MA DPhil FRS

Senior Research Associate, Novartis Institute for Medical Sciences, London;
Professor of Pharmacology, University College, London

M. M. Dale MB BCh PhD

Senior Teaching Fellow, Department of Pharmacology, University of Oxford;
Honorary Lecturer, Department of Pharmacology, University College, London

J. M. Ritter MA DPhil FRCP

Professor of Clinical Pharmacology, The Guy's, King's College and St Thomas' Hospitals' Medical and Dental School,
King's College, London

Illustrations by Peter Lamb

FOURTH EDITION

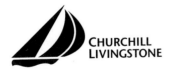

CHURCHILL LIVINGSTONE

EDINBURGH LONDON NEW YORK PHILADELPHIA SYDNEY TORONTO 1999

CHURCHILL LIVINGSTONE
A Division of Harcourt Publishers Limited

Churchill Livingstone, 1–3 Baxter's Place, Leith Walk, Edinburgh EH1 3AF

First edition 1987
Second edition 1991
Third edition 1995
Fourth edition 1999
Reprinted 2000

Standard edition ISBN 0443 059748
International edition ISBN 0443 059942
Reprinted 2000

British Library of Cataloguing in Publication Data
A catalogue record for this book is available from the British Library.

Library of Congress Cataloging in Publication Data
A catalog record for this book is available from the Library of Congress.

Medical knowledge is constantly changing. As information becomes available, changes in treatment, procedures, equipment and the use of drugs become necessary. The authors and publisher have, as far as it is possible, taken care to ensure that the information given in the text is accurate and up-to-date. However, readers are strongly advised to confirm that the information, especially with regard to drug usage, complies with current legislation and standard of practice.

The
publisher's
policy is to use
**paper manufactured
from sustainable forests**

Printed in China
GCC/01

Preface

For this fourth edition, as in the previous three, our approach has been not only to describe what drugs do, but to emphasise the mechanisms by which they act – where possible at the cellular and molecular level. Therapeutic agents have a high rate of obsolescence and many new ones are introduced each year; an appreciation of the mechanisms of action of the class of drugs to which a new agent belongs provides a good starting point for understanding and using it intelligently.

In this edition, we have changed colour – from angry red to cool blue. All our diagrams have been updated and redrawn, and many new figures have been added. Continuing the procedure used in earlier editions we have, wherever feasible, used real data in our diagrams rather than notional information. As before, we have put emphasis on the chemical structures of those drugs for which knowledge of structure/activity relationships enhances appreciation of how the drugs act, and we have omitted many chemical structures which do not add to pharmacological understanding in favour of diagrams which do.

All chapters have been updated. As regards new material, we have taken into account not only new agents but also recent extensions of basic knowledge which presage further drug development, and, where possible, we have given a brief outline of new treatments in the pipeline. To keep the book to the same manageable size, we have cut down sections of the previous edition that were growing obsolete.

There are two new chapters: on 'Obesity' and 'Gene therapy'.

The chapter on method and measurement in pharmacology includes more information on the assessment of drug effects in man, with a discussion of the principles of risk-benefit analysis.

Because many students feel overwhelmed by the number of drugs available and the plethora of drug names, we have sought to lighten the burden by providing a list of the most important agents as an appendix, divided into those of primary and those of secondary interest.

The section on molecular aspects of drug action – an area moving so fast it can quickly get out of sight – has been brought up to date and new information on signal transduction has been included. There has been significant revision of the following topics:

- cardiovascular pharmacology (reflecting the increasing and impressively evidence-based use of statins)
- peptides and proteins as mediators
- nitric oxide
- drugs acting on 5-HT receptors
- approaches to the treatment of HIV infection
- neurodegenerative disorders and approaches to their treatment.

In addition, we have emphasised the significant progress in the understanding of the biology of cancer (including the trendy new area of apoptosis) which is expected to lead to new anticancer therapies in the near future.

Inappropriate immune and inflammatory responses are involved in many if not most of the diseases which the clinician will meet, and the development of drugs to control these processes is a major concern of the pharmaceutical industry. Students of both pharmacology and medicine need to be aware of developments in these fields. Accordingly, the sections on inflammation and allergy and the drugs used in inflammatory and immune diseases have been substantially revised.

To make the book more manageable, we have split some of the chapters in earlier editions. For example, the chapter on 'Absorption, distribution and fate of drugs' in the third edition has been divided into two new chapters; 'Absorption and distribution' and Drug elimination and pharmacokinetics' while the material on endocrines has been dispersed into three chapters: 'The pituitary and adrenal cortex', 'The thyroid' and 'Bone metabolism'.

We have again incorporated short sets of key points, set off in boxes throughout the text. These are not intended to be comprehensive summaries but rather to highlight pharmacological information that we consider important. Factual knowledge in pharmacology is so extensive and expanding so rapidly that students can easily find the information load daunting. Our key point boxes are intended to make it easier for students to get to grips with the essentials of the subject.

As in the third edition, the therapeutic uses of drugs has been given prominence by setting it out in easily identified 'clinical boxes'.

Pharmacology is a lively scientific discipline in its own right, with an importance beyond that of providing a basis for the use of drugs in therapy. We have, therefore, where appropriate, included brief coverage of the use of drugs as probes for elucidating cellular and physiological functions, even when the compounds have no clinical uses. Above all, we hope to communicate some of our own unflagging enthusiasm for the science of pharmacology.

It was gratifying to find that many readers found helpful the short summaries of relevant physiological and biochemical processes which we had placed at the beginning of most chapters to form a basis for the subsequent discussion of pharmacological actions; we have therefore retained these. To cater for graduate students and university teachers who apparently found the previous editions useful, we have included fairly extensive sections on 'References and further reading' at the end of each chapter. Mindful of the fact that the medical curriculum now stresses project work and the preparation of special study modules, many references have been annotated to emphasise aspects of their coverage and make them easier for students to use.

We are grateful to the readers who have written appreciative letters about the book and particularly to those who made constructive comments, which we have done our best to incorporate. Comments on the new edition will be welcome.

ACKNOWLEDGEMENTS

We would like to thank the following for their help and advice in the preparation of this edition: Professor J. Mandelstam, Dr M. Weber, Dr T.C. Cunnane, Professor R.J.P. Williams, Sir John Vane and the staff of the Royal Society of Medicine Library.

London 1999

H. P. Rang
M. M. Dale
J. M. Ritter

Contents

SECTION 3
DRUGS AFFECTING MAJOR ORGAN SYSTEMS

SECTION 4
THE CENTRAL NERVOUS SYSTEM

GENERAL PRINCIPLES

1

How drugs act: general principles

Pharmacology can be defined as the study of the manner in which the function of living systems is affected by chemical agents. It is a rather young science, having first achieved independent recognition at the end of the 19th century in Germany. Long before this, of course, herbal remedies were widely used, but there was a surprising reluctance to apply anything resembling scientific principles to therapeutics. Even Robert Boyle, who laid the scientific foundations of chemistry in the middle of the 17th century, was content, when dealing with therapeutics (*A Collection of Choice Remedies*, 1692), to recommend concoctions of worms, dung, urine and the moss from a dead man's skull. Indeed, therapeutics only began to be influenced by science in the mid-19th century, at which time Virchow dismissed the subject thus: 'Therapeutics is in an empirical stage cared for by practical doctors and clinicians, and it is by means of a combination with physiology that it must rise to be a science, which today it is not.' At that time, knowledge of the normal and abnormal functioning of the body was too rudimentary to provide even a rough basis for understanding drug effects; at the same time disease and death were regarded as semi-sacred subjects, appropriately dealt with by authoritarian, rather than scientific, doctrines. Clinical practice often displayed an obedience to authority, and

ignored what appear to be easily ascertainable facts. Thus, cinchona bark was recognised as a specific and effective treatment for malaria, and a sound protocol for its use was laid down by Lind in 1765. In 1804, however, Johnson declared it to be unsafe until the fever had subsided, and he recommended instead the use of large doses of calomel in the early stages—a murderous piece of advice, which was nonetheless generally followed for the next 40 years.

DRUGS IN MEDICINE

Repeated attempts were made to construct systems of therapeutics, many of which produced even worse results than pure empiricism. One of these was *allopathy*, espoused by James Gregory (1735–1821). The favoured remedies included blood-letting, emetics and purgatives, used until the dominant symptoms of the disease were suppressed. Many patients died from such treatment, and it was in reaction against it that Hahnemann introduced the practice of *homoeopathy* in the early 19th century. The guiding principles of homoeopathy are:

- like cures like
- activity can be enhanced by dilution.

The system rapidly drifted into absurdity: for example, Hahnemann recommended the use of drugs at dilutions of $1:10^{60}$, equivalent to 1 molecule in a sphere the size of the orbit of Neptune.

Many other systems of therapeutics have come and gone, and the variety of dogmatic principles that they embodied have tended to hinder rather than advance scientific progress.*

---

*Therapeutic systems whose basis lies outside the domain of science are, of course, very much alive today, and they are even gaining ground under the general banner of 'alternative' or 'holistic' medicine. Mostly they reject the 'medical model' which attributes disease to an underlying derangement of normal function that can

Drugs have, for many years, been the most widely used form of therapeutic intervention available to doctors. Reliance on natural products, mainly from plants, predominated until, in the 1920s, synthetic chemicals were first introduced, and the modern pharmaceutical industry began to develop.* Natural products remain an important source of new drugs, but most are now synthetic chemicals.

Scientific understanding of drug action—the kind of understanding that enables us to predict the pharmacological effects of a novel chemical substance, or to design a chemical that will produce a specified therapeutic effect—is growing rapidly, but is still far from complete. Even so, certain generalisations are possible, and these are discussed in this chapter.

To begin with, we should gratefully acknowledge Paul Ehrlich for insisting early in this century that drug action should be understood in terms of conventional chemical interactions between drugs and tissues, and for dispelling the idea that the remarkable potency and specificity of action of some drugs put them somehow out of reach of chemistry and physics and required the intervention of magical 'vital forces'. Although it is the case that many drugs produce actions in doses and concentrations so small that the dimensions assume an almost astronomical remoteness, low concentrations still involve very large numbers of molecules. Thus one drop of a solution of a drug at only 10^{-10} mol/l still contains about 10^{10} drug-molecules, so there is no mystery in the fact that it may

produce an obvious pharmacological response. Some bacterial toxins (e.g. diphtheria toxin) act with such precision that a single molecule taken up by a target cell is sufficient to kill it.

THE BINDING OF DRUG MOLECULES TO CELLS

One of the basic tenets of pharmacology is that drug molecules must exert some chemical influence on one or more constituents of cells in order to produce a pharmacological response. In other words, drug molecules must get so close to these constituent cellular molecules that their function is altered. Of course, the molecules in the organism vastly outnumber the drug molecules and if the drug molecules were merely distributed at random, the chance of interaction with any particular class of cellular molecule would be negligible. Pharmacological effects therefore require, in general, the non-uniform distribution of the drug molecule within the body or tissue, which is the same as saying that drug molecules must be 'bound' to particular constituents of cells and tissues in order to produce an effect. Ehrlich summed it up thus: '*Corpora non agunt nisi fixata*' (in this context, 'A drug will not work unless it is bound').**

Understanding the nature of these binding sites, and the mechanisms by which the association of a drug molecule with a binding site leads to a physiological response, constitutes the major thrust of pharmacological research. Most drugs produce their effects by binding, in the first instance, to protein molecules. Even apparent exceptions, such as general anaesthetics (see Ch. 32), which have long been thought to produce their effects by an interaction with membrane lipid, now appear to interact mainly with membrane proteins (see Franks & Lieb 1994). The only important exception to proteins as target sites is DNA, on which a number of antitumour and antimicrobial drugs act (Ch. 41), as well as mutagenic and carcinogenic agents (Ch. 49).

PROTEIN TARGETS FOR DRUG BINDING

Four kinds of regulatory proteins are commonly involved as primary drug targets, namely:

- enzymes
- carrier molecules

be defined in biochemical or structural terms, detected by objective means, and influenced beneficially by appropriate chemical or physical interventions. They focus instead mainly on subjective malaise, which may be disease-associated or not. Abandoning objectivity in defining and measuring disease goes along with a similar departure from scientific principles in assessing therapeutic efficacy, with the result that principles and practices can gain acceptance without satisfying any of the criteria of validity that would convince a critical scientist, and that are required by law to be satisfied before a new drug can be introduced into therapy. Public acceptance, alas, has little to do with demonstrable efficacy.

*In recent years, biotechnology has emerged as a major source of new therapeutic agents in the form of antibodies, enzymes and various regulatory proteins, including hormones, growth factors and cytokines (see Buckel 1996). Though such biotechnology products are generally produced in a very different way from conventional drugs, the pharmacological principles are essentially the same. Gene therapy and cell-based therapies (see Ch. 50), though still in their infancy, will take therapeutics into a new domain. The principles governing the design, delivery and control of functioning artificial genes introduced into cells, or of engineered cells introduced into the body, are very different from those of drug-based therapeutics, and will require a different conceptual framework, which texts such as this will increasingly need to embrace if they are to stay abreast of modern medical treatment.

**There are, if one looks hard enough, exceptions to Ehrlich's dictum, drugs which act without being bound to any tissue constituent (for example osmotic diuretics, osmotic purgatives, antacids, heavy metal chelating agents). Nonetheless, the principle remains true for the great majority.

- ion channels
- receptors.

A few other types of protein (e.g. structural proteins such as tubulin, which specifically binds **colchicine**; Ch. 13) are known to function as drug targets, and it must be remembered that there exist many drugs whose sites of action are not yet known. Furthermore, many drugs are known to bind (in addition to their primary targets) to plasma proteins (see Ch. 4), as well as to cellular constituents, without producing any obvious physiological effect. Nevertheless, the generalisation that most drugs act on one or other of the four types of protein listed above serves as a good starting point.

Further discussion of the mechanisms by which such binding leads to cellular responses is given in Chapter 2.

A NOTE ON TERMINOLOGY

The term *receptor* tends to be used loosely, and can cause confusion. Some authors use it to mean *any* target molecule with which a drug molecule has to combine in order to elicit its specific effect, which can include any of the four types listed. Thus, the voltage-sensitive sodium channel of excitable membranes is sometimes referred to as the 'receptor' for local anaesthetics (see Ch. 40), or the enzyme dihydrofolate reductase as the 'receptor' for **methotrexate** (Ch. 42). In each case the drug molecule combines with and incapacitates the protein molecule, thus producing its effect. This is different from the situation where, for example, **adrenaline** acts on a receptor in the heart (see Ch. 8). In this case, the primary function of the receptor molecule is to serve as a recognition site for catecholamines. When adrenaline binds to the receptor, a train of reactions is initiated (see Ch. 2), leading to an increase in force and rate of the heartbeat. The receptor produces an effect only when adrenaline is bound; otherwise it is functionally silent.* This, in general, is true of all receptors for endogenous mediators (hormones, neurotransmitters, cytokines, etc.). There is a distinction between *agonists*, which 'activate' the receptors, and *antagonists*, which may combine at the same site without causing activation. Receptors of this type form a key part of the system of chemical communication that all multicellular organisms use to coordinate the activities of their cells and organs. Without them we would be no better than a bucketful of amoebae. The distinction between agonists and antagonists only exists for receptors with

this type of physiological regulatory role; we cannot usefully speak of 'agonists' for the noradrenaline carrier or for the voltage-sensitive sodium channel or for dihydrofolate reductase. In pharmacology it is best to reserve the term 'receptor' for interactions of the regulatory type, where the small molecule (*ligand*) may function either as an agonist or as an antagonist; in practice this limits use of the term to receptors which have a physiological regulatory function, and this usage will be observed in this book.** More details about the molecular nature of receptors, and the ways in which they influence cell function, are given in Chapter 2.

DRUG SPECIFICITY

For a drug to be useful as either a therapeutic or a scientific tool, it must act selectively on particular cells and tissues. In other words it must show a high degree of *binding-site specificity*. Conversely, proteins that function as drug targets generally show a high degree of *ligand specificity*; they will recognise only ligands of a certain precise type, and ignore closely related molecules.

These principles of binding-site and ligand specificity can be clearly recognised in the actions of a mediator such as angiotensin (Ch. 15). This peptide acts strongly on vascular smooth muscle, and on the kidney tubule, but has very little effect on other kinds of smooth muscle, or on the intestinal epithelium. Other mediators affect a quite different spectrum of cells and tissues, the pattern in each case being determined by the specific pattern of expression of the protein receptors for the various mediators. On the other hand, a small chemical change, such as conversion of one of the amino acids in angiotensin from L- to D-form, or removal of one amino acid from the chain, can inactivate the molecule altogether, since the receptor fails to bind the altered form. The complementary specificity of ligands and binding sites, which gives rise to the very exact molecular recognition properties of proteins, is central to explaining many of the phenomena of pharmacology. It is no exaggeration to say that the ability of proteins to interact in a highly selective way with other molecules—including other proteins—is the basis of living machines. Its relevance to the understanding of drug action will be a recurring theme in this book.

Finally, it must be emphasised that no drug acts with

---

*Actually some receptors, such as the benzodiazepine receptor (Ch. 33) show resting activity, which can be either increased or decreased when a ligand molecule binds (see p. 10).

**We break our own rule in Chapter 16 by referring to the 'LDL receptor', a term in common usage to describe a macromolecule—not strictly a receptor according to our definition—which plays a key role in lipoprotein metabolism.

complete specificity. Thus histamine antagonists (Ch. 13), although they can be shown to have a higher affinity for histamine receptors than for other sites, produce many effects, such as sedation and prevention of vomiting, which do not appear to depend on histamine antagonism. In general, the lower the potency of a drug, and the higher the dose needed, the more likely it is that sites of action other than the primary one will assume significance. In clinical terms, this is often associated with the appearance of unwanted side-effects, of which no drug is free.

A major aim of pharmacological research is to identify and characterise, in molecular terms, the protein targets of many different types of drug. This has revealed the mode of action of many drugs, such as **opiate analgesics** (Ch. 37), **cannabinoids** (Ch. 39), and **benzodiazepine tranquillisers** (Ch. 33), whose actions were described in exhaustive detail for many years without yielding any clues about the molecular basis of their effects. All have now been shown to target well-defined receptors, which have been fully characterised by gene-cloning techniques (see Ch. 2).

RECEPTOR CLASSIFICATION

Where the action of a drug can be associated with a particular receptor, this provides a valuable means for classification and refinement in drug design. For example, pharmacological analysis of the actions of histamine (see Ch. 12) showed that some of its effects (the H_1 effects, such as smooth muscle contraction) were strongly antagonised by the competitive histamine antagonists then known. Black and his colleagues, in 1970, suggested that the remaining actions of histamine, which included its stimulant effect on gastric secretion, might represent a second class of histamine receptor (H_2). Testing a number

of histamine analogues, they found that some were selective in producing H_2 effects, with little H_1 activity. By analysing which parts of the histamine molecule conferred this type of specificity, they were able to develop selective antagonists, which proved to be potent in blocking gastric acid secretion, a development of major therapeutic significance (Ch. 21). A third type of histamine receptor (H_3) has recently been defined.

This example illustrates the principle of receptor classification based on pharmacological criteria—receptors being classified on the basis of the effects of particular drugs—which continues to be a valuable and widely-used approach. Newer experimental approaches have subsequently revealed several different criteria on which to base receptor classification. The first of these was the direct measurement of ligand binding to receptors (see p. 11), which allowed many new receptor subclasses to be defined—subclasses only very dimly discernible from studies of drug effects. More recently, molecular cloning has revealed the amino acid sequence of many receptors (see Ch. 2), providing a completely new basis for classification at a much finer level of detail than can be reached through pharmacological analysis. Finally, analysis of the biochemical pathways that are activated in response to receptor activation (see Ch. 2) shows patterns that provide yet another basis for classification. The result of this data explosion has been that receptor classification has suddenly become very much more detailed, with a proliferation of receptor subtypes for all of the main types of ligand; more worryingly, alternative molecular and biochemical classifications began to spring up which were incompatible with the accepted pharmacologically defined receptor classes. Responding to this growing confusion, the International Union of Pharmacological Sciences (IUPHAR) has set up various expert working groups to produce agreed receptor classifications for the major types, taking into account the pharmacological, molecular and biochemical information available.* These wise men have a hard task; their conclusions will be neither perfect nor final, but are essential to ensure a consistent terminology. To the student, this may seem an arcane exercise in taxonomy, generating much detail but little illumination; the tedious lists of drug names, actions and side-effects that used to burden the subject are in danger of being replaced by exhaustive tables of receptors, ligands and transduction pathways. In this book, we have tried to avoid detail for its own sake, and include only such information on receptor classification as seems

---

Targets for drug action

- A drug is a chemical that affects physiological function in a *specific way*.
- Most drugs are effective because they bind to particular target proteins, namely:
  —enzymes
  —carriers
  —ion channels
  —receptors.
- Specificity is reciprocal: individual classes of drug bind only to certain targets, and individual targets recognise only certain classes of drug.
- No drugs are completely specific in their actions. In many cases, increasing the dose of a drug will cause it to affect targets other than the principal one, and lead to side-effects.

---

*Published as The IUPHAR compendium of receptor characterization and classification 1998. IUPHAR Media, London.

interesting in its own right, or is helpful in explaining the actions of important drugs. A useful summary of known receptor classes is now published annually (*Trends in Pharmacological Sciences, Receptor Supplement*).

QUANTITATIVE ASPECTS OF DRUG–RECEPTOR INTERACTIONS

The first step in drug action on specific receptors is the formation of a reversible drug–receptor complex, the reactions being governed by the Law of Mass Action. Suppose that a piece of tissue, such as heart muscle or smooth muscle, contains a total number of receptors N_{tot} for an agonist such as adrenaline. When the tissue is exposed to adrenaline at concentration x_A and allowed to come to equilibrium, a certain number N_A of the receptors will become occupied, and the number of vacant receptors will be reduced to $N_{tot} - N_A$. Normally the number of adrenaline molecules applied to the tissue in solution greatly exceeds N_{tot}, so that the binding reaction does not appreciably reduce x_A. The magnitude of the response produced by the adrenaline will be related (even if we do not know exactly how) to the number of receptors occupied, so it is useful to consider what quantitative relationship is predicted between N_A and x_A. The reaction can be represented by:

$$\begin{array}{cccc} A & + & R & \underset{k_{-1}}{\overset{k_{+1}}{\rightleftharpoons}} & AR \\ \text{drug} & & \text{free receptor} & & \text{complex} \\ (x_A) & & (N_{tot} - N_A) & & (N_A) \end{array}$$

The Law of Mass Action (which states that the rate of a chemical reaction is proportional to the product of the concentrations of reactants) can be applied to this reaction.

$$\text{Rate of forward reaction} = k_{+1}x_A(N_{tot} - N_A) \quad (1.1)$$

$$\text{Rate of backward reaction} = k_{-1}N_A \quad (1.2)$$

At equilibrium the two rates are equal:

$$k_{+1}x_A(N_{tot} - N_A) = k_{-1}N_A \quad (1.3)$$

The proportion of receptors occupied or 'occupancy', $p_A = N_A/N_{tot}$, which is independent of N_{tot}, is:

$$p_A = \frac{x_A}{x_A + k_{-1}/k_{+1}} \quad (1.4)$$

Defining the equilibrium constant for the binding reaction, $K_A = k_{-1}/k_{+1}$, equation (1.4) can be written:

$$p_A = \frac{x_A}{x_A + K_A} \quad \text{or} \quad p_A = \frac{x_A/K_A}{x_A/K_A + 1} \quad (1.5)$$

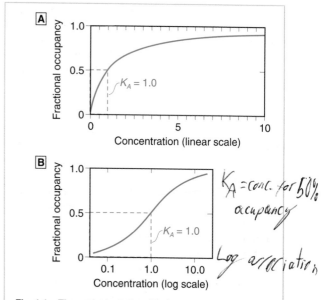

Fig. 1.1 **Theoretical relationship between occupancy and ligand concentration, plotted according to equation (1.5).** **A** Plotted with a linear concentration scale, this curve is a rectangular hyperbola. **B** Plotted with a logarithmic concentration scale, it is a symmetrical sigmoid curve.

[handwritten: $K_A = $ conc. for 50% occupancy]

[handwritten: Log association]

This important result is known as the *Hill–Langmuir equation.**

The equilibrium constant, K_A, is a characteristic of the drug and of the receptor; it has the dimensions of concentration and is numerically equal to the concentration of drug required to occupy 50% of the sites at equilibrium. (Verify from equation (1.5) that when $x_A = K_A$, $P_A = 0.5$.) The higher the *affinity* of the drug for the receptors, the lower will be K_A. Equation (1.5) describes the relationship between occupancy and drug concentration, and generates a characteristic curve known as a *rectangular hyperbola*, as shown in Figure 1.1A. It is common in pharmacological work to use a logarithmic scale of concentration; this converts the hyperbola to a symmetrical sigmoid curve (Fig. 1.1B).

AGONIST CONCENTRATION–EFFECT CURVES

The binding of drugs to their receptors in tissues can be measured directly (see p. 11) and shown to obey equation

---

*A. V. Hill first published it in 1909, when he was still a medical student. Langmuir, a physical chemist working on gas adsorption, derived it independently in 1916. Both subsequently won Nobel prizes. Until recently, it was known to pharmacologists as the Langmuir equation, even though Hill deserves the credit.

(1.5). Usually, however, it is a biological response, such as a rise in blood pressure, contraction or relaxation of a strip of smooth muscle in an organ bath, or the activation of an enzyme, that is actually measured and plotted as a *concentration–effect* or *dose–response curve*, as in Figure 1.2. Though they look similar to the theoretical concentration–occupancy curves in Figure 1.1B, they cannot be used to measure the affinity of agonist drugs for their receptors, since the physiological response produced is not, as a rule, directly proportional to occupancy. For an integrated physiological response, such as a rise in arterial blood pressure produced by adrenaline, many factors interact. Adrenaline (see Ch. 8) increases cardiac output and constricts some blood vessels while dilating others, and the change in arterial pressure itself evokes a reflex response which modifies the primary response to the drug. It is obviously unrealistic to expect that the final effect will be directly proportional to occupancy in this instance, and the same is true of most drug-induced effects.

A second difficulty in drawing inferences about agonist affinity from concentration–effect curves is that the concentration of the drug *at the receptors* is often not known, even though the concentration in the organ bath is simple to calculate. Thus agonists may be subject to rapid enzymic degradation or uptake by cells as they diffuse from the surface towards their site of action, and a steady state can be reached in which the agonist concentration at the receptors is very much less than the concen-

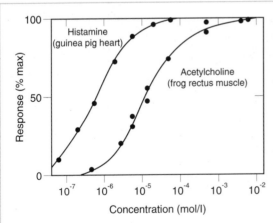

Fig. 1.2 Experimentally observed concentration–effect curves. Though the lines, drawn according to the binding equation (1.5), fit the points well, such curves do not give correct estimates of the affinity of drugs for receptors. This is because the relationship between receptor occupancy and response is usually non-linear.

Binding of drugs to receptors

- Binding of drugs to receptors necessarily obeys the Law of Mass Action.
- At equilibrium, *receptor occupancy* is related to *drug concentration* by the *Hill–Langmuir equation*.
- The higher the *affinity* of the drug for the receptor, the lower the concentration at which it produces a given level of occupancy.
- The same principles apply when two or more drugs compete for the same receptors; each has the effect of reducing the apparent affinity for the other.

tration in the bath. In the case of **acetylcholine**, for example, which is hydrolysed by cholinesterase present in most tissues (see Ch. 7), the concentration reaching the receptors can be less than 1% of that in the bath, and an even bigger difference has been found with **noradrenaline**, which is avidly taken up by sympathetic nerve terminals in many tissues (see Ch. 8). Thus, even if the concentration–effect curve looks just like a facsimile of the binding curve, as in Figure 1.2, it cannot be used directly to determine the affinity of the agonist for the receptors.

COMPETITIVE ANTAGONISM

Equation (1.5) describes the relationship between concentration and occupancy when a single drug is present. The treatment can easily be extended to describe the situation when two or more competing drugs are present. 'Competing' means that the receptor can bind only one drug molecule at a time. Applying the same Mass Action rules as before, the occupancy equation becomes:

$$p_A = \frac{x_A/K_A}{x_A/K_A + x_B/K_B + 1} \quad (1.6)$$

Comparing this result with equation (1.5) shows that adding drug B (the competitive antagonist), as expected, reduces the occupancy by drug A, if the concentration of A is kept the same. Alternatively, the concentration of A may be increased (to x_A' say) so as to restore p_A, to the value reached in the absence of the antagonist, the ratio r (= x_A'/x_A), by which the concentration will need to be increased, is given (from equations 1.5 and 1.6) by:

$$r = \frac{x_B}{K_B} + 1 \quad (1.7)$$

If it is assumed that the response of the test system depends only on the agonist occupancy p_A', then it is predicted from the theory given above that the effect of the competitive antagonist on the response can also

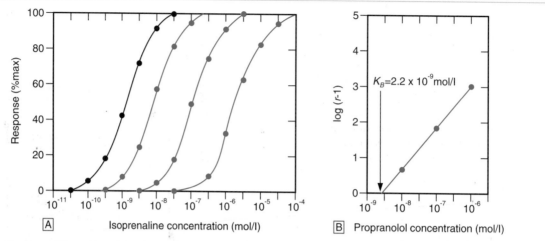

Fig. 1.3 **Competitive antagonism of isoprenaline by propranolol measured on isolated guinea-pig atria.** [A] Concentration–effect curves at various propranolol concentrations (indicated on the curves). Note the progressive shift to the right without a change of slope or maximum. [B] Schild plot (equation 1.8). The equilibrium constant (K) for propranolol is given by the abscissal intercept 2.2×10^{-9} mol/l. (Results from: Potter L T 1967 J Pharmacol 155: 91)

be overcome by increasing the agonist concentration r-fold. Equation (1.7) is therefore useful experimentally, because it should apply to measurements of biological responses as well as to direct measurements of agonist binding. Equation (1.7), which is often known as the *Schild equation* after its originator, predicts two characteristic properties of competitive antagonism:

- The dose ratio r depends *only* on the concentration and equilibrium constant of the antagonist, and not on the size of response that is chosen as a reference point for the measurements, nor on the equilibrium constant for the agonist. On a semi-logarithmic plot of effect against concentration, therefore, the effect of the competitive antagonist will be to shift the curve to the right without changing its slope or maximum, a characteristic that can easily be tested experimentally.
- The dose ratio achieved should increase linearly with x_B, and the slope of a plot of $(r-1)$ against x_B is equal to $1/K_B$.* This relationship, being independent of the characteristics of the agonist, should be the same for all agonists that act on the same population of receptors.

These equations have been verified for many examples of competitive antagonism (Fig. 1.3).

PARTIAL AGONISTS AND THE CONCEPT OF EFFICACY

So far, we have considered drugs either as *agonists*, which in some way 'activate' the receptor when they

occupy it, or as *antagonists*, which cause no activation. However, the ability of a drug molecule to activate the receptor is actually a graded, rather than an all-or-nothing, property. If a series of chemically related agonist drugs acting on the same receptors is tested on a given biological system, it is often found that the maximal response (the largest response that can be produced by that drug in high concentration) differs from one drug to another. Some compounds (known as *full agonists*) can produce a maximal response (the largest response that the tissue is capable of giving), whereas others (*partial agonists*) can only produce a submaximal response (Fig. 1.4). The difference between full and partial agonists lies in the relationship between occupancy and response.

Figure 1.5 shows the relationship between occupancy and concentration for drugs whose equilibrium constant is 1.0 μmol/l. Drug *a* is a full agonist, producing a

---

*Equation (1.7) can be expressed logarithmically in the form:

$$\log(r-1) = \log x_B - \log K_B \qquad (1.8)$$

Thus a plot of $\log(r-1)$ against $\log x_B$, usually called a *Schild plot*, should give a straight line with unit slope and an abscissal intercept equal to $\log K_B$. Following the pH and pK notation, antagonist potency can be expressed as a pA_2 value; under conditions of competitive antagonism $pA_2 = -\log K_B$. Numerically, pA_2 is defined as *the negative logarithm of the molar concentration of antagonist required to produce an agonist dose ratio equal to 2*. As with pH notation, its principal advantage is that it produces simple numbers, a pA_2 of 6.5 being equivalent to $K_B = 3.2 \times 10^{-7}$ mol/l.

Competitive antagonism

- *Reversible competitive antagonism* is the commonest and most important type of antagonism, and has two main characteristics:
  - in the presence of the antagonist, the agonist log-concentration–effect curve is shifted to the right without change in slope or maximum, the extent of the shift being a measure of the *dose ratio*
  - the dose ratio increases *linearly* with antagonist concentration; the slope of this line is a measure of the affinity of the antagonist for the receptor.
- Antagonist affinity, measured in this way, is widely used as a basis for receptor classification.

maximal response at about 0.2 µmol/l, the relationship between response and occupancy is shown by the steep curve in B. Comparable plots for a partial agonist are shown as the shallow curves in A and B, the essential difference being that the response at any given occupancy is much smaller for the partial agonist, which cannot produce a maximal response even at 100% occupancy. This can be expressed quantitatively in terms of *efficacy*, a parameter originally defined by Stephenson (1956) which describes the 'strength' of a single drug–receptor complex in evoking a response of the tissue. Subsequently, it was appreciated that characteristics of the

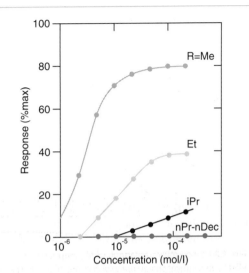

Fig. 1.4 Partial agonists. Concentration–effect curves for substituted methonium compounds on frog *rectus abdominis* muscle. The compounds were members of the decamethonium series (Ch. 7), R Me$_2$ N$^+$(CH$_2$)$_{10}$ N$^+$ Me$_2$ R. The maximum response obtainable decreases (i.e. efficacy decreases) as the size of R is increased. With R = nPr or larger, the compounds cause no response, and are pure antagonists. (Results from: Van Rossum J M 1958 Pharmacodynamics of cholinometic and cholinolytic drugs. St Catherine's Press, Bruges)

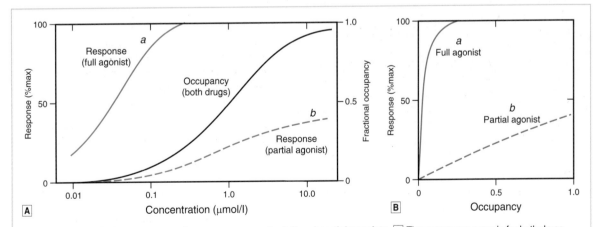

Fig. 1.5 Theoretical occupancy and response curves for full and partial agonists. [A] The occupancy curve is for both drugs, the response curves *a* and *b* are for full and partial agonist respectively. [B] The relationship between response and occupancy for full and partial agonist, corresponding to the response curves in A. Note that curve *a* produces maximal response at about 20% occupancy, while curve *b* produces only a submaximal response even at 100% occupancy.

tissue (e.g. the number of receptors that it possesses and the nature of the coupling between the receptor and the response; see Ch. 2), as well as of the drug itself, were important, and the concept of *intrinsic efficacy* was developed (see Jenkinson 1996, Kenakin 1993). The relationship between occupancy and response can thus be represented:

$$\text{Response} = f\left(\frac{\varepsilon N_{tot}\, x_A}{x_A + K_A}\right)$$

Characteristics of tissue

Characteristics of drug

In this equation, f represents the *transducer function* which describes the characteristics of the responding system; ε is the *intrinsic efficacy*, which is a characteristic of the drug–receptor complex. The importance of this formal representation is that it explains how differences in the transducer function and the density of receptors in different tissues can result in the same agonist, acting on the same receptor, appearing as a full agonist in one tissue and as a partial agonist in another. By the same token, the relative potencies of two agonists may be different in different tissues, even though the receptor is the same.

For a more detailed discussion of drug–receptor interactions, see Kenakin (1993), Jenkinson (1996).

It would be nice to be able to give a more concrete account of what efficacy means in physical terms, and to understand why one drug may be an agonist while another, chemically very similar, is an antagonist. As yet this cannot be done, but the simple scheme known as the *two-state model* (see Colquhoun 1973, Leff 1995) shown in Figure 1.6 provides a starting point. It is envisaged that the receptor can exist in two states, 'resting' (R) and 'activated' (R*), either of which can bind a drug molecule, the equilibrium constants being K and K^* respectively. A shift in the equilibrium between these two states in favour of R* initiates the response (see Ch. 2). Normally, when no ligand is present, the equilibrium favours the resting state. For binding of a drug molecule to shift the equilibrium in favour of R* (in other words, for a drug to be an agonist), the necessary condition is that the drug should have a higher affinity for R* than for R $(K > K^*)$. The larger the ratio K/K^*, the greater the drug's efficacy. If $K = K^*$, binding will leave the conformational equilibrium undisturbed, and the drug will be a pure competitive antagonist. This formalism is undoubtedly too simple, especially for receptors that act through more complex transduction machinery (see Ch. 2); more elaborate models are discussed by Kenakin (1993).

For some receptors, we now realise, an appreciable level of activation exists even when no ligand is present. Examples include the benzodiazepine receptor (see Ch. 33) and the dihydropyridine receptor (Ch. 15). Furthermore, receptor mutations occur, either spontaneously, in some disease states, or experimentally created (see Ch. 2), which result in appreciable activation in the absence of any ligand (*constitutive activation*). Recently, it has been found that simply over-expressing β-adrenoceptors can result in their constitutive activation (Bond et al. 1995), a result that may prove to have major pathophysiological implications. Under these conditions, a ligand which binds preferentially to the inactivated state (i.e. $K^* > K$) can shift the equilibrium towards this state. Such compounds are known as *inverse agonists*, since they reduce the level of constitutive activation (Fig. 1.7). Like cats, however, most receptors have a strong preference for the inactive state; for these, there is no practical difference between a competitive antagonist and an inverse agonist. Constitutive activation is a relatively recent discovery, however, and may prove to be of greater pharmacological significance than is realised at present (see Milligan et al. 1995).

Whatever its theoretical status, efficacy is a concept of great practical importance, since the ability of a drug to act as an agonist or antagonist on a particular type of receptor is often crucial for its therapeutic use.

Stephenson (1956), studying the actions of acetylcholine analogues in isolated tissues, found that many full agonists were capable of eliciting maximal responses at very low occupancies, often less than 1%. If a full

---

Agonists, antagonists and efficacy

- Drugs acting on receptors may be *agonists* or *antagonists*.
- Agonists initiate changes in cell function, producing effects of various types; antagonists bind to receptors without initiating such changes.
- Agonist potency depends on two parameters: *affinity* (i.e. tendency to bind to receptors) and *efficacy* (i.e. ability, once bound, to initiate changes which lead to effects).
- For antagonists, efficacy is zero.
- Full agonists (which can produce maximal effects) have high efficacy; *partial agonists* (which can produce only submaximal effects) have intermediate efficacy.
- According to the two-state model, efficacy reflects the relative affinity of the compound for the resting and activated states of the receptor. Agonists show selectivitiy for the activated state; antagonists show no selectivity.
- *Inverse agonists* show selectivity for the resting state of the receptor, this being of significance only in unusual situations where the receptors show constitutive activity.

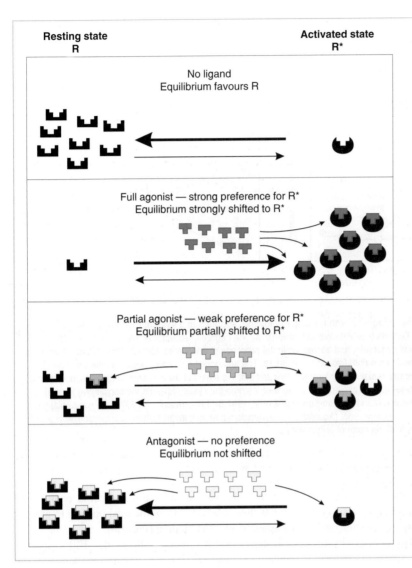

Fig. 1.6 Schematic representation of effects of ligands on receptor activation. In the resting state (no ligand) the equilibrium normally favours the resting state. A full agonist binds preferentially to the activated state, and shifts the equilibrium towards activation. A partial agonist shows a weaker preference, and shifts the equilibrium to a smaller extent, even when the receptors are fully occupied. An antagonist shows no preference, and does not shift the equilibrium, though it reduces the effect of an agonist by preventing the agonist from binding to the receptors.

response can occur when only a small fraction of the receptors is occupied, the system may be said to possess *spare receptors*, or a *receptor reserve*. This is common with drugs that elicit smooth muscle contraction, but less so for other types of receptor-mediated response, such as secretion, smooth muscle relaxation or cardiac stimulation, where the effect is more nearly proportional to receptor occupancy. The existence of spare receptors does not imply any actual subdivision of the receptor pool, but merely that the pool is larger than the number needed to evoke a full response. This surplus of receptors over the number actually needed might seem to be a somewhat profligate biological arrangement. It means,

however, that a given number of agonist–receptor complexes, corresponding to a given level of biological response, can be reached with a lower concentration of hormone or neurotransmitter than would be the case if fewer receptors were provided. Economy of hormone or transmitter secretion is thus achieved at the expense of providing more receptors.

DIRECT MEASUREMENT OF DRUG BINDING TO RECEPTORS

The binding of drugs to receptors can often be measured directly by the use of radioactive drug molecules (usually

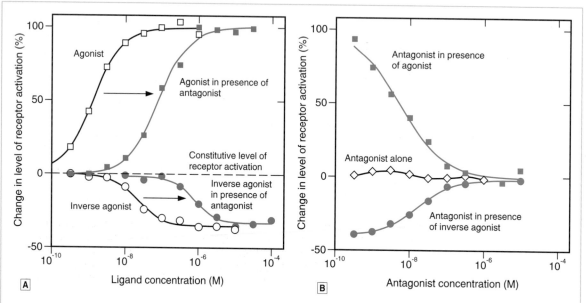

Fig. 1.7 The interaction of a competitive antagonist with normal and inverse agonists in a system that shows receptor activation in the absence of any added ligands (constitutive activation). [A] The degree of receptor activation (vertical scale) increases in the presence of an agonist (open squares), and decreases in the presence of an inverse agonist (open circles). Addition of a competitive antagonist shifts both curves to the right (closed symbols). [B] The antagonist on its own does not alter the level of constitutive activity (open symbols), since it has equal affinity for the active and inactive states of the receptor. In the presence of an agonist (closed squares) or an inverse agonist (closed circles), the antagonist restores the system towards the constitutive level of activity. These data (reproduced with permission from Newman-Tancredi A et al. 1997 Br J Pharmacol 120: 737–739) were obtained with cloned human 5-HT receptors expressed in a cell line. (Agonist: 5-carboxamidotryptamine; inverse agonist: spiperone; antagonist: WAY 100635; see Ch. 9 for information on 5-HT receptor pharmacology.)

with ^{3}H, ^{14}C or ^{125}I). The main requirements are that the radioactive ligand (which may be an agonist or antagonist) must bind with high affinity and specificity, and can be labelled to a sufficient specific radioactivity to enable minute amounts of binding to be measured. The usual procedure is to incubate samples of the tissue (or membrane fragments) with various concentrations of radioactive drug until equilibrium is reached. The tissue is then removed, or the membrane fragments separated by filtration or centrifugation, and dissolved in scintillation fluid for measurement of its radioactive content.

In such experiments there is invariably a certain amount of 'non-specific binding' (i.e. drug taken up by structures other than receptors) which obscures the specific component, and needs to be kept to a minimum. The amount of non-specific binding is estimated by measuring the radioactivity taken up in the presence of a saturating concentration of a (non-radioactive) ligand that inhibits completely the binding of the radioactive drug to the

receptors, leaving behind the non-specific component. This is then subtracted from the total binding to give an estimate of specific binding (Fig. 1.8).

If the specific binding follows the Hill–Langmuir equation (equation 1.5), the relationship between the amount bound (B) and ligand concentration (x) should be:

$$B = \frac{B_{max}x}{x + K} \qquad (1.9)$$

B_{max} is the total number of binding sites in the preparation (often expressed as pmol/mg protein) and K is the equilibrium constant (see equation 1.5). To display the results in linear form, equation (1.9) may be rearranged to:

$$\frac{B}{x} = \frac{B_{max}}{K} - \frac{B}{K} \qquad (1.10)$$

A plot of B/x against B (known as a Scatchard plot;

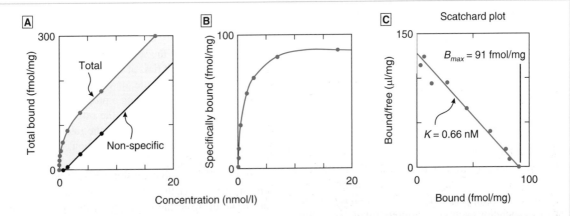

Fig. 1.8 Measurement of receptor binding (β-adrenoceptors in cardiac cell membranes). The ligand was ³H-cyanopindolol, a derivative of pindolol (see Ch. 8). **A** Measurements of total and non-specific binding at equilibrium. Non-specific binding is measured in the presence of a saturating concentration of a non-radioactive β-receptor agonist, which prevents the radioactive ligand from binding to β-receptors. The difference between the two lines (light blue) represents specific binding. **B** Specific binding plotted against concentration. The curve is a rectangular hyperbola (equation 1.9). **C** Scatchard plot (equation 1.10). This gives a straight line from which the binding parameters K and B_{max} can be calculated.

Fig. 1.8) gives a straight line from which both B_{max} and K can be estimated. Statistically, this procedure is not without problems, and it is now usual to estimate these parameters from the untransformed binding values by an iterative non-linear curve-fitting procedure.

Autoradiography can also be used to investigate the distribution of receptors in structures such as the brain, and direct labelling with ligands containing positron-emitting isotopes is now used to obtain images by *positron-emission tomography* (PET) of receptor distribution in humans. This technique has been used, for example, with schizophrenic patients, to measure the degree of dopamine receptor blockade produced by antipsychotic drugs under clinical conditions (see Ch. 34). When combined with pharmacological studies, binding measurements have proved very valuable. It has, for example, been confirmed that the spare receptor hypothesis for muscarinic receptors in smooth muscle is correct; agonists are found to bind, in general, with rather low affinity, and a maximal biological effect occurs at low receptor occupancy. It has also been shown, in skeletal muscle and other tissues, that denervation leads to an increase in the number of receptors in the target cell, a finding that accounts, at least in part, for the phenomenon of denervation supersensitivity. More generally, it appears that receptors tend to increase in number, usually over the course of a few days, if the relevant hormone or transmitter is absent or scarce, and

to decrease in number if it is in excess, a process of adaptation which produces gradual changes in responsiveness to drugs or hormones with continued administration (see p. 16).

Binding curves with agonists are more difficult to interpret than those with antagonists, since they often reveal an apparent heterogeneity among receptors. For example, agonist binding to muscarinic receptors (Ch. 7) and also to β-adrenoceptors (Ch. 8) suggests at least two populations of binding sites with different affinities. This may be due to the fact that receptors can exist either unattached or coupled within the membrane to another macromolecule, the G-protein (see Ch. 2), which constitutes part of the transduction system through which the receptor exerts its regulatory effect. Antagonist binding does not show this complexity, probably because antagonists, by their nature, do not lead to the secondary event of G-protein coupling. Agonist affinity has, indeed, proved to be a very elusive parameter to measure, a fact which has generated an algebraic paperchase in the pharmacological literature, with many enthusiastic followers.

DRUG ANTAGONISM

Frequently, the effect of one drug is diminished or completely abolished in the presence of another. One mechanism, competitive antagonism, was discussed earlier;

a more complete classification includes the following mechanisms:

- chemical antagonism
- pharmacokinetic antagonism
- antagonism by receptor block
- non-competitive antagonism, i.e. block of receptor–effector linkage
- physiological antagonism.

Chemical antagonism

Chemical antagonism refers to the uncommon situation where the two substances combine in solution, so that the effect of the active drug is lost. Examples include the use of chelating agents (e.g. **dimercaprol**) which bind to heavy metals and thus reduce their toxicity, and the use of neutralising antibodies against protein mediators, such as cytokines and growth factors. The latter strategy is currently limited to experimental use, but may be developed for therapeutic use in the near future (see Ch. 10).

Pharmacokinetic antagonism

Pharmacokinetic antagonism describes the situation in which the 'antagonist' effectively reduces the concentration of the active drug at its site of action. This can happen in various ways. The rate of metabolic degradation of the active drug may be increased (e.g. the reduction of the anticoagulant effect of **warfarin** when an agent that accelerates its hepatic metabolism, such as **phenobarbitone**, is given; see Chs 5 and 48). Alternatively, the rate of absorption of the active drug from the gastrointestinal tract may be reduced, or the rate of renal excretion may be increased. Interactions of this sort are discussed in more detail in Chapter 48. They have a tendency to occur unexpectedly in clinical situations, and are a major preoccupation of clinical pharmacologists.

Antagonism by receptor block

Receptor-block antagonism involves two important mechanisms:

- reversible competitive antagonism
- irreversible, or non-equilibrium, competitive antagonism.

Reversible competitive antagonism has been discussed in some detail earlier in this chapter. Its key features are *surmountability*, expressed in the parallel shift of the agonist log-concentration–effect curve without any reduction in the maximal response, and the *linear Schild plot* (see p. 8). These characteristics reflect the fact that the rate of dissociation of the antagonist molecules is sufficiently high that, on addition of the agonist, a new equilibrium is rapidly established. In effect, the agonist is able to displace the antagonist molecules from the receptors, although it has, of course, no power to evict a bound antagonist molecule, or vice versa. Displacement occurs because, by occupying a proportion of the vacant receptors, the agonist reduces the rate of association of the antagonist molecules, so that the rate of dissociation temporarily exceeds that of association, and the overall antagonist occupancy falls.

Irreversible, or non-equilibrium, competitive antagonism occurs when the antagonist dissociates very slowly, or not at all, from the receptors, with the result that no change in the antagonist occupancy takes place when the agonist is applied.*

The fractional occupancy by the agonist is thus reduced in proportion to the fraction of receptors not occupied by the antagonist. Thus, if the fraction of receptors blocked by the antagonist is p_B, the fraction accessible to the agonist is reduced to $(1 - p_B)$.

The antagonism is *non-surmountable* because no matter how high the agonist concentration, the agonist occupancy cannot exceed $(1 - p_B)$. The effects of reversible and irreversible antagonists are compared in Figure 1.9. In some cases (Fig. 1.10A), the theoretical effect is accurately reproduced, but the distinction between reversible and irreversible competitive antagonism (or even non-competitive antagonism; see p. 15) is not always so clear. This is because of the phenomenon of spare receptors (see p. 11); if the agonist occupancy required to produce a maximal biological response is very small (say 1% of the total receptor pool), then it is possible to block irreversibly nearly 99% of the receptors without reducing the maximal response. The effect of a lesser degree of antagonist occupancy will be to produce a parallel shift of the log-concentration–effect curve that is indistinguishable from reversible competitive antagonism (Fig. 1.10B). In fact, it was the finding that an irreversible competitive antagonist of histamine was able to reduce the sensitivity of a smooth muscle preparation to histamine nearly 100-fold without reducing the maximal response that first gave rise to the spare receptor hypothesis. Irreversible competitive antagonism occurs with drugs that possess reactive groups which form covalent bonds with the receptor. These are mainly used as experimental tools for investigating receptor function, and

---

*Some authors refer to this type of antagonism as non-competitive, but this term is best reserved for antagonism that does not involve occupation of the receptor site (see p. 15).

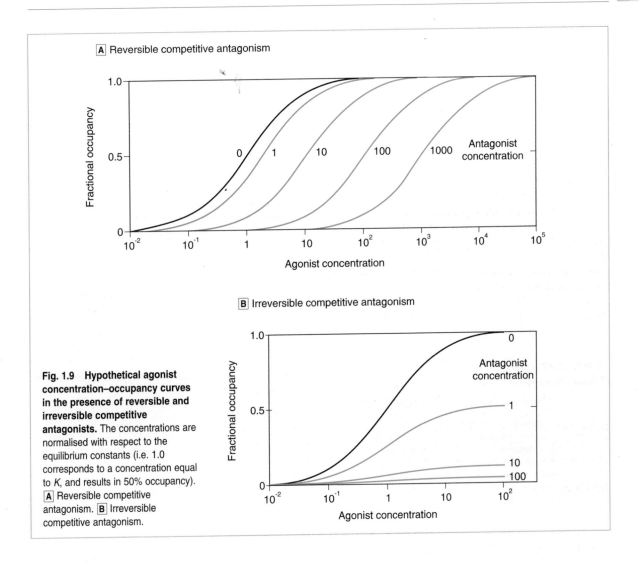

Fig. 1.9 Hypothetical agonist concentration–occupancy curves in the presence of reversible and irreversible competitive antagonists. The concentrations are normalised with respect to the equilibrium constants (i.e. 1.0 corresponds to a concentration equal to *K*, and results in 50% occupancy). **A** Reversible competitive antagonism. **B** Irreversible competitive antagonism.

few are used clinically. Irreversible enzyme inhibitors which act similarly are clinically used, however, and include drugs such as **aspirin** (Ch. 13), **omeprazole** (Ch. 21) and **monoamine oxidase inhibitors** (Ch. 35).

Non-competitive antagonism

Non-competitive antagonism describes the situation where the antagonist blocks at some point the chain of events that leads to the production of a response by the agonist. For example, drugs such as verapamil and nifedipine prevent the influx of calcium ions through the cell membrane (see Ch. 15) and thus block non-specifically the contraction of smooth muscle produced by other drugs. As a rule, the effect will be to reduce the

slope and maximum of the agonist log-concentration–response curve as in Figure 1.10B though it is quite possible for some degree of rightward shift to occur as well.

Physiological antagonism

Physiological antagonism is a term used loosely to describe the interaction of two drugs whose opposing actions in the body tend to cancel each other. For example, histamine acts on receptors of the parietal cells of the gastric mucosa to stimulate acid secretion, while omeprazole blocks this effect by inhibiting the proton pump; the two drugs can be said to act as physiological antagonists.

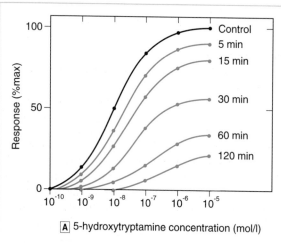
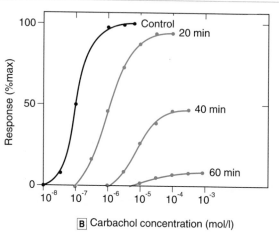

A 5-hydroxytryptamine concentration (mol/l)

B Carbachol concentration (mol/l)

Fig. 1.10   Effects of irreversible competitive antagonists on agonist concentration–effect curves. **A** Rat stomach smooth muscle responding to 5-hydroxytryptamine at various times after addition of methysergide (10^{-9} mol/l). **B** Rabbit stomach responding to carbachol at various times after addition of dibenamine (10^{-5} mol/l). (After: (A) Frankhuijsen A L, Bonta I L 1974 Eur J Pharmacol 26: 220; (B) Furchgott R F 1965 Adv Drug Res 3: 21)

Drug antagonism

Drug antagonism occurs by various mechanisms:

- chemical antagonism (interaction in solution)
- pharmacokinetic antagonism (one drug affecting the absorption, metabolism or excretion of the other)
- competitive antagonism (both drugs binding to the same receptors); the antagonism may be reversible or irreversible
- non-competitive antagonism (the antagonist interrupts receptor–effector linkage)
- physiological antagonism (two agents producing opposing physiological effects).

DESENSITISATION AND TACHYPHYLAXIS

Often, the effect of a drug gradually diminishes when it is given continuously or repeatedly. *Desensitisation* and *tachyphylaxis* are synonymous terms used to describe this phenomenon which often develops in the course of a few minutes. The term *tolerance* is conventionally used to describe a more gradual decrease in responsiveness to a drug, taking days or weeks to develop, but the distinction is not a sharp one. The term *refractoriness* is also sometimes used, mainly in relation to a loss of therapeutic efficacy. *Drug resistance* is a term used to describe the loss of effectiveness of antimicrobial or antitumour drugs (see Chs 41 and 43). Many different

mechanisms can give rise to this type of phenomenon. They include:

- change in receptors
- loss of receptors
- exhaustion of mediators
- increased metabolic degradation
- physiological adaptation
- active extrusion of drug from cells (mainly relevant in chemotherapy (see Chs 41 & 43).

Change in receptors

Among receptors directly coupled to ionic channels, desensitisation is often rapid and pronounced. At the neuromuscular junction (Fig. 1.11A), there is evidence that the desensitised state is caused by a slow conformational change in the receptor, resulting in tight binding of the agonist molecule without the opening of the ionic channel (see Changeux et al. 1987). A similar change has been described for the β-adrenoceptor (Fig. 1.11B), which becomes, on desensitisation, unable to activate adenylate cyclase, though it can still bind the agonist molecule. It is believed that phosphorylation of specific residues in the receptor protein is responsible for many types of desensitisation (see Ch. 2).

Loss of receptors

Prolonged exposure to agonists often results in a gradual decrease in the number of receptors as measured by

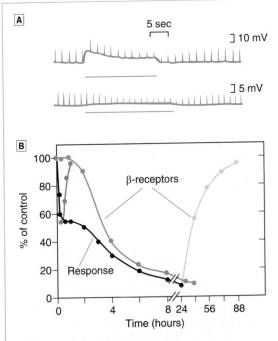

Fig. 1.11 Two kinds of receptor desensitisation.
A Acetylcholine (ACh) at the frog motor endplate. Brief depolarisations (upward deflections) are produced by short pulses of ACh delivered from a micropipette. A lung pulse (horizontal line) causes the response to decline with a time-course of about 20 seconds, owing to desensitisation, and it recovers with a similar time-course. B β-adrenoceptors of rat glioma cells in tissue culture. Isoprenaline (1 μM) was added at time zero, and the adenylate cyclase response and β-adrenoceptor density measured at intervals. During the early uncoupling phase, the response (black line) declines with no change in receptor density (dark blue line). Later, the response declines further concomitantly with disappearance of receptors from the membrane by internalisation. The grey and light blue lines show the recovery of the response and receptor density after the isoprenaline is washed out during the early or late phase. (From: (A) Katz B, Thesleff S 1957 J Physiol 138: 63; (B) Perkins J P 1981 Trends Pharmacol Sci 2: 326)

drug-binding studies. This occurs with β-adrenoceptors (Fig. 1.11B) and appears to be a slower process than the 'uncoupling' from adenylate cyclase mentioned above. In studies on cell cultures, the number of β-adrenoceptors can fall to about 10% of normal in 8 hours in the presence of a low concentration of **isoprenaline**. Recovery to normal takes several days. Similar changes have been described for other types of receptor, including those for various peptides. It is believed that the vanishing receptors are taken into the cell by endocytosis of patches of the membrane. This type of adaptation is common for hormone receptors, and has obvious relevance to the effects produced when drugs are given for extended periods. Receptor desensitisation is generally an unwanted complication, but it can be exploited clinically. For example, gonadotrophin-releasing hormone (see Ch. 26) is used to treat endometriosis or prostatic cancer; given continuously, this hormone paradoxically inhibits gonadotrophin release (in contrast to the normal stimulatory effect of the physiological secretion, which is pulsatile).

Exhaustion of mediators

In some cases, desensitisation is associated with depletion of an essential intermediate substance. Drugs such as **amphetamine**, which acts by releasing noradrenaline and other amines from nerve terminals (see Chs 8 and 28), show marked tachyphylaxis because the releasable stores of noradrenaline become depleted.

Increased metabolic degradation

Tolerance to some drugs, for example **barbiturates** (Ch. 33) and **ethanol** (Ch. 39), occurs partly because repeated administration of the same dose produces a progressively lower plasma concentration. The degree of tolerance that results is generally modest, and in both of these examples other mechanisms contribute to the substantial tolerance that actually occurs.

Physiological adaptation

Diminution of a drug's effect may occur because it is nullified by a homeostatic response. For example, the blood pressure-lowering effect of thiazide diuretics is limited because of a gradual activation of the renin–angiotensin system (see Ch. 15). Such homeostatic mechanisms are very common, and if they occur slowly the result will be a gradually developing tolerance. It is a common experience that many side-effects of drugs, such as nausea or sleepiness, tend to subside even though drug administration is continued. We may assume that some kind of physiological adaptation is occurring, though little is known about the mechanisms involved.

REFERENCES AND FURTHER READING

Bond R A, Leff P, Johnson T D et al. 1995 Physiological effects of inverse agonists in transgenic mice with myocardial overexpression of the β_2-adrenoceptor. Nature 374: 270–276 (*A study with important clinical implications, showing that overexpression of β-receptors results in constitutive receptor activation*)

Buckel P 1996 Recombinant proteins for therapy. Trends Pharmacol Sci 17: 450–456 (*Thoughtful review of the status of, and prospects for, protein-based therapeutics*)

Changeux J-P, Giraudat J, Dennis M 1987 The nicotinic acetylcholine receptor: molecular architecture of a ligand-regulated ion channel. Trends Pharmacol Sci 8: 459–465 (*One of the first descriptions of receptor action at the molecular level*)

Colquhoun D 1973 The relationship between classical and cooperative models for drug action. In: H P Rang (ed) Drug receptors. Macmillan, London (*An excellent, and still relevant, discussion of the relationship between 'allostain' and 'classical' models of agonist action*)

Franks N P, Lieb W R 1994 Molecular and cellular mechanisms of general anaesthesia. Nature 367: 607–614 (*A review of new ideas about the site of action of anaesthetic drugs*)

Jenkinson D H 1996 Classical approaches to the study of drug–receptor interactions. In: Foreman J C, Johansen T (eds) Textbook of receptor pharmacology. CRC Press, Boca Raton (*Good account of pharmacological analysis of receptor-indicated effects*)

Kenakin T 1993 Pharmacologic analysis of drug–receptor interactions, 2nd edn. Raven Press, New York (*Excellent and detailed textbook, covering most of the material in this chapter in greater depth*)

Lauence D R (ed) 1998 A dictionary of pharmacology and allied topics. Elsevier, Amsterdam (*An excellent compendium, strongly recommended. Incorporates fringe, as well as mainstream terminology*)

Leff P 1995 The two-state model of receptor activation. Trends Pharmacol Sci 16: 89–97 (*An update of the discussion by Colquhoun (1972) taking into account discoveries at the molecular level*)

Milligan G, Bond R A, Lee M 1995 Inverse agonism: pharmacological curiosity or potential therapeutic strategy? Trends Pharmacol Sci 16: 10–13 (*Excellent review of the significance of constitutive receptor activation, and the effects of inverse agonists*)

Sibley D R, Lefkowitz R J 1985 Molecular mechanisms of receptor desensitization using the β-adrenergic receptor-coupled adenylate cyclase system as a model. Nature 317: 124–129 (*Good discussion of the phenomenon and mechanisms of receptor desensitization*)

Stephenson R P 1956 A modification of receptor theory. Br J Pharmacol 11: 379–393 (*Classic analysis of receptor action, introducing the concept of efficacy*)

How drugs act: molecular aspects

In this chapter, we move from the general principles of drug action outlined in Chapter 1 to the molecules that are involved in recognising chemical signals and translating them into cellular responses. It is in the area of molecular pharmacology that the most rapid advances have been made in recent years. This new knowledge can seem impenetrably complex when couched in the terminology and style of modern molecular biology, but actually provides a simpler and more coherent framework for understanding drug action than existed previously, and it is this aspect, rather than the molecular detail, on which we focus here. Advances in molecular pharmacology are not only changing our understanding of drug action; they are also opening up many new therapeutic possibilities, further discussed in other chapters.

First, we consider the types of target proteins on which drugs commonly act, which were mentioned briefly in Chapter 1. Next, we will consider the main families of receptors which have been revealed by cloning and structural studies. Finally, we will discuss the various forms of receptor–effector linkage (*signal transduction mechanisms*) through which receptors are coupled to the regulation of cell function. The relationship between the molecular structure of a receptor and its functional linkage to a particular type of effector system is a principal theme. In this chapter, we go into more detail than

is necessary for understanding today's pharmacology at a basic level, but we are confident that tomorrow's pharmacology will rest solidly on the advances in cellular and molecular biology that are discussed here.

TARGETS FOR DRUG ACTION

The protein targets for drug action on mammalian cells (Fig. 2.1) which are described in this chapter can be broadly divided into:

- receptors
- ion channels
- enzymes
- carrier molecules.

Other types of protein targets for specific classes of drugs are also known. These include certain structural proteins, such as tubulin (the target for **colchicine**; see Ch. 13), intracellular proteins known as *immunophilins*, which are the target for various immunosuppressive drugs, such as **cyclosporin** (Ch. 13). Targets for chemotherapeutic drugs (Chs 41–47), where the aim is to suppress invading microorganisms or cancer cells, include DNA and cell wall constituents as well as other proteins.

Receptors
Receptors (Fig. 2.1A) form the sensing elements in the system of chemical communications that coordinates the function of all the different cells in the body, the chemical messengers being hormones, transmitter substances or other mediators, such as cytokines and growth factors. Many therapeutically useful synthetic drugs act, either as agonists or antagonists, on receptors for known endogenous mediators. Some examples are given in Table 2.1. In most cases, the endogenous mediator was discovered before—often many years before—the receptor was characterised pharmacologically and biochemically, but there are examples of receptors for synthetic drug

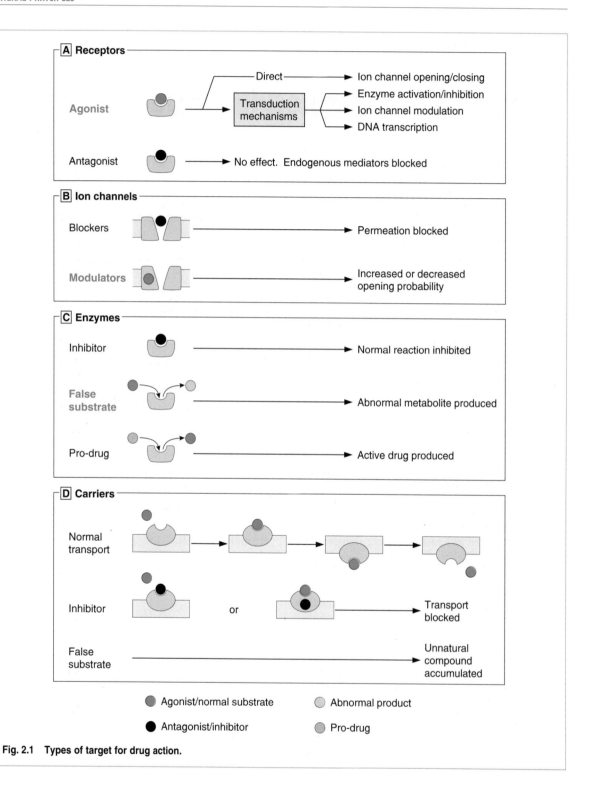

Fig. 2.1 Types of target for drug action.

Table 2.1 Some examples of targets for drug action

Type of target	Effectors		Refer to
Receptors	**Agonists**	**Antagonists**	
Nicotinic ACh receptor	Acetylcholine	Tubocurarine	Ch. 7
	Nicotine	α-bungarotoxin	
β-adrenoceptor	Noradrenaline	Propranolol	Ch. 8
	Isoprenaline		
Histamine (H$_1$ receptor)	Histamine	Mepyramine	Ch. 13
Histamine (H$_2$ receptor)	Impromidine	Ranitidine	Ch. 21
Opiate (μ-receptor)	Morphine	Naloxone	Ch. 37
5-HT$_2$ receptor	5-HT	Ketanserin	Ch. 9
Dopamine (D$_2$ receptor)	Dopamine	Chlorpromazine	Ch. 30
	Bromocriptine		
Insulin receptor	Insulin	Not known	Ch. 22
Oestrogen receptor	Ethinylestradiol	Tamoxifen	Ch. 26
Progesterone receptor	Norethisterone	Danazol	Ch. 26
Ion channels	**Blockers**	**Modulators**	
Voltage-gated Na$^+$ channels	Local anaesthetics	Veratridine	Ch. 40
	Tetrodotoxin		
Renal tubule Na$^+$ channels	Amiloride	Aldosterone	Ch. 20
Voltage-gated Ca^{2+} channels	Divalent cations (e.g. Cd^{2+})	Dihydropyridines	Ch. 14
		β-adrenoceptor agonists	Ch. 8
Voltage-gated K$^+$ channels	4-aminopyridine		Ch. 40
ATP-sensitive K$^+$ channels	ATP	Cromokalim	Ch. 15
		Sulphonylureas	Ch. 22
GABA-gated Cl$^-$ channels	Picrotoxin	Benzodiazepines	Ch. 29
Glutamate-gated (NMDA) cation channels	Dizocilpine, Mg^{2+} Ketamine	Glycine	Ch. 29
Enzymes	**Inhibitors**	**False substrates**	
Acetylcholinesterase	Neostigmine		Ch. 7
	Organophosphates		
Choline acetyltransferase		Hemicholinium	Ch. 7
Cyclo-oxygenase	Aspirin		Ch. 13
Xanthine oxidase	Allopurinol		Ch. 13
Angiotensin-converting enzyme	Captopril		Ch. 15
Carbonic anhydrase	Acetazolamide		Ch. 20
HMG-CoA reductase	Simvastatin		Ch. 16
Dopa decarboxylase		Methyldopa	Ch. 8
Monoamine oxidase-A	Iproniazid		Ch. 35
Monoamine oxidase-B	Selegiline		Ch. 31
Dihydrofolate reductase	Trimethoprim		Ch. 43
	Methotrexate		Chs 13, 42
DNA polymerase	Cytarabine	Cytarabine	Ch. 42
Enzymes involved in DNA synthesis	Azathiaprine		Ch. 13
Enzymes of blood clotting cascade	Heparin		Ch. 17
Plasminogen*			Ch. 17
Thymidine kinase	Acyclovir		Ch. 44
HIV protease	Saquinavir		Ch. 44
Reverse transcriptase	Didanosine (ddl)		Ch. 44
	Zidovudine		Ch. 44

Table 2.1 (continued)

Type of target	Effectors		Refer to
Carriers	**Inhibitors**	**False substrates**	
Choline carrier (nerve terminal)	Hemicholinium		Ch. 7
Noradrenaline uptake 1	Tricyclic antidepressants		Ch. 35
	Cocaine		Ch. 8
		Amphetamine	Ch. 8
		Methyldopa	Ch. 15
Noradrenaline uptake (vesicular)	Reserpine		Ch. 8
Weak acid carrier (renal tubule)	Probenecid		Ch. 20
$Na^+/K^+/2Cl^-$ co-transporter (loop of Henle)	Loop diuretics		Ch. 20
Na^+/K^+ pump	Cardiac glycosides		Ch. 15
Proton pump (gastric mucosa)	Omeprazole		Ch. 21
Others			
Immunophilins	Cyclosporin		Ch. 13
	Tacrolimus		
Tubulin	Colchicine		Ch. 13
	Taxol		Ch. 42

Note: Other biochemical targets for drugs used in chemotherapy are discussed in Chapters 41–47.
*Plasminogen activators: tissue plasminogen activator (TPA), APSAC (Ch. 17).

molecules (e.g. **benzodiazepines**, Ch. 33; and **sulphonylureas**, Ch. 22) for which no endogenous mediator has been identified. Receptors are discussed in more detail below (pp. 24–45).

Ion channels

Some ion channels (known as *ligand-gated* ion channels) are directly linked to a receptor, and open only when the receptor is occupied by an agonist, However, many other types of ion channel also serve as targets for drug action. The interaction can be indirect, involving a G-protein and other intermediaries (see below), or direct, where the drug itself binds to the channel protein and alters its function. The simplest type of interaction involves a physical blocking of the channel by the drug molecule (Fig. 2.1B), exemplified by the blocking action of **local anaesthetics** on the voltage-gated sodium channel (see Ch. 40), or the blocking of sodium entry into renal tubular cells by the diuretic **amiloride** (see Ch. 20). Channel function can also be modulated by drugs which bind to accessory sites on the channel protein; examples include the action of vasodilator drugs of the **dihydropyridine** type (see Ch. 15) on calcium channels. In this case, the opening of the channels, which normally occurs in response to depolarisation of the membrane, may be inhibited or facilitated according to the structure of the

dihydropyridine. The binding of the drug molecule thus influences the *gating* of the channel, a quite different mechanism from that of drugs which block *permeation* of the channel without greatly affecting its gating. Another example is that of the **benzodiazepine** tranquillisers (see Ch. 33). These drugs bind to a region of the GABA-receptor/chloride channel complex (an example of a direct ligand-gated channel; see above), this region being distinct from the GABA binding site. Most benzodiazepines are agonists (see Ch. 1), which act to facilitate the opening of the channel by the neurotransmitter GABA (see Ch. 29), but some inverse agonists are known that have the opposite effect, causing anxiety rather than tranquillity.

Another interesting example of drug action on ion channels concerns a special type of potassium channel in the membrane of the pancreatic β-cells, which secrete insulin when the plasma glucose concentration rises (see Ch. 22). These channels open when the intracellular ATP concentration drops (see Ashcroft 1988), and are blocked by drugs of the **sulphonylurea** class, which are used to treat diabetes (Ch. 22). Blocking these potassium channels causes the β-cell to depolarise, thus stimulating insulin secretion. The sulphonylureas do not block the channel physically, but modulate its gating by binding to an associated protein, the sulphonylurea receptor (see Panten et al. 1996). The same type of channel occurs also in smooth muscle cells, and is the target for a new type of vasodilator drug (**cromakalim**; see Ch. 15) which selectively opens such channels and hyperpolarises the cells.

Ion channel modulation by drugs, acting directly on the channel or indirectly, is one of the most important mechanisms by which pharmacological effects are produced at the cellular level. The development of the patch-clamp technique (see below), which enables ion channel function to be observed with dramatic clarity and directness, has contributed greatly to understanding in this area in recent years.

Enzymes

Many drugs are targeted on enzymes (Fig. 2.1C) examples being given in Table 2.1. Most commonly, the drug molecule is a substrate analogue that acts as a *competitive inhibitor* of the enzyme, either reversibly (e.g. **neostigmine**, acting on acetylcholinesterase; Ch. 7), or irreversibly (e.g. **aspirin**, acting on cyclo-oxygenase; Ch. 13). The immunophilin to which **cyclosporin** binds (see above) has enzymic activity as an isomerase which catalyses the *cis–trans* isomerisation of proline residues in proteins, a reaction that is important in allowing expressed proteins to fold correctly. Inhibition of this enzymic activity by cyclosporin appears to be one of the mechanisms by which it causes immunosuppression. Another type of interaction involves the drug as *a false substrate*, where the drug molecule undergoes chemical transformation to form an abnormal product which subverts the normal metabolic pathway. An example is the anticancer drug, **fluorouracil**, which replaces uracil as an intermediate in purine biosynthesis, but cannot be converted into thymidylate, thus blocking DNA synthesis and preventing cell division (Ch. 42).

It should also be mentioned that drugs may require enzymic degradation to convert them from an inactive form, the *pro-drug* (see Ch. 5), to an active form. Examples are given in Table 5.3. Furthermore, as discussed in Chapter 49, certain types of drug toxicity result from the enzymic conversion of the drug molecule to a reactive metabolite. As far as the primary action of the drug is concerned this is an unwanted side reaction, but it is of major practical importance.

Carrier molecules

The transport of ions and small organic molecules across cell membranes generally requires a carrier protein, since the permeating molecules are often too polar (i.e. in-sufficiently lipid soluble) to penetrate lipid membranes on their own. There are many examples of such carriers (Fig. 2.1D), including those responsible for the transport of glucose and amino acids into cells, the transport of ions and many organic molecules by the renal tubule, the transport of sodium and calcium ions out of cells and the uptake of neurotransmitter precursors (such as choline) or of neurotransmitters themselves (such as noradrenaline, 5-hydroxytryptamine, glutamate, and peptides) by nerve terminals. These transporters belong to a well-defined structural family, distinct from the corresponding receptors (see Giros & Caron 1993). The carrier proteins embody a recognition site that makes them specific for a particular permeating species, and these recognition sites can also be targets for drugs whose effect is to block the transport system. Some examples are given in Table 2.1.

RECEPTOR PROTEINS

Isolation and characterisation of receptors

In the 1970s, pharmacology entered a new phase when receptors, which had until then been treated largely as theoretical entities, began to emerge as biochemical realities, following the first successful receptor labelling experiments (see Ch. 1). If a tightly bound radioactive ligand is available, this makes it possible to extract and purify the radioactively labelled receptor material. This approach was first used successfully on the nicotinic acetylcholine receptor (see Ch. 7), where advantage was taken of two natural curiosities. The first is that the electric organs of many fish, such as rays (*Torpedo* sp.) and electric eels (*Electrophorus* sp.) consist of modified muscle tissue in which the acetylcholine-sensitive membrane is extremely abundant, and these organs contain much larger amounts of acetylcholine receptor than any other tissue. Secondly, the venom of snakes of the cobra family contains polypeptides which bind with very high specificity to nicotinic acetylcholine receptors. These substances, known as α-toxins, can be labelled and used to assay the receptor content of tissues and tissue extracts. The best-known is α-**bungarotoxin**, which is the main component of the venom of the Malayan banded krait (*Bungarus multicinctus*).* Treatment of muscle or

---

*Nature has had the good sense to keep these heavily-armed fishes and snakes well apart. Ironically enough, *B. multicinctus* is now officially an endangered species, threatened by scientists' demand for its venom. Evolution for survival can go one step too far.

electric tissue with non-ionic detergents is used to render the membrane-bound receptor protein soluble. It can then be purified by the technique of affinity chromatography in which a receptor ligand, bound covalently to the matrix of a chromatography column, is used to adsorb the receptor and separate it from other substances in the extract. The receptor can then be eluted from the column by flushing it through with a solution containing an antagonist, such as gallamine. Similar approaches have now been used to purify a great many hormone and neurotransmitter receptors, as well as ion channels, carrier proteins and other kinds of target molecules.

The impact of molecular biology

Once receptor proteins were isolated and purified, it was possible to analyse the amino acid sequence of a short stretch, allowing the corresponding base sequence of the mRNA to be deduced (with some ambiguity, because of degeneracy in the genetic code). Oligonucleotide probes were then synthesised and used to extract the full-length DNA sequence by conventional cDNA cloning methods, starting from a cDNA library obtained from a tissue source rich in the receptor of interest. The first receptor clones were obtained in this way, but now there are many alternative strategies. For example, *expression cloning* entails the use of a cDNA vector/host system that allows the production of the protein encoded by the cDNA. If the protein is expressed directly, in a bacterial cell, antibodies against the receptor protein may be used to detect bacterial clones carrying the correct cDNA. Otherwise, the cDNA may be transcribed artificially to produce mRNA, which is injected into a frog oocyte. The mRNA corresponding to the receptor protein is translated by the oocyte, and the protein is expressed on its surface, where its presence can be detected by recording changes in membrane potential or conductance in response to application of the relevant agonist. This technique, though laborious, is widely used, because it dispenses with the need to purify the receptor protein and obtain antibodies to it.

It is also possible to introduce foreign DNA into mammalian cell lines by transfection, and to monitor receptor expression by the appearance of specific ligand binding. This technique is often used to study the binding and pharmacological characteristics of the receptors that have been cloned by the approaches described above. In some cases it has been used as a cloning method itself (mainly for cytokine receptors), in conjunction with autoradiographic detection to identify the individual cells expressing the receptor.

Cloning strategies which require neither protein purifi-

cation nor expression systems, but only faith, have also been used successfully. These are based on anticipated sequence homologies between the receptor that is sought and those already known. A region of sequence homology allows, by the use of PCR (polymerase chain reaction) and RACE (rapid amplification of cDNA ends), replication of DNA molecules that contain that sequence. If the chosen sequence is, for example, one that is conserved in several dopamine receptors, what is amplified may well turn out to be another (novel) dopamine receptor, or it may turn out to be something quite different. Unexpected receptors (e.g. the cannabinoid receptor; see Ch. 39) are sometimes found by accident in this way, and there are several examples of 'orphan receptors'*— receptor-like structures for which no functional ligand is known.

The cloning of receptors has often brought to light molecular variants (subtypes) of known receptors, which had not been evident from pharmacological studies. This tends to produce some taxonomic confusion, but in the long term, molecular characterisation of receptors is essential. Barnard, one of the high priests of receptor cloning, is undaunted by the proliferation of molecular subtypes among receptors which pharmacologists had thought that they understood. He quotes Thomas Aquinas: 'Types and shadows have their ending, for the newer rite is here.' The newer rite, he confidently asserts, is molecular biology.

RECEPTOR FAMILIES: STRUCTURE AND SIGNAL TRANSDUCTION MECHANISMS

Receptors elicit many different types of cellular effect, some of which may be very rapid, such as those involved in synaptic transmission, which in general occupy a millisecond timescale. Other receptor-mediated effects, such as those produced by thyroid hormone or various steroid hormones, are very slow and occur over hours or days. There are also many examples of intermediate timescales—catecholamines, for example, usually act in a matter of seconds, whereas many peptides take rather longer to produce their effects. Not surprisingly, very different types of linkage between the receptor occupation and the ensuing response are involved. In terms of both molecular structure and the nature of the

---

*An oddly Dickensian term which seems inappropriately condescending, since we can assume that these receptors play defined roles in physiological signalling—their 'orphanhood' reflects our ignorance, not their status.

transduction mechanism, we can distinguish four receptor types, or *superfamilies* (see Figs 2.2 and 2.3):

- *Type 1: Channel-linked receptors.* These are also known as *ionotropic receptors.* They are membrane receptors which are coupled directly to an ion channel, and are the receptors on which fast neurotransmitters act. Examples include the nicotinic acetylcholine receptor (nAChR; see Ch. 7), the GABA_A receptor (see Ch. 29), the glutamate receptor (see Ch. 29).
- *Type 2: G-protein-coupled receptors.* These are also known as *metabotropic receptors*, or *7-transmembrane-spanning* receptors. They are membrane receptors which are coupled to intracellular effector systems via a G-protein (see below). Receptors for many hormones and slow transmitters, e.g. the muscarinic acetylcholine receptor (mAChR; see Ch. 7), adrenergic receptors (see Ch. 8) fall into this class.
- *Type 3: Kinase-linked receptors.* These are membrane receptors which incorporate an intracellular protein kinase domain (usually tyrosine kinase) within their structure. They include receptors for insulin and various cytokines and growth factors, (see Chs 12 and

22). Closely related are receptors linked to guanylate cyclase, such as the atrial natriuretic factor (ANF) receptor (Chs 14 and 15).
- *Type 4: Receptors that regulate gene transcription.* These are also known as *nuclear receptors*, though some are actually located in the cytosol rather than the nuclear compartment. They include receptors for steroid hormones (see Ch. 24), thyroid hormone (Ch. 27) and other agents such as retinoic acid and vitamin D.

Receptors of the first three categories are all membrane proteins, whereas Type 4 receptors are soluble cytosolic or intranuclear proteins.

The molecular organisation of typical members of each of these four receptor superfamilies is shown in Figure 2.3. Though individual receptors show considerable sequence variation in particular regions, and the lengths of the main intracellular and extracellular domains also vary from one to another within the same family, the overall structural patterns are remarkably consistent, and the identification of these superfamilies represents a major step forward in understanding how drugs act.

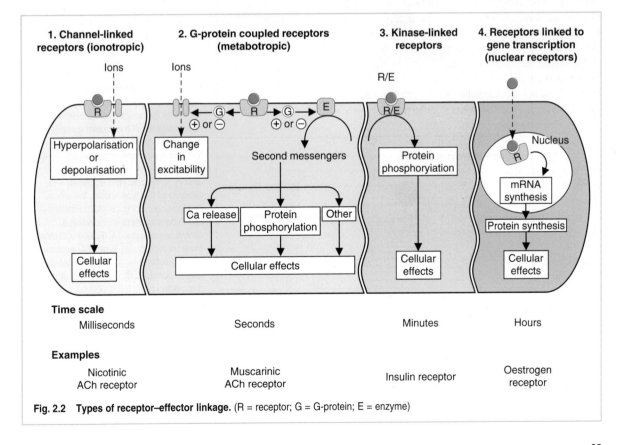

Fig. 2.2 Types of receptor–effector linkage. (R = receptor; G = G-protein; E = enzyme)

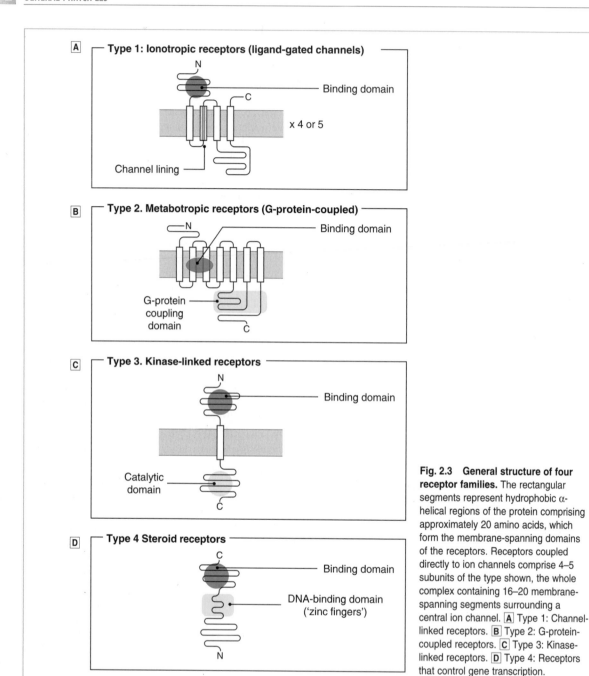

A ⌐ Type 1: Ionotropic receptors (ligand-gated channels) ¬

N

Binding domain

x 4 or 5

Channel lining

B ⌐ Type 2. Metabotropic receptors (G-protein-coupled) ¬

N

Binding domain

G-protein coupling domain

C

C ⌐ Type 3. Kinase-linked receptors ¬

N

Binding domain

Catalytic domain

C

D ⌐ Type 4 Steroid receptors ¬

C

Binding domain

DNA-binding domain ('zinc fingers')

N

Fig. 2.3   General structure of four receptor families. The rectangular segments represent hydrophobic α-helical regions of the protein comprising approximately 20 amino acids, which form the membrane-spanning domains of the receptors. Receptors coupled directly to ion channels comprise 4–5 subunits of the type shown, the whole complex containing 16–20 membrane-spanning segments surrounding a central ion channel. **A** Type 1: Channel-linked receptors. **B** Type 2: G-protein-coupled receptors. **C** Type 3: Kinase-linked receptors. **D** Type 4: Receptors that control gene transcription.

In the following section, we will discuss the structures and transduction mechanisms associated with each of these four receptor types in some detail. For many readers, this amount of detail may be unnecessary, but we include it as a pointer to the future.

CHANNEL-LINKED RECEPTORS

Molecular structure

The nicotinic acetylcholine receptor is typical of this family of receptors, and it has been studied in more detail

The four main types of receptor

	Type 1: Channel-linked receptors	Type 2: G-protein-coupled receptors	Type 3: Kinase-linked receptors	Type 4: Receptors that control gene transcription
Location	Membrane	Membrane	Membrane	Intracellular
Effector	Channel	Enzyme or channel	Enzyme	Gene transcription
Coupling	Direct	G-protein	Direct or indirect	Via DNA
Examples	nAChR	mAChR	Insulin receptor	Steroid/thyroid receptors
	GABA_A receptor	Adrenoceptors	Growth factor and cytokine receptors	
			ANF receptor	

Receptor structure

- There are four receptor 'superfamilies', whose members share a common architecture.
- Three of the superfamilies are transmembrane membrane receptors which respond to ligands outside the cell; the fourth type is intracellular.
- Membrane receptors contain one or more hydrophobic membrane-spanning α-helical segments, linking the extracellular ligand-binding region of the receptor to the intracellular domain which is involved in signalling.

than any other receptor (see Karlin 1993). The receptor consists of four different types of subunit, termed α, β, γ, δ each of M_r 40–58 kDa. The four subunits show marked sequence homology, and analysis of the hydrophobicity profile, which determines which sections of the chain are likely to form membrane-spanning α-helices, suggests that they are inserted into the membrane as shown in Figure 2.4. The oligomeric structure ($\alpha_2,\beta,\gamma,\delta$) possesses two acetylcholine binding sites, each lying at the interface between one of the two α-subunits and its neighbour. Both must bind acetylcholine molecules in order for the receptor to be activated. This receptor is sufficiently large to be seen in electron micrographs, and Figure 2.4 shows its structure, based mainly on a high resolution electron diffraction study (Unwin 1993, 1995). Each subunit spans the membrane four times, so the oligomer has no less than 20 membrane-spanning helices surrounding a central pore.

The long extracellular N-terminal tails of the subunits have, in common with many membrane proteins, sugar residues coupled to particular amino acids (glycosylation), but these do not appear to be essential for function. The two acetylcholine-binding sites lie on the N-termini of the two α-subunits. It appears that one of the transmembrane helices (M2) from each of the five subunits forms the lining of the ion channel (Fig. 2.4). The five M2 helices that form the pore are sharply kinked inwards halfway through the membrane, forming a constriction, and are believed to snap to attention when acetylcholine is bound, thus opening the channel.

The use of site-directed mutagenesis, which enables short regions, or single residues, of the amino acid sequence to be altered, has shown (see Galzi & Changeux 1994) that a mutation of a critical residue in the M2 helix changes the channel from being cation-selective (hence excitatory, in the context of synaptic function) to being anion-selective (typical of receptors for inhibitory transmitters, such as GABA). Other mutations affect properties such as gating and desensitisation of ligand-gated channels.

Other receptors for fast transmitters, such as the GABA_A receptor, the 5-H_{T3}-receptor (Ch. 9) and glutamate receptors are built on the same pattern (see Barnard 1992), and furthermore show considerable sequence homology with the nicotinic acetylcholine receptor;* the number of subunits that go to make up a functional receptor varies somewhat, but is usually four or five. Though the basic plan is constant, there are many sequence variations between receptors in different species, and between the receptor subtypes in the same species. Thus, the nicotinic acetylcholine receptors found in different brain regions differ among themselves, and differ from the muscle receptor. Molecular heterogeneity within a single class of receptors has become a recurring theme as sequence data have accumulated, but its functional significance remains elusive. Some of the known pharmacological

---

*Recently, an ATP-gated channel, the P_{2X}-receptor (see Ch. 9) has been found to have a different structure, with only two membrane-spanning helices in each subunit, a structure resembling that of various primitive sodium channels in other tissues (see Surprenant et al. 1995). Also glutamate-gated channels (Ch. 29) possess three rather than four, transmembrane helices, with a hairpin loop between M1 and M3, which forms the channel lining.

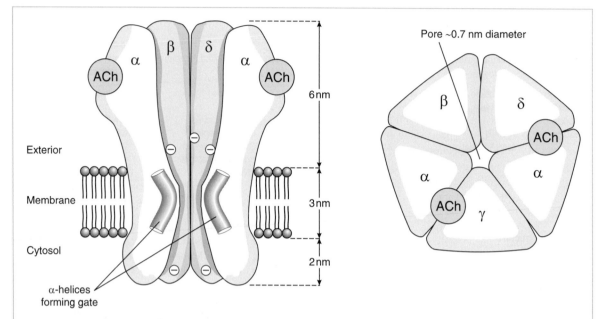

Fig. 2.4 Structure of the nicotinic acetylcholine receptor (a typical ligand-gated ion channel) in side-view (left) and plan-view (right). The five receptor subunits ($\alpha_2, \beta, \gamma, \delta$) form a cluster surrounding a central transmembrane pore, the lining of which is formed by the M2 helical segments of each subunit. These contain a preponderance of negatively charged amino acids, which makes the pore cation selective. There are two acetylcholine binding sites in the extracellular portion of the receptor, at the interface between the α- and the adjoining subunits. When acetylcholine binds, the kinked α-helices either straighten out, or swing out of the way, thus opening the channel pore. (Based on Unwin 1993, 1995)

differences (e.g. sensitivity to blocking agents) that are known to exist between muscle and brain acetylcholine receptors are now known to correlate with specific sequence differences; however, as far as we know, all nicotinic acetylcholine receptors respond to the same physiological mediator and produce the same kind of synaptic response, so why many variants should have evolved is still a puzzle.

The gating mechanism

Receptors of this type control the fastest synaptic events in the nervous system, in which a neurotransmitter acts

---

Channel-linked receptors

- These are sometimes called *ionotropic receptors*.
- They are involved mainly in fast synaptic transmission.
- They are oligomeric proteins containing about 20 transmembrane segments arranged around a central aqueous channel.
- Ligand binding and channel opening occur on a millisecond timescale.
- Examples include nACh, $GABA_A$, 5-HT_3-receptors.

---

on the postsynaptic membrane of a nerve or muscle cell and transiently increases its permeability to particular ions. Most excitatory neurotransmitters such as acetylcholine at the neuromuscular junction (Ch. 7) or glutamate in the central nervous system (Ch. 29) cause an increase in sodium and potassium permeability. This results in a net inward current carried mainly by sodium ions, which depolarises the cell and increases the probability that it will generate an action potential. The action of the transmitter reaches a peak in a fraction of a millisecond, and usually decays within a few milliseconds. The sheer speed of this response implies that the coupling between the receptor and the ionic channel is a direct one, and the molecular structure of the receptor/channel complex (see above) agrees with this. It is known that purified acetylcholine receptors can function as ionic gates in completely artificial membranes, which rules out the involvement of any biochemical intermediates (in the cell or within the membrane) in the transduction process.

A breakthrough by Katz & Miledi in 1972 made it possible for the first time to study the properties of individual receptor-operated ionic channels by the use of noise analysis. Studying the action of acetylcholine at the motor endplate they observed that small random fluctuations of membrane potential were superimposed on the steady depolarisation produced by acetylcholine (Fig. 2.5). These fluctuations arise because, in the presence of an agonist, there is a dynamic equilibrium between open and closed ion channels. In the steady state, the rate of opening balances the rate of closing, but from moment to moment the number of open channels will show random fluctuations about the mean. By measuring the amplitude of these fluctuations, the conductance of a single ion channel can be calculated, and by measuring their frequency (usually in the form of a spectrum in which the noise power of the signal is plotted as a function of frequency) the average duration for which a single channel stays open (*mean channel lifetime*) can be calculated. In the case of acetylcholine acting at the endplate, the channel conductance is about 20 picosiemens (pS), which is equivalent to an influx of about 10^7 ions per second through a single channel under normal physiological conditions, and the mean life-time is 1–2 milliseconds. The magnitude of the single channel conductance confirms that permeation occurs through a physical pore through the membrane, since the ion flow is too large to be compatible with a carrier mechanism. The channel conductance produced by different acetylcholine-like agonists is the same, whereas the mean channel lifetime varies. A simple scheme which accounts for these observations and also gives a physical explanation of efficacy for this type of drug response (see pp. 8–11) is as follows:

$$A + R \underset{k-1}{\overset{k+1}{\rightleftharpoons}} AR \underset{\alpha}{\overset{\beta}{\rightleftharpoons}} AR^* \qquad (2.1)$$

$$\underbrace{}_{\text{channel closed}} \qquad \underbrace{}_{\substack{\text{channel} \\ \text{open}}}$$

The conformation R*, representing the open state of the ion channel, is thought to be the same for all agonists, accounting for the finding that the channel conductance does not vary. Kinetically, the mean channel lifetime is determined mainly by the closing rate constant, α, and clearly varies from one drug to another. In this scheme, an agonist of high efficacy which activates a large proportion of the receptors that it occupies will be characterised by $\beta > \alpha$, whereas a drug of low efficacy will have the characteristic $\alpha > \beta$. For a pure antagonist, $\beta = 0$.

Studies on other transmitters that mediate fast synaptic responses show that although the ionic selectivity of the channel varies according to the nature of the synapse, as well as its conductance and mean lifetime, the basic

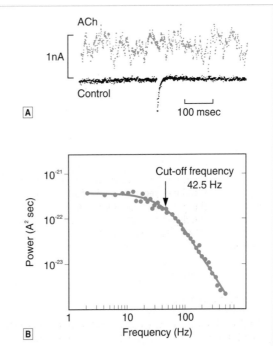

Fig. 2.5 Acetylcholine-induced noise at the frog motor endplate. [A] Records of membrane current recorded at high gain under voltage-clamp. The upper noise record was recorded during the application of ACh from a micropipette. The lower record was obtained in the absence of ACh, the blip in the middle being caused by the spontaneous release of a packet of ACh from the motor nerve. The steady (DC) component of the ACh signal has been removed by electronic filtering, leaving the high frequency noise signal. [B] Power spectrum of ACh-induced noise recorded in a similar experiment to that shown above. The spectrum is calculated by Fourier analysis and fitted with a theoretical (Lorentzian) curve which corresponds to the expected behaviour of a single population of channels whose lifetime varies randomly. The cut-off frequency (at which the power is half of its limiting low-frequency value) enables the mean channel lifetime to be calculated. (From: (A) Anderson C R, Stevens C F 1973 J Physiol 235: 655; (B) Ogden D C et al. 1981 Nature 289: 596)

mechanism of the scheme above appears to be quite general. The patch-clamp recording technique, devised by Neher and Sakmann, allows the very small current flowing through a single ionic channel to be measured directly (Fig. 2.6), and the results have fully confirmed the interpretation of channel properties based on noise analysis. This remarkable technique provides a view, unique in biology, of the physiological behaviour of individual protein molecules, and has given many new

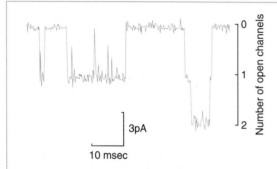

Fig. 2.6 Single acetylcholine-operated ion channels at the frog motor endplate recorded by the patch-clamp technique. The pipette, which was applied tightly to the surface of the membrane, contained 10 µmol/l ACh. The downward deflections show the currents flowing through single ion channels in the small patch of membrane under the pipette tip. Towards the end of the record two channels can be seen to open simultaneously. The conductance and mean lifetime of these channels agrees well with indirect estimates from noise analysis (see Fig. 2.5). (Figure courtesy of D Colquhoun and D C Ogden)

insights into the gating reactions and permeability characteristics of both the transmitter-operated channels discussed here (see Colquhoun 1987) and various voltage-gated channels (see Ch. 40). One observation is that some transmitters, most notably glutamate (see Ch. 29), cause individual channels to open to any one of several distinct conductance levels, a finding which clearly necessitates some revision of the simple scheme above in which only a single open state, R*, is represented. It is likely that residues lining the pore region of the channel, which control its conductance and ion selectivity, can change their position in a stepwise manner, producing these functional sub-states (the physiological significance of which is unknown).

G-PROTEIN-COUPLED RECEPTORS

This family comprises many of the receptors that are familiar to pharmacologists, such as muscarinic ACh receptors (mAChR), adrenoceptors, dopamine receptors, 5-HT receptors, opiate receptors, receptors for many peptides, purine receptors and many others, including the chemoreceptors involved in olfaction (see Ronnett & Snyder 1992). For most of these, a variety of subtypes has been defined on pharmacological grounds. Many of these numerous receptors have been cloned, revealing a remarkably coherent pattern of their molecular structure.

Like Greek amphitheatres, they are all very similar in their basic architecture.

Most neurotransmitters, with the exception of peptides, interact both with metabotropic and with ionotropic receptors (see above), allowing the same molecule to produce a wide variety of effects.

Molecular structure

The first receptor of this type to be fully characterised was the β-adrenoceptor (Ch. 8), which was cloned in 1986. Subsequently molecular biology caught up very rapidly with pharmacology, and most of the receptors that were identified on the basis of their pharmacological properties have now been cloned; what seemed re-volutionary in 1986 is now commonplace. Metabotropic receptors consist of a single polypeptide chain of 400–500 residues whose general anatomy is shown in Figure 2.3B. They all possess seven transmembrane α-helices, similar to those of the channel-linked receptors discussed above, and these regions are the most highly conserved among the various receptors in this class. Both the extracellular amino terminus and the intracellular carboxy terminus vary greatly in length and sequence; another highly variable region is the long third cyto-plasmic loop (Fig. 2.3B). The understanding of the func-tion of receptors of this type owes much to detailed studies of a closely related protein, *rhodopsin*, which is responsible for transduction in retinal rods. This protein is abundant in rods, and therefore much easier to study than receptor proteins (which are anything but abundant); it is built on an identical plan to that shown in Figure 2.3 (see Stryer 1986) and also produces a response in the rod (hyperpolarisation, associated with a switching off of a sodium conductance) through a mechanism involving a G-protein. The most obvious difference is that a photon, rather than an agonist molecule, produces the response. In effect, rhodopsin can be regarded as incorporating its own inbuilt agonist molecule, namely retinal, which isomerises from the *trans* (inactive) to the *cis* (active) form when it absorbs a photon.

Site-directed mutagenesis experiments show that the long third cytoplasmic loop, part of which shows a high degree of conservation among these receptors, is the region of the molecule that couples to the G-protein, since deletion or modification of this section results in receptors that still bind ligands but cannot associate with G-proteins or produce responses. Usually, a particular receptor subtype couples selectively with a particular G-protein, and it has been shown that swapping, by genetic engineering, of the third cytoplasmic loop between different receptors alters their G-protein selectivity.

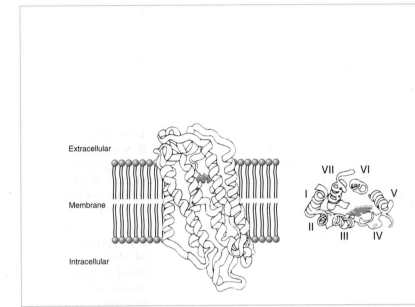

Fig. 2.7 Molecular model of a G-protein-coupled receptor (β-adrenoceptor) lying in the cell membrane, with a molecule of noradrenaline (blue) lying in its binding site. The arrangement of the seven transmembrane helices (I–VII), is based on the crystal structure of bacterial rhodopsin. The docking site for the agonist molecule is shown lying among the helices. The particular amino acid side-chains (not shown) that interact with the agonist molecule have been discovered by selective mutagenesis experiments in which individual residues have been mutated and the effect on agonist binding measured. Similar models are available for several different receptors. (Kindly provided by Dr C R Snell, Novartis Institute for Medical Sciences)

For small molecules, such as noradrenaline, the ligand-binding domain appears to reside not on the extracellular N-terminal region, as with the ion channel-coupled receptors (a region which, one might think, would be easily accessible to small hydrophilic molecules), but buried in the cleft between the α-helical segments within the membrane (Fig. 2.7), similar to the slot occupied by retinal in the rhodopsin molecule (see review by Hibert et al. 1993). Peptide ligands, such as substance P (Ch. 10) bind more superficially, as one might expect (see Schwartz & Rosenkilde 1996). By single site mutagenesis experiments, it is possible to map the ligand-binding domain of these receptors, and the hope is that it may soon be possible to design synthetic ligands based on knowledge of the receptor site structure—an important milestone for the pharmaceutical industry, which has relied up to now mainly on the structure of endogenous mediators (such as histamine) or plant alkaloids (such as morphine) for its chemical inspiration. So far, nobody has succeeded in obtaining a G-protein-coupled receptor in crystalline form, so the powerful technique of X-ray crystallography cannot yet be used to define the molecular structure of these receptors in detail. Until then, drug design will remain a somewhat hit-or-miss business.

Alternative mechanisms of receptor activation

Though activation of G-protein-coupled receptors is normally the consequence of agonist binding, it can occur by other mechanisms. Rhodopsin, mentioned earlier, is activated by light-induced *cis-trans* isomerisation of prebound retinal. Another example is that of thrombin, a protease involved in the blood clotting cascade (see Ch. 17), which also, surprisingly, initiates a variety of cellular response by binding to a G-protein-coupled receptor. Its protease activity is essential for this activity, and it has been found that it works by snipping off a length of 41 amino acids from the extracellular N-terminal tail of the receptor (Fig. 2.8; see Coughlin 1994). The exposed N-terminal residues then bind to receptor domains in the extracellular loops, functioning as a 'tethered agonist'. Other protease-activated receptors have also been described. One consequence of this type of activation is that the receptor can only be activated once, since the cleavage cannot be reversed, so continuous resynthesis of receptor protein is necessary. Inactivation occurs by desensitisation, involving phosphorylation (see below), after which the receptor is internalised and degraded, to be replaced by newly synthesised protein.

G-protein-coupled receptors may also be constitutively active, in the absence of any agonist (see Ch. 1). This was first shown for the β-adrenoceptor (see Ch. 8), where mutations in the third intracellular loop, or simply overexpression of the receptor result in constitutive receptor activation. This can be recognised, as discussed in Chapter 1, by the fact that an inverse agonist (but not a simple competitive antagonist) can reduce the level of activation. Several human disease states have been described (see below) which are associated either with

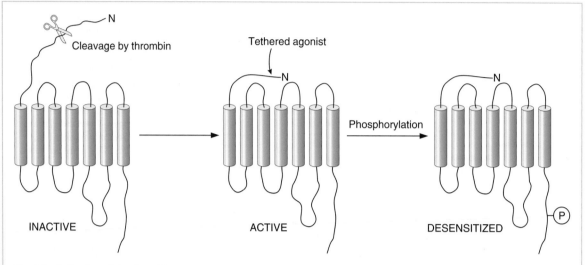

Fig. 2.8   Activation of the thrombin receptor by proteolytic cleavage of the N-terminal extracellular domain. Inactivation occurs by phosphorylation. Recovery requires resynthesis of the receptor.

spontaneous receptor mutations that result in constitutive activation of receptors, or with the production of auto-antibodies directed against the extracellular domain of receptors, which mimic the effect of agonists.

Desensitisation

The sequence of these receptors includes certain residues (serine and threonine) mainly in the C-terminal cyto-plasmic tail which act as *phosphorylation sites* where specific kinase enzymes catalyse the coupling of phos-phate groups. This has the effect of reducing the inter-action of the receptor with the G-protein, and is important as a mechanism of agonist-induced desensitisation (see Ch. 1). Some of these kinases are linked specifically to a particular receptor (e.g. the β-adrenoceptor kinase, BARK) and account for homologous (receptor-specific) desensitisation, whereas others, such as protein kinase A and protein kinase C (see below) are quite promis-cuous, and lead to heterologous (cross-) desensitisation (see review by Chuang et al. 1996). Following phos-phorylation, the receptors may either be reactivated by phosphatases, or internalised by endocytosis and then degraded, to be replaced by newly synthesised receptors (see Koenig & Edwardson 1997).

G-PROTEINS AND THEIR ROLE

G-proteins represent the level of middle management in the organisational hierarchy, able to communicate between the receptors—choosy mandarins alert to the faintest sniff of their own particular hormone—and the effector enzymes or ion channels—the blue collar brigade that gets the job done without any questions about what kind of hormone authorised the process. As we all know, middle management is where the real power resides. They are the go-between proteins, but were actually called G-proteins because of their interaction with the guanine nucleotides, GTP and GDP. They are currently the object of much interest (for recent reviews, see Dolphin 1996, Gudermann et al. 1996, Neer 1995).

G-proteins consist of three subunits, α, β and γ (Fig. 2.9). Guanine nucleotides bind to the α-subunit, which has enzymic activity, catalysing the conversion of GTP to GDP. The β- and γ-subunits remain associated as a βγ complex. All three subunits are anchored to the membrane through a fatty acid chain, attached to an amino acid residue through a reaction known as *prenylation*. G-proteins appear to be freely diffusible in the plane of the membrane, and it is a key aspect of their function that a single pool of G-protein in a cell can interact with several different receptors and effectors in an essentially promiscuous fashion. This has been demonstrated in experiments in which individual recep-tors and G-proteins are co-expressed in cells which normally lack one or other component. In the 'resting' state (Fig. 2.9), the G-protein exists as an unattached αβγ trimer, with GDP occupying the site on the α-subunit. When a receptor is occupied by an agonist molecule, a

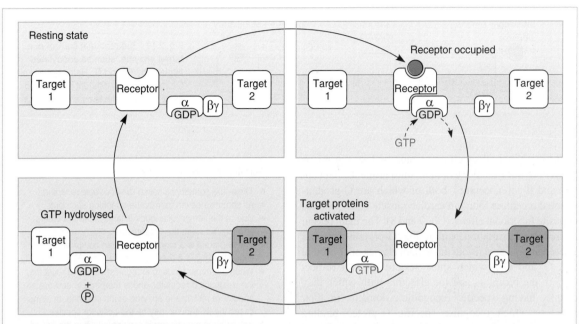

Fig. 2.9 The function of the G-protein. The G-protein consists of three subunits (α, β, γ), which are anchored to the membrane through attached lipid residues. Coupling of the α-subunit to an agonist-occupied receptor causes the bound GDP to exchange with intracellular GTP; the α-GTP complex then dissociates from the receptor and from the $\beta\gamma$ complex, and interacts with a target protein (Target 1, which may be an enzyme such as adenylate cyclase, or an ion channel). The $\beta\gamma$ complex may also activate a target protein (Target 2). The GTP-ase activity of the α-subunit is increased when the target protein is bound, leading to hydrolysis of the bound GTP to GDP, whereupon the α-subunit reunites with $\beta\gamma$. The activated state of the target proteins is shown in blue.

conformational change occurs, involving the cytoplasmic domain of the receptor (Fig. 2.3B), causing it to acquire high affinity for $\alpha\beta\gamma$. Association of $\alpha\beta\gamma$ with the receptor causes the bound GDP to dissociate and to be replaced with GTP (GDP/GTP exchange), which in turn causes dissociation of the G-protein trimer, releasing α-GTP and $\beta\gamma$-subunits; these are the 'active' forms of the G-protein, which diffuse in the membrane and can associate with various enzymes and ion channels, causing activation or inactivation as the case may be (Fig. 2.9).*

*Until recently it was thought that G-protein signalling occurred only through the α-subunit, and that the $\beta\gamma$ complex served merely as a chaperone to keep the flighty α-subunits out of range of the various effector proteins to which they might otherwise snuggle up. However, the $\beta\gamma$ complexes actually make assignations of their own, and control effectors in much the same way as the α-subunits (see Clapham & Neer 1997). In general, it appears that higher concentrations of $\beta\gamma$ complex than of α-subunits are needed, so $\beta\gamma$-mediated effects occur at higher levels of receptor occupancy than α-mediated effects. The control of ion channels by G-proteins, discussed on page 39, exemplifies the dual role of the α- and $\beta\gamma$-subunits.

The process is terminated when the hydrolysis of GTP to GDP occurs through the GTPase activity of the α-subunit. The resulting α-GDP then dissociates from the effector, and reunites with $\beta\gamma$, completing the cycle. Attachment of the α-subunit to an effector molecule actually increases its GTPase activity, the magnitude of this increase being different for different types of effector. Since GTP hydrolysis is the step that terminates the ability of the α-subunit to produce its effect, regulation of its GTPase activity by the effector protein means that the activation of the effector tends to be self-limiting. Mechanisms of this type in general result in amplification because a single agonist–receptor complex can activate several G-protein molecules in turn, and each of these can remain associated with the effector enzyme for long enough to produce many molecules of product. The product (see below) is often a 'second messenger', and further amplification occurs before the final cellular response is produced.

How is specificity achieved so that each kind of receptor produces a distinct pattern of cellular responses? With a common pool of promiscuous G-proteins linking the various receptors and effector systems in a cell it

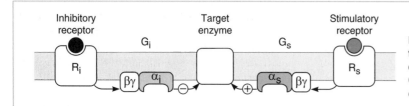

Fig. 2.10 Bidirectional control of a target enzyme, such as adenylated cyclase by G_s and G_i. Heterogeneity of G-proteins allows different receptors to exert opposite effects on a target enzyme.

might seem that all specificity would be lost, but this is clearly not the case. For example, muscarinic ACh receptors and β-adrenoceptors, both of which are G-protein-coupled receptors found in cardiac muscle cells, produce opposite functional effects (Chs 7 and 8). The main reason is molecular variation within the G-protein family.* These variants give rise to three main classes of G-protein (G_s, G_i and G_q), which show selectivity with respect to both the receptors and the effectors with which they couple, having specific recognition domains in their structure which recognise specific G-protein-binding domains in the receptor and effector molecules; G_s and G_i produce, respectively, stimulation and inhibition of the enzyme adenylate cyclase (Fig. 2.10), and a similar bidirectional control operates on other effectors, such as phospholipase C (see Gudermann et al. 1996). The G-proteins can be thought of as the intramembrane managers, bustling like stock exchange jobbers between receptors and effectors, controlling this microcosm but communicating very little with the world outside.

The α-subunits of these G-proteins differ in structure. One functional difference that has been useful as an experimental tool to distinguish which type of G-protein is involved in different situations, concerns the action of two bacterial toxins, *cholera toxin* and *pertussis toxin*. These toxins, which are enzymes, catalyse a conjugation reaction (ADP-ribosylation) on the α-subunit of G-proteins. Cholera toxin acts only on G_s, and it causes persistent activation. Many of the symptoms of cholera, such as the excessive secretion of fluid from the gastrointestinal epithelium, are due to the uncontrolled activation of adenylate cyclase that occurs. Pertussis toxin acts on G_i in a similar way.

*There are, to date, more than 20 known subtypes of G_α, 6 of G_β, and 12 of G_γ providing, in theory, about 1500 variants of the trimer. Even if only some are functional, there is plenty of scope for providing quite specific linkages between receptors and their effectors. By now, you will be unsurprised (even if somewhat bemused) by such a display of molecular heterogeneity, for it is the way of evolution.

G-protein-coupled receptors

- These are sometimes called *metabotropic receptors*.
- All comprise seven membrane-spanning segments.
- One of the intracellular loops is larger than the others and interacts with the G-protein.
- The G-protein is a membrane protein comprising three subunits (αβγ), the α-subunit possessing GTPase activity.
- When the trimer binds to antagonist-occupied receptor, the α-subunit dissociates and is then free to activate an effector (a membrane enzyme or ion channel). In some cases the βγ-subunit may be the activator species.
- Activation of the effector is terminated when the bound GTP molecule is hydrolysed, which allows the α-subunit to recombine with βγ.
- There are several types of G-protein, which interact with different receptors and control different effectors.
- Examples include mAChR, adrenoceptors and neuropeptide receptors.

Targets for G-proteins

We have discussed the receptors and the G-proteins in some detail. What happens next? The pioneering studies on receptor–effector coupling, which led to the discovery of the role of G-proteins, focused on the regulation of a key membrane enzyme, *adenylate cyclase*, which was known to be activated by catecholamines in many different cells. It is now known that other membrane enzymes, such as *phospholipase C* and *phospholipase A_2*, as well as a variety of ion channels, are similarly controlled (see Gudermann et al. 1996, Milligan 1995 for more details).

Three of these G-protein-coupled effector systems will now be considered in more detail. They are:

- the adenylate cyclase/cAMP system
- the phospholipase C/inositol phosphate system
- the regulation of ion channels.

The adenylate cyclase/cAMP system

The role of cAMP (cyclic 3′,5′-adenosine monophosphate) as a second messenger was first revealed by the work of Sutherland and his colleagues in the late 1950s. This discovery demolished at a stroke the barriers that existed between biochemistry and pharmacology, and introduced the concept of second messengers (see below) in signal transduction. Cyclic-AMP is a nucleotide synthesised within the cell from ATP by the action of a membrane-bound enzyme, adenylate cyclase. It is produced continuously and inactivated by hydrolysis to 5'-AMP, by the action of a family of enzymes known as phosphodiesterases. Many different drugs, hormones and neurotransmitters produce their effects by increasing or decreasing the catalytic activity of adenylate cyclase and thus raising or lowering the concentration of cAMP within the cell.

Cyclic AMP regulates many aspects of cellular function including, for example, enzymes involved in energy metabolism, cell division and cell differentiation, ion transport, ion channels, and the contractile proteins in smooth muscle. These varied effects are, however, all brought about by a common mechanism, namely the activation of various *protein kinases* by cAMP. These enzymes catalyse the phosphorylation of serine and threonine residues in different cellular proteins, using ATP as source of phosphate groups, and thereby regulate their function. Phosphorylation can either activate or inhibit target enzymes or ion channels. Figure 2.11 shows the ways in which increased cAMP production in response to β-adrenoceptor activation affects the various enzymes involved in glycogen and fat metabolism in liver, fat and muscle cells. The result is a coordinated

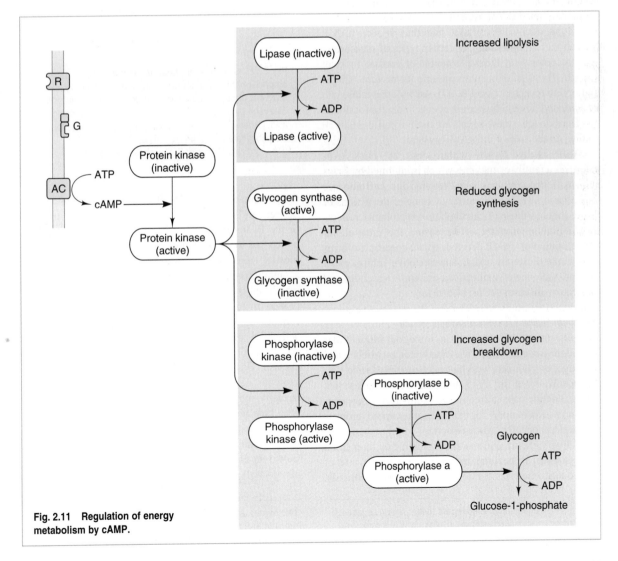

Fig. 2.11 Regulation of energy metabolism by cAMP.

response in which stored energy in the form of glycogen and fat is made available as glucose to fuel muscle contraction.

Other examples of regulation by cAMP-dependent protein kinases include the increased activity of voltage-activated calcium channels in heart muscle cells (see Ch. 14); phosphorylation of these channels increases the amount of calcium entering the cell during the action potential, and thus increases the force of contraction of the heart.

In smooth muscle, cAMP-dependent protein kinase phosphorylates (thereby inactivating) another enzyme, *myosin-light-chain kinase*, which is required for contraction. This accounts for the smooth muscle relaxation produced by many drugs which increase cAMP production in smooth muscle (see Ch. 15).

As mentioned above, receptors linked to G_i rather than G_s inhibit adenylate cyclase, and thus reduce cAMP formation. Examples include certain types of muscarinic ACh receptor (e.g. the M_2 receptor of cardiac muscle; see Ch. 7), α_2-adrenoceptors in smooth muscle (Ch. 8) and opioid receptors (see Ch. 37). Adenylate cyclase can be activated directly by certain agents, includin **forskolin** and fluoride ions; these agents are used experimentally in studies on the role of the cAMP system.

cAMP is hydrolysed within cells by *phosphodiesterases* a family of enzymes which is inhibited by drugs such as methylxanthines (e.g. **theophylline**, **caffeine**; see Chs 19 and 38). The similarity of some of the actions of these drugs to those of catecholamines probably reflects their common property of increasing the intracellular concentration of cAMP. Various tissue-specific isoforms of phosphodiesterase exist, and selective inhibitors of this enzyme have applications in cardiovascular and respiratory diseases* (Chs 14 and 19).

The phospholipase C/inositol phosphate system

The phosphoinositide system, an important intracellular second messenger system, was discovered by Michell and Berridge, biochemists working independently in the UK.

Michell noted in 1975 that many hormones that produce an increase in free intracellular calcium concentration (which include, for example, muscarinic agonists and α-adrenoceptor agonists acting on smooth muscle and salivary glands, and vasopressin acting on liver cells) also produce an accompanying increase in the rate of degradation of a class of minor membrane phospholipids,

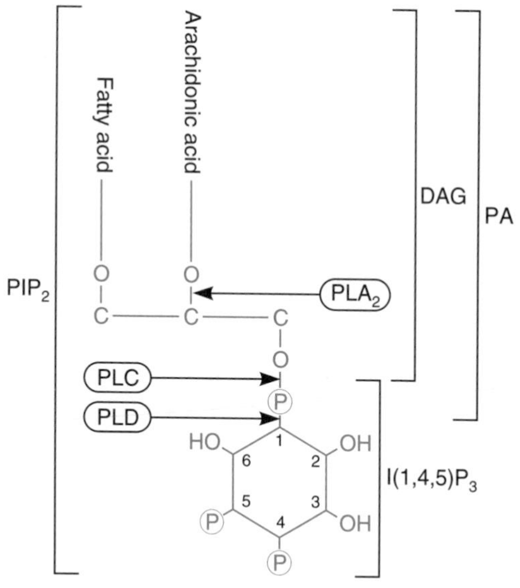

Fig. 2.12 Structure of phosphatidylinositol bisphosphate (PIP₂), showing sites of cleavage by different phospholipases to produce active mediators. Cleavage by phospholipase A_2 (PLA_2) yields arachidonic acid. Cleavage by phospholipase C (PLC) yields inositol tris-phosphate ($I(1,4,5)P_3$) and diacylglycerol (DAG). (PA = phosphatidic acid; PLD = phospholipase D)

the phosphatidylinositols (PI;** see Figs 2.12 and 2.13). Subsequently it was found that one particular member of the PI family, namely PI (4,5) *bis*-phosphate (PIP₂), which has additional phosphate groups attached to the inositol ring, plays a key role. PIP₂ is the substrate for a membrane-bound enzyme, phospholipase C_β (PLC_β), which splits it into *diacylglycerol* (DAG) and *inositol (1,4,5) tris-phosphate* (IP₃; Fig. 2.12), both of which function as second messengers as discussed below. The activation of PLC_β by various agonists is mediated through a G-protein in just the same way as adenylate cyclase, described above, though different G-protein subtypes are involved. A different isozyme PLC_γ can also be activated directly by receptors of the kinase-linked type (see above) through a quite separate mechanism, not involving a G-protein (see p. 41). Following cleavage of PIP₂ and release of IP₃ the status quo is restored as shown in Figure 2.13. DAG is phosphorylated to form phosphatidic acid (PA), while the IP₃ is dephosphorylated

---

*One such, of recent fame, is **sildenafil** (better known as viagra) which inhibits a phosphodiesterase insoform which is selectively expressed in blood vessels of the genitalia.

**Alternative abbreviations for these mediators are: PtdIns (PI); PtdIns (4,5)-P₂ (PIP₂); Ins (1,4,5)-P₃ (IP₃); Ins (1,3,4,5)-P₄ (IP₄). We use the shorter, more pronounceable abbreviations.

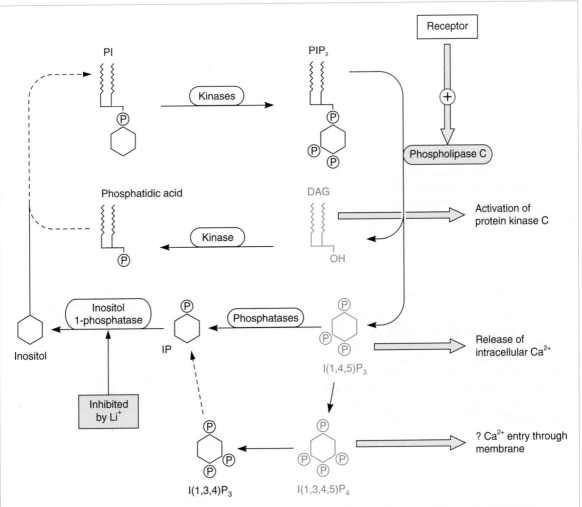

Fig. 2.13   The PI cycle. Receptor-mediated activation of phospholipase C results in the cleavage of PIP$_2$, forming DAG (which activates protein kinase C) and IP$_3$ (which releases intracellular calcium). The role of IP$_4$, which is formed from IP$_3$ and other inositol phosphates, is unclear, but it may facilitate calcium entry through the plasma membrane. IP$_3$ is inactivated by dephosphorylation to inositol. DAG is converted to phosphatidic acid, and these two products are used to regenerate PI and PIP$_2$.

and then recoupled with PA to form PI once again. **Lithium**, an agent used in psychiatry (see Ch. 35) blocks this recycling pathway (see Fig. 2.13).

The receptor-mediated activation of phospholipase A$_2$, leading to the production of arachidonic acid metabolites, appears to be basically similar to the activation of phospholipase C. The role of arachidonic acid and its metabolites as mediators is discussed further in Chapter 12. (See also Figs 12.4–12.7.) It is of interest that arachidonic acid and its metabolites have recently been shown to function as intracellular messengers, controlling potassium channel function in certain neurons (see

Piomelli 1997), in addition to their well-known role as local hormones communicating between cells.

Inositol phosphates and intracellular calcium

IP$_3$ acts by releasing calcium from intracellular stores. Intracellular calcium is stored in vesicles—the endoplasmic reticulum—which actively sequester calcium, keeping the free concentration in the cytosol to about 10^{-7} mol/l or less. IP$_3$ binds to a specific receptor present in the membrane of the endoplasmic reticulum, which is coupled to a calcium-selective ion channel, whose molecular structure is similar to that of the channel-linked

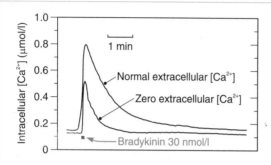

Fig. 2.14 **Increase in intracellular calcium concentration in response to receptor activation.** The records were obtained from a single rat sensory neuron grown in tissue culture. The cells were loaded with the fluorescent calcium indicator, Fura-2, and the signal from a single cell monitored with a fluorescence microscope. A brief exposure to the peptide bradykinin, which causes excitation of sensory neurons (see Ch. 37) causes a transient increase in $[Ca^{2+}]_i$ from the resting value of about 150 nmol/l. When calcium is removed from the extracellular solution, the bradykinin-induced increase in $[Ca^{2+}]$ is still present, but is smaller and briefer. The response in the absence of extracellular calcium represents the release of stored intracellular calcium, resulting from the intracellular production of IP_3. The difference between this and the larger response when calcium is present extracellularly is believed to represent calcium entry through receptor-operated ion channels in the cell membrane. (Figure kindly provided by G M Burgess and A Forbes, Novartis Institute for Medical Research)

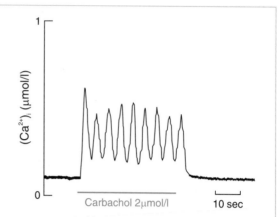

Fig. 2.15 **Oscillations of intracellular calcium in response to an agonist.** The recording was made from a single parotid gland cell, with Fura-2 as an intracellular calcium indicator, as in Figure 2.14. During the period indicated by the horizontal bar, the cell was exposed to 2 μmol/l carbachol (which elicits secretion from the salivary gland; see Ch. 7) which produced a sequence of regular oscillations in the intracellular calcium concentration. (From: Gray P T A 1988 J Physiol 406: 35–53)

receptors in the plasma membrane, discussed earlier. Opening these channels in the endoplasmic reticulum membrane releases a flood of calcium into the cell and raises the free concentration 10- to 100-fold (see Berridge 1993, 1997).

Two techniques have been particularly important in unravelling the role of inositol phosphates and intracellular calcium as messengers controlling hormone responses. One is the measurement of free intracellular calcium concentration by the use of fluorescence indicators, such as Fura-2. This dye can be introduced into cells and used to report moment-to-moment changes in calcium concentration within a single cell, or even in parts of a cell. Figure 2.14 shows the signal recorded in this way from a sensory neuron in response to application of bradykinin, a peptide that causes excitation of these cells (see Ch. 37).

Another useful technique is intracellular perfusion of cells by means of tight-seal pipettes, which enables different substances that do not cross the cell membrane, such as IP_3, to be introduced into a cell while the mem-

brane potential or conductance of the cell is recorded, or while monitoring intracellular calcium. As a refinement, potential messenger substances can be introduced into cells in an inactive ('caged') form and activated by photolysis, induced by an intense light flash.

Since the discovery of $(1,4,5)$-IP_3 as the major calcium-releasing messenger, a variety of other inositol phosphates have come on the scene (see Downes 1988) in which the phosphate groups appear to play musical chairs around the inositol molecule, and much effort has gone into trying to identify a physiological role for some of these products. There is some evidence (see Clapham 1995, Downes 1988) that the tetraphosphate $(1,3,4,5)$-IP_4 facilitates calcium entry through the cell membrane, thus helping to replenish the intracellular stores, but this remains controversial.

The use of intracellular calcium monitoring in single cells has shown, in many instances, the surprising result that calcium release in response to agonists or IP_3 injection does not occur continuously, but in a series of waves (Fig. 2.15; Berridge 1993, 1997). This is partly due to the fact that calcium itself can, in many types of cell, act to open calcium channels in the endoplasmic reticulum, producing a delayed surge of calcium triggered by the initial small response. Negative feedback may also occur, as calcium can activate kinases that phosphorylate, and hence desensitise, the receptors (see p. 32). This delayed feedback can give rise to an oscillatory response. Improvements in the spatial and temporal resolution of calcium-monitoring techniques have revealed that calcium release can occur in very discrete regions of cells and in very brief bursts (known to afficionados as *puffs* and *sparks*).

An increase in free intracellular calcium concentration occurs in many types of cell in response to a wide variety of agonists, and it is perhaps the most important pathway by which cellular effects are produced. (For general reviews on intracellular calcium regulation see Clapham 1995, Berridge 1993, 1997.) The range of cellular responses mediated by intracellular calcium is too broad to discuss in detail. Examples that are of particular pharmacological importance include:

- smooth muscle contraction (Ch. 15)
- increased force of contraction of cardiac muscle (Ch. 14)
- secretion from exocrine glands and transmitter release from neurons (Chs 6 and 28)
- hormone release (Chs 22 and 24)
- cytotoxicity (Ch. 31).

This list is far from complete. The actions of calcium depend on its ability to regulate various functional proteins, including enzymes, contractile proteins and ion channels. These proteins may bind calcium directly, or the effect may be mediated through other calcium-binding proteins, such as *calmodulin*, a ubiquitous cytosolic calcium-binding protein which controls a wide variety of effectors, including, for example, NO synthase (Ch. 11).

Diacylglycerol and protein kinase C. Diacylglycerol (DAG) is produced as well as IP_3 whenever receptor-induced PI hydrolysis occurs. The main effect of DAG is to activate a membrane-bound protein kinase, protein kinase C (PKC), which causes phosphorylation of serine and threonine residues of a variety of intracellular proteins (see Nishizuka 1986, Parker & Dekker 1996, Walaas & Greengard 1991). DAG, unlike the inositol phosphates, is highly lipophilic and remains within the membrane. It binds to a specific site on the protein kinase C molecule which is thought to migrate from the cytosol to the cell membrane in the presence of DAG, thereby becoming activated. At least 13 different types of PKC are now known to exist; they have distinct cellular distributions, and probably have different substrate specificities in terms of the proteins that are phosphorylated. They have in common the property of being activated by **phorbol esters** (highly irritant, tumour-promoting compounds produced by certain plants), which have been extremely useful in studying the functions of PKC. Interestingly, one of the subtypes is activated by arachidonic acid, which is a product of phospholipid hydrolysis by phospholipase A_2 (see above), so PKC activation can also occur with agonists that activate this enzyme. The role of protein phosphorylation in signal transduction is discussed further below.

The regulation of ion channels

G-protein-coupled receptors can control ion channel function by mechanisms that do not involve any second messengers such as cAMP or inositol phosphates; instead, the G-protein interacts directly with the channel, presumably in the same way as it interacts with membrane enzymes responsible for second messenger synthesis. This was first shown for cardiac muscle, but it now appears that this pattern of direct G-protein/channel interaction may be quite general (see Wickham & Clapham 1995). The clearest examples come from studies on potassium channels. In cardiac muscle, for example, muscarinic ACh receptors are known to enhance K permeability (thus hyperpolarising the cells and inhibiting electrical activity; see Ch. 14). Similar mechanisms are believed to operate in neurons, where opiate analgesics reduce excitability by opening potassium channels (see Ch. 37). These actions are produced by direct interaction between the G-protein subunit and the channel, without the involvement of second messengers. As shown in Figure 2.9, either the free α-subunit, or the βγ-subunit of the G-protein, may be the mediator which controls the channel.

The postulated roles of G-protein-coupled receptors in controlling enzymes and ion channels are summarised in Figure 2.16.

Agonist specificity

The linkage of a particular receptor to a particular signal transduction pathway depends mainly on the structure of the receptor, particularly in the region of the third intracellular loop, which confers specificity for a particular G-protein, from which the rest of the signal transduction pathway follows. It is known that mutations in this region, which do not affect the ligand-binding specificity of the receptor, can cause it to switch from one pathway (e.g. cAMP) to another (e.g. the inositol phosphate pathway), which it would not normally activate. In general, the nature of the agonist does not alter the signal transduction pathway, so all agonists acting on a particular receptor produce basically the same type of cellular response. Complications are beginning to appear, however, and there is now evidence (see Kenakin 1995) that different agonists may produce different activated forms of the receptor, and hence different cellular responses—a phenomenon termed *agonist trafficking*. Examples are

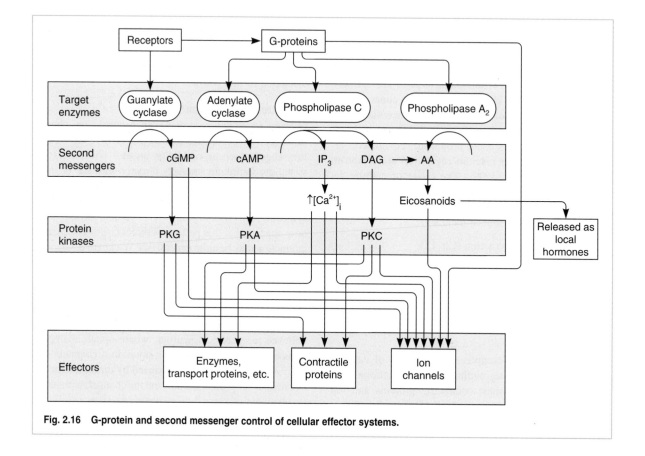

Fig. 2.16   G-protein and second messenger control of cellular effector systems.

Effectors controlled by G-proteins

Two key pathways are controlled by receptors, via G-proteins. Both can be activated or inhibited by pharmacological ligands, depending on the nature of the receptor and G-protein.

● Adenylate cyclase/cAMP:
  — AC catalyses formation of the intracellular messenger, cAMP.
  — cAMP activates various protein kinases which control cell function in many different ways by causing phosphorylation of various enzymes, carriers and other proteins.
● Phospholipase C/inositol tris-phosphate/diacylglycerol:
  — catalyses the formation of two intracellular messengers, IP_3 and DAG, from membrane phospholipid.

— IP_3 acts to increase free cytosolic calcium by releasing calcium from intracellular compartments.
— Increased free calcium initiates many events, including contraction, secretion, enzyme activation and membrane hyperpolarisation.
— DAG activates protein kinase C, which controls many cellular functions by phosphorylating a variety of proteins.

Receptor-linked G-proteins also control:

● phospholipase A, (and thus the formation of arachidonic acid and eicosanoids)
● ion channels (e.g. K^+ and Ca^{2+} channels, thus affecting membrane excitability, transmitter release, contractility, etc.).

---

rare, and the idea is currently controversial—indeed heretical to many pharmacologists, who are accustomed to think of agonists in terms of their affinity and efficacy and nothing else. If substantiated, it will add a new dimension to the way in which we think about drug specificity.

TYROSINE-KINASE- AND GUANYLATE-CYCLASE-LINKED RECEPTORS

Tyrosine-kinase-linked receptors are quite different in structure and function from either the channel-linked receptors or the G-protein-coupled receptors discussed above. They mediate the actions of a wide variety of growth factors and cytokines (see Ch. 12), and also of certain hormones, such as insulin (see Ch. 22) and leptin (Ch. 23). For more detail, see reviews by Barbacid (1996), Ihle (1995) and Mayer & Baltimore (1993). Guanylate-cyclase-linked receptors mediate the actions of certain peptides such as atrial natriuretic peptide (see Ch. 14).

The basic structure of these receptors is shown in Figure 2.3C. They comprise very large extracellular (ligand-binding) and intracellular (effector) domains, with about 400–700 residues in each. In the case of the insulin receptor, most of the extracellular domain consists of a separate polypeptide chain which is linked by disulphide bonds to the chain that forms the transmembrane and intracellular regions. In contrast, the growth factor receptors consist of a single long chain of over 1000 residues. Cytokine receptors are generally similar, but are often dimeric. In all cases the receptors trigger a *kinase cascade* (see below). With growth-factor and insulin receptors, the intracellular region possesses tyrosine kinase activity, and incorporates both ATP- and substrate-binding sites. Cytokine receptors do not usually have intrinsic kinase activity, but associate, when activated by ligand binding, with kinases known as *Jaks* (see below), which are the first step in the kinase cascade.

With only a single transmembrane helix linking the outer receptor domain with the inner kinase domain, a simple allosteric interaction seems unlikely as a mechanism by which the kinase is activated by ligand binding. Instead, ligand binding generally leads to dimerisation of pairs of receptors. The association of the two intracellular kinase domains allows an incestuous autophosphorylation of tyrosine residues in these two kinase domains to occur. The autophosphorylated tyrosine residues then serve as high-affinity binding sites for other intracellular proteins, which have in common a highly conserved sequence of about 100 amino acids, known as the SH2 domain (standing for Src-homology, since it was first identified in the Src oncogene product). Individual SH2-domain proteins, of which many are now known, bind very selectively to the phosphotyrosine residues of particular receptors, so the pattern of events triggered by particular growth factors is highly specific. The mechanism is summarised in Figure 2.17.

Protein phosphorylation and kinase cascade mechanisms

What happens after the SH2-containing protein binds to the phosphorylated receptor varies greatly according to the receptor that is involved; many SH2-containing

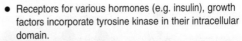

Kinase-linked receptors

- Receptors for various hormones (e.g. insulin), growth factors incorporate tyrosine kinase in their intracellular domain.
- Cytokine receptors have an intracellular domain which binds and activates cytosolic kinases when the receptor is occupied.
- The receptors all share a common architecture, with a large extracellular ligand-binding domain connected via a single α-helix to the intracellular domain.
- Signal transduction generally involves dimerisation of receptors, followed by autophosphorylation of tyrosine residues. The phosphotyrosine residues act as acceptors for the SH2 domains of a variety of intracellular proteins, thereby allowing control of many cell functions.
- They are involved mainly in events controlling cell growth and differentiation, and act indirectly by regulating gene transcription.
- Two important pathways are:
  — the Ras/Raf/MAP kinase pathway which is important in cell division, growth and differentiation
  — the Jak/Stat pathway activated by many cytokines, which controls the synthesis and release of many inflammatory mediators.
- A few hormone receptors (e.g. ANF) have a similar architecture, and are linked to guanylate cyclase.

proteins are enzymes, such as protein kinases or phospholipases. Some growth factors activate a specific subtype of phospholipase C (PLC$_\gamma$) thereby causing phospholipid breakdown, IP$_3$ formation and calcium release (see above). Other SH2-containing proteins are 'adaptors' which serve as a coupling between phosphotyrosine-containing proteins and a wide variety of other functional proteins, including many that are involved in the control of cell division and differentiation. The principal action of growth factors is to stimulate transcription of particular genes.

Two well-defined signal transduction pathways are summarised in Figure 2.17. The *Ras/Raf* pathway (Fig. 2.17A) mediates the effect of many growth factors and mitogens. Ras, which is a proto-oncogene product, functions like a G-protein, and conveys the signal (by GDP/GTP exchange) from the SH2-domain protein, *Grb*, which is phosphorylated by the receptor tyrosine kinase. Activation of Ras, in turn activates Raf, which is the first of a sequence of serine/threonine kinases, each of which phosphorylates, and activates, the next in line. The last of these, *MAP-kinase*, phosphorylates one or more transcription factors which initiate gene expression, resulting in a variety of cellular responses, including cell division. Many cancers are associated with

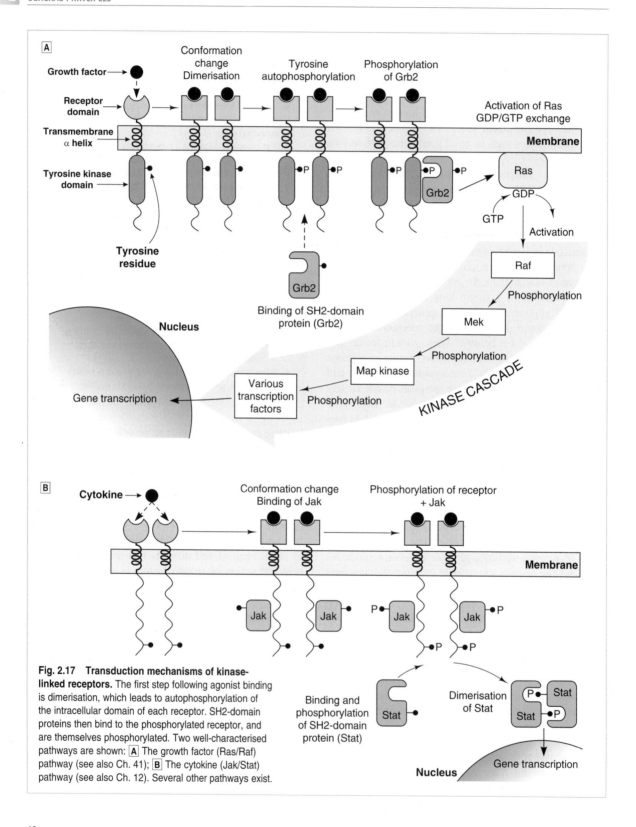

Fig. 2.17 Transduction mechanisms of kinase-linked receptors. The first step following agonist binding is dimerisation, which leads to autophosphorylation of the intracellular domain of each receptor. SH2-domain proteins then bind to the phosphorylated receptor, and are themselves phosphorylated. Two well-characterised pathways are shown: [A] The growth factor (Ras/Raf) pathway (see also Ch. 41); [B] The cytokine (Jak/Stat) pathway (see also Ch. 12). Several other pathways exist.

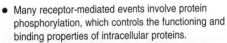

mutations in the genes coding for proteins involved in this cascade, leading to activation of the cascade in the absence of the growth factor signal (see Ch. 41). (For more details, see reviews by Avruch et al. 1994, Marshall 1996.)

A second pathway, the *Jak/Stat* pathway (Fig. 2.17B) is involved in responses to many cytokines. Dimerisation of these receptors occurs when the cytokine binds, and this attracts a cytosolic tyrosine kinase unit (Jak) to associate with, and phosphorylate, the receptor dimer. Jaks belong to a family of proteins, different members having specificity for different cytokine receptors. Among the targets for phosphorylation by Jak are a family of transcription factors (Stats). These are SH2-domain proteins which bind to the phosphotyrosine groups on the receptor–Jak complex, and are themselves phosphorylated. Thus activated, Stat migrates to the nucleus and activates gene expression (see Ihle 1995).

There has recently been an explosion of work on signal transduction pathways, leading to a bewildering profusion of molecular detail, often couched in a jargon which is apt to deter the faint-hearted. Perseverance will be rewarded, however, for there is no doubt that important new drugs, particularly in the areas of inflammation, immunology and cancer, will come from the targeting of some of these newly identified proteins (see Levitzki 1996).

It is interesting that the membrane-bound form of guanylate cyclase, the enzyme responsible for generating the second messenger cGMP in response to the binding of peptides such as atrial natriuretic peptide (ANP; see Chs 11 and 15), which intuitively one would have expected to resemble adenylate cyclase in its structure and regulation (see above), actually resembles the tyrosine kinase family, and is activated in a similar way by dimerisation when the agonist is bound (see Garbers & Lowe 1994). It is not known whether tyrosine phosphorylation is involved in the activation of the enzyme.

RECEPTORS THAT REGULATE GENE TRANSCRIPTION

The receptor-mediated regulation of DNA transcription is characteristic of steroid and thyroid hormones, and is quite different from the mechanisms described so far (see Evans 1988, Mangelsdorf et al. 1995 for reviews). The work of Jensen in Chicago, originally led to the recognition that the highly varied effects of different steroid drugs and hormones (which include numerous effects on the reproductive system, the kidney, the immune system, etc.) all operate through the same basic

---

Protein phosphorylation in signal transduction

- Many receptor-mediated events involve protein phosphorylation, which controls the functioning and binding properties of intracellular proteins.
- Receptor-linked tyrosine kinases, cyclic nucleotide-activated tyrosine kinases, and intracellular serine/threonine kinases comprise a 'kinase cascade' mechanism which leads to amplification of receptor-mediated events.
- There are many kinases, with differing substrate specificities, allowing specificity in the pathways activated by different hormones.
- Desensitisation of G-protein-coupled receptors occurs as a result of phosphorylation by specific receptor kinases, causing the receptor to become non-functional, and to be internalised.
- There is a large family of phosphatases which act to reverse the effects of kinases.

---

mechanism, namely by stimulating transcription of selected genes, leading to the synthesis of particular proteins and the production of cellular effects (see Ch. 24). Most receptors are located in the nucleus, and the ligands are all lipophilic compounds which can readily cross the cell membrane.* The basic structure of this family of receptors is shown in Figures 2.3D and 24.7. They are large monomeric proteins of 400–1000 residues, containing a highly conserved region of about 60 residues in the middle of the molecule, which constitutes the DNA-binding domain of the receptor. It contains two loops of about 15 residues each (*zinc fingers*), knotted together by a cluster of four cysteine residues surrounding a zinc atom; these structures occur in many proteins that regulate DNA transcription, and the fingers are believed to wrap around the DNA helix. The hormone-binding domain lies downstream of this central region, while upstream lies a variable region which is responsible for controlling gene transcription.

On binding a steroid molecule, the receptor changes its conformation, which facilitates the formation of receptor dimers. These dimers bind to specific sequences of the nuclear DNA, known as hormone-responsive elements, which lie about 200 base pairs upstream from the genes that are regulated. An increase in RNA polymerase activity and the production of specific mRNA occur within a few minutes of adding the steroid, though

---

*There are a few exceptions to the general rule that steroids act by controlling protein synthesis. Aldosterone, in particular, produces rapid, non-genomic effects on renal function that appear to be mediated by a membrane receptor (Ch. 20).

the physiological response may take hours or days to develop. The different steroid hormones are able induce or repress specific genes, and thus initiate completely different patterns of protein synthesis, and produce different physiological effects. For example, glucocorticoids inhibit transcription of the gene for cyclo-oxygenase-2 (COX-2), which may account for their anti-inflammatory properties (see Ch. 13), whereas mineralocorticoids stimulate the production of various transport proteins that are involved in renal tubular function (see Ch. 20). Specificity at the DNA level seems to be a function of the amino-terminal and DNA-binding domain of the receptor, rather than of the hormone-binding domain since chimaeric receptors consisting of the amino-terminus/DNA-binding part of one receptor (A) coupled to the hormone-binding part of another (B) will respond to hormone B but produce the effects associated with hormone A. More detail is given in the reviews mentioned above.

Other molecules which act in a similar way by binding to intracellular receptors of this family include *thyroid hormones* (Ch. 25), *vitamin D* (Ch. 27) and *retinoic acid*. Retinoic acid is an important regulator of embryonic development, and gradients of this substance arising during development play a key role in controlling the development of limbs and organs

Intracellular receptors of this type (of which more than 100 have been cloned) function generally as transcriptional regulators, but in many cases the ligand to which they respond has not been identified—such molecules have been termed *orphan receptors* (Laudet & Adelmant 1995).

There are also, as with the tyrosine kinase receptors, several examples of oncogene products which appear to be surrogates of steroid or thyroid hormone receptors, but do not require hormone binding for activation.

CONTROL OF RECEPTOR EXPRESSION

Receptor proteins are synthesised by the cells that express them, and the level of expression is itself controlled, via the pathways discussed above, by receptor-mediated events. We can no longer think of the receptors as the fixed elements in cellular control systems, responding to changes in the concentration of ligands, and initiating changes in the components of the signal transduction pathway—they are themselves subject to regulation. Short-term regulation of receptor function generally occurs through desensitisation, as discussed above. Long-term regulation occurs through an increase or decrease of receptor expression. Examples of this type of control (see review by Donaldson et al. 1997) include the proliferation of various postsynaptic receptors after denervation (see Ch. 5), the up-regulation of various G-protein-coupled and cytokine receptors in response to inflammation (see Ch. 12), and the induction of growth factor receptors by certain tumour viruses (see Ch. 41). Adaptive responses to long-term drug treatment are very common, particularly with drugs that act on the central nervous system. They may take the form of a very slow onset of the therapeutic effect (e.g. with antidepressant drugs; see Ch. 35), or the development of drug dependence (Ch. 39). Though the details are not yet clear, it is most likely that changes in receptor expression, secondary to the immediate action of the drug, are involved—a kind of 'secondary pharmacology' whose importance is only now becoming clearer.

RECEPTORS AND DISEASE

Increasing understanding of receptor function in molecular terms has revealed a number of disease states directly linked to receptor malfunction. The principal mechanisms involved are:

- autoantibodies directed against receptor proteins
- mutations in genes encoding receptors and proteins involved in signal transduction.

An example of the former is *myasthenia gravis* (see Ch. 7), a disease of the neuromuscular junction, due to autoantibodies which inactivate nicotinic acetylcholine receptors. Autoantibodies can also mimic the effects of agonists, as in many cases of thyroid hypersecretion,

---

Receptors that control gene transcription (intracellular receptors)

- Ligands include steroid hormones, thyroid hormones, vitamin D and retinoic acid.
- Receptors are intracellular proteins, so ligands must first enter cells.
- Receptors consist of a conserved DNA-binding domain attached to variable ligand-binding and transcriptional control domains.
- DNA-binding domain recognises specific base sequences, thus promoting or repressing particular genes.
- Pattern of gene activation depends on both cell type and nature of ligand, so effects are highly diverse.
- Effects are produced as a result of altered protein synthesis, and thus are slow in onset.

caused by activation of thyrotropin receptors. Activating antibodies have also been discovered in patients with severe hypertension (α-adrenoceptors), cardiomyopathy (β-adrenoceptors) and certain forms of epilepsy and neurodegenerative disorder (glutamate receptors). The list is growing steadily

Inherited mutations of genes encoding G-protein-coupled receptors account for various disease states (see Birnbaumer 1995). Mutated vasopressin and ACTH receptors (see Chs 20 and 24) can result in resistance to these hormones. Conditions in which receptor mutations result in permanently switched-on effector mechanisms

in the absence of agonist have also been described (see Lefkowitz 1993). One of these involves the receptor for thyrotropin, producing continuous oversecretion of thyroid hormone; another involves the receptor for luteinising hormone, and results in precocious puberty. There is also a rare form of hypoparathyroidism, which appears to result from defective G-protein coupling of the parathyroid hormone receptor to adenylate cyclase.

Mutations of the genes encoding growth factor receptors and many other proteins involved in signal transduction can result in malignant transformation of cells (see Ch. 42).

REFERENCES AND FURTHER READING

Ashcroft F M 1988 Adenosine 5'-triphosphate-sensitive potassium channels. Annu Rev Neurosci 11: 97–118 (*Review on an important type of K+ channel that regulates membrane properties in response to metabolic conditions within cells*)

Avruch J, Zhang X-F, Kyriakis J M 1994 Raf meets Ras: completing the framework of a signal transduction pathway. Trends Biochem Sci 19: 277–283 (*Review focusing on the linkage between two important pathways that link membrane receptors to intracellular events*)

Barbacid M 1996 Neurotrophic factors and their receptors. Curr Biol 7: 148–155 (*Useful review of neural growth factors and their associated tyrosine kinase-linked receptors*)

Barnard E A 1992 Receptor classes and the transmitter-gated ion channels. Trends Biochem Sci 17: 368–374 (*Short general review of the molecular biology of channel-linked receptors*)

Berridge M 1993 Inositol trisphosphate and calcium signalling. Nature 361: 315–325 (*Excellent general review*)

Berridge M 1997 Elementary and global aspects of calcium signalling. J Physiol 499: 291–306 (*Excellent general review*)

Birnbaumer M 1995 Mutations and diseases of G-protein-coupled receptors. R Receptor Sig Trans Res 15: 131–160 (*Focuses on the growing list of clinical disorders associated with receptor malfunction*)

Chuang T T, Iacovelli L, Sallese M, De Blasi A 1996 G protein-coupled receptors: heterologous regulation of homologous desensitization and its implications. Trends Pharmacol Sci 17: 416–421 (*Short review of desensitisation mechanisms*)

Clapham D E 1995 Calcium signaling. Cell 80: 259–268 (*Excellent general review*)

Clapham D, Neer E 1997 G-protein βγ subunits. Ann Rev Pharmacol Toxicol 37: 167–203 (*On the diversity and role in signalling of G-protein βγ-subunits—the poor relations of the α-subunits*)

Colquhoun D 1987 Affinity, efficacy and receptor classification: is the classical theory still useful? In: Black J W, Jenkinson D H, Gerskowitch V P (eds) Perspectives on receptor classification. Liss, New York (*Review written at the time of transition from the old to the new model of receptor activation*)

Coughlin S R 1994 Protease-activated receptors start a family. Proc Natl Acad Sci USA 91: 9200–9202 (*Discusses the growing family of receptors—such as the thrombin receptor—activated by proteolytic cleavage*)

Dolphin A C 1996 G-proteins. In: Foreman J C, Johansen G (eds) Textbook of receptor pharmacology. CRC Press, Boca Raton

Donaldson L F, Hanley M R, Villablanca A C 1997 Inducible receptors. Trends Pharmacol Sci 18: 171–181 (*Emphasises processes controlling receptor expression*)

Downes C P 1988 Inositol phosphates: a family of signal molecules. Trends Neurosci 11: 336–338

Evans R M 1988 The steroid and thyroid hormone receptor superfamily. Science 240: 889–895 (*Excellent general review*)

Galzi J-L, Changeux J-P 1994 Neurotransmitter-gated ion channels as unconventional allosteric proteins. Curr Opin Struct Biol 4: 554–565 (*Review focusing on molecular mechanisms of channel activation*)

Garbers D L, Lowe D G 1994 Guanylyl cyclase receptors. J Biol Chem 269: 30741–30744

Giros B, Caron M G 1993 Molecular characteristics of the dopamine transporter. Trends Pharmacol Sci 14: 43–49

Gudermann T, Kalkbrenner F, Schultz G 1996 Diversity and selectivity of receptor-G protein signalling. Annu Rev Pharmacol Toxicol 36: 429–459 (*Discusses how selectivity is achieved between many ligands, receptors and interlinking transduction pathways*)

Hibert M F, Trumpp-Kallmeyer S, Hoflack J, Bruinvels A 1993 This is not a G protein-coupled receptor. Trends Pharmacol Sci 14: 7–12 (*Discusses what can and cannot be inferred from molecular modelling of receptor structure and function*)

Ihle J N 1995 Cytokine receptor signalling. Nature 377: 591–594

Karlin A 1993 Structure of nicotinic acetylcholine receptors. Curr Opin Neurobiol 3: 299–309 (*Excellent general review*)

Kenakin, T 1995 Agonist-receptor efficacy II: agonist trafficking of receptor signals. Trends Pharmacol Sci 16: 232–238 (*Discusses whether and how different ligands acting on the same receptor might elicit different cellular responses*)

Koenig J A, Edwardson J M 1997 Endocytosis and recycling of G protein-coupled receptors. Trends Pharmacol Sci 18: 276–287 (*Excellent review of the complex life cycle of a receptor molecule*)

Laudet V, Adelmant G 1995 Lonesome receptors. Curr Biol 5: 124–127 (*Short review of 'orphan' receptors*)

Lefkowitz R J 1993 Turned on to ill effect. Nature 365: 603–605 (*Discussion of the pathological consequences of β-adrenoceptors that are activated without agonists being present*)

Levitzki A 1996 Targeting signal transduction for disease therapy. Curr Opin Cell Biol 8: 239–244 (*Points out therapeutic opportunities for targeting components of signal transduction pathways*)

Mangelsdorf D J, Thummel C, Beato M et al. 1995 The nuclear receptor superfamily: the second decade. Cell 83: 835–839

Marshall C J 1996. Ras effectors. Curr Opin Cell Biol 8: 197–204 (*Account of one of the most important signal transduction pathways*)

Mayer B J, Baltimore D 1993 Signalling through SH2 and SH3 domains. Trends Cell Biol 3: 8–13 (*Review of the recognition domains of proteins in the phosphorylation cascades that are responsible for achieving selectivity*)

Milligan G 1995 Signal sorting by G-protein-linked receptors. Adv Pharmacol 32: 1–29 (*More on the selectivity problem*)

Neer E 1995 Heterotrimeric G proteins: organisers of trans-membrane signals. Cell 80: 249–257 (*Excellent general review*)

Nishizuka Y 1986 Studies and perspectives of protein kinase C. Science 233: 305–312 (*Review on one of the main phosphorylating enzymes that plays a key role in receptor-mediated signalling*)

Nishizuka Y 1988 The molecular heterogeneity of protein kinase C and its implications for cellular regulation. Nature 334: 661–665 (*As above*)

Panten U, Schwanstecher M, Schwanstecher U 1996 Sulfonylurea receptors and mechanism of sulfonylurea action. Exp Clin Endocrinol Diabetes 104: 1–9 (*A special receptor system involved in regulation of ATP-sensitive K^+ channels*)

Parker P J, Dekker L (eds) 1996 Protein kinase C. Springer, Berlin (*Authoritative reviews for PKC aficionados*)

Piomelli D 1997 Arachidonic acid in cell signalling. Springer, New York (*Excellent account of role of arachidonic acid as intra- and extracellular mediator*)

Ronnett G V, Snyder S H 1992 Molecular messengers of olfaction. Trends Neurosci 15: 508–513 (*Outlines role of adenylate cyclase in olfactory signalling—close parallels with other receptor systems*)

Schwartz T W, Rosenkilde M M 1996 Is there a 'lock' for all agonist 'keys' in 7TM receptors? Trends Pharmacol Sci 17: 213–216 (*More on the selectivity problem*)

Stryer L 1986 Cyclic GMP cascade of vision. Annu Rev Neurosci 6: 87–119 (*Review by one of the pioneers, showing similarities of visual transduction and chemical receptor mechanisms*)

Surprenant A, Buell G, North R A 1995 P_{2X} receptors bring new structure to ligand-gated ion channels. Trends Neurosci 18: 224–229 (*Account of a new structural class of channel-linked receptors*)

Taga T, Kishimoto T 1992 Cytokine receptors and signal transduction. FASEB J 7: 3387–3396

Unwin N 1993 Nicotinic acetylcholine receptor at 9A resolution. J Mol Biol 229: 1101–1124 (*The first structural study of a channel-linked receptor*)

Unwin N 1995 Acetylcholine receptor channel imaged in the open state. Nature 373: 37–43 (*Refinement of 1993 paper, showing for the first time how channel opening occurs—a technical tour de force*)

Walaas S I, Greengard P 1991 Protein phosphorylation and neuronal function. Pharmacol Rev 43: 299–349 (*Excellent general review*)

Wickham K D, Clapham, D E 1995 G-protein regulation of ion channels. Curr Opin Neurobiol 5: 278–285 (*Discusses direct and indirect regulation of ion channels by G-protein-coupled receptors*)

3

Method and measurement in pharmacology

We emphasised in Chapters 1 and 2 that drugs, being molecules, produce their effects by interacting with other molecules. This interaction can lead to effects at all levels of biological organisation, from molecules to human populations* (Fig. 3.1). In this chapter, we consider the principles of metrication at the various organisational levels, concentrating on laboratory methods, and referring only briefly to the principles of clinical trials. Assessment of drug action at the population level is the concern of *pharmacoepidemiology* and *pharmacoeconomics* (see Walley & Haycocks 1997), disciplines which are beyond the scope of this book.

Methods for measuring drug effects are needed in order that we may compare the properties of different substances, or the same substance under different circumstances, requirements which are met by the techniques of *bioassay*. Nowadays, one of the main aims of bioassay is to provide information that will be predictive of the effect of the drug in the clinical situation (where the objective is improvement of function in the whole patient who is suffering from the effects of disease). The choice of laboratory test systems (*in vitro* and *in vivo* 'models') that provide this predictive link has received much attention, and advances in understanding the molecular basis of disease are opening up new possibilities (e.g. transgenic animal models; see below) in this area.

---

*Consider the effect of cocaine on organised crime, the effect of organophosphate 'nerve gases' on the stability of dictatorships, or the effect of anaesthetics on the feasibility of surgical procedures for examples of molecular interactions that affect the behaviour of populations and societies.

In the past, bioassay was often used to measure the concentration of drugs and other active substances in the blood or other body fluids, an application now superseded by analytical chemistry techniques.

BIOASSAY

Bioassay is defined as the estimation of the concentration or potency of a substance by measurement of the biological response that it produces.

The uses of bioassay are:

- to measure the pharmacological activity of new or chemically undefined substances
- to investigate the function of endogenous mediators
- to measure drug toxicity and unwanted effects
- to measure the concentration of known substances (now largely obsolete).

Clinical trials, used to assess the clinical effectiveness of drug treatments, embody the same principles as other types of bioassay, adapted to the special situation. Beyond the realm of bioassay lies *pharmacoeconomics*, a newly emerging discipline which seeks to measure drug effects in social and economic terms, and is becoming increasingly important in guiding government decisions on drug prescribing and health-care policies.

Bioassay is essential in the development of new drugs. The activity of a new compound must be compared in various test systems with that of known compounds. The choice of suitable test systems for this preliminary bioassay is important and not always easy. The tests must be simple and quick, and they must also be as specific as possible for the type of biological activity that is being sought. Sometimes this is straightforward; local anaesthetic activity, for example, can be measured reliably by the ability of a substance to block action potential propagation in an isolated length of peripheral nerve. The results obtained in this way correlate well with

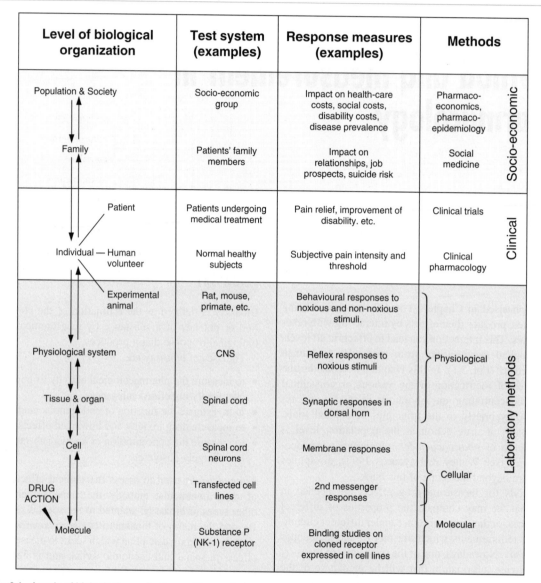

Level of biological organization	Test system (examples)	Response measures (examples)	Methods	
Population & Society	Socio-economic group	Impact on health-care costs, social costs, disability costs, disease prevalence	Pharmaco-economics, pharmaco-epidemiology	Socio-economic
Family	Patients' family members	Impact on relationships, job prospects, suicide risk	Social medicine	
Patient	Patients undergoing medical treatment	Pain relief, improvement of disability. etc.	Clinical trials	Clinical
Individual — Human volunteer	Normal healthy subjects	Subjective pain intensity and threshold	Clinical pharmacology	
Experimental animal	Rat, mouse, primate, etc.	Behavioural responses to noxious and non-noxious stimuli.	Physiological	Laboratory methods
Physiological system	CNS	Reflex responses to noxious stimuli		
Tissue & organ	Spinal cord	Synaptic responses in dorsal horn		
Cell	Spinal cord neurons	Membrane responses	Cellular	
DRUG ACTION	Transfected cell lines	2nd messenger responses		
Molecule	Substance P (NK-1) receptor	Binding studies on cloned receptor expressed in cell lines	Molecular	

Fig. 3.1   Levels of biological organisation and types of pharmacological measurement.

activity in clinical use, so the test has good predictive value. In other cases, appropriate test systems are not at all obvious. There is, for example, no reliable test system for assessing the activity of antipsychotic drugs, there being no 'animal model' equivalent (either naturally occurring or experimentally produced) of schizophrenia. Assessment of a new compound is usually based on a profile of activity in a range of test systems, in the expectation that clinical effectiveness will be associated with a particular pattern of activity in such a profile, rather than with activity in one particular test system.

In general, the less well we understand the mechanism of the therapeutic action of a drug, the more difficult it is to predict clinical effectiveness from the results of assays based on laboratory test systems. In many cases, it is not until the point of actual clinical trial that it is known for certain whether the drug even possesses therapeutic activity of the kind required.

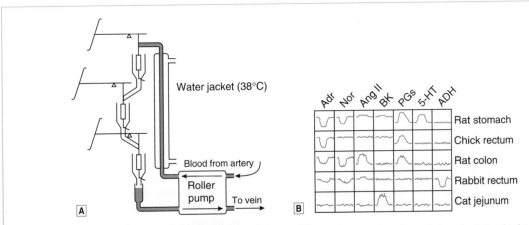

Fig. 3.2 Parallel assay by the cascade superfusion technique. [A] Blood is pumped continuously from the test animal over a succession of test organs, whose responses are measured by a simple transducer system. [B] The response of these organs to a variety of test substances (at 0.1–5 ng/ml) is shown. Each active substance produces a distinct pattern of responses, enabling unknown materials present in the blood to be identified and assayed. (Adr = adrenaline; Nor = noradrenaline; Ang II = angiotensin II; BK = bradykinin; PG prostaglandin; 5-HT = 5-hydroxytryptamine; ADH = antidiuretic hormone) (From: Vane J R 1969 Br J Pharmacol 35: 209–242)

In addition to its role in developing new therapeutic agents, bioassay is useful in the study of new hormonal or other chemically mediated control systems. Mediators in such systems are often first recognised by the biological effects that they produce. The first clue may be the finding that a tissue extract or some other biological sample produces an effect on an assay system. For example, the ability of extracts of the posterior lobe of the pituitary to produce a rise in blood pressure and a contraction of the uterus was observed at the turn of the century. These actions were made the basis of quantitative assay procedures and a standard preparation of the extract was established by international agreement in 1935. By use of these assays it was shown that two distinct peptides—**vasopressin** and **oxytocin**—were responsible, and they were eventually identified and synthesised in 1953. Biological assay had already revealed much about the synthesis, storage and release of the hormones, and was essential for their purification and identification. Nowadays, it does not take 50 years of laborious bioassays to identify new hormones before they are chemically characterised,* but bioassay still plays a key role.

Bioassays on different test systems may be run in parallel to reveal the profile of activity of an unknown mediator. This was developed to an almost Baroque splendour in the work of Vane and his colleagues, who studied the generation and destruction of endogenous active substances, such as **prostanoids** (see Ch. 12) by the technique of cascade superfusion (Fig. 3.2). In this technique the sample is run sequentially over a series of test preparations chosen to differentiate between different active constituents of the sample. The pattern of responses produced identifies effectively the active material, and the use of such assay systems for 'on line' analysis of biological samples has been invaluable in studying the production and fate of short-lived mediators such as prostanoids and the endothelium-derived relaxing factor (Ch. 11).

GENERAL PRINCIPLES OF BIOASSAY

The use of standards

J. H. Burn wrote in 1950: 'Pharmacologists today strain at the king's arm, but they swallow the frog, rat and mouse, not to mention the guinea pig and the pigeon.' He was referring to the fact that the 'king's arm' had been long since abandoned as a standard measure of length, whereas drug activity continued to be defined in terms of dose needed to cause, say, vomiting of a pigeon or cardiac arrest in a mouse. A plethora of 'pigeon units', 'mouse units' and the like, which no two laboratories

---

*In 1988, a Japanese group (Yanagisawa et al. 1988) described in a single paper, regarded as something of a *tour de force*, the bioassay, purification, chemical analysis and synthesis, and DNA-cloning of a new vascular peptide, *endothelin* (see Ch. 15).

could agree on, contaminated the literature.* Even if two laboratories cannot agree—because their pigeons differ—on the activity in pigeon units of the same sample of an active substance, they should nonetheless be able to agree that preparation X is, say, 3.5 times as active as standard preparation Y on the pigeon test. Biological assays are therefore designed to measure the relative potency of two preparations, usually a *standard* and an *unknown*. The best kind of standard is, of course, the pure substance, but it is often necessary to establish standard preparations of various hormones, natural products and antisera against which laboratory samples can be calibrated, even though the standard preparations are not chemically pure.

The design of bioassays

Given the aim of comparing the activity of two preparations, a standard (S) and an unknown (U) on a particular preparation, a bioassay must provide an estimate of the dose or concentration of U that will produce the same biological effect as that of a known dose or concentration of S. As Figure 3.3 shows, provided that the log-dose–effect curves for S and U are parallel, the ratio, M, of equiactive doses will not depend on the magnitude of response chosen. Thus, M provides an estimate of the potency ratio of the two preparations. A comparison of the magnitude of the effects produced by equal doses of S and U does not provide an estimate of M (see Fig. 3.3).

The main problem with all types of bioassay is that of biological variation, and the design of bioassays is aimed at:

- minimising variation
- avoiding systematic errors resulting from variation
- estimation of the limits of error of the assay result.

Many different experimental designs have been proposed to maximise the efficiency and reliability of bioassays (see Laska & Meisner 1987). Commonly, comparisons are based on analysis of dose–response curves, from which the matching doses of standard and unknown are calculated. Such calculations become much simpler if the dose–response curves are linear. In many cases this can be achieved (see Ch. 1) by using a logarithmic dose

scale and restricting observations to the middle region of the log-dose–effect curve, which is usually close to a straight line. The use of a logarithmic dose scale means that the curves for standard and unknown will normally be parallel, and the potency ratio (M) of the unknown, relative to the standard, is determined by the horizontal distance between the two curves (Fig. 3.3). Assays of this type are known as *parallel line assays*, the minimal design being the 2 + 2 assay, in which two doses of standard (S_1 and S_2) and two of unknown (U_1 and U_2) are used. The doses are chosen to give responses lying on the linear part of the log-dose–response curve, and are given repeatedly in randomised order, providing an inherent measure of the variability of the test system, which can be used, by means of straightforward statistical analysis, to estimate the confidence limits of the final result.

In practice, most bioassays will give results whose 5% confidence limits lie within ±20% and many will do better than this.

The 2 + 2 assay also detects whether or not the two log-dose–effect lines deviate significantly from parallelism. If the lines are not parallel, which may be the case if the assay is used to compare two drugs whose mechanism of action is not the same, it is not possible to define the relative potencies of S and U unambiguously in terms

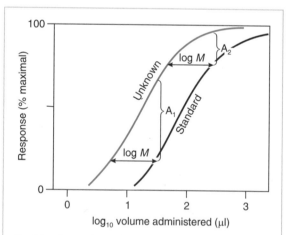

Fig. 3.3 Comparison of the potency of unknown and standard by bioassay. Note that comparing the magnitude of responses produced by the same dose (i.e. volume) of standard and unknown gives no quantitative estimate of their relative potency. (The differences, A_1 and A_2, depend on the dose chosen.) Comparison of equi-effective doses of standard and unknown gives a valid measure of their relative potencies. Since the lines are parallel, the magnitude of the effect chosen for the comparison is immaterial; i.e. log M is the same at all points on the curves.

---

*More picturesque examples of absolute units of the kind that Burn would have frowned upon are the PHI and the mHelen. PHI, cited by Colquhoun (1971), stands for 'purity in heart index' and measures the ability of a virgin pure-in-heart to transform, under appropriate conditions, a he-goat into a youth of surpassing beauty. The mHelen is a unit of beauty, 1 mHelen being sufficient to launch 1 ship.

of a simple ratio. The experimenter must then face up to the fact that there are qualitative as well as quantitative differences between the two, so that comparison requires measurement of more than a single dimension of potency. An example of this kind of difficulty is met when diuretic drugs (Ch. 20) are compared. Some ('low ceiling') diuretics are capable of producing only a small diuretic effect, no matter how much is given; others ('high ceiling') can produce a very intense diuresis (described as 'torrential' by authors with vivid imaginations). A comparison of two such drugs requires not only a measure of the doses needed to produce an equal low-level diuretic effect, but also a measure of the relative heights of the ceilings.

Quantal and graded responses

An assay may be based on a *graded response*, (e.g. change in blood glucose concentration, contraction of a strip of smooth muscle, change in the time taken for a rat to run a maze), or on *all-or-nothing responses* (e.g. death, loss of righting reflex, success in maze-running within a stipulated time). With the latter, known as a *quantal response* because it either happens or it doesn't, the proportion of animals responding will vary according to the dose used. The shape and slope of such a curve is governed by the individual variation between animals—the more uniform the population, the steeper the curve, and the more precise the assay. With graded responses, the steepness of the

---

Bioassay

- Bioassay is the measurement of concentration or potency of a drug from the magnitude of the biological effect that it produces.
- Bioassay normally involves comparison of the *unknown* preparation with a *standard*. Estimates that are not based on comparison with standards are usually unreliable and vary from laboratory to laboratory.
- Comparisons are best made on the basis of dose–response curves, which allow estimates of the equiactive concentrations of unknown and standard to be used as a basis for the potency comparison. *Parallel line assays* follow this principle.
- The biological response may be *quantal* (the proportion of tests in which a given all-or-nothing effect is produced) or graded. Different statistical procedures are appropriate in each case.
- Different approaches to metrication apply according to the level of biological organisation at which the drug effect needs to be measured. Approaches range through molecular and chemical techniques, in vitro and in vivo animal studies, clinical studies on volunteers and patients, to measurement of effects at the socioeconomic level.

---

dose–response curve is a property of the test system and has nothing to do with biological variation. Quantal responses can be used in essentially the same way as graded responses for the purposes of bioassay, though the appropriate statistical procedures are slightly different.

BIOASSAYS IN MAN

Studies involving human subjects fall into two distinct categories. *Human and clinical pharmacology* focuses on using human subjects (either healthy volunteers or patients) essentially as experimental animals, to check whether mechanisms that operate in other species also apply to man. The scientific principles underlying such measurements are the same, but the ethical and safety issues are paramount, and ethical committees associated with all medical research centres tightly control the type of experiment that can be done. *Clinical trials* aim to measure *therapeutic effectiveness* and constitute an important and highly specialised form of biological assay. The need to use patients for experimental purposes imposes many restrictions. Some of the basic principles involved in clinical trials are discussed in this section.

Any new drug that is intended for therapeutic use in man naturally has first to be tested experimentally in human subjects, according to the phases shown in Table 3.1, the first three of which constitute experimental studies of the kind that we are discussing in this chapter. These phases relate to the formal process that a pharmaceutical company must follow before a new compound is licensed to be sold for use in man. Many clinical trials, aimed at testing new therapeutic concepts, such as the use of existing drugs in new indications, or in combination with others, are undertaken as research projects independently of the drug development process, and not designated by phase.

An example of a trial to compare two analgesic drugs (see Ch. 37) is shown in Figure 3.4. Though many animal tests have been devised (for example, measuring the effect of different doses of an analgesic drug on the mean time taken for groups of mice to jump off a surface heated to a mildly painful temperature), they often fail to predict accurately the subjective relief of pain in man. More useful assessments of analgesic drugs have, therefore, been developed on the basis of subjective reports of relief from persistent pain, such as that of malignant disease. Figure 3.4 shows a comparison of **morphine** and **codeine** in which a modified 2 + 2 design was used. Each of the four doses was given on different occasions to each of the four subjects, the order being randomised and both subject and observer being unaware of the

Table 3.1 Phases of clinical testing of new compounds

Phase I	Measurement of pharmacological action, potency, pharmacokinetic characteristics, side-effects, etc. usually in normal volunteers (exceptionally in patients, e.g. anticancer drugs)
Phase II	Tests to establish whether or not a new drug has detectable efficacy in small groups of patients, and to establish dosage regime to be used for Phase III trials
Phase III	Large-scale comparative trials in patients, designed to establish efficacy, compare the new drug with other available treatments, establish optimal dosage, determine incidence of unwanted effects, etc., before the drug is licensed for marketing
Phase IV	Surveillance of the efficacy and incidence of unwanted effects of a new drug after it has been licensed and made available for prescription

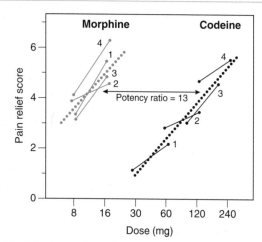

Fig. 3.4 Assay of morphine and codeine as analgesics in man. Each of four patients (numbered 1–4) was given, on successive occasions in random order, four different treatments (high and low morphine, and high and low codeine) by intramuscular injection and the subjective pain relief score calculated for each. The calculated regression lines gave a potency ratio estimate of 13 for the two drugs. (After: Houde R W et al. 1965 In: Analgetics. Academic Press, New York)

THE USE OF GENETIC STRAINS AND TRANSGENIC ANIMALS

By selective breeding, it is possible to obtain pure animal strains which express abnormalities closely resembling human disease conditions, and these are extremely useful for characterising drug effects that may be clinically relevant. Genetic models of this kind include spontaneously hypertensive rats, genetically obese mice, epilepsy-prone dogs and mice, rats with deficient vasopressin secretion, and many other examples.

More recently, deliberate genetic manipulation of the germ-line is increasingly used to generate transgenic animals with defined mutations as a means of replicating human disease states in experimental animals, and thereby providing animal models that are expected to be more predictive of therapeutic drug effects in man (see reviews by Maerki & Haerri 1996, Polites 1996). This technology, first reported in 1980, allows the inactivation of existing genes ('knock-outs') or the insertion of new

---

Transgenic animal models

- Transgenic animals are produced by introducing mutations into the germ cells of animals (usually mice) which allow new genes to be introduced ('knock-ins') or existing genes to be inactivated ('knock-outs') in the animals in a breeding colony.
- Insertion or deletion of certain genes results in phenotypic changes resembling human disease, and is an increasingly used approach to developing disease models for drug testing.
- The induced mutation operates throughout the development and lifetime of the animal, and may be lethal. The new technique of conditional mutagenesis is an advance which should allow the abnormal gene to be switched on or off at a chosen time.

---

dose given. Pain relief was assessed by questions from the trained observer, and the results showed morphine to be 13 times as potent as codeine. This, of course, does not prove its superiority, but merely shows that a smaller dose is needed to produce the same effect. Such a measurement is, however, an essential preliminary to assessing the relative therapeutic merits of the two drugs, for any comparison of other factors, such as side-effects, duration of action, tolerance or dependence, needs to be done on the basis of doses that are equiactive so far as analgesia is concerned.

genes ('knock-ins') in breeding colonies of animals. Examples of such models include transgenic mice that overexpress the amyloid precursor protein (APP; see Masliah et al. 1996), which is important in the pathogenesis of Alzheimer's disease (see Ch. 31). When they are a few months old, these mice develop pathological lesions and cognitive changes resembling Alzheimer's disease, and provide a very useful model, where none existed hitherto, with which to test possible new therapeutic approaches to the disease. Mice in which the gene for a particular adenosine receptor subtype has been inactivated show distinct behavioural and cardiovascular abnormalities, such as increased aggression, reduced response to noxious stimuli and raised blood pressure (Ledent et al. 1997). These findings serve to pinpoint the physiological role of this receptor whose function was hitherto unknown, and to suggest new ways in which agonists or antagonists for these receptors might be developed for therapeutic use (e.g. to reduce aggressive behaviour or to treat hypertension). Generating new transgenic animals is a substantial undertaking, but the technology is improving rapidly, and the use of such models in pharmacology will undoubtedly become widespread. There are several limitations. One is that the gene switch may cause the animals to die during gestation, or shortly after birth. A second is that adaptive changes may compensate for the lack, or overexpression, of a particular gene and complicate interpretation of the phenotypic changes seen in the transgenic animals. To overcome these problems, ways of achieving *conditional mutagenesis* are being developed (see Plueck 1996), whereby the introduced genes are engineered so that they are expressed only in particular cells (e.g. neurons), or so that they can be switched on or off by an external signal, such as administration of interferon, allowing the animal to develop normally up to this point. At present the technology is mainly confined to the mouse, which breeds quickly, but is inconveniently small for many experimental purposes. Despite this, its importance is growing rapidly.

CLINICAL TRIALS

A clinical trial is a method for comparing objectively, by a prospective study, the results of two or more therapeutic procedures. For new drugs, this is carried out during phase III of clinical development (Table 3.1). It is important to realise that, until about 30 years ago, methods of treatment were chosen on the basis of clinical impression and personal experience rather than objective testing.* Though many drugs, with undoubted effectiveness, remain in use without ever having been subjected to a controlled clinical trial, any new drug is now required to have been tested in this way before being licensed for general clinical use.**

General accounts of the principles and organisation of clinical trials are given by Friedman et al. (1997). A clinical trial aims to compare the response of a *test group* of patients receiving a new treatment (A) with that of a *control group* receiving an existing 'standard' treatment (B). Treatment A might be a new drug or a new combination of existing drugs, or any other kind of therapeutic intervention such as a surgical operation, diet, physiotherapy and so on. The standard against which it is judged (treatment B) might be a currently used drug treatment or (if there is no currently available effective treatment) a placebo or no treatment at all.

The use of controls is crucial in clinical trials. Claims of therapeutic efficacy based on reports that, for example, 16 out of 20 patients receiving drug X got better within 2 weeks are of no value without a knowledge of how 20 patients receiving no treatment, or a different treatment, would have fared. Usually, the controls are provided by a separate group of patients from those receiving the test treatment, but sometimes a cross-over design is possible in which the same patients are switched from test to control treatment or vice versa, and the results compared. *Randomisation* (see p. 54) is essential to avoid bias in assigning individual patients to test or control groups. Hence, the randomised controlled clinical trial is now regarded as the essential tool for assessing clinical efficacy of new drugs.

Concern inevitably arises over the ethics of assigning patients at random to an untreated control group when the doctor in charge believes the test treatment to have

---

*Not exclusively. James Lind conducted a controlled trial in 1753 on 12 mariners which showed that oranges and lemons offered protection against scurvy. However, 40 years passed before the British Navy acted on his advice, and a further century before the US Navy did.

**It is fashionable in some quarters to argue that to require evidence of efficacy of therapeutic procedures in the form of a controlled trial runs counter to the doctrines of 'holistic' medicine. This is a fundamentally anti-scientific view, for science advances only by generating predictions from hypotheses and by subjecting the predictions to experimental test. Standing up for the scientific approach is the recent *evidence-based medicine* movement (see Sackett et al. 1996), which sets out strict criteria for assessing therapeutic efficacy, based on randomised, controlled clinical trials, and urges scepticism about therapeutic doctrines whose efficacy have not been so demonstrated.

advantages. However, the reason for setting up a trial is that doubt exists in the minds of many doctors that the treatment is efficacious, so for these doctors there is no ethical dilemma. If individual doctors are personally convinced that the treatment is beneficial, they should clearly avoid participating in a controlled trial. All would agree on the principle of informed consent,* whereby each patient must be told the nature of the trial, and agree to participate on the basis that he or she will be randomly and unknowingly assigned to either the treated or the control group.

Unlike the kind of bioassay that we have been considering up to this point, the clinical trial does not normally give any information about potency or the form of the dose–response curve, but merely compares the response produced by two stipulated therapeutic regimes. The investigator must decide in advance what dose to use and how often to give it, and the trial will only reveal whether the chosen regime performed better or worse than the control treatment. It will not say whether increasing or decreasing the dose would have improved the response; another trial would be needed to ascertain that. The basic question posed by a clinical trial is thus simpler than that addressed by most conventional bioassays. However, the organisation of clinical trials, with the problem of avoiding bias, is immeasurably more complicated, time-consuming and expensive than that of any laboratory-based assay.

Avoidance of bias

There are two main strategies that aim to minimise bias in clinical trials, namely:

- randomisation
- the double-blind technique.

If two treatments are being compared on a series of selected patients, the simplest form of randomisation is to allocate each patient to A or B by reference to a series of random numbers. If the number of patients is large enough, roughly equal numbers will be assigned to each group. In a small series, however, the groups could end up poorly matched, and a compromise solution is to split the series into blocks of, say, eight patients, each block consisting of four of A and four of B arranged in random order. Another difficulty with simple randomisation is that the two groups may turn out to be

ill-matched with respect to characteristics such as age, sex, or disease severity. The chance of serious mismatching of the groups obviously decreases as the size of the series increases. With small-scale trials, *stratified randomisation* is often used to avoid the difficulty. Thus the subjects might be divided into age categories, random allocation to A or B being used within each category. It is possible to treat two or more characteristics of the trial population in this way. Thus, if it were important to balance the groups with respect to age and disease severity, it might be necessary to define three age bands, each being split into mild and severe cases, making six strata in all. It will be appreciated that the number of strata can quickly become large, and the process is self-defeating when the number of subjects in each becomes too small. As well as avoiding error resulting from imbalance of groups assigned to A and B, stratification can also allow more sophisticated conclusions to be reached. B might, for example, prove to be better than A in a particular group of patients even if it is not significantly better overall.

The double-blind technique, which means that neither subject nor investigator is aware at the time of the assessment which treatment is being used, is intended to minimise subjective bias. It has been repeatedly shown that, with the best will in the world, subjects and investigators both contribute to bias if they know which treatment is which, so the use of a double-blind technique is an important safeguard. It is not always possible, however. A dietary regime or a surgical operation, for example, can seldom be disguised, and even with drugs, pharmacological effects may reveal to the patient what he is taking and predispose him to report accordingly.** In general, however, the use of a double-blind procedure, with precautions if necessary to disguise such clues as the taste or appearance of the two drugs, is an important principle.

Maintaining the blind can be problematic. In an attempt to determine whether melatonin is effective in countering jet-lag, a pharmacologist selected a group of fellow pharmacologists attending a congress in Australia, providing them with unlabelled capsules of melatonin or placebo, with a jet-lag questionnaire to fill in when they arrived. Many of them (one of the authors included), with analytical resources easily to hand, opened the

---

*Even this can be contentious, since patients who are unconscious, demented or mentally ill are unable to give such consent, yet no-one would want to preclude trials that might offer improved therapies to these needy patients.

**The distinction between a true pharmacological response and a beneficial clinical effect produced by the knowledge (based on the pharmacological effects that the drug produces) that an active drug is being administered is not easy to draw, and we should not expect a mere clinical trial to resolve such a fine semantic issue.

capsules and consigned them to the bin on finding that they contained placebo. Even pharmacologists are only human.

The size of the sample

Both ethical and financial considerations dictate that the trial should involve the minimum number of subjects, and much statistical thought has gone into the problem of deciding in advance how many subjects will be required to produce a useful result. The results of a trial cannot, by their nature, be absolutely conclusive. This is because it is based on a sample of patients and there is always a chance that the sample was atypical of the population from which it came. Two types of erroneous conclusion are possible, referred to as *type I* and *type II errors*. A type I error occurs if a difference is found between A and B when none actually exists (false positive). A type II error occurs if no difference is found though A and B do actually differ (false negative). A major factor that determines the size of sample needed is the degree of certainty the investigator seeks in avoiding either type of error. The probability of incurring a type I error is expressed as the *significance* of the result. To say that A and B are different at the 0.05 level of significance means that the probability of obtaining a false positive result (i.e. incurring a type I error), is less than 1 in 20. For most purposes this level of significance is considered acceptable as a basis for drawing conclusions.

The probability of avoiding a type II error (i.e. failing to detect a real difference between A and B) is termed the *power* of the trial. We tend to regard type II errors more leniently than type I errors, and trials are often designed with a power of 0.8–0.9. To increase the significance and the power of a trial requires more patients. The second factor that determines the sample size required is the magnitude of difference between A and B that is regarded as clinically significant. For example, to detect that a given treatment reduces the mortality in a certain condition by 10 percentage points, say from 50% (in the control group) to 40% (in the treated group) would require 850 subjects, assuming that we wanted to achieve a 0.05 level of significance and a power of 0.9. If we were content to reveal a reduction only by 20 percentage points (and very likely miss a reduction by 10 points) only 210 subjects would be needed. In this example, missing a real 10-point reduction in mortality could result in abandonment of a treatment that would save 100 lives for every 1000 patients treated—an extremely serious mistake from society's point of view. This simple example emphasises the need to assess clinical benefit (which is often difficult to quantify) in parallel with statistical considerations (which are fairly straightforward), in planning trials.

Meta-analysis

It is possible, by the use of the statistical technique known as *meta-analysis* or *overview analysis*, to combine the data obtained in several individual trials (provided each has been conducted according to a randomised design) in order to gain greater power and significance. This can be very useful in arriving at a conclusion on the basis of several published trials, of which some claimed superiority of the test treatment over the control while others did not. As an objective procedure, it is certainly preferable to the 'take-your-pick' approach to conclusion-forming adopted by most human beings when confronted with contradictory data. It has several drawbacks, however (see Naylor 1997), the main one being 'publication bias', since negative studies are generally considered less interesting, and are therefore less likely to be published, than positive studies. Double counting, caused by the same data being incorporated into more than one trial report, is another problem.

Sequential trials

The purpose of sequential trials (see Armitage 1978) is to minimise the number of subjects used by computing the results continuously as the trial proceeds, and stopping it as soon as a result (at a predetermined level of significance) is achieved. In this type of trial, the subjects are usually paired, one subject receiving each treatment. (Alternatively, a cross-over design can be used in which each subject receives the treatments consecutively.) The result of each individual comparison is scored as *A better than B*, *B better than A*, or *no discernible difference*, and the analysis is performed graphically (Fig. 3.5). The example shown is a three-way comparison of **heroin**, **pholcodeine** and placebo used as cough suppressants in patients with chronic cough. Each patient was given the three treatments consecutively, in random order, and asked to rate them in order of effectiveness. The red line on the diagram represents the comparison between pholcodeine and heroin. If a subject preferred pholcodeine the line was extended upwards and to the right; if he preferred heroin the line was drawn downwards and to the right. Overall, the line was nearly horizontal, and after 24 subjects it crossed the boundary indicating that no significant difference could be demonstrated. The other two lines progress fairly steadily towards the boundaries indicating that both heroin (lower boundary) and pholcodeine (upper boundary) were better than the placebo. The position of the boundaries in such a diagram is calculated on the basis of the significance level and

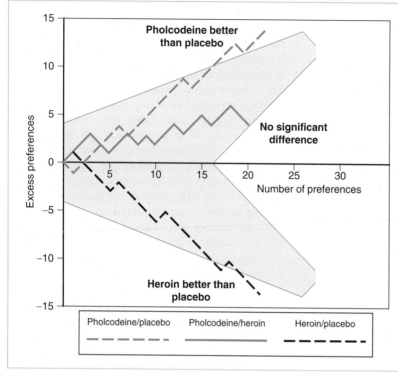

Fig. 3.5 Sequential clinical trial to compare pholcodeine, heroin and placebo as cough suppressants. Each of 27 patients was given, under double-blind conditions, the three treatments on successive occasions and asked to rank them in order of effectiveness. The stated preferences were then plotted on the diagram. The lines comparing either drug with placebo crossed the 0.05 significance limit after about 20 preferences had been expressed, showing both drugs to be significantly better than placebo. The line comparing heroin and pholcodeine failed to show a significant difference. The right-hand limit corresponds to power of 0.85 (i.e. a 15% chance that a real difference exists). (Redrawn from: Snell E S, Armitage P 1957 cited in Armitage P 1978 Sequential medical trials. Blackwell, Oxford)

power required. Sequential trials are not, as a rule, suitable where assessment of the result of treatment takes a long time (e.g. where death rates are being compared) since all the subjects will have been committed to the trial before any results are obtained.

Various 'hybrid' trial designs, which have the advantage of sequential trials in minimising the number of patients needed but do not require strict pairing of subjects, have been devised (see Friedman et al. 1997). Even with conventional trials, successive interim analyses of the accumulated data (by monitoring groups independent of the investigators) are generally made as the trial progresses, which allows the trial to be terminated as soon as a clear result is achieved. In a large-scale trial (Beta-blocker Heart Attack Trial Research Group 1982) of the value of long-term treatment with the β-adrenoceptor blocking drug **propranolol** (Ch. 8) following heart attacks, the interim results showed a significant reduction in mortality which led to the early termination of the trial.

The organisation of clinical trials

The organisation of large-scale clinical trials involving hundreds or thousands of patients at many different centres, is a massive and expensive undertaking, which makes up one of the major costs of developing a new drug, and can easily go wrong.

One large trial (Anturane Reinfarction Trial Research Group 1978) involved 1620 patients at 26 research centres in the US and Canada, 98 collaborating researchers, and a formidable list of organising committees, including two independent audit committees to check that the work was being carried out in conformity with the strict protocols established. The conclusion was that the drug under test (sulfinpyrazone) reduced by almost one-half the mortality from repeat heart attacks in the 8-month period after a first attack, and could save many lives. The US Food and Drug Administration, however, refused to grant a licence for the use of the drug, criticising the trial as unreliable and biased in several respects. Their independent analysis of the data showed the beneficial effect of the drug to be slight and insignificant. Further analysis and further trials, however, supported the original conclusion, but by then the efficacy of aspirin in this condition had been established, so the use of sulfinpyrazone never found favour.

Clinical trials

- A clinical trial is a special type of bioassay done to compare the clinical efficacy of new drug or procedure with that of a known drug or procedure (or a placebo).
- Generally the aim is a straight comparison of unknown (A) with standard (B) at a single dose level. The result may be: 'B better than A', 'B worse than A', or 'No difference detected'. *Efficacy, not potency* is compared.
- To avoid bias, clinical trials should be:
  — controlled (comparison of A with B, rather than study of A alone).
  — randomised (assignment of subjects to A or B on a random basis)
  — double-blind (neither subject nor assessor knows whether A or B is being used)
- *Type I errors* (concluding that A is better than B when the difference is actually due to chance) and *type II errors* (concluding that A is no better than B because a real difference has escaped detection) can occur; the likelihood of either kind of error gets less as the sample size and number of end-point events is increased.
- *Sequential trials* are appropriate in some cases and provide a way of limiting the number of subjects studied.
- Clinical trials require very careful planning and execution and are inevitably expensive.
- Meta-analysis is a statistical technique used to pool the data from several independent trials.

MEASUREMENT OF TOXICITY

Before any new compound is approved for testing in man, extensive toxicity testing is done in various animal species and with in vitro systems. The crudest type of toxicity test is the LD_{50} (lethal dose for 50% of a group of animals), in which various doses of the drug, estimated to cover the range from 0 to 100% lethality, are administered to groups of animals. The mortality in each group within a fixed period of time (say 2 days) is determined and used to construct a curve relating fractional mortality to dose, from which the LD_{50} can be estimated. This test, once regarded as essential for measuring toxicity, is now largely discredited, particularly in relation to drugs intended for therapeutic use. The problems with it are:

- It measures only mortality and not sublethal toxicity.
- The LD_{50} varies widely between species and cannot be safely extrapolated to man.
- It measures only acute toxicity produced by a single dose, and not long-term toxicity.
- It cannot measure idiosyncratic reactions (i.e. reactions

occurring at low dosage in a small proportion of subjects) though such reactions may be more relevant in practice than 'high dose' toxicity (see Chs 48 and 49).
- It requires the use of many animals, and entails suffering disproportionate to the knowledge gained.

An example of the weakness of the LD_{50} test as a measure of toxicity is shown in Figure 3.6. A single oral dose of **indomethacin** was given to groups of rats and the percentage mortality noted 24 hours and 14 days later. There was a nearly 30-fold difference in the LD_{50} according to the time at which the assessment was made, and a dose of indomethacin that was 100% lethal within 14 days caused no deaths within 24 hours. This example shows strikingly that the arbitrary choice of experimental conditions for the LD_{50} test can drastically alter the results obtained. An official UK report on the LD_{50} test concluded that although some rough measure of acute toxicity in animals was needed for many substances, a simple 'limit' test, aimed at determining the effect on animals of the largest dose likely to be administered to a human being, was generally preferable. This principle has now been accepted by regulatory authorities in most countries; the elimination of the formal requirement for LD_{50} tests has considerably reduced the number of animals used for toxicity testing (see Paton 1993 for an account of the practical and ethical issues involved).

Toxicity takes many forms and cannot be measured purely in terms of increased mortality. The battery of tests through which potential new drugs are put during

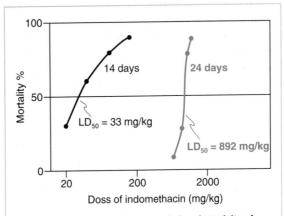

Fig. 3.6 Comparison of acute and chronic toxicity of indomethacin in mice. The LD_{50} measured 24 hours after dosing is 27 times larger than the LD_{50} measured at 14 days. Variability is also much less for the acute test, shown by the steeper red curve. (From: Beyer K H 1978 Discovery, development and delivery of new drugs. Spectrum Publications, Jamaica)

their development is designed to reveal many types of toxicity that are known to occur in man, and regulatory authorities require extensive and detailed studies of animal toxicity before they will grant a licence for testing in patients and eventual sale of a new drug. Public opinion is inclined to demand the unattainable, namely that before any drug is released for widespread use, there is certainty that it will lack toxicity when used under clinical conditions. As Witts has pointed out, however: 'The final test of the safety of a drug is in fact its release for general use. 'The only way that rare but serious toxicities can be detected is by clinical observation or by post-marketing surveillance (*Phase IV studies,* Table 3.1).

Studies on animals and human volunteers can never be a complete safeguard against toxicity in clinical use for two reasons. First, only such effects as are looked for are likely to be found. In 1960, when **thalidomide** was developed, the possibility of drug-induced foetal malformations (teratogenesis) had not yet been recognised, and the animal tests used at that time did not anticipate this form of toxicity; nor was there any likelihood of discovering it from studies on human volunteers. Discovery came only as a result of astute clinical detective work after the drug had been released and very successfully promoted. Once recognised, the effect can be tested for in animals and future disasters on the thalidomide scale* are highly unlikely. However, unsuspected types of toxicity will continue to appear, as exemplified by the syndrome of sclerosing peritonitis produced by **practolol** and the increased incidence of thrombotic disorders in women taking oral contraceptives.

Secondly, toxic effects may occur only in a very small proportion of patients. Thus an effect occurring in 1 in 1000 individuals will escape detection in a clinical trial on a few hundred patients, but may be of considerable clinical importance. For example, **phenylbutazone** (an anti-inflammatory drug; see Ch. 13) causes, as a rare side-effect, aplastic anaemia, which has a high mortality. Phenylbutazone is estimated to kill 22 patients out of every million treated with the drug. It is obvious that such an infrequent event could not be discovered in a clinical trial. In common with other types of idiosyncratic reaction, it does not seem to become any more frequent if the dose of the drug is increased, and thus would also escape detection in high-dose toxicity tests in animals.

The recognition that animal studies and clinical trials by no means eliminate the risk of toxic effects when

*An estimated 10 000 children born with severe malformations. See Sjostrom (1972).

the drug is released for general clinical use has led to the development of monitoring schemes in most countries which are intended to facilitate detection of toxicity. In the UK, the Medicines Commission runs a 'Yellow Card' scheme which relies on voluntary reporting by doctors and pharmacists of incidents that they think may be the result of adverse reactions to drugs. In Britain, over 15 000 such reports are received annually, and the aim is that classification of reported incidents by drug and by type of reaction will reveal rare forms of toxicity, such as the phenylbutazone example mentioned above. The dangers of high-oestrogen contraceptive pills, and of practolol (see above) were first detected in this way. Though useful, the Yellow Card system has serious weaknesses since it relies on voluntary reporting of incidents that are suspected to be drug-related. There are moves to supplement it with systematic computerised monitoring of prescriptions of new drugs together with medical incidents occurring in those patients. Such a system would be expected to reveal a correlation between the use of a drug and the occurrence of a particular adverse reaction long before a doctor's suspicions might be aroused to the point of submitting a Yellow Card.

The function of monitoring is to sound an alarm; because of the haphazard origin of the data, it cannot by itself provide convincing evidence of toxicity. The next stage is therefore an epidemiological study designed to discover whether or not the incidence of the suspected type of reaction is actually increased in patients treated with the drug.

Therapeutic index

Ehrlich recognised that a drug must be judged not only by its useful properties, but also by its toxic effects, and he expressed the *therapeutic index* of a drug in terms of the ratio between the average minimum effective dose and the average maximum tolerated dose in group of subjects, i.e.

$$Therapeutic\ index\ = \frac{Maximum\ non\text{-}toxic\ dose}{Minimum\ effective\ dose}$$

Unfortunately, the variability between individuals is not taken into account in this definition. Even if for any one subject there is a large margin between the maximum tolerated dose and minimum effective dose, individuals may vary widely in their sensitivity, so it is quite possible that the effective dose in some individuals will be toxic to others. A widely used definition which takes into account individual variation is:

$$Therapeutic\ index = LD_{50}/ED_{50}$$

Thus defined, therapeutic index gives some idea of the margin of safety in use of a drug, by drawing attention to the importance of the relationship between the effective and toxic doses, but it has obvious limitations and is therefore very rarely quoted as a number. Thus, it is not really a useful guide to the safety of a drug in clinical use. There are several reasons for this:

- LD_{50} is not a good guide to toxicity in the therapeutic setting (see above).
- ED_{50} is often not definable, since it depends on what measure of effectiveness is used. Analgesic drugs, for example, may need to be given in different dosages according to the nature and severity of the pain. The ED_{50} for **aspirin** used for a mild headache would be much lower than the value for aspirin as an antirheumatic drug.
- Some very important forms of toxicity are *idiosyncratic* (i.e. only a small proportion of individuals are susceptible; see Ch. 48). In other cases, toxicity depends greatly on the clinical state of the patient. Thus, **propranolol** is dangerous to an asthmatic patient in doses that are harmless to a normal individual. More generally, we can say that wide individual variation (see Ch. 48) in either the effective dose or the toxic dose of a drug makes it inherently less predictable, and therefore less safe, though this is not reflected in the therapeutic index.

These shortcomings mean that therapeutic index is of little value as a measure of the clinical usefulness of a drug; **digoxin**, for example, used in treating cardiac failure for many years, has a notably low therapeutic index. Therapeutic index has rather more relevance as a measure of the impunity with which an overdose may be given. Thus, one reason why the **benzodiazepines** replaced **barbiturates** as hypnotic drugs (see Ch. 33) is that their therapeutic index is much greater, so they are much less likely to kill when taken in accidental or deliberate overdose. Ironically, though, thalidomide— probably the most harmful drug ever marketed—was promoted specifically on the basis of its exceptionally high therapeutic index.

In summary, though therapeutic index expresses a valid general concept, it provides no quantitative measure of the actual usefulness of a drug. It is well to be suspicious of mathematically defined quantities that cannot be enumerated.

Benefit and risk

Alternative ways of quantifying the benefits and risks of drugs in clinical use have received much attention. One useful approach is to estimate from clinical trial data the proportion of test and control patients who will experience (a) a defined level of clinical benefit (for example, survival beyond 2 years, pain relief to a certain predetermined level, slowing of cognitive decline by a given amount), and (b) adverse effects of defined degree. These estimates of proportions of patients showing beneficial or harmful reactions can be expressed as '*number needed to treat*' (NNT; i.e. the number of patients who need to be treated in order for one to show the given effect, whether beneficial or adverse). For example, in a recent study of pain relief by antidepressant drugs compared with placebo, the findings were: for benefit (a defined level of pain relief), NNT = 3; for minor unwanted effects, NNT = 3; for major adverse effects, NNT = 22. Thus, of 100 patients treated, on average 33 will benefit from the drug, 33 will experience minor unwanted effects, and 4 or 5 will experience major unwanted effects, information that is helpful in guiding therapeutic choices. One advantage of this type of analysis is that it can take into account the underlying disease severity in quantifying benefit. Thus, if drug A halves the mortality of an often-fatal disease (reducing it from 50% to 25%, say), the NNT to save one life is 4; if drug B halves the mortality of a rarely fatal disease (reducing it from 5% to 2.5%, say), the NNT to save one life is 40. Notwithstanding other considerations, drug A is judged to be more valuable than drug B, even though both reduce mortality by a half. Furthermore, the clinician must realise that to save one life with drug B, 40 patients must be exposed to a risk of adverse effects, whereas only 4 are exposed for each life saved with Drug A.

Therapeutic index

- Therapeutic index (= LD_{50}/ED_{50}) provides a very crude measure of the safety of any drug as used in practice.
- Its main limitations are:
  - It is based on animal toxicity data, which may not reflect forms of toxicity that are important clinically.
  - It takes no account of idiosyncratic toxic reactions.
- More sophisticated measures of risk–benefit analysis for drugs in clinical use are coming into use, and include the 'number-needed-to-treat' (NNT) principle.

REFERENCES AND FURTHER READING

Anturane Reinfarction Trial Research Group 1978 Sulfinpyrazone in the prevention of cardiac death after myocardial infarction. N Engl J Med 298: 289–295 (*Example of a large-scale clinical trial*)

Armitage P 1978 Sequential clinical trials. Blackwell, Oxford (*Standard textbook*)

Beta-blocker Heart Attack Trial Research Group 1982 A randomised trial of propranolol in patients with acute myocardial infarction. 1. Mortality results. JAMA 247: 1707–1714 (*A trial that was terminated early when clear evidence of benefit emerged*)

Colquhoun D 1971 Lectures on biostatistics. Oxford University Press, Oxford (*Standard textbook*)

Friedman L M, Furberg C D, DeMets D L 1997 Fundamentals of clinical trials, 3rd edn. Mosby, St Louis, Missouri (*Standard textbook*)

Laska E M, Meisner M J 1987 Statistical methods and the applications of bioassay. Annu Rev Pharmacol 27: 385–397 (*Useful references for those concerned with statistical principles of assay design and analysis*)

Ledent C, Veaugois J-M, Schiffmann S N et al. 1997 Aggressiveness, hypoalgesia and high blood pressure in mice lacking the adenosine A_{2a} receptor. Nature 388: 674–676 (*Examples of the use of a transgenic model to study receptor function*)

Maerki U, Haerri A 1996 Transgenic technology: principles. Int J Exp Path 77: 247–250 (*Short review article*)

Masliah E, Sisk A, Mallory M, Mucke L, Schenk D, Games D 1996 Comparison of neurodegenerative pathology in transgenic mice overexpressing V717F beta-amyloid precursor protein and Alzheimer's disease. J Neurosci 16: 5795–5811 (*An example of a transgenic disease model*)

Naylor C D 1997 Meta-analysis and the meta-epidemiology of clinical research. Br Med J 315: 617–619 (*Thoughtful review on strengths and weaknesses of meta-analysis*)

Paton W D M 1993 Man and mouse: animals in medical research. Oxford University Press, Oxford (*Excellent and balanced account of issues surrounding animal experimentation*)

Plueck A 1996 Conditional mutagenesis in mice: the Cre/loxP recombination system. Int J Exp Path 77: 269–278 (*An emerging technology for allowing genes to be switched on or off during the lifetime of an animal*)

Polites H G 1996 Transgenic model applications to drug discovery. Int J Exp Path 77: 257–262 (*Useful general review*)

Sackett D L, Rosenburg W M C, Muir-Gray J A, Haynes R B, Richardson W S 1996 Evidence-based medicine: what it is and what it isn't. Br Med J 312: 71–72 (*Balanced account of the value of 'evidence-based medicine'—an important recent trend in medical thinking*)

Sjostrom N 1972 Thalidomide and the power of the drug companies. Penguin, London. (*Well-written polemical account of the thalidomide story*)

Walley T, Haycocks A 1997 Pharmacoeconomics: basic concepts and terminology. Br J Clin Pharmacol 43: 343–348 (*Useful introduction to analytical principles that are becoming increasingly important for therapeutic policy-makers*)

Yanagisawa M, Kurihara H, Kimura S et al. 1988 A novel potent vasoconstrictor peptide produced by vascular endothelial cells. Nature 332: 411–415 (*The first paper describing endothelin—a remarkably full characterisation of an important new mediator*)

4

Absorption and distribution of drugs

The action of any drug requires it to achieve an adequate concentration in the fluid bathing the target tissue, although the effects of 'hit and run' drugs (e.g. alkylating agents) outlast their presence in solution. The two fundamental processes that determine the concentration of a drug at any moment and in any region of the body are:

- *translocation of drug molecules*
- *chemical transformation.*

In this chapter we discuss drug translocation and the factors that determine absorption and distribution, with emphasis on different routes of administration. Chemical transformation by drug metabolism and other processes involved in drug elimination are described in Chapter 5.

TRANSLOCATION OF DRUG MOLECULES

Drug molecules move around the body in two ways:

- *bulk flow transfer* (i.e. in the bloodstream)
- *diffusional transfer* (i.e. molecule-by-molecule, over short distances).

The chemical nature of a drug makes no difference to its transfer by bulk flow. The cardiovascular system provides a very fast long-distance bulk flow distribution system. In contrast, *diffusional* characteristics differ markedly between different drugs. In particular, ability to cross hydrophobic diffusion barriers is strongly influenced by lipid solubility. Aqueous diffusion is also part of the overall mechanism of drug transport, since it is this process that delivers drug molecules to and from the non-aqueous barriers. The rate of diffusion of a substance depends mainly on its molecular size, the *diffusion coefficient* for small molecules being inversely proportional to the square root of molecular weight. Thus, large molecules diffuse more slowly than small ones, but the variation with molecular weight is relatively slight. Many drugs fall within the molecular weight range 200–1000, and variations in aqueous diffusion rate have only a small effect on their overall pharmacokinetic behaviour. For most purposes we can regard the body as a series of interconnected *well-stirred compartments* within each of which the drug concentration remains uniform. It is the movement between compartments, generally involving the penetration of non-aqueous diffusion barriers, that determines where, and for how long, a drug will be present in the body after it has been administered. The analysis of drug movements with the help of a simple compartmental model is discussed in Chapter 5.

THE MOVEMENT OF DRUG MOLECULES ACROSS CELL BARRIERS

The barriers between aqueous compartments in the body consist of cell membranes. A single layer of membrane separates the intracellular from the extracellular compartments. An *epithelial barrier*, such as the gastrointestinal mucosa or renal tubule, consists of a layer of cells tightly connected to each other so that molecules must traverse at least two cell membranes (inner and outer) to pass from one side to the other. *Vascular endothelium* is more complicated, its anatomical disposition and permeability varying from one tissue to another. Gaps between endothelial cells are packed with a loose matrix of proteins that act as filters, retaining large molecules and letting smaller ones through. The cut off of molecular size is not exact: water transfers rapidly whereas molecules of 80 000–100 000 daltons molecular weight transfer very slowly. In some organs, especially the central nervous system and the placenta, there are tight junctions between the cells, and penetration by drug molecules involves crossing endothelial cell membranes, an important feature that makes these vascular beds quite distinct from those of other organs and has major pharmacokinetic consequences. In other organs (e.g. the liver and spleen) endothelium is discontinuous, allowing free passage of cells. In the liver, hepatocytes form the barrier between intra- and extravascular compartments and take on several endothelial cell functions. Endothelial cells lining post-capillary venules have specialised functions relating to leukocyte migration and inflammation: the sophistication of the intercellular junction can be appreciated from the observation that leukocyte migration can occur without any detectable leak of water or small ions (see Ch. 12). *Fenestrated endothelium* in which the adlumenal and ablumenal membranes are apposed, giving a pock-marked appearance on scanning electron microscopy, occurs in exocrine glands such as the parotid.

There are four main ways by which small molecules cross cell membranes (Fig. 4.1):

- by diffusing directly through the *lipid*
- by diffusing through *aqueous pores* that traverse the lipid
- by combination with a transmembrane *carrier protein* that binds a molecule on one side of the membrane then changes conformation and releases it on the other
- by *pinocytosis*.

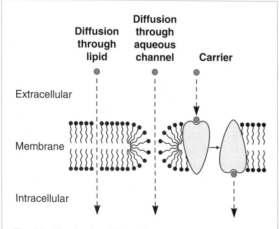

Fig. 4.1 Routes by which solutes can traverse cell membranes. (Molecules can also cross cellular barriers by pinocytosis.)

Of these routes, diffusion through lipid and carrier-mediated transport are particularly important in relation to pharmacokinetic mechanisms. Diffusion through aqueous pores is unimportant in this context, since these pores are too small in diameter (about 0.4 nm) to allow most drug molecules (which usually exceed 1 nm in diameter) to pass through. Pinocytosis involves invagination of part of the cell membrane and the trapping within the cell of a small vesicle containing extracellular constituents. The vesicle contents can then be released within the cell, or extruded from its other side. This mechanism appears to be important for the transport of some macromolecules (e.g. **insulin**, which crosses the blood–brain barrier by this process), but not for small molecules. Diffusion through lipid and carrier-mediated transport will now be discussed in more detail.

Diffusion through lipid

Non-polar substances (i.e. substances with molecules in which electrons are uniformly distributed) dissolve freely in non-polar solvents, such as lipids, and therefore penetrate cell membranes very freely by diffusion. The permeability coefficient, P, for a substance diffusing passively through a membrane is determined by the number of molecules crossing the membrane per unit area in unit time and the concentration difference across the membrane. Permeant molecules must be present within the membrane in sufficient numbers, and must be mobile within the membrane if rapid permeation is to occur. Thus two physicochemical factors contribute to P, namely solubility in the membrane (which can be expressed as a *partition coefficient* for the substance distributed between the membrane phase and the aqueous environment) and diffusivity, which is a measure of the mobility of molecules within the lipid and is expressed as a *diffusion coefficient*. Among different drug molecules the diffusion coefficient varies only slightly, as noted above, so the most important variable is the partition coefficient (see Fig. 4.2). Thus, there is a close correlation between lipid solubility and the permeability of the cell membrane to different substances. For this reason, lipid solubility is one of the most important determinants of the pharmacokinetic characteristics of a drug, and many properties, such as rate of absorption from the gut, penetration into the brain and other tissues, and the extent of renal elimination can be predicted from knowledge of a drug's lipid solubility.

pH and ionisation

One important complicating factor in relation to membrane permeation is that many drugs are weak acids or

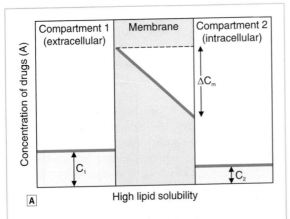

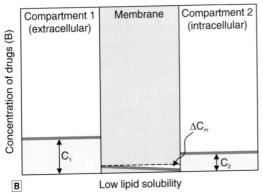

Fig. 4.2 The importance of lipid solubility in membrane permeation. [A] and [B] Figures show the concentration profile in a lipid membrane separating two aqueous compartments. A lipid-soluble drug (A) is subject to a much larger transmembrane concentration gradient (DC_m) than a lipid-insoluble drug (B). It therefore diffuses more rapidly even though the aqueous concentration gradient ($C_1 - C_2$) is the same in both cases.

bases and therefore exist in both unionised and ionised form, the ratio of the two forms varying with pH. For a weak base, the ionisation reaction is:

$$BH^+ \underset{}{\overset{K_a}{\rightleftharpoons}} B + H^+$$

and the dissociation constant pK_a is given by the Henderson–Hasselbalch equation:

$$pK_a = pH + \log_{10} \frac{[BH^+]}{[B]}$$

For a weak acid:

$$AH \underset{}{\overset{K_a}{\rightleftharpoons}} A^- + H^+$$

$$pK_a = pH + \log_{10} \frac{[AH]}{[A^-]}$$

In either case the ionised species, BH^+ or A^-, has very low lipid solubility and is virtually unable to permeate membranes except where a specific transport mechanism exists. The lipid solubility of the uncharged species, B or AH, will depend on the chemical nature of the drug; for many drugs the uncharged species is sufficiently lipid soluble to permit rapid membrane permeation, though there are exceptions (e.g. aminoglycoside antibiotics; see Ch. 43) where even the uncharged molecule is insufficiently lipid soluble to cross membranes appreciably. This is usually due to a preponderance of hydrogen-bonding groups, such as –OH, as in the sugar moiety in the aminoglycosides, that render the uncharged molecule hydrophilic.

pH partition and ion trapping

Ionisation affects not only the rate at which drugs permeate membranes, but also the steady-state distribution of drug molecules between aqueous compartments, if a pH difference exists between them. Figure 4.3 shows how a weak acid (e.g. **aspirin**, pK_a 3.5) and a weak base (e.g. **pethidine**, pK_a 8.6) would be distributed at equilibrium between three body compartments, namely plasma (pH 7.4), alkaline urine (pH 8) and gastric juice (pH 3). Within each compartment the ratio of ionised to unionised drug is governed by the pK_a and the pH of that compartment, according to the Henderson–Hasselbalch equation. It is assumed that the unionised species can cross the membrane, and therefore reaches an equal concentration in each compartment. The ionised species is assumed not to cross at all. The result is that at equilibrium the total (ionised + unionised) concentration of the drug will be different in the two compartments, with an acidic drug being concentrated in the compartment with high pH ('*ion trapping*'), and vice versa. The theoretical concentration gradients produced by ion trapping can be very large if there is a large pH difference between compartments. Thus, aspirin would be concentrated more than fourfold with respect to plasma in an alkaline renal tubule, and about 6000-fold in plasma with respect to the acidic gastric contents. Such large gradients are, however, unlikely to be achieved in reality for two main reasons. Firstly, the attribution of total impermeability to the charged species is not realistic, and even a small permeability will considerably attenuate the concentration difference that can be reached. Secondly, body compartments rarely approach equilibrium. Neither the gastric contents nor the renal tubular fluid stands still, and the resulting flux of drug molecules has the effect of reducing the concentration gradients well below the theoretical equilibrium conditions. The pH partition mechanism nonetheless correctly explains some of the

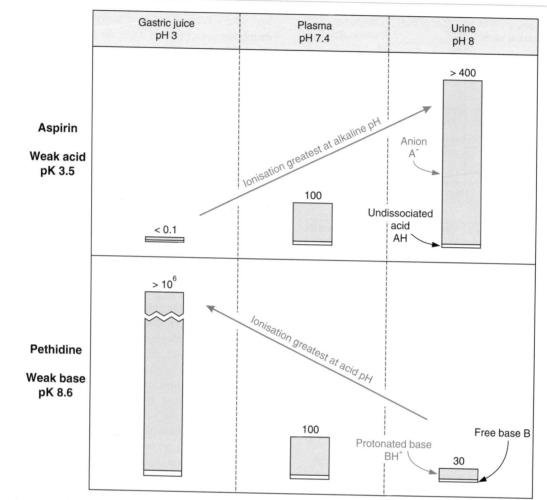

| Gastric juice pH 3 | Plasma pH 7.4 | Urine pH 8 |

Fig. 4.3 Theoretical partition of a weak acid (aspirin) and a weak base (pethidine) between aqueous compartments (urine, plasma and gastric juice) according to the pH difference between them. Numbers represent relative concentrations (total plasma concentration = 100). It is assumed that the uncharged species in each case can permeate the cellular barrier separating the compartments, and thus reaches the same concentration in all three. Variations in the fractional ionisation as a function of pH give rise to the large total concentration differences with respect to plasma.

qualitative effects of pH changes in different body compartments on the pharmacokinetics of weakly acidic or basic drugs, particularly in relation to renal excretion and penetration of the blood–brain barrier. pH partition is not the main determinant of the site of absorption of drugs from the gastrointestinal tract. This is because the enormous absorptive surface area of the villi and micro-villi in the ileum compared to the much smaller surface area in the stomach is of overriding importance. Thus, absorption of an acidic drug such as **aspirin** is promoted by drugs that accelerate gastric emptying (e.g. **meto-**

clopramide) and retarded by drugs that slow gastric emptying (e.g. **propantheline**), despite the fact that the acidic pH of the stomach contents favours absorption of weak acids. Values of pK_a for some common drugs are shown in Figure 4.4.

Some important consequences of the pH partition mechanism are:

● Urinary acidification accelerates excretion of weak bases and retards that of weak acids, while urinary alkalinisation has the opposite effect.

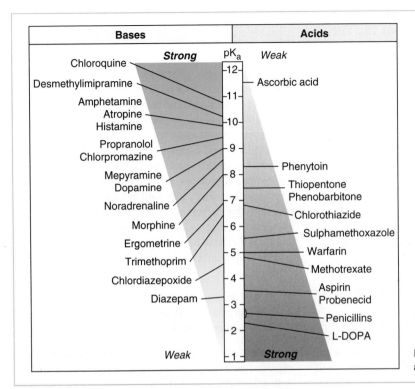

Fig. 4.4 pKa values for some acidic and basic drugs.

- Increasing plasma pH (e.g. by administration of sodium bicarbonate) causes weakly acidic drugs to be extracted from the central nervous system into the plasma. Conversely, reducing plasma pH (e.g. by administration of a carbonic anhydrase inhibitor such as **acetazolamide**; see p. 366) causes weakly acidic drugs to become concentrated in the central nervous system, increasing their neurotoxicity. This has practical consequences in choosing a means to alkalinise urine in treating **aspirin** overdose (see p. 367): either bicarbonate or acetazolamide increases urine pH and hence increases salicylate elimination, but bicarbonate is used since it reduces rather than increases distribution of salicylate to the central nervous system.

Carrier-mediated transport

Many cell membranes possess specialised transport mechanisms that regulate entry and exit of physiologically important molecules, such as sugars, amino acids, neurotransmitters and metal ions. Generally, such transport systems involve a carrier molecule, i.e. a transmembrane protein which binds one or more molecules or ions, changes conformation and releases them on the other side of the membrane. Such systems may operate purely passively, without any energy source; in this case they merely facilitate the process of transmembrane equilibration of the transported species in the direction of its electrochemical gradient and the mechanism is called *facilitated diffusion*. Alternatively, they may be coupled to an energy source, either directly to ATP hydrolysis or indirectly to the electrochemical gradient of another species such as Na^+; in this case transport can occur against an electrochemical gradient and is called *active transport*. Carrier-mediated transport, because it involves a binding step, shows the characteristic of *saturation*. With simple diffusion the rate of transport increases directly in proportion to the concentration gradient, whereas with carrier-mediated transport the carrier sites become saturated at high ligand concentrations and the rate of transport does not increase beyond this point. Furthermore, *competitive inhibition* of transport can occur if a second ligand that binds to the carrier is present.

Carriers of this type are ubiquitous and many pharmacological effects are the result of interference with them. Thus, nerve terminals have transport mechanisms for accumulating specific neurotransmitters, and there are many examples of drugs that act by inhibiting these transport mechanisms (see Chs 7, 8 and 28). From a pharmacokinetic point of view, though, there are only a few sites in the body where carrier-mediated drug transport is important, the main ones being:

- the renal tubule
- the biliary tract
- the blood–brain barrier
- the gastrointestinal tract.

P-glycoprotein (the drug transporter responsible for multidrug resistance in neoplastic cells, p. 680) has recently been found in renal tubular brush border membranes, in bile canaliculi, in astrocyte foot processes in brain microvessels and in the gastrointestinal tract. It may play an important part in absorption, distribution and elimination of many drugs. The characteristics of transport systems are discussed later when patterns of distribution and elimination in the body as a whole are considered more fully.

In addition to the processes so far described that govern the transport of drug molecules across the barriers between different aqueous compartments, two additional factors have a major influence on drug distribution and elimination. These are:

- binding to plasma proteins
- partition into body fat and other tissues.

Movement of drugs across cellular barriers

- To traverse cellular barriers (e.g. gastrointestinal mucosa, renal tubule, blood–brain barrier, placenta), drugs have to cross lipid membranes.
- Drugs cross lipid membranes mainly (a) by passive diffusional transfer and (b) by carrier-mediated transfer.
- The main factor that determines the rate of passive diffusional transfer across membranes is a drug's lipid solubility. Molecular weight is a less important factor.
- Many drugs are weak acids or weak bases, whose state of ionisation varies with pH according to the Henderson–Hasselbalch equation.
- With weak acids or bases, only the uncharged species (the protonated form for a weak acid; the unprotonated form for a weak base) can diffuse across lipid membranes; this gives rise to pH partition.
- pH partition means that weak acids tend to accumulate in compartments of relatively high pH, whereas weak bases do the reverse.
- Carrier-mediated transport (e.g. in the renal tubule, blood–brain barrier, gastrointestinal epithelium) is important for some drugs that are chemically related to endogenous substances.

BINDING OF DRUGS TO PLASMA PROTEINS

Many drugs exist in plasma mainly in bound form at therapeutic concentrations. The fraction of drug that is free in aqueous solution can be as low as 1%, the remainder being associated with plasma protein. The most important plasma protein in relation to drug binding is albumin, which binds many acidic drugs (for example **warfarin**, non-steroidal anti-inflammatory drugs, sulphonamides) and a smaller number of basic drugs (for example tricyclic antidepressants, **chlorpromazine**). Other plasma proteins, including β-globulin and an acid glycoprotein which, although present in much smaller amounts than albumin, is an acute phase protein that increases in disease, have also been implicated in the binding of certain basic drugs, such as **quinine**.

The amount of a drug that is bound to protein depends on three factors:

- the free drug concentration
- its affinity for the binding sites
- the protein concentration.

As a first approximation, the binding reaction can be regarded as a simple association of the drug molecules with a finite population of binding sites, exactly analogous to drug–receptor binding (see Ch. 1).

$$D \quad + \quad S \quad \rightleftharpoons \quad DS$$

free	binding	complex
drug	site	

The usual concentration of albumin in plasma is about 0.6 mmol/l (4 g/100 ml). With two sites per albumin molecule, the drug-binding capacity of plasma albumin would therefore be about 1.2 mmol/l. For most drugs the total plasma concentration required for a clinical effect is much less than 1.2 mmol/l, so with usual therapeutic doses the binding sites are far from saturation, and the concentration bound [DS] varies nearly in direct proportion to the free concentration [D]. Under these conditions the fraction bound, [DS]/([D] + [DS]), is independent of the drug concentration. However, some drugs, for example **tolbutamide** (Ch. 22) and some sulphonamides (Ch. 43), work at plasma concentrations at which the binding to protein is approaching saturation (i.e. on the flat part of the binding curve). This means that addition of more drug to the plasma will increase the free concentration disproportionately. Doubling the dose of such a drug can therefore more than double the free (pharmacologically active) concentration. This is shown for the anti-inflammatory drug **phenylbutazone** in Figure 4.5.

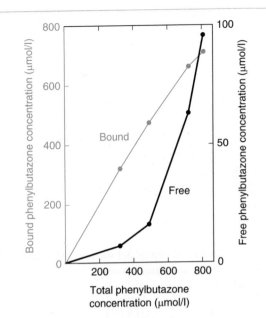

Fig. 4.5   Binding of phenylbutazone to plasma albumin.
The graph shows the disproportionate increase in free
concentration as the total concentration increases, due to the
binding sites approaching saturation. (Data from: Brodie B,
Hogben C A M 1957 J Pharm Pharmacol 9: 345)

The existence of binding sites on plasma albumin for
which many different drugs have an affinity means that
competition can occur between them, so that administration of drug B can reduce the protein binding, and
hence increase the free plasma concentration, of drug
A. To do this, drug B needs to occupy an appreciable
fraction of the binding sites. Few therapeutic drugs affect
the binding of other drugs because they occupy, at therapeutic plasma concentrations, only a tiny fraction of the

---

Binding of drugs to plasma proteins

- Plasma albumin is most important; β-globulin and acid
  glycoprotein also bind some drugs.
- Plasma albumin binds mainly acidic drugs (approximately
  two molecules per albumin molecule). Basic drugs may
  be bound by β-globulin and acid glycoprotein.
- Saturable binding sometimes leads to a non-linear
  relation between dose and free (active) drug
  concentration.
- Extensive protein binding slows drug elimination
  (metabolism and/or excretion by glomerular filtration).
- Competition between drugs for protein binding rarely
  leads to clinically important drug interactions.

---

available sites. **Sulphonamides** (Ch. 43) are an exception
because they occupy about 50% of the binding sites at
therapeutic concentrations, and so can cause unexpected
effects by displacing other drugs or, in premature babies,
bilirubin (Ch. 48). Much has been made of the importance of binding interactions of this kind as a source
of untoward drug interactions in clinical medicine, but
it is now appreciated that this type of competition is less
important than was once thought (see Ch. 48).

PARTITION INTO BODY FAT AND OTHER TISSUES

Fat represents a large, non-polar compartment. In practice this is important for only a few drugs, mainly because
the effective fat : water partition coefficient is relatively
low for most drugs. **Morphine**, for example, though quite
lipid-soluble enough to cross the blood–brain barrier,
has a lipid : water partition coefficient of only 0.4, so
sequestration of the drug by body fat is of little importance. With **thiopentone**, on the other hand (fat : water
partition coefficient approximately 10), accumulation
in body fat is considerable, and has important pharmacokinetic consequences when the drug is used as an intravenous anaesthetic agent (Ch. 32).

The second factor that limits the accumulation of
drugs in body fat is its low blood supply—less than 2%
of the cardiac output. Thus drugs are delivered to body
fat rather slowly, so that the theoretical equilibrium distribution between fat and body water is approached slowly.
For practical purposes, therefore, partition into body fat
when drugs are given acutely is important only for a few
highly lipid-soluble drugs (e.g. general anaesthetics;
Ch. 32). When lipid-soluble drugs are given chronically,
however, accumulation in body fat is often significant
(e.g. benzodiazepines; Ch. 33). Furthermore, there are
some environmental contaminants ('xenobiotics'), such
as insecticides, that are poorly metabolised. If ingested
regularly such xenobiotics accumulate slowly but progressively in body fat.

Body fat is not the only tissue in which drugs can accumulate. **Chloroquine**—an antimalarial drug (Ch. 46)
used additionally to treat rheumatoid arthritis (Ch. 13)—
has a high affinity for melanin and is taken up by tissues
such as retina that are rich in melanin granules, which
may account for the retinopathy that can occur during
prolonged treatment of patients with rheumatoid disease.
Tetracyclines (Ch. 43) accumulate slowly in bones and
teeth, because they have a high affinity for calcium,
and should not be used in children for this reason. Very
high concentrations of **amiodarone** (an antidysrhythmic
drug; Ch. 14) accumulate in liver and lung as well as fat.

DRUG DISPOSITION

We will now consider how the basic processes responsible for the translocation and distribution of drug molecules—diffusion, penetration of membranes, binding to plasma protein and partition into fat and other tissues—influence the overall behaviour of drug molecules in the body. Such drug disposition can be divided into four stages:

- absorption from the site of administration
- distribution within the body
- metabolism
- excretion.

Absorption and distribution are considered here, metabolism and excretion in Chapter 5. The main routes of drug administration and elimination are shown schematically in Figure 4.6.

DRUG ABSORPTION
ROUTES OF ADMINISTRATION

Absorption is defined as the passage of a drug from its site of administration into the plasma. It is therefore important for all routes of administration, except intravenous injection. There are instances, such as inhalation of a bronchodilator aerosol to treat asthma (Ch. 19), where absorption as just defined is not required for the drug to act, but in most cases the drug must enter plasma before reaching its site of action.

The main routes of administration are:

- oral
- sublingual
- rectal
- application to other epithelial surfaces (e.g. skin, cornea, vagina and nasal mucosa)
- inhalation

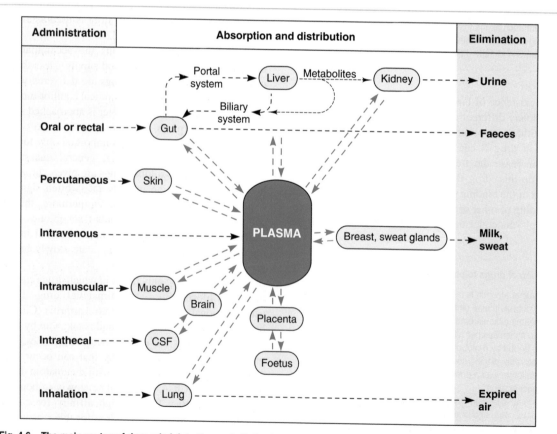

Fig. 4.6 The main routes of drug administration and elimination.

- injection
  —subcutaneous
  —intramuscular
  —intravenous
  —intrathecal.

Oral administration

Most drugs are taken by mouth and swallowed. Little absorption occurs until drug enters the small intestine.

Drug absorption from the intestine

The mechanism of drug absorption is the same as for other epithelial barriers, namely passive transfer at a rate determined by the ionisation and lipid solubility of the drug molecules. Figure 4.7 shows the absorption of a series of weak acids and bases as a function of pK_a. As expected, strong bases of pK_a 10 or higher are poorly absorbed, as are strong acids of pK_a less than 3, because they are fully ionised. Several clinically important drugs are strong bases, such as the muscle relaxants **vecuronium** and **suxamethonium** which are quaternary ammonium compounds and are poorly absorbed from the gastrointestinal tract; they are given intravenously (Ch. 7).

There are a few instances where intestinal absorption depends on carrier-mediated transport rather than simple lipid diffusion. Examples include **levodopa**, used in treating parkinsonism (see Ch. 31), which is taken up by the carrier that normally transports phenylalanine, and **fluorouracil** (Ch. 42), a cytotoxic drug that is transported by the system that carries natural pyrimidines (thymine

and uracil). Iron is absorbed via a specific carrier on the surface of mucosal cells in the jejunum, and calcium is absorbed by means of a vitamin D-dependent carrier system.

Factors affecting gastrointestinal absorption. Typically, about 75% of a drug given orally is absorbed in 1–3 hours, but numerous factors alter this, some physiological and some to do with the formulation of the drug. The main factors are:

- gastrointestinal motility
- splanchnic blood flow
- particle size and formulation
- physicochemical factors.

Gastrointestinal motility has a large effect. Many disorders (e.g. migraine, diabetic neuropathy) cause gastric stasis and slow drug absorption. Drug treatment can also affect motility, either reducing (e.g. drugs that block muscarinic receptors; see Ch. 7) or increasing it (e.g. **metoclopramide**, which is used in migraine to facilitate absorption of analgesic; see Ch. 9). Excessively rapid movement of gut contents can impair absorption. A drug taken after a meal is often more slowly absorbed because its progress to the small intestine is delayed. There are exceptions, however, and several drugs (e.g. **propranolol**) reach a higher plasma concentration if they are taken after a meal, probably because food *increases splanchnic blood flow*. Conversely, splanchnic blood flow is greatly reduced in hypovolaemic states, with a resultant slowing of drug absorption.

Particle size and formulation have major effects on absorption. In 1971, patients in a New York hospital were found to require unusually large maintenance doses of **digoxin** (Ch. 14). In a study on normal volunteers it was found that standard oral digoxin tablets from different manufacturers resulted in grossly different plasma concentrations (Fig. 4.8) even though the digoxin content of the tablets was the same, because of differences in particle size. Because digoxin is rather poorly absorbed, small differences in the pharmaceutical formulation can make a large difference to the extent of absorption.

Pharmaceutical preparations are formulated to produce desired absorption characteristics. Capsules may be designed to remain intact for some hours after ingestion in order to delay absorption, or tablets may have a resistant coating to give the same effect. In some cases, a mixture of slow- and fast-release particles is included in a capsule to produce rapid but sustained absorption. More elaborate pharmaceutical systems include various modified-release preparations (e.g. a long-acting form of **nifedipine** that permits once daily use). Such preparations not only

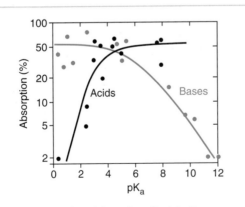

Fig. 4.7 Absorption of drugs from the intestine as a function of pK_a, for acids and bases. Weak acids and bases are well absorbed; strong acids and bases are poorly absorbed. (Redrawn from: Schanker L S et al. 1957 J Pharmacol 120: 528)

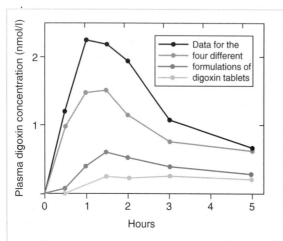

Fig. 4.8 Variation in oral absorption among different formulations of digoxin. The four curves show the mean plasma concentrations attained for the four preparations, each of which was given on separate occasions to four subjects. The large variation has caused the formulation of digoxin tablets to be standardised since this study was published. (From: Lindenbaum J et al. 1971 N Engl J Med 285: 1344)

increase the dose interval, but also reduce adverse effects related to high peak plasma concentrations following administration of a conventional formulation (e.g. flushing following regular nifedipine; Ch. 14). Osmotically driven 'mini-pumps' can be implanted experimentally, and some oral extended-release preparations that are used clinically use the same principle, the tablet containing an osmotically active core and being bounded by an impermeable membrane with a precisely engineered pore to allow drug to exit in solution as the tablet traverses the ileum. This results a form of drug delivery that approximates to a constant-rate infusion into the bowel lumen. Such preparations may, however, cause problems related to high local concentrations of drug in the intestine (an osmotically released preparation of the anti-inflammatory drug **indomethacin** had to be withdrawn because it caused small bowel perforation), and are subject to variations in small bowel transit time that occur during ageing and with disease.

Physicochemical factors (including some drug interactions; Ch. 48) affect drug absorption by influencing the state of the drug in the intestine. **Tetracycline** binds strongly to calcium ions, and calcium-rich foods (especially milk) prevent its absorption (Ch. 43). Bile-acid-binding resins such as **cholestyramine** (used to treat hypercholesterolaemia; Ch. 16) bind several drugs, for

example **warfarin** (Ch. 17) and **thyroxine** (Ch. 25) which should be administered at least 1 hour before or 4–6 hours after cholestyramine for this reason.

When drugs are administered by mouth, the intention is usually that they should be absorbed and cause a systemic effect, but there are exceptions. **Vancomycin** is very poorly absorbed and is administered orally to eradicate toxin-forming *Clostridium difficile* from the gut lumen in patients with pseudomembranous colitis (an adverse effect of treatment with broad-spectrum antibiotics caused by appearance of this organism in the bowel). **Mesalazine** is a formulation of 5-aminosalicylic acid in a pH-dependent acrylic coat that degrades in the terminal ileum and proximal colon and is used to treat inflammatory bowel disease affecting this part of the gut. **Olsalazine** is a pro-drug consisting of a dimer of two molecules of 5-aminosalicylic acid that is cleaved by colonic bacteria in the distal bowel and is used to treat patients with distal colitis.

Bioavailability. To get from the lumen of the small intestine into the systemic circulation a drug must not only penetrate the intestinal mucosa; it must also run the gauntlet of enzymes that may inactivate it in gut wall and liver. The term bioavailability is used to indicate the proportion of drug that passes into the systemic circulation after oral administration, taking into account both absorption and local metabolic degradation. It is a convenient term for making bland generalisations, but the concept creaks badly if attempts are made to use it with quantitative precision, or even to define it.* One problem is that it is not a characteristic solely of the drug preparation: variations in enzyme activity of gut wall or liver, in gastric pH or intestinal motility, all affect it. Because of this, one cannot speak strictly of the bio-availability of a particular preparation, but only of that preparation in a given individual on a particular occasion. Even with these caveats, the concept is of limited use because it relates only to the total proportion of the drug that reaches the systemic circulation, and ignores the rate of absorption. If a drug is completely absorbed in 30 minutes, it will reach a much higher peak plasma concentration (and have a more dramatic effect) than if it were absorbed more slowly. One rarely sees a numerical

---

*The definition of bioavailability offered by the US Food and Drug Administration is: 'The rate and extent to which the therapeutic moiety is absorbed and becomes available to the site of drug action'. You may be forgiven for finding this confusing. The double use of 'and' gives the definition four possible meanings, two of which are obfuscated by the uncertain meaning of the phrase 'becomes available to the site of drug action'.

value assigned to 'bioavailability', and it is well to be wary of ostensibly measurable quantities that are used impressionistically, but not actually given values. For these reasons, regulatory authorities—which have to make decisions about the licensing of products that are 'generic equivalents' of patented products—lay importance on evidence of bioequivalence, i.e. evidence that the new product behaves sufficiently similarly to the existing one to be substituted for it without causing clinical problems.

Sublingual administration

Absorption directly from the oral cavity is sometimes useful (provided the drug does not taste too horrible) when a rapid response is required, particularly when the drug is either unstable at gastric pH or rapidly metabolised by the liver. **Glyceryl trinitrate** is an example of a drug that is often given sublingually (see Ch. 14). Drugs absorbed from the mouth pass straight into the systemic circulation without entering the portal system, and so escape first-pass metabolism.

Rectal administration

Rectal administration is used either for drugs that are required to produce a local effect (e.g. anti-inflammatory drugs for use in ulcerative colitis), or to produce systemic effects. Absorption following rectal administration is often unreliable, but this route can be useful in patients who are vomiting or are unable to take medication by mouth (e.g. postoperatively). It is used to administer **diazepam** to children who are in *status epilepticus* (Ch. 36) in whom it is difficult to establish intravenous access.

Application to epithelial surfaces

Cutaneous administration

Cutaneous administration is used when a local effect on the skin is required (e.g. topically applied steroids). Appreciable absorption may nonetheless occur and lead to systemic effects.

Most drugs are absorbed very poorly through unbroken skin, because their lipid solubility is too low. However, a number of organophosphate insecticides (see Ch. 7), which need to penetrate an insect's cuticle in order to work, are absorbed through skin, and accidental poisoning occurs in farm workers. A case is recounted of a 35-year-old florist in 1932. 'While engaged in doing a light electrical repair job at a work bench he sat down in a chair on the seat of which some "Nico-Fume liquid" (a 40% solution of free nicotine) had been spilled. He felt the solution wet through his clothes to the skin over the left buttock, an area about the size of the palm of his hand. He thought nothing further of it and continued at his work for about fifteen minutes, when he was suddenly seized with nausea and faintness … and found himself in a drenching sweat. On the way to hospital he lost consciousness.' He survived, just, and then 4 days later: 'On discharge from the hospital he was given the same clothes that he had worn when he was brought in. The clothes had been kept in a paper bag and were still damp where they had been wet with the nicotine solution.' The sequel was predictable. He survived again, but felt thereafter 'unable to enter a greenhouse where nicotine was being sprayed.' Transdermal dosage forms of nicotine are now used to reduce the withdrawal symptoms that accompany stopping smoking (Ch. 39).

Such transdermal dosage forms, in which the drug is incorporated in a stick-on patch applied to an area of thin skin, are used increasingly, and several drugs—for example oestrogen for hormone replacement (Ch. 26)—are available in this form. Such patches produce a steady rate of drug delivery and avoid presystemic metabolism. However, the method is suitable only for relatively lipid-soluble drugs, and such preparations are relatively expensive.

A few peptide hormone analogues, for example of anti-diuretic hormone (ADH) and of gonadotrophin-releasing hormone (see Ch. 24) as well as calcitonin itself, are

---

> **Drug absorption and bioavailability**
>
> - Drugs of very low lipid solubility, including those that are strong acids or bases, are generally poorly absorbed from the gut.
> - A few drugs (e.g. levodopa) are absorbed by carrier-mediated transfer.
> - Absorption from the gut depends on many factors, including:
>   — gastrointestinal motility
>   — gastrointestinal pH
>   — particle size
>   — physicochemical interaction with gut contents (e.g. chemical interaction between calcium and tetracycline antibiotics).
> - Bioavailability is the fraction of an ingested dose of a drug that gains access to the systemic circulation. It may be low because absorption is incomplete, or because the drug is metabolised in the gut wall or liver before reaching the systemic circulation.
> - Bioequivalence implies that if one formulation of a drug is substituted for another no clinically untoward consequences will ensue.

given as nasal sprays. These peptides are inactive when given orally, as they are quickly destroyed in the gastro-intestinal tract, but enough is taken up from the nasal mucosa to provide a therapeutic effect. Such absorption is believed to take place through mucosa overlying nasal-associated lymphoid tissue which has similarities to the mucosa of Peyer's patches which is also uniquely permeable.

Eye drops

Many drugs are applied as eye drops, relying on absorption through the epithelium of the conjunctival sac to produce their effects. Desirable local effects within the eye can be achieved without causing systemic side-effects; for example, **dorzolamide** is a carbonic anhydrase inhibitor which is given as eye drops to lower intraoccular pressure in patients with glaucoma. It achieves this without affecting the kidney (see Ch. 20), thus avoiding the acidosis which inevitably accompanies chronic oral administration of **acetazolamide**. Some systemic absorption from the eye occurs, however, and can result in unwanted effects (e.g. bronchospasm in asthmatic patients using **timolol** eye drops for glaucoma).

Administration by inhalation

Inhalation is the route used for volatile and gaseous anaesthetics (see Ch. 32), the lung serving as the route both of administration and elimination. The rapid exchange resulting from the large surface area and blood flow makes it possible to achieve rapid adjustments of plasma concentration. The pharmacokinetic behaviour of inhalation anaesthetics is discussed more fully in Chapter 32.

Drugs used for their effects on the lung are also given by inhalation, usually as an aerosol. Glucocorticoids (e.g. **beclomethasone**) and bronchodilators, such as **salbutamol** (Ch. 19), are given in this way to achieve much higher concentrations in the lung than elsewhere in the body, thus minimising side-effects. Drugs given by inhalation for their action on the airways are usually partially absorbed into the circulation, and systemic side-effects (e.g. tremor following salbutamol) can occur. Chemical modification of a drug may minimise such absorption. Thus **ipratropium**, a muscarinic receptor antagonist (Chs 7 and 19), is a quaternary ammonium ion analogue of atropine. It is used as an inhaled bronchodilator because its poor absorption minimises systemic adverse effects.

Administration by injection

Intravenous injection is the fastest and most certain route of drug administration. If a single bolus injection

is given, it produces a very high concentration of drug, which will first reach the right heart and lungs and then the systemic circulation. The actual peak concentration reaching the tissues depends critically on the rate of injection. Administration by steady intravenous infusion avoids the uncertainties of absorption from other sites, while avoiding high peak plasma concentrations. Drugs given intravenously include **lignocaine** (Ch. 14), anaesthetic agents such as **propofol** (Ch. 32), and **diazepam** for patients with status epilepticus (Ch. 33).

Subcutaneous or *intramuscular injection* of drugs usually produces a faster effect than oral administration, but the rate of absorption depends greatly on the site of injection and on local blood flow.

The rate-limiting factors in absorption from the injection site are:

- diffusion through the tissue
- removal by local blood flow.

Absorption from a site of injection is increased either by hyaluronidase (an enzyme that breaks down intercellular matrix thereby increasing diffusion) or by increasing local blood flow. Conversely, absorption is reduced in patients with circulatory failure ('shock').

Methods for delaying absorption

It may be desirable to delay absorption, either to reduce the systemic actions of drugs that are being used to produce a local effect, or to prolong systemic action. Thus, addition of **adrenaline** or **noradrenaline** to a solution of local anaesthetic reduces absorption of the local anaesthetic into the general circulation. This usefully prolongs the anaesthetic effect, as well as reducing systemic toxicity.

Another method of delaying absorption from intramuscular or subcutaneous sites is to use a relatively insoluble 'slow-release' form, for example a poorly soluble salt, ester or complex, injected either as an aqueous suspension or an oily solution. **Procaine penicillin** (Ch. 43) is a poorly soluble salt of penicillin; when injected as an aqueous suspension it is slowly absorbed and exerts a prolonged action. Esterification of steroid hormones (e.g. **medroxyprogesterone acetate**, **testosterone propionate**; see Ch. 26) and antipsychotic drugs (e.g. **fluphenazine decanoate**; Ch. 34) increases their solubility in oil and slows their rate of absorption when they are injected in an oily solution.

The physical characteristics of a preparation may also be changed so as to influence its rate of absorption. Examples of this are the **insulin zinc suspensions** (see

Ch. 22); insulin forms a complex with zinc, the physical form of which can be altered by varying the pH. One form consists of a fine amorphous suspension which is relatively rapidly absorbed, and another consists of a suspension of large crystals which are slowly absorbed. These two preparations can be mixed to produce an immediate, but sustained, effect.

Another method used to achieve slow and continuous absorption of certain steroid hormones (e.g. **oestradiol**; Ch. 26) is the subcutaneous implantation of solid pellets. The rate of absorption is proportional to the surface area of the implant.

Intrathecal injection

Injection of a drug into the subarachnoid space via a lumbar puncture needle is used for some specialised purposes. **Methotrexate** (Ch. 42) is administered in this way in the treatment of certain childhood leukaemias to prevent relapse in the central nervous system. Regional anaesthesia can be produced by injecting a local anaesthetic such as **bupivacaine** (see Ch. 40) intrathecally; **opiate analgesics** can also be used in this way (Ch. 37). **Baclofen** (a GABA analogue, Ch. 36) has been administered by this route to minimise its adverse effects when treating patients with disabling muscle spasm caused by chronic neurological disease. Some antibiotics (e.g. aminoglycosides) cross the blood–brain barrier very slowly, and in rare clinical situations where they are essential (e.g. nervous system infections with bacteria resistant to other antibiotics) can be given intrathecally or directly into the cerebral ventricles via a reservoir.

DISTRIBUTION OF DRUGS IN THE BODY

BODY FLUID COMPARTMENTS

Body water is distributed into four main compartments as shown in Figure 4.9. The total body water as a percentage of body weight varies from 50–70%, being rather less in women than in men.

Extracellular fluid comprises the *blood plasma* (about 4.5% of body weight), *interstitial fluid* (16%) and *lymph* (1.2%). *Intracellular fluid* (30–40%) is the sum of the fluid contents of all cells in the body. *Transcellular fluid* (2.5%) includes the cerebrospinal, intraocular, peritoneal, pleural and synovial fluids and digestive secretions. The foetus may also be regarded as a special type of transcellular compartment. To enter the transcellular compartments from the extracellular compartment a drug must cross a cellular barrier, a particularly important example in the context of pharmacokinetics being the *blood–brain barrier*.

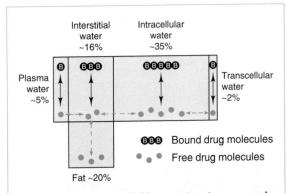

Fig. 4.9 The main body fluid compartments, expressed as a percentage of body weight. Drug molecules exist in bound or free form in each compartment, but only the free drug is able to move between the compartments.

The blood–brain barrier

The concept of the blood–brain barrier was introduced by Paul Ehrlich to explain his observation that intravenously injected dye stained most tissues yet the brain remained unstained. The barrier consists of a continuous layer of endothelial cells joined by tight junctions. The brain is consequently inaccessible to many systemically acting drugs, including many anticancer drugs and some antibiotics such as the aminoglycosides, whose lipid solubility is insufficient to allow penetration of the blood–brain barrier. However, inflammation, in the form of meningitis, can disrupt the integrity of the blood–brain barrier, allowing normally impermeant substances to enter the brain (Fig. 4.10), a fact that allows **penicillin** (Ch. 43) to be given systemically in the treatment of bacterial meningitis. Furthermore, in some parts of the central nervous system, including the chemoreceptor trigger zone, the barrier is leaky. This enables **domperidone**, a dopamine receptor antagonist (Ch. 34), to be used to prevent the nausea caused by dopamine agonists such as **apomorphine,** when these are used to treat advanced Parkinson's disease, without causing loss of efficacy by competition with dopamine receptors in the basal ganglia that are only accessible to drugs that have traversed the blood–brain barrier. Several peptides, including bradykinin and enkephalins, increase blood–brain barrier permeability by increasing pinocytosis, and there is interest in using this approach as a means of improving access of chemotherapy during treatment of brain tumours and other neurological disorders. In addition, extreme stress renders the blood–brain barrier permeable to drugs such as **pyridostigmine** (Ch. 7) that normally

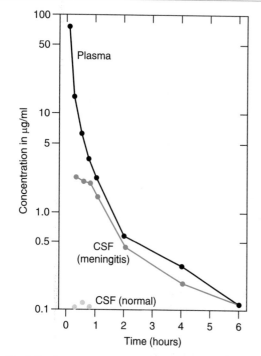

Fig. 4.10 Plasma and CSF concentrations of an antibiotic (thienamycin) following an intravenous dose (25 mg/kg). In normal rabbits, no drug reaches the CSF, but in animals with experimental *Escherichia coli* meningitis, the concentration of drug in CSF approaches that in the plasma. (From: Patamasucon & McCracken 1973 Antimicrob Agents Chemother 3: 270)

Volume of distribution

The apparent volume of distribution, V_d, is defined as the volume of fluid required to contain the total amount, Q, of drug in the body at the same concentration as that present in the plasma, C_p.

$$V_d = \frac{Q}{C_p} \qquad (4.1)$$

Values of V_d* have been measured for many drugs (Table 4.1). Some general patterns can be distinguished, but it is important to avoid identifying a given range of V_d too closely with a particular anatomical compartment. For example, insulin has a measured V_d similar to the volume of plasma water but exerts its effects on muscle, fat and liver via receptors that are exposed to interstitial fluid but not to plasma (Ch. 22).

Drugs confined to the plasma compartment

The plasma volume is about 0.05 l/kg body weight. A few drugs, such as **heparin** (Ch. 17), are confined to the plasma compartment because the molecule is too large to cross the capillary wall easily. More often, retention of a drug in the plasma following a single dose reflects strong binding to plasma protein. It is, nevertheless, the free drug in the interstitial fluid that exerts a pharmacological effect. Following repeated dosing, equilibration occurs and measured V_d increases. Some dyes, such as Evans blue, bind so strongly to plasma albumin that its distribution volume is used experimentally to measure plasma volume.

Drugs distributed in the extracellular compartment

The total extracellular volume is about 0.2 l/kg, and this is the approximate distribution volume for many polar compounds, such as **vecuronium** (Ch. 7), **gentamicin** and **carbenicillin** (Ch. 43). These drugs cannot easily enter cells because of their low lipid solubility, and do not normally cross the blood–brain or placental barriers.

Distribution throughout the body water

Total body water represents about 0.55 l/kg, and this distribution volume is achieved by relatively lipid-soluble

only act peripherally, a finding that has been invoked to explain the central symptoms of cholinesterase inhibition experienced by some soldiers during the Gulf War, who may have been exposed to low concentrations of cholinesterase inhibitors used as chemical weapons in the context of the stress of warfare.

Within each of these aqueous compartments, drug molecules usually exist both in free solution and in bound form; furthermore, drugs that are weak acids or bases will exist as an equilibrium mixture of the charged and uncharged forms, the position of the equilibrium depending on the pH (see p. 62).

The equilibrium pattern of distribution between the various compartments will thus depend on:

- permeability across tissue barriers
- binding within compartments
- pH partition
- fat : water partition.

*The experimental measurement of V_d is complicated by the fact that the amount of drug present in the body, Q, does not stay constant (because of metabolism and excretion of the drug) during the time that it takes for it to be distributed among the various body compartments that contribute to the overall V_d. It therefore has to be calculated indirectly from a series of measurements of plasma concentrations as a function of time. On the basis of a two-compartment model (see p. 90), the distribution volume of each compartment can be calculated, but the validity of such estimates necessarily depends on the validity of the kinetic model used.

Table 4.1 Distribution volumes for some drugs compared with volume of body fluid compartments

Volume (l/kg body weight)	Compartment	V_d (l/kg body weight)	
0.05	Plasma	0.05–0.1	Heparin Insulin
		0.1–0.2	Warfarin Sulphamethoxazole Glibenclamide Atenolol
0.2	Extracellular fluid	0.2–0.4 0.4–0.7	Tubocurarine Theophylline
0.55	Total body water		Ethanol Neostigmine Phenytoin
		1–2	Methotrexate Indomethacin Paracetamol Diazepam Lignocaine
		2–5	Glyceryl trinitrate Morphine Propranolol Digoxin Chlorpromazine
		> 10	Nortriptyline Imipramine

drugs that readily cross cell membranes, such as **phenytoin** (Ch. 36) and **ethanol** (Ch. 39). Binding of the drug anywhere outside the plasma compartment, as well as partitioning into body fat, can increase V_d beyond the absolute value for total body water. Thus there are many drugs with V_d greater than the total body volume such as **morphine** (Ch. 37), **tricyclic antidepressants** (Ch. 33) and **haloperidol** (Ch. 34). Such drugs are *not* efficiently removed from the body by haemodialysis, which is therefore unhelpful in managing overdose with such agents.

SPECIAL DRUG DELIVERY SYSTEMS

Several approaches are being explored in an attempt to improve drug delivery. They include:

- biologically erodable microspheres
- pro-drugs
- antibody–drug conjugates
- packaging in liposomes.

Drug distribution

- The major compartments are:
  —plasma (5% of body weight)
  —interstitial fluid (16%)
  —intracellular fluid (35%)
  —transcellular fluid (2%)
  —fat (20%).
- Volume of distribution (V_d) is defined as the volume of plasma that would contain the total body content of the drug at a concentration equal to that in the plasma.
- Lipid-insoluble drugs are mainly confined to plasma and interstitial fluids; most do not enter the brain following acute dosing.
- Lipid-soluble drugs reach all compartments, and may accumulate in fat.
- For drugs that accumulate outside the plasma compartment (e.g. in fat, or by being bound to tissues) V_d may exceed total body volume.

Biologically erodable microspheres. Microspheres of biologically erodable polymers can be engineered to adhere to mucosal epithelium in the gut. Such microspheres can be loaded with drugs, including high molecular weight substances, as a means of improving absorption, which occurs both through mucosal absorptive epithelium and also through epithelium overlying Peyer's patches. This approach has yet to be used clinically, but microspheres made from polyanhydride co-polymers of fumaric and sebacic acids by a technique known as phase inversion nanoencapsulation have been used to produce systemic absorption of **insulin** and of plasmid DNA following oral administration in rats. Since drug delivery is a critical problem in gene therapy (Ch. 51), this is potentially momentous!

Pro-drugs. Pro-drugs are inactive precursors which are metabolised to active metabolites, and are described in Chapter 5 on drug metabolism. Some of the examples in clinical use confer no obvious benefits, and have been found to be pro-drugs only retrospectively, not having been designed with this in mind. However, some do have advantages. For example, the cytotoxic drug **cyclophosphamide** (see Ch. 42) becomes active only after it has been metabolised in the liver, and can therefore be taken orally without causing serious damage to the gastrointestinal epithelium. **Levodopa** is absorbed from the gastrointestinal tract and crosses the blood–brain barrier via an amino acid transport mechanism before conversion to active dopamine in nerve terminals in the basal ganglia (Ch. 28). **Zidovudine** is phosphorylated to its active trisphosphate metabolite only in cells containing appropriate reverse transcriptase, hence conferring selective toxicity toward cells infected with the human immunodeficiency virus (Ch. 44). **Valaciclovir** and **famciclovir** are each ester pro-drugs *of* pro-drugs: respectively, of **aciclovir** and of **penciclovir**. Their bioavailability is greater than that of aciclovir and penciclovir, each of which is converted into active metabolites

in virally infected cells (Ch. 44). Other problems could theoretically be overcome by the use of suitable pro-drugs; for example instability of drugs at gastric pH, direct gastric irritation (**aspirin** was synthesised in the last century in a deliberate attempt to produce a pro-drug for salicylic acid that would be tolerable when taken by mouth), failure of drug to cross the blood–brain barrier and so on. Progress with this approach remains slow, however, and Albert (1965) warns the optimistic pro-drug designer: 'he will have to bear in mind that an organism's normal reaction to a foreign substance is to burn it up for food.'

Antibody–drug conjugates. One of the aims of cancer chemotherapy is to improve the selectivity of cytotoxic drugs (see Ch. 42). One interesting possibility is to attach the drug to an antibody directed against a tumour-specific antigen, which will bind selectively to tumour cells. Such approaches look promising in experimental animals, but it is still too early to say whether they will succeed in man.

Packaging in liposomes. Liposomes are minute vesicles produced by sonication of an aqueous suspension of certain phospholipids. They can be filled with non-lipid-soluble drugs or nucleic acid sequences (Ch. 51), which are retained until the liposome is disrupted. Liposomes are mainly taken up by reticuloendothelial cells, especially in the liver. They are also concentrated in malignant tumours and there is a possibility of achieving selective delivery of drugs in this way. **Amphotericin**, an antifungal drug used to treat systemic mycoses (Ch. 45), is available in a liposomal formulation that is less nephrotoxic and better tolerated than the conventional form, albeit considerably more expensive. In the future, it may also be possible to direct drugs or genes selectively by incorporating antibody molecules against specific tissue antigens into the surface of such particles.

REFERENCES AND FURTHER READING

Abbott N J, Romero I A 1996 Transporting therapeutics across the blood–brain barrier. Mol Med Today 2: 106–113 (*Strategies for overcoming/bypassing the blood–brain barrier*)

Audus K L, Chikhale P J, Miller D W, Thompson S E, Borchadt R T 1992 Brain uptake of drugs: chemical and biological factors. Adv Drug Res 23: 1–64 (*Highlights chemical and biological factors regulating permeability of the blood–brain barrier to drugs as a basis for drug delivery to the CNS*)

Brogden R N, McTavish D 1995 Nifedipine gastrointestinal therapeutic system (GITS). A review of its pharmacodynamic and pharmacokinetic properties and therapeutic efficacy in hypertension and angina pectoris. Drugs 50: 495–512 (*Novel formulation permitting once daily dosing and reduced*

adverse effects)

Chonn A, Cullis P R 1995 Recent advances in liposomal drug-delivery systems. Curr Opin Biotechnol 6: 698–708 (*Discusses delivery of recombinant proteins, antisense oligonucleotides and cloned genes*)

Fix J A 1996 Strategies for delivery of peptides utilizing absorption-enhancing agents. J Pharm Sci 85: 1282–1285 (*Brief review emphasising unresolved difficulties*)

Friedman A, Kaufer D, Shemer J, Hendler I, Soreq H, Tur-Kaspa I 1996 Pyridostigmine brain penetration under stress enhances neuronal excitability and induces early immediate transcriptional response. Nature Med 2: 1382–1385 (*Peripherally acting drugs administered during severe stress may unexpectedly penetrate the blood–brain barrier. See also* accompanying comment on 'The Gulf War, stress and a leaky blood brain barrier' by I Hanin, pp 1307–1308)

Keppler D, Arias I M 1996 Hepatic canalicular membrane. Introduction: transport across the hepatocyte cannalicular membrane FASEB J 11: 15–18 (Succinct review)

Koch-Weser J, Sellers E M 1976 Binding of drugs to serum albumin (2 parts). N Engl J Med 294: 311–316, 526–531 (Definitive)

Kremer J M H, Wilting J, Janssen L M H 1988 Drug binding to human α-1-acid glycoprotein in health and disease. Pharmacol Rev 40: 1–47

Langer R 1995 1994 Whittacker lecture: polymers for drug delivery and tissue engineering. Ann Biomed Eng 23: 101–111

Leveque D, Jehl F 1995 P-glycoprotein and pharmacokinetics. Anticancer Res 15: 331–336 (Update on impact of P-glycoprotein on drug disposition)

Mathiovitz E, Jacob J S, Jong Y S et al. 1997 Biologically erodable microspheres as potential oral drug delivery systems. Nature 386: 410–414 (Oral delivery of three model substances of different molecular size: dicoumarol, insulin and plasmid DNA)

Oliyai R, Stella V J 1993 Prodrugs of peptides and proteins for improved formulation and delivery. Ann Rev Pharmacol Toxicol 33: 521–544 (Review of pro-drug strategy for peptide absorption/delivery)

Partridge W M, Golden P L, Kang Y S, Bickel U 1997 Brain microvascular and astrocyte localization of P-glycoprotein. J Neurochem 68: 1278–1285 (Immunoreactive P-glycoprotein in brain microvasculature is localised to astrocyte foot processes and the role of P-glycoprotein in the blood–brain barrier)

Sayani A P, Chien Y W 1996 Systemic delivery of peptides and proteins across absorptive mucosae. Crit Rev Ther Drug Carrier Syst 13: 85–184 (Discusses insulin, enkephalin and calcitonin in particular)

Somogyi A 1996 Renal transport of drugs: specificity and molecular mechanisms. Clin Exp Pharmacol Physiol 23: 986–989 (Short review of selective organic anion and cation transporters in the proximal tubule)

Drug elimination and pharmacokinetics

Drug elimination is the irreversible loss of drug from the body, and occurs by two processes, metabolism and excretion. Excretion involves the loss of chemically unchanged drug, metabolism the conversion of one chemical entity to another. The main routes by which drugs and their metabolites leave the body are:

- the kidneys
- the hepatobiliary system
- the lungs (important for volatile/gaseous anaesthetics)

Most drugs leave the body in the urine, either unchanged or as polar metabolites. Some drugs are secreted into bile via the liver, but most are then reabsorbed from the intestine. There are, however, instances (e.g. **rifampicin**) where faecal loss accounts for the elimination of a substantial fraction of unchanged drug in healthy individuals, and faecal elimination of drugs such as **digoxin** that are normally excreted in urine becomes progressively more important in patients with advancing renal failure. Excretion via the lungs occurs only with highly volatile or gaseous agents (e.g. general anaesthetics). Drugs are also excreted in secretions such as milk or sweat. Elimination by these routes is quantitatively negligible compared with renal excretion, although excretion into milk can sometimes be important because of effects on the baby.

Lipophilic substances are not eliminated efficiently by the kidney (see below). Consequently, most lipophilic drugs are metabolised to more polar products which are then excreted in urine. Drug metabolism occurs predominantly in the liver, mainly by the *cytochrome P450* system. Some P450 enzymes are extrahepatic, and play an important part in several synthetic pathways including steroid biosynthesis in the adrenal gland and the biosynthesis of prostacyclin and thromboxanes (Ch. 12), but here we shall be concerned with catabolism of drugs by the hepatic cytochrome P450 system. In the first part of this chapter we consider this and other pathways of drug metabolism, and factors that influence renal elimination; in the second part we present a simple pharmacokinetic model that describes how absorption, distribution, metabolism and excretion determine the variation of drug concentration with time during dosing by various regimens.

DRUG METABOLISM

Animals have evolved complex systems that detoxify foreign chemicals, including carcinogens and toxins present in poisonous plants. Drugs, many of which were discovered by modifying the structure of plant alkaloids, are a special case of such foreign chemicals and, like alkaloids, they often exhibit distinct chirality (i.e. there is more than one stereoisomer). Drug metabolism involves two kinds of biochemical reaction known as *phase I* and *phase II* reactions. These often, though not invariably, occur sequentially.

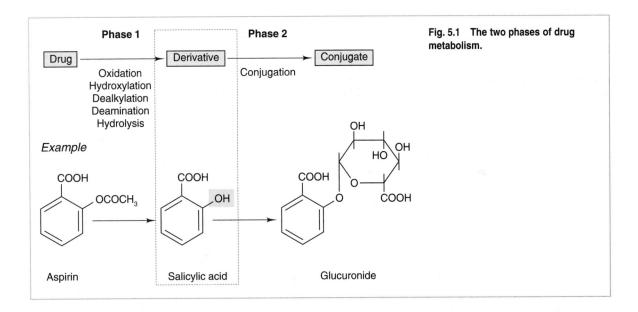

Fig. 5.1 The two phases of drug metabolism.

Phase I reactions consist of oxidation, reduction or hydrolysis, and the products are often more chemically reactive and hence, paradoxically, sometimes more toxic or carcinogenic than the parent drug. Phase II reactions involve conjugation, which normally results in inactive compounds (although there are exceptions, for example the active sulphate metabolite of **minoxidil**, a potassium channel activator used to treat severe hypertension; Ch. 15). Phase I reactions often introduce a relatively reactive group, such as hydroxyl, into the molecule (functionalisation). This functional group then serves as the point of attack for the conjugating system to attach a substituent such as glucunonide (Fig. 5.1). Both stages usually decrease lipid solubility, thus increasing renal elimination.

Phase I and phase II reactions take place mainly in the liver, though some drugs are metabolised in plasma (e.g. hydrolysis of **suxamethonium** by plasma cholinesterase; see Ch. 7), lung (e.g. various **prostanoids**; see Ch. 12), or gut (e.g. **tyramine**, **salbutamol**; Ch. 8). Many hepatic drug-metabolising enzymes, including cytochrome P450, are embedded in the smooth endoplasmic reticulum. They are often called 'microsomal' enzymes because, on homogenisation and differential centrifugation, the endoplasmic reticulum is broken into very small fragments that sediment only after prolonged high-speed centrifugation in the 'microsomal' fraction. To reach these metabolising enzymes in life, a drug must cross the hepatocyte plasma membrane. Polar molecules do this more slowly than non-polar molecules except where specific transport mechanisms exist, so hepatic metabolism is in general less important for polar drugs than for lipid-soluble drugs, and a greater proportion is excreted unchanged in the urine.

Stereoselectivity. Many clinically important drugs, such as **sotalol** (Ch. 14), **warfarin** (Ch. 17) and **cyclophosphamide** (Ch. 42), are mixtures of stereoisomers, the components of which differ not only in their pharmacodynamic activity but also in their metabolism, which may follow completely distinct pathways. Several clinically important drug interactions involve stereospecific inhibition of metabolism of one drug by another (Ch. 48). In some cases, drug toxicity appears to be due mainly to one of the stereoisomers, not necessarily the pharmacologically active one. Where practicable, regulatory authorities now urge that new drugs should consist of pure stereoisomers to avoid these complications.

PHASE I REACTIONS

THE P450 MONO-OXYGENASE SYSTEM

Nature and classification of P450 enzymes

Cytochrome P450 enzymes are haem proteins. They have unique redox properties that are fundamental to their diverse functions. These relate to the variable spin state (high/low) of the haem iron, which lies in an octahedral complex with six ligands and within which it can adopt either a penta- or hexa-coordinate configuration. P450 enzymes also have unique spectral properties and the reduced forms combine with carbon monoxide to form a pink compound (hence 'P') with absorption peaks near 450 nm (range 447–452 nm). The first evidence that there is more than one form of cytochrome P450 came from the observation that treatment of rats with 3-methyl-cholanthrene, an inducing agent (see below), caused a shift in the absorption maximum from 450 to 448 nm. It is now known that the hepatic cytochrome P450 system comprises a large family ('superfamily') of related but distinct enzymes, which differ from one another in amino acid sequence, in regulation by inhibitors and inducing agents, and in the specificity of the reactions that they catalyse. Different members of the family have distinct, but often overlapping, substrate specificities, with some enzymes acting on the same substrates as each other but at different rates. Purification of P450 enzymes and cDNA cloning form the basis of the current classification system, which is based on amino acid sequence similarities. 74 *CYP* gene families have so far been described, of which three main ones (*CYP1, 2* and *3*) are involved in drug metabolism in human liver. Some of the main enzymes are: CYP1A2, CYP2A6, CYP2C9, CYP2C19, CYP2D6, CYP2E1 and CYP3A4. Examples of therapeutic drugs that are substrates for these enzymes are shown in Table 5.1.

Table 5.1 Common therapeutic drugs that are substrates for P450 enzymes

P450	Drug
CYP1A1	Theophylline
CYP1A2	Caffeine, ondansetron, paracetamol, tacrine, theophylline
CYP2A6	Methoxyflurane
CYP2C8	Taxol
CYP2C9	Ibuprofen, mefenamic acid, phenytoin, tolbutamide, warfarin
CYP2C19	Omeprazole
CYP2D6	Clozapine, codeine, debrisoquine, metoprolol, tricyclic antidepressants
CYP2E1	Alcohol, enflurane, halothane
CYP3A4/5	Cyclosporin, erythromycin, ethinyloestradiol, losartan, lignocaine, midazolam, nifedipine, terfenadine

From: Pichard et al. (1995) Predictability of drug metabolism from in vitro studies. In: Alvan G et al. (eds) COST B1 conference on variability and specificity in drug metabolism. European Commission, Luxembourg, pp 45–56.

Mechanism of drug oxidation by P450

Drug oxidation by the mono-oxygenase system requires molecular oxygen, NADPH and a flavoprotein (NADPH-P450 reductase), in addition to drug substrate (DH) and P450 enzyme. The overall net effect of the reaction is the addition of one atom of oxygen (from molecular oxygen) to the drug to form a hydroxyl group (DOH), the other atom of oxygen being converted to water. The apparent simplicity of this overall reaction is deceptive, since the mechanism involves a complex catalytic cycle in which NADPH-P450 reductase supplies one or both electrons needed for the oxidation and restores the redox state of the P450. The cycle is illustrated in Figure 5.2 and involves cyclic oxidation/reduction of haem iron in conjunction with substrate binding and oxygen activation. The ferric iron in free P450 is mainly in a low spin form. After binding DH, a conformational change converts the ferric (Fe^{3+}) iron to the high spin state, making it easier to reduce. Reduction from Fe^{3+} to Fe^{2+} is achieved by a single electron which is relayed from NADPH (electron donor) to P450 via the flavoprotein NADPH-P450 reductase. Molecular oxygen binds the reduced $Fe^{2+} \cdot DH$ complex to form a $Fe^{2+}O \cdot DH$ complex. This then accepts a second electron from NADPH-P450 reductase (or alternatively from cytochrome b_5) and a proton, to yield a peroxide complex: $Fe^{2+}OOH \cdot DH$. Addition of a second proton cleaves the $Fe^{2+}OOH \cdot DH$ complex to yield water and a ferric oxene $(FeO)^{3+}$ drug complex: $(FeO)^{3+} \cdot DH$. $(FeO)^{3+}$ extracts a hydrogen atom from DH to form a pair of transient free radicals $D^{\bullet}$ and $Fe^{3+}OH^{\bullet}$. $D^{\bullet}$ acquires the bound $OH^{\bullet}$ radical to form hydroxylated drug (DOH) which is released from the complex with regeneration of P450 in its initial state.

P450 and biological variation

There are important variations in the expression and regulation of P450 enzymes between species. For instance, the activation pathways of certain dietary heterocyclic amines (formed when meat is cooked) to genotoxic products involves one member of the P450 superfamily (CYP1A2) which is constitutively present in humans and rats (which develop colon tumours after treatment with such amines), but not in cynomolgus monkeys (which do not). Such species differences have crucial implications for the choice of species to be used for toxicity and carcinogenicity testing during the development of new drugs for use in man.

Within human populations there are major sources of inter-individual variation in P450 enzymes that are of great importance in therapeutics. These include genetic

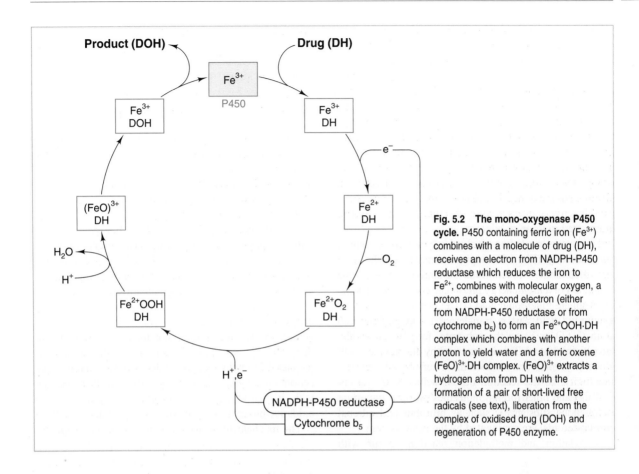

Fig. 5.2 The mono-oxygenase P450 cycle. P450 containing ferric iron (Fe^{3+}) combines with a molecule of drug (DH), receives an electron from NADPH-P450 reductase which reduces the iron to Fe^{2+}, combines with molecular oxygen, a proton and a second electron (either from NADPH-P450 reductase or from cytochrome b_5) to form an $Fe^{2+}OOH \cdot DH$ complex which combines with another proton to yield water and a ferric oxene $(FeO)^{3+} \cdot DH$ complex. $(FeO)^{3+}$ extracts a hydrogen atom from DH with the formation of a pair of short-lived free radicals (see text), liberation from the complex of oxidised drug (DOH) and regeneration of P450 enzyme.

polymorphisms: for example, one variant (*CYP2D6*) leads to poor and extensive hydroxylation of **debrisoquine**. Environmental factors (Ch. 48) are also important. Enzyme inhibitors and inducers are present in the diet and environment (e.g. grapefruit juice inhibits metabolism of **terfenadine**—see p. 84—whereas Brussels sprouts and cigarette smoke induce P450 enzymes).

Inhibition of P450

Inhibitors of P450 differ in their selectivity toward different isoforms of the enzyme, and are classified by their mechanism of action. Some drugs compete for the active site, but are not themselves substrates (e.g. **quinidine** is a potent competitive inhibitor of CYP2D6 but is not a substrate for it). Non-competitive inhibitors include drugs such as **ketoconazole** which forms a tight complex with the Fe^{3+} form of the haem iron of CYP3A4 causing reversible non-competitive inhibition. So-called mechanism-based inhibitors require oxidation by a P450 enzyme. Examples include **gestodene** (CYP3A4), **diethylcarbamate** (CYP2E1) and **furafylline** (CYP1A2). An oxidation product (e.g. a postulated epoxide intermediate of gestodene) binds covalently to the enzyme which then destroys itself ('suicide inhibition'). Many clinically important interactions between drugs are due to inhibition or induction of P450 enzymes (see Ch. 48).

OTHER PHASE I REACTIONS

Not all drug oxidation reactions exclusively involve the P450 system. For example, **ethanol** is metabolised by a soluble cytoplasmic enzyme, alcohol dehydrogenase in addition to CYP2E1. Other exceptions include xanthine oxidase, which inactivates **6-mercaptopurine** (Ch. 42), and monoamine oxidase which inactivates many biologically active amines (e.g. **noradrenaline**, **tyramine**, **5-HT**; see Chs 8 and 35).

Reductive reactions are much less common than oxidations, but some are important. For example **warfarin** (Ch. 17) is inactivated by conversion of a ketone to a hydroxyl group by CYP2A6.

Hydrolytic reactions do not involve hepatic microsomal enzymes, but occur in plasma and in many tissues. Both ester and amide bonds are susceptible to hydrolysis, the former more readily than the latter.

PHASE II REACTIONS

If a drug molecule has a suitable 'handle' (e.g. a hydroxyl, thiol or amino group), either in the parent molecule or in a product resulting from phase I metabolism, it is susceptible to conjugation, i.e. attachment of a substituent group. This synthetic step is called a phase II reaction. The resulting conjugate is almost always pharmacologically inactive and less lipid soluble than its precursor and is excreted in urine or bile.

The groups most often involved in conjugate formation are glucuronyl (Fig. 5.3), sulphate, methyl, acetyl, glycyl and glutathione. Glucuronide formation involves the formation of a high-energy phosphate compound, uridine diphosphate glucuronic acid (UDPGA), from which the glucuronic acid part is transferred to an electron-rich atom (N, O or S) on the substrate, forming an amide, ester or thiol bond. This is catalysed by an enzyme, UDP glucuronyl transferase, which has a very broad substrate specificity, so the reaction occurs with a wide variety of drugs and other foreign molecules. Several important endogenous substances, such as bilirubin and adrenal corticosteroids, are conjugated by the same system.

Acetylation and methylation reactions occur with acetyl-CoA and S-adenosyl methionine, respectively, acting as the donor compounds. Many of these conjugation reactions occur in the liver, but other tissues, such as lung and kidney, are also involved.

INDUCTION OF MICROSOMAL ENZYMES

A number of drugs such as **rifampicin** (Ch. 43), **ethanol** (Ch. 39), **carbamazepine** (Ch. 36), increase the activity of microsomal oxidase and conjugating systems when administered repeatedly. Many carcinogenic chemicals (e.g. benzpyrene, 3-methylcholanthrene) also have this effect, which can be substantial; Figure 5.4 shows a nearly 10-fold increase in the rate of benzpyrene metabolism 2 days after a single dose. The effect is referred to as induction, and is the result of increased synthesis of microsomal enzymes, rather than a change in the activity of existing enzyme via an allosteric effect.

Enzyme induction can increase as well as decrease drug toxicity. There are drugs, for example **paracetamol**, whose phase I metabolites are mainly responsible for their toxicity (see Chs 13 and 49), so that toxicity is increased following enzyme induction. The carcinogenic action of some polycyclic hydrocarbons is associated with increased hepatic formation of highly reactive oxidative products (e.g. epoxides) that can damage DNA.

The mechanism by which induction occurs is incom-

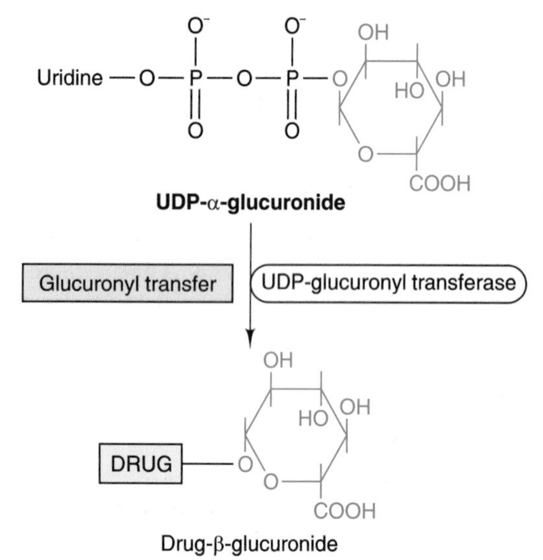

Fig. 5.3   The glucuronide conjugation reaction.

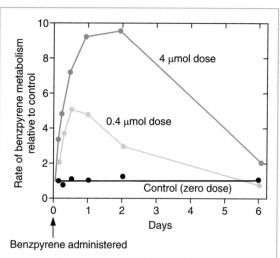

Fig. 5.4   Stimulation of hepatic metabolism of benzpyrene. Young rats were given benzpyrene (i.p.) in the doses shown, and the benzpyrene metabolising activity of liver homogenates measured at times up to 6 days. (From: Conney A H et al. 1957 J Biol Chem 228: 753)

pletely understood but is similar to that involved in the action of steroid and other hormones that bind to nuclear receptors (see Ch. 2). The most thoroughly studied inducing agents are polycyclic aromatic hydrocarbons. These bind to the ligand-binding domain of a soluble protein termed the aromatic hydrocarbon (Ah-) receptor. This complex is transported to the nucleus by an Ah-receptor nuclear translocator and binds Ah-receptor response elements in the DNA, thereby promoting transcription of the *CYP1A1* gene. In addition to enhanced transcription, some inducing agents (e.g. ethanol which induces CYP2E1 in man) also influence mRNA processing and may stabilise mRNA or P450 protein.

FIRST-PASS (PRESYSTEMIC) METABOLISM

The liver (or sometimes the gut wall) extracts and metabolises some drugs so efficiently that the amount reaching the systemic circulation is considerably less than the amount absorbed. This is known as *first-pass* or *presystemic metabolism*, and is important for many clinically important drugs (Table 5.2).

First-pass metabolism is generally a nuisance in practice, because:

- a much larger dose of the drug is needed when it is given orally than when it is given by other routes
- marked individual variations occur in the extent of first-pass metabolism of a given drug (see Ch. 48),

Table 5.2   Drugs undergoing substantial presystemic elimination

Aspirin	Lignocaine
Chlormethiazole	Metoprolol
Chlorpromazine	Morphine
Dextropropoxyphene	Nortriptyline
Glyceryl trinitrate	Pethidine
Imipramine	Propranolol
Isosorbide dinitrate	Salbutamol
Levodopa	Verapamil

resulting in unpredictability when such drugs are taken orally.

PHARMACOLOGICALLY ACTIVE DRUG METABOLITES

In some cases (see Table 5.3) a drug becomes pharmacologically active only after it has been metabolised. Thus **azathioprine**, an immunosuppressant drug (Ch. 13), is metabolised to **mercaptopurine**, and **enalapril**, an angiotensin-converting enzyme inhibitor (Ch. 15), is hydrolysed to its active form **enalaprilat**. Such drugs, in which the parent compound lacks activity of its own, are known as *pro-drugs*. These are sometimes designed deliberately to overcome problems of drug delivery (Ch. 4). Metabolism can alter the pharmacological actions of a drug qualitatively. **Aspirin** powerfully inhibits some

Table 5.3   Some drugs that produce active or toxic metabolites

Inactive (pro-drugs)	Active	Toxic
Heroin } Codeine }	→ Morphine	
Propranolol	→ 4-hydroxypropranolol	
Paracetamol		→ N-acetyl-p-benzo-quinone imine
Imipramine	→ Desmethylimipramine	
Amitriptyline	→ Nortriptyline	
Diazepam	→ Nordiazepam ────→ Oxazepam	
Cortisone	→ Hydrocortisone	
Prednisone	→ Prednisolone	
Cyclophosphamide	→ Phosphoramide mustard	
Chloral hydrate	→ Trichloroethanol	
Azathioprine	→ Mercaptopurine	
	Halothane	→ Trifluoroacetic acid
	Sulphonamides	→ Acetylated derivatives
	Methoxyflurane	→ Fluoride
Enalapril	→ Enalaprilat	
Zidovudine	→ Zidovudine triphosphate	

platelet functions and has anti-inflammatory activity (Ch. 13). It is hydrolysed to salicylic acid (Fig. 5.1), which has anti-inflammatory but not antiplatelet activity. **Terfenadine**, a non-sedating antihistamine, can cause serious cardiac arrhythmias. This seldom occurs, because in recommended doses it is largely converted by presystemic hepatic metabolism to an active carboxylic acid metabolite, which blocks H_1-receptors but lacks the effect of terfenadine on cardiac K^+ channels that is believed to cause arrhythmia. Metabolism of terfenadine is inhibited by grapefruit juice and by some antibiotics and antifungal drugs (see above), which increase its tendency to cause cardiac arrhythmia (see Ch. 48). The pharmacologically active non-toxic metabolite (**fexofenadine**) has now replaced terfenadine in the US, and is also available in the UK. In other instances, metabolites may have pharmacological actions similar to the parent compound (e.g. **benzodiazepines**, many of which form long-lived active metabolites that cause their effects to persist after the parent drug has disappeared). There are also cases in which metabolites are responsible for certain toxic effects. Hepatotoxicity of **paracetamol** is an example (see Ch. 49), as well as the bladder toxicity of **cyclophosphamide** which is caused by its toxic metabolite acrolein. Methanol and ethylene glycol both exert their toxic effects via metabolites formed by alcohol dehydrogenase. Poisoning with these agents is treated with ethanol (or with a more potent inhibitor), which competes for the active site of the enzyme. Hepatic necrosis is a rare but sometimes fatal complication of **halothane** anaesthesia. It is caused by immune sensitisation to new antigens formed by trifluoroacetylation of liver protein (Ch. 49). **Disulfiram** inhibits CYP2E1, and has recently been found to reduce substantially the formation of trifluoroacetic acid during halothane anaesthesia. This has raised the intriguing possibility that it could provide prophylaxis against halothane hepatitis.

RENAL EXCRETION OF DRUGS AND DRUG METABOLITES

Drugs differ greatly in the rate at which they are excreted by the kidney, ranging from **penicillin** (Ch. 43), which is cleared from the blood almost completely on a single transit through the kidney, to **diazepam** (Ch. 33), which is cleared extremely slowly. Most drugs fall somewhere in between, and the products of phase I and phase II metabolism are nearly always cleared more quickly than the parent compound. There are three basic processes that account for these wide differences in renal excretion:

- glomerular filtration
- active tubular secretion or reabsorption
- passive diffusion across tubular epithelium.

GLOMERULAR FILTRATION

Glomerular capillaries allow drug molecules of molecular weight below about 20 000 to diffuse into the glomerular filtrate. Plasma albumin (MW 68 000) is almost completely held back, but drugs—with the exception of macromolecular substances such as **heparin** (Ch. 17)—cross the barrier freely. If a drug binds appreciably to plasma albumin its concentration in the filtrate will be less than the total plasma concentration. If, like **warfarin** (Ch. 17), a drug is approximately 98% bound to albumin, the concentration in the filtrate is only 2% of that in plasma and clearance by filtration is correspondingly reduced.

TUBULAR SECRETION AND REABSORPTION

Up to 20% of renal plasma flow is filtered through the glomerulus, leaving at least 80% of delivered drug to pass on to the peritubular capillaries of the proximal tubule. Here drug molecules are transferred to the tubular lumen by two independent and relatively non-selective carrier systems. One of these transports acidic drugs (as well as various endogenous acids, such as uric acid), while the other handles organic bases. Some of the more important drugs that are transported by these two carrier systems are shown in Table 5.4. The carriers can transport drug molecules against an electrochemical gradient, and can, therefore, reduce the plasma concentration nearly to zero. Since at least 80% of the drug delivered to the kidney is presented to the carrier, tubular secretion is

---

Drug metabolism

- Phase I reactions: oxidation, reduction and hydrolysis:
  — usually form more chemically reactive products, sometimes pharmacologically active, toxic or carcinogenic
  — often involve mono-oxygenase system in which cytochrome P450 plays a key role.
- Phase II reactions: conjugation (e.g. glucuronidation) of a reactive group (often inserted during phase I reaction) usually forms inactive and readily excretable products.
- Induction of enzymes by other drugs and chemicals can greatly accelerate hepatic drug metabolism.
- Some drugs show rapid 'first-pass' hepatic metabolism, and thus poor oral bioavailability.

potentially the most effective mechanism for drug elimination by the kidney. Unlike glomerular filtration, carrier-mediated transport can achieve maximal drug clearance even when most of the drug is bound to plasma protein.* **Penicillin** (Ch. 43), for example, though about 80% protein bound and therefore cleared only slowly by filtration, is almost completely removed by proximal tubular secretion, and its overall rate of elimination is very high.

Many of the drugs that are excreted by the kidney share the same transport system (Table 5.4), and competition can occur between them leading to drug interactions. **Probenecid**, which was developed for the purpose of prolonging the action of penicillin by retarding its excretion, is an example.

Table 5.4 Some drugs and related substances that are actively secreted into the proximal renal tubule

Acids	Bases
Acetazolamide	Amiloride
p-aminohippuric acid	Dopamine
Aminosalicylic acid	Histamine
Cephaloridine	Mepacrine
Frusemide	Morphine
Glucuronic acid conjugates	Pethidine
Glycine conjugates	Quaternary ammonium
5-hydroxyindole acetic acid	compounds
Indomethacin	Quinine
Methotrexate	Serotonin
Penicillins	Tolazoline
Probenecid	Triamterene
Renal radiocontrast media	
Salicylic acid	
Sulphate conjugates	
Sulphinpyrazone	
Thiazide diuretics	
Uric acid	

*Because filtration involves isosmotic movement of both water and solutes, it will not affect the free concentration of drug in the plasma. Thus the equilibrium between free and bound drug will not be disturbed, and there will be no tendency for the bound drug to dissociate as the blood traverses the glomerular capillary. The rate of clearance of the drug by filtration is therefore reduced directly in proportion to the fraction that is bound. In the case of active tubular secretion, this is not so; secretion may be retarded very little even though the drug is mostly bound. This is because the carrier transports drug molecules unaccompanied by water. As free drug molecules are taken from the plasma, therefore, the free plasma concentration tends to fall. This causes a net dissociation of bound drug from the protein, so that effectively all of the drug, bound and free, is available to the carrier.

DIFFUSION ACROSS THE RENAL TUBULE

As glomerular filtrate traverses the tubule, water is reabsorbed, the volume of urine emerging being only about 1% of that of the filtrate. If the tubule is freely permeable to drug molecules, the drug concentration in the filtrate will remain close to that in the plasma, and some 99% of the filtered drug will be reabsorbed passively. Drugs with high lipid solubility, and hence high tubular permeability, are therefore excreted slowly. If the drug is highly polar, and therefore of low tubular permeability, filtered drug remains in the tubule, and its concentration rises until it is about 100 times as high in the urine as in the plasma. Drugs handled in this way include **digoxin**, and aminoglycoside antibiotics. Many drugs, being weak acids or weak bases, change their ionisation with pH (see p. 62), and this can markedly affect renal excretion. The ion-trapping effect means that a basic drug is more rapidly excreted in an acid urine, because the low pH within the tubule favours ionisation and thus inhibits reabsorption. Conversely, acidic drugs are most rapidly excreted if the urine is alkaline (Fig. 5.5). Urinary alkalinisation is used to accelerate the excretion of **aspirin** in treating selected cases of overdose.

DRUG ELIMINATION EXPRESSED AS CLEARANCE

Renal clearance, CL_r, is defined as the volume of plasma containing the amount of substance that is removed by the kidney in unit time. It is calculated from the plasma concentration, C_p, the urinary concentration, C_u, and the rate of flow of urine, V_u, by the equation:

$$CL_r = \frac{C_u V_u}{C_p} \tag{5.1}$$

CL_r varies greatly for different drugs, from a negligible value (less than 1 ml/min) to the theoretical maximum set by the renal plasma flow (about 700 ml/min). The main determinants, as explained above, are the rate of active tubular secretion and the rate of passive reabsorption. For a small but important group of drugs that are not inactivated by metabolism, the rate of renal elimination is the main factor that determines their duration of action (Table 5.5). These drugs have to be used with special care in individuals whose renal function may be impaired, including the elderly and patients with renal disease or any severe acute illness.

The clearance concept is also useful in quantifying the rate of metabolic degradation of drugs, since this can be expressed in terms of the volume of plasma containing the amount of drug that is metabolised in unit time.

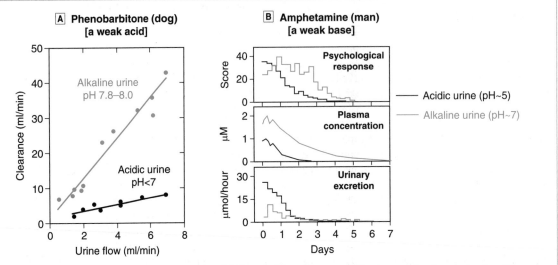

Fig. 5.5   The effect of urinary pH on drug excretion. [A] Phenobarbitone clearance in the dog as a function of urine flow. Because phenobarbitone is acidic, alkalinising the urine increases clearance about fivefold. [B] Amphetamine excretion in man. Acidifying the urine increases the rate of renal elimination of amphetamine, reducing its plasma concentration and its effect on the subject's mental state. (Data from: Gunne & Anggard 1974 In: Torrell T et al. (eds) Pharmacology and pharmacokinetics. Plenum, New York)

Table 5.5	Drugs that are excreted largely unchanged in the urine
100–75%	Amiloride, frusemide, chlorothiazide, gentamicin, methotrexate, atenolol, ampicillin (after i.v. dosing; less after oral dosing), digoxin, pyridostigmine
75–50%	Carbenicillin, benzylpenicillin, cimetidine, cephaloridine, oxytetracycline, neostigmine
~50%	Propantheline, tubocurarine

Thus the overall rate of metabolism can be denoted by CL_{met}.

BILIARY EXCRETION AND ENTEROHEPATIC CIRCULATION

Liver cells transfer various substances, including drugs, from plasma to bile by means of transport systems similar to those of the renal tubule and which also involve P-glycoprotein (see Ch. 4). Various hydrophilic drug conjugates (particularly glucuronides) are concentrated in bile and delivered to the intestine where the glucuronide is usually hydrolysed, releasing active drug once more; free drug can then be reabsorbed and the cycle repeated (enterohepatic circulation). The effect of this is to create a 'reservoir' of recirculating drug that can amount

> **Elimination of drugs by the kidney**
>
> - Most drugs, except those highly bound to plasma protein, cross the glomerular filter freely.
> - Many drugs, especially weak acids and weak bases, are actively secreted into the renal tubule, and thus more rapidly excreted.
> - Lipid-soluble drugs are passively reabsorbed by diffusion across the tubule, so are not efficiently excreted in the urine.
> - Because of pH partition, weak acids are more rapidly excreted in alkaline urine, and vice versa.
> - Several important drugs are removed predominantly by renal excretion, and are liable to cause toxicity in elderly persons and patients with renal disease.

to about 20% of total drug in the body and prolongs drug action. Examples where this is important include **morphine** (Ch. 37) and **ethinyloestradiol** (Ch. 26). Several drugs are excreted to an appreciable extent in bile. **Vecuronium** (a non-depolarising muscle relaxant; Ch. 7) is an example of a drug that is excreted mainly unchanged in bile. **Rifampicin** (Ch. 43) is absorbed from the gut and slowly deacetylated, retaining its biological activity. Both forms are secreted in the bile, but the deacetylated form is not reabsorbed, so eventually most of the drug leaves the body in this form, in the faeces.

PHARMACOKINETICS

The relationship between the administration of a drug, the time-course of its distribution and the magnitude of the concentration attained in different regions of the body is termed *pharmacokinetics* (what the body does to the drug), to distinguish it from *pharmacodynamics* (what the drug does to the body). The distinction is useful, though the words cause dismay to etymological purists. In this section a simple quantitative model is presented that synthesises the effects on drug concentration of the simultaneous operation of absorption, distribution, metabolism and excretion. This will, in particular, enable us to predict the time-course of drug action, which is extremely important from a clinical viewpoint.

SINGLE-COMPARTMENT MODEL

Consider first a highly simplified model of a human being, which consists of a single well-stirred compartment (of volume V_d) into which a quantity of drug Q is introduced rapidly by intravenous injection, and from which it can escape either by being metabolised or excreted (Fig. 5.6). The initial concentration, $C(0)$, will be Q/V_d. The concentration $C(t)$ at a later time t will depend on the rate of elimination of the drug. Most drugs exhibit first-order kinetics where the rate of elimination is directly proportional to drug concentration. Drug concentration then decays exponentially (Fig. 5.7), being described by the equation:

$$C(t) = C(0)\exp\frac{-CL_s}{V_d}\cdot t \qquad (5.2)$$

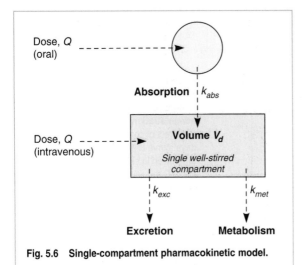

Fig. 5.6 Single-compartment pharmacokinetic model.

where CL_s is the total clearance of the drug, equal to the sum of the clearance by metabolism and by renal excretion. Taking logarithms:

$$\ln C(t) = \ln C(0) - \frac{CL_s}{V_d}\cdot t \qquad (5.3)$$

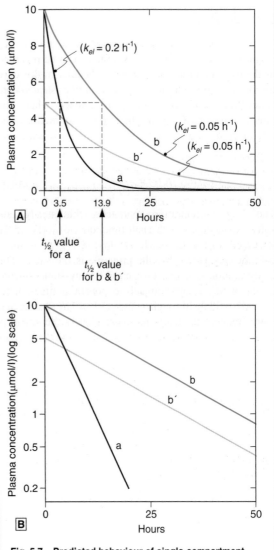

Fig. 5.7 **Predicted behaviour of single-compartment model following intravenous drug administration at time 0.** Drugs a and b differ only in their elimination rate constant, k_{el}. Curve b′ shows the plasma concentration time-course for a smaller dose of B. Note that $t_{1/2}$ (indicated by broken lines) does not depend on the dose. **A** Linear concentration scale. **B** Logarithmic concentration scale.

Thus, plotting $C(t)$ logarithmically against t yields a straight line with slope $-CL_s/V_d$. The inverse of this slope (CL_s/V_d) is the *elimination rate constant*, k_{el}. The *half-life*, $t_{1/2}$, is an easily conceptualised parameter inversely related to k_{el}. It is the time taken for $C(t)$ to decrease by 50% and is equal to $\ln2/k_{el}$ $(0.693/k_{el})$. The plasma half-life is therefore determined by the distribution volume V_d and clearance CL_s.

EFFECT OF REPEATED DOSAGE

Drugs are usually given as repeated doses rather than single injections. A continuous infusion can be regarded as the extreme of a repeated dose schedule. In this case the plasma concentration increases until a steady-state concentration, *C(steady state)*, is reached where the rate of infusion, X, equals the rate of elimination. The rate of elimination is equal to $Cl_s \times C(steady\ state)$, so that:

$$C(steady\ state) = \frac{X}{CL_s} \qquad (5.4)$$

The drug concentration approaches this steady-state value exponentially, with a half-time equal to $t_{1/2}$ (Fig. 5.8). Repeated injections (each of dose Q) give a more complicated pattern but the principle is the same. The concentration will rise to a mean steady-state concentration with an approximately exponential time-course but will oscillate (through a range Q/V_d). The smaller and more frequent the doses the more closely the situation approaches that of a continuous infusion and the smaller the swings in concentration. The exact dosage schedule, however, does not affect the *mean* steady-state concentration, nor the rate at which it is approached. In practice, a steady state is effectively achieved after three plasma half-times. Speedier attainment of the steady state can be achieved by starting with a larger dose. Such a *loading* dose is sometimes useful, for example when starting treatment of a patient with rapid atrial fibrillation with **digoxin** (Ch. 14). It must again be emphasised that the simple behaviour predicted for the single-compartment model only roughly corresponds to real life. Inclusion of other body compartments, particularly slowly equilibrating ones such as body fat, will result in additional exponential components in the overall kinetic behaviour. Pharmacokinetic studies in man show that to produce a realistic simulation the inclusion of two or three compartments is often necessary (see later).

EFFECT OF VARIATION IN RATE OF ABSORPTION

If a drug is absorbed slowly from the gut or from an injection site into the plasma, it is (in terms of a compartmental model) as though it were being injected slowly into the bloodstream. For the purpose of kinetic modelling, the transfer of drug from the site of administration to the central compartment can be represented approximately by a rate constant, k_{abs} (see Fig. 5.6). This assumes that the rate of absorption is directly proportional, at any moment, to the amount of drug still unabsorbed, which is at best a rough approximation to reality. The effect of slow absorption on the time-course

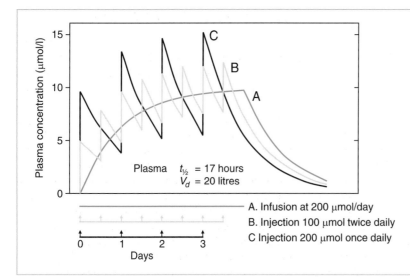

Plasma $t_{1/2}$ = 17 hours
V_d = 20 litres

A. Infusion at 200 μmol/day
B. Injection 100 μmol twice daily
C Injection 200 μmol once daily

Fig. 5.8 Predicted behaviour of single-compartment model with continuous or intermittent drug administration. Smooth curve A shows the effect of continuous infusion for 4 days; curve B the same total amount of drug given in eight equal doses; and curve C the same total amount of drug given in four equal doses. Note that in each case a steady state is effectively reached after about 2 days (about 3 × $t_{1/2}$), and that the mean concentration reached in the steady state is the same for all three schedules.

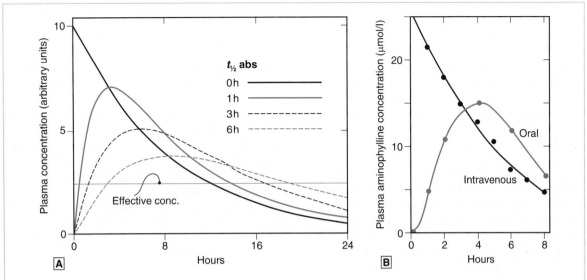

Fig. 5.9 The effect of slow drug absorption on plasma drug concentration. [A] Predicted behaviour of single-compartment model with drug absorbed at different rates from the gut or an injection site. The elimination half-time is 6 hours. The absorption half-times are marked on the diagram. (Zero indicates instantaneous absorption, corresponding to intravenous administration.) Note that the peak plasma concentration is reduced and delayed by slow absorption, and the duration of action somewhat increased.
[B] Measurements of plasma aminophylline concentration in man following equal oral and intravenous doses. (Data from: Swintowsky J V 1956 J Am Pharm Assoc 49: 395)

of the rise and fall of the plasma concentration is shown in Figure 5.9. The curves show the effect of spreading out the absorption of the same total amount of drug over different periods of time. In each case, all of the drug is absorbed, but the peak concentration appears later and becomes lower and less sharp if absorption is slow. Once absorption is complete, the plasma concentration declines with the same half-time, irrespective of the rate of absorption.

It can be shown that, for the kind of pharmacokinetic model discussed here, the *area* under the plasma concentration–time curve (often abbreviated to AUC, for *Area Under the Curve*) is directly proportional to the total amount of drug introduced into the plasma compartment, irrespective of the rate at which it enters. Comparison of the AUC following oral and intravenous administration can therefore be used to determine the fraction of the oral dose that enters the bloodstream, and thus to measure *bioavailability* (see p. 70). Incomplete absorption, or destruction by first-pass metabolism before the drug reaches the plasma compartment, will mean that the AUC for oral administration will be smaller than that for intravenous administration, whereas changes in the *rate* of absorption will not affect it. Again it is worth noting

that provided absorption is complete the relation between the rate of administration and the steady-state plasma concentration (equation 5.4) is unaffected by k_{abs}, though the size of the oscillation of plasma concentration with each dose will be reduced if absorption is slow.

MORE COMPLICATED KINETIC MODELS

So far we have considered a single-compartment pharmacokinetic model in which the rates of absorption, metabolism and excretion are all assumed to be directly proportional to the concentration of drug in the compartment from which transfer is occurring. This is a useful way to illustrate some basic principles, but is clearly a physiological oversimplification. The characteristics of different parts of the body, such as brain, body fat and muscle, are quite different in terms of their blood supply, partition coefficient for drugs and the permeability of their capillaries to drugs. These differences, which the single-compartment model ignores, can considerably affect the time-course of drug distribution and drug action, and much theoretical work has gone into the mathematical analysis of more complex models. Discussions can be found in specialised texts. They are beyond the scope of this book, and perhaps also beyond the limit of what is actually useful, for the experimental data on pharmacokinetic properties of drugs are seldom accurate or reproducible enough to enable complex models to be tested critically.

The two-compartment model, which introduces a separate 'peripheral' compartment to represent the tissues, in communication with the 'central' plasma compartment, more closely resembles the real situation without involving excessive complications.

TWO-COMPARTMENT MODEL

The two-compartment model is a widely used approximation in which the tissues are lumped together as a peripheral compartment which drug molecules can enter and leave only via the central compartment (Fig. 5.10) which normally represents the plasma (or plasma plus some extravascular space in the case of a few drugs that distribute especially rapidly). The effect of adding a second compartment to the model is to introduce a second exponential component into the predicted time-course of the plasma concentration, so that it comprises a fast and a slow phase. This pattern is often found experimentally, and is most clearly revealed when the concentration data are plotted semilogarithmically (Fig. 5.11). If, as is often the case, the transfer of drug between the central and peripheral compartments is relatively fast compared with the rate of elimination, then the fast phase (often called the α-phase) can be taken to represent the redistribution of the drug (i.e. drug molecules passing from plasma to tissues thereby rapidly lowering the plasma concentration). The plasma concentration reached when

the fast phase is complete, but before any elimination has occurred, allows a measure of the combined distribution volumes of the two compartments; the half-time for the slow phase (the β-phase) provides an estimate of the rate constant for elimination, k_{el}. If a drug is rapidly metabolised, the α- and β-phases are not well separated and the calculation of V_d and k_{el} is not straightforward. Problems also arise with drugs (e.g. very fat-soluble drugs) for which it is unrealistic to lump all the peripheral tissues together, so caution is needed in the interpretation of such pharmacokinetic data.

It is important to realise that the addition of extra compartments to the basic model affects only the predicted time-course of drug action, and not the steady state. Thus the relation between plasma concentration and dose derived for the single-compartment model (equation 5.4) still applies.

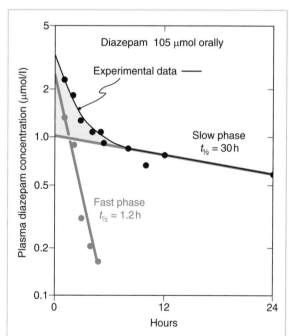

Fig. 5.11 Kinetics of diazepam elimination in man following a single oral dose. (The graph shows a semilogarithmic plot of plasma concentration versus time.) The experimental data (black symbols) follow a curve that becomes linear after about 8 hours (slow phase). Plotting the deviation of the early points (light blue shaded area) from this line on the same coordinates (blue symbols) reveals the fast phase. This type of two-component decay is consistent with the two-compartment model (Fig. 5.10) and is obtained with many drugs. (Data from: Curry S H 1980 Drug disposition and pharmacokinetics. Blackwell, Oxford)

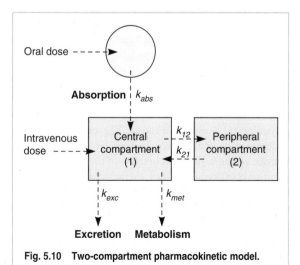

Fig. 5.10 Two-compartment pharmacokinetic model.

SATURATION KINETICS

In a few cases, such as **ethanol**, **phenytoin** and **salicylate**, the time-course of disappearance of drug from the plasma does not follow the exponential or biexponential pattern shown in Figures 5.7 and 5.11, but is initially linear (i.e. the drug is removed at a constant rate that is *independent* of plasma concentration). This is often called *zero-order kinetics* to distinguish it from the usual *first-order kinetics* which we have considered so far (terms that have their origin in chemical kinetic theory), though *saturation kinetics* is a better term. Figure 5.12 shows the example of ethanol. It can be seen that the rate of disappearance of ethanol from the plasma is constant at about 4 mmol/l per hour irrespective of its plasma concentration. The explanation for this is that the rate of oxidation by the enzyme alcohol dehydrogenase reaches a maximum at low ethanol concentrations because of limited availability of the cofactor, NAD^+ (see Ch. 39).

Saturation kinetics can have several important consequences (see Fig. 5.13). One is that the duration of action is more strongly dependent on dose than is the case with drugs that do not show metabolic saturation. Another consequence is that the relationship between dose and

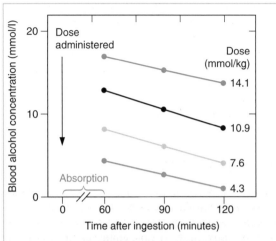

Fig. 5.12   Saturating kinetics of alcohol elimination in man. The blood alcohol concentration falls linearly rather than exponentially, and the rate of fall does not vary with dose. (From: Drew G C et al. 1958 Br Med J 2: 5103)

steady-state plasma concentration is steep and unpredictable, and does not obey the proportionality rule implicit in equation 5.4 for non-saturating drugs. The maximum

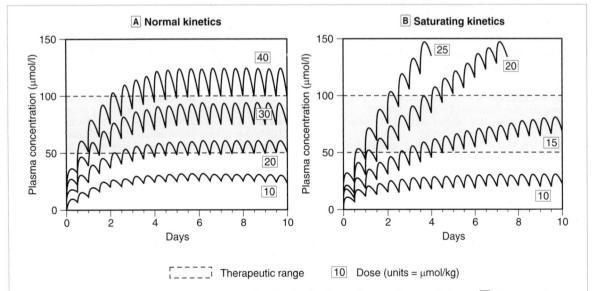

Fig. 5.13   Comparison of non-saturating and saturating kinetics for drugs given orally every 12 hours. [A] The curves show an imaginary drug, similar to the antiepileptic drug phenytoin at the lowest dose, but with linear kinetics. [B] The curves for saturating kinetics are calculated from the known pharmacokinetic parameters of phenytoin (see Ch. 36). Note (i) that no steady state is reached with higher doses of phenytoin and (ii) that a small increment in dose results after a time in a disproportionately large effect on plasma concentration. With linear kinetics the steady-state plasma concentration is directly proportional to dose. Curves were calculated with the 'Sympak' pharmacokinetic modelling program written by Dr J G Blackman, University of Otago.

rate of metabolism sets a limit to the rate at which the drug can be administered, and if this rate is exceeded, the amount of drug in the body will, in principle, increase indefinitely and never reach a steady state (Fig. 5.13). This does not actually happen because there is always some dependence of the rate of elimination on the plasma concentration (usually because other, non-saturating metabolic pathways or renal excretion contribute significantly at high concentrations). Nevertheless, the steady-state plasma concentration of drugs of this kind varies with dose more widely and less predictably than it does with non-saturating drugs. Similarly, variations in the rate of metabolism (e.g. through enzyme induction) also produce disproportionately large changes in the plasma concentration. These problems are well recognised for drugs such as **phenytoin**, an anticonvulsant whose plasma concentration needs to be closely controlled to achieve an optimal clinical effect (see Ch. 36).

Pharmacokinetics

- For many drugs, disappearance from the plasma follows an exponential time-course characterised by the plasma half-life.
- Plasma half-life, in the simple case, is directly proportional to the volume of distribution, and inversely proportional to the overall rate of clearance.
- With repeated dosage or sustained delivery of a drug, the plasma concentration approaches a steady value within 3–5 plasma half-lives.
- A two-compartment model is often needed. In this case the kinetics become biexponential. The two components roughly represent the processes of transfer between plasma and tissues (α-phase) and elimination from the plasma (β-phase).
- Some drugs show non-exponential 'saturation' kinetics, with important clinical consequences, especially a disproportionate increase in steady-state plasma concentration when daily dose is increased.

REFERENCES AND FURTHER READING

Benton R E, Honig P K, Zamani K, Cantilena L R, Woosley R L 1996 Grapefruit juice alters terfenadine pharmacokinetics, resulting in prolongation of repolarization on the electrocardiogram. Clin Pharmacol Ther 59: 383–388 (*Grapefruit juice sets the stage for a potentially fatal, albeit very uncommon, interaction between an over-the-counter pharmaceutical and a popular beverage. A regulatory nightmare!*)

Boobis A R, Edwards R J, Adams D A, Davies D S 1996 Dissecting the function of P450. Br J Clin Pharmacol 42: 81–89 (*Use of antipeptide antibodies directed against defined regions of human P450 enzymes*)

Gonzalez F J, Korzekwa K R 1995 Cytochromes P450 expression systems. Ann Rev Pharmacol Toxicol 35: 369–390 (*Catalytically active P450 enzymes can be expressed in bacterial, yeast or mammalian cells*)

Gooderham N J, Murray S, Lynch A M et al. 1996 Heterocyclic amines: evaluation of their role in diet associated human cancer. Br J Clin Pharmacol 42: 91–98 (*Heterocyclic amines are formed during cooking. They are absorbed after eating meat and converted into genotoxic hydroxylamines by CYP1A2 in human liver; they are both mutagenic and carcinogenic in bioassays. More nightmares!*)

Halpert J R 1995 Structural basis of selective cytochrome P450 inhibition. Ann Rev Pharmacol Toxicol 35: 29–53 (*Complementary properties of isoform-selective P450 inhibitors and their target enzymes determine inhibitor selectivity*)

Hutt A J, Tan S C 1996 Drug chirality and its clinical significance. Drugs 52 (suppl 5): 1–12 (*Short review*)

Kharasch E D, Hankins D, Mautz D, Thummel K E 1996 Identification of the enzyme responsible for oxidative halothane metabolism: implications for prevention of halothane hepatitis. Lancet 347: 1367–1371 (*Evidence that CYP2E1 is important in human oxidative halothane metabolism: 'single dose disulfiram may prove effective prophylaxis against halothane hepatitis'.*)

Murray M, Reidy G F 1990 Selectivity in the inhibition of mammalian cytochromes P450 by chemical agents. Pharmacol Rev 42: 85–101 (*Mechanisms of inhibition and development of preferential inhibitors of specific P450 enzymes*)

Nelson D R, Koymans L, Kamataki T et al. 1996 P450 superfamily: update on new sequences, gene mapping, accession numbers and nomenclature. Pharmacogenetics 6: 1–42 (*Classification of the superfamily of P450 enzymes*)

Park B K, Kitteringham N R, Pirmohamed M, Tucker G T 1996 Relevance of induction of human drug-metabolizing enzymes: pharmacological and toxicological implications. Br J Clin Pharmacol 41: 477–491 (*Reviews the mechanism and biological importance of enzyme induction, including implications for toxicity/carcinogenicity testing of new drugs*)

Raunio H, Pasanen M, Maenpaa J, Hakkola J, Pelkonen O 1995 Expression of extrahepatic cytochrome P450 in humans. In: Pacifici G M, Fracchia G M (eds) Advances in drug metabolism in man. European Commission, Luxembourg, pp 233–287 (*Reviews anabolic functions of P450 enzymes in man*)

Rowland M, Tozer T N 1995 Clinical pharmacokinetics: concepts and applications, 3rd edn. Williams & Wilkins, Baltimore (*Excellent text, over-modestly described by its authors as a 'primer'. Emphasises clinical applications*)

CHEMICAL MEDIATORS

Chemical mediators and the autonomic nervous system

INTRODUCTION

The network of chemical signals and associated receptors by which cells in the body communicate with one another provides many targets for drug action, and has always been a focus of attention for pharmacologists. Chemical transmission in the peripheral nervous system, and the various ways in which the process can be pharmacologically subverted, are discussed in this chapter. In addition to *neurotransmission*, we also consider briefly the less clearly defined processes, collectively termed *neuromodulation*, by which many mediators and drugs exert control over the function of the nervous system. The relative anatomical and physiological simplicity of the peripheral nervous system has made it the proving ground for most of the important discoveries about chemical transmission, though the same general principles apply to the central nervous system (see Ch. 28). For more detail than is given here, see Cooper et al. 1996. Studies

initiated on the peripheral nervous system have been central to the understanding and classification of many major types of drug action, so it is worth recounting a little history. An excellent account is given by Bacq (1975).

Experimental physiology became established as an approach to the understanding of the function of living organisms in the middle of the 19th century. The peripheral nervous system, and particularly the autonomic nervous system, received a great deal of attention. The fact that electrical stimulation of nerves could elicit a whole variety of physiological effects—from blanching of the skin to arrest of the heart—presented a real challenge to comprehension, particularly of the way in which the signal was passed from the nerve to the effector tissue. In 1877 Du Bois-Reymond was the first to put the alternatives clearly: 'Of known natural processes that might pass on excitation, only two are, in my opinion, worth talking about—either there exists at the boundary of the contractile substance a stimulatory secretion …; or the phenomenon is electrical in nature.' The latter view was more generally believed. In 1869 it had been shown that an exogenous substance, **muscarine**, could mimic the effects of stimulating the vagus nerve, and that **atropine** could inhibit the actions both of muscarine and of nerve stimulation. In 1905 Langley showed the same for **nicotine** and **curare** acting at the neuromuscular junction. Most physiologists interpreted these phenomena as stimulation and inhibition of the nerve endings, respectively, rather than as evidence for chemical transmission. Hence, the suggestion of T R Elliott, in 1904, that **adrenaline** might act as a chemical transmitter mediating the actions of the sympathetic nervous system was coolly received, until Langley, the Professor of Physiology at Cambridge, and a powerful figure at that time, suggested, a year later, that transmission to skeletal muscle involved the secretion by the nerve terminals of a substance related to nicotine.

One of the key observations for Elliott was that

degeneration of sympathetic nerve terminals did not abolish the sensitivity of smooth muscle preparations to **adrenaline** (which the electrical theory predicted) but actually enhanced it. The hypothesis of chemical transmission was put to direct test by Dixon in 1907, who tried to show that vagus nerve stimulation released from a dog's heart into the blood a substance capable of inhibiting another heart. The experiment failed, and the atmosphere of scepticism prevailed.

It was not until 1921, in Germany, that Loewi showed that stimulation of the vagosympathetic trunk to an isolated and cannulated frog's heart could cause the release into the cannula of a substance ('Vagusstoff') that, if the cannula fluid was transferred from the first heart to a second, would inhibit the second heart. This is a classic and much-quoted experiment that proved extremely difficult for even Loewi to perform reproducibly. In an autobiographical sketch, Loewi tells us that the idea of chemical transmission arose in a discussion that he had in 1903 but no way of testing it experimentally occurred to him until he dreamed of the appropriate experiment one night in 1920. He wrote some notes of this very important dream in the middle of the night, but in the morning could not read them. The dream obligingly returned the next night, and, taking no chances, he went to the laboratory at 3 a.m. and carried out the experiment successfully. Loewi's experiment may be, and was, criticised on numerous grounds (it could, for example, have been potassium rather than a neurotransmitter that was acting on the recipient heart), but a series of further experiments proved him to be right. His findings can be summarised as follows:

- Stimulation of the vagus caused the appearance in the perfusate of the frog heart of a substance capable of producing, in a second heart, an inhibitory effect resembling vagus stimulation.
- Stimulation of the sympathetic nervous system caused the appearance of a substance capable of accelerating a second heart. By fluorescence measurements, Loewi concluded later that this substance was adrenaline.
- **Atropine** prevented the inhibitory action of the vagus on the heart but did not prevent release of 'Vagusstoff'. Atropine thus prevented the effects, rather than the release, of the transmitter.
- When 'Vagusstoff' was incubated with ground-up frog heart muscle it became inactivated. This effect is now known to be due to enzymatic destruction of acetylcholine by cholinesterase.
- **Physostigmine** (eserine), which potentiated the effect of vagus stimulation on the heart, prevented destruc-

tion of 'Vagusstoff' by heart muscle, providing evidence that the potentiation is due to inhibition of cholinesterase which normally destroys the transmitter substance acetylcholine.

A few years later, in the early 1930s, Dale showed convincingly that acetylcholine was also the transmitter substance at the neuromuscular junction of striated muscle and at autonomic ganglia. One of the keys to Dale's success lay in the use of very highly sensitive bioassays, especially the leech dorsal muscle, for measuring acetylcholine release (see Ch. 3). Chemical transmission at sympathetic nerve terminals was demonstrated at about the same time as cholinergic transmission and by very similar methods. Cannon and his colleagues at Harvard first showed unequivocally the phenomenon of chemical transmission at sympathetic nerve endings, by experiments in vivo in which tissues made supersensitive to adrenaline by prior sympathetic denervation were shown to respond, after a delay, to the transmitter released by stimulation of the sympathetic nerves to other parts of the body. The chemical identity of the transmitter, tantalisingly like adrenaline, but not identical to it, caused confusion for many years, until in 1946 von Euler showed it to be the non-methylated derivative, noradrenaline.

For a more detailed account of the physiology and pharmacology of the autonomic nervous system, see Broadley (1996).

THE PERIPHERAL NERVOUS SYSTEM

The peripheral nervous system consists of the following principal elements:

- autonomic nervous system, which includes the enteric nervous system
- somatic efferent system, innervating skeletal muscle
- somatic and visceral afferent system.

In this chapter we are concerned mainly with the autonomic nervous system, which for a long time occupied centre stage in the pharmacology of chemical transmission. Aspects of the somatic efferent system are considered in Chapter 7. *Afferent* nerves (particularly the non-myelinated nerves subserving nociceptive and other functions; see Ch. 37) also have important *effector* functions in the periphery, mediated mainly by neuropeptides (Ch. 10). Many afferent fibres are present in autonomic nerves, and are anatomically part of the autonomic nervous system, but it is the efferent pathways that are the main concern of this chapter.

BASIC ANATOMY AND PHYSIOLOGY OF THE AUTONOMIC NERVOUS SYSTEM

The autonomic nervous system (see Appenzeller & Oribe 1997) consists of three main anatomical divisions, *sympathetic* and *parasympathetic* (see Fig. 6.1), and the *enteric nervous system*, consisting of the intrinsic nerve plexuses of the gastrointestinal tract, which are closely interconnected with the sympathetic and parasympathetic systems.

The autonomic nervous system conveys all of the outputs from the central nervous system to the rest of the body except for the motor innervation of skeletal muscle. The enteric nervous system has sufficient integrative capabilities to allow it to function independently of the central nervous system, but the sympathetic and parasympathetic systems are essentially agents of the central nervous system, and cannot function without it. The auto-

nomic nervous system is largely outside the influence of voluntary control. The main processes that it regulates are:

- contraction and relaxation of smooth muscle
- all exocrine and certain endocrine secretions
- the heartbeat
- certain steps in intermediary metabolism.

A degree of autonomic control influences many other processes, including the function of the immune system and the somatosensory system, though the physiological importance of autonomic control in such systems is not yet clear.

The main difference between the autonomic and the somatic efferent pathways is that the former consists of two neurons arranged in series, whereas in the latter a single motoneuron connects the central nervous system to the skeletal muscle fibre (Fig. 6.2). The two neurons in the autonomic pathway are known respectively as

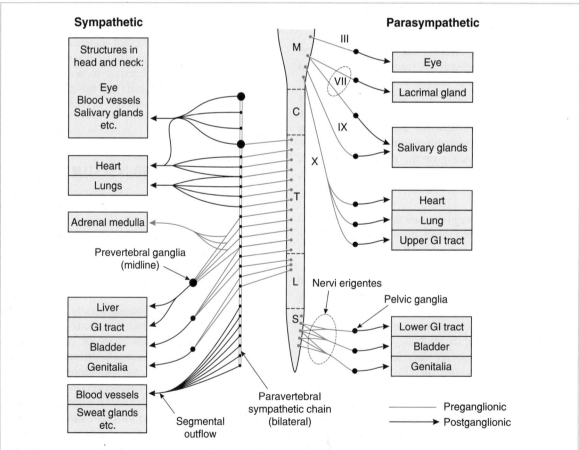

Fig. 6.1 Basic plan of the mammalian autonomic nervous system. (M = medullary; C = cervical; T = thoracic; L = lumbar, S = sacral)

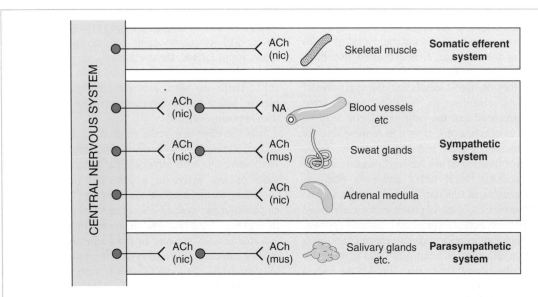

Fig. 6.2 Acetylcholine (ACh) and noradrenaline (NA) as transmitters in the peripheral nervous system. The main two types of acetylcholine receptor, nicotinic (n) and muscarinic (m) (see Ch. 7), are indicated.

preganglionic and *postganglionic*. In the sympathetic nervous system, the intervening synapses lie in *autonomic ganglia*, which are outside the central nervous system and contain the nerve endings of preganglionic fibres and the cell bodies of postganglionic fibres. In parasympathetic pathways, the postganglionic cells are mainly found in the target organs, and discrete parasympathetic ganglia are found only in head and neck.

The sympathetic preganglionic neurons have their cell bodies in the lateral horn of the grey matter of the thoracic and lumbar segments of the spinal cord, and the fibres leave the spinal cord in the spinal nerves as *thoracolumbar sympathetic outflow*. Just outside the spinal cord they leave the spinal nerve as filaments that run to the *paravertebral chain* of sympathetic ganglia, which lies bilaterally on either side of the spinal column. Each preganglionic nerve branches, and makes synaptic contact with ganglion cells in several sympathetic ganglia. These ganglia contain the cell bodies of the postganglionic sympathetic neurons, the axons of which rejoin the spinal nerve. Many of the postganglionic sympathetic fibres reach their peripheral destinations via the branches of the spinal nerves. Others, destined for abdominal and pelvic viscera, have their cell bodies in a group of unpaired *prevertebral ganglia* in the abdominal cavity. The only exception to the two-neuron arrangement is the innervation of the adrenal medulla,

which secretes catecholamines in response to activity in the nerves supplying it. The cells of the adrenal medulla are, in effect, modified postganglionic sympathetic neurons, and the nerves supplying the gland are equivalent to preganglionic fibres.

The parasympathetic nerves emerge from two separate regions of the central nervous system. The *cranial outflow* consists of preganglionic fibres in certain cranial nerves, namely the oculomotor nerve (carrying parasympathetic fibres destined for the eye), the facial and glossopharyngeal nerves (carrying fibres to the salivary glands and the nasopharynx) and the vagus nerve (carrying fibres to the thoracic and abdominal viscera). The ganglia lie scattered in close relation to the target organs; the postganglionic neurons are very short compared with those of the sympathetic system. Parasympathetic fibres destined for the pelvic and abdominal viscera emerge as the *sacral outflow* from the spinal cord in a bundle of nerves known as the *nervi erigentes* (since stimulation of these nerves evokes genital erection—a fact of some importance to those responsible for artificial insemination of livestock). These fibres synapse in a group of scattered pelvic ganglia, whence the short postganglionic fibres run to target tissues such as the bladder, rectum and genitalia. The pelvic ganglia carry both sympathetic and parasympathetic fibres, and the two divisions are not anatomically distinct in this region.

The enteric nervous system (reviewed by Furness & Costa 1987, Goyal & Hirano 1996) consists of the neurons whose cell bodies lie in the intramural plexuses in the wall of the intestine. It is estimated that there are more cells in this system than in the spinal cord, and functionally they do not fit simply into the sympathetic/ parasympathetic classification. Incoming nerves from both the sympathetic and the parasympathetic systems terminate on enteric neurons, as well as running directly to smooth muscle, glands and blood vessels. Some enteric neurons function as mechanoreceptors or chemo-receptors, providing local reflex pathways that can control gastrointestinal function without external inputs. The enteric nervous system is pharmacologically more complex than the sympathetic or parasympathetic systems, involving many neuropeptide and other transmitters (such as 5-hydroxytryptamine, NO and ATP) and is often de-scribed as a collection of 'little brains' outside the central nervous system, rather like those of many invertebrates.

Basic anatomy of the autonomic nervous system

- The autonomic nervous system comprises three divisions: *sympathetic, parasympathetic* and *enteric*.
- Basic (two-neuron) pattern of the sympathetic and parasympathetic systems consists of preganglionic neuron with cell body in CNS, postganglionic neuron with cell body in autonomic ganglion.
- Parasympathetic system is connected to the CNS via:
  —cranial nerve outflow (III, VII, IX, X)
  —sacral outflow.
- Parasympathetic ganglia usually lie close to or within the target organ.
- Sympathetic outflow leaves CNS in thoracic and lumbar spinal roots. Sympathetic ganglia form two paravertebral chains, plus some midline ganglia.
- The enteric nervous system consists of neurons lying in the intramural plexuses of the gastrointestinal tract. It receives inputs from sympathetic and parasympathetic systems, but can act on its own to control the motor and secretory functions of the intestine.

In some places (e.g. in the visceral smooth muscle of the gut and bladder and in the heart) the sympathetic and the parasympathetic systems produce opposite effects, but there are others where only one division of the autonomic system operates. The sweat glands and most blood vessels, for example, have only a sympathetic innervation, whereas the ciliary muscle of the eye has only a parasympathetic innervation. Bronchial smooth muscle has only a parasympathetic (constrictor) inner-vation (though its tone is highly sensitive to circulating adrenaline—acting probably to inhibit the constrictor

innervation rather than on the smooth muscle directly). Resistance arteries (see Chs 11 and 15) have a sympathetic vasoconstrictor innervation, but no parasympathetic innervation; instead, the constrictor tone is opposed by a background release of nitric oxide from the endothelial cells. There are other examples, such as the salivary glands, where the two systems produce similar, rather than opposing, effects.

It is therefore a mistake to think of the sympathetic and parasympathetic systems as physiological opponents. Each serves its own physiological function and can be more or less active in a particular organ or tissue according to the need of the moment. Cannon rightly emphasised the general role of the sympathetic system in evoking 'fight-or-flight' reactions in an emergency, but emergencies are rare in most animals. In everyday life, the autonomic nervous system functions continuously to control specific local functions, such as adjustments to postural changes or exercise (see Janig & MacLachlan 1992); the popular concept of a continuum from the extreme 'rest-and-digest' state (parasympathetic active, sympathetic quiescent) to the extreme emergency 'fight-or-flight' state (sympathetic active, parasympathetic quiescent) is a misleading oversimplification.

Table 6.1 lists some of the more important autonomic responses in humans.

Physiology of the autonomic nervous system

- The autonomic system controls: smooth muscle (visceral and vascular); exocrine (and some endocrine) secretions; rate and force of the heart; certain metabolic processes (e.g. glucose utilisation).
- Sympathetic and parasympathetic systems have opposing actions in some situations (e.g. control of heart rate, gastrointestinal smooth muscle); but not in others (e.g. salivary glands, ciliary muscle).
- Sympathetic activity increases in stress (fight-or-flight response) whereas parasympathetic activity predominates during satiation and repose. Both systems exert a continuous physiological control of specific organs under normal conditions, when the body is at neither extreme.

TRANSMITTERS IN THE AUTONOMIC NERVOUS SYSTEM

The two main neurotransmitters that operate in the autonomic system are acetylcholine and noradrenaline, whose sites of action are shown diagrammatically in Figure 6.2. This diagram also shows the type of post-synaptic receptor with which the transmitters interact at

Table 6.1 The main effects of the autonomic nervous system

Organ	Sympathetic	Adrenergic receptor type	Parasympathetic	Cholinergic receptor type
Heart				
SA node	Rate ↑	β_1	Rate ↓	M_2
Atrial muscle	Force ↑	β_1	Force ↓	M_2
AV node	Automaticity ↑	β_1	Cond. vel. ↓	M_2
			AV block	M_2
Ventricular muscle	Automaticity ↑	β_1	No effect	
	Force ↑			
Blood vessels				
Arterioles				
Coronary	Constriction	α		
Muscle	Dilatation	β_2	No effect	
Viscera				
Skin	Constriction	α	No effect	
Brain				
Erectile tissue	Constriction	α	Dilatation	? M_3
Salivary gland		α		
Veins	Constriction	α	No effect	
	Dilatation	β_2		
Viscera				
Bronchi				
Smooth muscle	No sympathetic innervation, but dilated by circulating adrenaline	β_2	Constriction	M_3
Glands	No effect		Secretion	M_3
GI tract				
Smooth muscle	Motility ↓	$\alpha_1, \alpha_2, \beta_2$	Motility ↑	M_3
Sphincters	Constriction	α_2, β_2	Dilatation	M_3
Glands	No effect		Secretion	M_3
			Gastric acid secretion	M_1
Uterus				
Pregnant	Contraction	α	Variable	
Non-pregnant	Relaxation	β_2		
Male sex organs	Ejaculation	α	Erection	? M_3
Eye				
Pupil	Dilatation	α	Constriction	M_3
Ciliary muscle	Relaxation (slight)	β	Contraction	M_3
Skin				
Sweat glands	Secretion (mainly cholinergic)	α	No effect	
Pilomotor	Piloerection	α	No effect	
Salivary glands	Secretion	α, β	Secretion	M_3
Lacrimal glands	No effect		Secretion	M_3
Kidney	Renin secretion	β_2	No effect	
Liver	Glycogenolysis	α, β_2	No effect	
	Gluconeogenesis			

The adrenergic and cholinergic receptor types shown are described more fully in Chapters 7 and 8. Transmitters other than acetylcholine and noradrenaline contribute to many of these responses (see Table 6.2).

the different sites. (discussed more fully in Chs 7 and 8). Some general rules apply:

- All motor nerve fibres leaving the central nervous system release acetylcholine, which acts on nicotinic receptors (although in autonomic ganglia a minor component of excitation is due to activation of muscarinic receptors (see Ch. 7)).
- All postganglionic parasympathetic fibres release acetylcholine, which acts on muscarinic receptors.
- All postganglionic sympathetic fibres (with one important exception) release noradrenaline, which may act on either α- or β-adrenoceptors (see Ch. 8). The exception, where transmission is due to acetylcholine acting on muscarinic receptors, is the sympathetic fibres suppling *sweat glands*. In some species, there is evidence for a cholinergic sympathetic nerve supply causing vasodilatation in skeletal muscle, but this does not exist in humans.

Acetylcholine and noradrenaline are the grandees among autonomic transmitters, and are central to understanding autonomic pharmacology. However, many other chemical mediators are also released by autonomic neurons (see below), and their functional significance is gradually becoming clearer.

SOME GENERAL PRINCIPLES OF CHEMICAL TRANSMISSION

DALE'S PRINCIPLE

Dale's principle, advanced rather tentatively by him in 1934, states, in its modern form: 'A mature neurone releases the same transmitter (or transmitters) at all of its synapses.' Dale considered it unlikely that a single neuron could store and release different transmitters at different nerve terminals, and his view has been substantiated by physiological and neurochemical evidence. It is known, for example, that the axons of motor neurons have branches that synapse on interneurons in the spinal cord, in addition to the main branch that innervates skeletal muscle fibres in the periphery. The transmitter at both the central and the peripheral nerve endings is acetylcholine, in accordance with Dale's principle. There is so far no known case of a neuron that releases different transmitters at different terminals.

Dale's principle does not imply that a neuron releases only one transmitter—indeed there are many examples to the contrary (see Co-transmission, below)—or that it cannot change its transmitter repertoire. For example, sympathetic neurons, during development, switch from being cholinergic to being noradrenergic. Moreover, recent evidence (see below) shows that the balance of the cocktail of mediators released by a nerve terminal can vary with stimulus conditions, and in response to presynaptic modulators. Though purists still defend the general validity of Dale's principle, which was, of course, framed before these complexities were discovered, it is beginning to look like an oversimplification.

DENERVATION SUPERSENSITIVITY

It is known, mainly from the work of Cannon on the sympathetic system, that if a nerve is cut and its terminals allowed to degenerate, the structure supplied by it becomes supersensitive to the transmitter substance released by the terminals. Thus skeletal muscle, which normally responds to injected acetylcholine only if a large dose is given directly into the arterial blood supply, will, after denervation, respond by contracture to much smaller amounts. Other organs, such as salivary glands and blood vessels show similar supersensitivity to acetylcholine and noradrenaline when the postganglionic nerves degenerate, and there is evidence that pathways in the central nervous system show the same phenomenon.

Several mechanisms are known to contribute to denervation supersensitivity, and the extent and mechanism of the phenomenon varies from organ to organ. Reported mechanisms include the following:

- *Proliferation of receptors.* This is particularly marked in skeletal muscle, in which the number of acetylcholine receptors increases 20-fold or more after denervation; the receptors are no longer localised on the endplate region of the fibres. Elsewhere, much smaller increases in receptor number (about twofold) have often been reported, but there are examples where no change occurs.

- *Loss of mechanisms for transmitter removal.* At noradrenergic synapses the loss of neuronal uptake of noradrenaline (see p. 145) contributes substantially to denervation supersensitivity. At cholinergic synapses a partial loss of cholinesterase occurs (see p. 131).
- *Increased postjunctional responsiveness.* In some cases the postsynaptic cells become supersensitive without a corresponding increase in the number of receptors. Thus, smooth muscle cells become partly depolarised and hyperexcitable, and this phenomenon contributes appreciably to their supersensitivity. The mechanism of this change and its importance for other synapses is not known.

Supersensitivity can occur, but is less marked, when transmission is interrupted by processes other than nerve section. Pharmacological block of ganglionic transmission, for example, if sustained for a few days, causes some degree of supersensitivity of the target organs, and long-term blockade of postsynaptic receptors also causes receptors to proliferate, leaving the cell supersensitive when the blocking agent is removed. Phenomena such as this are of importance in the central nervous system, where such supersensitivity can cause 'rebound' effects when drugs are given for some time and then stopped.

PRESYNAPTIC INTERACTIONS

The presynaptic terminals that synthesise and release transmitter in response to electrical activity in the nerve fibre, are often themselves sensitive to transmitter substances and to other substances that may be produced locally in tissues (for reviews see Starke et al. 1989, Vizi 1980). Such presynaptic effects most commonly act to inhibit transmitter release, but may enhance it. Figure 6.3 shows the inhibitory effect of adrenaline on the release of acetylcholine (evoked by electrical stimulation) from the postganglionic parasympathetic nerve terminals of the intestine. The release of noradrenaline from nearby sympathetic nerve terminals can also inhibit release of acetylcholine. Noradrenergic and cholinergic nerve terminals often lie close together in the myenteric plexus, so the opposing effects of the sympathetic and parasympathetic systems result not only from the opposite effects of the two transmitters on the smooth muscle cells, but also from the inhibition of acetylcholine release by noradrenaline acting on the parasympathetic nerve

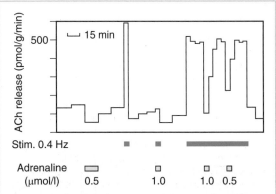

Fig. 6.3 Inhibitory effect of adrenaline on acetylcholine release from postganglionic parasympathetic nerves in the guinea-pig ileum. The intramural nerves were stimulated electrically where indicated, and the acetylcholine released into the bathing fluid determined by bioassay. Adrenaline strongly inhibits acetylcholine release. (From: Vizi E S 1979 Prog Neurobiol 12: 181)

terminals. A similar situation exists in the heart, where a mutual presynaptic inhibition has been demonstrated; noradrenaline inhibits acetylcholine release, as in the myenteric plexus, and acetylcholine also inhibits noradrenaline release. These are examples of *heterotropic* interactions, where one neurotransmitter affects the release of another. *Homotropic* interactions also occur, where the transmitter, by binding to *presynaptic autoreceptors*, affects the nerve terminals from which it is being released. There is evidence (see Starke et al. 1989) that this type of *autoinhibitory feedback* acts powerfully at noradrenergic nerve terminals. One of the strongest pieces of evidence is that the amount of noradrenaline released from tissues in response to repetitive stimulation of sympathetic nerves is increased 10-fold or more in the presence of an antagonist that blocks the presynaptic noradrenaline receptors (see Ch. 8). This suggests that the released noradrenaline can inhibit further release by at least 90%.

A similar state of affairs probably exists also at cholinergic nerve terminals, where release of transmitter can be increased considerably by antagonists that block the autoinhibitory action of acetylcholine on nerve terminals. In both the noradrenergic and cholinergic systems the presynaptic autoreceptors are pharmacologically distinct from the postsynaptic receptors (see Chs 7 and 8), so there are drugs that act selectively, as agonists or antagonists, on the pre- or postsynaptic receptors.

Cholinergic and noradrenergic nerve terminals respond not only to acetylcholine and noradrenaline, as described above, but also to other substances that are released as co-transmitters, such as ATP and neuropeptide Y or derived from other sources, including nitric oxide, prostaglandins, adenosine, dopamine, serotonin, gamma-aminobutyric acid (GABA), opioid peptides and many other substances. The physiological role and pharmacological significance of these various interactions

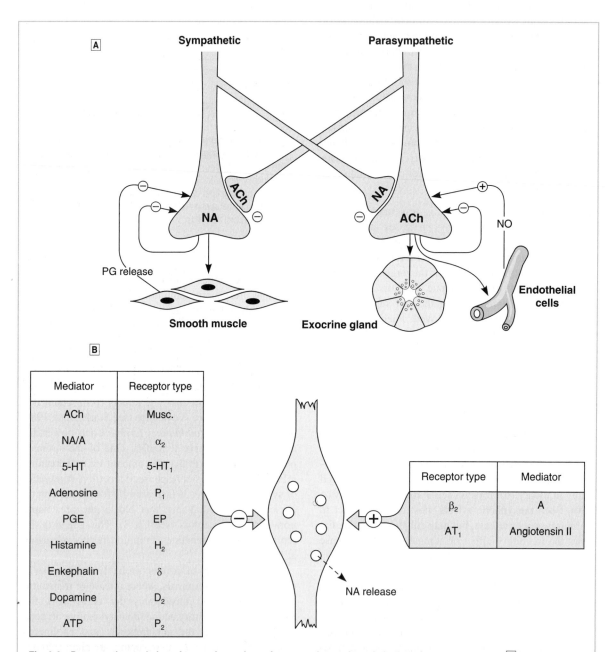

Fig. 6.4 Presynaptic regulation of transmitter release from noradrenergic and cholinergic nerve terminals. [A] Postulated homotropic and heterotropic interactions between sympathetic and parasympathetic nerves. [B] Some of the known inhibitory and facilitatory influences on noradrenaline release from sympathetic nerve endings. (ACh = acetylcholine; A = adrenaline; NA = noradrenaline; NO = nitric oxide; NPY = neuropeptide Y; PG = prostaglandin; PGE = prostaglandin E; 5-HT = 5 hydroxytryptamine)

is still unclear, but the description of the autonomic nervous system represented in Figure 6.1 is undoubtedly oversimplified. Figure 6.4 shows some of the main presynaptic interactions between autonomic neurons, and summarises the many chemical influences that regulate transmitter release from noradrenergic neurons.

Presynaptic receptors regulate transmitter release mainly by affecting calcium entry into the nerve terminal (see Stjarne 1989, Wu & Saggau 1997). When a nerve terminal is depolarised by an action potential, voltage-gated N-type calcium channels open (see Fig. 6.10), and the resulting ingress of calcium is the trigger for transmitter-containing vesicles to discharge their contents into the synaptic cleft. Regulation of these calcium channels occurs mainly by phosphorylation (see Ch. 2). Most presynaptic receptors are of the G-protein-coupled type and are linked to phosphorylation events by either phospholipase C (which inhibits calcium entry) or adenylate cyclase (which facilitates calcium entry). Other mechanisms may also contribute to presynaptic inhibition, such as an increased K^+-permeability, leading to hyperpolarisation of the terminal (analogous to the mechanism by which acetylcholine slows the heart; see Ch. 14), or impairment of the coupling between increased $[Ca^{2+}]_i$ and vesicle discharge (see Starke et al. 1989, Wu & Saggau 1997)

POSTSYNAPTIC MODULATION

Chemical mediators often act on postsynaptic structures, including neurons, smooth muscle cells, cardiac muscle cells, etc. in such a way that their excitability or spontaneous firing pattern is altered. In many cases, as with presynaptic modulation, the mechanisms appear to involve changes in calcium and/or potassium channel function mediated by a second messenger. We give only a few examples here:

- The slow excitatory effect produced by various mediators, including acetylcholine and peptides such as substance P (see Ch. 37), on many peripheral and central neurons results mainly from a *decrease* in K^+-permeability. On the other hand, the inhibitory effect of various opiates is mainly due to *increased* K^+-permeability.
- Neuropeptide Y (NPY), which is released as a co-transmitter with noradrenaline at many sympathetic nerve endings and enhances the vasoconstrictor effect of noradrenaline, thus greatly facilitating transmission (Fig. 6.5); the mechanism is not known.
- *Long-term potentiation* is a special and very long-lasting form of synaptic modulation associated with glutamate-mediated transmission in certain brain regions, and is believed to be important in memory. It is discussed further in Chapter 28.

Neuromodulation and presynaptic interactions

- As well as functioning directly as neurotransmitters, chemical mediators may regulate:
  —presynaptic transmitter release
  —neuronal excitability.
  Both are examples of neuromodulation, and generally involve second messenger regulation of membrane ion channels.
- Presynaptic receptors may inhibit or increase transmitter release, the former being more important.
- Inhibitory presynaptic autoreceptors occur on noradrenergic and cholinergic neurons, causing each transmitter to inhibit its own release (autoinhibitory feedback).
- Many endogenous mediators (e.g. GABA, prostaglandins, opioid and other peptides) as well as the transmitters themselves exert presynaptic control (mainly inhibitory) over autonomic transmitter release.

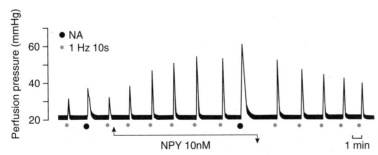

Fig. 6.5 Effect of neuropeptide Y (NPY) on noradrenergic transmission. Vasoconstriction (upward deflection) of the rabbit ear artery occurs in response to injections of noradrenaline (NA) (black symbols) or to a brief period of sympathetic nerve stimulation (blue symbols). Infusion of a low concentration of NPY greatly increases the response to both. (From: Rand M J et al. 1987 Cardiovasc Pharmacol 10 (suppl 12): S33–S44)

The pre- and postsynaptic effects described above are often described as *neuromodulation* (see Burnstock 1987, Kaczmarek & Levitan 1987) since the mediator acts to increase or decrease the efficacy of synaptic transmission without participating directly as a transmitter. Many neuropeptides, for example, affect membrane ion channels in such a way as to increase or decrease excitability, and thus control the firing pattern of the cell. Neuromodulation is a term with as many definitions as authors, and we cannot distinguish unequivocally, on functional, anatomical or biochemical grounds, exactly how a neurotransmitter differs from a neuromodulator. In general, though, neuromodulation involves slower processes (taking seconds to days) than neurotransmission (which occurs in milliseconds); furthermore, neuromodulation operates through cascades of intracellular messengers (Ch. 2), rather than directly on ligand-gated ion channels. Some aspects of this problem of terminology are discussed in Chapter 12.

TRANSMITTERS OTHER THAN ACETYLCHOLINE AND NORADRENALINE: NANC TRANSMISSION

As mentioned above, acetylcholine or noradrenaline are not the only autonomic transmitters. The rather grudging realisation that this was so, dawned many years ago when it was noticed that autonomic transmission in many organs could not be completely blocked by drugs that abolish responses to these transmitters. The dismal but tenacious term *non-noradrenergic non-cholinergic* (NANC) *transmission* was coined. Later, fluorescence and immunocytochemical methods showed that neurons,

including autonomic neurons, contain many potential transmitters, often several in the same cell. Compounds believed to function as NANC transmitters include *ATP*, *vasoactive intestinal peptide* (VIP), *neuropeptide Y* (NPY) and *nitric oxide* (see Fig. 6.6, Table 6.2), which function at postganglionic nerve terminals, as well as *substance P*, *5-hydroxytryptamine*, *γ-aminobutyric acid* (GABA) and *dopamine*, which play a role in ganglionic transmission (see Lundberg 1996 for a comprehensive review).

CO-TRANSMISSION

It is probably the rule rather than the exception that neurons release more than one transmitter or modulator (see Furness et al. 1989, Hokfelt et al. 1986, Lundberg 1996), each of which interacts with specific receptors and produces effects, often both pre- and postsynaptically. We are only just beginning to understand the functional implications of this (see Kupfermann 1991). The example of noradrenaline/ATP co-transmission at the sympathetic nerve endings is shown in Figure 6.6, and the best-studied examples and mechanisms are summarised in Table 6.2 and Figures 6.7 and 6.8.

What, one might well ask, could be the functional advantage of co-transmission, compared with a single transmitter acting on various different receptors? The possible advantages include:

- One constituent of the cocktail (e.g. a peptide) may be removed or inactivated more slowly than the other (e.g. a monoamine) and therefore reach targets further from the site of release, and produce longer-lasting

Tissue response

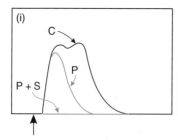
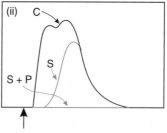

Fig 6.6 Noradrenaline/ATP co-transmission in the guinea-pig vas deferens. Contractions of the tissue are shown in response to a single electrical stimulus causing excitation of sympathetic nerve endings. With no blocking drugs present, a twin-peaked response is produced (C). The early peak is selectively abolished by the ATP antagonist, suramin (S), while the late peak is blocked by the α_1-adrenoceptor antagonist, prazosin (P). The response is completely eliminated when both drugs are present. (Reproduced with permission from: von Kugelgen & Starke 1991 Trends Pharmacol Sci 12: 319–324)

Table 6.2 Examples of NANC transmitters and co-transmitters in the peripheral nervous system

Transmitter	Location	Function
Non-peptides		
ATP	Postganglionic sympathetic neurons (e.g. blood vessels, vas deferens)	Fast depolarisation/contraction of smooth muscle cells
GABA, 5-HT	Enteric neurons	Peristaltic reflex
Dopamine	Some sympathetic neurons (e.g. kidney)	Vasodilatation
NO	Pelvic nerves	Erection
NO	Gastric nerves	Gastric emptying
Peptides		
Neuropeptide Y (NPY)	Postganglionic sympathetic neurons (e.g. blood vessels)	Facilitates constrictor action of NA Inhibits NA release
Vasoactive intestinal peptide (VIP)	Parasympathetic nerves to salivary glands	Vasodilatation Co-transmitter with ACh
	NANC innervation of airways smooth muscle	Bronchodilatation
GnRH	Sympathetic ganglia	Slow depolarisation Co-transmitter with ACh
Substance P	Sympathetic ganglia	Slow depolarisation
	Enteric neurons	Co-transmitter with ACh
CGRP	Non-myelinated sensory neurons	Vasodilatation Vascular leakage Neurogenic inflammation

effects. This appears to be the case, for example, with acetylcholine and GnRH in sympathetic ganglia (Jan & Jan 1983).

- The balance of the transmitters released may vary under different conditions. At sympathetic nerve terminals, for example, where noradrenaline and NPY are stored in separate vesicles, NPY is preferentially released at high stimulation frequencies (see Stjarne 1989), so that differential release of one or other mediator may result from varying impulse patterns. Differential effects of presynaptic modulators are also possible, for isoprenaline (a β-adrenoceptor agonist; see Ch. 8) inhibits ATP release, while enhancing noradrenaline release from sympathetic nerve terminals (Gonçalves et al. 1996).

MECHANISMS OF TRANSMITTER RELEASE

The principal mechanism of transmitter release (see Fig. 6.9), in both the peripheral and central nervous systems, and also in many hormone-secreting cells, is

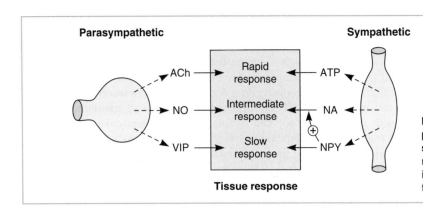

Fig 6.7 The main co-transmitters at postganglionic parasympathetic and sympathetic neurons. The different mediators generally give rise to fast, intermediate and slow responses of the target organ.

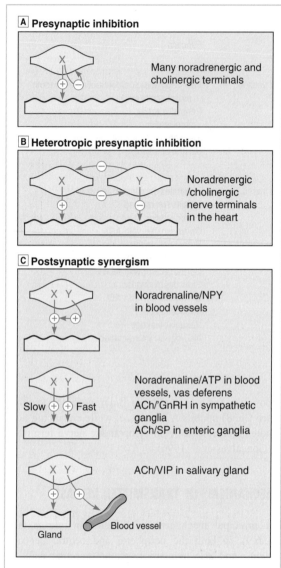

Fig. 6.8   Co-transmission and neuromodulation—some examples. [A] Presynaptic inhibition. [B] Heterotropic presynaptic inhibition. [C] Postsynaptic synergism. (ACh = acetylcholine; NPY = neuropeptide Y; GnRH = gonadotrophin-releasing hormone = LHRH; SP substance P; VIP = vasoactive intestinal peptide)

peptides, amino acids and purines, are all released in basically the same way. In neurons, the process is initiated by the arrival of an action potential, which depolarises the membrane, thereby opening voltage-activated calcium channels and causing calcium to enter the cell. Evidence in favour of this mechanism comes from many sources, the most compelling being the early discovery, by Katz and his colleagues, that acetylcholine release at the neuromuscular junction is 'quantal' (i.e. occurs in discrete multimolecular packets), the direct observation of vesicle fusion during transmitter release, by rapid-freeze electron microscopy, and the correlation of release with sudden steps in the electrical capacitance of the membrane (as the vesicle fuses and increases the surface area of the cell). There is also biochemical evidence showing that, in addition to the transmitter, other constituents of the vesicles are released at the same time. Exocytosis represents the climax of the *synaptic vesicle cycle*, shown in a simplified form in Figure 6.9 (see Calakos & Scheller 1996, Südhof 1995). The synaptic vesicles, loaded with transmitter, attach to docking sites located inside the synaptic membrane facing the synaptic cleft. These sites are closely associated with the calcium channels (see Stanley 1997), so the vesicles are optimally placed to respond by discharging their contents when the channel opens and calcium enters the nerve terminal. Having done so, the empty vesicle is recaptured by endocytosis, and returns to the interior of the terminal, where it fuses with the larger endosomal membrane. The endosome buds off new vesicles, which take up transmitter from the cytosol by means of specific transport proteins, and are again docked on the presynaptic membrane. This sequence, which typically takes several minutes, is controlled by various trafficking proteins associated with the plasma membrane (*synaptotaxin* and *SNAPs*) and the vesicles (e.g. *synaptobrevins* and *synaptotagmins*, or *SNARES*), as well as cytosolic proteins. Several of these proteins possess calcium-binding sites, providing a link between the primary trigger—calcium influx—and the response—exocytosis. So far, there are few examples of drugs which affect transmitter release by interacting with these trafficking proteins, though the *botulinum neurotoxins* (see Ch. 7) do so. It is likely to be a fertile area for future drug discovery efforts, however, so stay tuned.

If this neat and tidy picture of transmitter packets ready and waiting to pop obediently out of the cell in response to a puff of calcium seems a little too good to be true, rest assured that the picture is no longer quite so simple The bulk discharge of vesicle contents by exocytosis is not the whole story of neurosecretion. Recently, for example, it has been shown that vesicles may fuse

exocytosis, whereby the transmitter is stored in intracellular vesicles, which fuse transiently with the cell membrane and discharge their contents, in response to an increase in the intracellular calcium concentration (see Nicholls et al. 1992). Though it has been studied in most detail for cholinergic and noradrenergic synapses, there is good evidence that other transmitters, including

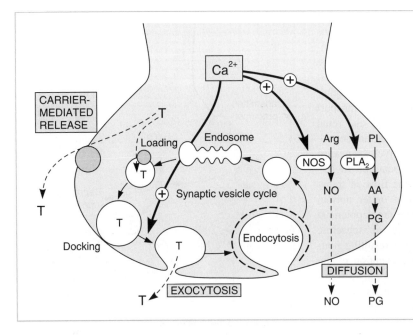

Fig. 6.9 Role of exocytosis, carrier-mediated transport and diffusion in mediator release. The main mechanism of release of monoamine and peptide mediators is by Ca^{2+}-mediated exocytosis, but carrier-mediated release from the cytosol also occurs.
T represents a typical amine transmitter, such as noradrenaline or 5-hydroxytryptamine.
   Nitric oxide (NO) and prostaglandins (PGs) are released by diffusion as soon as they are formed, from arginine (Arg) and arachidonic acid (AA) respectively, through the action of Ca^{2+}-activated enzymes, nitric oxide synthase (NOS) and phospholipase A_2 (see Chs 10 and 11 for more details).

Mechanisms of release of neurotransmitters and neuromodulators

- Most mediators are stored in presynaptic vesicles and released by exocytosis.
- Specialised synthetic enzymes and transport proteins are responsible for the uptake of precursors and synthesis and storage of individual mediators. These are often the targets for drugs that affect neurotransmission.
- Some important mediators (nitric oxide, prostaglandins) are synthesised 'on demand' and released by diffusion.
- Exocytosis, nitric oxide synthesis and prostaglandin synthesis are all activated by an increase in intracellular calcium concentration.
- Transmitter action is commonly terminated by reuptake of the transmitter into nerve terminals by a specific transport mechanism.

transiently with the cell membrane and release only part of their contents (see Neher 1993) before becoming disconnected. It is also known that acetylcholine and other mediators can leak out of nerve endings from the cytosolic compartment, independently of vesicle fusion, probably by utilising carriers in the plasma membrane (Fig. 6.9); the functional significance of this is unknown.

Nitric oxide (see Jaffrey & Snyder 1995, Yun et al. 1996, Ch. 11) and **arachidonic acid metabolites** (e.g. prostaglandins; see Piomelli, 1994; Fig 6.9; Ch. 12) are two important examples of mediator release that does not

involve vesicles and exocytosis, but relies on diffusion. The mediators are not stored, but escape from the cell as soon as they are synthesised. In both cases, the synthetic enzyme is activated by calcium, and the moment-to-moment control of the rate of synthesis depends on the intracellular calcium concentration. This kind of release is necessarily slower than the classical exocytotic mechanism, but in the case of nitric oxide, is fast enough for it to function as a true transmitter (see Ch. 11).

TERMINATION OF TRANSMITTER ACTION

Chemically transmitting synapses other than the peptidergic variety (Ch. 10) invariably incorporate a mechanism for rapidly disposing of the released transmitter, so that its action remains brief and localised. At cholinergic synapses (Ch. 7), the released acetylcholine is inactivated very rapidly in the synaptic cleft by acetylcholinesterase, but in most cases (see Fig. 6.10), transmitter action is terminated by active reuptake into the presynaptic nerve, or into supporting cells, such as glia. Such reuptake depends on transporter proteins, each being specific for a particular transmitter (see Borowsky & Hoffmann 1995). They belong to a distinct family of membrane proteins, each possessing 12 transmembrane helices. They all act as co-transporters of sodium ions, chloride ions and transmitter molecules, and it is the inwardly directed 'downhill' gradient for sodium that provides the energy for the inward 'uphill' movement of the transmitter. The simultaneous transport of ions along with the transmitter means that the process generates a net current across the membrane, which can be measured directly, and used to monitor the transport process (Brew & Attwell 1988). Very similar mechanisms are responsible for other physiological transport processes, such as glucose uptake (Ch. 22) and renal tubular transport of amino acids. Since it is the electrochemical gradient for sodium ions that drives the inward transport of transmitter molecules, a reduction of this gradient can reduce or even reverse the flow of transmitter. This is probably not important under normal conditions, but when the nerve terminals are depolarised or abnormally loaded with sodium (e.g. in ischaemic conditions; see Attwell et al. 1993) the resulting non-vesicular release of transmitter (and prevention of the normal synaptic reuptake mechanism) may play a significant role in the effects of ischaemia on tissues such as heart and brain (see Chs 14 and 31).

BASIC STEPS IN NEUROCHEMICAL TRANSMISSION—SITES OF DRUG ACTION

Figure 6.10 summarises the main processes that occur in a classical chemically transmitting synapse, and provides a useful basis for understanding the actions of the many different classes of drug, discussed in later chapters, which act by facilitating or blocking neurochemical transmission.

All of the steps shown in Figure 6.10 (except for transmitter diffusion, step 8) can be influenced by drugs. For example, the enzymes involved in synthesis or inactivation of the transmitter can be inhibited by drugs, as can the transport systems responsible for the neuronal uptake of the transmitter or its precursor. The actions of the great majority of drugs that act on the peripheral nervous system (Chs 7 and 8) and the central nervous system fit into this general scheme.

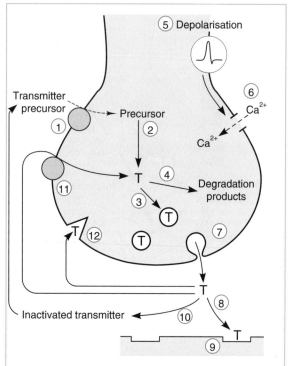

Fig 6.10 The main processes involved in synthesis, storage and release of amine transmitters: 1 = uptake of precursors; 2 = synthesis of transmitter; 3 = storage of transmitter in vesicles; 4 = degradation of surplus transmitter; 5 = depolarisation by propagated action potential; 6 = influx of Ca^{2+} in response to depolarisation; 7 = release of transmitter by exocytosis; 8 = diffusion to postsynaptic membrane; 9 = interaction with postsynaptic receptors; 10 = inactivation of transmitter; 11 = reuptake of transmitter or degradation products; 12 = interaction with presynaptic receptors. These processes are well characterised for many transmitters (e.g. acetylcholine, monoamines, amino acids, purines). Peptide mediators (see Ch. 10) differ in that they may be synthesised and packaged in the cell body rather than the terminals.

REFERENCES AND FURTHER READING

Appenzeller O, Oribe E 1997 The autonomic nervous system: an introduction to basic and clinical concepts. 5th edn. Elsevier, New York (*Comprehensive textbook*)

Attwell D, Barbour B, Szatkowski M 1993 Non-vesicular release of neurotransmitter. Neuron 11: 401–407 (*Summarises evidence for, and potential significance of non-vesicular release*)

Bacq Z M 1975 Chemical transmission of nerve impulses: a historical sketch. Pergamon Press, Oxford (*Lively account of the history of the discovery of chemical transmission*)

Borowsky B, Hoffmann B J 1995 Neurotransmitter transporters: molecular biology, function and regulation. Int Rev Neurobiol 38: 139–199 (*Detailed review article*)

Brew H, Attwell D I 1988 Electrogenic glutamate uptake is a major current carrier in the membrane of axolotl retinal ganglion cells. Nature 327: 707–709 (*Elegant physiological analysis of glutamate transport by neurons*)

Broadley K J 1996 Autonomic Pharmacology. Taylor & Francis, London (*Comprehensive textbook*)

Burnstock G 1987 Mechanisms of interaction of peptide and non-peptide vascular neuro-effector systems. J Cardiovasc Pharmacol 10 (suppl 12): 574–581 *(Review of co-autonomic transmission)*

Calakos N, Scheller R H 1996 Synaptic vesicle biogenesis, docking and fusion: a molecular description. Physiol Rev 76: 1–29 *(Summarises recent advances in mechanism of exocytosis)*

Cooper J C, Bloom F E, Roth R H 1996 The biochemical basis of neuropharmacology, 7th edn. Oxford University Press, New York *(Excellent general account, covering a broad area of neuropharmacology)*

Furness J B, Costa M 1987 The enteric nervous system. Churchill Livingstone, Edinburgh

Furness J B, Morris J L, Gibbins I L, Costa M 1989 Chemical coding of neurons and plurichemical transmission. Annu Rev Pharmacol Toxicol 29: 289–306 *(Excellent review of co-transmission)*

Gonçalves J, Bueltmann R, Driessen B 1996 Opposite modulation of cotransmitter release in guinea-pig vas deferens: increase of noradrenaline and decrease of ATP release by activation of prejunctional β-receptors. Naunyn-Schmiedebergs Arch Pharmacol 353: 184–192 *(Shows that presynaptic regulation can affect specific transmitters in different ways)*

Goyal R K, Hirano I 1996 The enteric nervous system. N Engl J Med 334: 1106–1115 *(Excellent review article)*

Hokfelt T, Fuxe K, Pernow B 1986 Coexistence of neuroactive substances in neurones: a new principle in chemical transmission. Progress in brain research. Elsevier, Amsterdam *(Early account of co-transmission, by pioneers in neuropeptide research)*

Jaffrey S R, Snyder S H 1995 Nitric oxide: a neuronal messenger. Ann Rev Cell Dev Biol 11: 417–440 *(Excellent review of the mediator role of NO in the nervous system)*

Jan Y N, Jan L Y 1983 A LHRH-like peptidergic neurotransmitter capable of 'action at a distance' in autonomic ganglia. Trends Neurosci 6: 320–325 *(Electrophysiological analysis of co-transmission)*

Janig W, McLachlan E M 1992 Characteristics of function-specific pathways in the sympathetic nervous system. Trends Neurosci 15: 475–481 *(Short article emphasising that the sympathetic system is far from being an all-or-none alarm system)*

Kaczmarek L, Levitan I 1987 Neuromodulation. Oxford University Press, New York *(Textbook reviewing recent developments in neurotransmission)*

Kupfermann I 1991 Functional studies of cotransmission. Physiol Rev 71: 683–732 *(Good review article)*

Lundberg J M 1996 Pharmacology of co-transmission in the autonomic nervous system: integrative aspects on amines, neuropeptides, adenosine triphosphate, amino acids and nitric oxide. Pharmacol Rev 48: 114–192 *(Detailed and informative review article)*

Neher E 1993 Secretion without full fusion. Nature 363: 497–498 *(Elegant techniques used to investigate the microphysiology of vesicular release)*

Nicholls J G, Martin A R, Wallace B G 1992 From neuron to brain. Sinauer, Sunderland, MA *(Excellent standard textbook)*

Piomelli D 1994 Eicosanoids in synaptic transmission. Crit Rev Neurobiol 8: 65–83 *(Discusses role of arachidonic acid metabolites as neural mediators)*

Stanley E E 1997 The calcium channel and the organization of the presynaptic transmitter release face. Trends Neurosci 20: 404–409 *(More on the microphysiology of vesicular release)*

Starke K, Gothert M, Kilbinger H 1989 Modulation of neurotransmitter release by presynaptic autoreceptors. Physiol Rev 69: 864–989 *(Comprehensive review article)*

Stjarne L 1989 Basic mechanisms and local modulation of nerve impulse-induced secretion of neurotransmitters from individual sympathetic nerve varicosities. Rev Physiol Biochem Pharmacol 112: 4–137 *(Excellent review on presynaptic regulation)*

Südhof T C 1995 The synaptic vesicle cycle: a cascade of protein–protein interactions. Nature 375: 645–653 *(Summarises recent advances in vesicular release at the molecular level)*

Vizi E S 1980 Presynaptic modulation of neurochemical transmission. Prog Neurobiol 12: 181–290 *(Early review on presynaptic regulation)*

Wu L-G, Saggau P 1997 Presynaptic inhibition of elicited neurotransmitter release. Trends Neurosci 20: 204–212 *(An update on the physiology of presynaptic inhibition)*

Yun H Y, Dawson V L, Dawson T M 1996 Neurobiology of nitric oxide. Crit Rev Neurobiol 10: 291–316 *(Useful review article)*

7

Cholinergic transmission

This chapter is concerned mainly with cholinergic transmission in the periphery, and the way in which drugs affect it. Cholinergic mechanisms in the CNS and their relevance to dementia are discussed in Chapters 28 and 31.

The discovery of the pharmacological action of **acetylcholine** (ACh) arose from work on adrenal glands. Adrenal extracts were known to produce a rise in blood pressure owing to their content of adrenaline. In 1900 Reid Hunt found that after adrenaline had been removed from such extracts, they produced a fall in blood pressure instead of a rise. He attributed the fall to their content of choline but later concluded that a more potent derivative of choline must be responsible. With Taveau he tested a number of choline derivatives and discovered that

acetylcholine was some 100 000 times more active than choline in lowering the rabbit's blood pressure. Although Hunt's studies suggested that acetylcholine was present in tissues, its physiological function was not apparent at that time and it remained a pharmacological curiosity until its transmitter role was discovered (see Ch. 6).

MUSCARINIC AND NICOTINIC ACTIONS OF ACETYLCHOLINE

In a study of the pharmacological actions of acetylcholine carried out in 1914, Dale distinguished two types of activity which he designated as *muscarinic* and *nicotinic*. The muscarinic actions of acetylcholine are those that can be reproduced by the injection of **muscarine**, the active principle of the poisonous mushroom *Amanita muscaria*, and can be abolished by small doses of **atropine**. On the whole, muscarinic actions correspond to those of parasympathetic stimulation, as shown in Table 7.1. After the muscarinic effects have been blocked by atropine, larger doses of acetylcholine produce another set of effects, closely similar to those of **nicotine**. They include:

- stimulation of all autonomic ganglia
- stimulation of voluntary muscle
- secretion of adrenaline from the adrenal medulla.

The muscarinic and nicotinic actions of acetylcholine are demonstrated in Figure 7.1 in an experiment on the blood pressure of an anaesthetised cat. Small and medium doses of acetylcholine produce a transient fall in blood pressure due to arteriolar vasodilatation and slowing of the heart—muscarinic effects which are abolished by atropine. A large dose of acetylcholine given after atropine produces nicotinic effects: an initial rise in blood pressure due to a stimulation of sympathetic ganglia and consequent vasoconstriction, and a secondary rise resulting from secretion of adrenaline.

Dale's classification was originally made on pharmaco-

Table 7.1 Subtypes of acetylcholine receptors

	Nicotinic		Muscarinic		
Type	Muscle-type	Neuronal-type	M_1 'neural'	M_2 'cardiac'	M_3 'glandular'
Main locations	Skeletal neuromuscular junction	Autonomic ganglia Sensory nerve terminal CNS (many regions)	*Neural* CNS (cortex, hippocampus) Ganglia (enteric, autonomic) *Gastric* Parietal cells	*Cardiac* Atria Conducting tissue *Neural* Presynaptic terminals	Exocrine glands Smooth muscle Vascular endothelium
Effects **Cellular**	Opening cation channels Membrane depolarisation (fast epsp)		$\uparrow IP_3$, DAG Depolarisation Excitation (slow epsp) ($\downarrow G_K$)	$\downarrow$ cAMP Inhibition ($\uparrow G_K$, $\downarrow I_{Ca}$) Slow ipsp	$\uparrow IP_3$ Stimulation ($\uparrow [Ca]_i$)
Functional	Neuromuscular transmission	Ganglionic transmission Presynaptic facilitation in CNS	CNS excitation (? memory) Gastric acid secretion Gastrointestinal motility	Cardiac inhibition Presynaptic inhibition Neural inhibition	Secretion Smooth muscle contraction Vasodilatation (via NO)
Agonists	Acetylcholine (ACh) Carbamylcholine (CCh)	ACh CCh Nicotine Lobeline Cytisine Epibatidine DMPP	ACh Oxotremorine McNA343	ACh CCh	ACh CCh
Antagonists	Tubocurarine Pancuronium Atracurium Vecuronium α-bungarotoxin	Trimetaphan Mecamylamine Hexamethonium	Atropine Pirenzepine Dicyclomine	Atropine Gallamine AF-DX 116	Atropine HHSD**

*DMPP = dimethylphenylpiperazinium
**HHSD = hexahydrosiladifenol

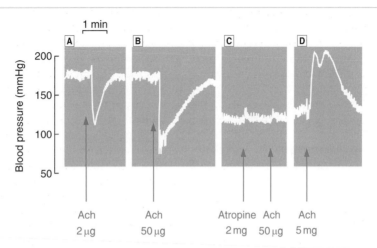

Fig. 7.1 Dale's experiment showing that acetylcholine produces two kinds of effect on the cat's blood pressure. Arterial pressure was recorded with a mercury manometer from a spinal cat. [A] ACh causes a fall in blood pressure due to vasodilatation. [B] A larger dose also produces bradycardia. Both A and B are muscarinic effects. [C] After atropine (muscarinic antagonist) the same dose of ACh has no effect. [D] Still under the influence of atropine, a much larger dose of ACh causes a rise in blood pressure (due to stimulation of sympathetic ganglia), accompanied by tachycardia, followed by a secondary rise (due to release of adrenaline from the adrenal gland). These effects result from its action on nicotinic receptors. (From: Burn J H 1963 Autonomic pharmacology. Blackwell, Oxford)

logical grounds, but it corresponds closely to the main physiological functions of acetylcholine in the body. The muscarinic actions correspond to those of acetylcholine released at postganglionic parasympathetic nerve endings, with two significant exceptions:

- Acetylcholine causes generalised vasodilatation, even though most blood vessels have no parasympathetic innervation. This is an indirect effect: acetylcholine (like many other mediators) acts on vascular endothelial cells to release *nitric oxide*; see Ch. 11) which relaxes smooth muscle. The physiological function of this is uncertain, since acetylcholine is not normally present in circulating blood.
- Acetylcholine evokes secretion from sweat glands, which are innervated by cholinergic fibres of the sympathetic nervous system (see Table 6.1).

The nicotinic actions correspond to those of acetylcholine acting on autonomic ganglia of the sympathetic and parasympathetic systems, the motor endplate of voluntary muscle and the secretory cells of the adrenal medulla.

ACETYLCHOLINE RECEPTORS

Though Dale himself dismissed the concept of receptors as sophistry rather than science, his classification pro-

vided the basis for distinguishing the two major classes of acetylcholine receptor (see Ch. 2).

NICOTINIC RECEPTORS

Nicotinic receptors fall into two classes, the *muscle* and *neuronal* types (Table 7.1). Muscle receptors occur at the skeletal neuromuscular junction (NMJ), whereas neuronal nicotinic receptors occur in autonomic ganglia, and also in the brain, where acetylcholine is a transmitter (Ch. 28). Both are ligand-gated ion channels (see Ch. 2). The molecular structure of these receptors, described in Chapter 2, is generally similar, but they differ pharmacologically (see Colquhoun et al. 1987). The muscle receptor has a pentameric structure ($\alpha\alpha\beta\gamma\varepsilon$ in the adult) made up of four distinct subunits. Neuronal receptors, particularly in the brain, are much more diverse (see McGehee & Role 1995), being built from various permutations of eight different subtypes of the α-subunit and four of the β-subunit. The functional significance of this diversity remains uncertain. In the periphery, the different action of agonists and antagonists on ganglionic and neuromuscular synapses is of practical importance, and mainly reflects the differences between the muscle and neuronal nicotinic receptors Table 7.1). Among the agonists, **decamethonium** (see below) is a potent depolarising agent (i.e. agonist) at the neuromuscular junction, but a weak antagonist on autonomic ganglia, whereas **epibatidine**, a substance extracted from in the skin of a South American frog, is an extremely potent and selective agonist at neuronal receptors. Antagonists also show strong selectivity. For example, α-bungarotoxin (see Ch. 2) blocks acetylcholine receptors at the neuromuscular junction at very low concentrations, but has no effect on autonomic ganglia. On the other hand, agents such as **mecamylamine** block neuronal, but not neuromuscular, acetylcholine receptors. The role of nicotinic receptors in the central nervous system is discussed in Chapters 28 and 39.

MUSCARINIC RECEPTORS

Gene cloning has revealed five distinct types of muscarinic receptor (see Wess 1996), but only four have been distinguished functionally and pharmacologically (see Goyal 1989). Three of these (M_1, M_2, M_3) are well characterised (Table 7.1). M_1-receptors ('neural') are found mainly on CNS and peripheral neurons and gastric parietal cells. They mediate excitatory effects, for example the slow muscarinic excitation mediated by acetylcholine in sympathetic ganglia (Ch. 6) and central neurons. This excitation is produced by a decrease in K^+-conductance, which causes membrane depolarisation. Deficiency of this kind of acetylcholine-mediated effect in the brain is possibly associated with dementia (see Ch. 31). M_1-receptors are also involved in the increase of gastric acid secretion following vagal stimulation (see Ch. 21).

M_2-receptors ('cardiac') occur in the heart, and also on the presynaptic terminals of peripheral and central neurons. They exert inhibitory effects, mainly by increasing K^+-conductance and by inhibiting calcium channels (see Ch. 2). M_2-receptor activation is responsible for the vagal inhibition of the heart, as well as presynaptic inhibition in the central nervous system and periphery (Ch. 6).

M_3-receptors ('glandular/smooth muscle') produce mainly excitatory effects, i.e. stimulation of glandular secretions (salivary, bronchial, sweat, etc.) and contraction of visceral smooth muscle. M_3-receptors also mediate relaxation of smooth muscle (mainly vascular), which results from the release of nitric oxide from neighbouring endothelial cells (Ch. 11). M_1-, M_2- and M_3-receptors occur also in specific locations in the CNS (see Ch. 24). M_4-receptors are largely confined to the CNS, and their functional role is not well understood.

The pharmacological classification of these receptor types relies on the existence of selective agonists and antagonists that can distinguish between them. Most agonists are non-selective, but two experimental compounds, **McNA343** and **oxotremorine**, are selective for M_1-receptors; **carbachol** is relatively inactive on these receptors. There is more selectivity amongst antagonists. Though most of the classical muscarinic antagonists (e.g. **atropine**, **hyoscine**) are non-selective, **pirenzepine** is selective for M_1-receptors. **Gallamine**, better known as a neuromuscular-blocking drug (see p. 125) is also a selective M_2-receptor antagonist, and recently other experimental drugs have been found that are selective for M_2- or M_3-receptors (Table 7.1).

Muscarinic receptors all belong to the family of G-protein-coupled receptors (Ch. 2). The odd-numbered members of the group (M_1, M_3, M_5) act through the inositol phosphate pathway (p. 37), while the even-numbered receptors (M_2, M_4) act by inhibiting adenylate cyclase and thus reducing intracellular cAMP (see Goyal 1989).

Acetylcholine receptors

- Main subdivision is into nicotinic (nAChR) and muscarinic (mAChR) subtypes.
- nAChRs are directly coupled to cation channels, and mediate fast excitatory synaptic transmission at the neuromuscular junction, autonomic ganglia, and at various sites in the CNS. Muscle and neuronal nAChR differ in their molecular structure and pharmacology.
- mAChRs are G-protein-coupled receptors, causing:
  — activation of phospholipase C (hence formation of IP_3 and DAG as second messengers)
  — inhibition of adenylate cyclase
  — activation of K^+-channels or inhibition of Ca^{2+}-channels.
- mAChR mediate ACh effects at postganglionic parasympathetic synapses (mainly heart, smooth muscle, glands), and contribute to ganglionic excitation. They occur in many parts of the CNS.
- Three main types of mAChR occur:
  — M_1-receptors ('neural'), producing slow excitation of ganglia. They are selectively blocked by pirenzepine.
  — M_2-receptors ('cardiac'), causing decrease in cardiac rate and force of contraction (mainly of atria). They are selectively blocked by gallamine. M_2 receptors also mediate presynaptic inhibition.
  — M_3-receptors ('glandular'), causing secretion, contraction of visceral smooth muscle, vascular relaxation.
- All mAChR are activated by ACh and blocked by atropine. There are also subtype-selective agonists and antagonists.

PHYSIOLOGY OF CHOLINERGIC TRANSMISSION

The physiology of cholinergic transmission is described in detail by Ginsborg & Jenkinson (1976) and Nicholls

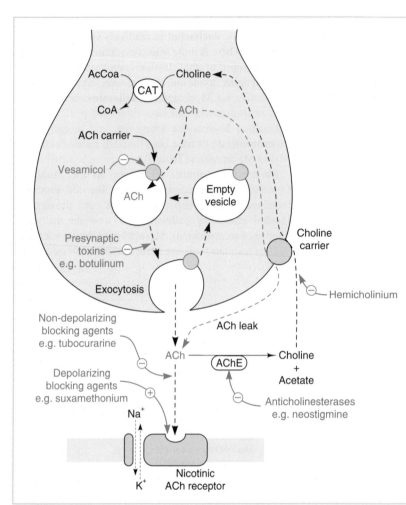

Fig. 7.2 Events and sites of drug action at a nicotinic cholinergic synapse. ACh is shown acting postsynaptically on a nicotinic receptor controlling a cation channel (e.g. at the neuromuscular or ganglionic synapse). There is evidence that a presynaptic nicotine receptor (not shown) can act to facilitate ACh release during sustained synaptic activity. The nerve terminal also contains acetylcholinesterase (not shown); when this is inhibited, the amount of free ACh, and the rate of leakage of ACh via the choline carrier, are increased. Under normal conditions, this leakage of ACh is insignificant.

At muscarinic cholinergic junctions (e.g. heart, smooth muscle, exocrine glands), both postsynaptic and presynaptic (inhibitory) receptors are of the muscarinic type.

et al. (1992). The main ways in which drugs can affect cholinergic transmission are shown in Figure 7.2.

ACETYLCHOLINE SYNTHESIS AND RELEASE

Acetylcholine metabolism is well reviewed by Parsons et al. (1993). Acetylcholine is synthesised within the nerve terminal from choline, which is taken up into the nerve terminal by an active transport system, similar to that which operates for transmitters such as noradrenaline (Ch. 8), 5-HT (Ch. 9) and amino acids (Ch. 29). The difference is that it transports the precursor, choline, not acetylcholine, so it is not important in terminating the action of the transmitter. The concentration of choline in the blood and body fluids is normally about 10 μmol/l, but in the immediate vicinity of cholinergic nerve terminals it increases, probably to about 1 mmol/l, when the released acetylcholine is hydrolysed, and more than 50% of this choline is normally recaptured by the nerve terminals. Free choline within the nerve terminal is acetylated by a cytosolic enzyme, *choline acetyltransferase* (CAT), which transfers the acetyl group from acetyl-CoA. The rate-limiting process in acetylcholine synthesis appears to be choline transport, the activity of which is regulated according to the rate at which acetylcholine is being released. Cholinesterase is present in the presynaptic nerve terminals and acetylcholine is continually being hydrolysed and resynthesised. Inhibition of the nerve terminal cholinesterase causes the accumulation of 'surplus' acetylcholine in the cytosol, which is not available for release by nerve impulses (though it is able to leak out via the choline carrier). Most of the acetylcholine synthesised, however, is packaged into synaptic vesicles, in which its concentration is very high (about 100 mmol/1), and from which release occurs by exocytosis, triggered by calcium entry into the nerve terminal (see Ch. 6).

Cholinergic vesicles accumulate acetylcholine actively, by means of a specific transport protein, a serpentine structure comprising 12 transmembrane helical regions, belonging to the general family of amine transporters which are responsible for transmitter accumulation both through the plasma membrane and through the synaptic vesicle membrane (see Liu & Edwards 1997, Usdin et al. 1995). Accumulation by the acetylcholine transporter is coupled to the large electrochemical gradient for protons that exists between intracellular organelles and the cytosol; it is blocked selectively by the experimental drug **vesamicol** (see Parsons et al. 1993), resulting in a slowly developing neuromuscular block. Following its release, the acetylcholine diffuses across the synaptic cleft* to combine with receptors on the postsynaptic cell. Some of it succumbs on the way to hydrolysis by acetyl-cholinesterase, an enzyme that is bound to the basement membrane of the nerve terminal, which lies between the pre- and postsynaptic membranes. At fast cholinergic synapses (e.g. the neuromuscular and ganglionic synapses), but not at slow ones (smooth muscle, gland cells, heart, etc.), the released acetylcholine is hydrolysed very rapidly (within 1 ms), so that it acts only very briefly. At the neuromuscular junction, which is a highly specialised synapse, a single nerve impulse releases about 300 synaptic vesicles (altogether about three million acetylcholine molecules) from the nerve terminals supplying a single muscle fibre, which contain altogether about three million synaptic vesicles. Approximately two million acetylcholine molecules combine with receptors, of which there are about 30 million on each muscle fibre, the rest being hydrolysed without reaching a receptor. The acetylcholine molecules remain bound to receptors for, on average, about 2 ms, and are quickly hydrolysed after dissociating, so that they cannot combine with a second receptor. The result is that transmitter action is very rapid and very brief, which is important for a synapse that has to initiate speedy muscular responses, and which may have to transmit signals faithfully at high frequency. Muscle cells are much larger than neurons, and require much more synaptic current to generate an action potential. Thus all of the chemical events happen

on a larger scale than at a neuronal synapse: the number of transmitter molecules in a quantum, the number of quanta released, and the number of receptors activated by each quantum are all 10–100 times greater. Our brains would be huge, but not very clever, if their synapses were built on the industrial scale of the neuromuscular junction.

Presynaptic modulation

Acetylcholine release is regulated by mediators, including acetylcholine itself, acting on presynaptic receptors, as discussed in Chapter 6. At postganglionic parasympathetic nerve endings, inhibitory M_2-receptors participate in autoinhibition of acetylcholine release (see Kilbinger 1984); other mediators, such as **noradrenaline**, also inhibit the release of acetylcholine (see Ch. 6). At the neuromuscular junction, on the other hand, presynaptic nicotinic receptors are believed to *facilitate* acetylcholine release (see Prior et al. 1995), a mechanism that may allow the synapse to function reliably during prolonged high-frequency activity. Facilitatory presynaptic nicotinic receptors also occur in the brain (see review by Wonnacott, 1997), and probably account for the central actions of nicotine (see Ch. 39).

ELECTRICAL EVENTS IN TRANSMISSION AT CHOLINERGIC SYNAPSES

Acetylcholine, acting on the postsynaptic membrane of a nicotinic (neuromuscular or ganglionic) synapse, causes a large increase in its permeability to cations, particularly to sodium and potassium ions, and to a lesser extent, calcium ions. Because of the large inwardly directed electrochemical gradient for sodium ions across the cell membrane, an inflow of sodium ions occurs, causing depolarisation of the postsynaptic membrane. This transmitter-mediated depolarisation is called an *endplate potential* (epp) in a skeletal muscle fibre (see Ginsborg & Jenkinson 1976), or a *fast excitatory postsynaptic potential* (fast epsp) at the ganglionic synapse (see Skok 1980). In a muscle fibre the localised epp spreads to adjacent, electrically excitable parts of the muscle fibre; if its amplitude reaches the threshold for excitation, an action potential is initiated, which propagates to the rest of the fibre and evokes a contraction.

In a nerve cell, depolarisation of the soma or a dendrite by the fast epsp causes a local current to flow. This depolarises the axon hillock region of the cell, where, if the epsp is large enough, an action potential is initiated. Figure 7.3 shows that **tubocurarine**, a drug that blocks postsynaptic acetylcholine receptors (see p. 125) reduces

---

*At postsynaptic parasympathetic nerve terminals (e.g. those supplying intestinal smooth muscle) there is often no clearly defined 'synaptic cleft', such as exists at the neuromuscular or ganglionic synapse, and the transmitter may have to diffuse tens of microns to its site of action.

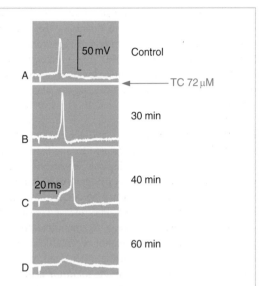

Fig. 7.3 Cholinergic transmission in an autonomic ganglion cell. Records were obtained with an intracellular microelectrode from a guinea-pig parasympathetic ganglion cell. The artefact at the beginning of each trace shows the moment of stimulation of the preganglionic nerve. Tubocurarine (TC), an acetylcholine antagonist, causes the epsp to become smaller. In record C it only just succeeds in triggering the action potential, and in D it has fallen below the threshold. Following complete block, antidromic stimulation (not shown) will still produce an action potential (cf. depolarisation block, Fig. 7.4). (From: Blackman J G et al. 1969 J Physiol 201: 723)

- A slow inhibitory (hyperpolarising) potential (slow ipsp) lasting 2–5 s. This mainly reflects a muscarinic (M_2) receptor-mediated increase in K^+-conductance, but other transmitters, such as dopamine and adenosine, also contribute.
- A slow epsp, which lasts for about 10 s. This is produced by acetylcholine acting on M_1-receptors, which close potassium channels.
- A late slow epsp, lasting for 1–2 minutes. This is thought to be mediated by a peptide co-transmitter, which may be substance P in some ganglia, and a GnRH-like peptide in others (see Ch. 6). Like the slow epsp, it is produced by a decrease in K^+-conductance.

Depolarisation block

Depolarisation block occurs at cholinergic synapses when the excitatory nicotinic receptors are *persistently* activated by nicotinic agonists, and it results from a decrease in the electrical excitability of the postsynaptic cell. This is shown in Figure 7.4. Application of **nicotine** to a sympathetic ganglion causes a depolarisation of the

---

the amplitude of the fast epsp until it no longer initiates an action potential, though the cell is still capable of responding when it is stimulated antidromically. Most ganglion cells are supplied by several presynaptic axons, and it requires simultaneous activity in more than one to make the postganglionic cell fire. At the neuromuscular junction, only one nerve fibre supplies each muscle fibre. Nevertheless, the amplitude of the epp is normally more than enough to initiate an action potential—indeed transmission still occurs when the epp is reduced by 70–80% and is said to show a large *margin of safety* so that fluctuations in transmitter release (e.g. during repetitive stimulation) do not affect transmission.

Transmission at the ganglionic synapse is more complex than at the neuromuscular junction. Though the primary event at both is the epp or fast epsp produced by acetylcholine acting on nicotinic receptors, this is followed in the ganglion by a succession of much slower postsynaptic responses, comprising:

Cholinergic transmission

- ACh synthesis:
  - Requires choline, which enters neuron via carrier-mediated transport.
  - Acetylation of choline, utilising acetylCoA as source of acetyl groups, involves choline acetyl transferase (CAT), a cytosolic enzyme found only in cholinergic neurons.
  - ACh is packaged into synaptic vesicles at high concentration by carrier-mediated transport.
- ACh release occurs by Ca^{2+}-mediated exocytosis. At the neuromuscular junction, one presynaptic nerve impulse releases 100–500 vesicles.
- At the NMJ, ACh acts on nAChR to open cation channels, producing a rapid depolarisation (endplate potential) which normally initiates an action potential in the muscle fibre. Transmission at other 'fast' cholinergic synapses (e.g. ganglionic) is similar.
- At 'fast' cholinergic synapses, ACh is hydrolysed within about 1 ms by acetylcholinesterase, so a presynaptic action potential produces only one postsynaptic action potential.
- Transmission mediated by mAChR is much slower in its timecourse, and synaptic structures are less clearly defined. In most cases ACh functions as a modulator rather than as a direct transmitter.
- Main mechanisms of pharmacological block: inhibition of choline uptake; inhibition of ACh release; block of postsynaptic receptors or ion channels; persistent postsynaptic depolarisation.

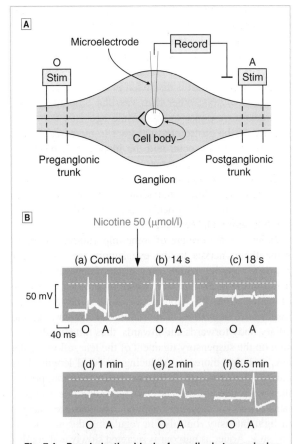

Fig. 7.4 Depolarisation block of ganglionic transmission by nicotine. [A] System used for intracellular recording from sympathetic ganglion cells of the frog, showing the location of orthodromic (O) and antidromic (A) stimulating electrodes. Stimulation at O excites the cell via the cholinergic synapse, whereas stimulation at A excites it by electrical propagation of the action potential. [B] The effect of nicotine: (a) Control records. The membrane potential is –55 mV (dotted line = 0 mV) and the cell responds to both O and A. (b) Shortly after adding nicotine the cell is slightly depolarised and spontaneously active, but still responsive to O and A. (c, d) The cell is further depolarised, to –25 mV, and produces only a vestigial action potential. The fact that it does not respond to A shows that it is electrically inexcitable. (e, f) In the continued presence of nicotine, the cell repolarises, and regains its responsiveness to A, but is still unresponsive to O, because the ACh receptors are desensitised by nicotine. (From: Ginsborg B L, Guerrero S 1964 J Physiol 172: 189)

also fail to produce an action potential. The main reason for the loss of electrical excitability during a period of maintained depolarisation is that the voltage-sensitive sodium channels (see Ch. 40) become inactivated (i.e. refractory) and no longer able to open in response to a brief depolarising stimulus.

A second type of effect is also seen in the experiment shown in Figure 7.4. After nicotine has acted for several minutes, the cell partially repolarises, and its electrical excitability returns, but, in spite of this, transmission remains blocked. This type of secondary, non-depolarising block occurs also at the neuromuscular junction when repeated doses of the depolarising drug, suxamethonium (see below) are used. The main factor responsible for the secondary block (known clinically as *phase II block*) appears to be *receptor desensitisation* (see Ch. 1). This causes the depolarising action of the blocking drug to subside, but transmission remains blocked because the receptors are desensitised to acetylcholine.

EFFECTS OF DRUGS ON CHOLINERGIC TRANSMISSION

Drugs can influence cholinergic transmission either by acting on acetylcholine receptors or by affecting the release or destruction of endogenous acetylcholine (Fig. 7.2).

Drugs that act on acetylcholine receptors may:

- mimic the action of acetylcholine (e.g. cholinergic agonists, such as **muscarine**, **nicotine** and various synthetic analogues of acetylcholine)
- block the action of acetylcholine (e.g. cholinergic antagonists, such as **atropine**, **tubocurarine** and similar agents).

Drugs that affect the release or destruction of acetylcholine may:

- enhance release (e.g. **4-aminopyridine** and related drugs, which affect the electrical properties of the presynaptic nerve terminals)
- inhibit cholinesterase, thereby increasing and prolonging the action of acetylcholine (e.g. **neostigmine**)
- inhibit acetylcholine release, by inhibiting synthesis (e.g. **hemicholinium**, which blocks choline uptake) or vesicular storage (e.g. **vesamicol**) or by inhibiting the release mechanism itself (e.g. **botulinum toxin, magnesium ion, aminoglycoside antibiotics**).

In the rest of this chapter we will consider the following

cell, which at first initiates action potential discharge. After a few seconds this discharge ceases, and transmission is blocked. The loss of electrical excitability at this time is shown by the fact that antidromic stimuli

groups of drugs, subdivided according to their physiological site of action:

- muscarinic agonists
- muscarinic antagonists
- ganglion-stimulating drugs
- ganglion-blocking drugs
- neuromuscular-blocking drugs
- anticholinesterases and other drugs that enhance cholinergic transmission.

DRUGS AFFECTING MUSCARINIC RECEPTORS

MUSCARINIC AGONISTS

Structure–activity relationships

Muscarinic agonists, as a group, are often referred to as *parasympathomimetic* because the main effects that they produce in the whole animal resemble those of parasympathetic stimulation. The structures of the most important compounds are given in Table 7.2. Acetylcholine itself and related choline esters are agonists at both muscarinic and nicotinic receptors, but act more potently on muscarinic receptors (see Fig. 7.1). Only bethanechol and pilocarpine are now used clinically.

The key features of the acetylcholine molecule that are important for its activity are the quaternary ammonium group, which bears a positive charge, and the ester group, which bears a partial negative charge, and is susceptible to rapid hydrolysis by cholinesterase. Variants of the choline ester structure (Table 7.2) have the effect of reducing the susceptibility of the compound to hydrolysis by cholinesterase, and altering the relative activity on muscarinic and nicotinic receptors.

Carbachol and **methacholine** are used as experimental tools. **Bethanechol**, which is a hybrid of these two molecules, is stable to hydrolysis and selective for muscarinic receptors, and is occasionally used clinically. **Pilocarpine** is a partial agonist, and shows some selectivity in stimulating secretion from sweat, salivary, lacrimal and bronchial glands, and contracting iris smooth muscle (see below), with weak effects on gastrointestinal smooth muscle and the heart.

Effects of muscarinic agonists

The main actions of muscarinic agonists are readily understood in terms of the parasympathetic nervous system.

Cardiovascular effects include cardiac slowing and a decrease in cardiac output. The latter action is due mainly to a decreased force of contraction of the atria, since the ventricles have only a sparse parasympathetic

innervation and a low sensitivity to muscarinic agonists (see Table 7.1). Generalised vasodilatation also occurs (an NO-mediated effect; see Ch. 11) and these two effects combine to produce a sharp fall in arterial pressure (Fig. 7.1). The mechanism of action of muscarinic agonists on the heart is discussed in Chapter 14.

Smooth muscle, other than vascular smooth muscle, contracts in response to muscarinic agonists. Peristaltic activity of the gastrointestinal tract is increased, which can cause colicky pain, and the bladder and bronchial smooth muscle also contract.

Sweating, lacrimation, salivation and *bronchial secretion* result from stimulation of exocrine glands. The combined effect of bronchial secretion and constriction can interfere with breathing.

Effects on the eye are of some importance. The parasympathetic nerves to the eye supply the *constrictor pupillae* muscle, which runs circumferentially in the iris, and the *ciliary muscle*, which adjusts the curvature of the lens (Fig. 7.5). Contraction of the ciliary muscle in response to activation of muscarinic receptors pulls the ciliary body forwards and inwards, thus relaxing the tension on the suspensory ligament of the lens, allowing the lens to bulge more and reducing its focal length. This parasympathetic reflex is thus necessary to accommodate the eye for near vision. The *constrictor pupillae* is important not only for adjusting the pupil in response to changes in light intensity, but also in regulating the intraocular pressure. Aqueous humour is secreted slowly and continuously by the cells of the epithelium covering the ciliary body, and it drains into the *canal of Schlemm* (Fig. 7.5) which runs around the eye close to the outer margin of the iris. The intraocular pressure is normally 10–15 mmHg above atmospheric, which keeps the eye slightly distended. Abnormally raised intraocular pressure (associated with glaucoma) damages the eye and is one of the commonest preventable causes of blindness. In acute glaucoma drainage of aqueous humour becomes impeded when the pupil is dilated because folding of the iris tissue occludes the drainage angle, causing the intraocular pressure to rise. Activation of the *constrictor pupillae* muscle by muscarinic agonists in these circumstances lowers the intraocular pressure, though in a normal individual it has little effect. The increased tension in the ciliary muscle produced by these drugs may also play a part in improving drainage by realigning the connective tissue trabeculae through which the canal of Schlemm passes.

Clinical use

The main use of muscarinic agonists is in treating glaucoma, by local instillation in the form of eye drops.

Table 7.2 Muscarinic agonists

Drug	Structure	Receptor specificity		Hydrolysis by AChE	Clinical uses
		Musc	*Nic*		
Acetylcholine		+++	+++	+++	None
Carbachol		++	+++	–	None
Methacholine		+++	+	++	None
Bethanechol		+++	–	–	Bladder* and GI hypotonia
Muscarine		+++	–	–	None[†]
Pilocarpine		++	–	–	Glaucoma
Oxotremorine		++	–	–	None

*Necessary to ensure that bladder neck is not obstructed.
[†]Cause of mushroom poisoning.

Pilocarpine is the most effective as, being a tertiary amine, it can cross the conjunctival membrane. It is a stable compound whose action lasts for about 1 day. A variety of drugs with different mechanisms of action are now available for the treatment of glaucoma, and are summarised in Table 7.3.

Bethanechol is very occasionally used to assist bladder emptying or to stimulate gastrointestinal motility (see Table 7.2). These effects are mediated mainly through M_1-receptors (see Table 7.1). In principle, a selective M_2 agonist would be useful for treating cardiac dysrhythmias but such drugs remain to be discovered.

MUSCARINIC ANTAGONISTS

Muscarinic receptor antagonists are often referred to as *parasympatholytic* because they selectively block the effects of parasympathetic nerve activity. All of them are competitive antagonists, and their chemical structures usually contain ester and basic groups in the same relationship as acetylcholine, but they have an aromatic group in place of the acetyl group. The two naturally occurring compounds, **atropine** and **hyoscine**, are alkaloids found in solanaceous plants. The deadly nightshade (*Atropa belladonna*) contains mainly atropine, whereas

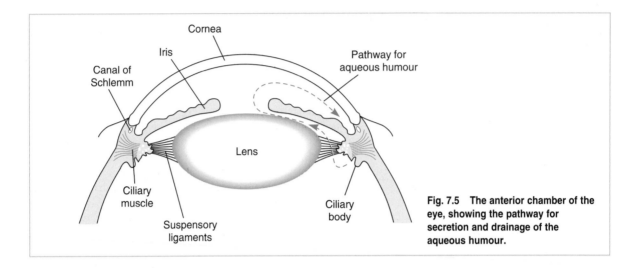

Fig. 7.5   The anterior chamber of the eye, showing the pathway for secretion and drainage of the aqueous humour.

Table 7.3   Drugs that lower intraocular pressure

Drug	Mechanism	Notes	Reference
Pilocarpine	Muscarinic agonist	Widely used as eye drops.	This chapter
Ecothiopate	Anticholinesterase	Widely used as eye drops. Can cause muscle spasm and systemic effects	This chapter
Timolol, carteolol	β-adrenoceptor antagonist	Given as eye-drops, but may still cause systemic side-effects: bradycardia, bronchoconstriction	Ch. 8
Acetazolamide, dorzolamide	Carbonic anhydrase inhibitor	Acetazolamide is given systemically. Side-effects, include diuresis, loss of appetite, tingling, neutropenia. Dorzolamide is used as eye drops. Side-effects include bitter taste and burning sensation	Ch. 20
Clonidine, apraclonidine, bromonidine	α_2-adrenoceptor agonist	Used as eye drops	Ch. 8
Latanoprost	Prostaglandin analogue	Can cause ocular pigmentation	Ch. 12

The most important drugs are shown in bold type.

the thorn apple (*Datura stramonium*) contains mainly hyoscine. These are tertiary ammonium compounds, which are sufficiently lipid soluble to be readily absorbed from the gut or conjunctival sac, and, importantly, to penetrate the blood–brain barrier. The quaternary derivative of atropine, **atropine methonitrate**, has peripheral actions very similar to those of atropine but, because of its exclusion from the brain, lacks central actions. **Ipratropium**, another quaternary ammonium compound, is used by inhalation as a bronchodilator. **Cyclopentolate** and **tropicamide** are tertiary amines developed for

ophthalmic use and administered as eye drops. **Pirenzepine** is a relatively selective M_1-receptor antagonist. Other subtype-specific antagonists, used experimentally but not yet clinically, include **AF-DX-116** (M_2-selective, acting mainly on the heart), and **himbacine** (M_4-selective, with mainly CNS effects).

Effects of muscarinic antagonists

All of the muscarinic antagonists produce basically similar peripheral effects, though some show a degree of selectivity, e.g. for the heart or the gastrointestinal tract, reflecting heterogeneity among muscarinic receptors (see p. 113).

The main effects of atropine are:

Inhibition of secretions. Salivary, lacrimal, bronchial and sweat glands are inhibited by very low doses of atropine, producing an uncomfortably dry mouth and skin. Gastric secretion is only slightly reduced. Mucociliary clearance in the bronchi is inhibited, so that residual secretions tend to accumulate in the lungs. **Ipratropium** lacks this effect.

Effects on heart rate. Atropine causes tachycardia, due to block of cardiac muscarinic receptors. The tachycardia is modest, up to 80–90 beats/min in humans. This is because there is no effect on the sympathetic system, but only inhibition of the existing parasympathetic tone. At very low doses, atropine causes a paradoxical bradycardia, which results from a central action, increasing vagal activity The response of the heart to exercise is unaffected. Arterial blood pressure is unaffected, since most resistance vessels have no cholinergic innervation.

Effects on the eye. The pupil is dilated (mydriasis)* by atropine administration, and becomes unresponsive to light. Relaxation of the ciliary muscle causes paralysis of accommodation (cycloplegia), so that near vision is impaired. Intraocular pressure may rise; though this is unimportant in normal individuals, it can be dangerous in patients suffering from narrow-angle glaucoma.

Effects on the GI tract. Gastrointestinal motility is inhibited by atropine, though this requires larger doses than the other effects listed, and is not complete. This is because excitatory transmitters other than acetylcholine are important in normal function of the myenteric plexus (see Chs 6, 9 and 21). Atropine is used in pathological conditions in which there is increased gastrointestinal motility; agents selective for M_3-receptors, which are being developed, may be preferable. **Pirenzepine**, owing to its selectivity for M_1-receptors, inhibits gastric acid secretion in doses that do not affect other systems.

Effects on other smooth muscle. Bronchial, biliary and urinary tract smooth muscle are all relaxed by atropine. Reflex bronchoconstriction (e.g. during anaesthesia) is prevented by atropine, whereas bronchoconstriction caused by local mediators, such as histamine and leuko-

trienes (e.g. in asthma; Ch. 19) is unaffected. Biliary and urinary tract smooth muscle are only slightly affected, probably because transmitters other than acetylcholine (see Ch. 6) are important in these organs; nevertheless, atropine and similar drugs commonly precipitate urinary retention in elderly men with prostatic enlargement.

Effects on the CNS. Atropine produces mainly excitatory effects on the central nervous system. At low doses this causes mild restlessness; higher doses cause agitation and disorientation. In *atropine poisoning*, which occurs mainly in young children who eat deadly nightshade berries, marked excitement and irritability result in hyperactivity and a considerable rise in body temperature, which is accentuated by the loss of sweating. These central effects are evidently the result of blocking muscarinic receptors in the brain, since they are opposed by anticholinesterase drugs such as **physostigmine**, which is an effective antidote to atropine poisoning. It is thus surprising that **hyoscine** has different central actions, causing marked sedation in low doses, though similar effects in high dosage. Hyoscine also has a useful antiemetic effect, and is used in treating motion sickness. Muscarinic antagonists also affect the extrapyramidal system, reducing the involuntary movement and rigidity of patients with Parkinson's disease (Ch. 31) and counteracting the extrapyramidal side-effects of many antipsychotic drugs (Ch. 34).

Drugs acting on muscarinic receptors

Muscarinic agonists
- Important compounds include ACh, carbachol, methacholine, muscarine and pilocarpine. They vary in muscarinic/nicotinic selectivity, and in susceptibility to cholinesterase.
- Main effects are: bradycardia and vasodilatation (endothelium-dependent), leading to fall in blood pressure; contraction of visceral smooth muscle (gut, bladder, bronchi, etc.); exocrine secretions, pupillary constriction and ciliary muscle contraction, leading to decrease of intraocular pressure.
- Main use is in treatment of glaucoma (esp. pilocarpine).

Muscarinic antagonists
- Most important compounds are atropine, hyoscine, ipratropium and pirenzepine.
- Main effects are: inhibition of secretions; tachycardia, pupillary dilatation and paralysis of accommodation; relaxation of smooth muscle (gut, bronchi, biliary tract, bladder); inhibition of gastric acid secretion (esp. pirenzepine); CNS effects (mainly excitatory with atropine; depressant, including amnesia, with hyoscine), including anti-emetic effect and anti-parkinsonian effect.

---

*The alluring quality of dilated pupils was well understood by Greek and Roman courtesans, whose cosmetic use of eye drops containing deadly nightshade berries led to the plant being called belladonna. Inability to see properly was evidently considered a price worth paying. The practice was also taken up by ballerinas, who, one might have thought, could easily have ended up hurtling off the stage.

Table 7.4 Muscarinic antagonists

Compound	Pharmacological properties	Clinical uses	Notes
Atropine	Non-selective antagonist Well absorbed orally CNS stimulant	• Adjunct for anaesthesia (reduced secretions, bronchodilatation) • Anticholinesterase poisoning • Bradycardia • GI hypermotility (antispasmodic)	Belladonna alkaloid Main side-effects: • urinary retention • dry mouth • blurred vision Dicyclomine is similar and used mainly as antispasmodic agent
Hyoscine (scopolamine)	Similar to atropine CNS depressant	As atropine • Motion sickness	Belladonna alkaloid Side-effects as atropine
Atropine methonitrate	Similar to atropine, but poorly absorbed and lacks CNS effects Significant ganglion-blocking activity	Mainly for GI hypermotility.	Quaternary ammonium derivative. Similar drugs include hyoscine butylbromide, propantheline
Ipratropium	Similar to atropine methonitrate Does not inhibit mucociliary clearance from bronchi	By inhalation for asthma, bronchitis	Quaternary ammonium compound
Tropicamide	Similar to atropine May raise intraocular pressure	Ophthalmic use to produce mydriasis and cycloplegia (as eye drops). Short-acting	
Cyclopentolate	Similar to tropicamide	As tropicamide (long-acting)	
Pirenzepine	Selective for M_1-receptors Inhibits gastric secretion by action on ganglion cells Little effect on smooth muscle or in CNS	Peptic ulcer	Fewer side effects than other muscarinic antagonists Largely superseded by other anti-ulcer drugs (see Ch. 21)

For chemical structures, see Hardman et al 1995.

Clinical uses of muscarinic antagonists

Cardiovascular
• Treatment of sinus bradycardia (e.g. after myocardial infarction; see Ch. 14): intravenous **atropine**.

Ophthalmic
• To dilate the pupil: e.g. **tropicamide eye drops** (relatively short-acting); **cyclopentolate eye drops** (long-acting).

Neurological
• Prevention of motion sickness: e.g. **hyoscine**, orally or transdermally.
• Parkinsonism (see Ch. 31), especially to counteract movement disorders caused by antipsychotic drugs (see Ch. 34): e.g. **benzhexol**, **benztropine**.

Respiratory
• Asthma (see Ch. 19): **ipratropium** by inhalation.

• Anaesthetic premedication to dry secretions: e.g. **atropine**, **hyoscine** by injection. Less commonly used nowadays since current anaesthetics are relatively non-irritant (see Ch. 32).

Gastrointestinal—to relax gastrointestinal smooth muscle ('antispasmodic' action) and suppress gastric acid secretion (see Ch. 21)
• To facilitate endoscopy and gastrointestinal radiology: e.g. **hyoscine butylbromide** intravenously.
• Irritable bowel syndrome, colonic diverticular disease: e.g. **dicyclomine** orally.
• Peptic ulcer disease; **pirenzepine** (M_1-selective, now less used since introduction of histamine H_2-antagonists and proton pump inhibitors).

The main uses of muscarinic antagonists are shown in Table 7.4 and the clinical box (p. 122).

DRUGS AFFECTING AUTONOMIC GANGLIA

GANGLION STIMULANTS

Most nicotinic receptor agonists affect both ganglionic and motor endplate receptors, but some show selectivity.

Nicotine (Table 7.5), **lobeline** and **dimethylphenyl-piperazinium** (DMPP) affect ganglionic nicotinic receptors preferentially. Nicotine and lobeline are tertiary amines found in the leaves of tobacco and lobelia plants respectively. Nicotine is well established in pharmacological folklore as it was the substance on the tip of Langley's paintbrush which he found would stimulate muscle fibres when applied to the endplate region, and which caused him to postulate in 1905 the existence of a 'receptive substance' on the surface of the fibres (Ch. 6). Both of these substances affect the neuromuscular junction in concentrations only slightly greater than those that affect ganglia. DMPP is a synthetic compound that is selective for ganglionic receptors.

These substances are not used clinically, but only as experimental tools. Nicotine is discussed in Chapter 39. They cause complex peripheral responses associated with generalised stimulation of autonomic ganglia. The effects of nicotine on the gastrointestinal tract and sweat glands are familiar to neophyte smokers (see Ch. 39), though usually insufficient to act as an effective deterrent.

GANGLION-BLOCKING DRUGS

Ganglion block can occur by several mechanisms:

- *By interference with acetylcholine release*, as at the neuromuscular junction (see p. 130 and Ch. 6). **Botulinum toxin**, **hemicholinium**, and magnesium ion all work in this way, causing skeletal muscle paralysis at the same time as ganglion block.
- *By prolonged depolarisation.* **Nicotine** (see Fig. 7.4) can block ganglia, after initial stimulation, in this way, as can acetylcholine itself if cholinesterase is inhibited so that it can exert a continuing action on the postsynaptic membrane. This type of block is of little importance at the ganglionic synapse.
- *By interference with the postsynaptic action of acetylcholine.* The few ganglion-blocking drugs of practical importance act by blocking neuronal nicotinic receptors or the associated ion channels.

50 years ago, Paton & Zaimis investigated a series of linear bis-quaternary compounds. Compounds with five or six carbon atoms (**hexamethonium**; Table 7.5) in the methylene chain linking the two quaternary groups produced ganglionic block, whereas compounds with

Table 7.5	Nicotinic receptor agonists and antagonists		
Drugs	Main site	Type of action	Notes
Agonists			
Nicotine	Autonomic ganglia	Stimulation then block	No clinical uses
	CNS	Stimulation	For CNS effects, see Ch. 39
Lobeline	Autonomic ganglia	Stimulation	
	Sensory nerve terminals	Stimulation	
Epibatidine	Autonomic ganglia, CNS	Stimulation	Isolated from frog skin. Highly potent. No clinical uses
Suxamethonium	Neuromuscular junction	Depolarisation block	Used clinically as muscle relaxant
Decamethonium	Neuromuscular junction	Depolarisation block	No clinical use
Antagonists			
Hexamethonium	Autonomic ganglia	Transmission block	No clinical use
Trimetaphan	Autonomic ganglia	Transmission block	Blood pressure lowering in surgery (rarely used)
Tubocurarine	Neuromuscular junction	Transmission block	Now rarely used
Pancuronium Atracurium Vecuronium	Neuromuscular junction	Transmission block	Widely used as muscle relaxants in anaesthesia

nine or ten carbon atoms (**decamethonium**) produced neuromuscular block.*

Hexamethonium deserves recognition as the first effective antihypertensive agent (see Ch. 15). Though no longer in clinical use, it is a valuable experimental tool. The only ganglion-blocking drug currently in clinical use is **trimetaphan** (Table 7.5; see below).

Effects of ganglion-blocking drugs

The effects of ganglion-blocking drugs are numerous and complex, as would be expected, since both divisions of the autonomic nervous system are blocked indiscriminately. The description by Paton of 'hexamethonium man' cannot be bettered:

He is a pink-complexioned person, except when he has stood in a queue for a long time, when he may get pale and faint. His handshake is warm and dry. He is a placid and relaxed companion; for instance he may laugh but he can't cry because the tears cannot come. Your rudest story will not make him blush, and the most unpleasant circumstances will fail to make him turn pale. His collars and socks stay very clean and sweet. He wears corsets and may, if you meet him out, be rather fidgety (corsets to compress his splanchnic vascular pool, fidgety to keep the venous return going from his legs). He dislikes speaking much unless helped with something to moisten his dry mouth and throat. He is long-sighted and easily blinded by bright light. The redness of his eyeballs may suggest irregular habits and in fact his head is rather weak. But he always behaves like a gentleman and never belches or hiccups. He tends to get cold and keeps well wrapped up. But his health is good; he does not have chilblains and those diseases of modern civilization, hypertension and peptic ulcer, pass him by. He gets thin because his appetite is modest; he never feels hunger pains and his stomach never rumbles. He gets rather constipated so that his intake of liquid paraffin is high. As old age comes on, he will suffer from retention

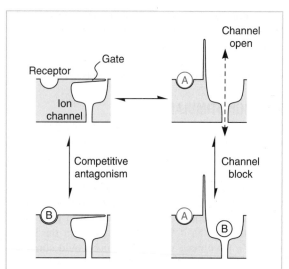

Fig. 7.6 Acetylcholine antagonism by receptor block (left) and channel block (right). The latter mechanism of action applies to many ganglion-blocking drugs. The gating mechanism shown is purely diagrammatic, and bears no resemblance to the molecular structure. (A = ACh molecule; B = blocking molecule)

of urine and impotence, but frequency, precipitancy and strangury will not worry him. One is uncertain how he will end, but perhaps if he is not careful, by eating less and less and getting colder and colder, he will sink into a symptomless, hypoglycaemic coma and die, as was proposed for the universe, a sort of entropy death.

In practice, the important effects are on the cardiovascular system. A marked fall in arterial blood pressure results mainly from block of sympathetic ganglia, which causes arteriolar vasodilatation. Most cardiovascular reflexes are blocked. In particular, the venoconstriction, which occurs normally when a subject stands up, and which is necessary to prevent the central venous pressure from falling sharply, is reduced. Standing thus causes a sudden fall in cardiac output and arterial pressure (*postural hypotension*) that can cause fainting. Similarly, the vasodilatation of skeletal muscle during exercise is normally accompanied by vasoconstriction elsewhere (e.g. splanchnic area) produced by sympathetic activity. If this adjustment is prevented, the overall peripheral resistance falls and the blood pressure also falls (*post-exercise hypotension*).

Clinical use

Ganglion-blocking drugs, because of their many side-effects, are now clinically obsolete, with the exception

---

*Because of the structural similarity of the methonium series of compounds to acetylcholine they were originally believed to act as competitive antagonists at the receptor sites. However, such drugs are now known to block, not the receptor, but the associated ion channel (see Ch. 2).

Tubocurarine (see p. 125) blocks ganglionic as well as neuromuscular transmission. On the ganglion its action is on the ion channel, whereas at the neuromuscular junction it binds mainly to the receptor, with only a minor component of channel block.

Channel block as a mechanism for regulating membrane excitability (Fig. 7.6) is discussed in relation to the heart (Ch. 14) and antiepileptic drugs (Ch. 36).

of **trimetaphan**, a very short-acting drug that can be administered as an intravenous infusion for certain types of anaesthetic procedure. Tilting of the operating table results in controlled hypotension, used to minimise bleeding during certain kinds of surgery. Trimetaphan can also be used to lower blood pressure as an emergency procedure.

Drugs acting on autonomic ganglia

Ganglion-stimulating drugs

- Compounds include nicotine, DMPP.
- Both sympathetic and parasympathetic ganglia are stimulated, so effects are complex, including: tachycardia and increase of blood pressure, variable effects on gastrointestinal motility and secretions, increased bronchial, salivary and sweat secretions. Additional effects result from stimulation of other neuronal structures, including sensory and noradrenergic nerve terminals.
- Ganglion stimulation may be followed by depolarisation block.
- Nicotine also has important CNS effects.
- No therapeutic uses.

Ganglion-blocking drugs

- Compounds include hexamethonium, trimetaphan, tubocurarine (also nicotine; see above).
- Block all autonomic ganglia and enteric ganglia. Main effects: hypotension and loss of cardiovascular reflexes, inhibition of secretions, gastrointestinal paralysis; impaired micturition.
- Clinically obsolete, except for occasional use of trimetaphan to produce controlled hypotension in anaesthesia.

NEUROMUSCULAR-BLOCKING DRUGS

The pharmacology of neuromuscular function is well reviewed by Bowman (1990). Drugs can block neuromuscular transmission either by acting presynaptically to inhibit acetylcholine synthesis or release, or by acting postsynaptically, the latter being the site of action of all of the clinically important drugs (except for **botulinum toxin**; see below).

Clinically, neuromuscular block is used only as an adjunct to anaesthesia, when artificial ventilation is available; it is not a therapeutic intervention. The drugs that are used all work by interfering with the postsynaptic action of acetylcholine. They fall into two categories:

- non-depolarising blocking agents (the majority), which act by blocking acetylcholine receptors (and, in some cases, also by blocking ion channels)
- depolarising blocking agents, which are agonists at acetylcholine receptors.

NON-DEPOLARISING BLOCKING AGENTS

In 1856 Claude Bernard, in a famous experiment, showed that 'curare' causes paralysis by blocking neuromuscular transmission, rather than by abolishing nerve conduction or muscle contractility. 'Curare' is a mixture of naturally occurring alkaloids found in various South American plants and used as arrow poisons by South American Indians. Many of these substances have neuromuscular-blocking activity, but the most important is **tubocurarine**, the structure of which was elucidated in 1935. Tubocurarine is now rarely used in clinical medicine, but a number of synthetic drugs with very similar actions have been developed, the most important ones being **pancuronium**, **vecuronium** and **atracurium** (Table 7.6), which differ mainly in their duration of action. **Gallamine** was the first useful synthetic successor to tubocurarine, but has been superseded by compounds with fewer side-effects. These substances are all quaternary ammonium compounds, which means that they are poorly absorbed and generally rapidly excreted. They also fail to cross the placenta, which is important in relation to their use in obstetric anaesthesia. The low oral absorption of tubocurarine allowed it to be used safely in the hunting of animals for food.

Mechanism of action

Non-depolarising blocking agents all act as competitive antagonists (see Ch. 1) at the acetylcholine receptors of the endplate, and this largely accounts for their actions. The amount of acetylcholine released by a nerve impulse normally exceeds by several-fold what is needed to elicit an action potential in the muscle fibre. It is therefore necessary to block 70–80% of the receptor sites before transmission actually fails. When this happens it is still possible to record a small endplate potential in the muscle fibre though its amplitude fails to reach threshold (Fig. 7.7). In any individual muscle fibre, transmission is all-or-nothing, so graded degrees of block represent a varying proportion of muscle fibres failing to respond. In this situation, where the amplitude of endplate potential in all of the fibres is close to threshold (just above in some, just below in others) small variations in the amount of transmitter released, or in the rate at which it is destroyed, will have a large effect on the proportion of fibres contracting, so the degree of block is liable to vary according to various physiological circumstances (e.g. stimulation frequency, temperature, cholinesterase

Table 7.6 Characteristics of neuromuscular-blocking drugs

Drug	Speed of onset	Duration of action	Main side-effects	Notes
Tubocurarine	Slow (>5 min)	Long (1–2 h)	Hypotension (ganglion block plus histamine release) Bronchoconstriction (histamine release)	Plant alkaloid, now rarely used Alcuronium is a semisynthetic derivative with similar properties but fewer side-effects
Gallamine	Slow	Long	Tachycardia (muscarinic antagonist)	100% renal excretion; therefore to be avoided in patients with poor renal function The first synthetic alternative to tubocurarine, now rarely used
Pancuronium	Intermediate (2–3 min)	Long	Slight tachycardia. No hypotension	The first steroid-based compound. Better side-effect profile than tubocurarine. Widely used Pipecuronium is similar
Vecuronium	Intermediate	Intermediate (30–40 min)	Few side-effects	Widely used. Occasionally causes prolonged paralysis, probably due to active metabolite Rocuronium is similar, with faster onset
Atracurium	Intermediate	Intermediate (<30 min)	Transient hypotension (histamine release)	Unusual mechanism of elimination (spontaneous non-enzymic chemical degradation in plasma). Degradation slowed by acidosis Widely used Doxacurium is chemically similar, but stable in plasma, giving it long duration of action Cisatracurium is the pure isomeric constituent of atracurium, similar but with less histamine release
Mivacurium	Fast (~2 min)	Short (~15 min)	Transient hypotension (histamine release)	New drug, chemically similar to atracurium, but rapidly inactivated by plasma cholinesterase (therefore longer acting in patients with liver disease or with genetic cholinesterase deficiency (see p. 129)
Suxamethonium	Fast	Short (~10 min)	Bradycardia (muscarinic agonist effect) Cardiac arrhythmias (increased plasma potassium concentration—avoid in patients with burns or severe trauma) Raised intraocular pressure (nicotinic agonist effect on extraocular muscles) Postoperative muscle pain	Acts by depolarisation of endplate (nicotinic agonist effect)—the only drug of this type still in use Paralysis is preceded by transient muscle fasciculations Short duration of action due to hydrolysis by plasma cholinesterase (prolonged action in patients with liver disease or genetic deficiency of plasma cholinesterase) Used for brief procedures (e.g. tracheal intubation, electroconvulsive shock therapy). Rocuronium has similar speed of onset and recovery with fewer unwanted effects

For chemical structures, see Hardman et al 1995.

inhibition, etc.) which normally have relatively little effect on the efficiency of transmission.

In addition to blocking receptors, some of these drugs also block ion channels in a manner similar to the ganglion-blocking drugs, though this is probably of little importance in practice. Furthermore (see Prior et al. 1995), some non-depolarising blocking agents also appear to block presynaptic autoreceptors, and thus

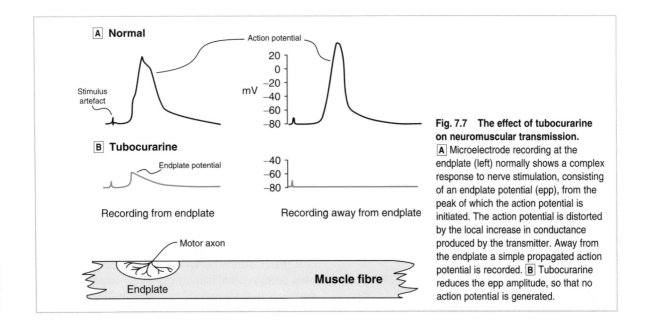

A Normal

Stimulus artefact

Action potential

Endplate potential

B Tubocurarine

Recording from endplate

Recording away from endplate

Motor axon

Endplate

Muscle fibre

Fig. 7.7 The effect of tubocurarine on neuromuscular transmission. **A** Microelectrode recording at the endplate (left) normally shows a complex response to nerve stimulation, consisting of an endplate potential (epp), from the peak of which the action potential is initiated. The action potential is distorted by the local increase in conductance produced by the transmitter. Away from the endplate a simple propagated action potential is recorded. **B** Tubocurarine reduces the epp amplitude, so that no action potential is generated.

inhibit the release of acetylcholine during repetitive stimulation of the motor nerve. This may play a part in causing the 'tetanic fade' seen with these drugs (see p. 129).

Effects of non-depolarising blocking drugs

The effects of non-depolarising neuromuscular-blocking agents are mainly due to motor paralysis, though some of the drugs also produce clinically significant autonomic effects. The first muscles to be affected are the extrinsic eye muscles (causing double vision) and the small muscles of the face, limbs and pharynx (causing difficulty in swallowing). Respiratory muscles are the last to be affected and the first to recover. An experiment in 1947 in which a heroic volunteer was fully curarised under artificial ventilation established this orderly paralytic march, and showed that consciousness and awareness of pain were quite normal even when paralysis was complete. The special characteristics of non-depolarising block, and the ways in which it differs from depolarisation block are described on page 129.

Unwanted effects

The main side-effect of tubocurarine is a fall in arterial pressure, mainly due to ganglion block. An additional cause is the release of histamine from mast cells (see Ch. 12), which can also give rise to bronchospasm in sensitive individuals. This is unrelated to nicotinic receptors, and is an effect common to many strongly

basic drugs. The other non-depolarising blocking drugs, especially vecuronium, cause less ganglion block and histamine release than tubocurarine, and hence less hypotension. Gallamine, and to a lesser extent pancuronium, block muscarinic receptors, particularly in the heart, which results in tachycardia.

Pharmacokinetic aspects

Neuromuscular-blocking agents are used mainly in anaesthesia to produce muscle relaxation. They are given intravenously, but differ in their rates of onset and recovery (Table 7.6, Fig. 7.8).

The non-depolarising blocking agents are mostly metabolised by the liver or excreted unchanged in the urine, exceptions being **atracurium**, which hydrolyses spontaneously in plasma, and **mivacurium**, which, like **suxamethonium**, is hydrolysed by plasma cholinesterase. Their duration of action varies between about 15 minutes and 1–2 hours (Table 7.6), by which time the patient regains enough strength to cough and breathe properly, though residual weakness may persist for much longer. The route of elimination is important, since many patients undergoing anaesthesia have impaired renal or hepatic function, which, depending on the drug used, can enhance or prolong the paralysis to an important degree. The action of gallamine, for example, may be dangerously prolonged in patients with renal failure.

Atracurium was designed to be chemically unstable at physiological pH (splitting into two inactive fragments

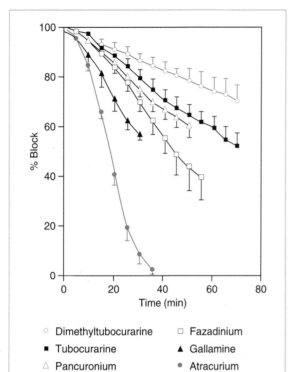

○ Dimethyltubocurarine ☐ Fazadinium
■ Tubocurarine ▲ Gallamine
△ Pancuronium ● Atracurium

Fig. 7.8 Rate of recovery from various non-depolarising neuromuscular-blocking drugs in man. Drugs were given intravenously to patients undergoing surgery, in doses just sufficient to cause 100% block of the tetanic tension of the indirectly stimulated adductor pollicis muscle. Recovery of tension was then followed as a function of time. (From: Payne J P, Hughes R 1981 Br J Anaesth 53: 45)

by cleavage at one of the quaternary nitrogen atoms), though indefinitely stable when stored at an acid pH. It has a short duration of action, which is unaffected by renal or hepatic function. Because of the marked pH-dependence of its degradation, however, its action becomes considerably briefer during respiratory alkalosis caused by hyperventilation.

DEPOLARISING BLOCKING AGENTS

This class of neuromuscular-blocking drugs was discovered by Paton & Zaimis in their study of the effects of symmetrical bisquaternary ammonium compounds. One of these, decamethonium, was found to cause paralysis without appreciable ganglion-blocking activity. Several features of its action showed it to be different from competitive blocking drugs such as tubocurarine. In particular it was found to produce a transient twitching

of skeletal muscle (fasciculation) before causing block, and when it was injected into chicks it caused a powerful extensor spasm, whereas tubocurarine simply caused flaccid paralysis. In 1951 Burns & Paton showed that its action was to cause a maintained depolarisation at the endplate region of the muscle fibre, which led to a loss of electrical excitability (see p. 117), and they coined the term 'depolarisation block'. The reason for the curious extensor spasm produced in birds is that they possess a special type of skeletal muscle, rare in mammals, that has many endplates scattered over the surface of each muscle fibre. A drug that causes endplate depolarisation produces a widespread depolarisation in such muscles, resulting in a maintained contracture. In normal skeletal muscle, with only one endplate per fibre, endplate depolarisation is too localised to cause contracture on its own. Fasciculation occurs because the developing endplate depolarisation initially causes a discharge of action potentials in the muscle fibre. This subsides after a few seconds as the electrical excitability of the endplate region of the fibre is lost.

Decamethonium itself was used clinically but has the disadvantage of too long a duration of action. Suxamethonium (Table 7.5) is closely related in structure to both decamethonium and acetylcholine (consisting of two acetylcholine molecules linked by their acetyl groups). Its action is shorter than that of decamethonium because it is quickly hydrolysed by plasma cholinesterase. Suxamethonium and decamethonium act on the motor endplate just like acetylcholine (i.e. they are agonists that increase the cation permeability of the endplate). The difference is that decamethonium and suxamethonium, when given as drugs, diffuse slowly to the endplate and the concentration at the endplate persists for long enough to cause loss of electrical excitability. Acetylcholine, in contrast, when released from the nerve, reaches the endplate in very brief spurts and is rapidly hydrolysed in situ, so it never causes sufficiently prolonged depolarisation to result in block. If cholinesterase is inhibited, however (see p. 135), it is possible for the circulating acetylcholine concentration to reach a level sufficient to cause depolarisation block.

Comparison of non-depolarising and depolarising blocking drugs

There are several differences in the pattern of neuromuscular block produced by these two mechanisms:

Anticholinesterase drugs are very effective in overcoming the blocking action of competitive agents. This is because the released acetylcholine, protected from hydrolysis, can diffuse further within the synaptic cleft, and so gains access to a wider area of postsynaptic membrane than it normally would. The chances of an acetylcholine molecule finding an unoccupied receptor before being hydrolysed are thus increased. This diffusional effect seems to be of more importance than a truly competitive interaction, for it is unlikely that appreciable dissociation of the antagonist can occur in the short time for which the acetylcholine is present. In contrast, depolarisation block is unaffected, or even increased, by anticholinesterase drugs.

The fasciculations seen with suxamethonium (see Table 7.6) as a prelude to paralysis do not occur with competitive drugs. There appears to be a correlation between the amount of fasciculation and the severity of the postoperative muscle pain that is often produced by suxamethonium.

'Tetanic fade' (a term used to describe the failure of muscle tension to be maintained during a brief period of nerve stimulation at a frequency high enough to produce a fused tetanus) is increased by non-depolarising blocking drugs, compared with normal muscle. This is probably due mainly to the block of presynaptic nicotinic receptors, which normally serve to sustain transmitter release during a tetanus (see Prior et al. 1995), and it does not occur with depolarisation block. This forms the basis of a simple test used by anaesthetists to discover which type of block is present. Electrodes are applied to the skin over a peripheral nerve, such as the ulnar nerve, and muscle contraction is observed during a short period of tetanic stimulation.

Unwanted effects and dangers of depolarising drugs

Suxamethonium, the only drug of this type in clinical use, can produce a number of important adverse effects (see Table 7.6).

Bradycardia. This is preventable by atropine and is probably due to a direct muscarinic action.

Potassium release. The increase in cation permeability of the motor endplates causes a net loss of potassium from muscle and, thus, a small rise in plasma potassium concentration. In normal individuals this is not important, but in cases of trauma, especially burns or injuries causing muscle denervation, it may be (Fig. 7.9). This is because denervation causes acetylcholine receptors to spread to regions of the muscle fibre away from the endplates (see Ch. 6), so that a much larger area of membrane is sensitive to suxamethonium. The resulting hyperkalaemia can be enough to cause serious ventricular dysrhythmia or even cardiac arrest.

Increased intraocular pressure. This results from contracture of extraocular muscles applying pressure to

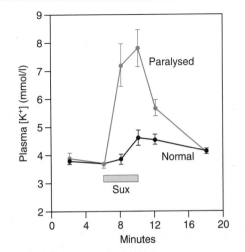

Fig. 7.9 Effect of suxamethonium on plasma potassium concentration in man. Blood was collected from veins draining paralysed and non-paralysed limbs of seven injured patients undergoing surgery. The injuries had resulted in motor nerve degeneration, and hence denervation supersensitivity of the affected muscles. (From: Tobey R E et al. 1972 Anaesthesiology 37: 322)

the eyeball. It is particularly important to avoid this if the eyeball has been injured.

Prolonged paralysis. The action of suxamethonium given intravenously normally lasts for less than 5 minutes because the drug is hydrolysed by plasma cholinesterase. Its action is prolonged by various factors that reduce the activity of this enzyme:

- Genetic variants in which plasma cholinesterase is abnormal (see Ch. 48). Severe deficiency, enough to increase the duration of action to 2 hours or more, occurs in only about 1 in 2000 individuals. Very rarely, the enzyme is completely absent and the paralysis lasts for many hours.
- Anticholinesterase drugs. The use of organophosphates to treat glaucoma (see Table 7.3) can inhibit plasma cholinesterase and prolong the action of suxamethonium. Competing substrates for plasma cholinesterase (e.g. procaine, propanidid) can also have this effect.
- Neonates and patients with liver disease may have low plasma cholinesterase activity and show prolonged paralysis with suxamethonium.

Malignant hyperthermia. This is a rare inherited condition, determined by an autosomal dominant gene (see Ch. 48), which results in intense muscle spasm and a dramatic rise in body temperature when certain drugs are given. The most commonly implicated drugs are suxamethonium and halothane, though it can be precipitated by a variety of other drugs. The condition carries a very high mortality (about 65%), and is treated by administration of **dantrolene**, a drug that inhibits muscle contraction by preventing calcium release from the sarcoplasmic reticulum.

DRUGS THAT ACT PRESYNAPTICALLY

Drugs that inhibit acetylcholine synthesis

The steps in the synthesis of acetylcholine in the presynaptic nerve terminals are shown in Figure 7.2. The rate-limiting process appears to be the transport of choline into the nerve terminal, and drugs (e.g. **hemicholinium** and **triethylcholine**) that inhibit acetylcholine synthesis do so by blocking this step. They are useful as experimental tools but have no clinical applications. Hemicholinium acts as a competitive inhibitor of choline uptake, but is not appreciably taken up itself. Triethylcholine, as well as inhibiting choline uptake, is itself transported and acetylated within the terminals, forming acetyltriethylcholine. This is stored in place of acetylcholine, and released as a false transmitter, but has no depolarising effect on the postsynaptic membrane. The blocking effect of these drugs develops slowly, as the existing stores of acetylcholine become depleted. **Vesamicol**, which acts by blocking acetylcholine transport into synaptic vesicles, has a similar effect.

Drugs that inhibit acetylcholine release

Acetylcholine release by a nerve impulse involves the entry of calcium ions into the nerve terminal; the increase in $[Ca^{2+}]_i$ stimulates exocytosis, and increases the rate of quantal release (Fig. 7.2). Agents that inhibit calcium entry include magnesium ion, and various aminoglycoside antibiotics (e.g. **streptomycin** and **neomycin**; see Ch. 43), which occasionally produce muscle paralysis as an unwanted side-effect when used clinically. Calcium antagonists (see Ch. 14), which block calcium entry into smooth muscle and cardiac cells, have little effect on the release of neurotransmitters, because the calcium channels involved in transmitter release are distinct from those responsible for calcium entry into smooth muscle cells.

Two potent neurotoxins, namely **botulinum toxin** and β-**bungarotoxin** act specifically to inhibit acetylcholine release. Botulinum toxin is a protein produced by the anaerobic bacillus *Clostridium botulinum*, an organism that can multiply in preserved food, and can cause botulism, an extremely serious type of food poisoning.

The potency of botulinum toxin is extraordinary, the minimum lethal dose in a mouse being less than 10^{-12} g— only a few million molecules. It belongs to the group of potent bacterial exotoxins that includes tetanus and diphtheria toxins. They possess two subunits, one of which binds to a membrane receptor and is responsible for cellular specificity. By this means the toxin enters the cell, where the other subunit produces the toxic effect (see Montecucco & Schiavo 1995). Botulinum toxin contains several components (A to G). They are peptidases which cleave specific proteins involved in exocytosis (synaptobrevins, syntaxins, etc.—see Ch. 6), thereby producing a long-lasting block of synaptic function. Each toxin component inactivates a different functional protein—a remarkably coordinated attack by a humble bacterium on a vital component of mammalian physiology.

Botulinum poisoning causes progressive parasympathetic and motor paralysis, with dry mouth, blurred vision and difficulty in swallowing, followed by progressive respiratory paralysis. Treatment with antitoxin is effective only if given before symptoms appear, for once the toxin is bound its action cannot be reversed. Mortality is high, and recovery takes several weeks. Anticholinesterases and drugs that increase transmitter release (see p. 137) are ineffective in restoring transmission. Among the more spectacular outbreaks of botulinum poisoning was an incident on Loch Maree in Scotland in 1922 when all eight members of a fishing party died after eating duck pâté for their lunch. Their ghillies, consuming humbler fare no doubt, survived. The inn-keeper committe suicide.

Botulinum toxin, injected locally into muscles, is used to treat a form of persistent and disabling eyelid spasm (blepharospasm) as well as other types of local muscle spasm, for example in spasticity (see Tsui, 1996).

β-bungarotoxin is a protein contained in the venom of various snakes of the cobra family, and has a similar action to botulinum toxin, though its active component is a phospholipase rather than a peptidase. The same venoms also contain α-bungarotoxin (see p. 23) which blocks postsynaptic acetylcholine receptors, so these snakes evidently cover all eventualities as far as causing paralysis of their victims is concerned.

DRUGS THAT ENHANCE CHOLINERGIC TRANSMISSION

Drugs that enhance cholinergic transmission act either by inhibiting cholinesterase (the main group) or by increasing acetylcholine release. In this chapter we focus on the peripheral actions of such drugs; drugs affecting cholinergic transmission in the central nervous system, used to treat senile dementia, are discussed in Chapter 31.

DISTRIBUTION AND FUNCTION OF CHOLINESTERASE

There are two distinct types of cholinesterase, namely acetylcholinesterase (AChE) and butyrylcholinesterase (BChE), closely related in molecular structure but differing in their distribution, substrate specificity and functions (see Chatonnet & Lockridge 1989). Both consist of globular catalytic subunits, which constitute the soluble forms found in plasma (BChE) and CSF (AChE). Elsewhere, the catalytic units are linked to collagen-like tails or to glycolipids, through which they are tethered, like a bunch of balloons, to the cell membrane or the basement membrane at various sites, such as the erythrocyte and the motor endplate.

Acetylcholinesterase is bound to the basement membrane in the synaptic cleft at cholinergic synapses, where its function is to hydrolyse the released transmitter.

The soluble form of AChE is also present in cholinergic nerve terminals, where it seems to have a role in regulating the free acetylcholine concentration, and from which it may be secreted; the function of the secreted enzyme is so far unclear. The membrane-bound form also occurs in unexpected places such as the erythrocyte, where its function is unknown. AChE is quite specific for acetylcholine and closely related esters such as methacholine. Certain neuropeptides, such as substance P (Ch. 10) are inactivated by AChE, but it is not known whether this is of physiological significance.

Butyrylcholinesterase (or pseudocholinesterase) has a widespread distribution, being found in tissues such as liver, skin, brain and gastrointestinal smooth muscle, as well as in soluble form in the plasma. It is not particularly associated with cholinergic synapses, and has a broader substrate specificity than AChE. It hydrolyses butyrylcholine more rapidly than acetylcholine, as well as other esters, such as **procaine**, **suxamethonium** and **propanidid** (a short-acting anaesthetic agent; see Ch. 32). The function of this enzyme is not known, but the plasma enzyme is important in relation to the inactivation of the drugs listed above. Genetic variants of BChE occur (see Ch. 48), and these partly account for the variability in the duration of action of these drugs. The very short duration of action of acetylcholine given intravenously (see Fig. 7.1) results from its rapid hydrolysis in the plasma. Normally AChE and BChE between them keep the plasma acetylcholine at an undetectably low level, so acetylcholine (unlike noradrenaline) is strictly a neurotransmitter and not a hormone.

AChE and BChE belong to the class of serine hydrolases, which includes many proteases, such as trypsin. The active site of AChE comprises two distinct regions (Fig. 7.10), an anionic site that possesses a glutamate residue, and an esteratic site in which a histidine imidazole ring and a serine –OH group are particularly important. Catalytic hydrolysis occurs by a mechanism common to other serine hydrolases, whereby the acetyl group is transferred to the serine –OH group, leaving (transiently) an acetylated enzyme molecule and a molecule of free choline. Spontaneous hydrolysis of the serine acetyl group occurs rapidly, and the overall turnover number of AChE is extremely high (over 10 000 molecules of acetylcholine hydrolysed per second by a single active site).

DRUGS THAT INHIBIT CHOLINESTERASE

Peripherally-acting anticholinesterase drugs fall into three main groups according to the nature of their interaction with the active site, which determines their duration of

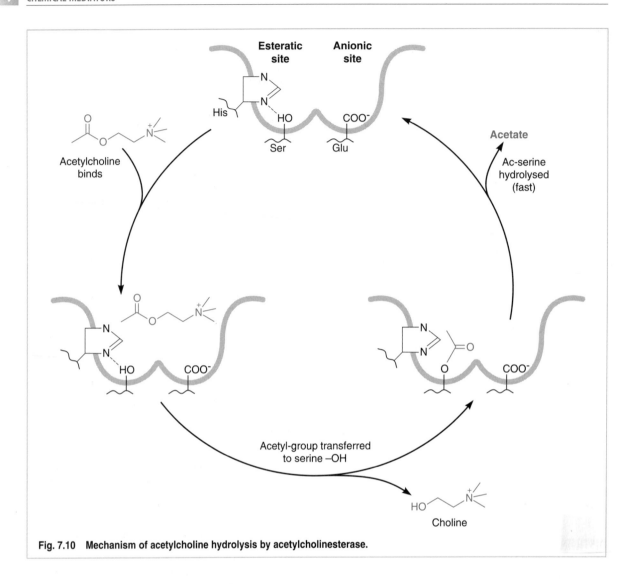

Fig. 7.10 Mechanism of acetylcholine hydrolysis by acetylcholinesterase.

action. Most of them inhibit AChE and BChE about equally. Centrally-acting anticholinesterases, developed for the treatment of dementia, are discussed in Chapter 31.

Short-acting anticholinesterases

The only important drug among the short-acting anticholinesterases is **edrophonium** (Table 7.7), a quaternary ammonium compound that binds to the anionic site of the enzyme only. The ionic bond formed is readily reversible and the action of the drug is very brief. It is used mainly for diagnostic purposes, since improvement of muscle strength by an anticholinesterase is characteristic of myasthenia gravis (see p. 136), but does not occur when muscle weakness is due to other causes.

Medium-duration anticholinesterases

The medium-duration anticholinesterases (Table 7.7) include **neostigmine** and **pyridostigmine**, which are quaternary ammonium compounds of clinical importance, and **physostigmine** (eserine), a tertiary amine, which occurs naturally in the Calabar bean.*

These drugs all possess strongly basic groups, which bind to the anionic site, but are carbamyl, as opposed to acetyl, esters. Transfer of the carbamyl group to the serine –OH of the esteratic site occurs as with acetylcholine, but

---

*Otherwise known as the ordeal bean. Extracts of these poisonous beans were once used to assess the guilt or innocence of suspected criminals and heretics; death implied guilt.

Table 7.7   Anticholinesterase drugs

Drug	Structure	Duration of action (long/med/short)	Main site of action	Notes
Edrophonium		S	NMJ*	Used mainly in diagnosis of myasthenia gravis Too short-acting for therapeutic use
Neostigmine		M	NMJ	Used i.v. to reverse competitive neuromuscular block Used orally in treatment of myasthenia gravis Visceral side-effects
Physostigmine		M	P	Used as eye drops in treatment of glaucoma
Pyridostigmine		M	NMJ	Used orally in treatment of myasthenia gravis Better absorbed than neostigmine, and has longer duration of action
Dyflos		L	P	Highly toxic organophosphate, with very prolonged action Has been used as eye drops for glaucoma
Ecothiopate		L	P	Used as eye drops in treatment of glaucoma Prolonged action; may cause systemic effects
Parathion		L	–	Converted to active metabolite by replacement of sulphur by oxygen Used as insecticide, but commonly causes poisoning in humans

*NMJ = neuromuscular junction; P = postganglionic parasympathetic junction

the carbamylated enzyme is very much slower to hydrolyse (Fig. 7.11), taking minutes rather than microseconds. The anticholinesterase drug is therefore hydrolysed, but at a negligible rate compared with acetylcholine, and the slow recovery of the carbamylated enzyme means that the action of these drugs is quite long-lasting.

Irreversible anticholinesterases

Irreversible anticholinesterases (Table 7.7) are penta-valent phosphorus compounds containing a labile group such as fluoride (in dyflos) or an organic group (in para-thion and ecothiopate). This group is released, leaving the residue of the molecule attached covalently through the phosphorus atom to the serine –OH group of the enzyme (Fig. 7.11). Most of these organophosphate compounds, of which there are many, developed as war gases and pesticides as well as for clinical use, interact only with the esteratic site of the enzyme and have no cationic group. Ecothiopate is an exception in having a quaternary nitrogen group designed to bind also to the anionic site.

The inactive phosphorylated enzyme is usually very

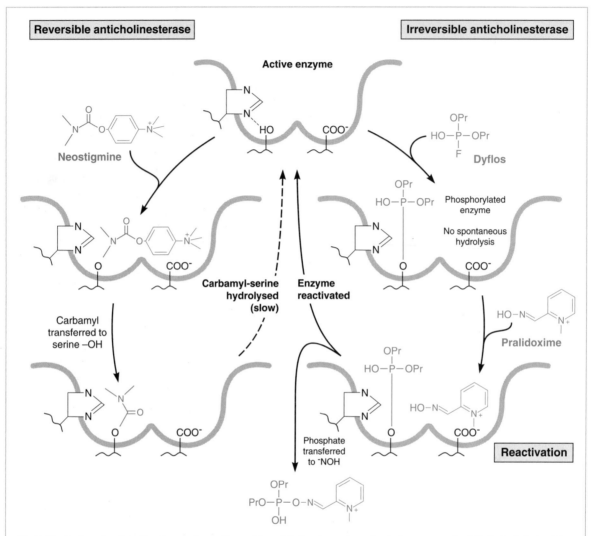

Fig. 7.11 **Action of anticholinesterase drugs.** *Reversible anticholinesterase* (neostigmine): recovery of activity by hydrolysis of the carbamylated enzyme takes many minutes. *Irreversible anticholinesterase* (dyflos); *reactivation of phosphorylated enzyme by pralidoxime.*

stable. With drugs such as dyflos no appreciable hydrolysis occurs, and recovery of enzymic activity depends on the synthesis of new enzyme molecules, a process that may take weeks. With other drugs such as ecothiopate slow hydrolysis occurs over the course of a few days, so that their action is not strictly irreversible. Dyflos and parathion are volatile non-polar substances of very high lipid solubility, and are rapidly absorbed through mucous membranes and even through unbroken skin and insect cuticles; the use of these agents as war gases or insecticides relies on this property. The lack of a specificity-

conferring quaternary group means that most of these drugs block other serine hydrolases (e.g. trypsin, thrombin) though their pharmacological effects result mainly from cholinesterase inhibition.

Effects of anticholinesterase drugs
Cholinesterase inhibitors affect:

- the autonomic cholinergic synapses
- the neuromuscular junction
- the central nervous system.

Some organophosphate compounds can produce, in addition, a form of neurotoxicity not associated with cholinesterase inhibition.

Effects on autonomic cholinergic synapses. These mainly reflect enhancement of acetylcholine activity at parasympathetic postganglionic synapses (i.e. increased secretions from salivary, lacrimal, bronchial and gastro-intestinal glands, increased peristaltic activity, broncho-constriction, bradycardia and hypotension, pupillary constriction, fixation of accommodation for near vision, fall in intraocular pressure). Large doses can stimulate, and later block, autonomic ganglia, producing complex autonomic effects. The block, if it occurs, is a depolari-sation block and is associated with a build-up of acetyl-choline in the plasma and body fluids. Neostigmine and pyridostigmine tend to affect neuromuscular trans-mission more than the autonomic system, whereas physo-stigmine and organophosphates show the reverse pattern. The reason is not clear, but therapeutic usage takes advantage of this partial selectivity.

Anticholinesterase poisoning (e.g. from contact with insecticides or war gases) causes severe bradycardia, hypotension and difficulty in breathing. Combined with a depolarising neuromuscular block, and central effects (see below), the result may be fatal.

Effects on the neuromuscular junction. The twitch tension of a muscle stimulated via its motor nerve is increased by anticholinesterases, owing to repetitive firing in the muscle fibre, associated with prolongation of the endplate potential. Normally, the acetylcholine is hydrolysed so quickly that each stimulus initiates only one action potential in the muscle fibre, but when AChE is inhibited, this is converted to a short train of action potentials in the muscle fibre, and hence greater tension. Much more important is the effect produced when transmission has been blocked by a competitive blocking agent, such as tubocurarine. In this case, addi-tion of an anticholinesterase can dramatically restore transmission. If a large proportion of the receptors are blocked, the majority of acetylcholine molecules will normally encounter, and be destroyed by, an AChE molecule before reaching a vacant receptor; inhibiting AChE will thus increase the number of acetylcholine molecules that will find a vacant receptor, and thus in-crease the endplate potential so that it reaches threshold. In myasthenia gravis (see below) transmission fails because there are too few acetylcholine receptors, and cholinesterase inhibition improves transmission just as it does in curarised muscle.

In large doses, such as can occur in poisoning, anti-cholinesterases initially cause twitching of muscles. This is because spontaneous acetylcholine release can give rise to endplate potentials that reach the firing threshold, and may later cause a paralysis due to depolarisation block, which is associated with the build-up of acetyl-choline in the plasma and tissue fluids.

Effects on the CNS. Tertiary compounds, such as physostigmine, and the non-polar organophosphates penetrate the blood–brain barrier freely and affect the brain. The result is an initial excitation, which can result in convulsions, followed by depression, which can cause unconsciousness and respiratory failure. These central effects result mainly from the activation of muscarinic receptors, and are antagonised by atropine. The potential use of brain-selective anticholinesterases to treat senile dementia is discussed in Chapter 31.

Neurotoxicity of organophosphates. Many organo-phosphates can cause a severe type of peripheral nerve demyelination, leading to slowly developing weakness and sensory loss. This is not a problem with clinically used anticholinesterases, but occasionally occurs with accidental poisoning. In 1931 an estimated 20 000 Americans were affected, some fatally, by contamina-tion of fruit juice with an organophosphate insecticide, and other similar outbreaks have been recorded. The

---

Cholinesterase and anticholinesterase drugs

- There are two main forms of cholinesterase: acetylcholinesterase (AChE), which is mainly membrane-bound, relatively specific for ACh, and responsible for rapid ACh hydrolysis at cholinergic synapses; butyrylcholinesterase (BuChE) or pseudocholinesterase, which is relatively non-selective, and occurs in plasma and many tissues. Both enzymes belong to the family of serine hydrolases.
- Anticholinesterase drugs are of three main types: short-acting (edrophonium); medium-acting (neostigmine, physostigmine); irreversible (organophosphates, dyflos, ecothiopate). They differ in the nature of their chemical interaction with the active site of ChE.
- Effects of antiChE drugs are due mainly to enhancement of cholinergic transmission at cholinergic autonomic synapses and at the neuromuscular junction. AntiChEs that cross the blood–brain barrier (e.g. physostigmine, organophosphates) also have marked CNS effects. Autonomic effects include bradycardia, hypotension, excessive secretions, bronchoconstriction, gastrointestinal hypermotility, decrease of intraocular pressure. Neuromuscular action causes muscle fasciculation and increased twitch tension, and can produce depolarisation block.
- AntiChE poisoning may occur from exposure to insecticides or nerve gases.

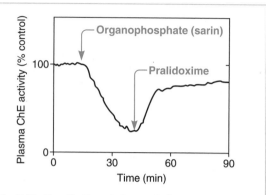

Fig. 7.12 Reactivation of plasma cholinesterase in a volunteer subject by intravenous injection of pralidoxime. (Redrawn from: Sim V M 1965 J Am Med Ass 192: 404)

mechanism of this reaction is only partly understood, but it seems to result from inhibition of an esterase (not cholinesterase itself) specific to myelin.

The main uses of anticholinesterases are summarised in the clinical box above.

Cholinesterase reactivation

Spontaneous hydrolysis of phosphorylated cholinesterase is extremely slow, a fact that makes poisoning with organophosphates very dangerous. **Pralidoxime** (Figs 7.11 and 7.12) reactivates the enzyme by bringing an oxime group into close proximity with the phosphorylated esteratic site. This group is a strong nucleophile and attracts the phosphate group from the serine –OH of the enzyme. The effectiveness of pralidoxime in reactivating plasma cholinesterase activity in a poisoned subject is shown in Figure 7.12. The main drawback to its use as an antidote to organophosphate poisoning is that within a few hours the phosphorylated enzyme undergoes a change ('ageing') that renders it no longer susceptible to reactivation, so that pralidoxime must be given early in order to work. Pralidoxime does not enter the brain, but related compounds have been developed to treat the central effects of organophosphate poisoning.

Myasthenia gravis

The neuromuscular junction is a remarkably robust structure which very rarely fails, myasthenia gravis being one of the very few disorders that specifically affects it (see reviews by Drachman 1981, Graus & De Baets 1993). This disease affects about 1 in 2000 individuals, who show muscle weakness and increased fatiguability resulting from a failure of neuromuscular transmission. The tendency for transmission to fail during repetitive activity can be seen in Figure 7.13. Functionally, it results in the inability of muscles to produce sustained contractions, of which the characteristic drooping eyelids of myasthenic patients are a sign. The effectiveness of anticholinesterase drugs in improving muscle strength in myasthenia was discovered in 1931, long before the cause of the disease was known.

The cause of the transmission failure is an autoimmune response which causes a loss of nicotinic acetylcholine receptors from the neuromuscular junction, first discovered in studies showing that the number of bungarotoxin-binding sites at the endplates of myasthenic patients was reduced by about 70% compared with that in normal subjects. It had been suspected that myasthenia had an immunological basis, for removal of the thymus gland (which often shows pathological changes in this disease) was frequently of benefit. The presence of antibody directed against the acetylcholine receptor protein was later discovered in the serum of myasthenic patients (see Drachman 1981). It was also found that immunisation of rabbits with purified acetylcholine receptor

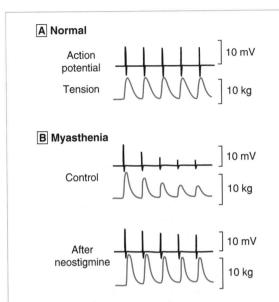

A Normal

Action potential] 10 mV

Tension] 10 kg

B Myasthenia

Control] 10 mV

] 10 kg

After neostigmine] 10 mV

] 10 kg

Fig. 7.13 Neuromuscular transmission in a normal and a myasthenic human subject. Electrical activity was recorded with a needle electrode in the adductor pollicis muscle, in response to ulnar nerve stimulation (3 Hz) at the wrist. **A** In normal subject, electrical and mechanical response is well sustained. **B** In myasthenic patient, transmission fails rapidly when nerve is stimulated. Treatment with neostigmine improves transmission. (From: Desmedt J E 1962 Bull Acad Roy Med Belg VII 2: 213)

caused, after a delay, symptoms very similar to those of human myasthenia gravis. The reason for the development of the autoimmune response in humans is still unknown.

The improvement of neuromuscular function by anti-

cholinesterase treatment (shown in Fig. 7.13) can be dramatic. It occurs because any given acetylcholine molecule released into the synaptic cleft is less likely to be destroyed by an encounter with cholinesterase, and therefore more likely to reach one of the few remaining receptors. If the disease progresses too far, the number of receptors remaining may become too few to produce an adequate endplate potential, and anticholinesterase drugs will then cease to be effective.

Alternative approaches to the treatment of myasthenia are to remove circulating antibody by plasma exchange, which is transiently effective, or, for a more prolonged effect, to inhibit antibody production with steroids (e.g. prednisolone) or immunosuppressant drugs (e.g. azathioprine; see Ch. 13).

OTHER DRUGS WHICH ENHANCE CHOLINERGIC TRANSMISSION

It was observed many years ago that **tetraethylammonium**, better known as a ganglion-blocking drug (see p. 123) could reverse the neuromuscular-blocking action of tubocurarine, and this was shown to be because it increases the release of transmitter evoked by nerve stimulation. Subsequently, **aminopyridines** (see Ch. 40), which block K^+-channels, and thus prolong the action potential in the presynaptic nerve terminal, were found to act similarly, and to be considerably more potent and selective in their actions than tetraethylammonium. These drugs are not selective for cholinergic nerves, but increase the evoked release of many different transmitters, so have too many unwanted effects to be useful in treating neuromuscular disorders.

REFERENCES AND FURTHER READING

Bowman W C 1990 Pharmacology of neuromuscular function. Wright, Bristol (*Detailed textbook*)

Burns B D, Paton W D M 1951 Depolarisation of the motor end-plate by decamethonium and acetylcholine. J Physiol 115: 41–73

Chatonnet A, Lockridge O 1989 Comparison of butyrylcholinesterase and acetylcholinesterase. Biochem J 260: 625–634 (*Short review on nature and functions of cholinesterases*)

Colquhoun D, Ogden D C, Mathie A 1987 Nicotinic acetylcholine receptors of nerve and muscle: functional aspects. Trends Pharmacol Sci 8: 465–472 (*Useful short review*)

Drachman D B 1981 The biology of myasthenia gravis. Annu Rev Neurobiol 4: 195–225 (*Review emphasising autoimmune nature of myasthenia*)

Ginsborg B L, Jenkinson D H 1976 Transmission of impulses from nerve to muscle. In: Zaimis E J (ed) Neuromuscular junction. Handbook of experimental pharmacology. Springer-

Verlag, Berlin, vol 42, pp 229–364 (*Excellent general account of neuromuscular physiology and pharmacology*)

Goyal R K 1989 Muscarinic receptor subtypes: physiology and clinical implications. New Engl J Med 321: 1022–1029 (*Good general review*)

Graus Y M, De Baets M H 1993 Myasthenia gravis: an autoimmune response against the acetylcholine receptor. Immunol Res 12: 78–100

Hardman J G, Limbird L E, Molinoff P B, Ruddon R W, Gilman A G (eds) 1995 Goodman & Gilman: the pharmacological basis of therapeutics, 9th edn. McGraw-Hill, New York (*Excellent authoritative textbook*)

Kilbinger H 1984 Presynaptic muscarinic receptors modulating acetylcholine release. Trends Pharmacol Sci 5: 103–105 (*Short review article*)

Liu Y, Edwards R H 1997 The role of vesicular transport proteins in synaptic transmission and neural degeneration. Annu Rev

Neurosci 20: 125–156 (*Review of recent ideas about functional role of transporters*)

McGehee D S, Role L W 1995 Physiological diversity of nicotinic acetylcholine receptors expressed by vertebrate neurons. Annu Rev Physiol 57: 521–546 (*Summarises molecular and physiological diversity among neuronal receptors in CNS and periphery*)

Montecucco C, Schiavo G 1995 Structure and function of botulinum neurotoxins. Q Rev Biophys 28: 423–472 (*Discusses the mode of action of an important group of presynaptic neurotoxins*)

Nicholls J G, Martin A R, Wallace B G 1992 From neuron to brain. Sinauer, Sunderland, MA (*Excellent general textbook*)

Parsons S M, Prior C, Marshall I G 1993 Acetylcholine transport, storage and release. Int Rev Neurobiol 35: 279–390 (*Useful review of the local metabolism of acetylcholine*)

Paton W D M 1954 The principles of ganglion block. Lectures on the scientific basis of medicine. Athlone Press, London, vol 2

Prior C, Tian L, Dempster J, Marshall I G 1995 Prejunctional actions of muscle relaxants: synaptic vesicles and transmitter mobilization as sites of action. Gen Pharmac 26: 659–666 (*Emphasises the role of presynaptic inhibition in the action of neuromuscular-blocking drugs*)

Skok V I 1980 Ganglionic transmission: morphology and physiology. In: Kharkevich D A (ed) Pharmacology of ganglionic transmission. Handbook of experimental pharmacology. Springer-Verlag, Berlin, vol 53, pp 9–39 (*Comprehensive account of ganglion-blocking drugs*)

Tsui J K C 1996 Botulinum toxin as a therapeutic agent. Pharmacol Ther 72: 13–24 (*A lethal toxin can be useful in therapeutics*)

Usdin T B, Eiden L E, Bonner T I, Erickson J D 1995 Molecular biology of the vesicular ACh transporter. Trends Neurosci 18: 218–224 (*Short review article*)

Wess J 1996 Molecular biology of muscarinic acetylcholine receptors. Crit Rev Neurobiol 10: 69–99 (*Describes receptor subtypes in detail*)

Wonnacott S 1997 Presynaptic nicotinic ACh receptors. Trends Neurosci 20: 92–98 (*Summarises evidence for a role of nicotinic ACh receptors as presynaptic regulators, most authors having postulated a postsynaptic excitatory role, which has proved elusive to pin down*)

Zaimis E 1976 Neuromuscular function. Handbook of experimental pharmacology. Springer-Verlag, Berlin, vol 42

8

Noradrenergic transmission

The noradrenergic neuron is an important target for drug action, both as an object for investigation in its own right and as a point of attack for many clinically useful drugs. For convenience a table summarising much of the pharmacological information is given at the end of the chapter (Table 8.3).

CLASSIFICATION OF ADRENOCEPTORS

In 1896 Oliver & Schafer demonstrated that injection of extracts of adrenal gland caused a rise in arterial pressure. Following the subsequent isolation of adrenaline as the active principle, it was shown by Dale in 1913 that adrenaline causes two distinct kinds of effect, namely vasoconstriction in certain vascular beds (which normally predominates and causes the rise in arterial pressure) and vasodilatation in others. Dale showed that the vasoconstrictor component disappeared if the animal was first

injected with an ergot derivative* (see Ch. 6), and noticed that adrenaline then caused a fall, instead of a rise, in arterial pressure. This result closely paralleled Dale's demonstration of the separate muscarinic and nicotinic components of the action of acetylcholine (see Ch. 7) and he pointedly avoided interpreting it in terms of a distinction between categories of receptor. Later pharmacological work, however, beginning with that of Ahlquist in 1948 showed clearly the existence of several subclasses of adrenoceptor. Ahlquist found that the rank order of the potencies of various catecholamines,** including **adrenaline**, **noradrenaline** and **isoprenaline** (a synthetic catecholamine; see Fig. 8.1), fell into two distinct patterns, depending on what response was being measured. He postulated the existence of two kinds of

---

*Dale was a new recruit in the laboratories of the Wellcome pharmaceutical company, and was responsible for checking the potency of adrenaline ampoules coming from the factory. He tested one batch at the end of a day's experimentation on a cat which he had earlier dosed with an ergot preparation. Because the adrenaline had such an unexpected effect, he advised that the whole expensive consignment should be destroyed. Unknown to him, the same sample was given to him again a few days later, and behaved perfectly normally. How Dale explained this to Wellcome's management is not recorded.

**Catecholamines are compounds containing a catechol nucleus (i.e. a benzene ring with two adjacent hydroxyl groups) and an amine-containing side-chain. Pharmacologically, the most important catecholamines (see Fig. 8.1) are:

- *Noradrenaline*, the transmitter substance released by postganglionic sympathetic neurons.
- *Adrenaline*, a hormone secreted, along with noradrenaline, by the adrenal medulla.
- *Dopamine*, the metabolic precursor of noradrenaline and adrenaline, which functions as a neurotransmitter in its own right in the brain (see Ch. 28), and possibly also in the periphery.
- *Isoprenaline*, a synthetic derivative of noradrenaline that is not found in the body.

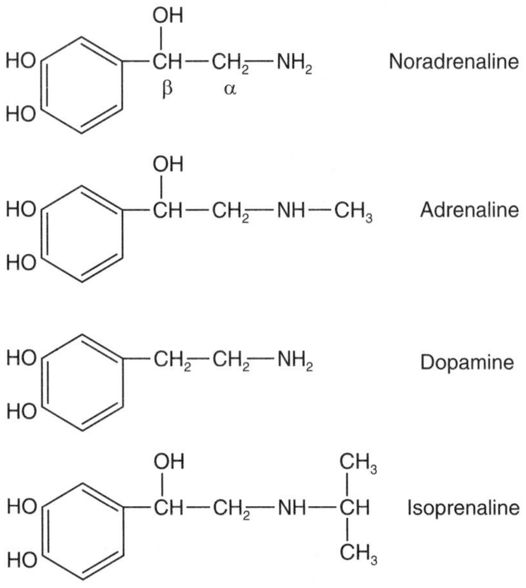

Fig. 8.1 Structures of the major catecholamines.

receptor, α and β, defined in terms of agonist potencies as follows:

Receptor	Order of agonist potency
α	Noradrenaline > adrenaline > isoprenaline
β	Isoprenaline > adrenaline > noradrenaline

It was then recognised that certain ergot alkaloids, which Dale had studied, act as selective α-receptor antagonists, and that Dale's adrenaline reversal experiment reflected the unmasking of the β effects of adrenaline by α-receptor blockade. Selective β-receptor antagonists were not developed until 1955, when their effects fully confirmed Ahlquist's original classification, and also suggested the existence of further subdivisions of both α- and β-receptors. It was first shown by Lands and his colleagues that different β-adrenoceptor agonists differ in their relative potency in eliciting different types of β-receptor-mediated effects in different tissues; subsequent studies with agonists and antagonists have confirmed the existence of two main α-receptor subtypes (α_1 and α_2) and three β-receptor subtypes (β_1, β_2 and β_3; Table 8.1). All are typical G-protein-coupled receptors, and cloning has revealed that α_1 and α_2 receptors each comprise at least three further subclasses, whose functions are, for the most part, still unclear (Bylund 1994, Insel 1996, Summers & McMartin 1993).

Each of these receptor classes is associated with a specific second messenger system (Table 8.1). Thus

α_1- and α_2-receptors are coupled to phospholipase C, and produce their effects mainly by the release of intracellular calcium; α_2-receptors are negatively coupled to adenylate cyclase, and reduce cAMP formation, as well as inhibiting Ca-channels; all three types of β-receptor act by stimulation of adenylate cyclase. The major effects that are produced by these receptors, and the main drugs that act on them are shown in Table 8.1.

The distinction between β_1- and β_2-receptors is an important one, for β_1-receptors are found mainly in the heart, where they are responsible for the positive inotropic and chronotropic effects of catecholamines (see Ch. 14). β_2-receptors, on the other hand, are responsible for causing smooth muscle relaxation in many organs. The latter is often a useful therapeutic effect, while the former is more often harmful; consequently, considerable efforts have been made to find selective β_2-agonists, which would relax smooth muscle without affecting the heart, and selective β_1 antagonists, which would exert a useful blocking effect on the heart without at the same time blocking β_2-receptors in bronchial smooth muscle (see Table 8.1). It is important to realise that the selectivity of these drugs is relative rather than absolute. Thus, compounds used as selective β_1 antagonists invariably have some action on β_2-receptors as well, which can

---

Classification of adrenoceptors

- Main pharmacological classification into α- and β-subtypes, based originally on order of potency among agonists, later on selective antagonists.
- There are two main α-adrenoceptor subtypes (α_1, α_2) and three β-adrenoceptor subtypes (β_1, β_2, β_3). Cloning studies show that all belong to the superfamily of G-protein-coupled receptors.
- Second messengers: α_1-receptors activate phospholipase C, thus producing IP_3 and DAG as second messengers; α_2-receptors inhibit adenylate cyclase, and thus decrease cAMP formation; all types of β-receptor stimulate adenylate cyclase.
- The main effects of receptor activation are:
  — α_1-receptors—vasoconstriction, relaxation of gastrointestinal smooth muscle, salivary secretion and hepatic glycogenolysis
  — α_2-receptors—inhibition of transmitter release (including NA and ACh release from autonomic nerves), platelet aggregation, contraction of vascular smooth muscle, inhibition of insulin release
  — β_1-receptors—increased cardiac rate and force
  — β_2-receptors—bronchodilatation, vasodilatation, relaxation of visceral smooth muscle, hepatic glycogenolysis and muscle tremor
  — β_3-receptors, lipolysis.

Table 8.1 Characteristics of adrenoceptors

	α_1	α_2	β_1	β_2	β_3
Tissues and effects					
Smooth muscle:					
Blood vessels	Constrict	Constrict		Dilate	
Bronchi	Constrict			Dilate	
GI tract	Relax	Relax (presynaptic effect)		Relax	
GI sphincters	Contract				
Uterus	Contract			Relax	
Bladder detrusor				Relax	
Bladder sphincter	Contract				
Seminal tract	Contract			Relax	
Iris (radial muscle)	Contract				
Ciliary muscle				Relax	
Heart					
Rate			Increase		
Force of contraction			Increase		
Skeletal muscle				Tremor	Thermogenesis
				Increased muscle mass and speed of contraction	
				Glycogenolysis	
Liver	Glycogenolysis			Glycogenolysis	
Fat					Lipolysis
					Thermogenesis
Pancreatic islets		Decrease insulin secretion			
Nerve terminals					
Adrenergic		Decrease release	Increase release		
Cholinergic		Decrease release			
Salivary gland	K$^+$ release		Amylase secretion		
Platelets		Aggregation			
Mast cells				Inhibition of histamine release	
Second messengers and effectors	PLC activation $\uparrow$ IP$_3$ $\uparrow$ DAG $\uparrow$ Ca^{2+}	$\downarrow$ cAMP $\downarrow$ Ca channels $\uparrow$ K channels	$\uparrow$ cAMP	$\uparrow$ cAMP	$\uparrow$ cAMP
Agonist potency order	A = NA $\gg$ ISO	A = NA $\gg$ ISO	ISO > A = NA	ISO > A $\gg$ NA	ISO = NA > A
Selective agonists	Phenylephrine, oxymetazoline	Clonidine, clenbuterol	Dobutamine, xamoterol	Salbutamol, terbutaline, salmeterol	BRL 37344
Selective antagonists	Prazosin, doxazocin	Yohimbine, idazoxan	Atenolol, metoprolol	Butoxamine	

A = adrenaline; cAMP = cyclic 3′,5′-adenosine monophosphate; DAG = diacylglycerol; ISO = isoprenaline; IP$_3$ = inositol (1,4,5) tris-phosphate; NA = noradrenaline; PLC = phospholipase C

cause unwanted effects, such as bronchoconstriction. Furthermore, the high degree of receptor specificity found for some compounds in laboratory animals is not invariably found in man. Also, it appears that both types of β-receptor contribute to some effects, such as the chronotropic action, with the relative contribution of each varying from species to species. It was originally thought that the effects mediated by α_1-receptors corresponded to the postsynaptic actions of adrenoceptor agonists, whereas α_2-receptors mediated only the presynatic inhibitory effects (see Ch. 6). However, α_2-receptors are widespread, and occur on liver cells, platelets and smooth muscle cells of blood vessels, as well as on presynaptic nerve terminals.

Partial agonist effects

Several drugs that act on adrenoceptors have the characteristics of partial agonists (see Ch. 1), i.e. they block receptors and thus antagonise the actions of full agonists, but also have a weak agonist effect of their own. Examples include **ergotamine** (α_1-receptors) and **clonidine** (α_2-receptors). Some β-adrenoceptor blocking drugs (e.g. **alprenolol**, **oxprenolol**) cause, under resting conditions, an increase of heart rate, while at the same time opposing the tachycardia produced by sympathetic stimulation. This has been interpreted as a partial agonist effect, though there is evidence that mechanisms other than β-receptor activation may contribute to the tachycardia.

The possible clinical significance of partial agonists is discussed under the headings of individual drugs later in this chapter. The pharmacology of ergot derivatives is discussed in Chapter 9.

PHYSIOLOGY OF NORADRENERGIC TRANSMISSION

THE NORADRENERGIC NEURON

Noradrenergic neurons in the periphery are postganglionic sympathetic neurons, whose cell bodies lie in sympathetic ganglia. They generally have long axons that end in a series of varicosities strung along the branching terminal network. These varicosities contain numerous synaptic vesicles, which are the sites of synthesis and release of noradrenaline. Fluorescence histochemistry, in which formaldehyde treatment is used to convert catecholamines to fluorescent quinone derivatives, shows clearly that noradrenaline is present at high concentration in these varicosities. Noradrenergic neurons contain a population of characteristic large dense-cored vesicles which are the storage organelles for noradrenaline, which is released by exocytosis. In most peripheral tissues, and also in the brain, the tissue content of noradrenaline closely parallels the density of the sympathetic innervation. With the exception of the adrenal medulla, sympathetic nerve terminals account for all of the noradrenaline

content of peripheral tissues. Organs such as the heart, spleen, vas deferens, and some blood vessels are particularly rich in noradrenaline (5–50 nmol/g of tissue) and have been widely used for studies of noradrenergic transmission. For detailed information on noradrenergic neurons, see Cooper et al. 1996, Fillenz 1990, Trendelenburg & Weiner 1988.

NORADRENALINE SYNTHESIS

The biosynthetic pathway for noradrenaline synthesis is shown in Figure 8.2. The metabolic precursor for noradrenaline is **L-tyrosine**, an aromatic amino acid present in the body fluids, which is taken up by adrenergic neurons. **Tyrosine hydroxylase**, the enzyme which catalyses the conversion of tyrosine to **dihydroxyphenylalanine** (DOPA) is found only in catecholamine-containing cells, probably free in the cytosol. It is a rather selective enzyme; unlike other enzymes involved in catecholamine metabolism, it does not accept indole derivatives as substrates, and so is not involved in 5-hydroxytryptamine metabolism. This first hydroxylation step is the main control point for noradrenaline synthesis. Tyrosine hydroxylase is inhibited by the end-product of the biosynthetic pathway, noradrenaline, and this provides the mechanism for the moment-to-moment regulation of the rate of synthesis; much slower regulation, taking hours or days, occurs by changes in the rate of production of the enzyme.

The tyrosine analogue α-**methyltyrosine** strongly inhibits tyrosine hydroxylase; it is used clinically in patients with the rare problem of inoperable phaeochromocytoma (see below), and may be used experimentally to block noradrenaline synthesis.

The next step, conversion of DOPA to dopamine, is catalysed by **DOPA decarboxylase**, a cytosolic enzyme that is by no means confined to catecholamine-synthesising cells. It is a relatively non-specific enzyme, and catalyses the decarboxylation of various other L-aromatic amino acids as well as L-DOPA, such as L-histidine and L-tryptophan, which are precursors in the synthesis of histamine and 5-HT, respectively. DOPA decarboxylase activity is not rate-limiting for noradrenaline synthesis. Though various factors, including certain drugs, affect the enzyme, it is not an effective means of regulating noradrenaline synthesis.

Dopamine-β-hydroxylase (DBH) is also a relatively non-specific enzyme, but its distribution is restricted to catecholamine-synthesising cells. It is located in synaptic vesicles, probably in membrane-bound form. A small amount of the enzyme is released from adrenergic nerve

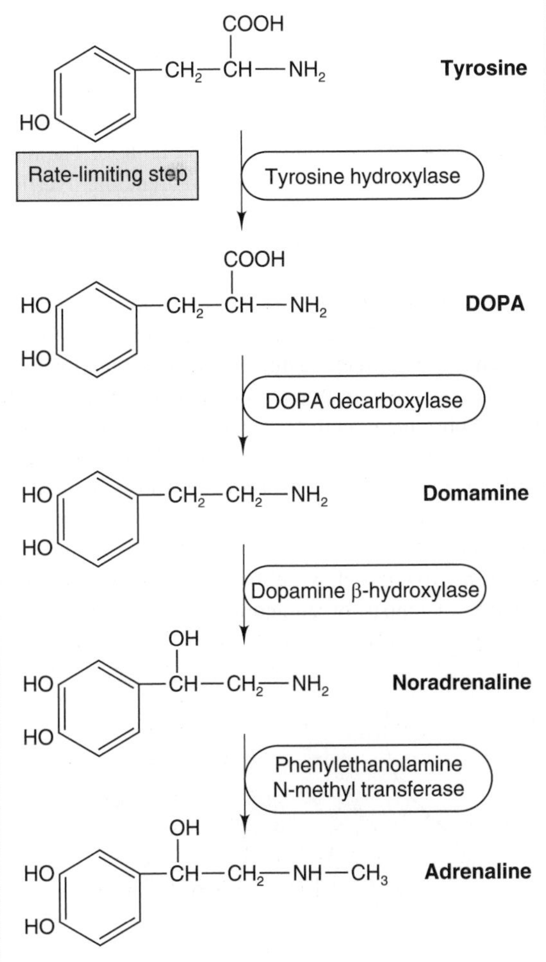

Fig. 8.2   Biosynthesis of catecholamines

terminals in company with noradrenaline; this presumably represents enzyme that is in a soluble form within the vesicle, since there is evidence that the membrane proteins of the vesicle are retained when the vesicle discharges its contents by exocytosis. Unlike noradrenaline, the released DBH is not subject to rapid degradation or uptake, so its concentration in plasma and body fluids can be used as an index of overall sympathetic nerve activity.

Many drugs inhibit DBH, including copper-chelating agents and **disulfiram** (a drug used mainly for its effect on ethanol metabolism; see Chs 5 and 39). Such drugs can cause a partial depletion of noradrenaline stores and interference with sympathetic transmission.

Phenylethanolamine N-methyl transferase (PNMT) catalyses the N-methylation of noradrenaline to adren-

aline. The main location of this enzyme is in the adrenal medulla, which contains a population of adrenaline-releasing (A) cells separate from the smaller proportion of noradrenaline-releasing (N) cells. The A cells, which appear only after birth, lie adjacent to the adrenal cortex, and there is evidence that the production of PNMT is induced by an action of the steroid hormones secreted by the adrenal cortex (see Ch. 24). PNMT is also found in certain parts of the brain, where there is some evidence that adrenaline may function as a transmitter. In these sites, also, PNMT formation is sensitive to steroid hormones, providing a possible mechanism whereby these hormones can affect brain function.

Noradrenaline turnover can be measured under steady-state conditions by measuring the rate at which labelled noradrenaline accumulates when a labelled precursor, such as tyrosine or DOPA, is administered. The turnover time is defined as the time taken for an amount of noradrenaline equal to the total tissue content to be degraded and resynthesised. In peripheral tissues the turnover time is generally about 5–15 h, but it becomes much shorter if sympathetic nerve activity is increased. Under normal circumstances the rate of synthesis closely matches the rate of release, so that the noradrenaline content of tissues is constant regardless of how fast it is being released.

NORADRENALINE STORAGE

Most of the noradrenaline in nerve terminals or chromaffin cells* is contained in vesicles; only a little is free in the cytoplasm under normal circumstances. The concentration in the vesicles is very high (0.3–1.0 mol/l), and is maintained by a transport mechanism similar to the amine transporter responsible for noradrenaline uptake into the nerve terminal, but using the transvesicular proton gradient as its driving force (see Liu & Edwards 1997). Certain drugs, such as **reserpine** (see below, Table 8.2) block this transport, and cause nerve terminals to become depleted of their noradrenaline stores. The vesicles contain two major constituents besides noradrenaline, namely ATP (about 4 molecules per molecule

---

*Chromaffin cells are catecholamine-containing non-neuronal cells derived from neural crest ectoderm, so called because they stain readily with various reagents that oxidise catecholamines to green or brown products. The largest group of chromaffin cells is in the adrenal medulla, but scattered cells are found elsewhere, e.g. in the wall of the intestine, sympathetic ganglia, carotid and aortic bodies. *Phaeochromocytoma* and *carcinoid tumour* are examples of chromaffin cell tumours.

of noradrenaline) and a protein called chromogranin A. These substances are released along with noradrenaline, and it is generally assumed that a reversible complex, depending partly on the opposite charges on the molecules of noradrenaline and ATP, is formed within the vesicle. This would serve both to reduce the osmolarity of the vesicle contents and also to reduce the tendency of noradrenaline to leak out of the vesicles within the nerve terminal.

ATP itself has a transmitter function at adrenergic synapses (see Lundberg 1996) being responsible for the fast excitatory synaptic potential and the rapid phase of contraction produced by sympathetic nerve activity in many smooth muscle tissues.

NORADRENALINE RELEASE

The processes linking the arrival of a nerve impulse at a noradrenergic nerve terminal to the release of noradrenaline are basically the same as those at other chemically transmitting synapses (see Ch. 6). Depolarisation of the nerve terminal membrane opens calcium channels in the nerve terminal membrane, and the resulting entry of calcium promotes the fusion and discharge of synaptic vesicles. A surprising feature of the release mechanism at the varicosities of noradrenergic nerves is that the probability of release, even of a single vesicle, when a nerve impulse arrives at a varicosity, is very low (less than 1 in 50; see Cunnane 1984). A single neuron possesses many thousand varicosities, so one impulse leads to the discharge of a few hundred vesicles, scattered over a wide area. This contrasts sharply with the cholinergic synapse, where the release probability at a single bouton is high, but the boutons are few in number; the total release is similar, but it is sharply localised.

Regulation of noradrenaline release

Noradrenaline release is affected by a variety of substances that act on *presynaptic receptors* (see reviews by Starke et al. 1989). Many different types of nerve terminal (cholinergic, noradrenergic, dopaminergic, 5-HT-ergic, etc.) are subject to this type of control, and many different mediators (e.g. acetylcholine, acting through muscarinic receptors, catecholamines acting through α- and β-receptors, angiotensin II, prostaglandins, purine nucleotides, neuropeptides, etc.) can act on presynaptic terminals. Presynaptic modulation represents an important physiological control mechanism throughout the nervous system.

Of particular interest is the evidence suggesting that

noradrenaline, by acting on presynaptic receptors, can regulate its own release, and also that of co-released ATP (see Ch. 6). This is believed to occur physiologically, so that released noradrenaline exerts a local inhibitory effect on the terminals from which it came—the so-called *autoinhibitory feedback mechanism* (Fig. 8.3). The main evidence comes from studies of noradrenaline overflow in which the amount of radioactivity is measured in the venous effluent from an organ whose stores of noradrenaline have been previously labelled by infusion of tritiated noradrenaline. It was shown many years ago that α-receptor blocking drugs increase (by 10-fold or more in some tissues) the amount of noradrenaline overflow that occurs in response to sympathetic nerve stimulation. Subsequent analysis has shown that most of this increase is due to an increase in noradrenaline release, resulting from the loss of the normal feedback regulation. The magnitude of the change in noradrenaline overflow implies that this regulatory mechanism can, in some tissues, act to damp down noradrenaline release by 90% or more. Agonists or antagonists affecting these pre-

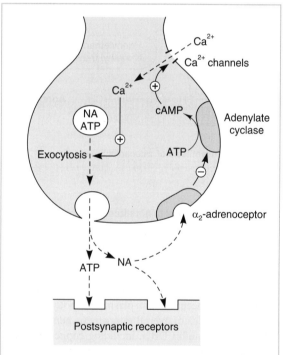

Fig. 8.3 Feedback control of noradrenaline release. The presynaptic α₂-receptor inhibits adenylate cyclase, thereby reducing intracellular cAMP. cAMP acts to promote Ca²⁺ influx in response to membrane depolarisation and hence to promote the release of noradrenaline and ATP.

synaptic receptors can, therefore, have large effects on sympathetic transmission. The physiological significance of presynaptic autoinhibition in the sympathetic nervous system is still somewhat contentious, and there is evidence that, in most tissues, it is less influential than measurements of transmitter overflow would imply. Thus, although large changes in noradrenaline overflow occur when the feedback mechanism is interfered with pharmacologically, the associated changes in *the tissue response* to sympathetic nerve activity are often rather small. This suggests that what is measured in overflow experiments may not be the physiologically important component of transmitter release.

The inhibitory feedback mechanism operates through α_2-receptors, which inhibit adenylate cyclase, and prevent the opening of calcium channels Sympathetic nerve terminals also possess β-receptors, coupled to activation of adenylate cyclase, which cause an increased noradrenaline release. Whether they have any physiological function is not yet clear.

UPTAKE AND DEGRADATION OF CATECHOLAMINES

Catecholamines differ markedly from acetylcholine in the way in which their action is terminated following release at the synapse. There is no synaptically located enzyme comparable with acetylcholinesterase that rapidly degrades catecholamines. Instead, reuptake of noradrenaline by noradrenergic nerve terminals, and by other cells, is the main mechanism for disposal of the released transmitter. Circulating adrenaline and noradrenaline are degraded enzymically, but much more slowly than acetylcholine. The two main enzymes responsible are both located intracellularly, so uptake into cells necessarily precedes metabolic degradation.

Uptake of catecholamines

Indirect evidence that sympathetic nerves can take up amines from the circulation and release them again as transmitter came originally from the work of Burn and his colleagues. In 1932 Burn found that the pressor effect of indirectly acting sympathomimetics (e.g. tyramine; see below) in whole animals was increased if the injection was preceded by injection of adrenaline, and he showed that this was because adrenaline was able to replenish the releasable amine stores of the nerve terminals. Later, it was demonstrated that tritiated noradrenaline was rapidly taken up from the circulation into tissues. Part of this uptake was by sympathetic neurons (for it disappeared when sympathetic nerves were allowed to degenerate), and the amine could be released again by

sympathetic nerve stimulation. In a study of noradrenaline uptake by isolated rat hearts, Iversen identified two distinct uptake mechanisms, each having the characteristics of a saturable active transport system capable of accumulating catecholamines against a large concentration gradient. These two mechanisms, called *uptake 1* and *uptake 2*, correspond to neuronal and extraneuronal uptake respectively. They have different kinetic properties as well as different substrate and inhibitor specificity, as summarised in Table 8.2.

The main differences are that uptake 1 is a high-affinity system with a relatively low maximum rate of uptake, whereas uptake 2 has low affinity for noradrenaline, but a much higher maximum rate. Also, uptake 1 is relatively selective for noradrenaline, whereas uptake 2 also accumulates adrenaline and isoprenaline. The effects of several important drugs that act on noradrenergic neurons depend on their ability either to inhibit uptake 1 or to enter the nerve terminal with its help (see Table 8.2). The uptake 1 transporter protein belongs to a family of neurotransmitter transporter proteins, which act as co-transporters of Na^+, Cl^- and the amine in question, using the electrochemical gradient for Na^+ as a driving force (see Ch. 6, Amara & Kuhar 1993, Brownstein & Hofmann 1994). Changes in this gradient can alter, or even reverse, the operation of uptake 1, with marked effects on the availability of the released transmitter at postsynaptic receptors.

Metabolic degradation of catecholamines

Endogenous and exogenous catecholamines are metabolised mainly by two enzymes, *monoamine oxidase* (MAO) and *catechol-O-methyl transferase* (COMT). MAO occurs within cells, bound to the surface membrane of mitochondria. It is abundant in noradrenergic nerve terminals, but is also present in many other places, such as liver and intestinal epithelium. MAO converts catecholamines to their corresponding aldehydes, which, in the periphery, are rapidly metabolised by *aldehyde dehydrogenase* to the corresponding carboxylic acid (Fig. 8.4). In the case of noradrenaline this yields *dihydroxymandelic acid* (DOMA). MAO can also oxidise other monoamines, important ones being dopamine and 5-HT. It is inhibited by various drugs (see Table 8.3), which are used mainly for their effects on the central nervous system, where these three amines all have transmitter functions (see Ch. 28). These drugs have important side-effects that are related to disturbances of peripheral adrenergic transmission. Within sympathetic neurons MAO controls the content of dopamine and noradrenaline, and the releasable store of noradrenaline increases

Table 8.2 Characteristics noradrenaline transport systems

	Uptake 1	Uptake 2	Vesicular
Transport of noradrenaline (rat heart)			
V_{max} (nmol/g per min)	1.2	100	
K_m (µmol/l)	0.3	250	~0.2
Specificity	NA > A > ISO	A > NA > ISO	NA = A ≫ ISO
Location	Neuronal membrane	Non-neuronal cell membrane (smooth muscle, cardiac muscle, endothelium)	Synaptic vesicle membrane
Other substrates	Methylnoradrenaline Dopamine 5-hydroxytryptamine Tyramine Adrenergic neuron blocking drugs (e.g. guanethidine)	(+)-noradrenaline Dopamine Serotonin Histamine	Dopamine 5-HT Guanethidine MPP$^+$ (see Ch. 31)
Inhibitors	Cocaine Tricyclic antidepressants (e.g. desipramine) Phenoxybenzamine Amphetamine	Normetanephrine Steroid hormones (e.g. corticosterone) Phenoxybenzamine	Reserpine Tetrabenazine

if the enzyme is inhibited. MAO and its inhibitors are discussed in more detail in Chapter 35.

The second major pathway for catecholamine metabolism involves methylation of one of the catechol –OH groups to give a methoxy derivative. COMT is a widespread enzyme that occurs in both neuronal and non-neuronal tissues. It acts on both the catecholamines themselves and the deaminated products, such as DOMA, that are produced by the action of MAO. The main final metabolite of adrenaline and noradrenaline is *3-methoxy-4-hydroxymandelic acid* (VMA). In patients with tumours of chromaffin tissue that secrete these amines (a rare cause of high blood pressure), the urinary excretion of VMA is markedly increased, this being used as a diagnostic test for this condition.

In the periphery, neither MAO nor COMT is primarily responsible for the termination of transmitter action, most of the released noradrenaline being quickly recaptured by uptake 1. Circulating catecholamines are usually inactivated by a combination of uptake 1, uptake 2 and

---

Noradrenergic transmission

- Transmitter synthesis:
  - L-tyrosine is converted to DOPA by tyrosine hydroxylase (rate-limiting step). Tyrosine hydroxylase occurs only in catecholaminergic neurons.
  - DOPA is converted to dopamine by dopa decarboxylase.
  - Dopamine is converted to NA by dopamine β-hydroxylase (DBH), located in synaptic vesicles.
  - In the adrenal medulla, NA is converted to adrenaline by phenylethanolamine N-methyl-transferase.
- Transmitter storage: NA is stored at high concentration in synaptic vesicles, together with ATP, chromogranin and DBH, all of which are released by exocytosis. Transport of NA into vesicles occurs by a reserpine-sensitive carrier. NA content of cytosol is normally low, due to monoamine oxidase in nerve terminals.

- Transmitter release occurs normally by Ca^{2+}-mediated exocytosis from varicosities on the terminal network. Non-exocytotic release occurs in response to indirectly acting sympathomimetic drugs (e.g. amphetamine) which displace NA from vesicles. NA escapes via uptake 1 (reverse transport).
- Transmitter action is terminated mainly by reuptake of NA into nerve terminals. This uptake (uptake 1) is blocked by tricyclic antidepressant drugs.
- NA release is controlled by autoinhibitory feedback, mediated by α_2-receptors.
- Co-transmission occurs at many noradrenergic nerve terminals, ATP and neuropeptide Y being frequently co-released with NA. ATP mediates the early phase of smooth muscle contraction in response to sympathetic nerve activity.

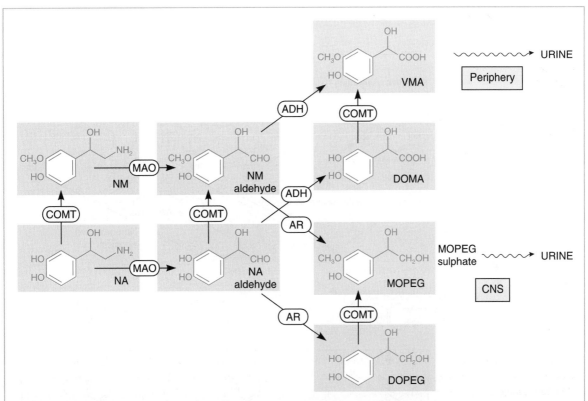

Fig. 8.4   The main pathways of noradrenaline metabolism in the brain and in the periphery. In the periphery, the oxidative branch (catalysed by ADH) predominates, giving VMA as the main urinary metabolite. In the brain, the reductive branch (catalysed by AR) predominates, producing MOPEG, which is conjugated to MOPEG sulphate before being excreted. (NA = noradrenaline; NM = normetanephrine; VMA = vanillylmandelic acid; DOMA = 3,4-dihydroxymandelic acid; MOPEG = 3-methoxy,4-hydroxyphenylglycol; DOPEG = 3,4-dihydroxyphenylglycol; MAO = monoamine oxidase; COMT catechol-O-methyl transferase; ADH aldehyde dehydrogenase; AR = aldehyde reductase)

COMT, the relative importance of these processes varying according to the agent concerned. Thus, circulating noradrenaline is removed mainly by uptake 1, whereas adrenaline is more dependent on uptake 2. Isoprenaline, on the other hand, is not a substrate for uptake 1, and is removed by a combination of uptake 2 and COMT.

The metabolism of noradrenaline in the central nervous system follows a different course (see Ch. 28 and Fig. 8.4). MAO is more important as a means of terminating transmitter action than it is in the periphery, and the resulting aldehydes are mainly reduced to the corresponding alcohols. The main excretory product of noradrenaline released in the brain is an ethyleneglycol derivative (MOPEG). Thus measurement of urinary VMA and MOPEG enables the central and peripheral release of noradrenaline to be quantified.

DRUGS ACTING ON ADRENOCEPTORS

STRUCTURE–ACTIVITY RELATIONSHIPS

The overall potency and receptor specificity of drugs that exert their effects by combining with adrenoceptors, depends on several factors:

- affinity for, and efficacy on, adrenoceptors
- interaction with neuronal uptake systems
- interaction with MAO
- interaction with COMT.

The relationship of these different factors with chemical structure is, not surprisingly, complex, but there are certain useful generalisations that can be made. The

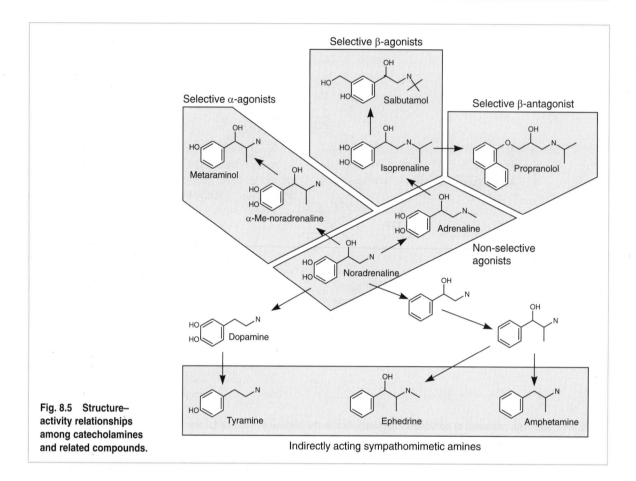

Fig. 8.5 Structure–activity relationships among catecholamines and related compounds.

noradrenaline molecule can be modified in several different ways to yield compounds that interact with adrenoceptors (Fig. 8.5).

- Increasing the bulkiness of substituents on the N-atom produces compounds (**adrenaline**, **isoprenaline** and **salbutamol**) of relatively greater potency as β-agonists, and less susceptible to uptake 1 and MAO.
- Addition of an α-methyl group (**α-methylnoradrenaline**, **metaraminol**) increases α_2-receptor selectivity and also renders compounds resistant to MAO, though they remain susceptible to uptake 1.
- Removal of the side-chain –OH group (**dopamine**) greatly reduces interaction with α- and β-adrenoceptors.
- Modification of the catechol –OH groups renders compounds resistant to COMT and uptake 1 (**salbutamol** and many β-receptor antagonists), which retain receptor activity.
- Removal of one or both –OH groups (**tyramine**, **am-**

phetamine, **ephedrine**) abolishes affinity for receptors, though these compounds are still indirectly acting sympathomimetic amines, as they are substrates for uptake 1.
- Extension of the alkyl side chain, with isopropyl substitution on the N-atom, and modification of catechol –OH groups (**propranolol**, **oxprenolol**, etc.) produces potent β-receptor antagonists.

These general rules account fairly well for the properties of many directly and indirectly acting sympathomimetic drugs and for β-receptor antagonists. α-receptor antagonists are much more heterogeneous, however, and defy such generalisations.

ADRENOCEPTOR AGONISTS

Examples of the main types of adrenoceptor agonist are given in Table 8.1 and the characteristics of individual drugs are summarised in Table 8.3.

Actions

The major physiological effects mediated by different types of adrenoceptor are summarised in Table 8.1.

Smooth muscle

All types of smooth muscle, except that of the gastro-intestinal tract, contract in response to stimulation of α_1-adrenoceptors. α-receptor stimulation causes a rise in the free intracellular calcium concentration, which activates the contractile mechanism. This is due mainly to calcium release from the endoplasmic reticulum, through the action of the second messenger, inositol trisphosphate (see Ch. 2). There may also be a link between the receptors and calcium channels in the membrane, though this is controversial.

When α-agonists are given systemically to experimental animals or man the most important action is on vascular smooth muscle, particularly in the skin and splanchnic vascular beds, which are strongly constricted. Large arteries and veins, as well as arterioles, are also con-stricted, resulting in decreased vascular compliance, increased central venous pressure and increased peripheral resistance, all of which contribute to an increase in systolic and diastolic arterial pressure. Some vascular beds (e.g. cerebral, coronary and pulmonary) are relatively little affected.

In the whole animal, baroreceptor reflexes are activated by the rise in arterial pressure produced by α-agonists, causing reflex bradycardia and inhibition of respiration.

Smooth muscle in the vas deferens, spleen capsule and eyelid retractor muscles (or nictitating membrane, in some species) is also stimulated by α-agonists and these organs are often used for pharmacological studies.

The α-receptors involved in smooth muscle con-traction are mainly α_1 in type, though vascular smooth muscle possesses both α_1- and α_2-receptors. It appears that α_1-receptors lie close to the sites of release (and are mainly responsible for neurally mediated vasoconstric-tion), while α_2-receptors lie elsewhere on the muscle fibre surface, and are activated by circulating catecholamines (see Broadley 1996, McGrath & Wilson 1988).

Stimulation of β-receptors causes relaxation of most kinds of smooth muscle by a mechanism involving an increase in intracellular cAMP concentration (see Ch. 2). cAMP appears to cause relaxation by activating a protein kinase, which, in turn, phosphorylates and inactivates *myosin-light-chain kinase*, thereby inhibiting contraction (see Fig. 15.1). β-receptor activation also enhances Ca^{2+} extrusion, and so reduces the intracellular calcium concentration. It also affects intracellular calcium binding, though the mechanism is uncertain. Relaxation is usually produced by β_2-receptors, though the receptor that is responsible for this effect in gastrointestinal smooth muscle is not clearly β_1 or β_2. In the vascular system, β_2-mediated vasodilatation is (particularly in humans) mainly endothelium-dependent and mediated by NO release (see Ch. 11). It occurs in many vascular beds and is especially marked in skeletal muscle.

The powerful inhibitory effect of the sympathetic system on gastrointestinal smooth muscle is produced by both α- and β-receptors, this tissue being unusual in that α-receptors cause relaxation in most regions. Part of the effect is due to stimulation of presynaptic α_2-receptors (see below), which inhibit the release of excitatory trans-mitters (e.g. acetylcholine) from intramural nerves, but there are also α-receptors on the muscle cells, stimulation of which hyperpolarises the cell (by increasing the membrane permeability to potassium) and inhibits action potential discharge. The sphincters of the gastrointestinal tract are contracted by α-receptor activation.

Bronchial smooth muscle is strongly dilated by activa-tion of β_2-adrenoceptors, and selective β_2-agonists are important in the treatment of asthma (see Ch. 19). Uterine smooth muscle responds similarly, and these drugs are also used to delay premature labour.

Nerve terminals

Presynaptic adrenoceptors are present on both cholin-ergic and adrenergic nerve terminals (see above and Ch. 6). The main effect (α_2-mediated) is inhibitory, but a weaker facilitatory action of β-receptors on adrenergic nerve terminals has also been described.

Heart

Catecholamines, acting on β_1-receptors, exert a powerful stimulant effect on the heart (see Ch. 14). Both the *heart rate* (*chronotropic effect*) and the *force of contraction* (*inotropic effect*) are increased, resulting in a markedly increased cardiac output and cardiac oxygen consump-tion. The *cardiac efficiency* (see Ch. 14) is reduced. Cate-cholamines can also cause *disturbance of the cardiac rhythm*, culminating in ventricular fibrillation. In normal hearts the dose required to cause marked dysrhythmia is greater than that which produces the chronotropic and inotropic effects, but in ischaemic conditions dys-rhythmias are produced much more readily. Figure 8.6 shows the overall pattern of cardiovascular responses to catecholamine infusions in humans, reflecting their actions on both the heart and vascular system.

Metabolism

Catecholamines encourage the conversion of energy stores (glycogen and fat) to freely available fuels (glucose

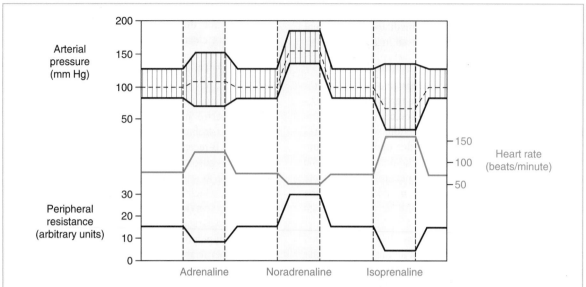

Fig. 8.6 Schematic representation of the cardiovascular effects of intravenous infusions of adrenaline, noradrenaline and isoprenaline in humans. Noradrenaline (predominantly α-agonist) causes vasoconstriction and increased systolic and diastolic pressure, with a reflex bradycardia. Isoprenaline (β-agonist) is a vasodilator, but strongly increases cardiac force and rate. Mean arterial pressure falls. Adrenaline combines both actions.

and free fatty acids), and cause an increase in the plasma concentration of the latter substances. The detailed biochemical mechanisms vary from species to species, but in most cases the effects on carbohydrate metabolism of liver and muscle (Fig. 8.7) are mediated through β₁-receptors (though hepatic glucose release can also be produced by α-agonists), and the stimulation of lipolysis is produced by β₃-receptors (see Table 8.1). Insulin secretion is also affected, the main influence being inhibitory, through α₂ receptors, an effect which further contributes to the hyperglycaemia. Adrenaline-induced hyperglycaemia in humans is blocked completely by a combination of α- and β-antagonists but not by either on its own. Selective β₃-receptor agonists (e.g. **BRL 37344**) have been developed, and may prove useful in the treatment of obesity, but are not yet approved for clinical use.

Other effects

Skeletal muscle is affected by adrenaline, acting on β₂-receptors, though the effect is far less dramatic than that on the heart. The twitch tension of fast-contracting fibres (white muscle) is increased by adrenaline, particularly if the muscle is fatigued, whereas the twitch of slow (red) muscle is reduced. These effects depend on an action on the contractile proteins, rather than on the membrane, and the mechanism is poorly understood. In man, **adrenaline** and other β₂-agonists cause a marked tremor, the

shakiness that accompanies fear, excitement or the excessive use β₂-agonists (e.g. **salbutamol**) in the treatment of asthma being examples of this. It probably results from an increase in muscle spindle discharge, coupled with an effect on the contraction kinetics of the fibres, these effects combining to produce an instability in the reflex control of muscle length. β-receptor antagonists are sometimes used to control pathological tremor. β₂-agonists also cause long-term changes in the expression of sarcoplasmic reticulum proteins that control contraction kinetics, and thereby increase the rate and force of contraction of skeletal muscle (see Zhang et al. 1996). **Clenbuterol**, an 'anabolic' drug used illicitly by sportsmen to improve performance, is a β₂-agonist which acts in this way.

Histamine release by human and guinea-pig lung tissue in response to anaphylactic challenge (see Ch. 12) is inhibited by catecholamines, acting apparently on β₂-receptors.

Lymphocytes are also sensitive to β-receptor agonists, both proliferation and lymphocyte-mediated cell killing being inhibited. The physiological and clinical importance of these effects has not yet been established.

Clinical use

The main clinical uses of adrenoceptor agonists are summarised in the clinical box (p. 152).

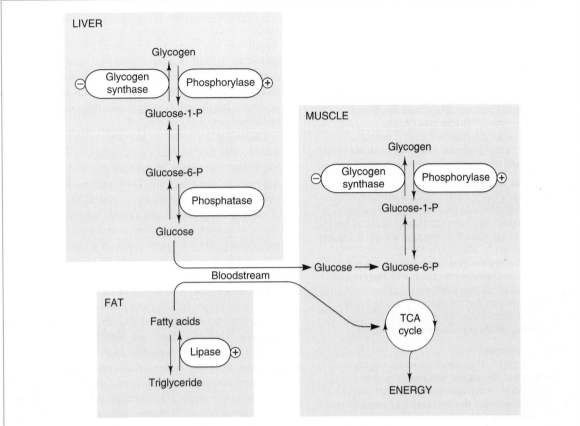

Fig. 8.7 **Regulation of energy metabolism by catecholamines.** The main enzymic steps that are affected by β-adrenoceptor activation are indicated by + and − signs, denoting stimulation and inhibition, respectively.

Adrenoceptor agonists

- Selective drugs exist for the main adrenoceptor subtypes, α_1, α_2, β_1, β_2 and β_3; NA itself shows some selectivity for α- over β-adrenoceptors; adrenaline shows little selectivity.
- Selective α_1-agonists include phenylephrine, oxymetazoline.
- Selective α_2-agonists include clonidine, α-methyl-noradrenaline. They cause a fall in blood pressure, partly by inhibition of NA release, and partly by a central action. Methylnoradrenaline is formed as a false transmitter from methyldopa, developed as a hypotensive drug (now largely obsolete).
- Selective β_1-agonists include dobutamine. Increased cardiac contractility may be useful clinically, but all β_1-agonists can cause cardiac dysrhythmias.
- Selective β_2-agonists include salbutamol, terbutaline and salmeterol, used mainly for their bronchodilator action in asthma.
- Selective β_3-agonists are being developed for the control of obesity.

ADRENOCEPTOR ANTAGONISTS

The main drugs in the adrenoceptor antagonist category are listed in Table 8.1, and further information is given in Table 8.3. In contrast to the situation with agonists, most adrenoceptor antagonists are selective for α- or β-receptors, and many are also subtype selective.

α-ADRENOCEPTOR ANTAGONISTS

The main groups of α-adrenoceptor antagonists are:

- non-selective α-receptor antagonists (e.g. **phenoxybenzamine, phentolamine**)
- α_1-selective antagonists (e.g. **prazosin, doxazosin, terazosin**)
- α_2-selective antagonists (e.g. **yohimbine, idazoxan**)
- ergot derivatives (e.g. **ergotamine, dihydroergotamine**). This group of compounds has

many actions in addition to α-receptor block, and is discussed in Chapter 9. Their action on α-adrenoceptors is of pharmacological interest (see p. 139) but not used therapeutically.

Non-selective αadrenoceptor antagonists

Phenoxybenzamine is not highly specific for α-receptors, and also antagonises the actions of acetylcholine, histamine and 5-hydroxytryptamine. It is long-lasting because it binds covalently to the receptor. **Phentolamine** is very similar, but it binds reversibly and its action is short-lasting. In humans, these drugs cause a fall in arterial pressure (because of block of α-receptor-mediated vasoconstriction) and postural hypotension. The cardiac output and heart rate are increased. This is a reflex response to the fall in arterial pressure, mediated through β-receptors. The concomitant block of α_2-receptors tends to increase noradrenaline release, which has the effect of enhancing the reflex tachycardia that occurs with any blood-pressure-lowering agent.

Labetalol is a mixed α- and β-receptor blocking drug, though clinically its effect on β-receptors predominates. Much has been made of the fact that it combines both activities in one molecule. To a pharmacologist, accustomed to putting specificity of action high on the list of pharmacological saintly virtues, labetalol may seem like a step backwards rather than forwards. It is used occasionally to treat hypertension in pregnancy.

α_1-selective antagonists

Prazosin was the first α_1-selective antagonist. Similar drugs with longer half-lives (e.g. **doxazosin, terazosin**), which have the advantage of allowing once-daily dosing, are now available. They are highly selective for α_1-receptors, and cause vasodilatation and fall in arterial pressure, but less tachycardia than occurs with non-selective α-receptor antagonists, presumably because they do not increase noradrenaline release from sympathetic nerve terminals. Some postural hypotension may occur.

α_1-receptor antagonists cause relaxation of the smooth muscle of the bladder neck and prostate capsule, which may be useful in cases of urinary retention associated with benign prostatic hypertrophy. **Tamsolusin**, an α_{1A}-receptor antagonist, shows some selectivity for the bladder, and causes less hypotension than drugs such as prazosin.

α_2-selective antagonists

Yohimbine is a naturally occurring alkaloid; various synthetic analogues have been made, such as idazoxan. These drugs are used experimentally to analyse α-receptor subtypes, and yohimbine, probably by virtue of its vasodilator effect, enjoys fame as an aphrodisiac (Dahl 1980), but they are not used therapeutically.

General clinical uses and unwanted effects of α-adrenoceptor antagonists

The main uses of α-adrenoceptor antagonists are related to their cardiovascular actions, and are summarised in the clinical box (p. 153). They have been tried for many purposes, but have only limited therapeutic applications.

In *hypertension*, non-selective α-blocking drugs are unsatisfactory, because of their tendency to produce tachycardia and cardiac dysrhythmias, and increased gastrointestinal activity. Selective α_1-receptor antagonists (especially the longer-acting compounds **doxazosin** and **terazosin**) are, however, useful. They do not affect cardiac function appreciably, and postural hypotension is less troublesome than with prazosin or non-selective α-receptor antagonists. There has been a recent resurgence in the use of these drugs to treat hypertension (see Ch. 15). Unlike other antihypertensive drugs, they cause a modest decrease in LDL, and an increase in HDL cholesterol (see Ch. 16), though the clinical importance of these ostensibly beneficial effects is uncertain. They are also used to control urinary retention in patients with benign prostatic hypertrophy.

Phaeochromocytoma is a catecholamine-secreting tumour of chromaffin tissue, and one of the effects is to cause episodes of severe hypertension. A combination of α- and β-receptor antagonists is the most effective way of controlling the blood pressure. The tumour may be surgically removable, and it is essential to block α- and β-receptors before surgery is begun, to avoid the effects of a sudden release of catecholamines when the tumour is disturbed mechanically. A combination of **phenoxybenzamine** and **atenolol** is effective for this purpose. Phenoxybenzamine should be given first, to avoid the risk of paradoxically worsening the hypertension by blocking β-receptor-mediated vasodilatation while β-receptor-mediated vasoconstriction is still operative.

Clinical uses of α-adrenoceptor antagonists

- Hypertension (see Ch. 15): α_1-selective antagonists. **Prazosin** is short-acting. Preferred drugs are longer-acting (e.g. **doxazosin, terazosin**), used either alone in mild hypertension, or in combination with other drugs.
- Benign prostatic hypertrophy (especially **tamsolusin**, a selective α_{1A}-receptor antagonist).
- Phaeochromocytoma: phenoxybenzamine used in conjunction with β-receptor antagonist in preparation for surgery.

β-ADRENOCEPTOR ANTAGONISTS

β-adrenoceptor antagonists comprise an important category of drugs. They were first discovered in 1958, 10 years after Ahlquist had postulated the existence of β-adrenoceptors. The first compound, **dichloroisoprenaline**, had fairly low potency, and was a partial agonist.

Further development led to **propranolol**, which is much more potent and a pure antagonist, with an equal blocking effect on β_1- and β_2-receptors. The potential clinical advantages of drugs with some partial agonist activity, and/or with selectivity for β_1-receptors, led to the development of **practolol** (selective for β_1-receptors, but no longer used clinically because of its toxicity), **oxprenolol** and **alprenolol** (non-selective with considerable partial agonist activity), and **atenolol** (β_1-selective with no agonist activity). Many very similar drugs have been developed, and the characteristics of the most important compounds are set out in Tables 8.1 and 8.3. Most β-receptor antagonists are inactive on β_3-receptors, so do not affect lipolysis.

Actions

The pharmacological actions of β-receptor antagonists can be deduced from Table 8.1. The effects produced in man depend on the degree of sympathetic activity, and are slight in subjects at rest. The most important effects are on the cardiovascular system and on bronchial smooth muscle.

In a subject at rest, **propranolol** causes little change in heart rate, cardiac output or arterial pressure, but reduces the effect of exercise or excitement on these variables (Fig. 8.8). Drugs with partial agonist activity, such as **oxprenolol**, increase the heart rate at rest, but reduce it during exercise. Maximum exercise tolerance is considerably reduced in normal subjects, partly because of the limitation of the cardiac response, and partly because the β-mediated vasodilatation in skeletal muscle is reduced. Coronary flow is reduced, but relatively less than the myocardial oxygen consumption, so oxygenation of the myocardium is improved, an effect of importance in the treatment of *angina pectoris* (see Ch. 14). In normal subjects, the reduction of the force of contraction of the heart is of no importance, but it may have serious consequences for patients with heart disease (see below).

An important, and somewhat unexpected, effect of β-receptor antagonists is their *antihypertensive action* (see Ch. 15). Patients with hypertension (though not normotensive subjects) show a gradual fall in arterial pressure that takes several days to develop fully. The mechanism is complex, and involves the following:

- reduction in cardiac output
- reduction of renin release from the juxtaglomerular cells of the kidney
- a central action, reducing sympathetic activity.

Blockade of the facilitatory effect of presynaptic β-

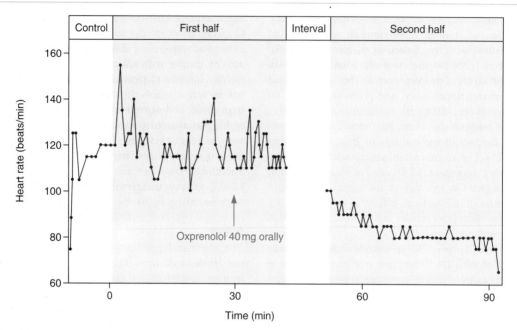

Fig. 8.8 **Heart rate recorded continuously in a spectator watching a live football match, showing the effect of the β-adrenoceptor antagonist, oxprenolol.** (From: Taylor S H, Meeran M K 1973 In: Burley et al. (eds) New perspectives in beta-blockade. CIBA Laboratories, Horsham)

receptors on noradrenaline release (see p. 145) may also contribute to the antihypertensive effect. The antihypertensive effect of β-receptor antagonists is clinically very useful. Because reflex vasoconstriction is preserved, postural and exercise-induced hypotension (see Ch. 15) are much less troublesome than with many other antihypertensive drugs.

Many β-receptor antagonists have an antidysrhythmic effect on the heart, which is of clinical importance (see Ch. 14).

Airways resistance in normal subjects is only slightly increased by β-receptor antagonists, and this is of no consequence. In asthmatic subjects, however, non-selective β-receptor antagonists (such as **propranolol**) can cause severe bronchoconstriction, which does not, of course, respond to the usual doses of drugs such as **salbutamol** or **adrenaline**. This danger is less with β_1-selective antagonists, but none are so selective that this danger can be ignored.

In spite of the involvement of β-receptors in the hyperglycaemic actions of adrenaline, β-receptor antagonists cause only minor metabolic changes in normal

Adrenoceptor antagonists

- Most antagonists are α- or β-adrenoceptor selective.
- Drugs that block α_1- and α_2-adrenoceptors (e.g. phenoxybenzamine, phentolamine) were once used to produce vasodilatation in treatment of peripheral vascular disease, now largely obsolete.
- Selective α_1-antagonists (e.g. prazosin, doxazosin, terazosin) are used in treating hypertension. Postural hypotension and impotence are unwanted effects.
- Yohimbine is a selective α_2-antagonist. It is not used clinically.
- β-adrenoceptor antagonists include propranolol, alprenolol, oxprenolol (non-selective between and β_1 and β_2), atenolol (β_1-selective). Some (alprenolol, oxprenolol) have partial agonist activity. Used mainly to treat hypertension, cardiac dysrhythmias, angina and myocardial infarction. They are also used to treat anxiety. Important hazards are bronchoconstriction, and bradycardia and cardiac failure (possibly less with partial agonists). Side-effects include cold extremities, insomnia, depression. Some show rapid first-pass metabolism, hence poor bioavailability.

subjects. They do not affect the onset of hypoglycaemia following an injection of insulin, but somewhat delay the recovery of blood glucose concentration. In diabetic patients, the use of β-receptor antagonists increases the likelihood of exercise-induced hypoglycaemia because the normal adrenaline-induced release of glucose from the liver is diminished.

Clinical use

The main uses of β-receptor antagonists are connected with their effects on the cardiovascular system, and are discussed in Chapters 14 and 15. They are as summarised in the clinical box below.

Unwanted effects

The main side-effects of β-receptor antagonists result from their receptor-blocking action.

Bronchoconstriction. This is of little importance in the absence of airways disease, but in asthmatic patients, this effect can be dramatic and life-threatening. It is

---

> **Clinical uses of β-adrenoceptor antagonists**
>
> **Cardiovascular system** (see Chs 14, 15)
> - Hypertension.
> - Angina pectoris.
> - Following myocardial infarction (protection against dysrhythmias and repeated infarctions). **Carvedilol**, which has vasodilator and antioxidant properties, may have advantages over other agents (see Ch. 15).
> - Cardiac dysrhythmias.
>
> **Other uses**
> - Glaucoma: e.g. **timolol**, used as eye drops. Fewer side-effects than anticholinesterases or muscarinic agonists (see Ch. 7).
> - Thyrotoxicosis (see Ch. 25), as adjunct to definitive treatment (e.g. preoperatively).
> - Anxiety states (see Ch. 33), to control somatic symptoms associated with sympathetic overactivity, such as palpitations and tremor.
> - Migraine prophylaxis (see Ch. 9).
> - Benign essential tremor (a familial disorder).
>
> - **Metoprolol** and **atenolol** are the most widely used.
> - The main risks and unwanted effects are:
>   - Bronchoconstriction—a serious hazard in asthmatic patients
>   - Aggravation of cardiac failure
>   - Bradycardia (heart block)
>   - Hypoglycaemia
>   - Physical fatigue
>   - Cold extremities
>   - Bad dreams.

---

also of clinical importance in patients with other forms of obstructive lung disease (e.g. chronic bronchitis, emphysema).

Cardiac failure. Patients with heart disease may rely on a degree of sympathetic drive to the heart to maintain an adequate cardiac output, and removal of this by blocking β-receptors will produce a degree of cardiac failure.* In theory, drugs with partial agonist activity (e.g. **oxprenolol**, **alprenolol**) offer an advantage since they can, by their own action, maintain a degree of β₁-receptor activation, while at the same time blunting the cardiac response to increased sympathetic nerve activity or to circulating adrenaline. Clinical trials so far, however, have not shown a clear advantage of these drugs measurable as a reduced incidence of cardiac failure.

Bradycardia. This can lead to life-threatening heart block and can occur in patients with coronary disease, particularly if they are being treated with anti-arrhythmic drugs that impair cardiac conduction (see Ch. 15).

Hypoglycaemia. Glucose release in response to adrenaline is a safety device that may be important to diabetic patients and to other individuals prone to hypoglycaemic attacks. The sympathetic response to hypoglycaemia produces symptoms (especially tachycardia) that warn patients of the urgent need for carbohydrate (usually in the form of a sugary drink). β-receptor antagonists reduce these symptoms, so incipient hypoglycaemia is more likely to go unnoticed by the patient. The use of β-receptor antagonists is generally to be avoided in patients with poorly controlled diabetes. There is a theoretical advantage in using β₁-selective agents, since glucose release from the liver is controlled by β₂-receptors.

Fatigue. Patients taking β-receptor blocking drugs often complain of fatigue, which is probably due to reduced cardiac output and reduced muscle perfusion in exercise.

Cold extremities. This results presumably from a loss of β-receptor-mediated vasodilatation in cutaneous vessels, and is a common side-effect. Again, β₁-selective drugs ought to be less likely to produce this effect, but it is not clear that this is so in practice.

Other side-effects associated with β-receptor antagonists are not obviously the result of β-receptor blockade. One

---

*Paradoxically, β-receptor antagonists in low doses and for long periods may actually be beneficial (in the sense of increasing ventricular function and survival) in patients with heart failure, though at the outset there is a danger of exacerbating the disease (see Pfeffer & Stevenson 1996).

is the occurrence of bad dreams, which occur mainly with highly lipid-soluble drugs such as propranolol, which enter the brain easily. **Practolol** was withdrawn from clinical use because it produced a serious *oculo-mucocutaneous syndrome*, as a rare idiosyncratic reaction (see Ch. 48).

DRUGS THAT AFFECT NORADRENERGIC NEURONS

Emphasis in this chapter is placed on peripheral sympathetic transmission. The same principles, however, are applicable to the central nervous system (see Ch. 28), where many of the drugs mentioned here also act.

DRUGS THAT AFFECT NORADRENALINE SYNTHESIS

Only a few clinically important drugs affect noradrenaline synthesis directly. Examples are α-**methyltyrosine**, which inhibits tyrosine hydroxylase and has been used in the treatment of phaeochromocytoma, and **carbidopa**, a hydrazine derivative of dopa, which inhibits dopa decarboxylase, and is used in the treatment of parkinsonism (see Ch. 31).

Methyldopa, a drug still occasionally used in the treatment of hypertension during pregnancy (see Ch. 15) is taken up by noradrenergic neurons, where it is decarboxylated and hydroxylated to form the false transmitter, α-methylnoradrenaline. This substance is not deaminated within the neuron by MAO, so it accumulates and displaces noradrenaline from the synaptic vesicles. The false transmitter is released in the same way as noradrenaline, but differs in two important respects in its action on adrenoceptors. α-methylnoradrenaline is somewhat less active than noradrenaline on α_1-receptors and thus is less effective in causing vasoconstriction. But it is more active on presynaptic (α_2) receptors, so the autoinhibitory feedback mechanism operates more strongly than normal, thus reducing transmitter release below the normal levels. Both of these effects (as well as a central effect, probably caused by the same cellular mechanism) contribute to the hypotensive action. It produces side-effects typical of centrally-acting antiadrenergic drugs (e.g. sedation) as well carrying a risk of immune haemolytic reactions and liver toxicity, so it is now little used, except for hypertension in late pregnancy.

6-hydroxydopamine (identical with dopamine except that it possesses an extra ring –OH group) is a neurotoxin of the Trojan horse kind. It is taken up selectively by noradrenergic nerve terminals, where it is converted to a reactive quinone, which destroys the nerve terminal, producing a 'chemical sympathectomy'. The cell bodies survive, and eventually the sympathetic innervation recovers. The drug is useful for experimental purposes, but has no clinical uses. If injected directly into the brain it selectively destroys those nerve terminals (i.e. dopaminergic, noradrenergic and adrenergic) that take it up, but it does not reach the brain if given systemically. MPTP (see Ch. 31) is a rather similar selective neurotoxin.

DRUGS THAT AFFECT NORADRENALINE STORAGE

Reserpine, an alkaloid of complex chemical structure, bearing no obvious relationship to catecholamines, comes from a shrub, *Rauwolfia*, which has been widely used in India for centuries as a medicine for the treatment of mental disorders. Reserpine, at very low concentration, blocks the transport of noradrenaline and other amines into synaptic vesicles, by binding to the transport protein (see Liu & Edwards 1997). Noradrenaline accumulates instead in the cytoplasm, where it is degraded by MAO. The noradrenaline content of tissues thus drops to a low level, and sympathetic transmission is blocked. Reserpine also causes depletion of 5-HT and dopamine from neurons in the brain in which these amines are transmitters (see Ch. 28). Reserpine is now only used experimentally, but was at one time used as an antihypertensive drug (see Ch. 15); its central effects, especially *depression*, which probably result from impairment of noradrenergic and 5-HT-mediated transmission in the brain (see Ch. 35) are a serious disadvantage.

DRUGS THAT AFFECT NORADRENALINE RELEASE

Drugs can affect noradrenaline release in four main ways:

- By preventing exocytosis from occurring in response to depolarisation of the nerve terminal (**noradrenergic neuron blocking drugs**).
- By evoking noradrenaline release in the absence of nerve terminal depolarisation (**indirectly acting sympathomimetic drugs**).
- By interacting with presynaptic receptors that inhibit or enhance depolarisation-evoked release (e.g. α_2-**agonists**, **angiotensin II**, **dopamine**, **prostaglandins**, etc.). Effects mediated through α_2-adrenoceptors are discussed elsewhere in this chapter; the importance of the numerous other endogenous substances known to affect sympathetic nerve terminals is not clear at present. It is likely that these mechanisms are more important in the central than in the peripheral nervous systems.
- By increasing or decreasing available stores of

noradrenaline (e.g. **reserpine**, see above; **monoamine oxidase inhibitors**). These drugs are discussed elsewhere in this chapter, and in Chapter 35, and are not considered further in this section.

Noradrenergic neuron blocking drugs

Noradrenergic neuron blocking drugs (e.g. **guanethidine**) were first discovered in the mid-1950s when alternatives to ganglion-blocking drugs, for use in the treatment of hypertension, were being sought. The main effect of guanethidine is to inhibit the release of noradrenaline from sympathetic nerve terminals. It has little effect on the adrenal medulla, and none on nerve terminals that release transmitters other than noradrenaline. Drugs very similar to it include bretylium, bethanidine, and debrisoquin (which is of interest mainly as a tool for studying drug metabolism; see Ch. 5).

Actions

Drugs of this class reduce or abolish the response of tissues to sympathetic nerve stimulation, but do not affect (or may potentiate) the effects of injected noradrenaline. Their ability to block noradrenaline release can be demonstrated by measurement, for example, of the release of radioactivity from organs such as the spleen or vas deferens, in response to stimulation of the sympathetic nerves after the transmitter stores have been labelled by infusion of radioactive noradrenaline.

The action of guanethidine on noradrenergic transmission is complex, and the subject of exhaustive research (see Broadley 1996). It is selectively accumulated by noradrenergic nerve terminals, being a substrate for uptake 1. Its initial blocking activity depends on impairment of impulse conduction in the nerve terminals due to this selective accumulation (Brock & Cunnane 1988). Its action is prevented by drugs, such as amphetamine (see below) which block uptake 1.

Guanethidine is also concentrated in synaptic vesicles by means of the vesicular transporter, possibly interfering with their ability to undergo exocytosis, and also displacing noradrenaline. In this way it causes a gradual and long-lasting depletion of noradrenaline in sympathetic nerve endings, similar to the effect of reserpine.

Given in large doses, guanethidine causes structural damage to noradrenergic neurons, which is probably due to the fact that the terminals accumulate the drug in high concentration. It can therefore be used as a selective neurotoxin.

Guanethidine is no longer used clinically. Though extremely effective in lowering blood pressure, it produces severe side-effects associated with the loss of sympathetic reflexes. The most troublesome are *postural hypotension, diarrhoea, nasal congestion* and *failure of ejaculation*. **Bretylium** is sometimes used to treat ventricular dysrhythmias resistant to other agents, during cardiac resuscitation (see Ch. 14); its mechanism of action in this setting is unknown.

INDIRECTLY ACTING SYMPATHOMIMETIC AMINES

Mechanism of action and structure–activity relationships

The most important drugs in the indirectly acting sympathomimetic amine category are **tyramine, amphetamine** and **ephedrine**, all of which are structurally related to noradrenaline (Fig. 8.5). They have only weak actions on adrenoceptors, but sufficiently resemble noradrenaline to be transported into nerve terminals by uptake 1. Once inside the nerve terminals they are taken up into the vesicles by the vesicular monoamine transporter, in exchange for noradrenaline, which escapes into the cytosol. Some of the cytosolic noradrenaline is degraded by MAO, while the rest escapes via uptake 1, in exchange for the foreign monoamine, to act on postsynaptic receptors (Fig. 8.9). Exocytosis is not involved in the release process, so their actions do not require the presence of calcium. They are not completely specific in their actions, and act partly by a direct effect on adrenoceptors, partly by inhibiting uptake 1 (thereby enhancing the effect of the released noradrenaline), and partly by inhibiting MAO.

As would be expected, the effects of these drugs are strongly influenced by other drugs that modify noradrenergic transmission. Thus, **reserpine** or **6-hydroxydopamine** abolishes their effects by depleting the terminals of noradrenaline. MAO inhibitors, on the other hand, strongly potentiate their effects, by preventing breakdown, within the terminals, of the transmitter displaced from the vesicles. MAO inhibition particularly enhances the action of **tyramine** because this substance is itself a substrate for MAO. Normally dietary tyramine is destroyed by MAO in the gut wall and liver before reaching the systemic circulation. When MAO is inhibited this is prevented, and ingestion of tyramine-rich foods, such as fermented cheese (e.g. ripe Brie) can then provoke a sudden and dangerous rise in blood pressure. Inhibitors of uptake 1, such as **imipramine** (see below) interfere with the effects of indirectly acting sympathomimetic amines by preventing their uptake into the nerve terminals.

These drugs, especially **amphetamine**, have important effects on the central nervous system (see Ch. 38), which depend on their ability to release, not only noradrenaline,

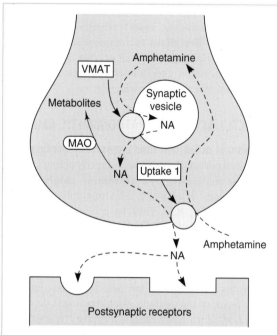

Fig. 8.9 The mode of action of amphetamine, an indirectly acting sympathomimetic amine. Amphetamine enters the nerve terminal via the NA carrier (uptake 1) and enters synaptic vesicles via the vesicular monoamine transporter, in exchange for NA, which accumulates in the cytosol. Some of the NA is degraded by MAO within the nerve terminal and some escapes, in exchange for amphetamine via uptake 1, to act on postsynaptic receptors. Amphetamine also reduces NA reuptake via uptake 1, so enhancing the action of the released NA.
(NA = noradrenaline; MAO = monoamine oxidase; VMAT = vesicular monoamine transporter)

but also 5-HT and dopamine from nerve terminals in the brain. An important characteristic of the effects of indirectly acting sympathomimetic amines is that marked tolerance develops. Repeated doses of amphetamine or tyramine, for example, produce progressively smaller pressor responses. This is probably caused by a depletion of the releasable store of noradrenaline, since the response can be restored, in experimental animals, by infusion of noradrenaline, which has the effect of replenishing the releasable store. A similar tolerance to the central effects also develops with repeated administration, which partly accounts for the liability of amphetamine and related drugs to cause dependence.

Actions

The peripheral actions of the indirectly acting sympathomimetic amines closely resemble those of noradrenaline,

namely *bronchodilatation, raised arterial pressure, peripheral vasoconstriction, increased force of myocardial contraction* and *inhibition of gut motility*, though they are longer-lasting. They have important central actions, which account for their significant abuse potential, and for their limited therapeutic applications (see Chs 38 and 39). Apart from **ephedrine**, which is still sometimes used as a nasal decongestant, since it has much less central action, these drugs are no longer used for their peripheral sympathomimetic effects.

INHIBITORS OF NORADRENALINE UPTAKE

Neuronal reuptake of released noradrenaline (uptake 1) is the most important mechanism by which its action is brought to an end. Many drugs inhibit this transport and thereby enhance the effects of both sympathetic nerve activity and injected noradrenaline. Uptake 1 is not responsible for clearing circulating adrenaline so these drugs do not affect responses to this amine.

The main class of drugs whose primary action is inhibition of uptake 1 are the **tricyclic antidepressants** (see Ch. 35), for example **desipramine**. These drugs have their major effect on the central nervous system, but also cause tachycardia and cardiac dysrhythmias, reflecting their peripheral effect on sympathetic transmission. **Cocaine**, known mainly for its abuse liability (Ch. 39) and local anaesthetic activity (Ch. 40), enhances sympathetic transmission, causing tachycardia and increased arterial pressure, by inhibiting uptake 1. Its central effects of euphoria and excitement (Ch. 38) are probably a manifestation of the same mechanism acting in the brain. It strongly potentiates the actions of noradrenaline in experimental animals or in isolated tissues provided the sympathetic nerve terminals are intact.

Many drugs that act mainly on other steps in sympathetic transmission also inhibit uptake 1 to some extent, presumably because the carrier molecule bears a steric relationship to other noradrenaline recognition sites, such as receptors and degradative enzymes. Examples include **amphetamine**, **phenoxybenzamine** and **guanethidine**.

Extraneuronal uptake (uptake 2), which is important in clearing circulating adrenaline from the bloodstream, is not affected by most of the drugs that block uptake 1. It is inhibited by **phenoxybenzamine**, however, and also by various corticosteroids (see Ch. 13). This action of corticosteroids may have some relevance to their therapeutic effect in conditions such as asthma, but is probably of minor importance.

The main sites of action of drugs that affect adrenergic transmission are summarised in Figure 8.10.

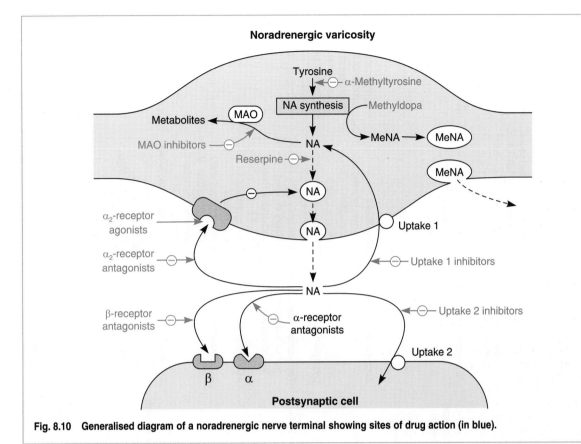

Fig. 8.10 Generalised diagram of a noradrenergic nerve terminal showing sites of drug action (in blue).

Drugs acting on noradrenergic nerve terminals

- Drugs that inhibit NA synthesis include:
  — α-methyltyrosine: blocks tyrosine hydroxylase, not used clinically
  — carbidopa: blocks dopa decarboxylase and is used in treatment of parkinsonism (see Ch. 31); not much effect on NA synthesis.
- Methyldopa gives rise to false transmitter (methyl-NA) which is a potent α₂-agonist, thus causing powerful presynaptic inhibitory feedback (also central actions). Occasionally used as antihypertensive agent.
- Reserpine blocks carrier-mediated NA accumulation in vesicles, thus depleting NA stores and blocking transmission. Effective in hypertension, but may cause severe depression.
- Noradrenergic neuron blocking drugs (e.g. guanethidine, bethanidine) are selectively concentrated in terminals (uptake 1), and in vesicles (vesicular transporter), and block

transmitter release, partly by local anaesthetic action. Effective in hypertension, but cause severe side-effects (postural hypotension, diarrhoea, nasal congestion, etc.) so now little used.
- 6-hydroxydopamine is selectively neurotoxic for noradrenergic neurons, because it is taken up and converted to a toxic metabolite. Used experimentally to eliminate noradrenergic neurons, not clinically.
- Indirectly acting sympathomimetic amines (e.g. amphetamine, ephedrine, tyramine) are accumulated by uptake 1 and displace NA from vesicles, allowing it to escape. Effect is much enhanced by MAO inhibition, which can lead to severe hypertension following ingestion of tyramine-rich foods by patients treated with MAO inhibitors.
- Drugs that inhibit uptake 1 include cocaine and tricyclic antidepressant drugs. Sympathetic effects are enhanced by such drugs.

Table 8.3 Summary of drugs that affect noradrenergic transmission

Type	Drug	Main action	Uses/function	Unwanted effects	Pharmacokinetic aspects	Notes
Sympathomimetic (directly acting)	Noradrenaline	α/β-agonist	Not used clinically. Transmitter at post-ganglionic sympathetic neurons, and in CNS. Hormone of adrenal medulla	Hypertension, vasoconstriction, tachycardia (or reflex bradycardia), ventricular dysrhythmias	Poorly absorbed by mouth. Rapid removal by tissues. Metabolised by MAO and COMT. Plasma $t_{1/2}$ ~2 min	
	Adrenaline	α/β-agonist	Asthma (emergency treatment), anaphylactic shock, cardiac arrest. Added to local anaesthetic solutions. Hormone of adrenal medulla	As noradrenaline	Given i.m. or s.c. As noradrenaline	See Chapter 19
	Isoprenaline	β-agonist (non-selective)	Asthma (obsolete). Not an endogenous substance	Tachycardia, dysrhythmias	Some tissue uptake, followed by inactivation (COMT). Plasma $t_{1/2}$ ~2 h	Now replaced by salbutamol in treatment of asthma (see Ch. 19)
	Dobutamine	β_1-agonist (non-selective)	Cardiogenic shock	Dysrhythmias	Plasma $t_{1/2}$ ~ 2 min. Given i.v.	See Chapter 14
	Salbutamol	β_2-agonist	Asthma, premature labour	Tachycardia, dysrhythmias, tremor, peripheral vasodilatation	Given orally or by aerosol. Mainly excreted unchanged. Plasma $t_{1/2}$ ~ 4 h	See Chaper 19
	Salmeterol	β_2-agonist	Asthma	As salbutamol	Given by aerosol. Long-acting	
	Terbutaline	β_2-agonist	Asthma	As salbutamol	Poorly absorbed orally. Given by aerosol. Mainly excreted unchanged. Plasma $t_{1/2}$ ~ 4 h	See Chapter 19
	Clenbuterol	β_2-agonist	'Anabolic' action to increase muscle strength	As salbutamol	Active orally. Long-acting	Illicit use in sport
	Phenylephrine	α_1-agonist	Nasal decongestion	Hypertension, reflex bradycardia	Given intranasally. Metabolised by MAO. Short plasma $t_{1/2}$	
	Methoxamine	α-agonist (non-selective)	Nasal decongestion	As phenylephrine	Given intranasally. Plasma $t_{1/2}$ ~ 1 h	
	Clonidine	α_2-partial agonist	Hypertension, migraine	Drowsiness, orthostatic hypotension, oedema and weight gain, rebound hypertension	Well absorbed orally. Excreted unchanged and as conjugate. Plasma $t_{1/2}$ ~ 12 h	See Chapter 15

Table 8.3 (continued)

Type	Drug	Main action	Uses/function	Unwanted effects	Pharmacokinetic aspects	Notes
Sympathomimetic (indirectly acting)	Tyramine	NA release	No clinical uses. Present in various foods	As noradrenaline	Normally destroyed by MAO in gut. Does not enter brain	See Chapter 35
	Amphetamine	NA release, MAO inhibitor, uptake 1 inhibitor, CNS stimulant	Used as CNS stimulant in narcolepsy, also (paradoxically) in hyperactive children. Appetite suppressant. Drug of abuse	Hypertension, tachycardia, insomnia. Acute psychosis with overdose. Dependence	Well absorbed orally. penetrates freely into brain. Excreted unchanged in urine. Plasma $t_{1/2} \sim$ 12 h, depending on urine flow and pH	See Chapter 38
	Ephedrine	NA release, β-agonist, weak CNS stimulant	Nasal decongestion	As amphetamine, but less pronounced	Similar to amphetamine	Contraindicated if MAO inhibitors are given
Adrenoceptor antagonists	Phenoxybenzamine	α-antagonist (non-selective, irreversible), uptake 1 inhibitor	Phaeochromocytoma	Hypotension, flushing, tachycardia, nasal congestion, impotence	Absorbed orally. Plasma $t_{1/2} \sim$ 12 h	Action outlasts presence of drug in plasma, because of covalent binding to receptor
	Phentolamine	α-antagonist (non-selective), vasodilator	Rarely used	As phenoxybenzamine	Usually given i.v. Metabolised by liver. Plasma $t_{1/2} \sim$2 h	Tolazoline is similar
	Prazosin	α_1-antagonist	Hypertension	As phenoxybenzamine	Absorbed orally. Metabolised by liver. Plasma $t_{1/2} \sim$4 h	Doxazosin, terazosin are similar but longer-acting. See Chapter 15
	Yohimbine	α_2-antagonist	Not used clinically. Claimed to be aphrodisiac	Excitement, hypertension		Idazoxan is similar
	Propranolol	β-antagonist (non-selective)	Angina, hypertension, cardiac dysrhythmias, anxiety tremor, glaucoma	Bronchoconstriction, cardiac failure, cold extremities, fatigue and depression, hypoglycaemia	Absorbed orally. Extensive first-pass metabolism. About 90% bound to plasma protein. Plasma $t_{1/2} \sim$4 h	Timolol is similar, and used mainly to treat glaucoma. See Chapter 14
	Alprenolol	β-antagonist (non-selective) (partial agonist)	As propranolol	As propranolol	Absorbed orally. Metabolised by liver. Plasma $t_{1/2} \sim$4 h	Oxprenolol and pindolol are similar. See Chapter 14
	Practolol	β_1-antagonist	Hypertension, angina, dysrhythmias	As propranolol, also oculomucocutaneous syndrome	Absorbed orally. Excreted unchanged in urine. Plasma $t_{1/2} \sim$4 h	Withdrawn from clinical use
	Metoprolol	β_1-antagonist	Angina, hypertension, dysrhythmias	As propranolol, less risk of bronchoconstriction	Absorbed orally. Mainly metabolised in liver. Plasma $t_{1/2} \sim$ 3 h	Atenolol is similar with a longer half-life. See Chapter 13

Table 8.3 (continued)

Type	Drug	Main action	Uses/function	Unwanted effects	Pharmacokinetic aspects	Notes
Adrenoceptor antagonists (continued)	Butoxamine	β_2-antagonist, weak α-agonist	No clinical uses			
	Labetalol	α/β-antagonist	Hypertension in pregnancy	Postural hypotension, bronchoconstriction	Absorbed orally. Conjugated in liver. Plasma $t_{1/2} \sim 4$ h	See Chapters 14 and 15
Drugs affecting noradrenaline synthesis	α–methyl-p-tyrosine	Inhibits tyrosine hydroxylase	Occassionally used in phaeochromocytoma		Absorbed orally. Does not enter brain	See Chapter 31
	Carbidopa	Inhibits dopa decarboxylase	Used as adjunct to L-dopa, to prevent peripheral effects			
	Methyldopa	False transmitter precursor	Hypertension in pregnancy	Hypotension, drowsiness, diarrhoea, impotence, hypersensitivity reactions	Absorbed slowly by mouth. Excreted unchanged or as conjugate. Plasma $t_{1/2} \sim 6$ h	See Chapter 15
	Reserpine	Depletes NA stores by inhibiting vesicular uptake of NA	Hypertension (obsolete)	As methyldopa. Also depression, parkinsonism, gynaecomastia	Poorly absorbed orally. Slowly metabolised. Plasma $t_{1/2} \sim 100$ h. Excreted in milk	Antihypertensive effect develops slowly, and persists when drug is stopped
Drugs affecting noradrenaline release	Guanethidine	Inhibits NA release. Also causes NA depletion, and can damage NA neurons irreversibly	Hypertension (obsolete)	As methyldopa. Hypertension on first administration	Poorly absorbed orally. Mainly excreted unchanged in urine. Plasma $t_{1/2} \sim 100$ h	Action prevented by uptake 1 inhibitors. Bethanidine and debrisoquin are similar
Drugs affecting noradrenaline uptake	Imipramine	Blocks uptake 1. Also has atropine-like action	Depression	Atropine-like side-effects. Cardiac dysrhythmias in overdose	Well absorbed orally. 95% bound to plasma protein. Converted to active metabolite (desmethylimipramine). Plasma $t_{1/2} \sim 4$ h	Desipramine and amitriptyline are similar. See Chapter 35
	Cocaine	Local anaesthetic. Blocks uptake 1, CNS stimulant	Rarely used local anaesthetic. Major drug of abuse	Hypertension, excitement, convulsions, dependence	Well absorbed orally	See Chapters 38 and 40

REFERENCES AND FURTHER READING

Amara S G, Kuhar M J 1993 Neurotransmitter transporters: recent progress. Annu Rev Neurosci 16: 73–93 (*Useful review on monoamine transporters*)

Broadley K J 1996 Autonomic pharmacology. Taylor & Francis, London (*Detailed textbook*)

Brock J A, Cunnane T C 1988 Studies on the mode of action of bretylium and guanethidine in post-ganglionic sympathetic nerve fibres. Naunyn-Schmiedebergs Arch Pharmacol 338: 504–509 (*Elegant electrophysiological analysis of action of sympathetic neuron-blocking drugs*)

Brownstein M J, Hofmann B J 1994 Neurotransmitter transporters. Recent Prog Hormone Res 49: 27–42 (*Good review article*)

Bylund D B 1994 Nomenclature of adrenoceptors. Pharmacol Rev 46: 121–136 (*Rationalisation of the taxonomy of adrenoceptors*)

Cooper J R, Bloom F E, Roth R H 1996 The biochemical basis of neuropharmacology. Oxford University Press, New York (*Excellent standard textbook*)

Cunnane T C 1984 The mechanism of neurotransmitter release from sympathetic nerves. Trends Neurosci 7: 248–253 (*Points out important differences between adrenergic and cholinergic neurons*)

Dahl R 1980 My Uncle Oswald. Penguin, Harmondsworth

Fillenz M 1990 Noradrenergic neurons. Cambridge University Press, Cambridge (*Comprehensive monograph*)

Insel P A 1996 Adrenergic receptors—evolving concepts and clinical implications. New Engl J Med 334: 580–585 (*Excellent review, focusing on applications*)

Liu Y, Edwards R H 1997 The role of vesicular transport proteins in synaptic transmission and neural degeneration. Annu Rev Neurosci 20: 125–156 (*Review of recent ideas about functional role of transporters*)

Lundberg J M 1996 Pharmacology of co-transmission in the autonomic nervous system: integrative aspects on amines, neuropeptides, adenosine triphosphate, amino acids and nitric oxide. Pharmacol Rev 48: 114–192 (*Comprehensive and informative review*)

McGrath J C, Wilson V 1988 α-adrenoceptor subclassification by classical and response-related methods: same question, different answers. Trends Pharmacol Sci 9: 162–165 (*Discusses problems of adrenoceptor taxonomy*)

Pfeffer M A, Stevenson L W 1996 β-adrenergic blockers and survival in heart failure. New Engl J Med 334: 1396–1397 (*Shows that β-adrenergic blockers in low doses can be beneficial in heart failure*)

Starke K, Göthert M, Kilbinger H 1989 Modulation of transmitter release by presynaptic autoreceptors. Physiol Rev 69: 864–989 (*Comprehensive review*)

Summers R J, McMartin L R 1993 Adrenoceptors and their second messenger systems. J Neurochem 60: 10–23 (*Short review article*)

Trendelenburg U, Weiner N 1988 Catecholamines. Handbook of experimental pharmacology. Springer-Verlag, Berlin, vol 90, parts 1, 2 (*Massive compilation of knowledge to date*)

Zhang K-M, Hu P, Wang S-W et al. 1996 Salbutamol changes the molecular and mechanical properties of canine skeletal muscle. J Physiol 496: 211–220 (*Surprising finding that salbutamol affects muscle function by non-receptor mechanisms*)

Other peripheral mediators: 5-hydroxytryptamine and purines

In this chapter we discuss two types of mediator, both of which play a role as neurotransmitters in the brain and periphery, and also probably function as local hormones. 5-hydroxytryptamine (5-HT) has a longer pharmacological history than purines, and there are more drugs in current use that act through 5-HT-mediated mechanisms than through purine-mediated mechanisms. In both cases, though, a combination of pharmacological and molecular biological approaches in recent years has uncovered a wide range of receptor subtypes, whose physiological significance—and hence therapeutic relevance—has yet to be clearly defined. We are in the phase where the pharmaceutical industry has seized on the opportunity offered by these potential new drug targets, and is producing a profusion of specific agonists and antagonists, which are in turn being used to clarify the physiological role of the various receptor systems. There is a sense of confident expectation of therapeutic advances on the horizon, but the student may be forgiven for finding the taxonomic niceties somewhat unrewarding at this stage. Useful reviews for the insatiable include Fredholm et al. 1994, Hoyer et al. 1994, North & Barnard 1997).

5-HYDROXYTRYPTAMINE

Serotonin was the name given in the last century to an unknown vasoconstrictor substance found in the serum after blood has clotted. It was identified chemically as 5-hydroxytryptamine (5-HT) in 1948, and shown to originate from the platelets. It was subsequently found in the gastrointestinal tract and central nervous system, and shown to function both as a neurotransmitter, and as a local hormone in the peripheral vascular system. This chapter deals with the metabolism, distribution and possible physiological roles of 5-HT in the periphery, and with the different types of 5-HT receptor and the drugs that act on them. Further information on the role of 5-HT in the brain, and its relationship to psychiatric disorders and the actions of psychotropic drugs, is presented in Chapters 28, 34 and 35. More detailed information on 5-HT in the CNS and in the periphery can be found in Cooper et al. (1996) and Fozard (1989).

DISTRIBUTION, BIOSYNTHESIS AND DEGRADATION

5-HT occurs in the highest concentrations in three situations in the body:

- *In the wall of the intestine.* About 90% of the total amount in the body is present in enterochromaffin cells, which are cells derived from the neural crest, similar to those of the adrenal medulla, that are interspersed with mucosal cells, mainly in the stomach and small intestine. Some 5-HT also occurs in nerve cells of the myenteric plexus, where it functions as an excitatory neurotransmitter (see Chs 6 and 21).
- *In blood.* 5-HT is present in high concentration in platelets, which accumulate it from the plasma by an active transport system, and release it when they aggregate at sites of tissue damage (see Ch. 17).
- *In the central nervous system.* 5-HT is a transmitter in the central nervous system (see Ch. 30) and is pre-

sent in high concentrations in localised regions of the midbrain. Its functional role is discussed in Chapter 30.

The biosynthesis of 5-HT follows a pathway similar to that of noradrenaline (see Ch. 8), except that the precursor amino acid is *tryptophan* instead of tyrosine (Fig. 9.1). 5-HT is present in the diet, but most is metabolised before entering the bloodstream. Tryptophan is converted to *5-hydroxytryptophan* (in chromaffin cells and neurons, but not in platelets) by the action of *tryptophan hydroxylase* (an enzyme confined to 5-HT-producing cells). The 5-hydroxytryptophan is then

decarboxylated to 5-HT, by the same amino acid decarboxylase that participates in the synthesis of catecholamines (Ch. 8) and histamine (Ch. 12). Platelets (and neurons) possess a high affinity 5-HT uptake mechanism, and platelets become loaded with 5-HT as they pass through the intestinal circulation, where the local concentration is relatively high. The mechanisms of synthesis, storage, release and reuptake of 5-HT are very similar to those of noradrenaline, and many drugs affect both processes indiscriminately (see Chs 8 and 35). Recent work has shown that 5-HT is often stored in neurons and chromaffin cells as a co-transmitter together with various peptide hormones, such as **somatostatin**, **substance P** or **vasoactive intestinal polypeptide** (VIP).

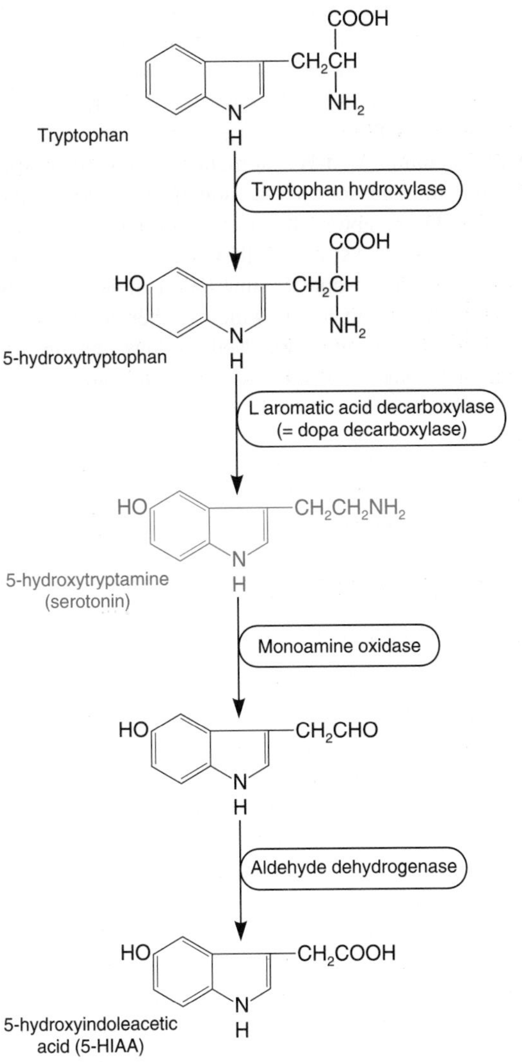

Degradation of 5-HT (Fig. 9.1) occurs mainly through oxidative deamination, catalysed by *monoamine oxidase*, followed by oxidation to *5-hydroxyindoleacetic acid* (5-HIAA), the pathway being exactly analogous to that of noradrenaline catabolism (Fig. 8.4). 5-HIAA is excreted in the urine, and serves as an indicator of 5-HT production in the body. This is used, for example, in the diagnosis of *carcinoid syndrome* (see below).

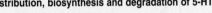

Fig. 9.1 Biosynthesis and metabolism of 5-HT.

Distribution, biosynthesis and degradation of 5-HT

- Structures rich in 5-HT are:
  — gastrointestinal tract (chromaffin cells and enteric neurons)
  — platelets
  — central nervous system.
- Metabolism closely parallels that of noradrenaline.
- Formed from dietary tryptophan, which is converted to 5-hydroxytryptophan by tryptophan hydroxylase, then to 5-HT by a non-specific decarboxylase.
- 5-HT is transported into 5-HT-containing cells by a specific transport system.
- Degradation occurs mainly by MAO, forming 5-HIAA, which is excreted in urine.

PHARMACOLOGICAL EFFECTS

The actions of 5-HT are numerous and complex, and show considerable species variation. This complexity reflects a profusion of 5-HT receptor subtypes which has been revealed in recent years (see below). The main sites of action are:

- *Gastrointestinal tract.* 5-HT causes increased gastrointestinal motility and contraction of isolated strips of intestine, this being partly due to a direct effect on the smooth muscle cells, and partly due to an indirect excitatory effect on enteric neurons. The peristaltic reflex, evoked by increasing the pressure within a segment of intestine, is mediated, partly at least, by the release of 5-HT from chromaffin cells in response to the mechanical stimulus. Chromaffin cells also respond to vagal stimulation by releasing 5-HT.

- *Smooth muscle* elsewhere in the body (e.g. *uterus* and *bronchial tree*) is also contracted by 5-HT in many species, but only to a minor extent in humans.
- *Blood vessels.* The effect of 5-HT on blood vessels depends on various factors, including the size of the vessel, the species, and the prevailing sympathetic activity. Large vessels, both arteries and veins, are usually constricted by 5-HT, though the sensitivity varies greatly. This is a direct action on vascular smooth muscle cells, mediated through 5-HT$_{2A}$-receptors (see below). 5-HT also causes vasodilatation by acting on 5-HT$_1$-receptors, partly by releasing nitric oxide from

endothelial cells (see Ch. 11), and partly by inhibiting noradrenaline release from sympathetic nerve terminals. Thus 5-HT$_{2A}$-receptors predominantly give rise to vasoconstriction, whereas 5-HT$_1$-receptors produce dilatation. When 5-HT$_{2A}$-receptors are blocked by ketanserin (see Table 9.1), the vasodilator effect is revealed (Fig. 9.2).

If 5-HT is injected intravenously, the blood pressure usually first rises, because of the constriction of large vessels, and then falls, because of arteriolar dilatation.

- *Platelets.* 5-HT causes platelet aggregation (see Ch. 17), via 5-HT$_{2A}$-receptors, and the platelets that collect in the vessel release more 5-HT. If the endothelium is intact, 5-HT release from adherent platelets causes vasodilatation, which helps to sustain blood flow; if it is damaged (e.g. by atherosclerosis), 5-HT causes constriction, and impairs blood flow further. These effects of platelet-derived 5-HT are thought to be important in vascular disease.
- *Nerve endings.* 5-HT stimulates nociceptive (pain-mediating) sensory nerve endings, an effect mediated by 5-HT$_3$-receptors. If injected into the skin it causes pain, and given systemically it elicits a variety of autonomic reflexes due to stimulation of afferent fibres in the heart and lungs, which further complicate the cardiovascular response. Nettle stings contain 5-HT, amongst other things. It also inhibits transmitter release

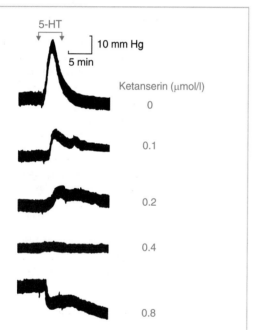

Fig. 9.2 Dual vascular effects of 5-HT. Dual effect of serotonin on blood vessels. The records show changes in the arterial perfusion pressure in a guinea-pig stomach preparation in response to 5-HT. The normal response to 5-HT is a strong vasoconstriction (*upper record*). Addition of increasing concentrations of the 5-HT$_{2A}$-receptor antagonist, ketanserin, reduces the vasoconstriction and reveals a vasodilator effect (*lower trace*), which is probably mediated by 5-HT$_1$-receptors. (From: van Nueten J M et al. 1981 J Pharmacol Exp Ther 218: 217)

Actions and functions of 5-HT

- Important actions are:
  — increased gastrointestinal motility (direct excitation of smooth muscle and indirect action via enteric neurons)
  — contraction of other smooth muscle (bronchi, uterus)
  — mixture of vascular constriction (direct and via sympathetic innervation) and dilatation (endothelium dependent)
  — platelet aggregation
  — stimulation of peripheral nociceptive nerve endings
  — excitation/inhibition of CNS neurons.
- Postulated physiological and pathophysiological roles include:
  — in periphery: peristalsis, vomiting, platelet aggregation and haemostasis, inflammatory mediator, sensitisation of nociceptors and microvascular control
  — in CNS: many postulated functions, including control of appetite, sleep, mood, hallucinations, stereotyped behaviour, pain perception and vomiting.
- Clinical conditions associated with disturbed 5-HT function include migraine, carcinoid syndrome, mood disorders and anxiety (see Chs 33 and 35).

from adrenergic neurons in the periphery, as discussed above.

• *Central nervous system.* 5-HT excites some neurons and inhibits others, and also acts presynaptically to inhibit transmitter release from nerve terminals. Different receptor types and different membrane mechanisms mediate these effects (see Table 9.1; Bobker & Williams 1990). The role of 5-HT in the central nervous system is discussed in Chapter 30.

CLASSIFICATION OF 5-HT RECEPTORS

It was long-ago realised that the actions of 5-HT are not all mediated by receptors of the same type, and various pharmacological classifications have come and gone. The most recent, if not the final, classification agreed at a summit meeting of 5-HT aficionados, and delivered with puffs of white smoke and much celebration, was presented and discussed in detail by Hoyer et al. (1994)

Table 9.1 The main 5-HT receptor subtypes

Receptor	Location	Main effects	Second messenger	Agonists	Antagonists
1A	CNS	Neuronal inhibition Behavioural effects: sleep, feeding, thermoregulation, anxiety	↓ cAMP	5-CT 8-OH-DPAT Buspirone (PA)	Spiperone Methiothepin Ergotamine (PA)
1B	CNS	Presynaptic inhibition Behavioural effects	↓ cAMP	5-CT	Methiothepin Ergotamine (PA)
1D	CNS Blood vessels	Cerebral vasoconstriction Behavioural effects: locomotion	↓ cAMP	5-CT Sumatriptan	Methiothepin Ergotamine (PA)
2A	CNS PNS Smooth muscle Platelets	Neuronal excitation Behavioural effects Platelet aggregation Smooth muscle contraction (gut, bronchi, etc.) Vasoconstriction/vasodilatation	↑ IP$_3$/DAG	α-Me 5-HT LSD (CNS)	Ketanserin Cyproheptadine Pizotifen (non-selective) LSD (periphery) Methysergide
2B	Gastric fundus	Contraction	↑ IP$_3$/DAG	α-Me 5-HT	
2C	CNS Choroid plexus	CSF secretion	↑ IP$_3$/DAG	α-Me 5-HT LSD	Methysergide
3	PNS CNS	Neuronal excitation (autonomic, nociceptive neurons) Emesis Behavioural effects: anxiety	None—ligand-gated cation channel	2-Me 5-HT Cl-phenyl biguanide	Ondansetron Tropisetron Granisetron
4	PNS (GI tract) CNS	Neuronal excitation GI motility	↑ cAMP	5-methoxy- tryptamine Metoclopramide	Various experimental Compounds (e.g. GR113808, SB207266)
5	CNS	Not known	Not known	Not known	Not known
6	CNS	Not known	Not known	Not known	Not known
7	CNS GI tract Blood vessels	Not known	↑ cAMP	5-CT, LSD No selective agonists	Various 5-HT$_2$ antagonists No selective antagonists

Abbreviations: 5-CT = 5-carboxamidotryptamine; 8-OH-DPAT = 8-hydroxy-2-(di n-propylamino)tetraline; α-Me 5-HT = α-methyl 5-HT; 2-Me 5-HT = 2-methyl 5-HT. For further details, see Eglen et al. 1997, Hoyer et al. 1994.
The list of agonists and antagonists includes only the better-known compounds. Many new selective 5-HT receptor ligands, known only by code numbers, are being developed. (PA) denotes partial agonist.

and is summarised in Table 9.1. This classification takes into account sequence data derived from cloning, signal transduction mechanisms and pharmacological specificity. Currently there are seven main receptor types, 5-HT$_{1-7}$, of which types 1 and 2 are further subdivided into 3 or 4 sub-categories, denoted A–D.

5-HT$_1$-receptors occur mainly in the brain, the subtypes being distinguished on the basis of their regional distribution and their pharmacological specificity. They function mainly as inhibitory presynaptic receptors, and are linked to inhibition of adenylate cyclase. The 5-HT$_{1A}$ subtype is particularly important in the brain, in relation to mood and behaviour (see Chs 29, 33 and 35). The 5-HT$_{1D}$ subtype, which is expressed in cerebral blood vessels, is believed to be important in migraine (see below), and is the target for **sumatriptan**, an agonist at 5-HT$_{1D}$-receptors, used to treat acute attacks. These vessels are unusual in that vasoconstriction is mediated by 5-HT$_1$-receptors; in most vessels, 5-HT$_2$-receptors are responsible. The hapless '5-HT$_{1C}$-receptor'—actually the first to be cloned—has been officially declared non-existent, having been ignominiously reclassified as the 5-HT$_{2C}$-receptor when it was found to be linked, not to adenylate cyclase, but to IP$_3$ production.

5-HT$_2$-receptors are more important in the periphery than in the CNS. The effects of 5-HT on smooth muscle and platelets, which have been known for many years, are mediated by the 5-HT$_{2A}$-receptor, as are some of the behavioural effects of agents such as lysergic acid diethylamide (LSD; see Table 9.1 and Ch. 38). 5-HT$_2$-receptors are linked to phospholipase C, which catalyses phosphatidylinositol hydrolysis; 5-HT$_2$ agonists thus stimulate IP$_3$ formation. The 5-HT$_{2A}$ subtype is functionally the most important, the others having a much more limited distribution and functional role. The role of 5-HT$_2$-receptors in normal physiological processes is probably a minor one, but it becomes more prominent in pathological conditions, such as asthma and vascular thrombosis (see Chs 16, 17 and 19).

5-HT$_3$-receptors occur mainly in the peripheral nervous system, particularly on nociceptive sensory neurons (see Ch. 37), and on autonomic and enteric neurons, on which 5-HT exerts a strong excitatory effect. 5-HT itself evokes pain when injected locally, and when given intravenously elicits a fine display of autonomic reflexes, which result from excitation of many types of vascular, pulmonary and cardiac sensory nerve fibre. The physiological role of this receptor is not known, but it has been postulated that excitation of vascular sensory nerve terminals by 5-HT released from platelets may be involved in the pathogenesis of migraine (see below). 5-HT$_3$-receptors

are exceptional in being directly linked to membrane ion channels (Ch. 2), and do not involve any second messenger step in their transduction mechanism. 5-HT$_3$-receptors also occur in the brain, particularly in the *area postrema*, a region of the medulla involved in the vomiting reflex, and selective 5-HT$_3$ antagonists are used as anti-emetic drugs (see Ch. 21).

5-HT$_4$-receptors have recently been identified as a sub-class distinct from 5-HT$_3$-receptors. They occur in the brain, as well as in peripheral organs, such as the gastrointestinal tract, bladder and heart. Their main physiological role appears to be in the gastrointestinal tract, where they produce neuronal excitation, and mediate the effect of 5-HT in stimulating peristalsis.

Little is so far known about the functions of the remaining types, 5, 6 and 7.

5-HT receptors

- Seven types (5-HT$_{1-7}$), with further subtypes (A–D) of 5-HT$_1$ and 5-HT$_2$. All are G-protein coupled receptors, except 5-HT$_3$ which is a ligand-gated cation channel.
- 5-HT$_1$-receptors occur mainly in CNS (all subtypes) and some blood vessels (5-HT$_{1D}$ subtype). Effects are neural inhibition and vasoconstriction. Act by inhibiting adenylate cyclase. *Specific agonists* include: sumatriptan (used in migraine therapy) and buspirone (used in anxiety). Ergotamine is a partial agonist. *Specific antagonists* include spiperone and methiothepin.
- 5-HT$_2$-receptors occur in CNS and many peripheral sites (especially blood vessels, platelets, autonomic neurons). Neuronal and smooth muscle effects are excitatory. Act through phospholipase C/inositol phosphate pathway. Specific ligands include LSD (agonist in CNS, antagonist in periphery). *Specific antagonists:* ketanserin, methysergide and cyproheptadine.
- 5-HT$_3$-receptors occur in peripheral nervous system, especially nociceptive afferent neurons and enteric neurons, and in CNS. Effects are excitatory, mediated via direct receptor-coupled ion channels. *Specific agonist:* 2-methyl-5-HT. *Specific antagonists:* ondansetron, tropisetron. Antagonists are used mainly as anti-emetic drugs, but may also be anxiolytic.
- 5-HT$_4$-receptors occur mainly in the enteric nervous system (also in CNS). Effects are excitatory, causing increased gastrointestinal motility. Act by stimulating adenylate cyclase. Specific agonists include metoclopramide (used to stimulate gastric emptying.
- Little is known so far about the function and pharmacology of 5-HT$_{5-7}$ receptors.
- Many new receptor-selective agonists and antagonists are being developed.

DRUGS ACTING ON 5-HT RECEPTORS

Table 9.1 lists some of the selective agonists and antagonists for the different receptor types. Many of these compounds have been useful as experimental tools for defining the receptor subtypes, but only a few have so far been developed for clinical use. The improved understanding of the location and function of the different receptor subtypes has, however, caused an upsurge of interest in developing compounds with improved receptor selectivity, and useful new drugs are likely to appear in the near future.

Important drugs that act on 5-HT receptors in the periphery include:

- 5-HT$_{1D}$-receptor agonists (e.g. **sumatriptan**) used for treating migraine (see below). Selective 5-HT$_{1A}$ agonists, such as 8-OH-DPAT (Table 9.1), are potent hypotensive agents, acting by a central mechanism, but are not used clinically.
- 5-HT$_3$-receptor antagonists (e.g. **ondansetron, granisetron, tropisetron**) used as anti-emetic drugs (see Ch. 21) particularly for controlling the severe nausea and vomiting that occurs with many forms of cancer chemotherapy—a major advance, since this side-effect is one of the main factors limiting the effective use of chemotherapy (Ch. 42).
- 5-HT$_2$-receptor antagonists (e.g. **dihydroergotamine, methysergide, cyproheptadine, ketanserin, ketotifen, pizotifen**). These 'classical' 5-HT antagonists act mainly on the 5-HT$_2$-receptor. They are, however, non-selective, and act also on other targets, such as α-adrenoceptors and histamine receptors. Dihydroergotamine and methysergide belong to the ergot family (see below) and are used mainly for migraine prophylaxis. Ketotifen is sometimes used to treat asthma (Ch. 19) but the role of 5-HT receptors in this condition is unclear. Other 5-HT$_2$ antagonists are used to control the symptoms of carcinoid tumours.
- 5-HT$_4$-receptor agonists (e.g. **metoclopramide, cisapride**), which stimulate coordinated peristaltic activity (known as a 'prokinetic action'), are used for treating gastrointestinal disorders (see Ch. 21).

5-HT is also important as a transmitter in the central nervous system, and several important antipsychotic and antidepressant drugs owe their actions to effects on these pathways (see Chs 30, 34 and 35). LSD is a relatively non-selective 5-HT receptor agonist or partial agonist, which acts centrally as a potent hallucinogen (see Ch. 38).

ERGOT ALKALOIDS

Ergot alkaloids constitute a hard-to-classify group of drugs that have preoccupied pharmacologists for more than a century. Many of them act on 5-HT receptors, but not selectively, and their actions are complex and diverse. Ergot alkaloids occur naturally in a fungus (*Claviceps purpurea*) that infests cereal crops. Epidemics of ergot poisoning have occurred, and still occur, when contaminated grain is used for food. The symptoms produced include mental disturbances and intensely painful peripheral vasoconstriction, leading to gangrene, which came to be known in the Middle Ages as *St Anthony's fire*, because it could be cured by a visit to the Shrine of St Anthony (which happened to be in an ergot-free region of France). Ergot contains many active substances, and it was the study of their pharmacological properties that led Dale to many important discoveries concerning acetylcholine, histamine and catecholamines.

Ergot alkaloids are complex molecules based on **lysergic acid** (a naturally occurring tetracyclic alkaloid). The important members of the group (Table 9.2) comprise various naturally occurring and synthetic derivatives containing different substituent groups attached to the basic nucleus. These compounds display many different types of pharmacological action, and it is difficult to discern any clear relationship between chemical structure and pharmacological properties.

Actions

Most of the effects of ergot alkaloids appear to be mediated through 5-HT receptors, adrenoceptors or dopamine receptors (Table 9.2) though some effects may be produced through other mechanisms. They all cause stimulation of smooth muscle, some being relatively selective for vascular smooth muscle, and others acting mainly on the uterus. **Ergotamine** and **dihydroergotamine** are respectively a partial agonist and an antagonist at α-adrenoceptors; **bromocriptine** is an agonist on dopamine receptors, particularly in the central nervous system; **methysergide** is an antagonist at 5-HT$_2$-receptors.

The main pharmacological actions and uses of these drugs are summarised in Table 9.2. As one would expect of drugs with so many actions, their physiological effects are complex, and rather poorly understood. Ergotamine, dihydroergotamine and methysergide are discussed here; further information on ergometrine and bromocriptine is given in Chapters 26, 28 and 31.

Vascular effects. When injected into an anaesthetised animal, **ergotamine** causes a sustained rise in blood pressure, caused by activation of α-adrenoceptors leading

Table 9.2 Properties of ergot alkaloids

Drug	5-HT receptor	α-adrenoceptor	Dopamine receptor	Uterine contraction	Main uses	Side-effects etc.
Ergotamine	Antagonist/partial agonist (5-HT₁)	Partial agonist (blood vessels) Antagonist (other sites)	Inactive	++	Migraine	Emesis Vasoconstriction (avoid in peripheral vascular disease) Avoid in pregnancy
Dihydro-ergotamine	Antagonist/partial agonist (5-HT₁)	Antagonist	Inactive	+	Migraine (largely obsolete)	Less emesis than ergotamine
Ergometrine	Antagonist/partial agonist (5-HT₁) (weak)	Weak antagonist/ partial agonist	Weak	+++	Prevention of postpartum haemorrhage	
Bromocriptine	Inactive	Weak antagonist	Agonist/partial agonist	–	Parkinson's disease (Ch. 31) Endocrine disorders (Ch. 24)	Emesis
Methysergide	Antagonist/partial agonist (5-HT₂)	–	–	–	Carcinoid syndrome Migraine (prophylaxis)	Retroperitoneal mediastinal fibrosis Emesis

to vasoconstriction. At the same time, ergotamine reverses the pressor effect of adrenaline (see Ch. 8). The vaso-constrictor effect of ergotamine is responsible for the peripheral gangrene of St Anthony's fire, and probably also for some of the effects of ergot on the central nervous system. Methysergide and dihydroergotamine have much less vasoconstrictor effect.

Actions on 5-HT receptors. Methysergide is a potent 5-HT₂-receptor antagonist, whereas ergotamine and dihydroergotamine act selectively on 5-HT₁-receptors. Though generally classified as antagonists, they show partial agonist activity in some tissues, and this may account for their activity in treating migraine attacks (see below).

Clinical use

The only use of ergotamine is in the treatment of attacks of migraine unresponsive to simple analgesics (see below). Methysergide is occasionally used for migraine prophylaxis, but its main use is in treating the symptoms of carcinoid tumours (see below). All of these drugs can be used orally or by injection.

Unwanted effects

Ergotamine often causes nausea and vomiting, and it must be avoided in patients with peripheral vascular

disease, because of its vasoconstrictor action. Methysergide also causes nausea and vomiting, but its most serious side-effect, which restricts its clinical usefulness considerably, is retroperitoneal and mediastinal fibrosis, which can impair the functioning of the gastrointestinal tract, kidneys, heart and lungs. The mechanism of this

---

Ergot alkaloids

- Active substances produced by a fungus infecting cereal crops, responsible for occasional poisoning incidents.
- The most important compounds are:
  — **ergotamine, dihydroergotamine**, used in migraine
  — **ergometrine**, used in obstetrics to prevent postpartum haemorrhage
  — **methysergide**, used to treat carcinoid syndrome, and occasionally for migraine prophylaxis
  — **bromocriptine**, used in parkinsonism and endocrine disorders.
- Main sites of action are 5-HT receptors, dopamine receptors and adrenoceptors (mixed agonist, antagonist and partial agonist effects.
- Unwanted effects include nausea and vomiting, vasoconstriction (contraindicated in patients with peripheral vascular disease).

is unknown, but it is noteworthy that similar fibrotic reactions also occur in carcinoid syndrome (see below) in which there is a high circulating level of 5-HT.

CLINICAL CONDITIONS IN WHICH 5-HT PLAYS A ROLE

In this section, we discuss two situations in which the peripheral actions of 5-HT are believed to be important, namely *migraine* and *carcinoid syndrome*. Further information is reviewed by Houston & Vanhoutte (1986). The possible role of 5-HT in vomiting, and the usefulness of $5-HT_3$ antagonists in treating drug-induced emesis, are discussed in Chapter 21. Interference with 5-HT-mediated transmission in the central nervous system is probably a factor in the actions of antidepressant and antipsychotic drugs (see Chs 30, 34 and 35).

MIGRAINE AND ANTIMIGRAINE DRUGS

Migraine is a common and debilitating condition, affecting 10–15% of people, the causation of which is not well understood (see Blau 1987, Moskowitz 1992). The classical pattern of events in a migraine attack consists of an initial visual disturbance (the *aura*), in which an area of the visual field is typically lost, and the surrounding area displays a shimmering pattern. This visual disturbance is followed, about 30 minutes later, by a severe throbbing headache, starting unilaterally, often with photophobia, nausea, vomiting and prostration, which lasts for several hours.

Pathophysiology

Views differ as to whether the primary event in migraine is a humoral disturbance, leading to vascular responses which in turn disturb brain function and elicit pain, or a neurological disturbance originating in the brain or meninges, of which pain and vasomotor changes are consequences. The classical view, proposed 50 years ago by Wolff, implicated an initial humorally mediated intracerebral vasoconstriction causing the aura and visual disturbances, and an ensuing extracerebral vasodilatation phase causing the headache. This hypothesis has not, however, been generally supported by more recent blood flow studies involving non-invasive monitoring techniques in migraine patients (see Moskowitz 1992, Olesen et al. 1990).

There is indeed a biphasic change in cerebral blood flow (Fig. 9.3), with a reduction of about 30% preceding the premonitory aura, followed by a highly variable increase of similar magnitude. However, the headache often begins during the initial vasoconstrictor phase, and blood flow changes of similar magnitude caused by other factors do not produce symptoms. Furthermore, the vasoconstriction starts posteriorly and gradually spreads forwards over the rest of the hemisphere, suggesting a neural rather than a humoral cause. Headache is believed to result from stimulation of sensory nerve terminals in extracerebral structures, such as the meninges or large arteries, and some studies (Friberg et al. 1991) have shown a unilateral widening of the middle cerebral artery on the side of the headache. Overall, however, the evidence suggesting that the headache is associated with vasodilatation is weak, and vascular changes are not established as the primary event in migraine.

A second hypothesis (see Lauritzen 1987) is that the underlying abnormality is neuronal, and is a process similar to cortical spreading depression. This is a dramatic, though poorly understood, phenomenon, thought to occur in concussion, and triggered by local trauma to the cortex. This causes an advancing wave of profound neural inhibition, which progresses slowly over the

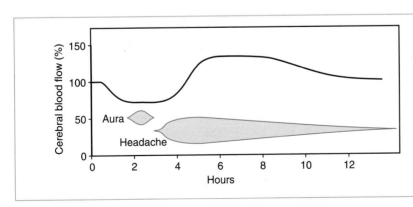

Fig 9.3 Cerebral blood flow changes during migraine. (After Olesen et al. 1990)

cortical surface at a rate of about 2 mm/min. In the depressed area the ionic balance is grossly disturbed, with an extremely high extracellular potassium concentration, and the blood flow is reduced.

A third hypothesis (see Moskowitz 1992) suggests that migraine is initiated by activity in peptidergic nerve terminals in the meningeal vessels, leading to pain, which becomes reinforced by inflammatory changes caused by the released neuropeptides (neurogenic inflammation; see Ch. 10). There is evidence that one of these peptides is released into the meningeal circulation during a migraine attack.

All of these hotly contested theories have difficulty in explaining the link between the cerebral vasoconstriction associated with the aura, and the later extracerebral change which causes headache, and the religious wars continue.

Whether one inclines to the view that migraine is a vascular disorder, a form of epilepsy, a platelet disorder, an inflammatory disease, a kind of spontaneous concussion, or just a bad headache, there is strong evidence to implicate 5-HT in its pathogenesis.

- There is a sharp increase in the urinary excretion of the main 5-HT metabolite, 5-HIAA, during the attack. The blood concentration of 5-HT falls, probably because of depletion of platelet 5-HT.
- Many of the drugs that are effective in treating migraine are 5-HT receptor agonists or antagonists. See the clinical box on this page for further information.

A shaky compromise between the neurogenic and vascular theories (Fig. 9.4) suggests that a primary neuronal disturbance leads to hyperactivity of noradrenergic and 5-HT-releasing neurons in the brainstem, causing intracerebral vasoconstriction. Release of 5-HT also leads to a local inflammatory response around the extracerebral vessels, associated with the local release of other mediators, particularly bradykinin and prostaglandins (see Ch. 12). 5-HT and these other mediators act on, among other things, nociceptive nerve terminals (see Ch. 37), causing pain and also releasing a variety of neuropeptides, which further reinforce and prolong the pain response. It is suggested that afferent nerve terminals in the wall of blood vessels may become hypersensitive to vascular distension, thus accounting for the fact that many of the drugs that are effective are vasoconstrictors.

Antimigraine drugs

The main drugs used to treat migraine are summarised in the clinical box on this page and their postulated sites of action are shown in Figure 9.4. It is important to

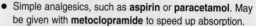

Drugs used for migraine

Acute attack

- Simple analgesics, such as **aspirin** or **paracetamol**. May be given with **metoclopramide** to speed up absorption.
- **Ergotamine** (5-HT$_{1D}$-receptor partial agonist). Various routes of administration (e.g. suppositories, sublingual tablets, inhaled spray) used to achieve absorption when patient is vomiting.
- **Sumatriptan** (5-HT$_{1D}$ agonist) is highly effective, but short-acting. Used instead of ergotamine. Contraindicated in patients with ischaemic heart disease because of tendency to cause chest pain owing to coronary artery spasm. Given by mouth (poorly absorbed) or subcutaneous injection. Short-acting (half-life about 2 hours). Newer compounds, e.g. **zolmitriptan**, **alnitidan**, are claimed to be faster-acting by mouth, and not to cause chest pain.

Prophylaxis (in cases with more than one severe attack per month)

- **Pizotifen** (adverse effects include weight gain, antimuscarinic effects).
- β-adrenoceptor antagonists (e.g. **propranolol**, **metoprolol**; see Ch. 8). Mechanism of action is not clear.
- Tricyclic antidepressants (e.g. **amitriptyline**; see Ch. 35). May be effective even though patients are not depressed.
- **Methysergide** (5-HT$_2$-receptor antagonist). Effective, but has dangerous and insidious adverse effects, especially retroperitoneal fibrosis and renal failure, so not generally used.
- α$_2$-adrenoceptor agonist (**clonidine**; see Ch. 8). Has been used, but efficacy is doubtful.
- Calcium antagonists (e.g. **dihydropyridines**, **verapamil**; see Ch. 15) cause headaches as a common side-effect, but paradoxically may reduce frequency of migraine attacks. Mechanism of action is not clear.
- **Cyproheptadine** (5-HT$_2$-receptor antagonist, also has antihistamine and calcium antagonist actions) sometimes used in refractory cases.

distinguish between drugs used to treat acute attacks of migraine (appropriate when the attacks are fairly infrequent, and prophylaxis is not justified), and drugs used for prophylaxis.

CARCINOID SYNDROME

Carcinoid syndrome (see Creutzfeld & Stockmann 1987) is a rare disorder associated with malignant tumours of enterochromaffin cells, usually arising in the small intestine and metastasising to the liver. These tumours secrete a variety of hormones. 5-HT is the most important, but neuropeptides, such as substance P (Ch. 10),

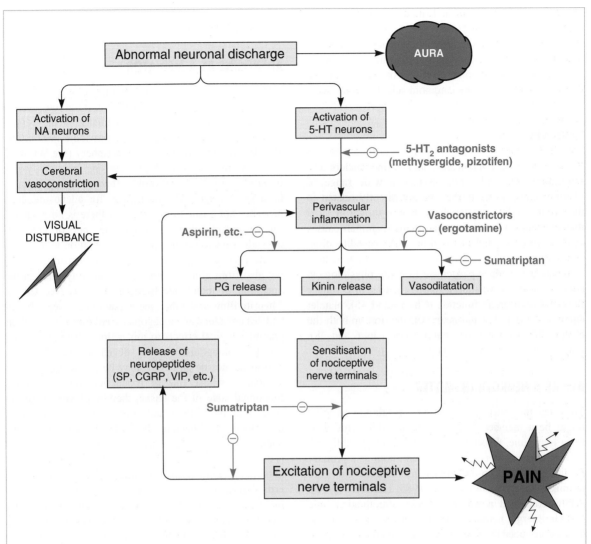

Fig. 9.4 Postulated pathogenesis of migraine. The initiating event is assumed to be an abnormal neuronal discharge, the cause and location of which is uncertain; it is probably set off by emotional or biochemical disturbances, but the details are unclear. An alternative view suggests that the primary event is excitation (cause unknown) of nociceptive nerve terminals in the meningeal vessels, leading to the cycle of neurogenic inflammation shown in the lower part of the diagram. (PG = prostaglandins; SP = substance P; CGRP = calcitonin gene-related peptide; VIP = vasoactive intestinal peptide)

and other agents, such as prostaglandins and bradykinin (Ch. 12), are also produced. The release of these substances into the bloodstream results in various unpleasant symptoms, including flushing, diarrhoea and bronchoconstriction, as well as hypotension, which may cause dizziness or fainting. Stenosis of heart valves also occurs, which can result in cardiac failure. The relationship of this to hormone secretion is not understood.

The syndrome is readily diagnosed by measuring the excretion of 5-HIAA, the main metabolite of 5-HT, in the urine, the level of which may increase 20-fold, and is raised even during periods when the tumour is asymptomatic.

5-HT$_2$ antagonists, such as **cyproheptadine**, are effective in controlling some of the symptoms of carcinoid syndrome. **Methysergide** is also effective, but is liable to cause retroperitoneal and mediastinal fibrosis, a potentially serious side-effect.

A complementary therapeutic approach is to use a long-acting analogue of somatostatin, namely **octreotide**, which suppresses hormone secretion from various neuro-endocrine cells, including carcinoid cells (see Ch. 24).

PURINES

Purines, especially *adenosine*, and purine nucleotides, especially *ADP* and *ATP*, produce a wide range of pharmacological effects that are not directly related to their role in energy metabolism. It was shown in 1929 that adenosine injected into anaesthetised animals causes cardiac slowing, a fall in blood pressure, vasodilatation, and inhibition of intestinal movements, and there is now evidence that purines participate in many physiological control mechanisms, such as the regulation of coronary flow and myocardial function (Chs 14 and 15), platelet aggregation (Ch. 17) and neurotransmission, in both the central and peripheral nervous system (Chs 6 and 28). For reviews, see Stone (1991), Williams (1987).

ATP AS A NEUROTRANSMITTER

The idea that such a work-a-day metabolite as ATP might be a member of the neurotransmitter elite was, for a long time, resisted, but is now firmly established. ATP is a transmitter in the periphery, both as a primary mediator and as a co-transmitter in noradrenergic nerve terminals (see Burnstock 1981, 1985, Lundberg 1996). ATP is contained in synaptic vesicles of both adrenergic and cholinergic neurons, and accounts for many of the actions produced by stimulation of autonomic nerves that are not due to acetylcholine or noradrenaline (see Ch. 6). These include effects such as relaxation of intestinal smooth muscle evoked by sympathetic stimulation, and contraction of the bladder produced by parasympathetic nerves. Burnstock and his colleagues have shown that ATP is released, in a calcium-dependent fashion, on nerve stimulation, and that exogenous ATP in general mimics the effects of nerve stimulation in various pre-parations. Furthermore, **suramin**, a drug recently shown to block ATP receptors (developed many years ago for treating trypanosome infections), blocks these synaptic responses. Recent work has also shown ATP to function as a conventional 'fast' transmitter in the CNS and in autonomic ganglia (Edwards & Gibb 1993).

The role of *intracellular* ATP in controlling membrane K^+ channels, which is important in the control of vascular

smooth muscle (Ch. 14) and of insulin secretion (Ch. 22), is quite distinct from its transmitter function.

ADENOSINE AS A MEDIATOR

Adenosine produces many pharmacological effects, both in the periphery and in the central nervous system (see below). It functions as a mediator in the central nervous system (see Brundege & Dunwiddie 1997, Stone 1991), and probably also in the periphery (see Williams 1987). Many tissues produce adenosine, but mainly as a by-product of ATP breakdown; there does not seem to be a special synthetic mechanism for adenosine. It is probably not a true transmitter, for there is no evidence for vesicular storage of adenosine, nor of calcium-dependent release in response to stimulation in the brain or the periphery; it is released not only from neurons, but also from glia and other cells, possibly through the operation of membrane transport systems (see Ch. 6). **Theophylline** and other methylxanthines (see Chs 19 and 38) are adenosine antagonists, and owe some of their pharmacological effects to this action. More potent and selective antagonists are in development. The main role of adenosine and ADP may be as local regulatory substances whose rate of production varies with the functional state of the tissue, thereby playing a role in controlling blood flow, and in protecting tissues against the effects of ischaemia. The role of adenosine in the phenomenon of 'ischaemic preconditioning' in the heart is discussed in Chapter 14, and a similar protective effect in brain ischaemia is also postulated (Ch. 31). Adenosine is destroyed or taken up within a few seconds when given intravenously (as in the treatment of supraventricular tachycardias—see Ch. 14), but longer-lasting analogues have been discovered which also show greater receptor selectivity. Adenosine uptake is blocked by **dipyridamole**, a vasodilator and antiplatelet drug (see Ch. 17).

PURINE RECEPTORS

Adenosine receptors and actions

The effects of *adenosine* are mediated by A_1, A_2 and A_3 receptors. All are G-protein-coupled receptors linked to the inhibition or stimulation of adenylate cyclase (Collis & Hourani 1993). These adenosine receptors are not sensitive to nucleotides such as AMP, ADP or ATP. Methylxanthines, especially analogues of **theophylline** (Ch. 19) are A_1/A_2-receptor antagonists; however, they also increase cAMP by inhibiting phosphodiesterase, which contributes to their pharmacological actions independently of adenosine receptor antagonism. Certain derivatives of theophylline are claimed to show greater selectivity for adenosine receptors over phosphodiesterase.

The main effects of adenosine, and the receptors involved are:

- Vasodilatation, including coronary vessels (A_2), except in the kidney, where A_1-receptors produce vasoconstriction. Adenosine infusion causes a fall in blood pressure.
- Inhibition of platelet aggregation (A_2).
- Block of cardiac AV conduction (A_1), and reduction of force of contraction.
- Bronchoconstriction, especially in asthmatic subjects (A_1). The anti-asthmatic effect of methylxanthines may partly reflect A_1-receptor antagonism.
- Release of mediators from mast cells (A_3). This contributes to bronchoconstriction.
- Stimulation of nociceptive afferent neurons, especially in the heart (A_2). Adenosine release in response to ischaemia has been suggested as a mechanism of anginal pain (Ch. 14). Carotid body afferents are also stimulated, causing reflex hyperventilation.
- Inhibition of transmitter release at many peripheral and central synapses (A_1). In the central nervous system, adenosine generally exerts a pre- and postsynaptic depressant action. It reduces motor activity, depresses respiration, induces sleep, and reduces anxiety, all of which effects are the opposite of those produced by methylxanthines (Ch. 38).
- Neuroprotection, in cerebral ischaemia, probably through inhibition of glutamate release through A_1-receptors (see Rudolphi et al. 1992; Ch. 31).

Uses of adenosine

Because of its inhibitory effect on cardiac conduction, adenosine may be used as an intravenous bolus injection, to terminate supraventricular tachycardia (Ch. 14). It is safer than alternative drugs such as β-adrenoceptor antagonists or verapamil, because of its short duration of action.

Otherwise adenosine is not used therapeutically, though longer-lasting A_1-receptor agonists could prove useful in various conditions (e.g. hypertension, ischaemic heart disease, stroke, etc.). Selective adenosine receptor antagonists could also have advantages over theophylline in the treatment of asthma (see Ch. 19).

ATP receptors and actions

ATP receptors respond to various adenine nucleotides, generally preferring ATP to ADP or AMP. They fall into two main classes, P_{2X} and P_{2Y} (each comprising several subtypes; see Boarder et al. 1995, North & Barnard 1997), the former being ligand-gated cation channels

and the latter, G-protein-coupled receptors, linked mainly to phosphoinositide hydrolysis, but also to adenylate cyclase in some cases. The role of ATP as a fast transmitter (see above), involves P_{2X} receptors, which are blocked by drugs, such as **suramin** and a purine analogue, **PPADS** (see North & Barnard, 1997). The other actions of ATP are mediated through P_{2Y} receptors, which are linked to various second messenger systems, and for which no specific antagonists are known. An important exception to the rule that P_2 receptors are relatively selective for ATP occurs in the platelet, which expresses a different receptor (P_{2T}) which responds selectively to ADP. ADP causes platelet aggregation, the opposite effect to that of adenosine (see above), and its action is actually antagonised by ATP. ADP released from platelets and from the vascular endothelium promotes thrombosis (see Ch. 17).

Drugs acting selectively on ATP and ADP receptors have not yet been developed for clinical purposes.

Purines as mediators

- ATP functions as a neurotransmitter (or co-transmitter) at peripheral neuroeffector junctions and central synapses. It also functions as an intracellular mediator, inhibiting the opening of membrane potassium channels.
- ATP acts on two types of purinoceptor (P_2), one of which (P_{2X}) is a ligand-gated ion channel responsible for fast synaptic responses. The other (P_{2Y}) is coupled to various second messengers. Suramin blocks the P_{2X} receptor.
- Adenosine affects many cells and tissues, including smooth muscle and nerve cells. It is not a conventional transmitter, but may be important as local hormone or modulator.
- ADP acts selectively on platelets, causing aggregation. This is important in thrombosis.
- Adenosine acts through A_1-, A_2- and A_3-receptors, coupled to inhibition or stimulation of adenylate cyclase. A_1- and A_2-receptors are blocked by xanthines, such as theophylline.
- The main effects of adenosine are:
  — hypotension (A_2) and cardiac depression (A_1)
  — inhibition of AV conduction (antidysrhythmic effect, A_1)
  — inhibition of platelet aggregation (A_2)
  — bronchoconstriction (probably secondary to mast cell activation, A_3)
  — presynaptic inhibition in CNS (responsible for neuroprotective effect, A_1).
- Adenosine is very short-acting and is sometimes used for its antidysrhythmic effect.
- New adenosine agonists and antagonists are in development, mainly for treatment of ischaemic heart disease and stroke.

REFERENCES AND FURTHER READING

Blau J N (ed) 1987 Migraine. Chapman & Hall, London *(Clinical textbook which also discusses physiology and pharmacology)*

Boarder M R, Weisman G A, Turner J T, Wilkinson G F 1995 G-protein-coupled P_2 purinoceptors: from molecular biology to functional responses. Trends Pharmacol Sci 16: 133–139 *(Review on G-protein-coupled purine receptors)*

Bobker D H, Williams J T 1990 Ion conductances affected by 5-HT receptor subtypes in mammalian neurons. Trends Neurosci 13: 169–173 *(Functional role of neuronal 5-HT receptors at the cellular level)*

Brundege J M, Dunwiddie T V 1997 Role of adenosine as a modulator of synaptic activity in the central nervous system. Adv Pharmacol 39: 353–391 *(Good review article)*

Burnstock G 1981 Purinergic receptors. Chapman & Hall, London *(Textbook by the main pioneer in this field)*

Burnstock G 1985 Purinergic mechanisms broaden their sphere of influence. Trends Neurosci 8: 5–6 *(Ideas about the functional role of purinergic transmission)*

Collis M G, Hourani S M O 1993 Adenosine receptor subtypes. Trends Pharmacol Sci 14: 360–366 *(Short review)*

Cooper J R, Bloom F E, Roth R H 1996 The biochemical basis of neuropharmacology. Oxford University Press, New York *(Excellent general textbook)*

Creutzfeld W, Stockmann F 1987 Carcinoids and carcinoid syndrome. Am J Med 82 (suppl 58): 4–16

Edwards F A, Gibb A J 1993 ATP—a fast neurotransmitter. FEBS Letters 325: 86–89

Eglen R M, Jasper J R, Chang D J, Martin G R 1997 The 5-HT$_7$ receptor: an orphan found. Trends Pharmacol Sci 18: 104–107

Fozard J R (ed) 1989 The peripheral actions of 5-hydroxytryptamine. Oxford University Press, Oxford *(Useful compilation of articles on 5-HT pharmacology)*

Fredholm B B, Abbrachio M B, Burnstock G et al. 1994 Nomenclature and classification of purinoceptors. Pharmacol Rev 46: 143–156 *(Useful review)*

Friberg L, Olesen J, Iversen H K, Sperling B 1991 Migraine pain associated with middle cerebral artery dilatation: reversal by sumatriptan. Lancet 338: 13–17 *(Clinical study on mode of action of sumatriptan)*

Green A R (ed) 1985 Neuropharmacology of serotonin. Oxford University Press, Oxford

Houston D S, Vanhoutte P M 1986 Serotonin and the vascular system: role in health and disease, and implications for therapy. Drugs 31: 149–163

Hoyer D, Clarke D E, Fozard J R et al. 1994 VII International Union of Pharmacology classification of receptors for 5-hydroxytryptamine. Pharmacol Rev 46: 157–203 *(The official view on 5-HT receptor classification)*

Lauritzen M 1987 Cerebral blood flow in migraine and cortical spreading depression. Acta Neurol Scand Suppl 113: 140 *(Review of clinical measurements of cerebral blood flow in migraine, which overturn earlier hypotheses)*

Lundberg J M 1996 Pharmacology of co-transmission in the autonomic nervous system: integrative aspects on amines, neuropeptides, adenosine triphosphate, amino acids and nitric oxide. Pharmacol Rev 48: 114–192 *(Comprehensive and informative review)*

Moskowitz M A 1992 Neurogenic versus vascular mechanisms of sumatriptan and ergot alkaloids in migraine. Trends Pharmacol Sci 13: 307–311 *(Discussion of controversies about pathophysiology of migraine)*

North R A, Barnard E A 1997 Nucleotide receptors. Curr Opin Neurobiol 7: 346–357 *(Update on purinergic receptors)*

Olesen J, Friberg J, Olsen T S 1990 Timing and topography of cerebral blood flow, aura and headache during migraine attacks. Ann Neurol 28: 791–798 *(Clinical studies with non-invasive blood-flow measurements)*

Rudolphi K A, Schubert P, Parkinson F E, Fredholm B B 1992 Neuroprotective role of adenosine in cerebral ischaemia. Trends Pharmacol Sci 13: 439–445 *(Argues that adenosine protects neurons against ischaemic damage—important therapeutic implications)*

Stone T W (ed) 1991 Adenosine in the nervous system. Academic Press, London *(Useful compilation of articles)*

Williams M 1987 Purine receptors in mammalian tissues: pharmacology and functional significance. Annu Rev Pharmacol Toxicol 27: 315–345 *(General review)*

10

Peptides and proteins as mediators

Today's pharmacology is based mainly on signalling molecules that are of low molecular weight, and non-peptide in nature. What has become plain, mainly in the last 20 years, is that peptides are at least as important, and possibly much more so, as signalling molecules. Yet, the pharmacological manipulation of peptide signalling is still far less advanced than that of, say, the cholinergic, adrenergic or 5-HT systems (Chs 7–9). Pharmacology, one could say, has some catching up to do.

Historically, there are two main reasons why pharmacology has a strong bias towards non-peptides. One is that the subject began with the analysis of the actions of natural (mainly plant) products thought to have medicinal properties. Very few of these were peptides, and they did not, for the most part, interact with peptide signalling systems. The second reason is that the methodology required to study peptides is of more recent origin. Key methodological advances were the introduction of solid phase peptide synthesis, the use of antibodies, both for radioimmunoassay and for immunocytochemical localisation of peptides, and the use of molecular biology approaches for studying the expression of peptides and their precursors. These technologies were unknown to chemists and pharmacologists until about 35 years ago, and very few were dogged enough to tackle peptide chemistry by classical methods.

In 1953, du Vigneaud made history, and earned a Nobel Prize, by determining the structure, and carrying out the synthesis, of oxytocin—the first peptide mediator to be characterised and the first to be synthesised commercially for use in medicine. There were many other examples of mediators, for example substance P, bradykinin (Ch. 12) and angiotensin (Ch. 15), which had been identified as peptides in the 1930s, but whose structure remained unknown for many years. All are small peptides of 11 residues or fewer, but determination of their structure, and their chemical synthesis, was a major task; the structure of bradykinin was not known until 1960, while that of substance P was published in 1970. By contrast, the use of the newer, now routine, methods enabled endothelin (a much larger peptide; see Ch. 15 and below) to be fully characterised, synthesised and its gene cloned within about a year, the complete information being published in a single paper (Yanagisawa et al. 1988). Protein mediators, such as cytokines (Ch. 12) and growth factors (Chs 12 and 18) containing 50 or more residues, are still very difficult to synthesise chemically, and the major advances in the last two decades have relied very largely on molecular biological approaches. The use of recombinant proteins as therapeutic agents—a development driven mainly by the emergent biotechnology industry—is rapidly gaining ground.

The purpose of this chapter is to give an overview of the main characteristics of peptides and proteins as mediators and as drugs, and to bring out the contrasts between these and non-peptides. For reviews, with more detail than can be provided here, see Buckel (1996), Cooper et al. (1996), Hökfelt (1991), Hökfelt et al. (1994).

GENERAL PRINCIPLES OF PEPTIDE PHARMACOLOGY

ROLE OF MOLECULAR BIOLOGY

Because peptide structures are represented directly in the

genome, molecular biology has been the key to most of the recent advances in knowledge. It is used in several ways:

- Cloning of the genes encoding peptide precursors (see below) has shown how various active peptides can arise from a single precursor protein.
- In some cases (e.g. calcitonin gene-related peptide, CGRP) new peptides have been discovered.
- Cloning of the genes encoding peptide receptors (see Ch. 2) has shown that they conform, in general, to the pattern of other receptors. There are no major surprises, but (particularly in the cytokine and chemokine field) many new receptors and subtypes have been discovered.*
- The control of precursor synthesis can be studied by measuring mRNA, for which highly sensitive and specific assays have been developed. The technique of *in situ hybridisation* enables the location and abundance of the mRNA to be mapped at microscopic resolution.

STRUCTURE OF PEPTIDES

Peptide and protein mediators vary from 3 to about 200 amino acids (Fig. 10.1), the arbitrary dividing line between peptides and proteins being about 50 residues. For convenience, in this chapter, we use the term 'peptides' to cover both classes. Peptides generally undergo post-translational modifications, such as C-terminal amidation, glycosylation, acetylation, carboxylation, sulphation or phosphorylation of specific residues. They often contain intramolecular disulphide bonds, so that the molecule adopts a partially cyclic conformation, and they may comprise two or more separate chains linked by disulphide bonds. The conformation of peptides in solution is generally ill-defined (see Milner-White 1989). Most peptides less than about 40 residues have proved impossible to crystallise, which precludes the use of X-ray diffraction methods to study their conformation, and methods for examining conformational structure in solution, such as nuclear magnetic resonance spectroscopy, have generally shown these molecules to be highly flexible. To imagine them fitting into a receptor site in a precise 'lock-and-key' mode is to imagine that you can

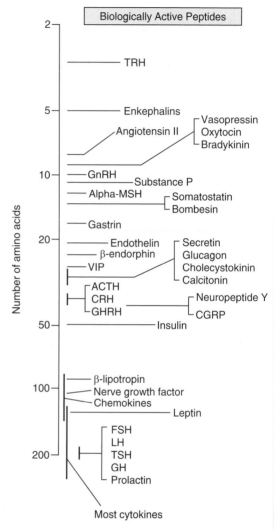

Fig. 10.1 Some typical peptide mediators.
(TRH = thyrotrophin-releasing hormone; GHRH = growth hormone-releasing hormone; Sub P = substance P; Alpha-MSH = α-melanocyte-stimulating hormone; VIP = vasoactive intestinal peptide; ACTH = adrenocorticotrophic hormone; CGRP = calcitonin gene-related peptide; CRH = corticotrophin-releasing hormone; GnRH = gonadotrophin-releasing hormone; FSH = follicle-stimulating hormone; LH = luteinising hormone; TSH = thyroid-stimulating hormone; GH = growth hormone)

*Recently, an orphan receptor (called ORL₁), closely resembling known opioid receptors, was identified by homology screening of brain cDNA libraries. Searching in an extract of brain peptides for possible ligands led to the identification of a hitherto unknown neuropeptide, christened *nociceptin* (Meunier et al. 1995). Its function remains unknown.

unlock your front door with a length of cooked spaghetti. Larger proteins adopt more restricted conformations, but because of their size, they generally interact with multiple sites on the receptor. These facts have greatly impeded the rational design of non-peptide analogues ('peptidomimetics') that mimic the structure of peptides and interact with peptide receptors. The use of random screening methods (somewhat to the chagrin of the rationalists) has nevertheless led in recent years to the discovery of many non-peptide ligands for peptide receptors (see below; Betancur et al. 1997).

TYPES OF PEPTIDE MEDIATOR

The soluble peptide mediators in the body, which are secreted by cells, and act on surface receptors of other cells, can be very broadly divided into (a) neuroendocrine mediators (discussed further in this chapter), (b) mediators of the immune system (**cytokines** and **chemokines**; see Ch. 12), (c) growth factors, which are produced by many different cells and tissues, and control cell growth and differentiation (see Chs 12 and 18), (d) other types of mediator, including plasma-derived peptides, notably **angiotensin** (Ch. 15), and **bradykinin** (Ch. 12), and substances such as **endothelin** (see Ch. 15), and **atrial natriuretic peptide** (see Ch. 15).

Some important examples of peptide and protein mediators are shown in Figure 10.1.

Peptides in the nervous system: comparison with conventional transmitters

In most respects, neuropeptide-mediated transmission closely resembles transmission by classical non-peptide mediators. In the 1970s and 1980s, when the abundance of neuropeptides in the brain and elsewhere was coming to light, they were thought to be fundamentally different from the conventional chemical transmitters in their organisation and function. However, the mechanisms for the storage and release (summarised in Fig. 10.2), and the receptor mechanisms through which their effects are produced (Ch. 2), are essentially the same for peptide and non-peptide transmitters. As with other chemical mediators, their effects may be excitatory or inhibitory, pre- or postsynaptic, and exerted over short or long distances from the site of release. There are, however, certain monopolies of function between peptide and non-peptide mediators. For example, peptides do not activate ligand-gated ion channels, and thus do not function as fast neurotransmitters in the manner of non-peptides, such as acetylcholine, glutamate, glycine or GABA (see Chs 7 and 28). Instead, they serve (as do many non-peptides) as 'neuromodulators' (Ch. 6), by activating G-protein-coupled receptors. On the other hand, the ligands for tyrosine-kinase-linked receptors (see Ch. 2) are all peptides or proteins.

In summary, the similarities in function between pep-tide and non-peptide mediators are much more striking than the differences. The main difference is constitutional rather than functional, and stems from the fact that peptides, being gene products, represent variations on a single theme—a linear string of amino acids. Evolution, of course, plays many tunes on this theme, far more than are played on the structure of non-peptide mediators. As a result the number of known peptide mediators now greatly exceeds that of non-peptides. As Iversen pointed out in 1983: 'almost overnight, the number of putative transmitters in the mammalian nervous system has jumped from the ten or so monoamine and amino acid candidates to more than 40'. Since then, no new monoamine transmitters have appeared, but there are at least another 40 peptides.

Peptides as co-transmitters are discussed in Chapter 6. Two well-documented examples (reviewed by Lundberg 1996) are the parasympathetic nerves supplying salivary glands (where the secretory response is produced by acetylcholine and the vasodilatation partly by **vasoactive intestinal peptide**) and the sympathetic innervation to various tissues, which involves release of the vaso-constrictor **neuropeptide Y** in addition to noradrenaline.

The distinction between neuropeptides and peripherally acting hormones is useful, but not watertight. Thus, **insulin, angiotensin, atrial natriuretic peptide** and **oxytocin** are best known as hormones that are formed, released, and act, in the periphery. They are, however, also found in the brain, though their role there is uncertain. Similarly, **endothelin** was first discovered in blood vessels, but is now know to occur extensively in the brain as well.

Multiple physiological roles of peptides

In common with many non-peptide mediators, such as noradrenaline, dopamine, 5-HT or acetylcholine, the same peptides are often found, and presumably function as mediators, in several different parts of the body. Intriguingly, there often appears to be some connection between the effects of a peptide at different sites, in terms of coordinated physiological functions. Thus angiotensin acts on the cells of the hypothalamus to release **vaso-pressin**, which in turn causes water retention; it also acts elsewhere in the brain to promote drinking behaviour and to increase blood pressure by activation of the sympathetic system; in addition, it releases aldosterone which causes salt and water retention, and it acts directly to constrict blood vessels. Each of these effects plays a part in the overall response of the body to water deprivation and reduced circulating volume. There are other examples of what appears to be an orchestrated functional response produced by the various actions of

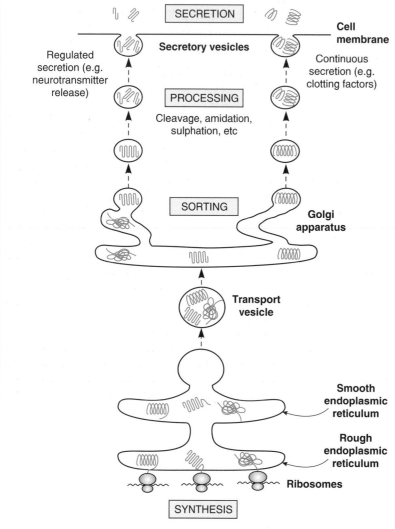

Fig. 10.2 Cellular mechanisms for peptide synthesis and release. Proteins synthesised by ribosomes are threaded through the membrane of the rough endoplasmic reticulum, whence they are conveyed via transport vesicles to the Golgi apparatus, where they are sorted and packaged into secretory vesicles. Processing (cleavage, glycosylation, amidation, sulphation, etc.) occurs within the transport and secretory vesicles, and the products are released from the cell by exocytosis. Constitutive secretion (e.g. secretion of plasma proteins, clotting factors, etc. by liver cells) occurs continuously, and little material is stored in secretory vesicles. Regulated secretion, (e.g. neurosecretion or cytokine secretion) occurs in response to increased $[Ca^{2+}]_i$ or other intracellular signals, and material is typically stored in significant amounts in an accumulation of secretory vesicles.

Structure and function of peptide mediators

- Size varies from three to several hundred amino acids; conventionally, molecules of fewer than 50 residues are called peptides, larger molecules being proteins.
- Neural and endocrine mediators range in size from 3 to over 200 residues. Cytokines, chemokines and growth factors are generally larger than 100 residues.
- Most known peptide mediators come from the nervous system and endocrine organs. However, some are formed in the plasma, and many occur at other sites (e.g. vascular endothelium, heart, cells of the immune system, etc.). The same peptide may occur in several places, and serve different functions.

- Small peptides and chemokines act mainly on G-protein-coupled receptors, and act through the same second messenger systems as those used by other mediators. Cytokines and growth factors generally act through tyrosine-kinase-linked membrane receptors.
- Peptides frequently function in the nervous system as co-transmitters with other peptides or with non-peptide transmitters.
- The number of known peptide mediators now greatly exceeds that of non-peptides.

a single mediator, but there are many more examples where the multiple effects just seem to be multiple effects.

So far, the cataract of new information about neuropeptides over the past 20 years has led to few useful generalisations about their functional role. A few new drugs with clinical uses have been developed, however, and more are likely in the future (see below).

BIOSYNTHESIS AND REGULATION OF PEPTIDES

Peptide structure is directly coded in the genome, in a way that the structure of, say, acetylcholine is not. It is in some ways simpler for a cell to produce a peptide than a conventional neurotransmitter. To do the latter, it must produce a series of carrier molecules (to collect the necessary precursors and store the product) and enzymes to perform the synthesis. To make a peptide (Fig. 10.3), it produces a precursor protein in which the peptide sequence is embedded, along with specific proteolytic enzymes that excise the active peptide, a process of sculpture rather than synthesis. The precursor protein is packaged into vesicles at the point of synthesis, and the active peptide is formed in situ ready for release (Fig. 10.2). Thus there is no need for special uptake mechanisms for procuring the starting materials, and there

are in general no mechanisms for recapturing released mediators, such as are important for non-peptides.

PEPTIDE PRECURSORS

Since the mid-1970s, cloning techniques have been used to define the structures of 30 or more peptide precursors (*preprohormones*). The general pattern (see Burger 1988; Fig. 10.3) is that the precursor protein, usually 100–250 residues in length, consists of an N-terminal *signal sequence*, followed by a variable stretch of unknown function, followed by a peptide-containing region in which several copies of active peptide fragments are contained. Often, several different peptides are found in one precursor, but sometimes there is only one in multiple copies. An extreme example occurs in the invertebrate *Aplysia*, in which the precursor contains 28 copies of the same short peptide. The signal peptide is strongly hydrophobic, which is important for insertion of the protein into the endoplasmic reticulum; it is cleaved off at an early stage, to form the *prohormone*. The active peptides are usually demarcated within the prohormone sequence by pairs of basic amino acids (Lys–Lys or Lys–Arg), which are cleavage points for the various trypsin-like proteases that act to release the peptides. This endoproteolytic cleavage generally occurs in the Golgi apparatus, or in the secretory vesicles. The enzymes

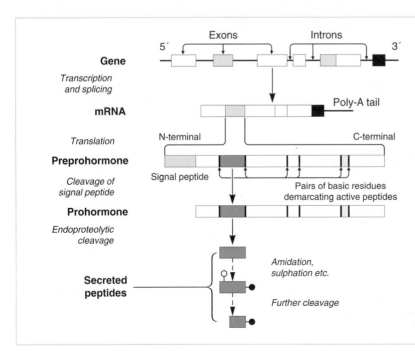

Fig. 10.3 Synthesis of a peptide mediator. The coding regions of the gene (exons) are transcribed and spliced to give rise to mRNA, segments of which are translated to produce the preprohormone. Cleavage of the N-terminal signal peptide produces the prohormone, from which endopeptidases excise peptide fragments. These may be active as such or they may undergo further post-translational processing (amidation, etc.).

responsible are known as *prohormone convertases*, of which two subtypes (PC1 and PC2) have been studied in detail (see Cullinan et al. 1991). Inspection of the prohormone sequence has often revealed likely cleavage points that demarcate unknown peptides. In some cases (e.g. CGRP; see below) new peptide mediators have been discovered in this way, but there are many examples where no function has yet been assigned. Whether they are, like strangers at a funeral, peptides waiting to declare their purpose, or merely functionless relics, remains a secret. There are also large stretches of the prohormone sequence lying between the active peptide fragments, for which no function is known. They may just be molecular rubbish, but few would bet on it.

The levels of mRNA coding for different prepro-hormones, which reflect the level of gene expression, are very sensitive to physiological conditions, and this type of transcriptional control is one of the main mechanisms by which peptide expression and release are regulated over the medium-to-long term. Inflammation, for example, increases the expression, and hence the release, of various cytokines by immune cells (see Ch. 12). Sensory neurons respond to peripheral inflammation by increased expression of tachykinins, which is important in the genesis of inflammatory pain (see Ch. 37).

DIVERSITY WITHIN PEPTIDE FAMILIES

Peptides commonly occur in families, with sequences and actions that are basically similar. Opioid peptides (see Ch. 37) provide a good example of the representation of such a family at the genomic level. Cloning studies have shown that opioid peptides, defined as peptides with opiate-like pharmacological effects, are coded by three distinct genes, whose products are respectively *preproopiomelanocortin* (POMC), *preproenkephalin* and *preprodynorphin*. Each of these precursors contains the sequences of a number of opioid peptides (Fig. 10.4). Hughes & Kosterlitz, who discovered the enkephalins in 1972, noticed that the sequence of metenkephalin is contained within that of a pituitary hormone, β-lipotropin. About this time, three other peptides with morphine-like actions were discovered, α-, β- and γ-endorphin, which also comprised stretches of the β-lipotropin molecule, and it was then found that the enkephalins actually come from the other gene products, proenkephalin and prodynorphin, POMC itself serving as a source of ACTH, melanocyte-stimulating hormones (MSH) and β-endorphin, but not of enkephalins. The expression of the precursor proteins varies greatly in different tissues and brain areas. For example, POMC and its derived

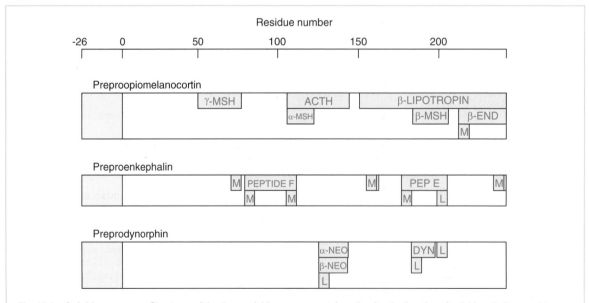

Fig. 10.4 Opioid precursors. Structures of the three opioid precursor proteins, showing the location of opioid and other peptides within the sequence. These contained peptides are bounded by pairs of basic amino acids, which form points of attack for enzymic cleavage. (MSH = melanocyte-stimulating hormone; ACTH = adrenocorticotrophic hormone; β-END = β-endorphin; M = methionine enkephalin; L= leucine enkephalin; DYN = dynorphin; NEO = neoendorphin)

peptides are found mainly in the pituitary and hypothalamus, whereas enkephalins and their precursors are found throughout the central and peripheral nervous systems, and also in other organs such as the adrenal medulla. Studies with immunofluorescence show that these peptides and precursors are clearly restricted to individual cells, and distinct patterns of processing, leading to production of different peptides from the same precursor, can also be recognised in different tissues and brain areas. In the brain, β-endorphin occurs mainly in neurons that project from the hypothalamus to the thalamus and brainstem, while the enkephalins are found mainly in short interneurons, in many brain areas.

In many cases, as with opioid peptides, the members of a peptide family are represented independently in the genome, but diversity can also arise by gene-splicing, or during post-translational processing of the prohormone.

Gene splicing as a source of peptide diversity

Genes contain coding regions (exons) interspersed with non-coding regions (introns). The DNA forming the gene is initially transcribed *in toto* to form RNA (hnRNA), which is then *spliced* to remove the introns, and some of the exons, forming the mRNA that is translated. Control of the splicing process allows a measure of cellular control over the peptides that are produced. The best examples of this are **calcitonin/calcitonin gene-related peptide** (CGRP) and **substance P/substance K**.

The calcitonin gene codes for calcitonin itself (Ch. 27) and also for a completely dissimilar peptide, CGRP. Differential splicing allows cells to produce either procalcitonin (expressed in thyroid cells) or pro-CGRP (expressed in many neurons) from the same gene.

Substance P and substance K are two closely related tachykinins belonging to the same family that are encoded on the same gene. Differential splicing results in the production of two precursor proteins—one of these includes both peptides, the other includes only substance P, and the ratio of the two varies widely between tissues, which correspondingly produce either one or both peptides. The control of the splicing process is not well understood.

Post-translational modifications as a source of peptide diversity

Many peptides, such as tachykinins and peptides related to ACTH (see Ch. 24) are converted enzymatically to amides, by amidation at the carboxy terminus, and this is important for their biological activity. Another common pattern is for tissues to generate peptides of varying length from the same primary sequence, by the action of specific peptidases that cut the chain at different points. Thus

procholecystokinin (pro-CCK) contains the sequences of at least five CCK-like peptides ranging in length from 4 to 58 amino acids, all with the same carboxy-terminal sequence. CCK itself (33 residues) is the main peptide produced by the intestine, whereas the brain produces mainly CCK-8. The opioid precursor, *prodynorphin*, similarly gives rise to several peptides with a common terminal sequence (see Fig. 10.4), the proportions of which vary in different tissues and in different neurons in the brain. In some cases (e.g. the inflammatory mediator, bradykinin; Ch. 12) peptide cleavage occurring after release gives rise to a new active peptide (Des–Arg^9-bradykinin), which acts on a different receptor, both peptides contributing to the inflammatory response.

PEPTIDE TRAFFICKING AND SECRETION

The basic mechanisms by which peptides are synthesised, packaged into vesicles, processed and secreted are summarised in Figure 10.2 (see review by Perone et al. 1997). Two secretory pathways exist, for *constitutive* and *regulated* secretion respectively. Constitutively secreted proteins (e.g. plasma proteins, clotting factors)* are not stored in appreciable amounts, and secretion is controlled by the rate of synthesis. Regulated secretion is controlled mainly by intracellular calcium, as described for amine transmitters in Chapter 6, and appreciable amounts of releasable peptides are present in cytoplasmic vesicles. Specific protein–protein interactions appear to be responsible for the sorting of different proteins into different vesicles, and for their selective release. Though the details are not fully understood, it seems clear that peptide and protein secretion by cells utilises essentially the same mechanisms as the release of conventional neurotransmitters and hormones. Identification of the specific 'trafficking' proteins involved in particular secretory pathways should yield novel drug targets for the selective control of secretion, but the prospect is still some way off, and conventional receptor-based pharmacology will be the basis for shorter-term therapeutic developments.

PEPTIDE ANTAGONISTS

Selective antagonists are known for the great majority of non-peptide receptors. In many cases they have come from nature (e.g. tubocurarine, atropine, strychnine, ergot

---

*Some clotting factors (e.g. factor Va, fibrinogen; see Ch. 17) are also stored in platelets, and undergo regulated secretion.

> ### Biosynthesis and release of peptides
>
> - The genetically coded *preprohormone* is a large protein comprising a *signal sequence* (involved in transfer of the protein across the membrane) plus the prohormone, which contains the embedded sequences of one or more active peptides.
> - The active peptides are produced intracellularly by selective enzymic cleavage, centred on pairs of adjacent Arg or Lys residues; in most cases the active peptides are stored (often in vesicles) in a releasable form.
> - A single precursor gene may give rise to several peptides, either by selective DNA splicing before transcription, by selective cleavage of the prohormone, or by post-translational modification.
> - There are many examples of closely related peptides, presumably produced by divergent evolution from a single gene, with different locations and physiological functions.
> - Peptides and proteins are located in intracellular vesicles, which are budded off from the endoplasmic reticulum and Golgi apparatus.
> - After sorting and post-translational processing of the peptide products, the vesicles differentiate into secretory vesicles, which discharge their contents by exocytosis.
> - With *constitutive release*, (e.g. plasma proteins, clotting factors) secretory vesicles are discharged as soon as they are formed, and secretion is continuous. With *regulated release* (neuropeptides and endocrine peptides), exocytosis is controlled by intracellular calcium, as with release of conventional transmitters.

derivatives), but synthetic chemistry has also succeeded in producing them in abundance, either by accident (e.g. antipsychotic drugs later identified as dopamine antagonists; Ch. 34) or by design (e.g. β-adrenoceptor antagonists, Ch. 8; 5-HT$_3$ antagonists, Ch. 9). For many years, peptide antagonists (apart from opiate antagonists; Ch. 37) remained elusive, and only a few are so far in clinical use, though their therapeutic potential is considerable (see Betancur et al. 1997). Recently, though, progress has been made in what had seemed to be a rather sterile area. Substitution of unnatural amino acids, particularly D-amino acids, into the sequence yields antagonists to various peptides, such as substance P, angiotensin and bradykinin. For reasons discussed below, however, such peptides are of little use therapeutically, so effort has gone into discovering non-peptides which bind to peptide receptors. One rational approach was to modify the peptide backbone, while retaining as far as possible the disposition of the side-chain groups that are responsible for binding to the receptor. Such compounds,

sometimes known as 'peptoids', have been developed for several peptide receptors (such as cholecystokinin and neuropeptide Y). In other cases, brute force—the random screening of large compound libraries—has succeeded where rational approaches failed, resulting in highly potent and selective antagonists that are in use, or under development, as therapeutic agents (see Table 10.1). Few if any agonists have been discovered in this way, and morphine-like compounds remain the only examples of non-peptide agonists at peptide receptors. Understanding of what makes non-peptides chemically recognisable by peptide receptors remains elusive, much to the frustration of medicinal chemists who would dearly like to be able to design such compounds de novo. Examples of peptide mediators for which peptide or non-peptide antagonists are known are given in Table 10.1. There remain many peptide mediators for which no antagonists are known, but strenuous efforts are being made to fill this gap, in the hope of developing new therapeutic agents.

Not surprisingly, it has proved easier to find synthetic compounds that block receptors for small peptides (e.g. most neuropeptides), which have only a few points of attachment, than for large peptides and proteins (e.g. cytokines and growth factors), which interact with the receptor at many points. These receptors are not easily fooled by small molecules, and efforts to target them therapeutically rely on protein-based approaches (see below).

PROTEINS AND PEPTIDES AS DRUGS

Some proteins, such as antibodies, cytokines, enzymes, clotting factors, etc., are used as therapeutic agents in specific conditions, and are invariably given by injection (see Table 10.2 for some examples; Bristow 1991, Buckel 1996 for further information). Apart from vaccines and clotting factors, most of the proteins currently in therapeutic use are functional human proteins prepared by recombinant technology,* which are used to supplement the action of endogenous mediators. Though their preparation requires advanced technology, such proteins are relatively straightforward and quick to develop as drugs, since they rarely cause toxicity, and have a more predictable therapeutic effect than synthetic drugs. The

---

*The use of recombinant material avoids the risk of transmitting viruses (e.g. hepatitis, AIDS), or prion infections (particularly Creutzfeld–Jakob disease; see Ch. 31) with human-derived material. Human blood products are widely used, nonetheless.

Table 10.1 Peptide antagonists

Mediator	Receptor types*	Antagonists		Further information
		Peptides or modified peptides	Non-peptides[†]	
Angiotensin	AT_1, AT_2	Saralasin Others known	Losartan, valsartan, etc. (AT_1-selective) AT_2-selective, and mixed antagonists known	Ch. 15

Bradykinin	B_1, B_2	Des–Arg[9], Leu[8]–BK
		  (B_1-selective)
		Icatibant (= HOE140,
		  B_2-selective)
		Others known
			No B_1 antagonists
			B_2 antagonists known
				Chs 12, 37

Calcitonin gene-related peptide	CGRP	CGRP[8–37]	Not known	Ch. 12
Cholecystokinin	CCK_A, CCK_B	Selective antagonists known	Devazepide, lorglumide (CCK_A-selective) CCK_B-selective compounds known	Ch. 30
Corticotrophin-releasing factor	CRF_1, CRF_2	Not known	CRF_1-selective antagonists known	Chs 24, 30
Endothelin	ET_1, ET_2	Selective compounds known	Bosentan (non-selective) Selective antagonists known	Ch. 15
Opioid peptides	μ, δ, κ	Selective antagonists known for μ, δ	Naloxone, naltrexone (non-selective) Naltrindole (δ-selective)	Ch. 37
Oxytocin/vasopressin	V_1, V_2, OT	Selective antagonists known	Selective antagonists known	Chs 20, 26
Tachykinins	NK_1, NK_2, NK_3	Selective antagonists known	Selective antagonists known	Chs 21, 37

*For further information on peptide receptor subtypes, see TIPS Receptor Nomenclature Supplement, 1996.
[†]For details of non-peptide compounds, see Betancur et al. (1997).
Antagonists of larger peptide and protein mediators (e.g. insulin, cytokines, growth factors) are not known.

next stage will be to develop 'designer proteins'—genetically engineered variants of natural proteins—for specific purposes. One example is the production of fusion proteins consisting of an antibody (targeted, for example, at a tumour antigen), or a peptide (for example bombesin or somatostatin, which bind to receptors on tumour cells) linked to a toxin (such as ricin or diphtheria toxin) to kill the cells (see Ch. 42). Another example is the soluble extracellular domain of the human immunoglobulin receptor, intended to control allergic diseases by acting as a decoy to capture circulating immunoglobulins, in order to prevent them from attaching to cellular receptors. Many ingenious ideas are being explored, and some prophets anticipate the dawn of a new era of therapeutics, as the dominion of small-molecule therapeutics begins to fade. Pharmacologists, needless to say, are somewhat sceptical, but nobody can afford to ignore the potential of biotechnology-based therapeutics in the future.

Smaller peptides are used therapeutically but, in general, peptides make bad drugs; there are several reasons for this:

- They cannot be given orally, either because they are hydrolysed in the gut or because they are not absorbed. Most are given by injection, some by nasal spray. (An important exception is **cyclosporin**, discussed in Ch. 13, which contains so many unnatural amino acids that no peptidase will touch it.)
- They are expensive to manufacture.
- They are usually quickly hydrolysed by plasma and tissue peptidases, and so have a short biological half-life, though there are exceptions to this.
- They do not penetrate the blood–brain barrier.

A list of therapeutic proteins and peptides is given in Table 10.2 (see also Bristow 1991, Buckel 1996).

Table 10.2 Peptides and protein as drugs

Drug	Use	Route
Peptides		
Captopril/enalapril (peptide-related)	Hypertension	Oral
	Heart failure (Ch. 15)	
Vasopressin	Diabetes insipidus (Ch. 24)	Intranasal, injection
Desmopressin		
Lypressin		
Oxytocin	Induction of labour (Ch. 26)	Injection
GnRH analogues (e.g. buserelin)	Infertility, suppression of ovulation (Ch. 26)	Intranasal, injection
	Prostate and breast tumours	
ACTH	Diagnosis of adrenal insufficiency (Ch. 24)	Injection
TSH/TRH	Diagnosis of thyroid disease (Ch. 25)	Injection
Calcitonin	Paget's disease of bone (Ch. 27)	Intranasal, injection
Insulin	Diabetes (Ch. 22)	Injection
Somatostatin, octreotide	Acromegaly, GI tumours (Ch. 24)	Intranasal, injection
Growth hormone	Dwarfism (Ch. 24)	Injection
Cyclosporin	Immunosuppression (Ch. 13)	Oral
F(ab) fragment	Digoxin overdose	Injection
Proteins		
Streptokinase, tissue plasminogen activator	Thromboembolism (Ch. 17)	Injection
Asparaginase	Tumour chemotherapy (Ch. 12)	Injection
DNAse	Cystic fibrosis (Ch. 19)	Inhalation
Interferons	Tumour chemotherapy (Chs 13, 42)	Injection
Erythropoietin, G-CSF, etc.	Anaemia (Ch. 18)	Injection
Clotting factors	Clotting disorders (Ch. 17)	Injection
Antibodies, vaccines, etc.	Infectious diseases	Injection or oral

---

Peptides and proteins as drugs

- In spite of the large number of known peptide mediators, only a few peptides are, as yet, useful as drugs, most of these being close analogues of endogenous peptide mediators.
- In most cases, peptides:
  - are poorly absorbed when given orally
  - have a short duration of action because of rapid degradation in vivo
  - fail to cross the blood–brain barrier
  - are expensive to manufacture.
- Peptide antagonists were slow to be discovered, but many are now available, and in development as therapeutic agents.
- Protein-based therapeutic agents are limited in number, and include hormones (e.g. insulin, growth hormone), clotting factors, cytokines, antibodies and enzymes. In many cases, recombinant technology is used to produce them.
- 'Designer proteins' prepared by recombinant methods, are expected to play an increasing therapeutic role in the future.

CONCLUDING REMARKS

The physiology and pharmacology of peptides—particularly neuropeptides—has stimulated a large amount of research over the last two decades, and the flow of data continues unabated. Cooper et al. (1996) advise peptide-watchers: 'Don't blink'. With more than a dozen major families of peptides, and a host of minor players, it is beyond the scope of this book to cover them individually or in detail. Instead, we will introduce information on peptide pharmacology wherever it has relevance to the physiology and pharmacology under discussion (e.g. bradykinin in inflammation, Ch. 12; endothelins and angiotensin in cardiovascular regulation, Ch. 15; tachykinins in asthma, Ch. 19; tachykinins and opioid peptides in nociception, Ch. 37; leptin and neuropeptide Y in obesity, Ch. 23). Useful general references on peptide pharmacology include Hokfelt et al. (1994), Cooper et al. (1996), Sherman et al. (1989).

Amino acids							
Side-chain type	Name	3-letter code	Single letter code	Side-chain type	Name	3-letter code	Single letter code
● **Basic**	Lysine	Lys	K	● **Hydrophobic**	Alanine	Ala	A
	Arginine	Arg	R		Valine	Val	V
	Histidine	His	H		Isoleucine	Ile	I
					Leucine	Leu	L
● **Uncharged polar**	Serine	Ser	S		Methionine	Met	M
	Threonine	Thr	T		Phenylalanine	Phe	F
	Asparagine	Asn	N		Tyrosine	Tyr	Y
	Glutamine	Gln	Q		Tryptophan	Trp	W
● **Acidic**	Aspartic acid	Asp	D				
	Glutamic acid	Glu	E	● **Special types**	Cysteine	Cys	C
					Glycine	Gly	G
					Proline	Pro	P

REFERENCES AND FURTHER READING

Betancur C, Azzi M, Rostene W 1997 Nonpeptide antagonists of neuropeptide receptors. Trends Pharmacol Sci 18: 372–386 (Describes success in finding non-peptide antagonists—for long elusive—and their possible therapeutic uses)

Bristow A F 1991 The current status of therapeutic peptides and proteins. In: Hider R C, Barlow D (eds) Polypeptide and protein drugs. Ellis Horwood, Chichester (Review article)

Buckel P 1996 Recombinant proteins for therapy. Trends Pharmacol Sci 17: 450–456 (Good account of therapeutic proteins)

Burger E 1988 Peptide hormones and neuropeptides: proteolytic processing of the precursor regulatory peptides. Arz Forsch 38: 754–761 (Describes the pattern of synthesis and processing that is common to all peptide hormones and transmitters)

Cooper J R, Bloom F E, Roth R H 1996 Biochemical basis of neuropharmacology. Oxford University Press, New York (Excellent standard textbook)

Cullinan W E, Day N C, Schafer M K et al. 1991 Neuroanatomical and functional studies of peptide precursor-processing enzymes. Enzyme 45: 285–300 (Review of enzyme mechanisms involved in neuropeptide processing)

Hökfelt T 1991 Neuropeptides in perspective: the last ten years. Neuron 7: 867–879 (Excellent overview by a neuropeptide pioneer)

Hökfelt T, Castel M-N, Morino P, Zhang X, Dagerlind A 1994 General overview of neuropeptides. In: Bloom F E, Kaplan D J (eds) Psychopharmacology: the fourth generation of progress. Raven Press, New York (Good general review)

Iversen L L, Iversen S D, Snyder S H (eds) 1983 Neuropeptides. Handbook of psychopharmacology. Plenum, New York, vol 16

Lundberg J M 1996 Pharmacology of co-transmission in the autonomic nervous system: integrative aspects on amines, neuropeptides, adenosine triphosphate, amino acids and nitric oxide. Pharmacol Rev 48: 114–192

Meunier J-C, Mollereau C, Toll L et al. 1995 Isolation and structure of the endogenous agonist of opioid receptor-like ORL$_1$ receptor. Nature 377: 532–535 (Describes a new opioid-like peptide—a ligand for a hitherto 'orphan' receptor)

Milner-White E J 1989 Predicting the biologically active conformations of short polypeptides. Trends Pharmacol Sci 10: 70–74 (Shows how difficult it is)

Perone M J, Windeatt S, Castro M G 1997 Intracellular trafficking of prohormones and proneuropeptides: cell type-specific sorting and targeting. Exp Physiol 82: 609–628 (Excellent review of mechanisms by which cells manage to avoid getting their many neuropeptides mixed up)

Sherman T G, Akil H, Watson S J 1989 The molecular biology of neuropeptides. Disc Neurosci 6: 1–58 (General review)

Yanagisawa M, Kurihara H, Kimura S et al. 1988 A novel potent vasoconstrictor peptide produced by vascular endothelial cells. Nature 332: 411–415 (The discovery of endothelin—a remarkable tour de force)

11

Nitric oxide

Nitric oxide (NO), a free radical gas, is formed in the atmosphere during lightning storms. Less dramatically, but with far-reaching biological consequences, it is also formed in an enzyme-catalysed reaction between *molecular oxygen* and *L-arginine* in mammals as well as more primitive species. The convergence of several lines of research led to the realisation that NO acts as a key signalling mechanism in the *cardiovascular* and *nervous* systems, and has a role in *host defence*. This rapidly evolving picture has been one of the most astonishing recent revelations of physiology.

A physiological function of NO was first discovered in the vasculature when it was shown that the *endothelium-derived relaxing factor* described by Furchgott & Zawadzki in 1980 could be quantitatively accounted for by the formation of NO by endothelial cells (Fig. 11.1). It was discovered independently that NO is the endogenous activator of soluble guanylate cyclase, leading to the formation of cyclic GMP (cGMP) which functions as a second messenger in many cells including nerves, smooth muscle, monocytes and platelets. Nitrogen and oxygen are neighbours in the periodic table, and NO shares several properties with O_2, in particular a high affinity for haem and other iron–sulphur groups. This is important for activation of guanylate cyclase, which contains a haem group, and for the inactivation of NO by haemoglobin.

The role of NO in various specific settings is touched on or described more fully in other chapters: the endothelium in Chapter 15, the autonomic nervous system in Chapter 6, as a chemical transmitter and mediator of excitotoxicity in the central nervous system in Chapters 28–31, and in the innate mediator-derived reactions of acute inflammation and the immune response in Chapter 12. Therapeutic uses of organic nitrates and of **nitroprusside** (NO donors) are described in Chapters 14 and 15. In the present chapter, we concentrate on general principles involved in the biosynthesis of NO and its pharmacological control and also touch on clinical conditions where disordered biosynthesis of NO is believed to play a part. There is a brief consideration of the therapeutic implications of these observations in terms of possible uses of drugs that potentiate or donate NO, and of inhibitors of NO synthesis.

BIOSYNTHESIS OF NITRIC OXIDE AND ITS CONTROL

NO synthase (NOS) enzymes are central to the control of NO biosynthesis. There are three known isoforms of NOS: an *inducible* form (expressed in macrophages and Kupffer cells, neutrophils, fibroblasts, vascular smooth muscle and endothelial cells in response to pathological stimuli such as invading microorganisms) and two so-called '*constitutive*' forms that are present under physiological conditions in endothelium and in neurons. These are referred to as iNOS (or mNOS or NOS-II), eNOS (or ecNOS or NOS-III) and nNOS (or ncNOS or NOS-I) respectively. eNOS is not restricted to endothelium, also being present in cardiac myocytes, renal mesangial cells, osteoblasts and osteoclasts and, in small amounts, in platelets. The constitutive enzymes generate small amounts of NO (picomolar), whereas the activity of iNOS is approximately a thousand times greater.

All three NOS isoforms are dimeric enzymes. They are structurally and functionally complex, bearing similarities to the cytochrome P450 enzymes (described in Ch. 5) that are so important in drug metabolism. Each

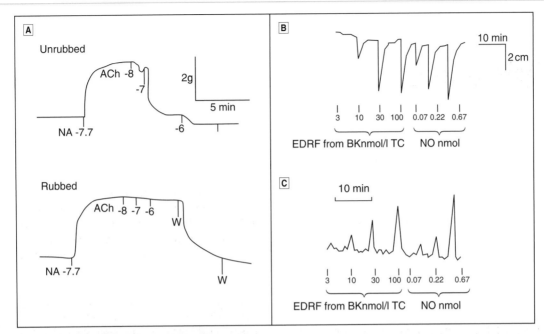

Fig. 11.1 Endothelium-derived relaxing factor is closely related to NO. [A] Acetylcholine relaxes a strip of rabbit aorta precontracted with noradrenaline if the endothelium is intact, but not if it has been removed by gentle rubbing. The numbers are logarithms of molar drug concentrations. [B] Endothelium-derived relaxing factor (EDRF) is released from a column of cultured endothelial cells by bradykinin (Bk 3–100 nmol) applied through the column of cells (TC) and relaxes a de-endothelialised precontracted bioassay strip, as does authentic NO. [C] A chemical assay of NO based on chemiluminescence shows that similar concentrations of NO are present in the EDRF released from the column of cells as in equiactive authentic NO solutions. (From: (A) Furchgott R F, Zawadzki J V 1980 Nature 288: 373–376; (B and C) Palmer et al. 1987 Nature 327: 524–526)

isoform contains iron protoporphyrin IX (haem), flavin adenine dinucleotide (FAD), flavin mononucleotide (FMN) and tetrahydrobiopterin as bound prosthetic groups. They also contain binding sites for L-arginine, NADPH and calcium–calmodulin. These prosthetic groups and ligands control the assembly of the enzyme into the active dimer. eNOS is dually acylated by N-myristoylation and cysteine palmitoylation. These post-translational modifications lead to its association with membranes in the Golgi apparatus and in *caveolae*—specialised microdomains in the plasma membrane derived from the Golgi apparatus in which eNOS is associated with *caveolin*, a transmembrane protein that is a key structural protein of caveolae involved in signal transduction.

The nitrogen atom in NO is derived from the terminal guanidino group of L-arginine. Details of the reaction mechanism are controversial and beyond the scope of this book, but it is known that NOS enzymes are functionally 'bimodal' in that they combine oxygenase and reductase activities associated with distinct structural domains. The oxygenase domain contains haem, while the reductase domain binds calcium–calmodulin, FMN, FAD and NADPH. By analogy with cytochrome P450, it is believed that the flavins accept electrons from NADPH and transfer them to the haem iron which binds O_2 and catalyses the stepwise oxidation of L-arginine to NO and citrulline. Uncoupled forms of the enzyme transfer electrons to other substrates, such as molecular oxygen, leading to the synthesis of superoxide anion rather than NO. L-arginine is usually present in excess in endothelial cytoplasm, so the rate of production of NO is determined by the activity of the enzyme rather than by substrate availability. Nevertheless, very high doses of L-arginine are able to restore endothelial NO bio-synthesis in some pathological states (e.g. hypercholes-terolaemia; see below) in which endothelial function is impaired. Possible explanations for this paradox include the existence of a distinct pool of substrate accessible to enzyme, which can become depleted despite apparently plentiful total cytoplasmic arginine concentrations; competition with endogenous inhibitors of NOS such as asymmetric dimethyl arginine (ADMA; see below) that might be increased in hypercholesterolaemia; and reassembly/reactivation of enzyme in which transfer of electrons has become uncoupled from L-arginine as mentioned above.

The activity of the constitutive isoforms of NOS is controlled by intracellular calcium–calmodulin (Fig. 11.2). The most important stimuli controlling endothelial NO synthesis in resistance vessels under physiological conditions are probably *mechanical*, pulsatile flow and shear stress being important. In addition, endothelial cells possess receptors for several vasodilators including acetylcholine, substance P and bradykinin, occupation of which increases $[Ca^{2+}]_i$ thereby stimulating endothelial

NO biosynthesis. Not all of these agonists are believed to be physiologically important, although they are useful as experimental tools for investigating endothelial function. Calcium ionophores (e.g. A23187) and polycations (e.g. poly-L-lysine) also cause endothelium-dependent relaxation. Several drugs with principal actions on other tissues (e.g. **propofol**, an intravenous anaesthetic agent— see Ch. 32—and **nebivolol**, a β-adrenoceptor antagonist) also release NO from endothelium by mechanisms that remain to be established. The resulting vasodilatation may contribute to their therapeutic or adverse effects.

In contrast to the constitutive isoforms of NOS, the activity of iNOS is independent of $[Ca^{2+}]_i$. Though iNOS contains a binding site for calcium–calmodulin, the very high affinity of this site for its ligand, means that iNOS is activated even at the low values of $[Ca^{2+}]_i$ present under

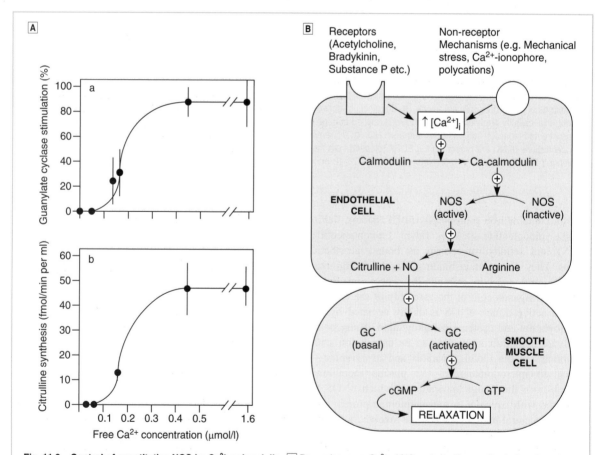

Fig. 11.2 Control of constitutive NOS by Ca²⁺–calmodulin. [A] Dependence on Ca^{2+} of NO and citrulline synthesis from L-arginine by rat brain synaptosomal cytosol. Rates of synthesis of NO from L-arginine were determined by stimulation of guanylate cyclase (a) or by synthesis of $^3[H]$-citrulline from L-$[^3H]$arginine (b). [B] Regulation of guanylate cyclase in smooth muscle by NO formed in adjacent endothelium (paracrine regulation). (From: (A) Knowles R G et al. 1989 Proc Natl Acad Sci USA 86: 5159–5162)

resting conditions. The enzyme is induced by bacterial lipopolysaccharide (LPS) and/or cytokines synthesised in response to LPS, notably interferon γ, whose antiviral effect is accounted for by this action. Tumour necrosis factor-α (TNF-α) and interleukin-1 (IL-1), unlike interferon γ, are not effective in inducing iNOS expression in their own right, but they each synergise with interferon γ in this regard (see Ch. 12). Induction is inhibited by glucocorticoids and by several cytokines, including transforming growth factor-β (TGF-β). There are important species differences in the inducibility of iNOS, which is less readily induced in human than in mouse cells. It is, however, produced by human macrophages in response to IgE after they have been treated with IL-4 which causes them to express CD23 receptors.

DEGRADATION AND CARRIAGE OF NITRIC OXIDE

NO reacts with oxygen to form N_2O_4, which combines with water to produce a mixture of nitrite and nitrate anions. Nitrite ions are oxidised to nitrate by oxyhaemoglobin. These reactions are summarised:

$$2NO + O_2 \rightarrow N_2O_4 \qquad (11.1)$$

$$N_2O_4 + H_2O \rightarrow NO_3^- + NO_2^- + 2H^+ \qquad (11.2)$$

$$NO_2^- + HbO \rightarrow NO_3^- + Hb \qquad (11.3)$$

Low concentrations of NO are relatively stable in air because equation (11.1) is a second-order reaction. Consequently, small amounts of NO produced in the lung escape degradation and can be detected in exhaled air. In contrast, NO reacts very rapidly with even low concentrations of superoxide anion (O_2^-) to produce peroxynitrite anion (ONOO⁻) which is responsible for some of its toxic effects.

NO diffuses freely across cell membranes, accounting adequately for its local paracrine actions on vascular smooth muscle or on monocytes or platelets adhering to the endothelium. The potential for action at a distance is, however, neatly demonstrated by *Rhodnius prolixus*, a blood-sucking insect that produces a salivary vasodilator/platelet inhibitor with the properties of a nitrovasodilator. This consists of a mixture of nitrosylated haemoproteins which bind NO in the salivary glands of the insect but subsequently release it in the tissues of its prey. The resulting local vasodilatation and inhibition of platelet activation presumably facilitates extraction of the bug's meal in liquid form.

The possibility that analogous carrier mechanisms

(e.g. cysteine- and/or –SH-containing proteins) operate in mammals, and allow NO to act at a distance from its site of biosynthesis has recently attracted intense interest, especially in the context of haemoglobin. When NO diffuses from endothelium into the blood, it reacts rapidly with haem, which has an affinity for NO >10 000 times greater than for O_2. In the absence of oxygen, NO bound to haemogobin is relatively stable but in the presence of oxygen NO is immediately converted to nitrate and the haem iron oxidised to methaemoglobin. In addition to this inactivation reaction, it has recently been shown that NO can also bind *reversibly* to globin via the reactive sulphydryl groups of a cysteine residue. It is suggested that the resulting S-nitrosylated haemoglobin may be involved in the transduction of NO-related activities such as the control of vascular resistance and blood pressure, possibilities that are currently hotly debated.

Nitric oxide: synthesis, inactivation and carriage

- NO is synthesised from L-arginine and molecular O_2 by NO synthase (NOS).
- NOS exists in three isoforms: inducible, and constitutive endothelial and neuronal forms (respectively iNOS, eNOS and nNOS). NOSs are dimeric flavoproteins, contain tetrahydrobiopterin and have homology with cytochrome P450. The constitutive enzymes are activated by Ca^{2+}–calmodulin.
- iNOS is induced in macrophages and other cells by interferon-γ.
- nNOS is present in CNS (see Chs 28–31) and in NANC nerves (see Ch. 6).
- eNOS is present in platelets and other cells in addition to endothelium.
- NO is unstable but can form more stable nitrosothiols, particularly with a cysteine residue in globin so that red cells can act as a kind of NO buffer. It is inactivated by combination with the haem of haemoglobin or by oxidation to nitrite and nitrate which is excreted in urine.

EFFECTS OF NITRIC OXIDE

Some physiological and pathological roles of NO are shown in Table 11.1. NO activates guanylate cyclase by combining with its haem group, and the physiological effects of low concentrations of NO produced under normal conditions by the constitutive enzymes are mediated by cGMP. In contrast, cytotoxic and/or cytoprotective effects of higher concentrations of NO relate to its chemistry as a free radical (see Ch. 31).

Table 11.1 Postulated* roles of endogenous NO

System	Role		
	Physiological	Pathological	
		Excess production	Inadequate production or action
Cardiovascular			
Endothelium/vascular smooth muscle	Control of regional blood flow; ?control of blood pressure	Hypotension (septic shock)	Atherogenesis, thrombosis, vasospasm (e.g. in ? hypercholesterolaemia, ? diabetes mellitus, ? essential hypertension)
Platelets	? limitation of adhesion/aggregation		
Host defence			
Macrophages, neutrophil leucocytes	Defence against viruses, bacteria, fungi, protozoans, metazoan parasites		
Nervous			
Central	Neurotransmission; long-term potentiation; plasticity (? memory, appetite control, nociception)	Excitotoxicity (Ch. 31) (e.g. ischaemic stroke, Huntington's disease, AIDS dementia)	
Peripheral	Neurotransmission (e.g. gastric emptying, penile erection)		Hypertrophic pyloric stenosis ? Impotence in diabetes mellitus

*Evidence is incomplete (see Moncada & Higgs 1993).

Biochemical and cellular aspects

Pharmacological effects of NO have been studied using NO gas dissolved in balanced salt solution that has been thoroughly deoxygenated by gassing with an inert gas such as helium. More conveniently, but less directly, various chemical donors of NO such as **nitroprusside** or **S-nitroso-acetylpenicillamine** ('SNAP') have been used as surrogates.

NO can activate guanylate cyclase in the same cells that produce it—an *autocrine* effect. Endothelial NO production influences albumin permeability, implying an autocrine effect within the endothelium, and there is also evidence of an autocrine effect within platelets (see below). However, more commonly NO functions as a *paracrine* rather than as an autocrine mediator, diffusing from its site of synthesis and activating guanylate cyclase in neighbouring cells. The resulting increase in cGMP affects protein kinases, cyclic nucleotide phosphodiesterases, ion channels and possibly other proteins. These effects lead to reduced $[Ca^{2+}]_i$ responses to contractile and proaggregatory agonists in, respectively, vascular smooth muscle and platelets, without markedly influencing basal $[Ca^{2+}]_i$. Additionally, NO causes hyperpolari-

sation of vascular smooth muscle in some circumstances as a consequence of K^+-channel activation. cGMP inhibits monocyte adhesion and migration, and inhibits smooth muscle and fibroblast proliferation, actions that contribute to the antiatherogenic role of NO.

When large amounts of NO are produced as a result of induction of NOS or of excessive stimulation of NMDA receptors in the brain, it can cause chemical effects (either directly or via peroxynitrate anions). These are involved in host defence and in the neuronal destruction that occurs when there is overstimulation of NMDA receptors by glutamate (see Chs 29 and 31). Paradoxically, NO is also cytoprotective under some circumstances (see Ch. 31).

Vascular effects (see also Ch. 15)

The endothelial L-arginine/NO pathway is tonically active in resistance vessels, providing a physiological vasodilator mechanism that influences peripheral vascular resistance and hence systemic blood pressure. Mutant mice that lack the gene coding for eNOS are hypertensive. *Increased* endothelial NO generation may contribute to the generalised vasodilatation that occurs during healthy pregnancy.

Platelets and leukocytes

NO potently inhibits adhesion and aggregation of platelets, neutrophil leukocytes and monocytes. These actions within the microenvironment of the vessel wall may be important in protecting against atherogenesis and thrombosis.

Neuronal effects (see Chs 6 and 30)

NO is a non-noradrenergic non-cholinergic (NANC) neurotransmitter in many tissues (Ch. 6), and is important in man in the gastrointestinal tract and upper airways (Ch. 19). It is implicated in the control of neuronal development and of synaptic plasticity in the central nervous system. Mice carrying a mutation disrupting the gene coding nNOS are viable and fertile but have grossly distended stomachs with histologic appearances similar to those in hypertrophic pyloric stenosis (a human disease which occurs in approximately 1 in 150 male infants and can be fatal if not corrected surgically in infancy, in which hypertrophy of the pylorus of the stomach causes obstruction to gastric outflow into the duodenum). They are resistant to neural stroke damage following middle cerebral artery ligation, and display grossly increased aggressive and sexually inappropriate behaviour.

Host defence (see Ch. 12)

Cytotoxic and/or cytostatic effects of NO are implicated in non-specific host defence against numerous pathogens and tumour cells including bacteria, fungi, protozoa, and metazoan parasites. The importance of this mechanism is evidenced by uniform susceptibility to *Leishmania major* (a protozoan parasite to which wild-type mice are highly resistant) of mice lacking iNOS. Mechanisms whereby NO damages invading pathogens include nitrosylation

---

Actions of nitric oxide

- NO exerts effects by:
  - activating guanylate cyclase, thereby indirectly influencing $[Ca^{2+}]_i$
  - cytotoxic effects via combination with superoxide anion to yield peroxynitrite anion.
- Actions of NO include:
  - vasodilatation; inhibition of platelet and monocyte adhesion and aggregation; inhibition of smooth muscle proliferation; protection against atherogenesis
  - synaptic effects in the peripheral and central nervous system (see Chs 6 and 28–31)
  - host defence and cytotoxic effects on pathogens (see Ch. 12)
  - cytoprotective effects.

---

of nucleic acids and combination with haem-containing enzymes including those involved in cell respiration.

THERAPEUTIC USE OF NITRIC OXIDE AND NITRIC OXIDE DONORS

Nitric oxide

Inhalation of high concentrations of NO (as occurred when cylinders of nitrous oxide, N_2O, for anaesthesia were accidentally contaminated) causes acute pulmonary oedema and methaemoglobinaemia, but concentrations below 50 ppm do not appear to be toxic. NO at 5–300 ppm inhibits bronchoconstriction in guinea pigs, but the main action of inhaled NO is pulmonary vasodilatation. Two distinctive features make this action potentially therapeutically important. First, it is *limited to the pulmonary circulation*. Second, since NO is administered in inspired air it *acts preferentially on ventilated alveoli*. These properties have raised hopes that inhaled NO may be therapeutically useful in disorders such as adult respiratory distress syndrome (see p. 349). This condition has a high mortality and is caused by diverse insults of which infection is the most common. It is characterised by intrapulmonary 'shunting' (i.e. pulmonary arterial blood entering the pulmonary vein without passing through capillaries in contact with ventilated alveoli) resulting in arterial hypoxaemia, and by acute pulmonary arterial hypertension. Inhaled NO causes vasodilatation specifically in ventilated alveoli, and thus reduces shunting. Early experience with NO in this condition has been encouraging, but it is unknown whether it improves long-term survival in these severely ill patients.

Nitric oxide donors

In contrast to the recent experimental use of NO as a therapeutic gas, nitrovasodilators have been used therapeutically for over a century. It is now appreciated that the common mode of action of these drugs, which are discussed in Chapters 14 and 15, is as a source of NO. There is considerable interest in the potential for selectivity of these agents: for instance, **glyceryl trinitrate** is more potent on vascular smooth muscle than on platelets whereas **S-nitroso glutathione** selectively inhibits platelet function.

INHIBITION OF NITRIC OXIDE

There are many potential mechanisms by which drugs can inhibit NO synthesis or action. Currently the most

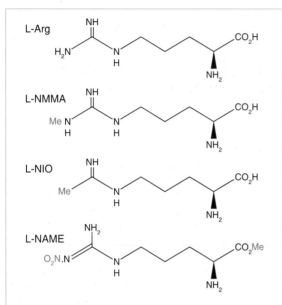

Fig. 11.3 L-arginine and some analogues that compete with it for NOS and inhibit NO formation. Groups that differ from arginine are shown in blue. (L-Arg = L-arginine; L-NMMA = N^G-monomethyl-L-arginine; L-NIO = N-iminoethyl-L-ornithine; L-NAME = N^G-nitro-L-arginine methyl ester)

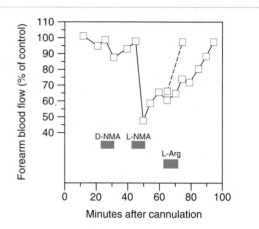

Fig. 11.4 Basal blood flow in the human forearm is influenced by NO biosynthesis. Forearm blood flow is expressed as a percentage of the flow in the non-cannulated control arm (which does not change). Brachial artery infusion of D-NMMA has no effect. L-NMMA causes vasoconstriction. L-arginine accelerates recovery from such vasoconstriction (dashed line). (From: Vallance et al. 1989 Lancet ii: 997–1000)

useful strategy remains the use of arginine analogues (see Fig. 11.3). Several such compounds, e.g. **N^G-monomethyl-L-arginine (L-NMMA)** and **N^G-nitro-L-arginine methyl ester (L-NAME)**, have proved of great value as experimental tools. Some of them, in particular *asymmetric dimethyl arginine (ADMA)*, have been detected in human urine, raising the possibility that they influence the L-arginine/NO pathway under pathological conditions (see above). Recently, an endogenous protein inhibitor of nNOS (termed 'PIN') has been discovered, which works by destabilising the NOS dimer.

Intravenous administration of L-NMMA increases blood pressure in several species, including humans. Increased blood pressure caused by L-NMMA in conscious rats is accompanied by vasoconstriction in renal, mesenteric, carotid and hindquarters vascular beds. Infusion of L-NMMA into human brachial artery causes vasoconstriction (Fig. 11.4). These observations can be explained on the basis of inhibition of the *basal* production of NO that occurs in these vascular beds under physiological conditions of flow and pulsatility.

There is interest in selective inhibitors of different forms of NOS, although high (>100-fold) selectivity has yet to be established. **N-iminoethyl-L-ornithine (L-NIO)** is a potent and irreversible inhibitor of iNOS in activated macrophages. **7-nitroindazole** inhibits mouse cerebellar NOS and, following intraperitoneal administration, inhibits *nociception* without altering arterial blood pressure; this selectivity apparently results from an incompletely understood pharmacokinetic effect related to access of the drug to NOS in brain and in endothelium.

Inhibition of the L-arginine/nitric oxide pathway

- Glucocorticoids inhibit biosynthesis of inducible (but not constitutive) NOS.
- Synthetic arginine analogues, e.g. L-NMMA, L-NAME compete with arginine and are useful experimental tools. L-NMMA has therapeutic potential in septic shock.
- Endogenous NOS inhibitors include ADMA and PIN (a protein which inhibits NOS dimerisation).
- Isoform selective inhibitors are being sought.

CLINICAL CONDITIONS IN WHICH NITRIC OXIDE MAY PLAY A PART

The wide distribution of NOS and diverse actions of NO have suggested that abnormalities in this pathway could be involved in the pathophysiology of numerous clinical disorders. Either increased or reduced production could play a part in disease states, and hypotheses abound. Evidence is harder to come by but has been sought using various indirect approaches including:

- Analysis of nitrate or of cGMP in urine. These approaches are bedevilled by the presence of nitrate in the diet, and by stimuli to membrane-bound guanylate cyclase such as the natriuretic peptides (see Ch. 14). Recently, the method has been refined by using mass spectrometry to measure the enrichment of ^{15}N- over naturally abundant ^{14}N-nitrate in urine following intravenous infusion of ^{15}N-labelled arginine.
- Measurement of vasoconstrictor effects of NOS inhibitors (e.g. **L-NMMA**).
- Comparison of vascular responses to endothelium-dependent agonists (e.g. acetylcholine) with endothelium-independent agonists that work through the same effector mechanism (e.g. nitroprusside).
- Measurement of the dilator response to increased blood flow in the brachial artery, which is partly NO-mediated.
- Study of histochemical appearances and pharmacological responses of tissue in vitro.

All such methods have limitations, and the dust is far from settled. Nevertheless, it seems clear that the L-arginine/NO pathway is indeed a player in the pathogenesis of several important diseases, opening the way to new therapeutic approaches including the use of selective NO donors as 'replacement' therapy and dietary supplementation with antioxidants (to reduce superoxide anion formation and hence stabilise NO) or with L-arginine.

We touch only briefly on these clinical conditions, and would caution the reader that not all of these exciting possibilities are likely to withstand the test of time! Some postulated pathological roles of excessive or reduced NO production are summarised in Table 11.1.

Nitric oxide in pathophysiology

- NO is synthesised under physiological and pathological circumstances.
- Either reduced or increased NO production can contribute to disease processes.
- Underproduction of neuronal NO is reported in babies with hypertrophic pyloric stenosis. Endothelial NO production is reduced in patients with hypercholesterolaemia and some other risk factors for atherosclerosis, and may contribute to atherogenesis.
- Overproduction of NO may be important in neurodegenerative diseases (see Ch. 31) and in septic shock.

---

iNOS

Sepsis can lead to multiple organ failure by a complex series of events. It is likely that whereas NO is of benefit in host defence early in this sequence by contributing to microbial killing, subsequent excessive NO production can cause harmful hypotension. Chronic low-grade endotoxaemia occurs in patients with cirrhosis of the liver, many of whom are systemically vasodilated. Urinary excretion of cGMP is increased in such patients, and the vasodilatation may be caused by induction of NOS leading to increased vascular NO synthesis.

L-NMMA may be of therapeutic use in patients with severe hypotension and multiple organ failure secondary to sepsis: preliminary clinical experience has been encouraging, but considerable caution is needed because NO biosynthesis in this setting has some advantageous effects (preservation of splanchnic and renal blood flow, as well as microbial killing). Animal models of sepsis suggest that the dose of inhibitor will be critical, with low doses of L-NMMA conferring benefit but higher doses increasing mortality. A clinical trial is in progress to determine if there is an effect on survival of critically ill patients with sepsis syndrome.

Constitutive NOS isoforms

eNOS

There is suggestive evidence of reduced NO biosynthesis in patients with *hypercholesterolaemia* and some other disorders that predispose to atheromatous vascular disease including *cigarette smoking* and *diabetes mellitus*. In hypercholesterolaemia, evidence of blunted NO release in forearm and coronary vascular beds is supported by evidence that this can be corrected by treating hyperlipidaemia or by supplementation with L-arginine. Low-dose chronic treatment of cholesterol-fed rabbits with an inhibitor of NOS markedly potentiates atherogenesis without increasing blood pressure or influencing plasma lipid concentrations. This implies that the endothelial dysfunction caused by dyslipidaemia and other cardiovascular risk factors could be of great importance in the pathogenesis of the accelerated atherosclerosis that is the cause of the excess morbidity and mortality associated with these conditions (see Ch. 16).

Endothelial dysfunction in diabetic patients with impotence occurs in tissue from the corpora cavernosum of penis studied in vitro,* as evidenced by blunted

---

*Such tissue was obtained during surgical insertion of penile prostheses, a treatment for impotence now largely superseded; see Ch. 15.

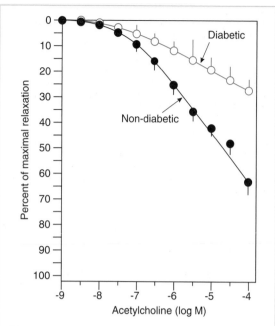

Fig. 11.5   Impaired endothelium-mediated relaxation of penile smooth muscle from diabetic men with impotence.
Mean (± SE) relaxation responses to acetylcholine in corpora cavernosa tissue (obtained at the time of performing surgical implants to treat impotence) from 16 diabetic men and 22 non-diabetics. (Data from: Saenz de Tejada et al. 1989 New Engl J Med 320: 1025–1030)

relaxation to acetylcholine despite preserved responses to nitroprusside (Fig. 11.5). Vasoconstrictor responses to intra-arterial **L-NMMA** are reduced in forearm vasculature of insulin-dependent diabetics, especially in patients with traces of albumin in their urine (early evidence of glomerular endothelial dysfunction), suggesting that basal NO synthesis may be reduced throughout their circulation. It has been hypothesised that a failure to increase endogenous NO biosynthesis underlies pre-eclampsia, a hypertensive disorder of pregnancy that accounts for many of the maternal deaths in economically developed societies and in which the normal vaso-dilatation seen in healthy pregnancy is lost.

nNOS

Excessive NMDA receptor activation contributes to several forms of neurological damage (see Ch. 31). nNOS is absent in pyloric tissue from babies with ideopathic hypertrophic pyloric stenosis.*

Clinical uses of NO donors and NO as a therapeutic gas, and of inhibition of the L-arginine/NO system are summarised in the clinical box below.

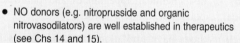

Nitric oxide in therapeutics

- NO donors (e.g. nitroprusside and organic nitrovasodilators) are well established in therapeutics (see Chs 14 and 15).
- Inhaled NO has therapeutic potential in adult respiratory distress syndrome but its effects on mortality are not known.
- Inhibition of NO biosynthesis (e.g. by L-NMMA) may be beneficial in patients with hypotension from multiple organ failure. It is a two-edged sword and dose will probably be critical.

---

*Are such individuals 'nNOS gene knockout humans'? What of their subsequent development?

REFERENCES AND FURTHER READING

Cockcroft J R, Chowienczyk P J, Brett S E et al. 1995 Nebivolol vasodilates human forearm vasculature: evidence for an L-arginine/NO-dependent mechanism. J Pharmacol Exp Therap 274: 1067–1071 (*This highly β1-selective antagonist vasodilates human resistance vasculature through the L-arginine/NO pathway*)

Elliott T G, Cockcroft J R, Groop P-H, Viberti G C, Ritter J M 1993 Inhibition of nitric oxide synthesis in forearm vasculature of insulin dependent diabetic patients. Clin Sci 85: 687–693 (*Blunted vasoconstrictor response to L-NMMA in diabetics, most marked in patients with microalbuminuria*)

Griffith O W, Stuehr D J 1995 Nitric oxide synthases: properties and catalytic mechanism. Ann Rev Physiol 57: 707–736 (*Mechanistic aspects of NOS catalysis*)

Gustafsson L E, Leone A M, Persson M G, Wiklund N P,

Moncada S 1991 Endogenous nitric oxide is present in the exhaled air of rabbits, guinea-pigs and humans. Biochem Biophys Res Commun 181: 852–857

Hobbs A J 1997 Soluble guanylate cyclase: the forgotten sibling. Trends Pharmacol Sci 18: 484–491 (*'Forgotten' in comparison to its illustrious sibling adenylate cyclase*)

Huang P L, Huang Z, Mashimo H et al. 1995 Hypertension in mice lacking the gene for endothelial nitric oxide synthase. Nature 377: 239–242 (*Absent EDRF activity in aorta, and hypertension in the mutant mice*)

Jaffrey S R, Snyder S 1996 PIN: an associated protein inhibitor of neuronal nitric oxide synthase. Science 274: 774–777 (*Works by destabilising the nNOS dimer*)

Jia L, Bonaventura C, Bonaventura J, Stamler J S 1996 S-nitrosohaemoglobin: a dynamic activity of blood involved in vascular control. Nature 380: 221–226 (*Controversial and fascinating paper that seriously challenges the orthodox view of NO as a paracrine mediator operating exclusively over a short range. See also accompanying editorial comment by Perutz M F pp 205–206*)

Karupiah G, Xie Q, Buller M L, Nathan C, Duarte C, MacMicking J D 1993 Inhibition of viral replication by interferon—induced nitric oxide synthase. Science 261: 1445–1448

Liu J, Garcia-Cardena G, Sessa W C 1996 Palmitoylation of endothelial nitric oxide synthase is necessary for optimal stimulated release of nitric oxide: implications for caveolae localization. Biochemistry 35: 13277–13281 (*N-myristoylation of eNOS is necessary for its association and targeting into the Golgi complex whereas palmitoylation influences its targeting to caveolae*)

Moncada S, Higgs A 1993 Mechanisms of disease: the L-arginine–nitric oxide pathway. N Engl J Med 329: 2002–2012 (*Excellent review of human/clinical aspects*)

Moncada S, Palmer R M J, Higgs E A 1991 Nitric oxide: physiology, pathophysiology and pharmacology. Pharmacol Rev 43: 109–142 (*Comprehensive basic review*)

Moore P K, Handy R C L 1997 Selective inhibitors of nitric oxide synthase—is no NOS really good NOS for the nervous system? Trends Pharmacol Sci 18: 204–211 (*Emphasis on compounds with selectivity for the neuronal isoform*)

Nelson R J, Demas G E, Huang P L et al. 1995 Behavioural abnormalities in male mice lacking neuronal nitric oxide synthase. Nature 378: 383–386 (*'A large increase in aggressive behaviour and excess, inappropriate sexual behaviour in nNOS-mice.'*)

Ribiero J M C, Hazzard J M H, Nussenzveig R H, Champagne D E, Walker F A 1993 Reversible binding of nitric oxide by a salivary haem protein from a blood sucking insect. Science 260: 539–541 (*Indisputable action at a distance*)

Snyder S H 1993 Janus faces of nitric oxide. Nature 364: 577 (*Discusses the cytoprotection/cytotoxicity paradox*)

Stuehr D J 1997 Structure–function aspects in the nitric oxide synthases. Ann Rev Pharmacol Toxicol 37: 339–359

Vallance P, Leone A, Calver A, Collier J, Moncada S 1992 Accumulation of endogenous inhibitor of nitric oxide synthesis in chronic renal failure. Lancet 339: 572–575 (*ADMA etc.; potential for pathogenic importance*)

Vanderwinden J-M, Mailleux P, Schiffmann S N, Vanderhaeghen J-J, De Laet M-H 1992 Nitric oxide synthase activity in infantile hypertrophic pyloric stenosis. N Engl J Med 327: 511–515

Wei X-q, Charles I G, Smith A et al. 1995 Altered immune responses in mice lacking inducible nitric oxide synthase. Nature 375: 408-411. (*Homozygotes lacking iNOS were uniformly susceptible to infection by* Leishmania major)

12

Local hormones, inflammation and allergy

Definitions of some terms applied to chemical mediators

The word *hormone*, as introduced by Bayliss & Starling, referred to a chemical substance that was secreted, without benefit of duct, directly into the bloodstream and which acted at long range, often slowly, on distant organs or tissues. When the role of some chemical substances in nervous transmission was established, *neurotransmitters* were held to be different from hormones in that they were released by neurons, not endocrine glands, and acted rapidly, briefly and at short range on an adjacent neuron or target cell. However, these tidy categories conferred a spurious order on the classification of the body's chemical messengers; in terms of defining and categorising them we have moved from orderly inexactitude towards a confused precision.

It was realised several years ago that some substances which were not neurotransmitters nevertheless acted briefly at short range on adjacent target cells (e.g. histamine from mast cells), and these were classed as *local hormones* or *paracrine secretions*; and one must now consider as local hormones the *autocrine secretions*, which act on the cells which secrete them, as, for example, many cytokines do. It has also become clear that some substances defined as true hormones in the Bayliss & Starling sense (e.g. insulin), as well as some substances categorised initially as 'local hormones' (e.g. 5-hydroxytryptamine in platelets) are also neurotransmitters in the CNS (see Ch. 31); and conversely that neurons in what is indubitably a part of the CNS—the hypothalamus—release peptides and possibly amino acids into the bloodstream for action on distant target cells (see Ch. 24).

Further complexity has been added to the problem of defining these terms by the finding that many of the substances, including several considered as hormones (e.g. insulin, corticotrophin, chorionic gonadotrophin and somatostatin), as well as others regarded as neurotransmitters (acetylcholine, catecholamines) are found in unicellular organisms such as protozoa and bacteria. Some have biological effects in these organisms: adrenaline stimulates adenylate cyclase in protozoa (an effect blocked by propranolol), and opioid peptides alter the behaviour of amoebae (an effect blocked by naloxone).

It seems to be the case that the basic biochemical mechanisms involved in cell-to-cell communication arose very early in evolution and have been highly conserved; and that, in higher organisms, these basic elements have been adapted for more complex communication requirements. The chemical messengers themselves can be used differently in different circumstances.

It is evident that in classifying the physiologically active chemical substances in man, the original concept of separate categories of hormones and transmitters has given way to the idea of a spectrum of agents in which some substances are predominantly neurotransmitters at one end (e.g. acetylcholine) and some are predominantly hormones at the other (e.g. the sex steroids), with a range of substances in between in which these characteristics may overlap. Operational definitions are necessary, rather than definitions based on rigid, separate categories. Many of the intermediate substances may be considered to be *local hormones* or *paracrine secretions*.

The first part of this chapter deals with the ways in which cells and chemical messengers interact when the body is under threat from invading pathogens (disease-causing organisms; see Ch. 41) or other noxious agents. The process to be considered is the *inflammatory reaction* (with the associated *immune response*) with emphasis on the chemical substances that act as local hormones in this context. Many inflammatory mediators (e.g. histamine and the prostaglandins) also have other functions in the body; these are also discussed briefly. Drugs which modify the action of the cells and mediators involved in these reactions are dealt with in Chapter 13.

These topics are dealt with simply in *Textbook of Immunopharmacology* (Dale et al. 1994).

Consideration of the term 'local hormone'

- 'Hormones', 'neurotransmitters' and 'local hormones' (also termed 'autocoids' or 'paracrine secretions') were once considered to be separate categories in terms of function and locus of action, but it is now clear that these categories overlap.
- Most chemical mediators in the body can be considered to be part of a spectrum, with substances which are predominantly neurotransmitters at one end (e.g. acetylcholine) and substances which are predominantly hormones at the other (e.g. sex steroids).
- The chemical mediators of inflammation are intermediates in this spectrum and are considered to be *paracrine secretions* or *local hormones*.

THE ACUTE INFLAMMATORY REACTION AND THE IMMUNE RESPONSE

A mammalian organism facing an invasion by a pathogen can call on a prodigious array of powerful defensive responses; the deployment of these constitutes the *acute inflammatory reaction*. When these defences are lacking (as for example in AIDS) or are suppressed by drugs,

organisms that are not normally pathogens can cause disease. However, in some circumstances these defensive responses may be brought into play inappropriately against innocuous substances from outside the body (e.g. pollen) or against the tissues of the body itself, and the responses themselves may then produce damage and may indeed constitute part of the disease process (either acutely as, for example, in anaphylaxis, or chronically as, for example, in asthma (Ch. 19), rheumatoid arthritis (Ch. 13), or atherosclerosis (Ch. 16). It is for these sorts of conditions that anti-inflammatory or immuno-suppressive drugs are used. Chemical mediators control or modulate these defensive responses of the host, and an understanding of the action of drugs which affect the inflammatory and the immune responses depends on an appreciation of the way in which the cells and the mediators interact with each other. An outline of these interactions is given below. Simple descriptions of the various topics covered will be found in Dale et al. (1994).

The acute inflammatory reaction consists of two components:

- an innate, non-immunological response, thought to have been developed early in evolution, and present in some form or other in most multicellular organisms
- the acquired, *specific* immune response.

The actions of cells and mediators that participate in the innate response can be sharpened and made much more effective by the immunological mechanisms of the acquired response.

We shall consider first the innate reactions, then the immune response and finally the outcome of the acute inflammation—either healing or progress to chronic inflammation.

It should be noted that there are many 'back-up' systems, so that a response to a pathogen can be produced in several ways, which is important for a reaction with survival value.

The outline given below will of necessity be a very general one. It may help if, in reading it, you keep in mind a picture of a boil, which is a local acute inflammatory reaction caused by staphylococci, since most (but not all) of the events described will apply to it.

At the macroscopic level, the inflamed area is *reddened, swollen, hot* and *painful*, and there is *interference* with, or *alteration* of, *function*. Examples of this latter characteristic are the spasm of bronchiolar smooth muscle which occurs in asthma, or the restriction of movement in an inflamed joint.

INNATE REACTIONS

In terms of what is happening locally within the tissues, the changes can be divided into *vascular* and *cellular* events. Mediators are generated both from plasma and from cells during the vascular events, and these mediators in turn modify and regulate the vascular and cellular events.

VASCULAR EVENTS AND THE MEDIATORS DERIVED FROM PLASMA

The vascular events are: an initial *dilatation* of the small arterioles resulting in *increased blood flow* followed by slowing and then *stasis* of the blood and an *increase in the permeability* of the postcapillary venules with *exudation* of fluid. The vasodilatation is brought about by various mediators (histamine, prostaglandins E_2 and I_2, and so on) produced by the interaction of the microorganism with tissue. Some of these mediators (e.g. histamine and platelet-activating factor) are also responsible for the initial phase of increased vascular permeability.

The fluid exudate contains a variety of mediators which influence the cells in the vicinity and the blood vessels themselves. These include the components for four proteolytic enzyme cascades: the complement system, the coagulation system, the fibrinolytic system, the kinin system. The components of these cascades are proteases that are inactive in their native form; they are activated by proteolytic cleavage, each activated component then activating the next.

The exudate is carried by lymphatics to local lymph glands or lymphoid tissue where the products of the invading microorganism can initiate an immune response.

The *complement system* comprises nine major components, designated C1 to C9. Activation of the cascade can be initiated by substances derived from microorganisms, such as yeast cell walls, endotoxins, etc. This pathway of activation is termed 'the alternative pathway' (Fig. 12.1). (The 'classical pathway' involves antibody and is dealt with below.) One of the main events is the enzymic splitting of *C3* which gives rise to various peptides, one of which, *C3a* (termed an 'anaphylatoxin'), can stimulate mast cells to secrete chemical mediators, and can also directly stimulate some smooth muscle, while another, *C3b* (termed an 'opsonin'), can attach to the surface of a microorganism and facilitate its ingestion by white blood cells (see below). Enzymic action on a later component, *C5*, releases *C5a* which—in addition to causing release of mediators from mast cells—is powerfully chemotactic (i.e. acts as a chemical attractant) for white blood cells, and also activates them. Some actions of these complement-derived mediators are considered below. Assembly of the last components in the sequence (*C5* to *C9*) on the cell membranes of certain bacteria leads to the lysis of these organisms (see Ch. 41). Hence, complement can mediate the destruction of invading bacteria or damage multicellular parasites; but it may sometimes cause injury to the host's own cells. The main event in the complement cascade—the splitting of C3—can also be brought about directly, by the principal enzymes of the coagulation and fibrinolytic cascades, thrombin and plasmin, and by enzymes released from white blood cells.

The *coagulation system* and the *fibrinolytic system* are described in Chapter 17. Factor XII is activated to XIIa (e.g. by collagen), and the end product is fibrin, which when laid down in the tissues during a host–pathogen interaction can serve to limit the extension of the infection. The main enzyme of the coagulation system, thrombin, is involved in the activation of the complement and kinin systems (Fig. 12.1) and, indirectly, in fibrinolysis (see Ch. 17).

The *kinin system* is another enzyme cascade; it results in the production of several mediators of inflammation, in particular bradykinin (Fig. 12.1) which is dealt with in more detail on page 221.

CELLULAR EVENTS

Of the cells involved in inflammation, some (vascular endothelial cells, mast cells and tissue macrophages) are normally present in tissues, while others (platelets and

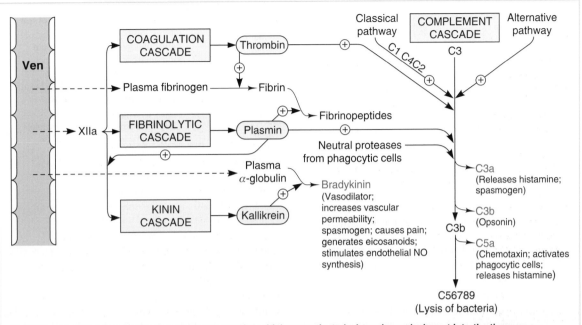

Fig. 12.1 Diagram showing the four enzyme cascades which are activated when plasma leaks out into the tissues as a result of the increased vascular permeability in an area of inflammation. Mediators generated are shown in dark blue. Complement components are indicated by C1, C2, etc. When plasmin is formed it tends to increase kinin formation and decrease the coagulation cascade. (Ven = postcapillary venule) (Adapted from: Dale et al. 1994)

leukocytes) gain access from the blood. The *leukocytes*, are actively motile cells and are of two classes:

- *Polymorphonuclear cells** (cells with many-lobed nuclei), which are subdivided into *neutrophils*, *eosinophils* and *basophils*, according to the staining properties of the granules in their cytoplasm. These cells may also be referred to as *granulocytes*.
- *Mononuclear cells* (or cells with single-bodied nuclei), which are subdivided into *monocytes* and *lymphocytes*.

Mast cells

The mast cell membrane has receptors both for a special class of antibody (IgE) and for complement components C3a and C5a. The cell can be activated to secrete mediators through these receptors and also by direct physical damage.

One of the main substances released by the mast cells is histamine (see below, p. 210); others are heparan or heparin (see Ch. 17), leukotrienes (p. 217), prostaglandin D_2 (p. 215), platelet-activating factor (p. 219), nerve growth factor (p. 225) and some interleukins (p. 224). For a simple overview of mast cells see Chapter 2 in Dale et al. (1994).

Polymorphonuclear leukocytes (polymorphs*)

Neutrophil polymorphs are the first of the blood leukocytes to enter the area of the inflammatory reaction (Fig. 12.2). They adhere to the vascular endothelial cells, a process which requires the interaction between adhesion molecules on the endothelial cell, e.g. the selectin and ICAM (**i**ntercellular **a**dhesion **m**olecule) families, with corresponding molecules on the neutrophil, e.g. the integrin family (see Horwitz 1997). The neutrophils then migrate through the wall of the vessel to the site of the invading pathogen, attracted by chemicals termed 'chemotaxins'—some released by the microorganism, such as formyl-Met–Leu–Phe; some produced locally, such as C5a (see above), leukotriene B_4 (p. 218) and various chemokines, in particular interleukin-8.

Neutrophils are capable of engulfing, killing and digesting microorganisms. They, and the eosinophils, have receptors on their membranes for the complement product, C3b, which acts as an 'opsonin' (see above), i.e. it forms a link between neutrophil and invading bacterium. (An even more effective link may be made by

---

*Some authors reserve the term 'polymorph' for neutrophils.

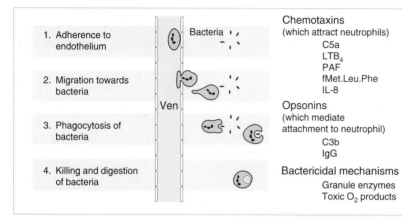

Fig. 12.2 Simplified diagram of the interaction of mediators and neutrophil leukocytes in an acute inflammatory reaction. Adherence involves interaction between the adhesion molecules on the endothelial cell and those on the neutrophil. (Ven = postcapillary venule; LTB_4 = leukotriene B_4; PAF = platelet-activating factor; C5a and C3b are complement components; fMet.Leu.Phe is a bacterial peptide; IgG = immunoglobulin G; IL-8 = interleukin-8)

Diagram labels:
1. Adherence to endothelium
2. Migration towards bacteria
3. Phagocytosis of bacteria
4. Killing and digestion of bacteria

Bacteria
Ven

Chemotaxins (which attract neutrophils)
C5a
LTB_4
PAF
fMet.Leu.Phe
IL-8

Opsonins (which mediate attachment to neutrophil)
C3b
IgG

Bactericidal mechanisms
Granule enzymes
Toxic O_2 products

antibody; see below.) The killing process involves the generation of toxic oxygen products, and the components of the microorganism are then broken down by enzymes—neutral proteases—in the neutrophil granules.

When the neutrophil is inappropriately activated, the toxic oxygen products and enzymes can cause damage to the host's own tissues. (For a simple overview see Muid et al. 1994.)

Eosinophils have similar capacities to neutrophils and, in addition, are armed with a number of potent granule constituents which, when released extracellularly, can damage multicellular parasites (e.g. helminths). They include eosinophil cationic protein, a peroxidase, the eosinophil major basic protein and a neurotoxin. The eosinophil is now considered to be of primary importance in the pathogenesis of the late phase of asthma, in which its granule proteins cause damage to bronchiolar epithelium (see p. 342 and Fig. 19.3). (For a simple overview see Wardlaw et al. 1994.)

Basophils are very similar in many respects to mast cells.

Monocytes/macrophages

The monocytes enter the area at a later stage of the reaction, several hours after the polymorphs. Adhesion to endothelium and migration into the tissue follow a pattern similar to that of the neutrophils (see above), though chemotaxis of monocytes involves additional chemokines, for example *MCP-1*,* which, reasonably enough, stands for 'monocyte chemoattractant protein-1' and *RANTES** which (wait for it—immunological

*The HIV-1 virus binds to the surface CD4 glycoprotein (see below) on monocyte/macrophages but is only able to penetrate the cell after binding to the receptors for these chemokines.

nomenclature has excelled itself here) stands for 'reglated upon activation, normal T cell expressed and secreted'.

In the tissues, monocytes become transformed into macrophages (literally 'big eaters', as compared to the neutrophil polymorphs which were originally called microphages or 'little eaters'). Similar cells, all belonging to the mononuclear phagocyte system, are normally present in various tissues, probably all derived originally from blood-borne monocytes. The macrophage has a remarkable range of abilities, being not only a Jack-of-all-trades but also master of many—particularly when activated by lymphocytes to participate in the specific immunological response (see below).

In *innate* reactions, macrophages bind lipopoly-saccharide (LPS)—a constituent of the outer membrane of Gram-negative bacteria (see Ch. 43)—by means of specific cell surface receptors. The binding stimulates generation and release of cytokines that act on vascular endothelial cells to increase vascular permeability, attract other leukocytes to the area and give rise to fever.

In areas of inflammation they engulf tissue debris and dead cells as well as microorganisms, and they are able to kill many (but not all) of these latter (see below). When stimulated by **glucocorticoids**, they secrete lipo-cortin (a polypeptide which modulates the inflammatory response; see Ch. 24).

Vascular endothelial cells (see also Chs 15 and 17)

The vascular endothelial cells—originally considered as passive lining cells—are now known to play an active part in inflammation. The endothelial cells in the small arterioles, by secreting nitric oxide—which causes relaxation of the underlying smooth muscle (see Ch. 11)—have a role in vasodilatation and thus in the delivery of plasma and blood cells to the area of inflammation, while the cells of the postcapillary venules have a regulatory role in the flow of exudate and thus in the delivery of plasma-derived mediators (see Fig. 12.1).

On the luminal surface, vascular endothelial cells express several adhesion molecules (the ICAM and selectin families; see above, p. 201 and Fig. 12.2) as well as a variety of receptors including those for histamine, acetylcholine, interleukin-1, etc.

In addition to nitric oxide, the cells can synthesise and release the vasodilator agent, prostacyclin (p. 216), the vasoconstrictor agent, endothelin (Ch. 15), plasminogen activator (Ch. 17), platelet-activating factor (p. 219), and several cytokines. Endothelial cell function is also involved in *angiogenesis*, i.e. the growth of new blood vessels, which occurs in repair processes, chronic inflammation and cancer.

Platelets

Platelets are involved primarily in coagulation and thrombotic phenomena (see Ch. 17) but may also play a part in inflammation. They have low-affinity receptors for IgE (see below) and are believed to contribute to the first phase of asthma (Fig. 19.3). In addition to generating thromboxane A_2 and platelet-activating factor (Ch. 17), they can generate free radicals and pro-inflammatory cationic proteins. Platelet-derived growth factor contributes to the repair processes which follow inflammatory responses or damage to blood vessels. (For a simple overview of platelets see Page 1994.)

Neurons

The cell types that contribute to the inflammatory reaction include a subset of sensory neurons that, in addition to relaying impulses to the central nervous system, release inflammatory neuropeptides when appropriately stimulated. These neurons are fine afferents (capsaicin-sensitive C and Aδ fibres) with specific receptors at their peripheral terminals (Szolcsànyi 1996). Chemical mediators generated during injury and inflammation—kinins, 5-hydroxytryptamine (5-HT), etc. (discussed below)—act on the receptors, stimulating the release of neuropeptides, particularly two tachykinins (neurokinin A, substance P) and calcitonin gene-related peptide (CGRP). Neuropeptides are considered below and in Chapter 10; see also Dray (1996).

Natural killer cells

Natural killer (NK) cells are specialised lymphocytes (see below) that are active in innate *non-immunological* reactions. In an unusual version of a receptor-mediated reaction, they kill target cells (virus-infected cells, tumour cells) that *lack* ligands for *inhibitory* receptors on the NK cells themselves. The ligands that are necessary are the major histocompatibility complex (MHC) molecules: NK cells attack any cell unless it expresses these molecules—the mother turkey strategy.* If the inhibitory receptors recognise MHC molecules on the target cell, the NK cell refrains from cytolytic attack. MHC molecules are proteins expressed on the surface of most host cells and, in simple terms, are specific for that individual, enabling the NK cells to avoid damaging host cells. They have other functions in the immune response as explained below.

MEDIATORS DERIVED FROM CELLS

When inflammatory cells are stimulated or damaged, another major mediator system is called into play—the *eicosanoids* (p. 213). Many of the current anti-inflammatory drugs act, at least in part, by interfering with synthesis of the eicosanoids. Other important inflammatory mediators derived from cells are *histamine, platelet-activating factor, nitric oxide, neuropeptides* and the *cytokines.***

The innate components of the inflammatory reaction

- The innate (non-immunological) components consist of vascular events and cellular events.
- Mediators are derived both from plasma and from cells, and in turn modify the vascular and cellular events.
- Vascular events:
  — vasodilatation
  — increased vascular permeability with exudation. The fluid exudate contains the components of enzyme cascades, the main ones being the kinin system and the complement system, both of which give rise to inflammatory mediators.
- Cellular events:
  — stimulation of release of mast cell mediators by complement components
  — accumulation in the tissues of white blood cells in response to chemoattractant molecules, and activation of these cells by non-immunological stimuli
  — engulfment and killing of microorganisms by phagocytic white blood cells.

---

*Richard Dawkins in *River out of Eden*, citing the zoologist, Schliedt, explains that 'the rule of thumb a mother turkey uses to recognise nest robbers is a dismayingly brusque one; in the vicinity of the nest, attack anything that moves, unless it makes a noise like a baby turkey.' (Quoted by Kärre & Welsh 1997.)

**The term 'cytokine' refers to a group of peptide cell regulators which includes lymphokines, chemokines, interleukins, interferons; see page 223.

Before describing these mediators, we must consider the process which makes the innate components of the inflammatory response to invading pathogen immeasurably more efficient—the specific immunological response.

THE SPECIFIC IMMUNOLOGICAL RESPONSE

The specific immunological response to an invading organism makes the host's defensive response not only substantially more efficient but more *specific* for the invading pathogen. It is a complex response, detailed consideration of which is beyond the scope of this book. A simplified version will be given here, stressing only those aspects which are relevant for an understanding of current anti-inflammatory and immunosuppressant drugs and potential new therapeutic agents. (For more detailed coverage, see Janeway & Travers 1996, or Roitt 1997.)

The key cells are the *lymphocytes* of which there are three main groups:

- *B cells*, which are responsible for antibody production, i.e. the humoral immune response (Fig. 12.3)
- *T cells*, which are important in the induction phase of the immune response and are responsible for cell-mediated immune reactions (Fig. 12.3)
- *natural killer cells* (Nk cells); these are specialised non-T, non-B lymphoid cells that are active in the non-immunological, *innate* response (considered above).

The involvement of lymphocytes in the specific immune response involves two phases: an *induction phase* and an *effector phase*, the latter consisting of two components—a humoral (antibody-mediated) component and a cell-mediated component.

We give, first, a brief overview of the events. During the induction phase, T cells are involved in complex ways with B cells and other T cells. On first contact with an antigen (foreign protein or polysaccharide), the lymphocytes that 'recognise' it, by means of surface receptors, initiate a series of cell divisions, giving rise to a large clone of cells that all have the capacity to recognise and respond to that particular antigen. These latter cells are responsible eventually for the effector phase; they either differentiate into plasma cells which go on to produce antibodies (if they are B cells) or are involved in cell-mediated immune responses (if they are T cells). Others will form an increased population of antigen-sensitive *memory* cells; a second exposure to the antigen will then result in a much multiplied response. The body does not

normally mount an immune response against its own tissues because *tolerance* to self antigens is produced during foetal life by deletion of those clones of T cells that would have recognised and reacted against its own tissues.

THE INDUCTION PHASE

A simplified outline of the main interactions between cells and mediators is given in Figure 12.3.

Antigenic molecules (e.g. bacterial products from the site of an infection, or experimentally injected proteins) reach the local lymph nodes via the lymphatics. The antigen is presented to lymphocytes on the surface of large dendritic cells called *antigen-presenting cells* (APCs). The APCs ingest and process the antigen and present it to uncommitted (naive) CD4-positive* T helper lymphocytes** in association with major histocompatibility complex (MHC) molecules.***

These naive T cells then develop interleukin-2 receptors as well as generating interleukin-2, a cytokine which has autocrine action, causing proliferation of the cells that release it—giving rise to a clone of *activated* T cells (sometimes termed Th0 cells)—which in turn give rise to two different subsets of helper cells: Th1 cells and Th2 cells. The action of specific interleukins determines whether Th1 or Th2 cells develop, IL-12 determining progress down the Th1 pathway, IL-4 determining progress down the Th2 pathway.

Each subset of Th cells then produces its own profile of cytokines that control a unique set of immune responses—the Th1 pathway controlling mainly *cell-mediated responses* and the Th2 pathway *antibody-mediated responses*.**** The cytokines serve as autocrine

---

*CD4 and CD8 are protein markers on lymphocytes—defined by monoclonal antibodies. Dendritic cells and macrophages also carry surface CD4 proteins.

**Sometimes termed T-helper precursor (Thp) cells.

***The main reason that it is difficult to transplant organs such as kidneys from one person to another is that their respective MHC molecules are different. Lymphocytes in the recipient of the transplant will be reactive to non-self (allogeneic) MHC molecules in the transplanted tissue, which is thus likely to be rejected by a rapid and powerful immunological reaction. CD4 cells and NK cells recognise MHC-I molecules, CD8 cells recognise MHC-II.

****Some authorities think that the above division of labour between Th1 and Th2 responses is an oversimplification since there is evidence that Th1 cytokines also have a role in some antibody-mediated responses, particularly in the production of opsonising and complement-activating antibodies (Abbas et al. 1996).

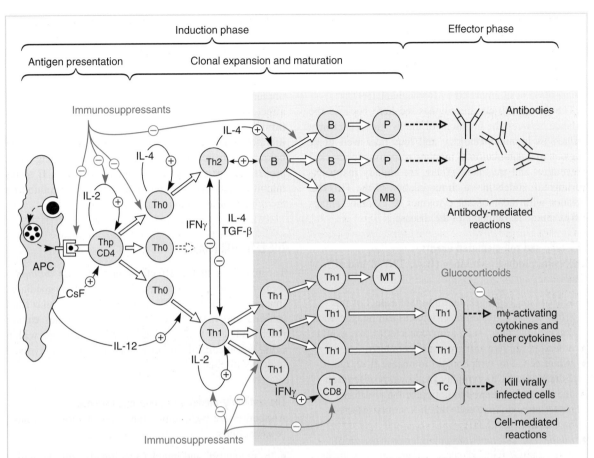

Fig. 12.3 Simplified diagram of the induction and effector phases of lymphocyte activation with the sites of action of immunosuppressants. Antigen-presenting cells (APC) ingest and process antigen (●) and present fragments of it (●) to naive, uncommitted CD4+ T-helper precursor (Thp) cells in conjunction with major histocompatibility complex molecules (⊏) and co-stimulatory factors (CSF). The Thp cells synthesise and express interleukin-2 (IL-2) receptors and release IL-2 which stimulates the cells by autocrine action, causing generation and proliferation of T-helper nought (Th0) cells. Autocrine cytokines (e.g. IL-4) cause proliferation of some Th0 cells to give Th2 cells—which are responsible for the development of antibody-mediated immune responses. These Th2 cells cooperate with and activate B cells to proliferate and to give rise eventually to memory B cells (MB) and plasma cells (P) that secrete antibodies. Autocrine cytokines (e.g. IL-2) cause proliferation of some Th0 cells to give Th1 cells (responsible for cell-mediated immune reactions). Some Th1 cells secrete macrophage (mφ)-activating cytokines and other cytokines; some secrete IFN-γ which activates CD8+ T cells to become cytotoxic cells (Tc) that can then kill virally infected host cells. IL-4 derived from Th1 cells inhibits Th2 cell function; IFN-γ derived from Th2 cells inhibits Th1 cell function.

growth factors for their own subset of T cells and have cross-regulatory actions on the development of the other subset (Abbas et al. 1996).

Knowledge of the subsets and their functions is leading to a better understanding not only of normal immune responses but also the pathogenesis of several diseases in that some pathological conditions are associated with Th1 responses and some with Th2. Diseases in which Th1 responses are dominant include insulin-dependent diabetes mellitus (Ch. 22), multiple sclerosis, *Helicobacter*-

induced peptic ulcer (Ch. 21), aplastic anaemia (Ch. 18) and rheumatoid arthritis (see Ch. 13). Th1 responses are implicated in allograft* rejection, and conversion of these Th1 responses to Th2 responses at the maternal/foetal interface prevents rejection of the foetal 'allograft'. Th2 responses are dominant in allergic conditions. AIDs

---

*An allograft is a tissue or organ graft between individuals that are genetically different but of the same species.

progression is associated with loss of Th1 cells and is facilitated by Th2 responses. Progression of some diseases is associated with the Th1/Th2 balance; for example, in tuberculoid leprosy, Th1 responses predominate, in lepromatous leprosy Th2 predominate. (Th1/Th2 polarisation is summarised by Romagnani 1997.)

The T cell subsets are emphasised here because the balance between the functions of the two subsets clearly influences immunopathology and thus may well point the way to manipulation of immune responses for disease prevention and treatment. There are already many experimental models in which modulation of the Th1/Th2 balance with recombinant cytokines or cytokine antagonists alters the outcome of the disease.

Th1 cells and cell-mediated events

Th1 cells produce cytokines (IL-2, TNF-β and IFN-γ) that:

- activate macrophages; an important aspect of this effect is that activated macrophages can phagocytose and kill microbes (such as mycobacteria) that would otherwise survive and grow intracellularly
- stimulate CD8+ lymphocytes to release IL-2; the IL-2 drives the CD8+ lymphocytes' own proliferation and then subsequent maturation of the proliferated clone into cytotoxic cells that kill virally infected host cells (Fig. 12.3)
- *inhibit Th2 cell functions* (by interferon-γ action).

Th2 cells and antibody-mediated events

Th2 cells produce cytokines (IL-4, TGF-β, IL-10) that:

- stimulate B cells to proliferate; the clone so produced then matures into plasma cells that produce antibodies, particularly IgE—the antibody that fixes to mast cells and eosinophils
- stimulate differentiation and activation of eosinophils
- *inhibit Th1 cell functions**, i.e. the activation of inflammatory cells and the cell-mediated reactions produced by Th1 cytokines.

The induction of antibody-mediated responses varies with the type of antigen. With most (but not all) antigens,

---

*'Suppressor' cells have not been mentioned. It is clear that there is cytokine-mediated antagonism (suppression?) between Th1 and Th2 cells and there is some evidence that, in some circumstances, CD8+ cells can inhibit (suppress) the action of some Th cells by secreting specific cytokines such as tumour necrosis factor-β (TNF-β), but whether dedicated, professional 'suppressor' cells exist, as was originally thought, is now controversial (see Roitt 1997).

a cooperative process between Th2 cells and B cells is necessary. B cells can also bind and present antigen to the T cell and the T cell then releases cytokines that act on the B cell.

The **anti-inflammatory steroids** (see Ch. 24) and the immunosuppressive drug, **cyclosporin** (see Ch. 13), affect the events at the stage of induction. The cytotoxic **immunosuppressive drugs** (see Ch. 13) inhibit the proliferative phase of both B and T cells. Eicosanoids (see below) are believed to play a part in controlling these processes. For example, prostaglandins of the E series inhibit lymphocyte proliferation, probably by inhibiting the release of interleukin-2.

THE EFFECTOR PHASE

The reactions in the effector phase may be *antibody-mediated* or *cell-mediated*. The antibody-mediated (humoral) response is effective in the extracellular fluid (plasma and tissue fluid). However, antibodies cannot reach and deal with pathogens when these are within cells; cell-mediated immune mechanisms have evolved to deal with this.

The antibody-mediated (humoral) response

Antibodies are γ-globulins (immunoglobulins) that have two functions:

- to 'recognise' and interact specifically with particular antigens, i.e. proteins or polysaccharides foreign to the host
- to activate one or more of the host's defence systems.

The foreign substances may be part of an invading organism (the coat of a bacterium) or released by such an organism (a bacterial toxin), or they may be materials introduced experimentally in the laboratory in studies of the immune response (e.g. the injection of egg albumin into the guinea pig).

An antibody is a Y-shaped protein molecule in which the arms of the Y (the 'Fab' portions) are the recognition sites for specific antigens, and the stem of the Y (the 'Fc' portion) activates host defence mechanisms. B lymphocytes, the cells which are responsible for antibody production, 'recognise' foreign molecules by means of receptors on their surfaces, the receptor being essentially the immunoglobulin which that B cell clone will eventually produce. The mammalian organism possesses a vast number of clones of B cells producing different antibodies with recognition sites for different antigens. It is a miraculous fact that we come equipped with the ability to make antibodies that can recognise and react with virtually all foreign proteins that we are likely to encounter during our lifetime.

The ability to make antibodies has survival value; children born without this ability suffer repeated infections—pneumonia, skin infections, tonsillitis, etc. Before the days of antibiotics, they died in early childhood, and even today they require regular replacement therapy with immunoglobulin (see Ch. 13).

There are five classes of antibodies—IgG, IgM, IgE, IgA and IgD—which differ from each other in certain structural respects. See Janeway & Travers (1996) or Roitt (1997) for details.

Antibodies markedly improve the host's response to an invading pathogen. Apart from their ability to interact *directly* with invading pathogens such as viruses or with bacterial toxins, thus impairing their capacity for damage, antibodies can multiply many-fold the effectiveness and specificity of the host's defence reaction in several ways, as follows:

Antibodies and the complement sequence. When antibodies react with antigenic material on the pathogen, the antigen–antibody reaction leads to the exposure, on the Fc portion, of a binding site for complement. This results in activation of the complement sequence with its biological repercussions—production of anaphylatoxin (C3a), chemotactic factor (C5a) and opsonin (C3b), and eventually the development of lytic potential (p. 200 and Figs 12.1 and 12.2). This route to C3 activation is referred to as 'the classical pathway' (because it was investigated first) to distinguish it from the 'alternative pathway' described above. The classical pathway provides an especially selective way of activating complement in response to a particular pathogen, since the antigen–antibody reaction which initiates it constitutes not only a highly specific recognition event but occurs in close association with the pathogen. The lytic property of complement can be used therapeutically: monoclonal antibodies and complement together can be used to clean bone marrow of cancer cells as an adjunct to chemotherapy or radiotherapy (see Ch. 42). Complement lysis is also implicated in the action of **antilymphocyte immunoglobulin** (Ch. 13, p. 244).

Antibodies and the ingestion of bacteria. Antibodies can attach to the particular antigenic moieties on the surface of microorganisms which have been 'recognised' by their Fab portions, leaving the Fc part of the molecule projecting. Phagocytic cells (neutrophils and macrophages) have receptors on their membranes for these projecting Fc portions of antibody. Antibody thus forms a very specific link between microorganism and phago-

cyte and is more effective than C3b as an opsonin in facilitating phagocytosis (see Fig. 12.2).

Antibodies and cellular cytotoxicity. In some cases, for example in the case of parasitic worms, the invader may be too big to be ingested by phagocytes. Antibody molecules can form a link between parasite and the host's white cells (in this case, eosinophils), which are then able to damage or kill the parasite by surface or extracellular actions.

Antibodies and mast cells or basophils. Mast cells and basophils have receptors for a particular form of antibody—IgE—which can become attached to the cell membrane. When antigen reacts with this cell-fixed antibody, a whole panoply of pharmacologically active mediators is secreted. A complex reaction such as this, found widely throughout the animal kingdom, is unlikely to have been developed and retained during evolution unless it had survival value for the host. However, its precise biological significance in defence is not clear, though it may be of importance in association with eosinophil activity in reactions against parasitic worms. When inappropriately triggered by substances not inherently damaging to the host, it is implicated in certain types of allergic reaction (see below and Ch. 19) and contributes to illness rather than survival.

Normal human immunoglobulin derived from pooled human plasma can be used as a replacement therapy in antibody deficiency states and to protect susceptible subjects against infections with hepatitis A virus, measles or rubella (German measles).

The cell-mediated immune response

The lymphocytes involved in cell-mediated responses are both cytotoxic T cells (derived from CD8+ cells) and inflammatory (cytokine-releasing) Th1 cells (see Fig. 12.3). They move into an inflammatory area by a process similar to that described for neutrophils and macrophages, namely interaction between adhesion molecules on both the endothelial cell and the lymphocyte.

Cytotoxic T cells

When a virus infects a mammalian cell (which can be virtually any of the cells in the body) there are two aspects to the resulting immune response. The first step, signalling that the cell is infected, is the expression on the cell surface of peptides derived from the pathogens in association with MHC molecules. The second step is the recognition of the peptide–MHC complex by CD8 proteins on cytotoxic (CD8+) T cells; these cells then destroy the virus-infected cell. Cooperation with macrophages may be required for the kill.

Cytokine-releasing Th1 cells

In areas of inflammation, the main role of these cells is to activate macrophages. Some pathogens (e.g. mycobacteria, listeria) have evolved strategies for surviving and multiplying within macrophages after ingestion. A complex of microorganism-derived peptide plus MHC molecule is expressed on the macrophage surface and is recognised by cytokine-releasing Th1 cells which generate cytokines that enable the macrophage to kill the intracellular microorganisms.

Activated macrophages (with or without intracellular pathogens) are virtually factories for the production of chemical mediators and can generate and secrete not only many cytokines, but toxic oxygen metabolites and neutral proteases that can kill extracellular organisms (e.g. *Pneumocystis carinii** and various helminths), complement components, eicosanoids (see p. 213), nitric oxide (see below and Ch. 11), a fibroblast-stimulating factor, pyrogens and the 'tissue factor' which starts the extrinsic pathway of the coagulation cascade (Ch. 17), as well as various other coagulation factors. They are also important in repair processes. Among the cytokines secreted is IL-12—which has a positive feedback effect, driving the development of further Th1 cells.

It is primarily the cell-mediated reaction that is responsible for the rejection of transplanted non-self tissue (allografts).

The specific immunological response, cell-mediated or humoral, is thus superimposed on the immunologically non-specific vascular and cellular reactions described previously, making them not only markedly more effective but much more **specific** *for particular invading organisms.* An important aspect of the specific immunological response is that the clone of lymphocytes that are programmed to respond to the antigens of the invading organism is greatly expanded after the first contact with the organism, and now contains 'memory cells'. Thus, subsequent exposure results in a greatly accelerated and more effective response. In some cases the response becomes so prompt and so efficient that, after the first exposure which initiates the specific immune response, some microorganisms can virtually never gain a foothold in the host's tissues again. Immunisation procedures make use of this fact.

The general events of the inflammatory and hypersensitivity reactions specified above vary in some tissues. Thus in the inflammation that underlies asthma, eosinophils and neuropeptides have a particularly significant

role—see Ch. 19. In inflammation in the CNS there is less infiltration of neutrophils, and monocyte infiltration is delayed—possibly owing to lack of adhesion molecule expression on CNS endothelium and deficient generation of chemotaxins (discussed by Perry 1995). It has long been known that some tissues—the CNS parenchyma, the anterior chamber of the eye and the testis—are privileged sites in that a foreign antigen introduced directly does not provoke an immune reaction. However, introduction elsewhere of an antigen already in the CNS parenchyma allows development of immune/inflammatory responses in the CNS (Matyszak et al. 1997).

SYSTEMIC RESPONSES IN INFLAMMATION

In addition to the local changes in an inflammatory area, there are often various general responses such as a rise in temperature (see p. 231) and an increase in blood leukocytes, termed 'leukocytosis' (or neutrophilia if the

---

The specific immunological response

- The specific immunological response vastly improves the effectiveness of the innate, non-immunological responses; It has two phases: the induction phase and the effector phase; the latter consisting of (i) antibody-mediated and (ii) cell-mediated components.
- In the induction phase, T helper lymphocytes (Th cells) regulate the further development of the immune response: Th1 cells regulating development of cell-mediated responses, Th2 antibody-mediated responses.
- Antibodies provide:
  — neutralisation of some viruses and of some bacterial toxins
  — more selective activation of the complement cascade
  — more effective ingestion of microorganisms
  — more effective attachment to multicellular parasites, facilitating their killing.
- Cell-mediated reactions involve:
  — CD8+ cytotoxic T cells interacting with and killing virus-infected cells
  — CD4+ T cells release cytokines, (e.g. interferon-γ) which enable macrophages to kill intracellular pathogens such as the tubercle bacillus. A variety of cytokines, acting on other cells, are released by both CD4+ T cells and macrophages.
- Inappropriately deployed immune reactions are termed hypersensitivity reactions; these underlie the autoimmune diseases, i.e. diseases due to immune reactions directed at the host's own tissues.
- Anti-inflammatory drugs and immunosuppressive agents are used when the normally protective inflammatory and/or immune responses are inappropriately deployed.

---

*This organism can cause pneumonia in AIDS patients and other immunosuppressed patients.

increase is in the neutrophils only). There is also an increase in certain plasma proteins termed 'acute phase proteins' (see Richards & Gauldie 1994). These include C-reactive protein, α_2-macroglobulin, fibrinogen (see Fig. 12.1), α_1-antitrypsin, and some complement components. C-reactive protein binds to certain microorganisms and the resulting complex activates complement.

UNWANTED INFLAMMATORY AND IMMUNE RESPONSES

The responses described above can, in some circumstances, be inappropriately triggered by substances which are innocuous or even endogenous, as occurs in autoimmune* disease. It is when this happens that it becomes necessary to use **anti-inflammatory** or **immunosuppressive drugs**. Unwanted immune responses are termed *allergic* or *hypersensitivity reactions* and have been classified into four types. See Roitt (1997, Ch. 16).

Type 1: Immediate or anaphylactic hypersensitivity

Type I hypersensitivity occurs when antigenic material that is not in itself noxious (such as grass pollen, products from dead house-dust mites, certain foodstuffs or some drugs) evokes the production of antibodies of the IgE type, which fix to mast cells and, in the lung, to eosinophils. Subsequent contact with the material causes the release of histamine (p. 210), platelet-activating factor (p. 219), eicosanoids (p. 213), and cytokines (p. 223) from mast cells. The effects may be localised to the nose (hay fever), the bronchial tree (the initial phase of asthma), the skin (urticaria) or the gastrointestinal tract. In some cases the reaction is more generalised and produces anaphylactic shock.

Roughly speaking, this type of hypersensitivity represents mainly inappropriate deployment of the processes outlined above in the section entitled 'Antibodies and mast cells or basophils' in the discussion of the humoral immune response (see p. 206). Some important unwanted effects of drugs are due to anaphylactic hypersensitivity responses (see Ch. 49).

Type II: Antibody-dependent cytotoxic hypersensitivity

Type II hypersensitivity occurs when the mechanisms outlined above (in the section entitled 'Antibodies and cellular cytotoxicity'; see p. 207) are directed against

*Autoimmune diseases are diseases caused by the host's immune system attacking his/her own tissue, i.e. they are due to inappropriately deployed immune responses.

cells within the host, which are, or which appear to be, foreign; for example after incompatible blood transfusions or the alteration of the host's cells by drugs. The antigens form part of the surface of these cells and evoke antibodies. The antigen–antibody reaction initiates the complement sequence (with its repercussions) and can provide a basis for the attack by killer cells.

Examples of this latter class are the alteration by drugs of neutrophil polymorphs which may lead to agranulocytosis (see Ch. 49), and of platelets which may lead to thrombocytopenic purpura (Ch. 18). Class II reactions are implicated in some types of autoimmune thyroiditis (e.g. Hashimoto's disease; see Ch. 25).

Type III: Complex-mediated hypersensitivity

Type III hypersensitivity occurs when antibody reacts with *soluble* antigen. The antigen–antibody complexes can activate complement (see above) or attach to mast cells and stimulate the release of mediators (see above). An experimental example of type III hypersensitivity is a reaction termed the *Arthus reaction*, which occurs if a foreign protein is injected subcutaneously into a rabbit or guinea pig which has a high concentration of circulating antibody against that protein. The area becomes red and swollen 3–8 hours later. This is because the antigen–antibody complexes settle in the small blood vessels, complement is activated, and neutrophils are attracted and activated (by C5a) to generate toxic O_2 products and secrete enzymes. Mast cells are also stimulated by C3a to release mediators. Damage caused by this process is involved in the reaction to mouldy hay, known as 'farmer's lung', and in certain types of autoimmune kidney and arterial disease. Type III hypersensitivity is also implicated in lupus erythematosus (a chronic, autoimmune inflammatory disease of connective tissue).

Type IV: Cell-mediated hypersensitivity

The prototype of type IV hypersensitivity (also known as delayed hypersensitivity) is the *tuberculin reaction*—the reaction seen when proteins derived from cultures of the tubercle bacillus are injected into the skin of a person who has been sensitised to the bacillus by a previous infection or by immunisation. After 24 hours, the area becomes reddened and thickened. An 'inappropriate' cell-mediated immune response (see above, p. 207) has been stimulated and there has been infiltration of mononuclear cells and the release of various cytokines. Cell-mediated hypersensitivity is the basis of the reaction seen with some rashes (e.g. in mumps and measles) and with mosquito and tick bites. It is also important in the skin reactions to drugs or industrial chemicals (see

Ch. 49), and in these cases the chemical combines with proteins in the skin to form the 'foreign' substance which evokes the cell-mediated immune response (Fig. 12.3). A substance acting in this way is called a *hapten*.

In essence, inappropriately deployed T cell activity underlies all types of hypersensitivity, being the initiating factor in Types I, II and III and being involved in both the initiation and effector phase in Type IV.

The hypersensitivity reactions given above are the basis of the clinically important group of *autoimmune* diseases. For a simple overview, see Steinman (1993). Some examples of autoimmune conditions have been given above; other examples, held to have a marked component of cell-mediated hypersensitivity, are rheumatoid arthritis (p. 237), multiple sclerosis and insulin-dependent diabetes (p. 391).

Immunosuppressive drugs and/or **glucocorticoids** are employed as part of the treatment of some autoimmune diseases, and the use of cytokines and of antibodies to T cell surface antigens (e.g. the CD4 receptor) is being explored.

THE OUTCOME OF THE INFLAMMATORY RESPONSE

After this outline of the specific immune response, we need to return to a consideration of the host–pathogen interaction—the local acute inflammatory response. It should be clear that this may consist of the innate, immunologically non-specific vascular and cellular events described initially, together with a varying degree of participation of the specific immunological response (either humoral or cell-mediated) the degree depending on several factors such as the nature of the pathogen and the organ or tissue involved. What is the final result of the interaction? If the pathogen has been dealt with adequately, there may be complete healing and the tissue may be virtually normal thereafter. If there has been damage (death of cells, pus formation, ulceration), repair is usually necessary and may result in scarring. If the pathogen persists, the condition is likely to proceed to *chronic* inflammation, a slow smouldering reaction which continues for months or even years and involves destruction of tissue as well as local proliferation of cells and connective tissue. The principal cell types found in areas of chronic inflammation are *mononuclear* cells and abnormal cells derived from macrophages. In areas of healing and chronic inflammation there is angiogenesis (growth of new blood vessels) and also greatly increased activity of *fibroblasts* which lay down fibrous

tissue. The response to some microorganisms has the characteristic of chronicity from the start; examples are syphilis, tuberculosis and leprosy.

The components of the chronic inflammatory response to microorganisms are also seen in many if not most chronic autoimmune conditions.

Mediators of importance in healing, repair processes and chronic inflammatory reactions are, amongst others, platelet-derived growth factor (p. 320), vascular endothelial growth factor, transforming growth factor, and various fibroblast growth factors.

MEDIATORS OF INFLAMMATION AND ALLERGY

In the highly complex repertoire of reactions which constitutes the host response to invading pathogen, the precise role of the various mediators has not been completely clarified. A putative mediator should fulfil certain criteria, modified from those outlined by Sir Henry Dale in 1933 for neurotransmitters. The degree to which the known inflammatory mediators fulfil these criteria is considered by Dale 1994, pp 206–207.

The mediators of pharmacological significance will be described below. Drugs which affect the inflammatory and immune responses will be considered in the next chapter.

HISTAMINE

Most of the early studies on the biological actions of this amine were carried out by Sir Henry Dale and his colleagues. Dale had shown that a local anaphylactic reaction (a Type I or 'immediate hypersensitivity reaction'; see above) was the result of an antigen–antibody reaction in sensitised tissue, and he subsequently demonstrated that histamine could largely mimic both the in vitro and in vivo anaphylactic responses. After the first generation of antihistamine drugs was produced, following the work of Bovet and his co-workers, it became clear (as a result of careful quantitative studies by Schild) that there were two types of histamine receptor in the body and that this first generation of antihistamine drugs affected only one type—the H_1-receptors. The second type, termed H_2-receptors and important particularly in gastric acid secretion, was unaffected. Black and his colleagues, following up the classification proposed by Schild, developed the second generation of antihistamine drugs— the H_2-receptor antagonists. Subsequently, Sir James Black was awarded the Nobel prize for his work on H_2-receptors (and β-adrenoceptors; Ch. 8). Later, evidence for the existence of a third type of histamine receptor—the H_3-receptor—was produced by Arrang et al. (1983).

Synthesis and storage of histamine

Histamine is a basic amine, 2-(4-imidazolyl)-ethyl-amine (see Table 12.1a), and is formed from histidine by histidine decarboxylase. It is found in most tissues of the body, but is present in high concentrations in the lungs and the skin and in particularly high concentrations in the gastrointestinal tract. At the cellular level, it is found largely in mast cells and basophils, associated with heparin, but non-mast-cell histamine occurs in 'histaminocytes' in the stomach and in histaminergic neurons in the brain (see Ch. 30). The basophil content of the tissues is negligible—except in certain parasitic infections and hypersensitivity reactions (p. 209)—and basophils form only 0.5% of circulating white blood cells.

In mast cells and basophils, histamine is held in intracellular granules in a complex with an acidic protein and a heparin of high molecular weight, termed macroheparin. Together these comprise the matrix of the granule in which the basic molecule histamine is held by ionic forces. The molar ratio for histamine, heparin and protein in mast cells is $1 : 3 : 6$ and the histamine content is approximately 0.1–0.2 pmol per mast cell, and 0.01 pmol per basophil.

Histamine release

Histamine is released from mast cells by exocytosis during inflammatory or allergic reactions. As explained earlier in this chapter, stimuli include the interaction of complement components C3a and C5a with specific receptors on the cell surface, or the interaction of antigen with cell-fixed IgE antibodies. Secretion is initiated by a rise in cytosolic calcium. Some neuropeptides, such as substance P, release histamine, though the concentrations required are fairly high. Various basic drugs, such as **morphine** and **tubocurarine** release histamine by non-receptor action.

Agents which increase cAMP formation (e.g. β-**adrenoceptor agonists**; see Ch. 8) inhibit histamine secretion; thus in these cells, cAMP-dependent protein kinase is an intracellular 'braking' mechanism. Replenishment of the histamine content of mast cell or basophil, after secretion, is a slow process which may take days or weeks, whereas turnover of histamine in the gastric 'histaminocyte' is very rapid.

Histamine is metabolised by histaminase and/or by the methylating enzyme imidazole N-methyl-transferase.

Histamine receptors

Histamine produces its action by an effect on specific histamine receptors, which are of three main types, H_1, H_2 and H_3, distinguished by means of selective antagonist drugs. Some details of the actions of antagonist and agonist drugs used to investigate and define the three types of histamine receptor are given in Tables 12.1a and 12.1b. Selective antagonists at H_1-, H_2- and H_3-receptors are **mepyramine**, **cimetidine** and **thioperamide** respectively. Selective agonists for H_2- and H_3-receptors are **dimaprit** and **(R)-methyl histamine**.

Histamine H_1 antagonists have clinical uses (see Chs 13 and 21), as do histamine H_2 antagonists (Ch. 21), but at present agents acting at H_3-receptors are used mainly as research tools.

Table 12.1a Details of some agonist drugs used to define the three types of histamine receptors*

Drug	Structure	Relative activity in vitro (histamine 100%)		
		H_1-receptors (ileum contraction)	H_2-receptors (stimulation of atrial rate)	H_3-receptors (histamine release from brain tissue)
Histamine		100	100	100
Dimaprit		< 0.0001	71	0.0008
(R) α-methylhistamine		0.49	1.02	1550

Table 12.1b   Details of some antagonist drugs used to define the three types of histamine receptors*

Drug	Structure	H_1 (K_B M)	H_2 (K_B M)	H_3 (K_B M)
Mepyramine		0.4×10^{-9}	–	$> 3 \times 10^{-6}$
Cimetidine		4.5×10^{-4}	0.8×10^{-6}	3.3×10^{-5}
Thioperamide		$> 10^{-4}$	$> 10^{-5}$	4.3×10^{-9}

*Data derived from Black J W et al 1972 Nature 236: 385–390; Ganellin C R 1982 In: Ganellin C R, Parson M E (eds) Pharmacology of histamine receptors. pp. 11–102; Arrang J M et al 1987 Nature 327: 117–123; van der Werf J F, Timmerman H 1989 Trends Pharmacol Sci 10: 159–162

Actions

Gastric secretion

Histamine stimulates the secretion of gastric acid by action on H_2-receptors. In clinical terms, this is the most important action of histamine, since it is implicated in the pathogenesis of peptic ulcer. It is considered in detail in Chapter 21.

Smooth muscle effects

Histamine, acting on H_1-receptors, causes contractions of the smooth muscle of the ileum, the bronchi and bronchioles, and the uterus.

The effect on the ileum is not as marked in man as it is in the guinea pig.* Histamine is one of the main mediators causing reduction of air flow in the first phase of bronchial asthma (see Ch. 19 and Fig. 19.3). Uterine muscle in most species is contracted. In humans this is only significant if a massive release of histamine is produced by anaphylaxis during pregnancy, since this may lead to abortion.

Cardiovascular effects

Histamine dilates blood vessels in man by an action on H_1-receptors; the effect is partly endothelium-dependent in some vascular beds. It increases the rate and the

output of the heart by action on cardiac H_2-receptors; this is a direct effect which may be coupled to an indirect, reflex response if there is a fall in blood pressure.

Injected intradermally, histamine causes a reddening of the skin and a wheal with a surrounding flare—the 'triple response' described by Sir Thomas Lewis over 50 years ago. The reddening is due to vasodilatation of the small arterioles and precapillary sphincters, and the wheal is due to increased permeability of the post-capillary venules. These effects are mainly due to activation of H_1-receptors. (Contrary to popular belief and the statements in some pathology textbooks, histamine does not increase *capillary* permeability. Its locus of action in increasing permeability is on the postcapillary *venules*, as was clearly demonstrated by Majno & Palade and their colleagues in 1961.) The flare is due to an 'axon reflex' which involves stimulation of sensory nerve fibres and the passage of antidromic impulses through neighbouring branches of the same nerve with release of a vasodilator mediator, probably calcitonin gene-related peptide (see above, p. 213, and Chs 10 and 15).

Itching

Itching occurs if histamine is injected into the skin or applied to a blister base, and is due to stimulation of sensory nerve endings.

CNS effects

Histamine is a transmitter in the CNS (discussed in Ch. 21, p. 370, and Ch. 28, p. 465).

*The response of guinea-pig ileum is the basis of the standard bioassay for histamine, familiar to students of experimental pharmacology.

It will be clear from the above that histamine is released in inflammation and is capable of producing many of the effects of inflammation and hypersensitivity—vasodilatation, increased vascular permeability and the spasm of smooth muscle. However, histamine H_1 antagonists do not have much effect on the acute inflammatory response per se; probably because histamine is a mediator of importance only in some sorts of type I hypersensitivity reaction, such as allergic rhinitis and urticaria. The use of H_1 antagonists in these and other conditions is dealt with in Chapter 13.

The main pathophysiological role of endogenous histamine is as a mediator of some types of vomiting by an action in the CNS (Ch. 21) and a stimulant of gastric acid secretion by an action on H_2-receptors (Ch. 21). It also has a physiological function as an inhibitor of neurotransmitter release, particularly in the CNS and the gastrointestinal tract.

Histamine

- Histamine is a basic amine, stored in granules within mast cells and basophils and secreted when complement components C3a and C5a interact with specific membrane receptors, or when antigen interacts with cell-fixed IgE.
- It produces effects by acting on H_1-, H_2- or H_3-receptors on target cells.
- The main actions in humans (and the receptors involved) are:
  — stimulation of gastric secretion (H_2)
  — contraction of most smooth muscle other than that of blood vessels (H_1)
  — cardiac stimulation (H_2)
  — vasodilatation (H_1)
  — increased vascular permeability (H_1).
- Injected intradermally it causes the 'triple response': local *vasodilatation* and *wheal* by direct action on blood vessels, and surrounding *flare* due to vasodilatation resulting from an 'axon' reflex in sensory nerves releasing a peptide mediator.
- The main pathophysiological roles of histamine are:
  — as a stimulant of gastric acid secretion (treated with H_2-receptor antagonists)
  — as a mediator of type 1 hypersensitivity reactions such as urticaria and hay fever (treated with H_1-receptor antagonists).
- H_3-receptors occur at presynaptic sites and inhibit the release of a variety of neurotransmitters.

EICOSANOIDS

Eicosanoids, unlike histamine, are not found preformed in the tissues; they are generated de novo from phospho-lipids. They are implicated in the control of many physiological processes and are among the most important mediators and modulators of the inflammatory reaction (Fig. 12.4).

Interest in eicosanoids arose in the 1930s after reports that semen contained a substance which contracted uterine smooth muscle. The substance was believed to originate in the prostate and was saddled with the misnomer, *prostaglandin*. Later it became clear that prostaglandin was not just one substance but a whole family of compounds, that they were generated in many if not most tissues and that they were derived from arachidonic acid.

Structure and biosynthesis

The main source of the eicosanoids is *arachidonic acid* (5,8,11,14-eicosatetraenoic acid), a 20-carbon unsaturated fatty acid containing four double bonds (hence 'eicosa' referring to the 20 carbon atoms, and 'tetraenoic' referring to the 4 double bonds). Arachidonic acid is found esterified in the phospholipids, usually in the 2 position (Fig. 12.5). The principal eicosanoids are the *prostaglandins*, the *thromboxanes* and the *leukotrienes*, though other derivatives of arachidonate, for example the *lipoxins*, are also produced. (The term *prostanoid* will be used here to encompass both prostaglandins and thromboxanes.) The initial and rate-limiting step in eicosanoid synthesis is the liberation of arachidonate, either in a one-step process or a two-step process (Fig. 12.6). The one-step process involves phospholipase A_2, the two-step process involves either phospholipase C and then diacylglycerol lipase, or phospholipase D then phospholipase A_2. Note that there are two forms of phospholipase A_2 (PLA_2)—one found intracellularly in the cytosol, and one present in the extracellular fluids. It is mainly the intracellular form which is implicated in the generation of inflammatory mediators, and its action can give rise not only to arachidonic acid and thus the eicosanoids, but also to lysoglyceryl-phosphoryl-choline (lyso-PAF), which is the precursor of another mediator of inflammation—*platelet-activating factor* (see Figs 12.4 and 12.11).

Many stimuli can liberate arachidonic acid, and they vary with the cell type, for example thrombin in platelets, C5a in neutrophils, bradykinin in fibroblasts and antigen–antibody reactions on mast cells. General cell damage also starts the process.

The free arachidonic acid is metabolised by several pathways—by one of two fatty acid cyclo-oxygenases (see below) which initiate the biosynthesis of the prostaglandins and thromboxanes, and by various lipoxygenases (p. 217) which initiate the synthesis of the leukotrienes,

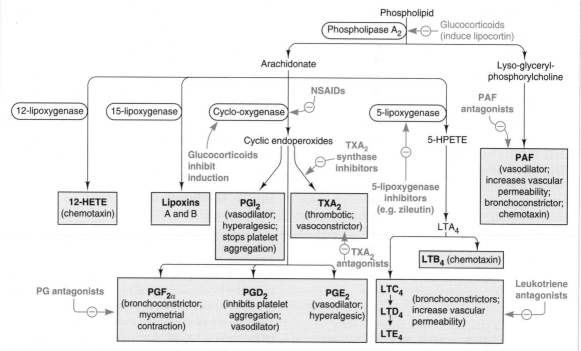

Fig. 12.4 Summary diagram of mediators derived from phospholipids and their actions, and the sites of action of anti-inflammatory drugs. The arachidonate metabolites are 'eicosanoids'. The glucocorticoids inhibit transcription of the gene for cyclo-oxygenase-2, which is induced in inflammatory cells by inflammatory mediators. The effects of PGE_2 depend on which of the three receptors for this prostanoid are activated; see text. (PG = prostaglandin; PGI_2 = prostacyclin; TX = thromboxane; LT = leukotriene; HETE = hydroxyeicosatetraenoic acid; HPETE = hydroperoxyeicosatetraenoic acid; PAF = platelet-activating factor; NSAIDs = non-steroidal anti-inflammatory drugs; see Ch. 13)

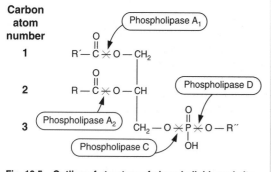

Fig. 12.5 Outline of structure of phospholipids and site of action of phospholipases—indicating how arachidonate can be released by a one-step process. The numbering of the carbon atoms in the glycerol 'backbone' is given on the left. Unsaturated fatty acids, such as arachidonic acid, are usually located at R on the second carbon. This figure shows O-acyl residues on carbon atoms 1 and 2, but O-alkyl residues can occur (see Fig. 12.10). (R″ = choline, ethanolamine, serine, inositol or hydrogen)

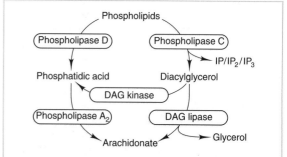

Fig. 12.6 Pathways of release of arachidonate from phospholipids by two-step processes. (IP = inositol phosphate; DAG = diacylglycerol) (See also Fig. 12.5 and Fig. 2.13.)

Mediators derived from phospholipids

- The main phospholipid-derived mediators are the eicosanoids (prostanoids and leukotrienes) and platelet-activating factor.
- The eicosanoids are derivatives of arachidonate which can be released from phospholipid by phospholipase (PL) action, either in one step by PLA$_2$, or by two steps— PLC then diacylglycerol lipase. Arachidonate can be metabolised either by one of two cyclo-oxygenases to give rise to various prostanoids, or by 5-lipoxygenase to give rise to various leukotrienes.
- Platelet-activating factor (PAF) is derived from phospholipid by PLA$_2$ giving rise to lyso-PAF which is acetylated to give PAF.

the lipoxins and other compounds (Figs 12.4, 12.7 and 12.8).

The anti-inflammatory action of the **glucocorticoids** (Ch. 24) is due largely to inhibition of *induction* of cyclo-oxygenase. These drugs may also stimulate production of the phospholipase A$_2$ inhibitor, lipocortin (Fig. 12.4).

The anti-inflammatory action of the **non-steroidal anti-inflammatory drugs** is due mainly to the fact that they inhibit the action of the fatty acid cyclo-oxygenases (Figs 12.4 and 12.7). Other compounds which act selectively on the cyclo-oxygenase induced in inflammatory cells or at specific sites of eicosanoid synthesis (e.g. inhibitors of 5-lipoxygenase, and thromboxane synthetase) are under test, as are specific antagonists of the prostaglandins and leukotrienes (Fig. 12.4).

PROSTANOIDS: PRODUCTS OF THE CYCLO-OXYGENASE PATHWAY

Cyclo-oxygenase (COX) exists in two forms—COX-1 and COX-2. COX-1 is found in most cells as a constitutive enzyme (i.e. it is always present) and it is thought that the prostanoids it produces are involved in normal homeostasis (e.g. regulating vascular responses and co-

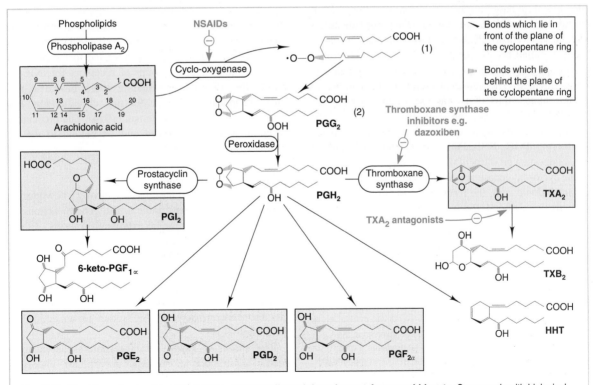

Fig. 12.7   The biosynthesis of prostaglandins, prostacyclin and thromboxane from arachidonate. Compounds with biological action are shown in boxes. There are two forms of cyclo-oxygenase (COX): one (COX–I) is constitutive and occurs in most cell types, and the other (COX–II) is induced in inflammatory cells by inflammatory stimuli. The current NSAIDs act mainly on COX–I. (PG = prostaglandin; TX = thromboxane; NSAIDs = non-steroidal anti-inflammatory drugs; HHT = 17-hydroxy-heptadecatrienoic acid; IFNγ = interferon γ)

ordinating the actions of circulating hormones). COX-2 is induced in inflammatory cells by an inflammatory stimulus. This has relevance for the mechanism of action of present and future **NSAIDs**.

Cyclo-oxygenase is found bound to the endoplasmic reticulum. It has two actions:

- an endoperoxide synthase action that first oxygenates arachidonate (step 1 in Fig. 12.7), followed by cyclisation to give the cyclic endoperoxide PGG_2 (step 2 in Fig. 12.7)
- a peroxidase action that converts PGG_2 to another cyclic endoperoxide, PGH_2 (see Fig. 12.7).*

Subsequent steps in arachidonate metabolism differ in different cells. In platelets, the pathway leads to *thromboxane A_2* synthesis, in vascular endothelium it leads to *prostacyclin* synthesis and in macrophages it leads mainly to synthesis of *prostaglandin E_2* (PGE_2). Mast cells synthesise *PGD_2*.

The confusing nomenclature of the eicosanoids derives from the fact that the names of the first two prostaglandins were based on the separation procedure—**PGE** partitioned into **E**ther, and PGF into the phosphate buffer (**F**osfat in Swedish). PGA and PGB (which are artefacts) were so called because of their stability or otherwise in **A**cids and **B**ases. Thereafter other letters of the alphabet were filled in. The subscripts refer to the number of double bonds; thus PGE_2 has two double bonds. The Greek letter subscript, the α in $PGF_{2\alpha}$, refers to the orientation of the hydroxyl above or below the plane of the ring. PGE_2, PGI_2, PGD_2, TXA_2 and $PGF_{2\alpha}$ are the most important products of the cyclo-oxygenase pathway. If the cyclo-oxygenase acts on eicosatrienoic acid instead of arachidonic acid, the resulting prostanoids have only a single double bond, for example PGE_1.

Catabolism of the prostanoids

Several intracellular enzymes are involved in inactivation of the prostaglandins. After carrier-mediated uptake there is rapid inactivation by 'prostaglandin-specific' enzymes, then slow inactivation by general fatty-acid-oxidising

---

*An autocatalytic mechanism is believed to be involved in the action of cyclo-oxygenase. The enzyme first produces a lipid peroxide—the formation of a peroxy radical at C11, compound (1) in Figure 12.7. This is followed by isomerisation, and also introduction of a hydroperoxy group at C15 to give PGG_2, compound (2) in Figure 12.7. It has been said that the lipid peroxide enhances the subsequent reactions of the enzyme, and that the continued presence of this (or other peroxides) is needed to sustain cyclo-oxygenase activity (although excess peroxide can inactivate the enzyme). See Lands (1981).

enzymes. The metabolites of the prostaglandins are excreted in the urine. The prostaglandin-specific enzymes are present in high concentration in the lung, and 95% of infused PGE_2, PGE_1 or $PGF_{2\alpha}$, is inactivated on first passage. The $t_{1/2}$ of most prostaglandins in the circulation is less than 1 minute.

PGI_2 is not taken up into cells by the transport system in the lung, and thus survives passage through the lung. However, it is very short-lived ($t_{1/2} < 5$ min), being hydrolysed to 6-keto $PGF_{1\alpha}$ (Fig. 12.7).

Thromboxane A_2 hydrolyses rapidly to the biologically inactive TXB_2 ($t_{1/2} = 30$ s).

Prostanoid receptors

A classification of prostanoid receptors has been proposed by Coleman et al. (1993). Using data of the rank order of potency of five natural prostanoids on a range of different preparations, five main prostanoid receptors have been defined, one each for the natural prostanoids, PGD_2, $PGF_{2\alpha}$, PGI_2, TXA_2 and PGE_2, termed DP-, FP-, IP-, TP- and EP-receptors respectively. Synthetic analogues of the natural prostanoids support and extend this classification, which has been further confirmed as receptor antagonists have become available. Data obtained with the synthetic compounds have led to the proposal that there are three subgroups of receptors for PGE_2—termed EP_1, EP_2 and EP_3. Binding studies have also provided supportive evidence for this classification. For a simple overview, see Coleman (1994). The prostanoid receptors have been cloned and all belong to the G-protein-coupled family.

Actions of the prostanoids

The prostanoids affect most tissues, having a bewildering variety of effects. Nevertheless, the general actions of the prostanoids can now be expressed in terms of their actions on their respective receptors as follows.

The action of PGD_2 on DP-receptors causes vasodilatation, inhibition of platelet aggregation, relaxation of gastrointestinal muscle, uterine relaxation, modification of release of hypothalamic/pituitary hormones. (Its bronchoconstrictor effect is due to an action on TP-receptors.)

The action of $PGF_{2\alpha}$ on FP-receptors causes myometrial contraction in humans (see Ch. 26), luteolysis in some species (e.g. cattle) and bronchoconstriction in other species (cats and dogs). (The receptors involved in $PGF_{2\alpha}$-mediated release of gonadotrophins and prolactin are not yet known.)

The action of PGI_2 (prostacyclin) on IP-receptors causes vasodilatation, inhibition of platelet aggregation (see Ch. 17), renin release and natriuresis via effects on tubular reabsorption of Na^+.

The action of TXA_2 on TP-receptors causes vaso-constriction, platelet aggregation (see Ch. 17) and bronchoconstriction (the last more marked in guinea pig than in humans).

The actions of PGE_2 are as follows:

- On EP_1-receptors it causes contraction of bronchial and gastrointestinal smooth muscle.
- On EP_2-receptors it causes bronchodilatation, vaso-dilatation, stimulation of intestinal fluid secretion and relaxation of gastrointestinal smooth muscle.
- On EP_3-receptors it causes contraction of intestinal smooth muscle, inhibition of gastric acid secretion (see Ch. 21 and Fig. 21.2), increased gastric mucus secretion, inhibition of lipolysis, inhibition of auto-nomic neurotransmitter release and stimulation of contraction of the pregnant human uterus (Ch. 26).

The role of the prostanoids in inflammation

The inflammatory response is always accompanied by the release of prostanoids, the predominant product being PGE_2, though PGI_2 can also be found. In areas of acute inflammation PGE_2 and PGI_2 are generated by the local tissues and blood vessels, and mast cells release PGD_2. In chronic inflammation, cells of the monocyte–macrophage series also release PGE_2 and TXA_2.

The prostanoids have a sort of Yin-Yang action in inflammation—stimulating some responses and decreasing others as follows.

PGE_2, PGI_2 and PGD_2 are powerful *vasodilators* in their own right and synergise with other inflammatory vasodilators such as histamine and bradykinin. It is this combined dilator action on precapillary arterioles which contributes to the redness and increased blood flow in areas of acute inflammation. These prostanoids do not directly increase the permeability of the post-capillary venules, but they potentiate this effect of hista-mine and bradykinin. Similarly, they do not themselves produce pain, but *potentiate* the effect of bradykinin by sensitising afferent C fibres (see Ch. 30). The anti-inflammatory effects of the **NSAIDs** are due largely to prevention of these actions of the prostaglandins.

Prostaglandins of the E series are also implicated in the production of fever. High concentrations are found in the CSF in infections, and there is evidence that the increase in temperature generated by endogenous fever-inducing cytokines is mediated by PGE_2. The antipyretic action of **NSAIDs** (Ch. 13) is due partly to inhibition of the synthesis of PGE_2 in the hypothalamus.

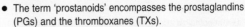

Prostanoids

- The term 'prostanoids' encompasses the prostaglandins (PGs) and the thromboxanes (TXs).
- Cyclo-oxygenase (COX) acts on arachidonate to produce cyclic endoperoxides (PGG_2, PGH_2).
- These can give rise to:
  — PGI_2 (prostacyclin) predominantly from vascular endothelium; it acts on IP-receptors. Main effects: vasodilatation and inhibition of platelet aggregation.
  — TXA_2 predominantly from platelets; it acts on TP-receptors. Main effects: platelet aggregation and vasoconstriction.
  — PGE_2. Main effects: on EP_1-receptors—contraction of bronchial and GIT smooth muscle; on EP_2-receptors—relaxation of bronchial, vascular and GIT smooth muscle; on EP_3-receptors—inhibition of gastric acid secretion, increased gastric mucus secretion, contraction of pregnant uterus and of GIT smooth muscle, inhibition of lipolysis and of autonomic neurotransmitter release. PGE_2 is a mediator of fever.
  — $PGF_{2\alpha}$ acts on FP-receptors which are found in smooth muscle and corpus luteum. Main effects in humans: contraction of uterus.
  — PGD_2, derived particularly from mast cells, acts on DP-receptors. Main effects: vasodilatation and inhibition of platelet aggregation.
- There are two forms of cyclo-oxygenase: COX-1, a constitutive enzyme, and COX-2, which is induced in inflammatory cells by inflammatory stimuli.

In addition to the pro-inflammatory mediator function mentioned above, prostaglandins have been shown to have a significant *anti-inflammatory* modulator role on inflammatory cells, *decreasing* their activities. Thus PGE_2 decreases lysosomal enzyme release and the generation of toxic oxygen metabolites from neutrophils and histamine release from mast cells. It also inhibits macrophage activation, lymphocyte activation (Fig. 12.3) and the generation and secretion of some cytokines.

Several prostanoids are available for clinical use (see the box on this page).

LEUKOTRIENES: PRODUCTS OF THE LIPOXYGENASE PATHWAYS

The lipoxygenases, soluble enzymes located in the cyto-sol, are found in lung, platelets, mast cells and white blood cells. The main enzyme in this group is 5-lipoxygenase—the first enzyme in the biosynthesis of the *leukotrienes* ('leuko' because they are found in white cells and 'trienes' because they contain a conjugated triene system of double bonds; see Fig. 12.8). On cell activation this enzyme translocates to the cell membrane where it becomes associated with a protein termed the 'five-lipoxygenase activating protein' (FLAP), which is necessary for leukotriene synthesis in intact cells. The 5-lipoxygenase adds a hydroperoxy group to C5 in arachidonic acid (Fig. 12.8). The next step in the pathway is the synthesis of *leukotriene A₄* (LTA_4). This compound may be converted enzymically to *LTB_4* and is also the precursor for an important class of cysteinyl-containing leukotrienes—*LTC_4, LTD_4, LTE_4* and *LTF_4* (also referred to as the sulphidopeptide leukotrienes). The first three of this latter group together constitute 'slow-reacting substance of anaphylaxis (SRS-A)', a substance shown many years ago to be generated in guinea-pig lung during anaphylaxis. LTB_4 is produced mainly by neutrophils, and the cysteinyl-leukotrienes mainly by eosinophils, mast cells, basophils and macrophages.

Lipoxins and other active products are also produced from arachidonate (Fig. 12.8).

Metabolism of the leukotrienes

LTB_4 can be converted to 20-hydroxy-LTB_4 by a unique membrane-bound P450 enzyme which occurs in the neutrophil, and then further oxidised to 20-carboxy-LTB_4. LTC_4 and LTD_4 are metabolised to LTE_4 which is excreted in the urine.

Actions and receptors* of the leukotrienes

LTB_4. LTB_4 acts on specific LTB_4-receptors defined by selective agonists and antagonists, the transduction mechanism being IP_3 generation and increase of cytosolic $[Ca^{2+}]_i$. It is a powerful chemotactic agent for both neutrophils and macrophages (see Fig. 12.2), acting in picogram amounts. On neutrophils, it also causes up-regulation of the membrane adhesion molecules and increases the production of toxic oxygen products and the release of granule enzymes. On macrophages and lymphocytes it stimulates proliferation and cytokine release.

Cysteinyl-leukotrienes. On the basis of the rank order of potency, there appear to be receptors for both LTD_4 and LTC_4, but there are few specific agonists for either compound. However, specific receptors for LTD_4 have been defined on the basis of numerous selective antagonists.

Cysteinyl-leukotrienes have actions on:

- *The respiratory system.* They are potent spasmogens, causing dose-related contraction of human bronchiolar muscle in vitro. LTE_4 is less potent than LTC_4 and LTD_4, but its effect is much longer-lasting. All cause an increase in mucus secretion. Given by aerosol in vivo to human volunteers they cause marked reduction in specific airway conductance and in maximum expiratory flow rate, the effect being more protracted than that produced by histamine (Fig. 12.9).
- *The cardiovascular system.* Small amounts of LTC_4 or LTD_4 given intravenously cause a rapid, short-lived fall in blood pressure, and significant constriction of small coronary resistance vessels. Given subcutaneously they are equipotent with histamine in causing wheal and flare. Given topically in the nose, LTD_4 increases nasal blood flow and increases local vascular permeability.

The role of leukotrienes in inflammation

LTB_4 can be found in inflammatory exudates and is present in the tissues in many inflammatory conditions, including rheumatoid arthritis, psoriasis (a chronic skin disease) and ulcerative colitis. The cysteinyl-leukotrienes are present in the sputum of chronic bronchitis in amounts

---

*Receptors for the leukotrienes are termed LT-receptors—BLT for the class exemplified by LTB_4 and CysLT for the cysteinyl-leukotrienes. LTC_4, LTD_4 and LTE_4 all act on the same CysLT-receptor.

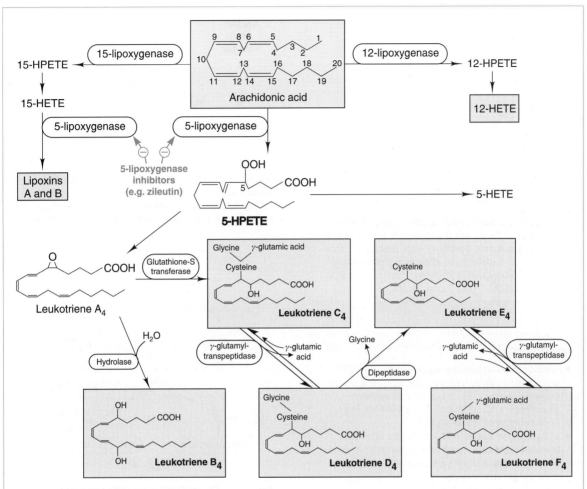

Fig. 12.8   The biosynthesis of leukotrienes from arachidonic acid. It is not clear whether LTF$_4$ occurs in vivo. Compounds with biological action are shown in grey boxes. (HETE = hydroxyeicosatetraenoic acid; HPETE = hydroperoxyeicosatetraenoic acid)

which are biologically active. On antigen challenge they are released from samples of human asthmatic lung in vitro and into nasal lavage fluid in vivo in subjects with allergic rhinitis. There is evidence that they contribute to the underlying bronchial hyper-reactivity in asthmatics and it is thought that they are among the main mediators of both the early and late phases of asthma (p. 340, Fig. 19.2). Several CysLT-receptor antagonists have shown promise in the treatment of asthma (see Ch. 19). It is also possible that cysteinyl-leukotrienes have a role in the cardiovascular changes of acute anaphylaxis.

Agents which inhibit the enzymes that generate the leukotrienes—5-lipoxygenase inhibitors—are under development as anti-asthmatic agents (e.g. **zileutin**; see Ch. 19) and anti-inflammatory agents.

PLATELET-ACTIVATING FACTOR (PAF)

Platelet-activating factor, which is also variously termed *PAF-acether* and *AGEPC* (acetyl-glyceryl-ether-phosphorylcholine), is a biologically active lipid which can produce effects at exceedingly low concentrations (less than 10^{-10} mol/l). The name platelet-activating factor is misleading, since PAF has actions on a variety of different target cells and is believed to be an important mediator in both acute and persisting allergic and inflammatory phenomena.

PAF (Fig. 12.10) is derived from its precursor, acyl-PAF, by phospholipase A_2 activity, resulting in 'lyso-PAF' which is then acetylated to give PAF, which in turn can be deacetylated to lyso-PAF (Fig. 12.11).

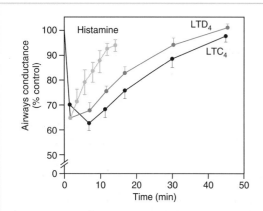

Fig. 12.9   The time-course of action on specific airways conductance of the cysteinyl-leukotrienes and histamine, in six normal subjects. Specific airways conductance was measured in a constant volume whole body plethysmograph and the drugs were given by inhalation. (From: Barnes P J, Piper P J, Costello J K 1984 Thorax 39: 500)

Leukotrienes (LTs)

- 5-lipoxygenase acts on arachidonate to give 5-HPETE which is converted by a dehydrase to LTA_4. This can be converted to either LTB_4 or to a series of cysteinyl-leukotrienes, LTC_4, LTD_4 and LTE_4, which have amino acids incorporated in their structure.
- LTB_4, acting on specific receptors, causes adherence, chemotaxis and activation of polymorphs and monocytes, and stimulates proliferation and cytokine production from macrophages and lymphocytes.
- The cysteinyl-leukotrienes cause:
  — contraction of bronchial muscle
  — vasodilatation in most vessels, but coronary vasoconstriction.
- LTB_4 is an important mediator in all types of inflammation; the cysteinyl-leukotrienes are of particular importance in asthma.

Sources of PAF

PAF is generated and released from most inflammatory cells when these are stimulated. Thus it is released from neutrophil polymorphs on phagocytosis of opsonised particles, from activated macrophages and eosinophils, from mast cells and basophils on interaction with antigen and from platelets on stimulation with thrombin.

Actions and role in inflammation

Acting on specific receptors, PAF has a wide range of pathophysiological actions and is capable of producing

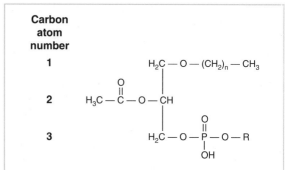

Fig. 12.10   The structure of PAF (platelet-activating factor). An O-alkyl residue is attached to carbon atom 1 (cf. Fig. 12.5). It may be hexadecyl or octadecyl; compounds containing either of these have PAF activity. (R = choline)

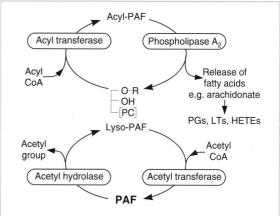

Fig. 12.11   The synthesis and breakdown of platelet-activating factor (PAF). (PC = phosphorylcholine; PG = prostaglandin; LT = leukotriene; HETE = hydroxyeicosatetraenoic acid)

many of the phenomena of inflammation. In doses of 0.02–200 pmol injected locally, it produces not only local *vasodilatation* and thus erythema, but also *increased vascular permeability* and wheal formation. Higher doses produce *hyperalgesia*. It is a potent *chemotaxin* for neutrophils and monocytes and is important in *recruiting eosinophils* into the bronchial mucosa in the late phase of asthma (Fig. 19.2). It can activate phospholipase A_2 with generation of eicosanoids.

On platelets, it causes *shape change* and the release of the contents of dense granules and of α_1 and α_2 granules. This effect is associated with metabolism of arachidonate and thromboxane A_2 generation and is important in haemostasis and thrombosis (see Ch. 17). PAF is also a *spasmogen* on both bronchial and ileal smooth muscle; its spasmogenic activity for human bronchial muscle may be due either to PLA_2 activation with resultant generation of cysteinyl-leukotrienes and/or be dependent on the presence of platelets.

The anti-inflammatory actions of the **glucocorticoids** are due, at least in part, to inhibition of PAF synthesis by virtue of the inhibitory effect of lipocortin on phospholipase A_2 (Fig. 12.4).

Competitive antagonists of the actions of PAF and/or specific inhibitors of lyso-PAF acetyl transferase could well be useful anti-inflammatory drugs. The former have been under test as anti-asthmatic agents (see Ch. 19).

Platelet-activating factor (PAF)

- PAF is released indirectly from many activated inflammatory cells by PLA_2 activity and acts on specific receptors in many cell types.
- Pharmacological actions: causes vasodilatation, increases vascular permeability, is chemotactic for leukocytes (especially eosinophils), activates leukocytes, activates and aggregates platelets and is spasmogenic for smooth muscle.
- It is a mediator in many types of inflammation and is implicated in bronchial hyper-responsiveness and in the delayed phase of asthma.

BRADYKININ

Bradykinin and the closely related peptide *kallidin* are vasoactive peptides formed by the action of enzymes on protein substrates termed *kininogens*. The two peptides are virtually identical (see Fig. 12.13), kallidin possessing one additional amino acid.

Source and formation of bradykinin

An outline of the formation of bradykinin is given in Figure 12.12. Prekallikrein is present in plasma as the inactive precursor of the proteolytic enzyme kallikrein. The substrate is *kininogen*—a plasma α-globulin. There are two forms of kininogen in plasma: high-molecular-weight kininogen (M_r 110 000) and low-molecular weight kininogen (M_r 70 000). Prekallikrein can be converted to the active enzyme (which is a serine protease) in a variety of ways. One of the physiological activators, particularly in the context of inflammation, is Hageman factor (factor XII of the blood clotting sequence; see Ch. 18 and Fig. 12.1). Hageman factor is normally in an inactive form in the plasma and is activated by contact

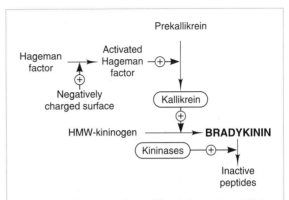

Fig. 12.12 The generation and breakdown of bradykinin. HMW-kininogen = high-molecular-weight kininogen; this substance probably acts both as a substrate for kallikrein and as a cofactor in the activation of prekallikrein.

with surfaces having a negative charge, such as collagen, basement membrane, bacterial lipopolysaccharides, urate crystals and so on. As a result of the increased vascular permeability which occurs in inflammation, Hageman factor, prekallikrein and the kininogens leak out of the vessels with the plasma (see Fig. 12.1). Contact with the negatively charged surfaces promotes the interaction of prekallikrein and Hageman factor, and this leads to kinin generation, bradykinin being clipped out of the high-molecular-weight kininogen molecules by the enzyme, which acts at two sites to release the nonapeptide (Fig. 12.13). Kallikrein can also activate the complement system, and can convert plasminogen to plasmin (see Fig. 12.1 and Ch. 18).

In addition to the plasma kallikrein described above, there are other kinin-generating kallikreins found in pancreas, salivary glands, colon and skin. Tissue kallikreins act on both high- and low-molecular-weight kininogens and generate mainly lysyl-bradykinin (or kallidin), a peptide with actions similar to those of bradykinin.

Inactivation of bradykinin

The main enzymes which inactivate bradykinin and related kinins are called *kininases* (Figs 12.12 and 12.13). One of these, *kininase II*, is the same as *angiotensin-converting enzyme* (see Ch. 15). This is a peptidyl dipeptidase which removes the two C-terminal amino acids from the kinin and inactivates it (Fig. 12.13). The enzyme is bound to the luminal surface of endothelial cells and is found mostly in the lung. It also cleaves the two C-terminal amino acids from the inactive peptide, angiotensin I, converting it to the active vasoconstrictor pep-

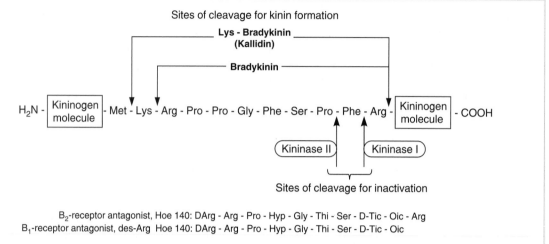

Fig. 12.13 **Structure of bradykinin and some bradykinin antagonists.** The sites of proteolytic cleavage for formation of kallidin and bradykinin by kallikrein from HMW-kininogen are shown in the upper half of the figure; the sites of cleavage for bradykinin inactivation are shown in the lower half. The B_2-receptor antagonist, icatibant (Hoe 140), has a pA_2 of 9, and the competitive B_1-receptor antagonist, des-Arg Hoe 140, has a pA_2 of 8. The Hoe compounds contain unnatural amino acids: Thi, D-Tic and Oic, which are analogues of phenylalanine and proline.

tide, angiotensin II (see Chs 15 and 20). Thus, the enzyme inactivates a vasodilator and activates a vasoconstrictor.

Kinins are also inactivated by the less specific *kininase I*, a carboxypeptidase present in serum (Fig. 12.13). It removes the C-terminal arginine from bradykinin, generating des-Arg^9-bradykinin, which is a specific agonist at one of the two main classes of bradykinin receptor (see below).

Actions and role of bradykinin in inflammation

Bradykinin (BK) causes vasodilatation and increased vascular permeability. Its vasodilator action is partly due to generation of PGI_2 (Fig. 12.4), and the release of nitric oxide (Ch. 11). It is a potent pain-producing agent (Ch. 37), an effect that is potentiated by the prostaglandins (see Ch. 37, Fig. 37.6, p. 586).

Bradykinin is *spasmogenic* for several types of smooth muscle including that of the intestine and the uterus; bronchial muscle is also contracted in some species. The contraction is slow and sustained in comparison with that produced by histamine (hence *brady* which means 'slow').

The pathophysiological function of bradykinin is still a matter of conjecture. The release of bradykinin by tissue kallikrein may be of importance in controlling blood flow to certain exocrine glands, and thus influencing the secretions of the glands. It is known to stimulate ion transport and fluid secretion by various epithelia,

including that of the intestine, the airways and the gall bladder. Excessive bradykinin production is probably a factor in causing diarrhoea in many gastrointestinal disorders, and in stimulating nasopharyngeal secretion in allergic rhinitis. It also plays a part in pancreatitis.

On the basis of experimental observations, it is capable of producing many of the phenomena seen in the inflammatory reaction—pain, vasodilatation, increased vascular permeability and spasm of smooth muscle, but its role in inflammation and allergy has not been clearly defined, not least because its effects are often part of a complex cascade of events which includes other mediators.

Bradykinin receptors

There is more than one type of bradykinin receptor; B_1 and B_2 subtypes are currently recognised, and the existence of other subtypes has been proposed. The effects mediated by B_1- and B_2-receptors are very similar.

The characterisation of the B_1-receptor is based on the fact that BK_{1-8} (des-Arg-BK, which is the product of kininase I action; see Fig. 12.13) is active only on a small subset of bradykinin-sensitive tissues, and that its effect is antagonised by selective peptide antagonists, such as Leu^{8}BK$_{1-8}$ and des-Arg Hoe 140 (pA_2:8; Fig. 12.13). B_1-receptors are often not seen when isolated tissues are first set up, but appear to be synthesised and expressed slowly over several hours. A similar process of induction is believed to occur during persistent inflammatory reactions. B_1-receptors are thought to be implicated in persistent inflammatory hyperalgesia.

The B_2-receptor is a catch-all category, consisting of virtually all bradykinin receptors which are not B_1 and subsuming most of the effects of bradykinin. They desensitise rapidly after activation and are not activated by BK_{1-8}. B_2-receptors belong to the family of G-protein-coupled receptors. Selective B_2-receptor antagonists have been developed, for example the peptide **icatibant** (Hoe 140, pA_2:9; see Fig. 12.13); and some non-peptide antagonists are in the pipeline. Such agents could well prove to be of value not only as investigative tools but also in the therapy of various disease states; for example some allergic conditions, carcinoid syndrome (see Ch. 9, p. 172), some gastrointestinal disorders and, possibly, also in acute pancreatitis (in which kinins released by pancreatic kallikrein contribute to the severe pain and the fluid exudation into the peritoneal cavity).

Bradykinin (BK)

- Bradykinin is a nonapeptide. It is clipped out of kininogen, a plasma α-globulin, by a proteolytic enzyme, kallikrein.
- It is converted by kininase I, to an octapeptide, BK_{1-8} (des-Arg-BK), which is inactivated by angiotensin-converting enzyme in the lung.
- Pharmacological actions:
  — vasodilatation (largely endothelial cell-dependent, due both to generation of NO and activation of PLA_2 with release of PGI_2)
  — increased vascular permeability
  — stimulation of pain nerve endings
  — stimulation of epithelial ion transport and fluid secretion in airways and GIT
  — contraction of intestinal and uterine smooth muscle.
- There are two main subtypes of BK receptors: B_1 and B_2; most BK effects in humans are due to action on B_2-receptors.
- There are selective competitive antagonists for both B_1-receptors (des-Arg Hoe 140; pA_2:8) and B_2-receptors (icatibant, pA_2:9).

NITRIC OXIDE

Nitric oxide (NO) is dealt with in detail in Chapter 11; here we consider only its role in inflammation.

It is mainly the inducible form of NO synthase (iNOS) that is involved in inflammatory reactions. Virtually all inflammatory cells express the inducible form of the enzyme in response to cytokine stimulation. NO synthase is also present in the bronchial epithelium of asthmatic subjects, in the mucosa of the colon in patients with ulcerative colitis and in synoviocytes in inflammatory joint disease. NO has mainly *pro-inflammatory* actions: it is a potent vasodilator, it increases vascular permeability and it increases the production of pro-inflammatory prostaglandins. It, or compounds derived from it, have cytotoxic action against bacteria, fungi, virus and metazoan parasites and is thought to enhance local defence mechanisms, but, produced in excess, it can be harmful to host cells. Some of its actions are, however, anti-inflammatory since, released from endothelial cells, it inhibits adhesion of neutrophils and platelets and platelet aggregation.

Inhibitors of iNOS are under investigation for treatment of inflammatory conditions. Patients with septic shock have benefited from inhibitors of iNOS, and in experimental arthritis, iNOS inhibitors have significantly reduced disease activity.*

NEUROPEPTIDES

Neuropeptides released from sensory neurons contribute to inflammatory reactions—constituting the phenomenon known as 'neurogenic inflammation'. The main peptides involved are substance P, neurokinin A and calcitonin gene-related peptide. Substance P and neurokinin A (members of the tachykinin family) act on mast cells, releasing histamine and other mediators, and produce smooth muscle contraction and mucus secretion; calcitonin gene-related peptide is a potent vasodilator. (See Chs 10, 15, 19 and 37.) Neurogenic inflammation is implicated in the pathogenesis of several inflammatory conditions including the delayed phase of asthma, allergic rhinitis, inflammatory bowel disease and some types of arthritis. See Maggi (1996).

CYTOKINES

Cytokines are peptides released from inflammatory tissue, connective tissue and immune system cells; they act by autocrine and paracrine mechanisms. They were once considered by many pharmacologists to be beyond the pale of respectable pharmacology—messy, ill-defined molecules whose actions were not only confusing, but were different when studied in different laboratories. Their very structures appeared to vary according to the method of extraction used, and each masqueraded under a plethora of different names. But recombinant DNA

---

*When it comes to inhibition of the *non*-inducible form of NOS, it is not the case that no NOS is good NOS.

technology has clarified the muddle, and cytokines can now be produced in pure form and the range of their individual activities can be properly established. Some order has been produced in the diffuse and chaotic nomenclature and it now even seems possible that they, (or, more probably, their non-peptide analogues) and/or their antagonists, might in the future be added to the list of useful therapeutic agents.

More than 50 cytokines have been identified, and the cytokine superfamily includes interleukins, chemokines, colony-stimulating factors (see Ch. 18), growth factors,* interferons, and the transforming growth factor (TGF*) and tumour necrosis factor families. Here we emphasise mainly the cytokines implicated in inflammatory and immune conditions. These cytokines are produced mainly from macrophages and lymphocytes but also from other leukocytes, endothelial cells and fibroblasts. Most are not produced constitutively but are synthesised *de novo* on cell activation. Most act locally by paracrine and/or autocrine mechanisms; exceptions being IL-1 (see below) and TNF-α. On the target cell, cytokines act on specific, high-affinity receptors, which, in most cases, are up-regulated in the cell when it is stimulated.

In addition to their own direct actions on cells, some cytokines induce formation of other cytokines (which could constitute a necessary amplification cascade), some induce the receptors for other cytokines, and some have complicated synergistic or antagonistic interactions with other cytokines. Cytokines have been likened to a complex signalling language with the final response of a particular cell involved being determined by a number of different messages received concurrently at the cell surface. The details of the functioning of this complex cytokine network are not yet fully understood. However, it is becoming clear that they are important pathophysiological mediators and are implicated in the pathogenesis of numerous disease states.

Various classifications of the cytokines can be found in the literature** as can a multitude of diagrams depicting complex networks of cytokines interacting with each other and with a range of target cells. A comprehensive coverage of this area is not possible here. For the purposes of this chapter we will divide cytokines into two main groups:

- those involved in the induction of the immune response—described above and outlined in Figure 12.3
- those involved in the effector phase of the immune/inflammatory response, which we will consider now.

The effector phase cytokines include both pro-inflammatory and anti-inflammatory peptides. The primary pro-inflammatory cytokines are tumour necrosis factor-α (TNF-α) and interleukin-1 (IL-1); these are released from macrophages and many other cells and can start a cascade of secondary cytokines amongst which are the *chemokines*—a subfamily of cytokines that attract and activate motile inflammatory cells.

There are at least 28 chemokines, subdivided into two groups: the α or C-X-C group in which the first two cysteine residues are separated by an intervening amino acid, and the β or C-C group in which they are not (Adams & Lloyd, 1997). The α chemokines (main example IL-8; see p. 201, Fig. 12.2) act on neutrophils and are predominantly involved in *acute inflammatory responses*. The β chemokines (main examples MCP-1*** and RANTES,*** see p. 202) act on monocytes, eosinophils and other cells, and are involved predominantly in *chronic inflammatory responses*.

The anti-inflammatory cytokines include TGF-β, IL-4, IL-10 and IL-13; these can inhibit the production of chemokines and the last three can inhibit responses mediated by Th1 cells (see above, p. 206).

Various growth factors (e.g. platelet-derived growth factor, fibroblast growth factor, vascular endothelial growth factor) are important in repair processes and are implicated in chronic inflammation.

For most cytokines the signal transduction mechanisms in the target cell involve the Jak/Stat pathway but the chemokines act through G-protein-coupled receptors (Ch. 2).

Some cytokines thought to be of particular importance in inflammatory and immune conditions—the interleukin-1 family, the interferons and nerve growth factor—are considered in more detail below; the colony-stimulating factors are considered in Chapter 18.

INTERLEUKIN-1 (IL-1)

Interleukin-1 is the term given to a family of three cytokines consisting of two *agonists*, IL-1α, IL-1β and an endogenous IL-1-receptor *antagonist* (IL-1ra).

---

*For insulin-like growth factor (IGF-1) see Chapter 27, page 455; for TGF-β see Fig. 42.2.

**The cytokine aficionado can find classification tables in Casciari et al. (1996) and Roitt (1997, p. 181).

***For the importance of these chemokines in HIV-1 infection, see Chapter 44, pages 709–713.

Interleukin-1 molecules are produced in infection and injury or on antigenic challenge, the primary source being the activated macrophage. IL-1α remains cell-associated and is active mainly during cell-to-cell contact, while the soluble IL-1β is the predominant form in biological fluids. All interleukin-1 molecules act on specific receptors on target tissues.

IL-1* is a significant pro-inflammatory cytokine, being important particularly in the systemic responses of inflammation (e.g. fever). It synergises with tumour necrosis factor-α (TNF-α) for many of the latter actions, and its synthesis is stimulated by TNF-α. It is implicated in the pathogenesis of rheumatoid arthritis, inflammatory bowel disease, septic shock and several autoimmune diseases. A local imbalance between IL-1 and IL-1ra, may underlie the development and progress of some of these conditions.

INTERFERONS

Interferons are a group of inducible cytokines synthesised in response to viral and other stimuli. There are three classes of interferon (IFN), termed IFN-α, IFN-β and IFN-γ. IFN-α is not a single substance but a family of 15 proteins with similar activities.

The interferons can be induced by other cytokines and IFN-α and IFN-β are produced in many cell types—macrophages, fibroblasts, endothelial cells, osteoblasts, etc., being strongly induced by viruses, and less strongly by other microorganisms and bacterial products. IFN-γ, also termed immune interferon, is produced mainly in antigen-activated T cells (see p. 204 and Fig. 12.3).

Actions of interferons. All interferons have antiviral activity, all can induce fever and all possess antitumour effects in vitro. In addition, IFN-γ has an important role in induction of Th1 responses (p. 204, Fig. 12.3; see also Abbas et al. 1996).

The production of interferon-γ during infections is beneficial in that it assists in overcoming the infection, but it can promote some allergic and autoimmune conditions.

Clinical use of interferons. Interferons are being used in cancer therapy (Ch. 42) and to treat virus infections (Ch. 44). Interferon-γ is undergoing trials for the therapy of hepatitis, leishmaniasis and leprosy, and interferon-β is being tried for the treatment of the relapsing–remitting form of multiple sclerosis.

NERVE GROWTH FACTOR (NGF)

This growth factor, which is usually known as a trophic factor on neurons, has recently been shown to be, in addition, an important mediator of inflammation (Levi-Montalcini et al. 1996). It is synthesised and released by mast cells and T cells and has autocrine actions on these cells. Its synthesis is strongly induced by the pro-inflammatory cytokines, IL-1 and TNF-α. It influences T and B cell proliferation and is chemotactic for neutrophils. It maintains the survival and sensitivity of the nociceptive neurons that release inflammatory neuropeptides and plays a part in the hyperalgesia that can accompany inflammation.

POTENTIAL THERAPIES BASED ON MANIPULATION OF THE IMMUNE RESPONSE

The use of naked DNA

It has recently been found that vaccination with naked DNA coding for particular proteins can induce long-continued cell-mediated and antibody-mediated immune responses to those proteins, a strategy that can be used to produce immunity to a range of viral, bacterial and parasitic pathogens. Thus, when a plasmid** containing the gene for influenza protein was injected into muscle tissue in mice, 90% of the animals so treated survived viral challenge, as compared with 20% of the controls.

Animal diseases in which DNA vaccination has proved effective include tuberculosis and rodent malaria in mice and hepatitis B in chimpanzees. Prevention of these infections involves *activation of protective* Th1 responses (see p. 206). In a further 30 or more experiments in a variety of animals, vaccination with naked DNA has been successful in inducing immune responses and/or conferring protection against pathogen challenge; in particular, it induces a cytotoxic lymphocytes response more effectively than other techniques (more details are given in Donnelly et al. 1997).

Suppression of unwanted autoimmune Th1 responses in mice with accentuation of Th2 responses (immune deviation) is also possible. Thus vaccination of mice with DNA encoding a particular portion of the T cell receptor that is critical in the development of experimental allergic encephalitis (EAE), resulted in reduced Th1 cytokines, elevated Th2 cytokines and prevention of the development of EAE when the antigen*** was

---

*The term IL-1 will be used for the agonist interleukin-1 molecules.

**Plasmids are described on page 658 (Ch. 41).

***The antigen used to produce EAE is myelin basic protein peptide.

injected. This approach may, in the future, be of value in the therapy of Th1-mediated conditions such as multiple sclerosis, juvenile diabetes and rheumatoid arthritis.

For short overviews of this area see Kumar & Sercarz 1996, McCarthy 1996.

Cytokines, cytokine receptors and T cell surface proteins as targets for new drugs

Cytokines are peptides and, as outlined in Chapter 10, there are problems involved in using peptides in therapy. Nevertheless various possibilities are being explored, amongst which are the following:

Modification of IL-10 function. IL-10 down-regulates Th1 responses (p. 224, Fig. 12.3). Systemic administration in rodents has suppressed T-cell-mediated inflammatory bowel disease, delayed hypersensitivity reactions and experimental autoimmune encephalomyelitis.

Modification of IL-2 function. IL-2 and IFN-γ have been used to stimulate cell-mediated immunity in lepromatous leprosy. Antibodies against a portion of the IL-2-receptor as well as complexes of IL-2 with toxins (e.g. diphtheria toxin) have shown promise in experimental IL-2-receptor-expressing leukaemias and lymphomas.

Modification of IL-1ra function. Recombinant IL-1ra (the IL-1-receptor antagonist) is being evaluated in the treatment of conditions in which IL-1 is known to be implicated in tissue damage. Inhibitors of the synthesis and release of IL-1 have shown efficacy in animal models of inflammation.

Modification of T cell function. Agents that block the co-receptors involved in T cell activation are under investigation as are peptides derived from MCH molecules, these last being in phase II clinical trial.

About 15 new agents for treating multiple sclerosis are being investigated, all affecting the immune system in some way. One example (*bovine myelin formulation*, an autoantigen that induces tolerance) is in phase III trial.

Anti-integrin drugs are under development for the potential treatment of inflammatory conditions; see Featherstone (1996). An antisense drug that prevents expression of the intracellular adhesion molecule, ICAM-1, is in phase II trial.

Further consideration of potential new therapies is given in Chapters 13 and 19.

Cytokines

- Cytokines are peptides that, in immune and inflammatory reactions, are released from and regulate the action of inflammatory and immune system cells.
- The cytokine superfamily includes the interferons, numerous interleukins, tumour necrosis factor (TNF), various growth factors, the chemokines and the colony-stimulating factors.
- They act in a complex interconnecting network on leukocytes, vascular endothelial cells, mast cells, fibroblasts, haemopoietic stem cells and osteoclasts, controlling proliferation, differentiation and/or activation through autocrine or paracrine mechanisms.
- Interleukin-1 and tumour necrosis factor-α are important primary inflammatory cytokines, inducing the formation of other cytokines.
- The three interferons (α, β and γ) have antiviral activity and interferon-γ has significant immunoregulatory function.

REFERENCES AND FURTHER READING

Abbas A K, Murphy K M, Sher A 1996 Functional diversity of helper lymphocytes. Nature 383: 787–793 (*Excellent review, helpful diagrams*)

Adams D H, Lloyd A R 1997 Chemokines: leucocyte recruitment and activation cytokines. Lancet 349: 490–495 (*Commendable review*)

Adorini L, Sinigaglia F 1997 Pathogenesis and immunotherapy of autoimmune disease. Trends Immunol 18: 209–211

Arai K, Lee F, Miyajima A et al. 1990 Cytokines: coordinators of immune and inflammatory responses. Annu Rev Biochem 59: 783–836 (*Early review; comprehensive*)

Arrang J M, Garbarg M, Schwartz J C 1983 Autoinhibition of brain histamine release mediated by a novel class (H₃) of histamine receptor. Nature 302: 832–834

Arrang J M, Garbarg M et al. 1987 Highly potent and selective ligands for histamine H₃ receptors. Nature 327: 117–123

Bancherau J, Steinman R M 1998 Dendritic cells and the control of immunity. Nature 392: 245–352 (*Good coverage of important cells*)

Barnes P J, Karin M 1997 Nuclear factor-κB—a pivotal transcription factor in chronic inflammatory diseases. N Engl J Med 336: 1066–1071

Black J W, Duncan W A M, Durant G J et al. 1972 Definition and antagonism of histamine H₂-receptors. Nature 236: 385–390 (*Definitive, seminal article on H₂-receptors*)

Borden E C 1992 Interferons—expanding therapeutic roles. N Engl J Med 326: 1491–1493

Buckley C D, Simmons D L 1997 Cell adhesion: a new target for therapy. Mol Med Today (Oct): 449–456

Burshtyn D N, Long E O 1997 Regulation through inhibitory receptors: lessons from natural killer cells. Trends Cell Biol 7: 473–478

Carlos T M, Harlan J M 1994 Leucocyte–endothelial adhesion molecules. Blood 84: 2068–2101 (*Comprehensive review*)

Casciari J J, Sato H et al. 1996 Tabular lexicon of cytokine structure and function. In: Chabner B A, Longo D N (eds) Cancer chemotherapy and biotherapy, 2nd edn. Lippincott-Raven, Philadelphia, pp 787–793

Coleman R 1994 Eicosanoid receptors. In: Dale M M, Foreman J C, Fan T-P (eds) Textbook of immunopharmacology, 3rd edn. Blackwell Scientific Publications, Oxford, ch 12, pp 143–154

Coleman R A, Humphrey P A, Kennedy I, Lumley P 1984 Prostanoid receptors: the development of a working classification. Trends Pharmacol Sci 5: 303–306

Coleman R A, Humphrey P A et al. 1993 Prostanoid receptors: their function and classification. In: Vane J, O'Grady J (eds) Therapeutic applications of prostaglandins. Edward Arnold, London, ch 2, pp 15–36 (Useful coverage; includes structures of prostanoids, their analogues and antagonists)

Dale M M 1994 Summary of section on mediators. In: Dale M M, Foreman J C, Fan T-P (eds) Textbook of immunopharmacology, 3rd edn. Blackwell Scientific Publications, Oxford, pp 206–207 (Considers which mediators meet the defined criteria)

Dale M M, Foreman J C, Fan T-P (eds) 1994 Textbook of immunopharmacology, 3rd edn. Blackwell Scientific Publications, Oxford (Simple textbook written with second and third year medical and science students in mind)

Dinarello C A 1997 Interleukin-1. Cytokine and Growth Factor Rev 8: 232–265

Donnelly J J, Ulmer J B, Liu M A 1997 Minireview: DNA vaccines. Life Sci 60: 163–172 (Minireview)

Dray A 1996 Afferent responses of sensory neurones. In: Geppetti P, Holzer P (eds) Neurogenic inflammation. CRC Press, London, ch 6, pp 69–79

Dwyer J M 1992 Manipulating the immune system with immune globulin. N Engl J Med 326: 107–116

Engelhard V H 1994 How cells process antigens. Scientific American (August): 44–51

Fearon D T, Locksley R M 1996 The instructive role of innate immunity in the acquired immune response. Science 272: 50–53 (Succinct review)

Featherstone C 1996 Anti-integrin drugs developed to treat inflammation. Lancet 347: 1106–1107

Foreman J C 1994 Mast cells and basophil leucocytes. In: Dale M M, Foreman J C, Fan T-P (eds) Textbook of immunopharmacology, 3rd edn. Blackwell Scientific Publications, Oxford, ch 2, pp 21–34

Hawkins R E, Llewelyn M B, Russell S J 1992 Adapting antibodies for clinical use. Br Med J 305: 1348–1352

Hill S J 1990 Distribution, properties, and functional characteristics of three classes of histamine receptor. Pharmacol Rev 42: 46–81

Horwitz A F 1997 Integrins and health. Scientific American (May): 68–75

Jaffe H S, Bucalco L R, Sherwin S A 1992 Anti-infective applications of interferon-gamma. Marcel Dekker, New York

Janeway C A, Travers P 1996 Immunobiology: the immune system in health and disease, 2nd edn. Churchill Livingstone, Edinburgh (Excellent textbook, good diagrams)

Johnson H J, Bazer F W et al. 1994 How interferons fight disease Scientific American (May): 40–47

Kärre K, Welsh R M 1997 Viral decoy vetoes killer cell. Nature 386: 446–447

Kumar V, Sercarz E 1996 Genetic vaccination: the advantages of going naked. Nature Med 2: 857–859

Lands W E 1981 Actions of anti-inflammatory drugs. Trends Pharmacol Sci 2: 78–80

Levi-Montalcini R, Skaper S D et al. 1996 Nerve growth factor: from neuropeptides to neurokine. Trends Neurosci 19: 514–519

(Clear coverage)

Lewis R A, Austen K F, Soberman R J 1990 Leukotrienes and other products of the 5-lipoxygenase pathway. N Engl J Med 323: 645–655

Luster A D 1998 Mechanisms of disease: chemokines—chemotactic cytokines that mediate inflammation. N Engl J Med 338: 436–445 (Excellent review; outstanding diagrams)

McCarthy M 1996 DNA vaccination: a direct line to the immune system. Lancet 348: 1232

Maggi C A 1996 Pharmacology of the efferent function of primary sensory neurones. In: Geppetti P, Holzer P (eds) Neurogenic inflammation. CRC Press, London, ch 7, pp 81–91 (Worthwhile)

Mantovani A, Bussolino F, Introna M 1997 Cytokine regulation of endothelial cell function: from molecular level to the bedside. Immunol Today 5: 231–239 (Pathophysiology of endothelial cell/cytokine interactions; detailed diagrams)

Matyszak M K, Townsend M J, Perery V H et al. 1997 Ultrastructural studies of an immune-mediated inflammatory response in the CNS parenchyma directed against a non-CNS antigen. Neuroscience 78: 549–560

Muid R E, Twomey B M, Dale M M 1994 The neutrophil leucocyte. In: Dale M M, Foreman J C, Fan T-P (eds) Textbook of immunopharmacology, 3rd edn. Blackwell Scientific Publications, Oxford, ch 3, pp 35–48

Page C P 1994 The platelet. In: Dale M M, Foreman J C, Fan T-P (eds) Textbook of immunopharmacology, 3rd edn. Blackwell Scientific Publications, Oxford, Ch 4, pp 49–54

Perry V H 1995 Novel aspects of inflammation in the central nervous system. EOS-Rivista di Immunolgia ed Immunopharmacologia 13: 92–95

Richards C D, Gauldie J 1994 The acute-phase protein response. In: Dale M M, Foreman J C, Fan T-P (eds) Textbook of immunopharmacology, 3rd edn. Blackwell Scientific Publications, Oxford, ch 24, pp 269–276

Roitt 1997 Essential immunology, 9th edn. Blackwell Science, Oxford, pp 476 (Excellent textbook; well illustrated)

Romagnani S 1996 Short analytical review: Th1 and Th2 in human diseases. Clin Immunol Immunopathol 80: 225–235 (Covers pathophysiology of Th1 and Th2 responses)

Romagnani S 1997 The Th1/Th2 paradigm. Immunol Today 18: 263–265 (Very good, succinct review)

Roth J, LeRoith D et al. 1982 The evolutionary origins of hormones, neurotransmitters and other extracellular chemical messengers. N Engl J Med 306: 523–527

Samuelsson B 1983 Leukotrienes: mediators of immediate hypersensitivity reactions and inflammation. Science 220: 568–575

Serhan C N, Haeggström J Z, Leslie C C 1996 Lipid mediator networks in cell signalling: update and impact of cytokines. FASEB J 10: 1147–1158

Steinman L 1993 Autoimmune disease. Scientific American 269: 74–83

Steranka L R, Farmer S G, Burch R M 1989 Antagonists of B_2 bradykinin receptors. FASEB J 3: 2019–2025

Strom T B, Kelly V R, Murphy J R, Nichols J 1993 Interleukin-2 receptor-directed therapies: antibody- or cytokine-based targeting molecules. Annu Rev Med 44: 343–353

Szolcsànyi J 1996 Neurogenic inflammation: reevaluation of the axon reflex theory. In: Geppetti P, Holzer P (eds) Neurogenic inflammation. CRC Press, London, Ch. 3, pp 33–42 (Good coverage of the basis of neurogenic inflammation)

Vane J R 1971 Inhibition of prostaglandin synthesis as a mechanism of action for aspirin-like drugs. Nature New Biol 231: 232–239 (Definitive, seminal article)

Vane J, O'Grady J (eds) 1993 Therapeutic applications of prostaglandins. Edward Arnold, London

Wardlaw A J, Moqbel R, Kay A B 1994 The eosinophil leucocyte. In: Dale M M, Foreman J C, Fan T-P (eds) Textbook of immunopharmacology, 3rd edn. Blackwell Scientific Publications, Oxford, Ch 5, pp 55–63

Winter G, Harris W J 1993 Humanised antibodies. Trends Pharmacol Sci 14: 139–143

Witt P L, Linder D J et al. 1996 Pharmacology of interferons: induced proteins, cell activation, and antitumour activity. In: Chabner B A, Longo D L (eds) Cancer chemotherapy and biotherapy. Lippincott-Raven, Philadelphia, ch 25, pp 585–607 *(Comprehensive review)*

13

Anti-inflammatory and immunosuppressant drugs

The main *anti-inflammatory agents* are the **glucocorticoids** and the **non-steroidal anti-inflammatory drugs**. The glucocorticoids are dealt with in detail in Chapter 24 and their immunosuppressive actions are discussed briefly at the end of this chapter; the non-steroidal anti-inflammatory drugs (NSAIDs) are dealt with below. Other anti-inflammatory drugs considered in this chapter are the **antirheumatoid agents** and **drugs used to treat gout**; the **histamine H_1-receptor antagonists** are also dealt with under this heading. The main *drugs affecting the immune response* are the immunosuppressants; agents which increase or modify the immune response are also briefly described.

NON-STEROIDAL ANTI-INFLAMMATORY DRUGS (NSAIDS)

Non-steroidal anti-inflammatory drugs are among the most widely used of all therapeutic agents. Some important examples are listed in Table 13.1. They are frequently prescribed for 'rheumatic' musculoskeletal complaints and are often taken without prescription for minor aches and pains. There are now more than 50 different NSAIDs on the market and none of these is ideal in controlling or modifying the signs and symptoms of inflammation, particularly those that occur in the common inflammatory joint diseases. Virtually all currently available NSAIDs can have significant unwanted effects, especially in the elderly. This situation is likely to improve as a result of recent research findings.

PHARMACOLOGICAL ACTIONS

NSAIDs include a variety of different agents of different chemical classes. Most of these drugs have three major types of effect:

- *anti-inflammatory effects:* modification of the inflammatory reaction
- *analgesic effect:* reduction of certain sorts of pain
- *antipyretic effect:* lowering of a raised temperature.

In general, all of these effects are related to the primary action of the drugs—inhibition of arachidonate cyclo-oxygenase (COX) and thus inhibition of the production of prostaglandins and thromboxanes—though some aspects of the action of individual drugs may occur by different mechanisms.

There are two types of COX enzyme, namely COX-1 and COX-2. COX-1 is a constitutive enzyme expressed in most tissues, including blood platelets, and is involved in cell–cell signalling and in tissue homeostasis. COX-2 is induced in inflammatory cells when they are activated and the primary inflammatory cytokines—interleukin-1 and tumour necrosis factor-α (see Ch. 12, p. 224)—are important in this regard. Thus COX-2 is responsible for the production of the prostanoid mediators of inflammation (Vane & Botting 1996). Most NSAIDs in current use are inhibitors of both isoenzymes, though they vary in the degree of inhibition of each (Griswold & Adams 1996). Clearly the anti-inflammatory action of the NSAIDs is mainly related to their inhibition of COX-2 and it is probable that, when used as anti-inflammatory agents, their unwanted effects are due largely to their inhibition of COX-1. New compounds with a selective action on

Table 13.1 Comparison of some commonly used NSAIDs

Drug	Plasma $t_{1/2}$ (hours)	Comments
Aspirin	3–5	See text, page 234
Diflunisal	8–13	Less GIT irritation than aspirin. Long-acting
Ibuprofen	2	First choice drug. Lowest incidence of unwanted effects
Fenbufen	10	A pro-drug, activated in the liver. Less risk of GIT, reactions, more risk of skin reactions
Naproxen	14	The same chemical class as ibuprofen but rather more potent; reasonable efficacy, moderate risk of adverse reactions
Mefenamic acid	4	Only moderate anti-inflammatory action. Diarrhoea likely. Haemolytic anaemia has been reported. Possible interaction with warfarin. Skin reactions can occur
Nabumetone	24*	A pro-drug, activated in the liver. Adverse effects less marked than with aspirin, antipyretic action more marked
Paracetamol	2–4	See text, page 236
Diclofenac	1–2	Moderate potency. Moderate risk of adverse GIT effects
Sulindac	7(18)*	A pro-drug interconvertible with active sulphide metabolite. Moderate risk of side-effects. Chemically related to indomethacin but less potent
Indomethacin	2	Potent inhibitor of COX in vitro. High incidence of non-GIT side-effects;[†] headache, dizziness, etc.
Tolmetin	5	Efficacy as for ibuprofen. Moderate risk of adverse effects
Piroxicam	45	GIT irritation in 20% of patients. Tinnitus. Rashes
Tenoxicam	72	Steady-state plasma concentration only after 2 weeks
Etodalac	7	New compound; so far few side-effects
Meloxicam	?	New compound; Weak action on COX-1 in GIT
Nimuselide	?	New compound. Markedly less GIT toxicity

*Half-life of metabolite. See also Table 13.2 for more detail on adverse reactions.
[†]See MacDonald et al. 1997.

COX-2 are in the pipeline and might well transform the approach to the treatment of inflammatory conditions.*

Assessing the COX selectivity of currently used drugs has proved to be a problem, since different assay systems can give different values for the same compound (see Griswold & Adams 1996). Furthermore, some agents (e.g. indomethacin, flurbiprofen) have time-dependent action, others (e.g. piroxicam, ibuprofen) do not.**

At best, the selectivity can only be approximated. The following values are taken mostly from Vane & Botting (1996) and are based on measurements of the IC_{50} (μM) in intact cells (unless otherwise stated), the ratio of COX-2 to COX-1 being given in brackets:

- Relatively selective for COX-1: **aspirin** (166), **indomethacin** (60), **sulindac** (100), **piroxicam** (250), **tolmetin** (175)
- Less selective for COX-1: **ibuprofen** (15), **paracetamol** (7.5)
- Equipotent on both enzymes: **naproxen** (0.6), **flurbiprofen** (1.3), **diclofenac** (0.7), **nabumetone***** (1.4)
- More selective for COX-2: **nimuselide***** (0.018), and celecoxib and rofecoxib, the latter two having been recently approved for the treatment of arthritis.

Not all NSAIDs manifest the three types of actions specified above to the same extent. Virtually all are analgesic and antipyretic, but the degree of anti-inflammatory activity varies: some (**indomethacin**, **piroxicam**) are strongly anti-inflammatory, most are moderately anti-inflammatory (**ibuprofen** and **nabumetone** being less so than the others), some (**paracetamol**) have minimum anti-inflammatory action.

In addition to these three categories of action, **aspirin**,

*It has been shown, in early clinical trials, that several new selective COX-2 inhibitors are anti-inflammatory and analgesic but have no adverse gastric action; see Vane & Botting (1998a).

**All four compounds listed inhibit both enzymes instantly—COX-1 more than COX-2, indomethacin being the most potent; but after 30-min incubation, indomethacin and flurbiprofen each shows significantly increased inhibition (indomethacin again being more potent), and each is equiactive on the two enzymes, their effect on COX-1 being partially reversible.

***Measurements on recombinant enzyme (Griswold & Adams 1996)

in particular, has other, qualitatively different pharmacological actions (see below, p. 234).

The main pharmacological actions and the common side-effects of the NSAIDs are outlined below, followed by a more detailed coverage of the salicylates and paracetamol and finally the clinical applications of the group as a whole.

Antipyretic effect

Normal body temperature is regulated by a centre in the hypothalamus which ensures a balance between heat loss and heat production. Fever occurs when there is a disturbance of this hypothalamic 'thermostat' that leads to the set-point of body temperature being raised. NSAIDs reset the thermostat. Once there has been a return to the normal set-point, the temperature-regulating mechanisms (dilatation of superficial blood vessels, sweating, etc.) then operate to reduce temperature. Normal temperature is not affected by NSAIDs.

The mechanism of the antipyretic action of the NSAIDs is thought to be due largely to inhibition of prostaglandin production in the hypothalamus. During an inflammatory reaction, bacterial endotoxins cause the release from macrophages of a pyrogen—interleukin-1 (IL-1; Ch. 12) —which stimulates the generation, in the hypothalamus, of E-type prostaglandins and these, in turn, cause the elevation of the set-point for temperature (reviewed by Foreman 1994). There is some evidence that prostaglandins are not the only mediators of fever; hence NSAIDs may have an additional antipyretic effect by mechanisms as yet unknown.

Analgesic effect

NSAIDs are mainly effective against pain associated with inflammation or tissue damage because they decrease production of the prostaglandins that sensitise nociceptors to inflammatory mediators such as bradykinin (see Chs 12 and 37). Therefore they are effective in arthritis, bursitis, pain of muscular and vascular origin, toothache, dysmenorrhoea, the pain of postpartum states and the pain of cancer metastases in bone—all conditions that are associated with increased prostaglandin synthesis. In combination with opioids, they decrease postoperative pain and in some cases can reduce the requirement for opioids by as much as one-third. Their ability to relieve headache may be related to the abrogation of the vasodilator effect of prostaglandins on the cerebral vasculature.

There is some evidence that they have a central effect—by an action mainly in the spinal cord.

Clinical data indicate that certain NSAIDs (e.g. **indomethacin, diflunisal, naproxen**) are effective in the control of some types of severe pain unrelated to inflammation (Rainsford 1984).

Anti-inflammatory effects

As has been described in Chapter 12, there are many chemical mediators of the inflammatory and allergic response. Each facet of the response—vasodilatation, increased vascular permeability, cell accumulation, etc.—can be produced by several different mechanisms. Furthermore, different mediators may be of particular importance in different inflammatory and allergic conditions and some mediators have complex interactions with others; thus, for example, small amounts of nitric oxide stimulates COX activity, large amounts inhibit it.

Drugs such as the NSAIDs reduce mainly those components of the inflammatory and immune response in which the products of COX-2 action play a significant part, namely:

- vasodilatation
- oedema (by an *indirect* action—the vasodilatation facilitates and potentiates the action of mediators such as histamine which increase the permeability of postcapillary venules; see p. 213)
- pain (see above).

COX inhibitors, per se, have no effect on those processes (lysosomal enzyme release, toxic O_2 radical production) that contribute to *tissue damage* in chronic inflammatory conditions such as rheumatoid arthritis, vasculitis and nephritis. In fact, because some prostaglandins (e.g. PGE_2 and PGI_2) *decrease* lysosomal enzyme release, *reduce* the generation of toxic O_2 products and *inhibit* lymphocyte activation, NSAIDs could actually exacerbate tissue damage in the long term.* Indeed a study in 105 osteoarthritis patients indicated that the arthritis progressed more quickly in patients treated with a strong inhibitor of cyclo-oxygenase (indomethacin) than in those treated with azapropazone, a weak inhibitor (Rashad et al. 1989).

MECHANISM OF ACTION

The main action of NSAIDs is, as stated above, *inhibition of arachidonate cyclo-oxygenase* (see Figs 12.4 and 12.7), as described originally by Vane in 1971.

---

*Certain NSAIDs can, in fact, be shown to *increase* pro-inflammatory stimuli (e.g. IL-1 generation; Bahl et al. 1994) and tissue-damaging processes (e.g. toxic oxygen radical production; Twomey & Dale 1992) by direct action on the relevant cells.

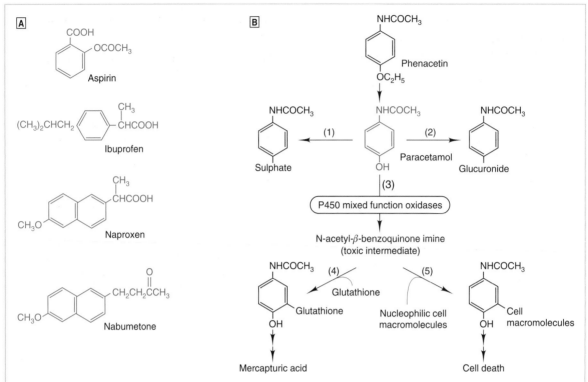

Fig. 13.1 **A** **The structure of some NSAIDs;** **B** **the metabolism of phenacetin and paracetamol.** With normal therapeutic doses, paracetamol is metabolised by pathways 1 and 2, and with higher doses, by pathways 3 and 4. When glutathione is depleted, the toxic intermediate interacts with proteins and there is cell damage (reaction 5). More details on the events which can follow from reaction 5 are given in Chapter 49.

COX is a bifunctional enzyme, having two distinct activities—the main cyclo-oxygenase action (steps 1 and 2 in Fig. 12.7) which gives PGG$_2$, and a peroxidase action which converts PGG$_2$ to PGH$_2$. Different NSAIDs inhibit the enzyme by different mechanisms, but all act at the first of the two sites.

The mechanism whereby NSAIDs inhibit cyclo-oxygenase is gradually being elucidated as a result of X-ray crystallographic analysis of the enzyme and its interaction with drugs, the initial work being done on COX-1. This has shown that in COX-1, the main cyclo-oxygenase site (as distinct from the peroxidase site) is a long hydrophobic channel. **Aspirin** (Fig. 13.1) causes *irreversible inactivation* of the enzyme by acetylating a serine residue at the apex of this channel thereby excluding arachidonate (Picot et al. 1994). Other NSAIDs (e.g. **flurbiprofen**) bind to other sites in the channel, producing the same effect; but aspirin is the only NSAID to cause covalent modification of the enzyme.

Paracetamol has analgesic and antipyretic activity but minimal anti-inflammatory effects.* It is possible that its antipyretic action is due to a selective effect on a specific COX isoenzyme in the CNS.

Other actions besides inhibition of cyclo-oxygenase may contribute to the anti-inflammatory effects of some NSAIDs. Reactive oxygen radicals produced by neutrophils and macrophages are implicated in tissue damage in some conditions, and NSAIDs that have particularly strong O$_2$-radical-scavenging effects as well as cyclo-oxygenase-inhibitory activity (such as **sulindac**) may decrease tissue damage.

COMMON UNWANTED EFFECTS

NSAIDs are responsible for nearly a quarter of the adverse drug reactions reported officially in the UK, and they also feature in the reports of drug-related deaths.

*Some authors state that paracetamol has significant anti-inflammatory action (see Skjelbred et al. 1984).

Non-steroidal anti-inflammatory drugs (NSAIDs)

NSAIDs have three major actions, all of which are due mainly to the inhibition of arachidonic acid cyclo-oxygenase in inflammatory cells (the COX-2 isoenzyme), and the resultant decrease in prostanoid synthesis.

- An anti-inflammatory action: the decrease in vasodilator prostaglandins (PGE_2, PGI_2) means less vasodilatation and, indirectly, less oedema. Accumulation of inflammatory cells is not reduced.
- An analgesic effect: decreased prostaglandin generation means less sensitisation of nociceptive nerve endings to inflammatory mediators such as bradykinin and 5-hydroxytryptamine. Relief of headache is probably due to decreased prostaglandin-mediated vasodilatation.
- An antipyretic effect: this is partly due to a decrease in the mediator prostaglandin (which is generated in response to the inflammatory pyrogen, interleukin-1) that is responsible for elevating the hypothalamic set-point for temperature control in fever.

Some important examples are aspirin, ibuprofen, naproxen, indomethacin, piroxicam, paracetamol. (The last agent has analgesic and antipyretic effects but little anti-inflammatory action.)

Table 13.2 Reports of serious unwanted reactions to NSAIDs*

Drug	Number of prescriptions (million)	Serious GIT reactions[†]	Serious reactions other than GIT[†]
Ibuprofen	5.47	6.6	6.6
Naproxen	4.67	32.8	8.4
Flurbiprofen	3.35	27.4	8.4
Fenbufen	1.57	35.7	33.8
Indomethacin (slow-release)[‡]	0.44	386.4	18.2
Sulindac	1.38	23.9	18.2
Piroxicam	9.16	58.7	9.4
Diflunisal	3.13	33.5	13.7

*Taken from the CSM Update by the Committee on Safety of Medicines (1986) in Br Med J 292: 1190. The data refer to prescription-related reports on the drugs during their first 5 years of marketing. See also MacDonald et al. 1997.
[†]Per million prescriptions
[‡]This formulation now withdrawn.

Although this may be partly because NSAIDs are used extensively in the elderly, the inherent toxicity of these drugs is clearly a contributory factor. When NSAIDs are used in joint diseases (which usually necessitates fairly large doses and long-continued use) there is a high incidence of side-effects—more particularly in the gastrointestinal tract but also in liver, kidney, spleen, blood and bone marrow (see Rainsford & Velo 1992). Table 13.2 outlines the risks of serious unwanted effects specific for the main NSAIDs.

Gastrointestinal disturbances

Adverse gastrointestinal events are the commonest unwanted effects of the NSAIDs, the relative risk being on average three times that in the population of non-NSAID users. Common gastrointestinal side-effects are dyspepsia, diarrhoea (but sometimes constipation), nausea and vomiting. It has been estimated that one in five *chronic* users of NSAIDs will have gastric damage, which can be silent but which carries a small but definite risk of serious haemorrhage and/or perforation. Patients using **piroxicam** have the highest risk of gastric bleeding; there is less risk with **diclofenac, meloxicam** and **naproxen**, less still with **ibuprofen** (Bateman 1994) and least with **nimuselide**.

NSAID-induced gastric damage is due mainly to the inhibition of COX-1 which is responsible for the synthesis of the prostaglandins that normally inhibit acid secretion, as well as having a protective action on the mucosa and modulating its blood flow (see Ch. 21, p. 371 and Fig. 21.2). Oral administration of prostaglandin analogues such as **misoprostol** (Ch. 12, clinical box on p. 218) can diminish NSAID-induced gastric damage.

Skin reactions

Skin reactions are the second most common unwanted effects of NSAIDs, particularly with **mefenamic acid** (10–15% frequency) and **sulindac** (5–10% frequency). The type of skin condition seen varies from mild rashes, urticaria, and photosensitivity reactions to more serious and potentially fatal diseases (which are fortunately rare).

Adverse renal effects

Therapeutic doses of NSAIDs in healthy individuals pose little threat to kidney function, but in some, susceptible patients, they cause acute renal insufficiency, which is reversible on stopping the drug. The basis of this effect is the inhibition of the biosynthesis of those prostanoids (PGE_2, PGI_2) involved in the maintenance of renal blood dynamics, and more particularly in the PGE_2-mediated compensatory vasodilatation that occurs in response to the action of noradrenaline or angiotensin II (see Ch. 20, p. 359).

Chronic NSAID consumption can cause 'analgesic nephropathy' which comprises chronic nephritis and renal papillary necrosis. Phenacetin (see Fig. 13.1), now withdrawn, was regarded as the main culprit. It is rapidly metabolised to another NSAID, **paracetamol** (see Fig. 13.1), and there is now a suggestion that paracetamol (and possibly some other NSAIDs) taken regularly in high doses over a long period, could increase the risk of similar renal disease. However, the daily use of small doses of aspirin, on its own, is not reported to be hazardous for the kidney.

More detail on the toxic effects of NSAIDs on the kidney is given in Chapter 49, pages 762–764; see also De Broe & Elseviers (1998).

Other unwanted effects

Other, much less common, unwanted effects of NSAIDs include bone marrow disturbances and liver disorders, the latter more likely if there is already renal impairment. Overdose of paracetamol causes liver failure (see below). NSAIDs (in particular, aspirin) may precipitate asthma in NSAID-sensitive asthmatic patients (see Ch. 19).

General unwanted effects of NSAIDs

Unwanted effects are common, particularly in the elderly, and include:

- Dyspepsia, nausea and vomiting; also gastric damage in chronic users, with risk of haemorrhage, due to abrogation of the protective effect of PGE_2 on gastric mucosa.
- Skin reactions.
- Reversible renal insufficiency (in individuals who have noradrenergic- or angiotensin-mediated vasoconstriction) due to lack of compensatory PGE_2-mediated vasodilatation.
- 'Analgesic-associated nephropathy'; this can occur following long-continued high doses of NSAIDs (e.g. paracetamol), and is often irreversible.
- Less commonly, liver disorders, bone marrow depression.
- Bronchospasm in 'aspirin-sensitive' asthmatics.

THE SALICYLATES AND PARACETAMOL

The salicylates

Natural products that contain precursors of salicylic acid, such as willow bark (which contains the glycoside salicin) and oil of wintergreen (which contains methyl-salicylate) have long been used for the treatment of rheumatism. Salicylic acid and acetylsalicylic acid (**aspirin**) were amongst the earliest drugs synthesised, and aspirin is now one of the most commonly consumed drugs, world-wide. **Sodium salicylate** is a salt of salicylic acid that has two-thirds of the potency of aspirin. Aspirin itself is relatively insoluble but its sodium and calcium salts are readily soluble. **Methylsalicylate** is used only in topical application. A newer member of this group is **diflunisal** (Table 13.1).

Aspirin in non-inflammatory conditions

It is becoming increasingly clear that aspirin—previously thought of as an old anti-inflammatory workhorse—is now approaching the status of wonder drug in that it is of benefit not only in inflammation but in an increasing number of other conditions:

- As a result of its antiplatelet action (Ch. 17, p. 321) low-dose aspirin is effective in cardiovascular disorders* (see Ch. 17, p. 324).
- Epidemiological studies have suggested that regular and sustained use of aspirin reduces (virtually halves) the risk of cancer of the colon and possibly also rectal cancer (which between them cause 25 000 deaths a year in the UK).
- There is preliminary evidence that aspirin reduces the risk (and retards the onset) of Alzheimer's disease (Ch. 31).
- Aspirin has been used to treat radiation-induced diarrhoea.

Pharmacokinetic aspects

As salicylates are weak acids, they are largely unionised in the acid environment of the stomach and their absorption is thus facilitated. However, most absorption occurs in the ileum because of the extensive surface area of the microvilli. Aspirin is hydrolysed by esterases in the plasma and the tissues—particularly the liver—yielding salicylate.** With low therapeutic doses most of the salicylate in the plasma is protein-bound. With high concentrations, however, relatively less is bound and more is available for action in the tissues. Approximately 25% of the salicylate is oxidised, some is conjugated to give the glucuronide or sulphate before excretion and

---

*Clinicians increasingly now classify aspirin as a cardiovascular drug and do not regard it as an NSAID.

**A possible basis for the selectivity of aspirin for platelet COX (as compared with vascular endothelium COX), is that platelet COX is acetylated in the portal circulation whereas the systemic vasculature is only exposed to salicylate as it emerges from the liver, and salicylate lacks antiplatelet action.

about 25% is excreted unchanged. The rate of urinary excretion is higher in alkaline than in acid urine since more of the unchanged salicylate will be ionised and therefore less will be reabsorbed in the tubules (see Ch. 4).

Because of partial saturation of the hepatic enzymes, the plasma half-life of aspirin will depend on the dose. With low dosage the $t_{1/2}$ is approximately 4 hours, and elimination follows first-order kinetics. With high doses (more than 4 g per day), elimination follows saturation kinetics (see Ch. 4) and the drug persists for more than 15 hours. (Note that the duration of action is not directly related to the plasma $t_{1/2}$ because of the irreversible nature of the action of the drug.)

Unwanted effects

Salicylates may produce local and systemic toxic effects.

Local effects. In the stomach, aspirin can cause gastritis with focal erosions and bleeding due to inhibition of the gastric mucosal cyclo-oxygenase with consequent loss of the mucosal-protecting action of the prostaglandins (see 'Unwanted effects' above). A study of 200 individuals with normal digestive tracts, who were given aspirin, showed that most lost 2–6 ml of blood per day in the faeces; some lost a good deal more. In addition to the action on gastric mucosal cyclo-oxygenase, an inhibitory effect on platelet cyclo-oxygenase, specific to aspirin, with consequent decrease of platelet aggregation (see Ch. 17) would contribute to the bleeding.

Systemic effects. Salicylates have many of the general unwanted effects of NSAIDs outlined above (pp. 232–234). In addition there are certain unwanted effects that occur specifically with salicylates.

Salicylism can occur with repeated ingestion of fairly large doses of salicylate. It is a syndrome consisting of tinnitus (a high-pitched buzzing noise), vertigo (a sensation of spinning, akin to being drunk), decreased hearing and sometimes also nausea and vomiting.

Other unwanted systemic effects include skin rashes and worsening of asthma in aspirin-sensitive patients. There is an association between aspirin intake and Reye's syndrome, which is a rare disorder in children. It is a combination of liver disorder and encephalopathy (CNS disturbances) that can follow an acute viral illness and it has a 20–40% mortality. It is not entirely clear to what extent aspirin is in fact implicated in its causation but the drug is best avoided in children with viral infections.

Salicylates can also cause various metabolic changes, the nature of which depends on the dose. Large therapeutic doses of salicylate *alter the acid–base balance and the electrolyte balance* and toxic doses have serious effects on these functions. The sequence of events with high doses is as follows: salicylates uncouple oxidative phosphorylation (mainly in skeletal muscle) leading to increased O_2 consumption and thus increased production of CO_2. This stimulates respiration. Salicylates also stimulate respiration by a direct action on the respiratory centre. The resulting hyperventilation causes a respiratory alkalosis that is normally compensated for by renal mechanisms, involving increased bicarbonate excretion. This condition of *compensated respiratory alkalosis* can occur in patients receiving high therapeutic doses of salicylates. Larger doses can cause a depression of the respiratory centre, which leads eventually to retention of CO_2 and thus an increase in plasma CO_2. Since this is superimposed on a reduction in plasma bicarbonate, an *uncompensated respiratory acidosis* will occur. This may be complicated by a *metabolic acidosis*, which is due to the accumulation of metabolites of pyruvic, lactic and acetoacetic acids (an indirect consequence of interference with carbohydrate metabolism) and the acid load associated with the salicylate itself.

Hyperpyrexia is likely to be present owing to the increased metabolic rate, and dehydration may follow from excessive vomiting.

With toxic doses of salicylates, *disturbance of haemostasis* can also occur, mainly as a result of an action on platelet aggregation. The effect of these doses on the CNS is, initially, stimulation with excitement but eventually coma and respiratory depression.

Salicylate poisoning, with the signs and symptoms outlined above, occurs more commonly, and is more serious, in children than in adults. The acid–base disturbance seen in children is usually a metabolic acidosis whereas that in adults is a respiratory alkalosis. Salicylate poisoning constitutes a medical emergency and the treatment requires correction of the acid–base disturbance, therapy for the dehydration and hyperthermia, and maintenance of kidney function. Gastric lavage and forced alkaline diuresis are used for removal of the drug (the latter procedure only if there is adequate circulatory and renal function).

Some important interactions with other drugs

Aspirin causes a potentially hazardous increase in the effect of warfarin, partly by displacing it from plasma proteins (Ch. 49) and partly because its effect on platelets interferes with haemostatic mechanisms (see Ch. 17). Sodium salicylate does not have this effect. Aspirin interferes with the effect of uricosuric agents such as **probenecid** and **sulphinpyrazone**, and since low doses of aspirin may, on their own, reduce urate excretion, aspirin should not be used in gout.

Paracetamol

Paracetamol (called acetaminophen in the USA) is one of the most commonly used non-narcotic analgesic–antipyretic agents. It has only weak anti-inflammatory activity. Its mechanism of action and the possible explanation of its differential actions on pain and inflammation are discussed above.

Pharmacokinetic aspects

Paracetamol is given orally and is well absorbed; peak plasma concentrations are reached in 30–60 minutes. A variable proportion is bound to plasma proteins and the drug is inactivated in the liver, being conjugated to give the glucuronide or sulphate (reactions 1 and 2 in Fig. 13.1). The plasma half-life of paracetamol with therapeutic doses is 2–4 hours but with toxic doses it may be extended to 4–8 hours.

Unwanted effects

With therapeutic doses, side-effects are few and uncommon, though allergic skin reactions sometimes occur. It is thought that regular intake of large doses over a long period may increase the risk of kidney damage (see above, p. 233).

Toxic doses (i.e. two to three times the maximum therapeutic dose) cause a serious, potentially fatal hepato-

toxicity. Renal toxicity can also occur. These toxic effects occur when the liver enzymes catalysing the normal conjugation reactions are saturated, causing the drug to be metabolised by the mixed function oxidases (reaction 3 in Fig. 13.1). The resulting toxic metabolite, N-acetyl-p-benzoquinone imine is inactivated by conjugation with glutathione (reaction 4 in Fig. 13.1), but when glutathione is depleted the toxic intermediate accumulates and reacts with nucleophilic constituents in the cell. This causes necrosis in the liver and also in the kidney tubules (reaction 5 in Fig. 13.1).

The initial symptoms of acute paracetamol poisoning are nausea and vomiting, the hepatotoxicity being a delayed manifestation that occurs 24–48 hours later. Treatment entails gastric lavage followed by oral activated charcoal. Further details of the toxic effects of paracetamol are given in Chapter 49. If the patient is seen sufficiently soon after ingestion, the liver damage can be prevented by giving agents that increase glutathione formation in the liver (**acetylcysteine** intravenously, or **methionine** orally).

If more than 12 hours have passed since the ingestion of a large dose, the antidotes, which themselves can cause adverse effects (nausea, allergic reactions) are less likely to be useful.

The clinical uses of the NSAIDs are summarised on page 237.

ANTIRHEUMATOID DRUGS

Rheumatoid disease is one of the commonest chronic inflammatory conditions in developed countries and rheumatoid arthritis is a common cause of disability. One in three patients with rheumatoid arthritis is likely to be severely disabled in 20 years. The primary inflam-

- For analgesia in painful conditions (e.g. headache, dysmenorrhoea, backache, bony metastases of cancers, postoperative pain):
  — The drugs of choice for short-term analgesia are aspirin, paracetamol and ibuprofen; more potent, longer-acting drugs (diflunisal, naproxen, piroxicam) are useful for chronic pain.
  — The requirement for narcotic analgesics can be markedly reduced by NSAIDs in some patients with bony metastases or postoperative pain.
- For anti-inflammatory effects in chronic or acute inflammatory conditions (e.g. rheumatoid arthritis and related connective tissue disorders, gout and soft tissue diseases). With many NSAIDs, the dosage required for chronic inflammatory disorders is usually greater than for simple analgesia and treatment may need to be continued for long periods; thus side-effects and toxic effects are likely to be seen. Treatment could be initiated with an agent known to have a low incidence of side-effects, such as ibuprofen. If this proves unsatisfactory, more potent agents (see Table 13.1) should be used.
- To lower temperature. Paracetamol is preferred because it lacks gastrointestinal side-effects and, unlike aspirin, has not been associated with Reye's syndrome in children.
- There is substantial individual variation in clinical response to NSAIDs and considerable unpredictable patient preference for one drug rather than another.

matory cytokines, interleukin-1 (IL-1) and tumour necrosis factor-α (TNF-α), have a major role in pathogenesis. The drugs used in therapy are the NSAIDs and the disease-modifying antirheumatoid drugs (DMARDs)—the latter so called to point up the comparison with the NSAIDs—which reduce the symptoms of rheumatoid disease but do not retard the progress of the disease (some, indeed, may make it worse).

DMARDs improve symptoms and can reduce disease activity in rheumatoid arthritis as measured by reduction in number of swollen and tender joints, pain score, disability score, articular index on radiology, and the serum concentration of acute-phase proteins and of rheumatoid factor (an IgM antibody against host IgG);[*] however, whether they halt the long-term progress of the disease is controversial, so the term 'disease-modifying' may be over-optimistic.

*The American College of Rheumatology has recommended specific criteria for defining improvement in rheumatoid arthritis (Felson et al. 1995).

The term DMARD is a latex concept that can be stretched to cover a variety of agents with different chemical structures and mechanisms of action. Included in this category are the **gold compounds**, **penicillamine**, **sulphasalazine**, **methotrexate** (see Ch. 42, p. 675) and some 4-aminoquinoline drugs—**chloroquine** and **hydroxychloroquine**. The antirheumatoid action of these agents was discovered, some more than 20 years ago, by serendipity and clinical intuition. When introduced, nothing was known about their mechanism of action in these conditions, and decades of in vitro experiments have resulted in bewilderment rather than understanding.

DMARDs may also be referred to as 'second-line drugs', and some have a place in the treatment of other chronic inflammatory diseases. The effects of this group of drugs on rheumatoid conditions are slow in onset and some (e.g. penicillamine) are not thought to have a general anti-inflammatory action.

Antirheumatoid agents for which, unlike the DMARDs, the mechanism of action *is* known are some immunosuppressants (e.g. **azathioprine**, **cyclosporin**) (see below, p. 242, and Ch. 42) and the **glucocorticoids** (covered in Ch. 24).

Mechanisms of action of DMARDs are reviewed by Bondeson (1997) and clinical applications of antirheumatoid drugs are reviewed by Porter & Sturrock (1993).

Cytokine-targeted therapies for rheumatoid conditions are coming on line (discussed below, p. 245).

Sulphasalazine

Sulphasalazine, commonly a first choice DMARD in the UK, produces remission in active rheumatoid arthritis. It is also used for chronic inflammatory bowel disease.

The mode of action of sulphasalazine is not clearly known but there is evidence that it can scavenge toxic oxygen metabolites produced by neutrophils.

This drug is a combination of sulphonamide (sulphapyridine) with a salicylate. It is split into its component parts by bacteria in the colon. Both moieties may be important but 5-amino-salicylic acid is the radical scavenger. It is poorly absorbed after oral administration. The common side-effects are gastrointestinal disturbances, malaise and headache. Skin reactions and leukopenia can occur but are reversible on stopping the drug. The absorption of folic acid is sometimes impaired; this can be countered by giving folic acid supplements. A reversible decrease in sperm count has also been reported. As with other sulphonamides, blood dyscrasias and anaphylactic-type reactions may occur in a few patients.

Gold compounds

The gold compounds used are **sodium aurothiomalate** and **auranofin**.

Actions and mechanism of action

The effect develops slowly, the maximum action occurring after 3–4 months. Pain and joint swelling subside and the progression of bone and joint damage diminishes.

The *mechanism of action* is not fully understood. In experimental studies, gold compounds inhibit mitogen-induced lymphocyte proliferation, reduce both the release and the activity of lysosomal enzymes, decrease the production of toxic O_2 metabolites from phagocytes, inhibit chemotaxis of neutrophils and reduce the release of mast cell mediators. Auranofin, but not aurothiomalate, inhibits the induction of IL-1 and TNF-α.

Pharmacokinetic aspects

Sodium aurothiomalate is given by deep intramuscular injection; auranofin is given orally. Peak plasma concentrations of aurothiomalate are reached in 2–6 hours. The compounds gradually become concentrated in the tissues, not only in synovial cells in joints (where the concentration is 50% of the plasma concentration) but also in macrophages throughout the body, and in liver cells, kidney tubules and the adrenal cortex. The gold complexes remain in the tissues for some time after treatment is stopped. Excretion is mostly renal, but some is excreted in the gastrointestinal tract. The $t_{1/2}$ is 7 days initially but increases with treatment, so the drug is usually given first at weekly then at monthly intervals.

Unwanted effects

Unwanted effects with aurothiomalate are seen in about one-third of patients treated, and serious toxic effects in about 1 patient in 10. Unwanted effects with auranofin are less frequent and less severe.

Important unwanted effects are skin rashes (which can be severe), mouth ulcers, proteinuria and blood dyscrasias. Encephalopathy, peripheral neuropathy and hepatitis can occur. If therapy is stopped when the early symptoms appear, the incidence of serious toxic effects is relatively low.

Penicillamine

Penicillamine is dimethylcysteine and is one of the substances produced by hydrolysis of penicillin. The D-isomer is used in the therapy of rheumatoid disease.

Actions and mechanism of action

About 75% of patients with rheumatoid arthritis respond to penicillamine. The effects take weeks to start and the main response is not seen for several months.

Penicillamine is thought to modify rheumatoid disease partly by decreasing IL-1 generation and/or partly by an effect on collagen synthesis, preventing the maturation of newly synthesised collagen. This latter action occurs at a late stage of collagen cross-linking.

The mechanism of action is still a matter of conjecture. The drug is known to have metal-chelating properties, an effect that is made use of in the treatment of hepatolenticular degeneration (Wilson's disease), in which there is copper accumulation in liver, kidneys and brain.

Penicillamine is a highly reactive thiol compound, and in addition to chelating metals, can substitute for cysteine (cys) in cysteine disulphide (cystine, cys–S–S–cys), the resulting complex being very much more soluble. This is the basis of its use in cystinuria—an inheritable disorder in which there is a defect in the transport of certain amino acids, associated with a very high concentration of cystine in the urine.

Pharmacokinetic aspects

Penicillamine is given orally and only half the dose administered is absorbed. It reaches peak plasma concentrations in 1–2 hours and is excreted in the urine. Dosage is started low and increased only gradually to avoid unwanted effects.

Unwanted effects

Unwanted effects occur in about 40% of patients treated and may necessitate cessation of therapy. Anorexia, nausea and vomiting and disturbances of taste (the latter related to the chelation of zinc) are seen but often disappear with continued treatment. In 20% of patients proteinuria occurs. Rashes and stomatitis are the most common unwanted effects and may resolve if the dosage is lowered, as may dose-related thrombocytopenia. Other bone marrow disorders (leukopenia, aplastic anaemia) are absolute indications for stopping therapy, as are the various autoimmune conditions (e.g. thyroiditis, myasthenia gravis) that sometimes supervene.

Penicillamine is a metal chelator and so should not be given with gold compounds.

Chloroquine

Chloroquine is a 4-aminoquinoline drug used mainly to treat malaria (Ch. 46). It has been shown to cause remission of rheumatoid arthritis but it does not retard the progression of bone damage. It is also used in both systemic and discoid lupus erythematosus.

Actions and the mechanism of action

Pharmacological effects do not come on until a month or more after the drug is started, and about half the patients treated respond.

The mechanism of action of chloroquine in rheumatoid disease is not fully understood. The drug inhibits mitogen-induced lymphocyte proliferation and decreases leukocyte chemotaxis, lysosomal enzyme release and generation of toxic oxygen metabolites. It also reduces the generation of IL-1. Some of these effects may follow from the fact that it has a lysosomotrophic action, being concentrated in and raising the pH of lysosomes, particularly in phagocytic cells such as macrophages, and thus interfering with the action of the acid hydrolases.

Some effects may result from the fact that it inhibits phospholipase A$_2$ and therefore reduces the formation of the eicosanoids and also PAF (p. 219). It may also intercalate in the DNA and inhibit DNA and RNA synthesis, as it does in microorganisms.

Pharmacokinetic aspects and unwanted effects

The pharmacokinetic aspects and unwanted effects of chloroquine are dealt with in Chapter 46.

Methotrexate

Methotrexate, a folic acid antagonist with cytotoxic and immunosuppressant activity (see below and Chs 41 and 42) and potent antirheumatoid action. It is commonly a first choice DMARD in the UK and the USA—though it is not actually licensed for this indication in either country. It has a more rapid onset of action than other DMARDs. It is also said to have fewer adverse effects (Bondeson 1997), though pulmonary fibrosis may be a problem. More than 50% of patients continue with it for 5 years or more, whereas about half stop other DMARDs within 2 years because of unwanted effects and lack of efficacy.

DRUGS USED IN GOUT

Gout is a genetically determined metabolic disease in which there is overproduction of purines. It is characterised by intermittent attacks of acute arthritis produced by the deposition of crystals of sodium urate (a product of purine metabolism) in the synovial tissue of joints. An inflammatory response is evoked, involving activation of the kinin, complement and plasmin systems (see Ch. 12 and Fig. 12.1), generation of lipoxygenase products such as LTB$_4$ (Fig. 12.8) and local accumulation of neutrophil granulocytes (Fig. 12.2). These engulf the crystals by phagocytosis, which causes generation of tissue-damaging toxic oxygen metabolites and subsequently lysis of the cells with release of proteolytic enzymes. Urate crystals also induce the production of IL-1 (Ch. 12, p. 224).

Drugs used to treat gout may act in the following ways:

- by inhibiting uric acid synthesis (**allopurinol**)
- by increasing uric acid excretion (uricosuric agents: **probenecid**, **sulphinpyrazone**)
- by inhibiting leukocyte migration into the joint (**colchicine**)
- by general anti-inflammatory and analgesic effects (**NSAIDs**; see p. 231).

Allopurinol

Allopurinol reduces the synthesis of uric acid by inhibiting xanthine oxidase (Fig. 13.2). It is an analogue of hypoxanthine and inhibits the enzyme mainly by substrate competition. Some degree of inhibition of de novo purine synthesis also occurs. Allopurinol is converted to alloxanthine by xanthine oxidase and this metabolite, which remains in the tissue for a considerable time, is an effective non-competitive inhibitor of the enzyme. The pharmacological action of allopurinol is largely due to alloxanthine.

Allopurinol reduces the concentration of the relatively insoluble urates and uric acid in tissues, plasma and urine, while increasing the concentration of the more soluble xanthines and hypoxanthines. The deposition of urate

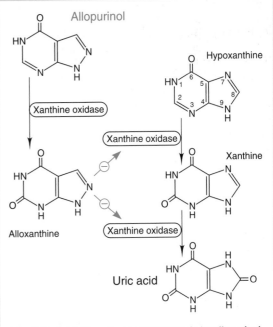

Fig. 13.2 Inhibition of uric acid synthesis by allopurinol. (See text for details.)

crystals in tissues ('tophi') is reversed and the formation of renal stones is inhibited.

Allopurinol is the drug of choice in the long-term treatment of gout, but it is ineffective in the treatment of an acute attack and indeed makes this worse.

Pharmacokinetic aspects

Allopurinol is given orally and is well absorbed in the gastrointestinal tract. Its half-life is 2–3 hours; it is converted to alloxanthine (Fig. 13.2) which has a half-life of 18–30 hours. Renal excretion is a balance between glomerular filtration and probenecid-sensitive tubular reabsorption.

Unwanted effects

Unwanted effects are few. Gastrointestinal disturbances and allergic reactions (mainly skin rashes) can occur, but disappear if the drug is stopped. Acute attacks of gout sometimes occur during the early stages of therapy.

Some important drug interactions. Allopurinol increases the effect of **mercaptopurine**, an antimetabolite that may be used in cancer chemotherapy, and also that of **azathioprine** (an immunosuppressant used to prevent transplant rejection; see below) which is metabolised to mercaptopurine. Allopurinol also enhances the effect of another anticancer drug, **cyclophosphamide** (Ch. 42). The effect of **oral anticoagulants** is increased owing to inhibition of their metabolism.

Uricosuric agents

Uricosuric agents are drugs that increase uric acid excretion by a direct action on the renal tubule. Examples are **probenecid** and **sulphinpyrazone** and the *uricosuric diuretics* derived from ethacrynic acid (discussed in Ch. 20, p. 361).

Colchicine

Colchicine has a specific effect in gouty arthritis and can be used both to prevent and to relieve acute attacks. It prevents migration of neutrophils into the joint by binding to *tubulin*, resulting in the depolymerisation of the microtubules and interfering with cell motility. Colchicine-treated neutrophils develop a 'drunken walk'. Colchicine may also prevent the production of a putative inflammatory glycoprotein by neutrophils that have phagocytosed urate crystals.

Pharmacokinetic aspects

Colchicine is given orally, is well absorbed and reaches peak concentrations in about an hour. It is excreted partly in the gastrointestinal tract and partly in the urine.

Unwanted effects

The unwanted effects of colchicine are largely gastro-intestinal—nausea, vomiting and abdominal pain. Severe diarrhoea may be a problem and with large doses may be associated with gastrointestinal haemorrhage and kidney damage. Rashes sometimes occur, also peripheral neuropathy. Long courses of treatment have occasionally resulted in blood dyscrasias.

ANTAGONISTS OF HISTAMINE

There are three classes of histamine antagonists: H_1-, H_2- and H_3-receptor antagonists. The former group was introduced first by Bovet and his colleagues in the 1930s, at a time when the classification of the histamine receptors had not been elucidated. (Indeed, the elucidation was possible only because these agents were available.) The term 'antihistamine' conventionally refers to the H_1-receptor antagonists, which affect various inflammatory and allergic mechanisms. These drugs are discussed in this section. The more recently developed H_2-receptor antagonists, the main clinical effect of which is on gastric secretion, are discussed in Chapter 21. H_3-receptor antagonists (Table 12.1b) are at present mainly used as investigational tools.

H_1-receptor antagonists (H_1-antihistamines)

Details of some characteristic H_1-receptor antagonists are shown in Table 13.3. All are lipid soluble and all contain a substituted ethylamine moiety.

Actions

Many of the pharmacological actions of the H_1-receptor antagonists follow from the actions of histamine outlined in Chapter 12. Thus in vitro they decrease histamine-mediated contraction of the smooth muscle of the bronchi, the intestine and the uterus. They inhibit histamine-induced bronchospasm in the guinea pig in vivo but are of little value in allergic bronchospasm in man. They reduce the increased vascular permeability caused by histamine.

Some of the actions of these drugs do not appear to be related to blockade of H_1-receptors and may well be due to antagonist effects at other receptors such as those for 5-HT, α_1-agonists and muscarinic agonists, both peripherally and in the CNS.

Some H_1-receptor antagonists have pronounced effects in the CNS. These are usually listed as 'side-effects' but they may be more clinically useful than the peripheral H_1-antagonist effects and should be recognised as such.

Table 13.3 Comparison of some commonly used H_1-receptor antagonists

Drug	$t_{1/2}$	Sedative action	Comments
Diphenhydramine	7 h	++	Some local anaesthetic activity and marked muscarinic-receptor antagonism. Used in motion sickness
Promethazine	12 h	++	Some local anaesthetic action and fairly marked muscarinic-receptor antagonism. Weak α_1-adrenoceptor antagonism. Anti-emetic. Injection can be painful
Chlorpheniramine	23 h	+	Potent H_1-receptor antagonism. If injected it can cause transient CNS stimulation
Mequitazine	38 h	Nil	Potent H_1-receptor antagonism; has minimal muscarinic-receptor antagonism. Peak plasma concentration after 6 h. High doses can impair CNS function
Astemizole	5 days (10 days)*	Nil	Has minimal muscarinic-receptor antagonism. Steady-state concentration not reached for several weeks: accumulation likely. Weight gain can occur. Very high doses can cause ventricular arrhythmias.

*$t_{1/2}$ of active metabolite

Some are fairly strong sedatives and may be used for this action (e.g. **promethazine**, a phenothiazine compound; see Table 13.3). Several are anti-emetic and are used to prevent motion sickness (e.g. **cyclizine**, **dimenhydrinate**, **cinnarizine**; see Ch. 21, Fig. 21.6).

Many H_1-receptor antagonists (e.g. **diphenhydramine**) also show significant antimuscarinic effects, though their affinity is much lower for muscarinic than for histamine receptors. (As measured on the guinea-pig ileum, the pA_2 of **mepyramine**, the prototype antihistamine for the H_1-receptors, is 9.2, and for the muscarinic receptors, 5.0). For circumstances in which selective H_1-receptor antagonism is desired, untrammelled by CNS effects, newer drugs have been developed, such as **astemizole**, **mequitazine** (see Table 13.3) and **terfenadine**. These non-sedating antihistamines, terfenadine in particular, can cause potentially fatal cardiac arrhythmias (see Ch. 5, p. 81, Ch. 48, p. 754, and Woosley 1996). The risk is extremely low—only about 0.25 adverse reactions reported per million doses sold daily (Lindquist & Edwards 1997)—but is increased if grapefruit juice or agents that inhibit cytochrome P450 in the liver are taken concomitantly (see Ch. 5). The non-toxic, pharmacologically active metabolite of terfenadine, **fexofenadine**, is now available.

Other, newer drugs which lack sedative action are **loratadine** and **cetirizine**.

Several H_1-receptor antagonists show weak blockade at α_1-adrenoceptors (an example is the phenothiazine, **promethazine**). **Cyproheptadine** (see Ch. 9) is a 5-HT antagonist as well as being an H_1-receptor antagonist. There are many other H_1-receptor antagonists in clinical use.

Clinical use of H_1-receptor antagonists

H_1-receptor antagonists can be used:

- For allergic reactions (see Ch. 12) including allergic rhinitis (hay fever), urticaria, insect bites, drug hypersensitivities. Drugs that lack sedative or muscarinic-receptor antagonist actions (e.g. fexofenadine or cetirizine) are preferred.
- As anti-emetics for the prevention of motion sickness or other causes of nausea, especially those associated with vertigo (e.g. labyrinthine disorders). Muscarinic-receptor antagonist actions of some antihistamines (e.g. cinnarizine, cyclizine) probably contribute to efficacy but also cause side-effects.
- For sedation: some H_1–receptor antagonists (e.g. promethazine; see Table 13.3) are fairly strong sedatives and may be used for this action.

The clinical uses of H_1-receptor antagonists are summarised in the clinical box above.

Pharmacokinetic aspects

Most H_1-receptor antagonists are given orally, are well absorbed, reach their peak effect in 1–2 hours and are effective for 3–6 hours, though there are exceptions (see Table 13.3). Most appear to be widely distributed throughout the body, but some do not penetrate the blood–brain barrier, for example the non-sedative drugs (see Table 13.3). They are metabolised in the liver and excreted in the urine.

Unwanted effects

What is defined as 'unwanted' will depend to a certain extent on what the drugs are used for. When used for purely peripheral actions, all the CNS effects are unwanted. When used for their sedative or anti-emetic actions, some of the CNS effects such as dizziness, tinnitus and fatigue are unwanted. Excessive doses can cause excitation and may produce convulsions in children.

The peripheral antimuscarinic actions are always unwanted. The commonest of these is dryness of the mouth, but blurred vision, constipation and retention of urine can also occur.

Unwanted effects not related to the drugs' pharmacological actions are also seen; thus gastrointestinal disturbances are fairly common while allergic dermatitis can follow topical application.

IMMUNOSUPPRESSANT DRUGS

Most immunosuppressants act in the induction phase of the immunological response (see Fig. 12.3). reducing lymphocyte proliferation; some also inhibit aspects of the effector phase. The drugs used for immunosuppression can be roughly divided into agents that:

- inhibit interleukin-2 (IL-2) production or action, e.g. **cyclosporin,*** **tacrolimus**, **rapamycin** (also known as sirolimus)

---

*Known as ciclosporine in Europe and cyclosporine in the USA.

- inhibit cytokine gene expression, e.g. the **corticosteroids**
- act by cytotoxic mechanisms, e.g. **cyclophosphamide**, **chlorambucil**
- inhibit purine or pyrimidine synthesis, e.g. **azathioprine**, **myclophenolate mofetil**, various newer agents under investigation (see below)
- block the T cell surface molecules involved in signalling, e.g. immunoglobulins—polyclonal and monoclonal antibodies.

Immunosuppressants are used in the therapy of autoimmune disease and to prevent and/or treat transplant rejection. Because they impair immune responses, they carry the hazard of a decreased response to infections and may facilitate the emergence of malignant cells. However, the relationship between these adverse effects and potency in preventing graft rejection varies in different drugs (see Morris 1996).

Cyclosporin

Cyclosporin is a fungal peptide with potent immunosuppressive activity but no effect on the acute inflammatory reaction per se. It was discovered by Borel and his co-workers in 1976 in the course of screening fungal products for antifungal activity and soon revolutionised the field of organ transplantation, significantly reducing the morbidity and the incidence of rejection. For a detailed review, see Borel et al. (1996).

It is a cyclic peptide of 11 amino acids, several of which are N-methylated and one of which was previously unknown.

Mechanism of action

Cyclosporin has numerous actions on various cell types, and its actions appear to be different when it is used in models of transplantation rejection as compared to autoimmune models; but, in general, the actions of relevance for immunosuppression are:

- decreased clonal proliferation of T cells, primarily by inhibiting interleukin-2 release and possibly also by decreasing expression of interleukin-2 receptors.
- reduced induction of and clonal proliferation of cytotoxic T cells from CD8+ precursor T cells
- reduced function of the effector T cells that mediate cell-mediated responses (e.g. decreased delayed-type hypersensitivity)
- some reduction of T-cell-dependent B cell responses.

The main action is a relatively selective effect on IL-2 gene transcription. Normally, interaction of antigen with a Th cell receptor results in an increase of intra-cellular Ca^{2+} (Ch. 2). Ca^{2+} (with calmodulin) stimulates a phosphatase, calcineurin,* that activates various transcription factors;** these, in turn, set in motion the transcription of the gene for IL-2. Cyclosporin binds with a cytosolic protein, termed 'cyclophilin' (a member of a group now called 'immunophilins';*** the drug/immunophilin complex binds to and inhibits calcineurin and thus interferes with activation of Th cells and production of IL-2 (Fig. 12.3).

Pharmacokinetic aspects

Cyclosporin can be given orally or by intravenous infusion. Absorption from the gastrointestinal tract is rather poor and varies in different individuals but peak plasma concentrations are usually attained in about 3–4 hours. Alternative formulations with improved oral absorption are now available. The plasma half-life is ~24 hours. Metabolism occurs in the liver and most of the metabolites (of which 14 have been identified) are excreted in the bile. It accumulates in most tissues at concentrations three to four times that seen in the plasma. Some of the drug remains in lymphomyeloid tissue and later in fat depots for some time after administration has stopped. Other drugs (e.g. ketoconazole) may increase the plasma concentration of cyclosporin.

Unwanted effects

The commonest and most serious unwanted effect of cyclosporin is nephrotoxicity—which is not thought to be associated with calcineurin inhibition. It may be a limiting factor in the use of the drug in some patients (see also Ch. 49). Hepatotoxicity and hypertension can also occur. Less important unwanted effects are anorexia, lethargy, hirsutism, tremor, paraesthesia (tingling sensation), gum hypertrophy and gastrointestinal disturbances. Cyclosporin has no depressant effects on the bone marrow.

---

*Calcineurin also activates nitric oxide synthase and may be implicated in nitric oxide transmitter function and NMDA-mediated neurotoxicity in the CNS (Snyder & Sabatini 1995).

**For example NF/AT, the 'nuclear factor of activated T cells'.

***The term 'immunophilin' was coined to describe the intracellular proteins that function as receptors for immunosuppressants such as cyclosporin, tacrolimus and rapamycin. It is now known that immunophilin molecules are implicated in several signal transduction mechanisms. Recent work has shown that the immunodeficiency virus, HIV-1 (see Ch. 44), also binds to intracellular cyclophilins and it has been suggested that this may be related to the mechanism whereby the virus interferes with Th cells.

Tacrolimus

Tacrolimus, originally termed FK506, is a macrolide antibiotic with a very similar mechanism of action to cyclosporin, the main difference being that the internal receptor for this drug is not cyclophilin but FK-binding protein (FKBP). The tacrolimus/FKBP complex inhibits calcineurin with the effects described above.

Tacrolimus is active at lower concentrations than cyclosporin.

Pharmacokinetic aspects and unwanted effects

Tacrolimus can be given orally or by intravenous injection. It is 99% metabolised by the liver and has a half-life of ~7 hours.

The unwanted effects of tacrolimus are similar to those of cyclosporin but less severe. Nephrotoxicity and hypertension have so far not been a serious problem. Neurotoxicity, gastrointestinal upsets and metabolic disturbances can occur. Thrombocytopenia and hyperlipidaemia have been reported but are reversible by reducing the dosage.

Glucocorticoids

Immunosuppression by glucocorticoids involves both their effects on the immune response and their anti-inflammatory actions. These are described in Chapter 24, p. 418, and the sites of action of the agents on cell-mediated immune reactions are indicated in Fig. 12.3.

Glucocorticoids are immunosuppressant mainly because, like cyclosporin, they restrain the clonal proliferation of Th cells, through decreasing transcription of the gene for IL-2; but also because they decrease the transcription of many other cytokine genes (including those for TNF-α, interferon-γ, IL-1 and many other interleukins) in both the induction and effector phases of the immune response. These effects on transcription are due to inhibition of the action of transcription factors, such as AP-1 and NF-κB (see p. 422)

Azathioprine

Azathioprine (Fig. 13.3) interferes with purine synthesis and is cytotoxic. It is widely used for immunosuppression particularly for control of tissue rejection in transplant surgery. This drug is metabolised to give **mercaptopurine**, a purine analogue that inhibits DNA synthesis (see Ch. 42).

Both cell-mediated and antibody-mediated immune reactions are depressed by this drug since it inhibits clonal proliferation in the induction phase of the immune response (see Fig. 12.3) by a cytotoxic action on dividing cells.

As is the case with mercaptopurine itself, the main

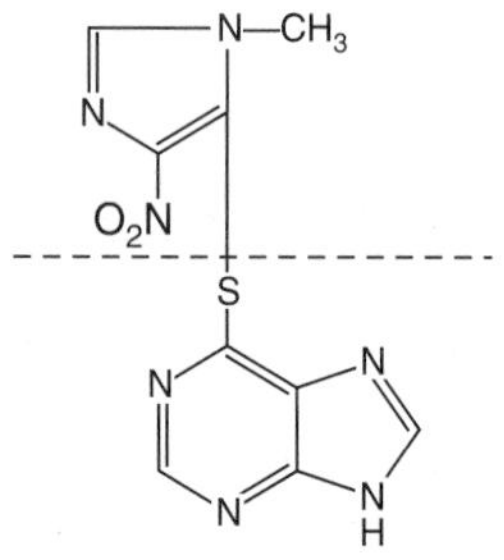

Fig. 13.3 Azathioprine. The dotted line indicates where the molecule is cleaved to release mercaptopurine.

unwanted effect is depression of the bone marrow. Other toxic effects are nausea and vomiting, skin eruptions and a mild hepatotoxicity.

Cyclophosphamide

Cyclophosphamide is a cytotoxic agent with powerful immunosuppressive effects. It is an alkylating agent with a particular action on lymphocytes. Its structure is given and its mechanism of action described in Chapter 42. As an immunosuppressant it affects the clonal proliferative phase of the immune response and reduces both antibody-mediated and cell-mediated immune reactions (Fig. 12.3).

Chlorambucil

Chlorambucil, another alkylating cytotoxic agent (see Ch. 42), is also used for immunosuppression and has effects similar to those of cyclophosphamide.

Mycophenolate mofetil

Mycophenolate mofetil is a semisynthetic derivative of a fungal antibiotic. In the body it is converted to myco-phenolic acid which restrains proliferation of both T and B lymphocytes and reduces production of cytotoxic T cells by inhibiting inosine monophosphate dehydrogenase, an enzyme crucial for de novo purine biosynthesis. T and B cells are particularly dependent on this pathway* so the drug has a fairly selective action on these cells.

Pharmacokinetic aspects and unwanted effects

It is given orally and well absorbed. Magnesium and aluminium hydroxides impair absorption and choles-tyramine reduces plasma concentrations. The metabolite, mycophenolic acid, undergoes enterohepatic cycling and

---

*Most cells obtain the purines needed for synthesising DNA not by the de novo synthesis pathway—as T and B cells do—but by an alternative pathway.

is eliminated by the kidney as the inactive glucuronide. Unwanted gastrointestinal effects are common.

Used with cyclosporin and steroids, it has proved to have effective immunosuppressant action in several clinical trials of kidney transplant rejection. See Lipsky (1996).

Immunoglobulins

Antibodies against human lymphocytes or their surface proteins can have significant immunosuppressant action. These antibodies are raised by immunising horses or rabbits, or from mice using hybridoma technology. Their disadvantage is that the foreign antibodies themselves elicit an immune response. To avoid this, animal immuno-globulins can now be 'humanised' by genetic engineering to combine the antigen-binding (Fab) site of a mouse monoclonal antibody with human immunoglobulin.

Polyclonal antibodies

Antilymphocyte immunoglobulin (ALG) and *antithymo-cyte immunoglobulin* (ATG) are obtained by immunising horses with human lymphocytes or with foetal thymic tissue respectively. These antibodies interact with multiple surface proteins implicated in T cell signal transduction and have indiscriminate action against both useful T cells and those that produce unwanted effects.

The immunoglobulin 'recognises' and binds to pro-tein on the lymphocyte surface causing the exposure of the complement-binding site on the Fc portion of the immunoglobulin; this activates the complement system (Ch. 12, p. 200) leading to the lysis of the lymphocyte.

The *unwanted effects* are mainly those to be expected with injection of foreign protein. Antibodies against the foreign immunoglobulin can be produced, anaphylactic reactions can occur (p. 209) and the complexes formed from the foreign protein with the human antibody can localise in the glomerulus of the kidney (p. 209).

Monoclonal antibodies

Monoclonal antibodies directed against surface compo-nents of T cells include immunoglobulins targeting the complex of CD3 protein with antigen receptor (muromonab-CD3, OKT3), the CD4 co-receptor and the IL-2 receptor. Some are currently being used, some are being assessed.

Initial doses of OKT3 can cause fever, hypotension, pulmonary oedema, nephropathy and encephalopathy, which is thought to be due to cytokine release; pretreat-ment with steroids diminishes these effects.

Rapamycin (sirolimus)

This is a macrolide antibiotic that, like tacrolimus, binds to the intracellular immunophilin, FKBP. However, the complex does not bind calcineurin nor does it affect IL-2 gene transcription; it interferes with the IL-2 *signal transduction pathway*, blocking the cell cycle (Ch. 42) of activated T cells in G_1 phase by inhibiting a novel kinase termed mTOR. Rapamycin competes with tacrolimus for FKBP in vitro but their effects are additive in vivo. This drug also reduces smooth muscle proliferation.

Phase I and II clinical trials of rapamycin supplementation of cyclosporin regimes are under way. Nephrotoxicity and hypertension have not been serious problems and hyperlipidaemia and thrombocytopenia have responded to reduction in drug dosage.

Clinical use of immunosuppressants

Immunosuppressants are used for three main purposes:

- to suppress rejection of transplanted organs and tissues (kidneys, bone marrow, heart, liver, etc.)
- to suppress graft-versus-host disease (i.e. the response of lymphocytes in the graft to host antigens) in bone marrow transplants
- to treat a variety of conditions which, while not completely understood, are believed to have an important autoimmune component in their pathogenesis. These include idiopathic thrombocytopenic purpura, some forms of haemolytic anaemia and of glomerulonephritis, myasthenia gravis, systemic lupus erythematosus, rheumatoid arthritis, psoriasis and ulcerative colitis.

Therapy for this third category often involves a combination of glucocorticoid and cytotoxic agents. For transplantation of organs or bone marrow, cyclosporin is usually combined with a glucocorticoid, or a cytotoxic drug, or antilymphocyte immunoglobulin.

Immunosuppressants

- Cyclosporin, tacrolimus, glucocorticoids:
  — Their main common action is to decrease clonal proliferation of Th cells by inhibiting transcription of IL-2; they achieve this by different mechanisms.
  — Cyclosporin and tacrolimus, given orally or i.v.; common adverse effect is nephrotoxicity, less severe with tacrolimus.
- For glucocorticoids see pp. 418–425.
- Azathioprine: is converted to mercaptopurine which inhibits DNA synthesis.
- Mycophenolate mofetil: limits DNA synthesis by inhibiting de novo purine synthesis.
- Antibodies against lymphocyte surface proteins: polyclonal antilymphocyte immunoglobulins bind non-specifically to lymphocytes; monoclonal antibodies are more specific.
- Rapamycin: inhibits IL-2 signal transduction.

The clinical use of immunosuppressants is summarised on this page.

POSSIBLE FUTURE DEVELOPMENTS

Rapid advances are being made in this area.

Immunosuppressive agents
New potential immunosuppressants under investigation include:

Brequinar sodium, an antimetabolite that inhibits de novo pyrimidine synthesis.

Mizoribine, an inhibitor of purine biosynthesis. This drug has been in use in transplantation treatment in Japan since 1984 and, compared with azathioprine, is more immunosuppressive but less myelotoxic or hepatotoxic.

Monoclonal antibodies. Potential targets for immunosuppressive monoclonal antibodies (apart from those specified above, p. 244) are cytokines, cytokine receptors, cell adhesion molecules, and lymphocyte differentiation molecules (Waldman & Cobbold 1993, Winter & Harris 1993).

Drugs that induce specific tolerance to donor antigens are being investigated for use in organ transplantation; these include agents that block the co-receptors involved in T cell activation, agents that promote T cell apoptosis, and peptides derived from MHC molecules. The last named compounds block T cell signalling and are in phase II trial.

Antirheumatoid agents
Leflunomide, a new, synthetic orally active pro-drug with immunosuppressant action is in phase III trial for antirheumatoid therapy.

Cytokine-targeted therapies under investigation include the anti-THF-α antibodies (monoclonal antibody cA2 against TNF-α, soluble THF-α fused to the Fc portion of human IgG), soluble TNF receptor (to mop up TNF-α), soluble IL-1 receptor (to mop up IL-1), recombinant IL-1ra, and synovial cells genetically altered to express IL-1ra (see Bondeson 1997, Firestein & Zvaifler 1997).

5-lipoxygenase inhibitors
Several agents that inhibit 5-lipoxygenase have been developed (see Ch. 19). These compounds prevent the conversion of arachidonate to 5-HPETE (Fig. 12.11) and hence inhibit synthesis of all the leukotrienes; an example is zileuton, which is in clinical trial. Their main application is likely to be as anti-asthmatic drugs (Ch. 19), where their reduction of the generation of LTC_4, LTD_4

and LTE_4 could be of value. It is also possible that, combined with suitable cyclo-oxygenase inhibitors, they could have many of the anti-inflammatory effects of the glucocorticoids without the toxic effects of these steroids.

Phosphodiesterase (PDE) inhibitors

An increase in cytosolic cyclic AMP reduces the activation of most inflammatory cells. Phosphodiesterase converts cyclic AMP to $5'$AMP. There are seven families of PDE isoenzymes, PDE_4 being of particular importance in neutrophils, eosinophils, mast cells and basophils, and PDE_3 in monocytes/macrophages and lymphocytes. Many PDE_4 inhibitors are under test as anti-inflammatory drugs (see Ch. 19, p. 348).

More information on potential new therapies is given in Chapters 12, p. 225, and 19.

REFERENCES AND FURTHER READING

Antel J P, Becher B, Owens T 1996 Immunotherapy for multiple sclerosis. Nature Med 2: 1074–1075 *(New approach to treatment)*

Bahl A K, Dale M M, Foreman J C 1994 The effect of non-steroidal anti-inflammatory drugs on the accumulation and release of interleukin-1-like activity by peritoneal macrophages from the mouse. Br J Pharmacol 113: 809–814

Bateman D N 1994 NSAIDs: time to re-evaluate gut toxicity. Lancet 343: 1051–1052

Bennett W M, De Broe M E 1989 Analgesic nephropathy a preventable renal disease. N Engl J Med 320: 1269–1271

Bondeson J 1997 The mechanisms of action of the disease-modifying antirheumatic drugs: a review with emphasis on macrophage signal transduction and the induction of inflammatory cytokines. Gen Pharmacol 29: 127–150 *(Comprehensive review)*

Borel J F, Baumann G et al. 1996 In vivo pharmacological effects of ciclosporin and some analogues. Adv Pharmacol 35: 115–246

Cash J M, Klippel J M 1994 Second-line drug therapy for rheumatoid arthritis. N Engl J Med 330: 1368–1376 *(Good review of DMARDs—disease-modifying antirheumatoid drugs)*

Chatenaud L 1998 Tolerogenic antibodies and fusion proteins to prevent graft rejection and treat autoimmunity. Mol Med Today (January): 25–30

Dale M M, Foreman J C, Fan T-P (eds) 1994 Textbook of immunopharmacology, 3rd edn. Blackwell Scientific Publications, Oxford *(Simple textbook intended for second and third year medical and science students)*

De Broe M E, Elseviers M M 1998 Current concepts: analgesic nephropathy. N Engl J Med 338: 446–452 *(Useful review)*

Emmerson B T 1996 The management of gout. N Engl J Med 334: 445–452 *(Clinical treatment of gout)*

Featherstone C 1996 HLA-derived peptides in clinical trial for allografts. Mol Med Today (November): 447 *(Possible new approach to treatment)*

Felson D T, Anderson J J et al. 1995 American College of Rheumatology, preliminary definition of improvement in rheumatoid arthritis. Arthritis Rheum 38: 727–735

Firestein G S, Zvaifler G S 1997 Anticytokine therapy for rheumatoid arthritis. N Engl J Med 337: 195–197 *(Editorial: possible new approach to treatment of rheumatoid arthritis)*

Foreman J C 1994 Pyrogenesis. In: Dale M M, Foreman J C, Fan T-P (eds) Textbook of immunopharmacology, 3rd edn. Blackwell Scientific Publications, Oxford, ch 21

Frolich J C 1997 A classification of NSAIDs according to the relative inhibition of cyclooxygenase enzymes. Trends Pharmacol Sci 18: 30–34

Ganellin C R, Parsons M E (eds) 1982 Pharmacology of histamine receptors. Wright, Bristol

Griswold D E, Adams J L 1996 Constitutive cyclooxygenase (COX-1) and inducible cyclooxygenase (COX-2): rationale for selective inhibition and progress to date. Med Res Rev 16: 181–206 *(Good review; emphasis on biochemistry)*

Lands W E M 1985 Mechanisms of action of antiinflammatory drugs. Adv Drug Res 14: 147–163

Lanza R P, Cooper D K C 1998 Xenotransplantation of cells and tissues: application to a range of diseases, from diabetes to Alzheimer's. Mol Med Today (January): 39–45

Lindquist M, Edwards I R 1997 Risks of non-sedating antihistamines Lancet 349: 1322

Lipsky J J 1996 Mycophenolate mofetil. Lancet 348: 1357–1359

MacDonald T M, Morant S V et al. 1997 Association of upper gastrointestinal toxicity of non-steroidal anti-inflammatory drugs with continued exposure: cohort study. Br Med J 315: 1333–1338

Marcus A J 1995 Aspirin as prophylaxis against colorectal cancer. N Engl J Med 333: 656–657

Morris R E 1995 Mechanisms of action of new immunosuppressive drugs. Therapeutic Drug Monitoring 17: 564–569 *(Succinct, edifying review)*

Morris R E 1996 Beware: shifting paradigms ahead. Lancet 348 (suppl. II): 26

Picot D, Lill P J, Garavito R M 1994 The X-ray crystal structure of the membrane protein prostaglandin H_2 synthase-1. Nature 367: 243–249

Porter D R, Sturrock R D 1993 Medical management of rheumatoid arthritis. Br Med J 307: 425–428

Rainsford K D 1984 Aspirin and the salicylates. Butterworth, London

Rainsford K D 1994 Nonsteroidal anti-inflammatory drugs. In: Dale M M, Foreman J, Fan T-P D (eds) Textbook of immunopharmacology, 3rd edn. Blackwell Scientific Publications, Oxford

Rainsford K D, Velo G P (eds) 1992 Side-effects of antiinflammatory/analgesic drugs. Kluwer Academic Publishers, Lancaster

Rankin A C 1997 Non-sedating antihistamines and cardiac arrhythmias. Lancet 350: 1115–1116

Rashad S, Hemingway A, Rainsford K et al. 1989 Effect of nonsteroidal anti-inflammatory drugs on the course of osteoarthritis. Lancet 2: 519–522

Rodriguez L A G, Jick H 1994 Risk of gastrointestinal bleeding and perforation associated with non-steroidal anti-inflammatory drugs. Lancet 343: 769–772

Simons F E R, Simons K J 1994 Drug therapy: the pharmacology and use of H_1-receptor-antagonist drugs. N Engl J Med 23: 1663–1670 *(Effective coverage)*

Skjelbred P, Lokken P, Skoglund L A 1984 Post-operative administration of acetaminophen to reduce swelling and other inflammatory events. Curr Ther Res 35: 377–385

Snyder S H, Sabatini D M 1995 Immunophilins and the nervous system. Nature Med 1: 32–37 (*Good coverage of mechanism of action of cyclosporin and related drugs*)

Suthantharin M, Morris R E, Strom T 1996 Immunosuppressants: cellular and molecular mechanisms of action. Am J Kidney Dis 28: 159–172 (*In-depth review*)

Twomey B, Dale M M 1992 Cyclooxygenase-independent effects of non-steroidal anti-inflammatory drugs on the neutrophil respiratory burst. Biochem Pharmacol 43: 413–418

Vane J R 1971 Inhibition of prostaglandin synthesis as a mechanism of action for aspirin-like drugs. Nature New Biol 231: 232–239 (*Definitive, seminal article*)

Vane J R, Botting R M 1996 Overview—mechanisms of action of anti-inflammatory drugs. In: Vane J, Botting J H, Botting R M (eds) Improved non-steroid anti-inflammatory drugs: COX-2 enzyme inhibitors. Kluwer Academic Publishers, London, ch. 1, pp 1–27 (*Valuable overview*)

Vane J, Botting J 1998a Mechanism of action of anti-inflammatory drugs: an overview. In: Vane J, Botting J (eds) Selective COX-2 inhibitors: pharmacology, clinical effects and therapeutic potential. Kluwer Academic Publishers, London

Vane J, Botting J (eds) 1998b Selective COX-2 inhibitors: pharmacology, clinical effects and therapeutic potential. Kluwer Academic Publishers, London (*Proceedings of a conference held in 1997. Fourteen articles by various authorities. Excellent up-to-date coverage*)

Vincent F, Kirkman R et al. 1998 Interleukin-2-receptor blockade with daclizaumab to prevent acute rejection in renal transplantation. N Engl J Med 338: 161–165

Waldmann H, Cobbold S 1993 The use of monoclonal antibodies to achieve immunological tolerance. Trends Pharmacol Sci 14: 143–147

Weinblatt M E 1995 Methotrexate for chronic diseases in adults. N Engl J Med 332: 330–331

Winter G, Harris W J 1993 Humanised antibodies. Trends Pharmacol Sci 14: 139–143

Wollheim F A 1997 Disease modifying drugs in rheumatoid arthritis: encouraging signs but effects not proved. Br Med J 314: 766–767

Woosley R L 1996 Cardiac actions of the antihistamines Annu Rev Pharmacol Toxicol 36: 233–252

DRUGS AFFECTING MAJOR ORGAN SYSTEMS

The effects of drugs on the heart will be considered under three main headings:

- rate and rhythm
- myocardial contraction
- metabolism and blood flow.

The effects of drugs on these three aspects of cardiac function are not, of course, independent of each other. For example, if a drug affects the electrical properties of the myocardial cell membrane, it is likely to influence both cardiac rhythm and myocardial contraction. Similarly, a drug that affects contraction will inevitably alter metabolism and blood flow as well. Nevertheless, from a therapeutic point of view, these three classes of effect represent distinct clinical objectives in relation to the treatment, respectively, of cardiac dysrhythmias, cardiac failure and coronary insufficiency. We also give a short account of natriuretic peptides made in the heart and secreted into the blood. We shall first consider functional aspects to provide a basis for understanding the effects of drugs on the heart and their place in treating cardiac disease.

PHYSIOLOGY OF CARDIAC FUNCTION

CARDIAC RATE AND RHYTHM

Cardiac myocytes owe their electrical excitability to a transient increase in membrane Na^+ and/or Ca^{2+} permeability in response to membrane depolarisation, leading to inward currents. Repolarisation occurs as a result of a delayed increase in K^+ permeability, leading to outward K^+ current, possibly supported by inward movement of Cl^-. The proteins that control these ion fluxes are beginning to be understood (see Ch. 40), and it is now known that voltage-dependent ion channels are glycosylated proteins which evolved from a common monomeric ancestral protein in prokaryotes over approximately 1.4 billion years. Na^+ and Ca^{2+} channels are heteromultimeric proteins in which α- and α_1-subunits (large tetrameric proteins) form the voltage-dependent ion-selective (Na^+ or Ca^{2+} respectively) channels. Electrophysiological features of cardiac muscle that distinguish it from other excitable tissues include:

- the spontaneous, intrinsic rhythm generated by specialised cells of the sinoatrial (SA) and atrioventricular (AV) nodes (i.e. pacemaker activity)
- absence of the fast Na^+ current in the SA and AV nodes; slow inward Ca^{2+} current is responsible for initiation and propagation of the action potential in these regions
- the long duration of the action potential and long refractory period
- the large influx of Ca^{2+} (the 'slow inward current') during the plateau of the action potential.

Thus several of the special features of cardiac rhythm relate to Ca^{2+} currents. There are two distinct kinds of Ca^{2+} channel in the heart: *intracellular channels* (e.g. the large ryanodine receptors and smaller inositol trisphosphate-activated Ca^{2+} channels that are discussed below in the section on myocardial contractility) and *voltage-dependent plasma membrane Ca^{2+} channels* which are important in the present context. The latter are expressed in many distinct types (including L-, T-, N-, P-, Q- and R-types) in different tissues, classified by their electrophysiological properties and responses to drugs (e.g.

dihydropyridines; see below), toxins (e.g. ω-agatoxin, ω-conotoxin) and ions (e.g. Ni^{2+}, Cd^{2+}). The main type in adult working myocardium is the L-type channel, which is also important in vascular smooth muscle; L-type channels are important in specialised conducting regions as well as in working myocardium, but here T-channels also play a role. T-channels are also prominent during foetal development and during cardiac myocyte proliferation, as well as being abundant in the central nervous system. The diversity of calcium channels in the cardiovascular system is reviewed by Katz (1996).

The action potential of an idealised cardiac muscle cell is shown in Figure 14.1A, and is divided into five phases:

Phase 0, rapid depolarisation, occurs when the membrane potential reaches the critical firing threshold (about −60 mV) at which the inward current of sodium ions flowing through the voltage-dependent sodium channels becomes large enough to produce a regenerative ('all-or-nothing') depolarisation. This mechanism is the same as that responsible for action potential generation by the membrane of nerve cells (see Ch. 40). The activation of these sodium channels by membrane depolarisation is transient, and if the membrane remains depolarised for more than a few milliseconds, they close again (inactivation). They are therefore closed during the plateau of the action potential, and remain unavailable for the initiation of another action potential until the membrane repolarises.

Phase 1, partial repolarisation occurs as the Na^+ current is inactivated. There may also be a transient voltage-sensitive outward current.

Phase 2, the plateau, results from an inward calcium current. Calcium channels show a pattern of voltage-sensitive activation and inactivation qualitatively similar to fast sodium channels, but with a much slower time-course. The plateau is assisted by a special property of the cardiac muscle membrane, known as inward-going rectification, which means that the potassium conductance falls to a low level when the membrane is depolarised. Because of this, there is little tendency for outward potassium current to restore the resting membrane potential during the plateau, so a relatively small inward calcium current suffices to maintain the plateau.

Phase 3, repolarisation, occurs as the calcium current inactivates and a delayed outwardly rectifying potassium current (analogous to but much slower than the potassium current that causes repolarisation in nerve fibres; Ch. 40) activates, causing outward potassium current. This is augmented by another potassium current which is activated by the high $[Ca^{2+}]_i$ during the plateau, and sometimes also by other potassium currents as well, including

one through channels activated by acetylcholine (see below) and another that is activated by arachidonic acid which is liberated under pathological conditions such as myocardial infarction.

Phase 4, the pacemaker potential, is a gradual depolarisation during diastole. Pacemaker activity is normally found only in nodal and conducting tissue. The pacemaker potential is caused by a combination of *increasing inward currents* and *reduced outward currents* during diastole. It is usually most rapid in cells of the SA node, which therefore acts as pacemaker for the whole heart. Cells in the SA node have a greater background conductance to sodium ions than do atrial or ventricular myocytes, leading to a greater background *inward current*. In addition, inactivation of voltage-dependent Ca^{2+} channels wears off during diastole resulting in increasing inward Ca^{2+} current during late diastole. Activation of T-type calcium channels during late diastole contributes to pacemaker activity in the SA node. The negative membrane potential early in diastole activates a cation channel which is permeable to Na^+ and K^+, giving rise to another inward current called I(f).*

Several voltage- and time-dependent *outward currents* play a part as well: delayed rectifier K^+ current (IK), which is activated during the action potential, is turned off by the negative membrane potential early in diastole. Current from the electrogenic Na^+/K^+ pump also contributes to the outward current during the pacemaker potential.

Figure 14.1B shows the action potential configuration in different parts of the heart. Phase 0 is absent in the nodal regions, where the conduction velocity is correspondingly slow (~5 cm/s) compared with other regions such as the Purkinje fibres (conduction velocity ~200 cm/s) which have the function of propagating the action potential rapidly to both ventricles. Regions that lack a fast inward current have a much longer refractory period than fast-conducting regions. This is because recovery of the slow inward current following its inactivation during the action potential takes a considerable time (a few hundred milliseconds), and the refractory period outlasts the action potential. With fast-conducting fibres, recovery from inactivation of the sodium current is quick, and the cell becomes excitable again as soon as it is repolarised.

Normally, the cardiac action potential is conducted in an orderly sequence: SA node, atrium, AV node, bundle of His, ventricle. This pattern can become disrupted either

---

*If for 'funny', because it is unusual for cation channels to be activated by hyperpolarisation; electrophysiologists are renowned for their peculiar sense of humour!

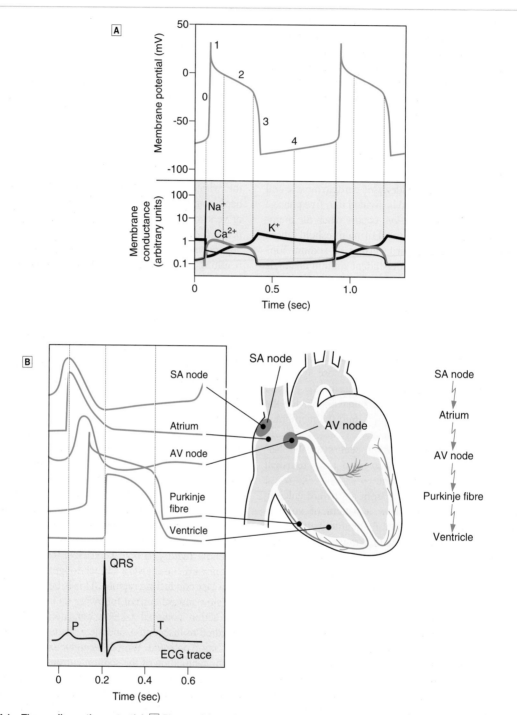

Fig. 14.1 The cardiac action potential. **A** Phases of the action potential (as recorded from a cardiac Purkinje fibre): 0 = rapid depolarisation; 1 = partial repolarisation; 2 = plateau; 3 = repolarisation; 4 = pacemaker depolarisation. The lower panel shows the accompanying changes in membrane conductance for Na^+, K^+ and Ca^{2+} ions. **B** Conduction of the impulse through the heart, with the corresponding ECG trace. Note that the longest delay occurs at the AV node, where the action potential has a characteristically slow waveform. (Adapted from: (A) Noble D 1975 The initiation of the heartbeat. Oxford University Press, Oxford)

by heart disease or by the action of drugs or circulating hormones, and an important therapeutic use of drugs is to restore a normal cardiac rhythm where it has become disturbed. The commonest cause of cardiac dysrhythmia is ischaemic heart disease, and many deaths following acute myocardial infarction result from ventricular fibrillation rather than directly from contractile failure.

Disturbances of cardiac rhythm

Clinically, dysrhythmias are generally classified according to:

- the site of origin of the abnormality—atrial, junctional or ventricular
- whether the rate is increased (tachycardia) or decreased (bradycardia).

It is often unclear which of the various mechanisms discussed below are responsible. These physiological mechanisms nevertheless provide a useful starting point for understanding how antidysrhythmic drugs work. Four basic mechanisms underlie pathological or drug-induced disturbances of cardiac rhythm:

- delayed after-depolarisation
- re-entry
- abnormal pacemaker activity
- heart block.

These will now be described in more detail.

Delayed after-depolarisation

Normal pacemaker activity, as described above, involves a spontaneous diastolic depolarisation, which initiates an action potential when it reaches threshold. Non-pacemaker cells do not normally undergo this diastolic depolarisation and remain quiescent if not excited by the arrival of an impulse from elsewhere in the heart. Under certain circumstances, however, a phenomenon called delayed after-depolarisation occurs, which can lead to a repetitive discharge that does not depend on the arrival of an impulse from elsewhere (Fig. 14.2). After-depolarisation follows an action potential if $[Ca^{2+}]_i$ increases excessively. It is accentuated if the extracellular calcium concentration (and hence the amount of calcium entering the cell during the plateau) is increased, and also by agents such as cardiac glycosides, noradrenaline or phosphodiesterase inhibitors that increase intracellular calcium. After-depolarisation is the result of a net inward current (known as the *transient inward current*). How does a rise in $[Ca^{2+}]_i$ cause an inward current? One possibility is that it activates sodium–calcium exchange (see Fig. 14.4). This transfers one Ca^{2+} ion out of the cell in exchange for entry of three Na^+ ions, resulting in

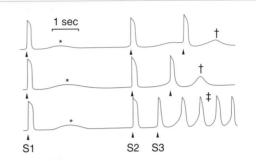

Fig. 14.2 After-depolarisation in cardiac muscle recorded from a dog coronary sinus in the presence of noradrenaline. The first stimulus (S1) causes an action potential followed by a small after-depolarisation. As the interval S2–S3 is decreased, the after-depolarisation gets larger (†) until it triggers an indefinite train of action potentials (‡). (Adapted from: Wit A L, Cranefield P F 1977 Circulation Res 41: 435)

a net influx of one positive charge and hence membrane depolarisation. Additionally, calcium opens non-selective cation channels in the plasma membrane, allowing entry of sodium and other ions analogous to the endplate potential at the neuromuscular junction (Ch. 7).

Re-entry

In normal cardiac rhythm, the conducted impulse dies out after it has activated the ventricles because it is surrounded by refractory tissue which it has just traversed. Re-entry describes the situation in which the impulse succeeds in re-exciting regions of the myocardium after the refractory period has subsided. A simple ring of tissue can give rise to a re-entrant rhythm if a transient or unidirectional conduction block is present (Fig. 14.3). Normally, an impulse originating at any point in the ring will propagate in both directions and die out when the two impulses meet, but if a damaged area causes either a transient block (so that one impulse is blocked but the second can get through; Fig. 14.3) or a unidirectional block, continuous circulation of the impulse can occur. This phenomenon is known as circus movement and was first demonstrated experimentally on rings of jellyfish tissue many years ago.

The 'ring' of tissue sometimes represents an anatomically distinct anomaly such as an accessory pathway linking atria and ventricles, as in patients with Wolff–Parkinson–White syndrome. Such pathways are increasingly accessible to ablation by various minimally invasive surgical techniques. However, more commonly the 'ring' of tissue is not anatomically distinct, but only functionally separate. If it retains a connection with the

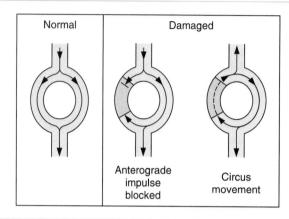

Fig. 14.3 Generation of a re-entrant rhythm by a damaged area of myocardium. The damaged area (grey) conducts in one direction only. This disturbs the normal pattern of conduction and permits continuous circulation of the impulse to occur.

Normal

Damaged

Anterograde impulse blocked

Circus movement

rest of the heart, it can act as a focus for high frequency re-excitation of the whole atrium or ventricle. The re-entrant rhythm will persist only if the time taken for propagation round the ring exceeds the refractory period, so it may be halted by drugs that prolong the refractory period (see below). On the other hand, myocardial damage may cause extreme slowing of action potential propagation, which favours re-entry. This slowing is often associated with the attenuation or disappearance of the sodium current responsible for the fast upstroke of the action potential. This current is reduced because the compromised cells are partly depolarised during diastole, so that fast sodium channels remain partly or completely inactivated, leaving only the slow inward current to support propagation of the action potential.

Re-entry underlies many types of dysrhythmia, the pattern depending on the site of the re-entrant circuit which may be in the atria, ventricles or nodal tissue.

Abnormal pacemaker activity

Under pathological conditions, pacemaker activity can arise in other parts of the heart than the SA node and conducting tissues. The main predisposing factors are:

- catecholamine action
- partial depolarisation, such as may occur in ischaemic damage.

Catecholamines, acting on β_1-adrenoceptors (see below), increase the rate of depolarisation during phase 4, and can cause normally quiescent parts of the heart to take on a spontaneous rhythm. Several tachyarrhythmias (e.g. paroxysmal atrial fibrillation) can be triggered by circumstances associated with increased sympathetic activity. Pain (e.g. during myocardial infarction) increases sympathetic discharge and releases adrenaline from the adrenal

gland. Partial depolarisation resulting from ischaemic damage is probably due to decreased activity of the electrogenic sodium pump, and also causes abnormal pacemaker activity.

Heart block

The AV node may be damaged (e.g. by infarction or fibrosis) so that it fails to conduct, the atria and ventricles beating independently of one another (complete AV block) at rates determined by their own pacemakers. Sporadic complete failure of AV conduction causes sudden periods of unconsciousness (Stokes–Adams attacks), and is treated by implanting an artificial pacemaker.

Cardiac dysrhythmias

- Dysrhythmias arise because of:
  - delayed after-depolarisation, which triggers ectopic beats
  - re-entry, resulting from partial conduction block
  - ectopic pacemaker activity
  - heart block.
- Delayed after-depolarisation is due to an inward current associated with abnormally raised $[Ca^{2+}]_i$.
- Re-entry is facilitated when parts of the myocardium are depolarised, conduction then depending on the Ca^{2+}-mediated 'slow response'.
- Ectopic pacemaker activity is encouraged by sympathetic activity.
- Heart block results from damage to the AV node or ventricular conducting system.
- Clinically, dysrhythmias are divided:
  - according to their site of origin (supraventricular and ventricular)
  - according to whether the heart rate is increased or decreased (tachycardia or bradycardia).

CARDIAC CONTRACTION

Cardiac output depends both on intrinsic and extrinsic factors. *Intrinsic factors* regulate *myocardial contractility* via intracellular calcium and ATP, and are sensitive to a variety of drugs and pathological processes. Cardiac output is also determined by *extrinsic circulatory factors*, including the contractile state of arterioles and veins, which are also influenced by drugs and/or disease.

Myocardial contractility and viability

The contractile machinery of the myocardial cell is basically the same as that of striated muscle. The interaction between actin and myosin filaments is normally blocked by the presence of *tropomyosin* bound to the actin filament. Tropomyosin forms part of the *troponin complex*, one component of which, troponin C, has binding sites for three or four calcium ions. When calcium is bound, the conformation of the troponin complex changes with the result that tropomyosin shifts out of the way, permitting binding of myosin cross-bridges to actin and initiating the contractile process. These changes are produced when the intracellular ionised calcium concentration $[Ca^{2+}]_i$ exceeds about 10^{-7} mol/l and the system is fully activated at about 10^{-6} mol/l.

The main mechanisms responsible for controlling $[Ca^{2+}]_i$ are summarised in Figure 14.4. The major route of calcium entry is via L-type voltage-sensitive calcium channels in the surface membrane. Calcium enters the cell by this route with each action potential and causes an immediate rise in $[Ca^{2+}]_i$. Activation of the contractile machinery is due in minor part directly to this influx but mainly to a secondary release of calcium from the sarcoplasmic reticulum which is triggered by small localised increases in cytoplasmic calcium concentration ('calcium sparks') subjacent to the T-tubule membrane. These tubules extend inward from the surface membrane and are close to the sub-sarcolemmal cisternae of the sarcoplasmic reticulum. The local rise in $[Ca^{2+}]_i$ acts on large calcium channels in the cisternae, called *ryanodine receptors* because they interact with this plant alkaloid (they are also activated by **caffeine** at high concentrations). These open to release large amounts of calcium ions from within the cisternae (where calcium is bound to a binding protein called calsequestrin) into the cytoplasm where they interact with troponin C.*

Calcium entry is balanced by removal of calcium from the cell, mainly by the *calcium–sodium exchange pump* mentioned above in connection with after-depolarisation. The imported sodium ions are in turn extruded, in exchange for potassium ions, by the *sodium–potassium pump*. This interconnection between sodium and calcium movements across the membrane means that changes in $[Na^+]_i$ affect $[Ca^{2+}]_i$ in the same direction. Thus, inhibition of the sodium–potassium pump (e.g. by cardiac glycosides; see below) raises $[Na^+]_i$ and slows sodium–calcium exchange. This leads to increased calcium stored in the sarcoplasmic reticulum, and hence to increased contraction. More than 99% of the total cell calcium is normally sequestered by intracellular organelles (mitochondria as well as sarcoplasmic reticulum), so a small shift of calcium between these stores and the cytosol can cause a large change in $[Ca^{2+}]_i$.

Many effects of drugs on cardiac contractility can be explained in terms of actions on $[Ca^{2+}]_i$, secondary to effects on voltage-sensitive calcium channels in plasma membrane or sarcoplasmic reticulum or on the sodium–potassium pump. Other factors that affect the force of contraction are the availability of oxygen and a source of metabolic energy such as glucose. Myocardial 'stunning'—contractile dysfunction that persists after ischaemia and reperfusion despite restoration of blood flow and absence of cardiac necrosis—is incompletely understood but can be clinically important. Its converse is known as 'ischaemic preconditioning': this means an improved ability to withstand ischaemia following previous ischaemic episodes. This potentially clinically beneficial syndrome is demonstrable experimentally in many species and could occur in several clinical settings in man. There is some evidence that it is mediated by *adenosine* (see Ch. 9), which accumulates as ATP is depleted. Adenosine inhibits adenylate cyclase (via an inhibitory G-protein) and activates other potential effectors such as phospholipase C and ATP-sensitive potassium channels. Exogenous adenosine affords a degree of protection similar to that caused by ischaemic preconditioning, and blockade of adenosine receptors prevents the protective effect of preconditioning. There is considerable interest in developing strategies to minimise bad effects of ischaemia (stunning) while maximising good ones (preconditioning).

---

*This mechanism involving calcium sparks contrasts with skeletal muscle where L-type calcium channels in T-tubules act *directly* as voltage sensors to control the ryanodine-sensitive receptors in the sarcoplasmic reticulum. It also contrasts with the situation in smooth muscle where smaller inositol trisphosphate-activated Ca^{2+} channels are responsible for coupling the contractile responses to agonist stimulation, Ch. 2; this type of channel is of less importance in cardiac myocytes, but may contribute to diastolic tone.

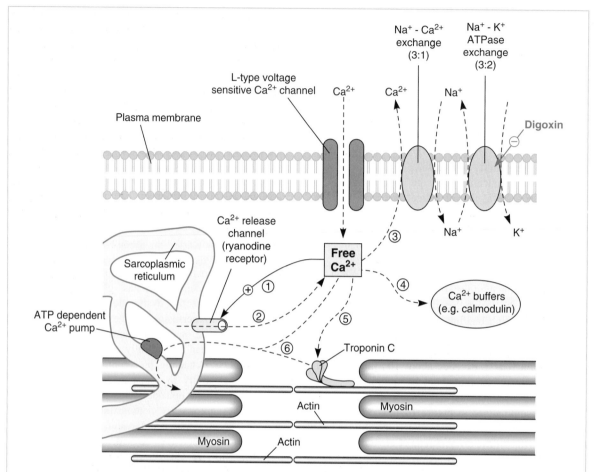

Fig. 14.4 The control of intracellular calcium in the cardial myocyte. Depolarisation of the plasma membrane during the action potential activates L-type voltage sensitive Ca^{2+} channels and Ca^{2+} diffuses into the cell, increasing free Ca^{2+} which acts (①) on Ca^{2+}-release channels (ryanodine receptors) in the sarcoplasmic reticulum to release Ca^{2+} (②) further increasing free Ca^{2+}, some of which is extruded from the cell by Na^{2+} exchange (③) some is bound to intracellular buffers (e.g. calmodulin (④), some binds to troponic C (⑤) thereby initiating contraction, and some being pumped back into the sarcoplasmic reticulum by an ATP-dependent Ca^{2+} pump (⑥) lowering cytoplasmic Ca^{2+} and initiating relaxation. (Based on Hafozzart, Ion channel and cardiac function, pp 211–224, in Molecular Cardiovascular Medicine.)

Ventricular function curves and heart failure

The force of contraction of the heart is determined partly by its intrinsic *contractility* (which, as described above, depends on the availability of intracellular calcium and ATP) and partly by extrinsic factors that affect *end-diastolic volume* and, hence, the resting length of the muscle fibres. The end-diastolic volume is determined largely by the end-diastolic pressure, and its effect on the stroke work of the heart is expressed in the Frank–Starling Law of the Heart, which reflects an inherent property of the contractile system. The Frank–Starling Law can be represented as a *ventricular function curve* (Fig. 14.5).

The *stroke work* of the ventricle is measured by the area enclosed by the pressure–volume curve during the cardiac cycle. It is approximated by the product of stroke volume and mean arterial pressure. As Starling showed, factors extrinsic to the heart can affect its performance in various ways, two patterns of response to increased load being particularly important:

- Increased cardiac filling pressure (*pre-load*), whether caused by increased blood volume or by venocon-striction, increases ventricular end-diastolic volume. This increases stroke volume and hence cardiac output

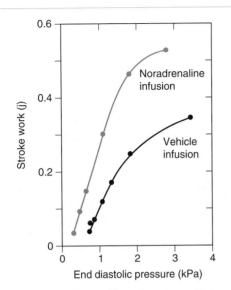

Fig. 14.5 Ventricular function curves in the dog. Intrinsic control (in this case increased myocardial contractility) is exemplified by the effect of noradrenaline infusion. Extrinsic control (the effect of external circulatory factors on the force of contraction of the heart) is shown by the relationship between stroke work and diastolic pressure. (Redrawn from: Sarnoff S J et al. 1960 Circ Res 8: 1108)

and mean arterial pressure. Cardiac work and cardiac oxygen consumption both increase.

- Peripheral arteriolar vasoconstriction increases *after-load*. End-diastolic volume, and hence stroke work, are initially unchanged but constant stroke work in the face of increased vascular resistance causes reduced stroke volume and hence increased end-diastolic volume. This in turn increases stroke work, until a steady state is re-established with increased end-diastolic volume and the same cardiac output as before. As with increased pre-load, cardiac work and cardiac oxygen consumption both increase.

Normally the filling pressure is only a few centimetres of water above zero, on the steep part of the ventricular function curve, so a large increase in stroke work can be achieved with only a small increase in filling pressure. The Starling mechanism plays little part in controlling cardiac output in healthy subjects (e.g. during exercise), because changes in contractility, mainly due to changes in sympathetic activity, achieve the necessary regulation without any increase in ventricular filling pressure (Fig. 14.5).

By contrast, in patients with heart failure (see Ch. 15)

the heart may be unable to deliver as much blood as the tissues require even when its contractility is increased by sympathetic activity. Heart failure has several causes, including myocardial disease (usually ischaemic), valvular disease, and severe hypertension (where excessive peripheral vascular resistance increases the cardiac work required to maintain adequate tissue perfusion). Under these conditions the basal (i.e. at rest) ventricular function curve is greatly depressed, and there is insufficient reserve, in the sense of extra contractility that can be achieved by sympathetic activity, to enable cardiac output to be maintained during exercise without a large increase in central venous pressure (Fig. 14.5). Oedema, which can affect peripheral tissues (causing swelling of the legs) and the lungs (causing breathlessness) is an important consequence of cardiac failure. It is caused by the increased venous pressure, and retention of sodium ions (see Ch. 20), rather than by the inadequate cardiac output per se.

Myocardial contraction

- Controlling factors are:
  —intrinsic contractility
  —extrinsic circulatory factors.
- Contractility depends critically on control of intracellular Ca^{2+}, and hence on:
  —Ca^{2+} entry across the cell membrane
  —Ca^{2+} storage in the sarcoplasmic reticulum.
- The main factors controlling Ca^{2+} entry are:
  — activity of voltage-gated Ca^{2+} channels
  — $[Na^+]_i$, which affects Ca^{2+}/Na^+ exchange.
  Many things affect these two processes, including catecholamines and drugs affecting the Na^+ pump.
- Extrinsic control of cardiac contraction is due to the dependence of stroke work on the end-diastolic volume, expressed in the Frank–Starling Law.
- Cardiac work is affected independently by after-load (i.e. peripheral resistance) and pre-load (i.e. central venous pressure).
- 'Heart failure' describes the condition in which the cardiac output is insufficient to meet the circulatory needs of the body (at rest or during exercise).

MYOCARDIAL OXYGEN CONSUMPTION AND CORONARY BLOOD FLOW

Relative to its large metabolic needs, the heart is one of the most poorly perfused tissues in the body. Coronary flow is, under normal circumstances, closely related to myocardial oxygen consumption, and both change over a nearly 10-fold range between conditions of rest and maximal exercise.

Physiological factors

The main physiological factors that regulate coronary flow are:

- physical factors
- vascular control by metabolites
- neural and humoral control.

Physical factors

During systole the pressure exerted by the myocardium on vessels that pass through it equals or exceeds the perfusion pressure, so coronary flow occurs only during diastole. Diastole is shortened more than systole during tachycardia, reducing the period available for myocardial perfusion. During diastole, the effective perfusion pressure is equal to the difference between the aortic and ventricular pressures (Fig. 14.6). If diastolic aortic pressure falls or diastolic ventricular pressure increases, then perfusion pressure falls and so (unless other control mechanisms can compensate) does coronary blood flow. Stenosis of the aortic valve produces both of these effects, and often causes ischaemic chest pain ('angina') even in the absence of coronary artery disease.

Vascular control by metabolites/mediators

Vascular control by metabolites is the most important mechanism by which coronary flow is regulated. A reduction in arterial P_{O_2} causes marked vasodilatation of coronary vessels in situ, but has little effect on isolated strips of coronary artery. This suggests that it is a change in the pattern of metabolites produced by the myocardial cells, rather than the change in P_{O_2} per se that controls the state of the coronary vessels, the most popular candidate for the dilator metabolite being *adenosine* (see Ch. 9).

Neural and humoral control

Coronary vessels have a dense sympathetic innervation, but sympathetic nerves (like circulating catecholamines) exert only a small direct effect on the coronary circulation. Large coronary vessels possess α-adrenoceptors that mediate vasoconstriction, whereas smaller vessels have β_2-adrenoceptors that have a dilator effect. Coronary vessels are also innervated by purinergic, peptidergic and nitrergic nerves. Normally, neural and endocrine effects on coronary vasculature are overshadowed by the vascular response to altered mechanical and metabolic activity.

Coronary atherosclerosis and its consequence

Partial occlusion of coronary vessels by atheromatous deposits occurs in at least 75% of the adult population of developed countries, but is asymptomatic for most of the natural history of the disease (see Ch. 15). Important consequences of coronary atherosclerosis are:

- angina (ischaemic chest pain)
- myocardial infarction.

Angina

Angina occurs when the oxygen supply to the myocardium is insufficient for its needs. The pain has a

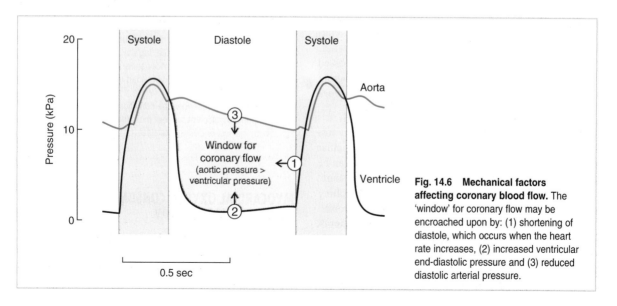

Fig. 14.6 Mechanical factors affecting coronary blood flow. The 'window' for coronary flow may be encroached upon by: (1) shortening of diastole, which occurs when the heart rate increases, (2) increased ventricular end-diastolic pressure and (3) reduced diastolic arterial pressure.

characteristic distribution in the chest, arm and neck, and is brought on by exertion or excitement when myocardial perfusion is reduced, as explained above, and the oxygen demands of the heart are increased. It is unpleasant in its own right as well as providing an important diagnostic pointer to the need for investigation and treatment of coronary atheromatous disease, and is an important target for therapeutic intervention (see below). A similar type of pain occurs in skeletal muscle when it is made to contract while its blood supply is interrupted, and Lewis showed many years ago that chemical factors released by ischaemic muscle are responsible. Possible candidates include *potassium ions, hydrogen ions, bradykinin* (Ch. 11) and *adenosine*, all of which stimulate nociceptors (see Ch. 37). It is possible that the same mediator that causes coronary vasodilatation is responsible, at higher concentration, for initiating pain.

Three kinds of angina are recognised clinically. *Stable angina* is characterised by predictable pain on exertion. It is produced by an increased demand on the heart and is due to a fixed narrowing of the coronary vessels, almost always by atheroma. Symptomatic therapy is directed at altering cardiac work with organic nitrates, β-adrenoceptor antagonists and/or calcium antagonists as described below, together with treatment of the underlying atheromatous disease (Ch. 16) and prophylaxis against thrombosis with **aspirin** (Ch. 17). *Unstable angina* is characterised by pain that occurs with less and less exertion, culminating in pain at rest. The pathology is basically the same as that involved in myocardial infarction, namely platelet–fibrin thrombus associated with a ruptured atheromatous plaque, but without complete occlusion of the vessel. The risk of infarction is substantial, and the main aim of therapy is to reduce this. **Aspirin** approximately halves the risk of myocardial infarction in this setting, and **heparin** is also effective (Ch. 17). *Variant angina* is uncommon. It occurs at rest and is caused by coronary artery spasm, again usually in association with atheromatous disease. Therapy is with coronary artery vasodilators (e.g. organic nitrates, calcium antagonists).

Myocardial infarction

Infarction of a segment of myocardium occurs when a coronary vessel becomes blocked by thrombosis. This may be fatal, and is the commonest cause of death in many parts of the world, usually as a result of mechanical failure of the ventricle or from dysrhythmia. Cardiac myocytes rely on aerobic metabolism, and if the supply of oxygen remains below a critical value a sequence of events leading to cell death by *necrosis*

ensues. Recently, however, it has been appreciated that the process of *apoptosis* may be initiated in cardiac myocytes under conditions of ischaemia as an alternative to necrosis (see Ch. 42 for a fuller account of apoptosis). This is an orderly gene-directed process of cell suicide which can be activated via various membrane receptors, including the receptor for tumour necrosis factor (TNF-α) which works through sphingosine as its second messenger. Each of these receptors activates interleukin-1-converting enzyme (ICE)-related proteases which inactivate poly-[ADP-ribose]-polymerase (PARP). This process is inhibited by 'anti-death' genes such as *bcl*-2. PARP repairs DNA damage by catalysing ADP-ribosylation of nucleoproteins at sites of DNA strand breaks, and if it is inhibited nuclear DNA becomes fragmented in a distinctive ladder pattern and the cell dies despite persistent integrity of the plasma and organelle membranes.

The relative importance of necrosis and apoptosis in myocardial cell death in clinically distinct settings of ischaemia is unknown, but it has been suggested that apoptosis may be an adaptive process in hypoperfused regions, sacrificing some jeopardised myocytes but thereby avoiding the arrhythmogenic disturbance of membrane function inherent in necrosis. Consequently it is currently unknown if pharmacological approaches to promote or inhibit this pathway could be clinically beneficial. The sequences of events leading from vascular occlusion to cell death via the two pathways are illustrated in Figure 14.7. Prevention of irreversible ischaemic damage following an episode of coronary thrombosis is an important therapeutic aim, and drug treatment aimed at protecting myocardial cells is currently being studied intensively. The main possibilities among existing therapeutic drugs, shown in Figure 14.7, are:

- thrombolytic and antiplatelet drugs to open the blocked artery: see Ch. 17
- oxygen
- opioids to prevent pain and reduce excessive sympathetic activity
- β-adrenoceptor antagonists
- angiotensin-converting enzyme inhibitors.

The latter two classes of drugs reduce cardiac work, and thereby the metabolic needs of the heart. β-adrenoceptor antagonists had only a small beneficial effect when given acutely to patients with acute myocardial infarction in the ISIS-1 study (although they have an important longer-term benefit during chronic treatment in reducing arrhythmic deaths), but are widely used in an attempt to reduce ischaemic damage in patients with unstable angina. Experimental studies have shown that

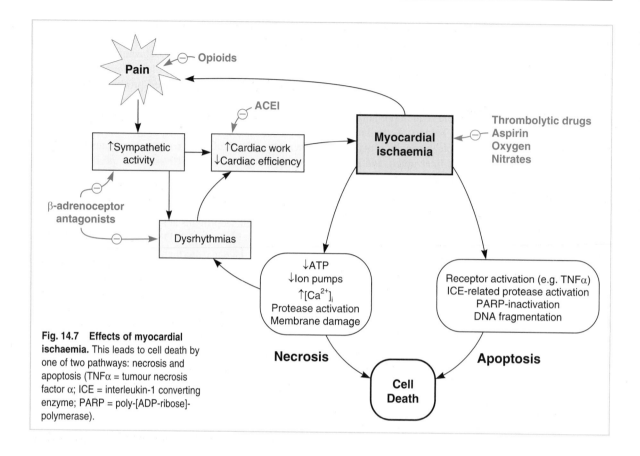

Fig. 14.7 Effects of myocardial ischaemia. This leads to cell death by one of two pathways: necrosis and apoptosis (TNFα = tumour necrosis factor α; ICE = interleukin-1 converting enzyme; PARP = poly-[ADP-ribose]-polymerase).

chronic treatment with **captopril** and other angiotensin-converting enzyme inhibitors improves survival and haemodynamics in rat models of myocardial infarction, and several clinical trials have confirmed that various angiotensin-converting enzyme inhibitors improve survival if given to patients shortly after myocardial infarction, especially if there is even a modest degree of myocardial dysfunction (e.g. reduced left ventricular ejection fraction estimated by echocardiography), without clinical signs of heart failure. Their peripheral haemodynamic effects are probably important in limiting undesirable changes in cardiac structure that follow myocardial infarction, but inhibition of the cardiac renin–angiotensin system has also been postulated as a mechanism.

Organic nitrates, despite being attractive candidates as drugs that could reduce ischaemic damage (since they also reduce cardiac work), and despite several small trials that appeared encouraging, proved disappointing in a large randomised controlled trial ('ISIS-4') in which they did not improve outcome in patients with myocardial infarction, although they are useful in preventing or treating anginal pain (see below). *Calcium antagonists*, which

reduce both cardiac work (via arteriolar vasodilatation and after-load reduction) and Ca^{2+} entry into cardiac myocytes, have been disappointing, although they have

---

Coronary flow, ischaemia and infarction

- The heart has a smaller blood supply in relation to its oxygen consumption than most organs.
- Coronary flow is controlled mainly by:
  — physical factors, including transmural pressure during systole
  — vasodilator metabolites.
  Autonomic innervation is less important.
- Coronary ischaemia is usually due to atherosclerosis, and causes anginal pain. Sudden ischaemia is usually due to thrombosis, and may cause cardiac infarction.
- Coronary spasm sometimes causes angina (variant angina).
- Cellular calcium overload results from ischaemia, and may be responsible for:
  —cell death
  —initiation of dysrhythmias.

not been fully evaluated (see below). Several clinical trials of short-acting dihydropyridines (e.g. **nifedipine**) were halted when adverse trends were evident. Calcium antagonists *are* useful in preventing anginal pain.

ATRIAL NATRIURETIC PEPTIDE (ANP) AND B TYPE NATRIURETIC PEPTIDE

Atrial cells have a specialised endocrine function in relation to the cardiovascular system. They contain secretory granules, and store and release a 28-amino-acid peptide (ANP) which has powerful effects on the kidney and vascular system. Release of ANP occurs in response to stretching of the atria by increased central venous pressure, signalling volume overload of the circulation. Saline infusion is sufficient to evoke ANP release. Two related natriuretic peptides (B and C, found respectively in ventricular muscle and vascular endothelium) are also known.

The main effects of natriuretic peptides are to increase Na^+ and water excretion by the kidney, relax vascular smooth muscle (except efferent arterioles of renal glomeruli which constrict), increase vascular permeability and inhibit the release and/or actions of several hormones and mediators including aldosterone, angiotensin II, endothelin and ADH. They exert their effects by combining with membrane receptors (which exist in at least two subtypes designated A and B).* NPR-A and NPR-B both incorporate a catalytic guanylate cyclase moiety. Binding of one of the natriuretic peptides to either receptor leads to generation of cGMP within the cell. This is the same response as that produced by organic nitrates (see later) and endothelium-derived NO (Ch. 11), which, however, achieve this by interacting with soluble rather than membrane-bound guanylate cyclase. Renal glomerular afferent arterioles are dilated by ANP but efferent arterioles are constricted, so filtration pressure is increased, leading to increased glomerular filtration and enhanced Na^+ excretion. Elsewhere, natriuretic peptides cause vasorelaxation especially of capacitance vessels, as do organic nitrates, and cause a fall in blood pressure. Their therapeutic potential is considered in Chapter 15.

DRUGS THAT AFFECT CARDIAC FUNCTION

Drugs that have a major action on the heart can be divided into the following groups:

- Drugs that *directly* affect myocardial cells. These include:
  —autonomic neurotransmitters and related drugs
  —cardiac glycosides and other inotropic agents
  —antidysrhythmic drugs
  —miscellaneous agents, including certain endogenous substances.
  The last are discussed elsewhere (e.g. glucagon, Ch. 22).
- Drugs that affect cardiac function indirectly, through actions elsewhere in the vascular system. Some antianginal drugs (e.g. nitrates) fall into this category, as do most drugs that are used to treat heart failure (e.g. diuretics and angiotensin-converting enzyme inhibitors).
- Ca^{2+} antagonists act both directly on myocardial cells and also affect cardiac function indirectly by relaxing arterioles.

AUTONOMIC TRANSMITTERS AND RELATED DRUGS

Many aspects of autonomic pharmacology have been discussed in Chapters 6, 7 and 8; here we mention only aspects that particularly concern the heart.

Autonomic control of the heart

Both sympathetic and parasympathetic systems normally exert a tonic effect on the heart at rest.

Sympathetic system
The main effects of sympathetic activity on the heart are:

- increased force of contraction (*positive inotropic effect*; Fig. 14.8)
- increased heart rate (*positive chronotropic effect*; Fig. 14.9)
- increased *automaticity*
- *repolarisation* and restoration of function following generalised cardiac depolarisation
- reduced *cardiac efficiency* (i.e. O_2 consumption is increased more than cardiac work).

These effects all result from activation of β_1-receptors. The β_1-effects of catecholamines on the heart, though complex, are probably all due to an increase in the

---

*The nomenclature of natriuretic peptides and their receptors is peculiarly obtuse. The peptides are named 'A' for atrial, 'B' for brain—despite being present mainly in cardiac ventricle—and 'C' for A,B,C...; the natriuretic peptide receptors (NPR) are named 'NPR-A' which preferentially binds ANP, 'NPR-B' which binds *C* natriuretic peptide preferentially, and 'NPR-C' for 'clearance' receptor, since until recently clearance via cellular uptake and degradation by lysosomal enzymes was the only definite known function of this binding site.

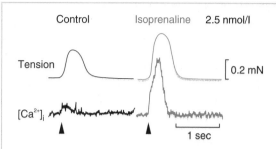

Fig. 14.8   The calcium transient in frog cardiac muscle.
A group of cells was injected with the phosphorescent Ca^{2+} indicator, aequorin, which allows $[Ca^{2+}]_i$ to be monitored optically. Isoprenaline causes a large increase in the Ca^{2+} transient in response to an electrical stimulus (▲) and in the tension produced. (From: Allen D G, Blinks J R 1978 Nature 273: 509)

intracellular concentration of cAMP (see Ch. 2). cAMP activates protein kinase A which phosphorylates sites on Ca^{2+} channels, including the α_1-subunits. This increases the probability that the channels will open, increasing inward Ca^{2+} current and hence force of cardiac contraction (Fig. 14.8). β_1-receptor activation also increases the Ca^{2+} sensitivity of the contractile machinery, possibly by phosphorylating troponin C; furthermore, it facilitates Ca^{2+} capture by the sarcoplasmic reticulum, thereby increasing the amount of Ca^{2+} stored intracellularly

available for release by the action potential. The net result of catecholamine action is to elevate and steepen the ventricular function curve (Fig. 14.5). The increase in heart rate results from an increased slope of the pacemaker potential (Figs 14.1 and 14.9) owing to a shift in the voltage-dependence of the conductances underlying the pacemaker currents so that they are switched on, and reach the firing threshold, earlier. Increased calcium entry also causes increased automaticity because of the effect of $[Ca^{2+}]_i$ on the transient inward current, which can result in a train of action potentials following a single stimulus (Fig. 14.2).

β_1-receptor activation causes hyperpolarisation of damaged or hypoxic myocardium. This is due to stimulation of the Na^+/K^+ pump, which generates a net outward sodium current. Such repolarisation may restore function if asystole has occurred following myocardial infarction, and adrenaline is administered intravenously during asystolic cardiac arrest.

The reduction of cardiac efficiency by catecholamines is important because it means that the oxygen requirement of the myocardium increases even if the work of the heart is unchanged. Myocardial infarction causes sympathetic activation (Fig. 14.7), which has the undesirable effect of increasing the oxygen needs of the damaged myocardium.

The actions and uses of drugs that act on β-receptors are described in Chapter 8.

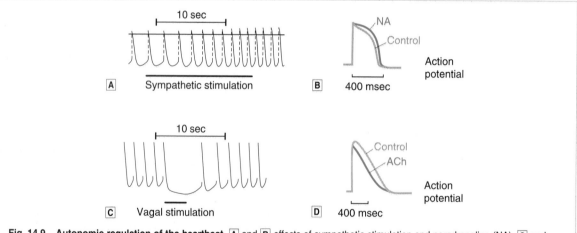

Fig. 14.9   Autonomic regulation of the heartbeat. [A] and [B] effects of sympathetic stimulation and noradrenaline (NA). [C] and [D] effects of parasympathetic stimulation and acetylcholine (ACh). Sympathetic stimulation (A) increases the slope of the pacemaker potential and increases heart rate whereas parasympathetic stimulation (C) abolishes the pacemaker potential, hyperpolarises the membrane and temporarily stops the heart (frog sinus venosus). NA (B) prolongs the action potential, while ACh (D) shortens it (frog atrium). (From: (A and C) Hutter O F, Trautwein W 1956 J Gen Physiol 39: 715; (B) Reuter H 1974 J Physiol 242: 429; (D) Giles W R, Noble S J 1976 J Physiol 261: 103)

Parasympathetic system

Parasympathetic activity produces effects that are, in general, opposite to those of sympathetic activation, namely:

- cardiac slowing and reduced automaticity
- decreased force of contraction (mainly in atria)
- inhibition of AV conduction.

These effects result from occupation of muscarinic (M_2) acetylcholine receptors, which are abundant in nodal and atrial tissue but sparse in the ventricle. These receptors are negatively coupled to adenylate cyclase, and thus reduce cAMP formation, acting to inhibit the slow calcium current, in opposition to β_1-adrenoceptors. M_2-receptors also open a potassium channel (called K_{ACh}) via G-protein coupling. The resulting increase in potassium permeability produces a hyperpolarising current that opposes the inward pacemaker current, slowing the heart and reducing automaticity (see Fig. 14.9).

The negative inotropic effect of parasympathetic stimulation in the atria is associated with marked shortening of the action potential (Fig. 14.9). Increased K^+ permeability and reduced Ca^{2+} current both contribute to the conduction block at the AV node, where propagation is dependent on the Ca^{2+} current. The shortening of the atrial action potential reduces the refractory period which can, paradoxically, increase the probability of re-entrant arrhythmias. Vagal activity is often increased during myocardial infarction, both in association with vagal afferent stimulation, and also as a side-effect of opioids used to control the pain. Coronary *vessels* lack cholinergic innervation.*

As well as producing opposite effects on myocardial

cells, the sympathetic and parasympathetic systems also interact presynaptically. The terminals of sympathetic and parasympathetic nerves are often closely related, and there is evidence for mutual inhibition of transmitter release by the two systems.

The actions and uses of drugs that act on muscarinic receptors are described in Chapter 7.

CARDIAC GLYCOSIDES

Cardiac glycosides come from plants of the foxglove family (*Digitalis* spp.). Their effectiveness in cardiac failure was described by Withering in 1775, who wrote on the use of the foxglove 'it has a power over the motion of the heart to a degree yet unobserved in any other medicine …'. Cardiac glycosides are still widely used for the treatment of cardiac failure in association with rapid atrial fibrillation, but the effectiveness of angiotensin-converting enzyme inhibitors in prolonging survival in patients with heart failure (Ch. 15) has led to decreased use of cardiac glycosides in patients with heart failure who are in sinus rhythm. Nevertheless, recent studies have shown that while digoxin does not reduce mortality it does reduce hospitalisation when added to diuretics and angiotensin-converting enzyme inhibitors in patients with chronic heart failure. Theoretical interest remains strong, because of evidence of an endogenous digitalis-like factor closely similar to **ouabain**. This is of uncertain physiological significance.

Chemistry

Foxgloves contain several cardiac glycosides with similar actions. **Digoxin** is the most important therapeutically. **Ouabain** is similar but shorter-acting; its sugar moiety consists of rhamnose, not found generally in mammals. The basic chemical structure of glycosides (Fig. 14.10) consists of three components, a *sugar moiety*, a *steroid* and a *lactone*. The sugar moiety consists of 1–4 linked monosaccharides, some of which are not found elsewhere in nature. The lactone ring is essential for activity, and substituted lactones can retain biological activity even when the steroid moiety is removed.

Actions

The main effects of glycosides are on the heart, but some of their extracardiac actions cause unwanted effects, such as nausea, vomiting and diarrhoea. The cardiac effects are:

- cardiac slowing and reduced rate of conduction through the AV node

---

> **Autonomic control of the heart**
>
> - Sympathetic activity, acting through β_1-adrenoceptors, increases heart rate, contractility and automaticity, but reduces cardiac efficiency (in relation to oxygen consumption).
> - β_1-adrenoceptors act by increasing cAMP formation, which increases calcium currents.
> - Parasympathetic activity, acting through M_2 muscarinic receptors, causes cardiac slowing, decreased force of contraction (atria only) and inhibition of AV conduction.
> - M_2-receptors inhibit cAMP formation, and also open K^+ channels, causing hyperpolarisation.

---

*The creator has, however, thoughtfully provided coronary *endothelium* with muscarinic *receptors* linked to NO synthesis, presumably for the delectation of vascular pharmacologists.

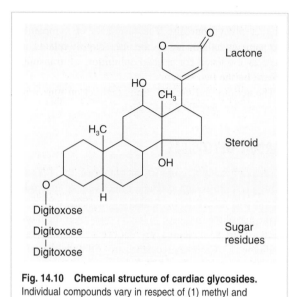

Fig. 14.10 Chemical structure of cardiac glycosides. Individual compounds vary in respect of (1) methyl and hydroxyl groups on the steroid nucleus, and (2) sugar residues.

- increased force of contraction
- disturbances of rhythm, especially:
  —block of AV conduction
  —increased ectopic pacemaker activity.

Adverse effects are common and can be severe. One of the main drawbacks of glycosides in clinical use is the narrow margin between effectiveness and toxicity.

Mechanism of action

The basic mechanisms of action of cardiac glycosides are increased vagal activity and inhibition of the Na^+/K^+ pump, which results from binding to a site on the extracellular aspect of the α-subunit of this α-β heterodimeric ATPase.

Rate and rhythm. Cardiac glycosides *slow AV conduction* by increasing vagal activity via an action on the central nervous system. Their beneficial effect in established rapid atrial fibrillation is mediated by this action on AV conduction. If ventricular rate is excessively rapid, the time available for diastolic filling is inadequate. Increasing the refractory period of the AV node is beneficial under these conditions, because it increases the minimum interval between impulses and reduces ventricular rate. The atrial dysrhythmia is unaffected, but the pumping efficiency of the heart improves owing to improved ventricular filling. Supraventricular tachycardia can be terminated by cardiac glycosides by slowing

AV conduction, although other drugs are usually employed for this indication (see below).

Larger doses of glycosides cause disturbances of rhythm. These may occur at plasma concentrations within, or only slightly above, the therapeutic range. Slowing of AV conduction can progress to AV block. In addition to depressing AV conduction, glycosides cause ectopic beats. Because Na^+/K^+ exchange is electrogenic (that is, it pumps more Na^+ ions out than K^+ ions in and thus generates a net hyperpolarising current), inhibition of the pump by glycosides causes depolarisation, predisposing to disturbances of cardiac rhythm. Furthermore, the increased cytoplasmic Ca^{2+} causes increased afterdepolarisation, leading first to coupled beats (bigeminy), in which a normal ventricular beat is followed by an ectopic beat; this is followed by ventricular tachycardia where there is a continuous succession of such triggered ectopic beats, and eventually by ventricular fibrillation.

Force of contraction. Glycosides cause a large increase in twitch tension in isolated preparations of cardiac muscle. Unlike catecholamines they do not accelerate relaxation (compare Fig. 14.8 with Fig. 14.11). Increased tension is caused by an increased intracellular calcium transient (Fig. 14.11). The action potential is only slightly affected and the slow inward current little changed, so the increased calcium transient probably reflects a greater release of calcium from intracellular stores. The most likely mechanism for this is as follows (see also Fig. 14.4):

- Glycosides bind to an extracellular site on the α-subunit of Na^+/K^+-ATPase on the plasma membrane of cardiac myocytes, and thus inhibit the Na^+/K^+ pump.
- Increased $[Na^+]_i$ slows extrusion of Ca^{2+}. This is

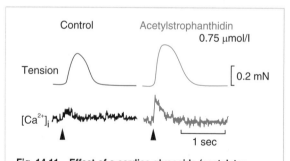

Fig. 14.11 Effect of a cardiac glycoside (acetylstrophanthidin) on the Ca^{2+} transient and tension produced by frog cardiac muscle. The effect was recorded as in Figure 14.8. (From: Allen D G, Blinks J R 1978 Nature 273: 509)

because extrusion of Ca^{2+} is by Na^+/Ca^{2+} exchange. Increasing $[Na^+]_i$ reduces the inwardly directed gradient for Na^+; the smaller this gradient the slower is extrusion of Ca^{2+} by Na^+/Ca^{2+} exchange.

- Increased $[Ca^{2+}]_i$ is stored in the sarcoplasmic reticulum, and thus increases the amount of $[Ca^{2+}]$ released by each action potential.

Interaction with extracellular K^+

Effects of cardiac glycosides are increased if plasma $[K^+]$ decreases, because of reduced competition with K^+ for their binding site on the Na^+/K^+-ATPase. This is clinically important because diuretics (Ch. 20) are often used together with glycosides to treat heart failure, and most of them decrease plasma $[K^+]$ thereby increasing the risk of arrhythmia.

Clinical aspects

Clinical use and unwanted effects of **digoxin** are summarised on this page.

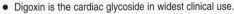

Cardiac glycosides

- Act by inhibiting Na^+/K^+ pump, thus increasing $[Na^+]_i$. This results in reduced Na^+/Ca^{2+} exchange, causing secondary rise in Ca^{2+} accumulation by sarcoplasmic reticulum.
- Main effect is increased force of contraction.
- Additional important effects are:
  —increase of ectopic pacemaker activity
  —impairment of AV conduction
  —increased vagal activity, causing bradycardia.
- Effects are increased by hypokalaemia.

OTHER DRUGS THAT INCREASE MYOCARDIAL CONTRACTILITY

Certain β_1-adrenoceptor agonists, e.g. **dobutamine**, are used to treat acute but potentially reversible heart failure (e.g. following cardiac surgery, or in some cases of cardiogenic shock) on the basis of their positive inotropic action. Dobutamine, for reasons that are not well understood, produces less tachycardia than other β_1-agonists. It is administered intravenously. Attempts to use orally-active β-agonists to treat chronic heart failure have been disappointing. **Xamoterol**, a partial agonist, causes modest haemodynamic improvement in mild heart failure but is deleterious in more severe disease, which makes its use problematic in a disorder whose natural history is to progress unpredictably from mild to severe.

Clinical uses of digoxin

- Digoxin is the cardiac glycoside in widest clinical use.
- Uses include:
  — slowing ventricular rate in rapid atrial fibrillation
  — treatment of heart failure in patients who remain symptomatic despite optimal use of diuretics (Ch. 20) and angiotensin-converting enzyme inhibitors (Ch. 15).
- Adverse effects include nausea, vomiting, cardiac arrhythmias, confusion.
- Administration is oral or, in urgent situations, intravenous.
- Elimination is mainly by renal excretion; elimination half-time is approximately 36 hours in patients with normal renal function, considerably longer in elderly patients and those with overt renal failure in whom reduced doses are needed.
- A loading dose is used in urgent situations.
- The therapeutic range of plasma concentrations, below which digoxin is unlikely to be effective and above which the risk of toxicity increases substantially, is fairly well defined. Determination of plasma digoxin concentration is useful when lack of efficacy or toxicity is suspected.
- Clinically important interactions occur with drugs that reduce plasma K^+ (e.g. loop diuretics) or which simultaneously reduce digoxin excretion and tissue binding (e.g. amiodarone, verapamil).

Inhibitors of a heart-specific subtype (type III) of phosphodiesterase, the enzyme responsible for the intracellular degradation of cAMP, increase contractility. They increase intracellular cAMP concentration, as do β-adrenoceptor agonists, and are pro-arrhythmic for the same reason. Compounds in this group include **amrinone** and **milrinone**, which are chemically and pharmacologically very similar. As with xamoterol, they improve haemodynamic indices in patients with heart failure but paradoxically worsen survival, presumably because of their pro-arrhythmic effect. This dichotomy has had a sobering effect on clinicians and drug regulatory authorities.

ANTIDYSRHYTHMIC DRUGS

A classification of antidysrhythmic drugs in terms of their electrophysiological effects was proposed by Vaughan Williams in 1970; this provides a useful basis for discussing their mechanisms of action, although many of the most useful drugs for treating dysrhythmias do not fit neatly into this classification (Table 14.1). Furthermore, emergency treatment of serious dysrhythmias is usually by physical means (e.g. pacing or electrical cardioversion

Table 14.1 Antidysrhythmic drugs unclassified in the Vaughan Williams' system

Drug	Use
Atropine	Sinus bradycardia
Adrenaline	Cardiac arrest
Isoprenaline	Heart block
Digoxin	Rapid atrial fibrillation
Adenosine	Supraventricular tachycardia
Calcium chloride	Ventricular tachycardia due to hyperkalaemia
Magnesium chloride	Ventricular fibrillation, digoxin toxicity

by applying a direct current shock to the chest) rather than drugs.

The classes (see Table 14.2) are:

- *Class I*: drugs that block voltage-sensitive sodium channels. They are subdivided: Ia, Ib and Ic (see below).
- *Class II*: β-adrenoceptor antagonists.
- *Class III*: drugs that prolong the cardiac action potential, thereby increasing the refractory period and suppressing ectopic and re-entrant activity.
- *Class IV*: calcium antagonists.

The phase of the action potential on which each of these classes of drug have their main effect is shown in Figure 14.12.

Mechanisms of action

Class I drugs

Class I drugs act by *blocking sodium channels*, just as local anaesthetics do, by binding to sites in the α-subunit of the sodium channel (see Ch. 40). Because this inhibits action potential propagation in many excitable cells, it has been referred to as 'membrane stabilising' activity, a phrase best avoided now that the ionic mechanism is well understood. Their characteristic effect on the action potential is to reduce the maximum rate of depolarisation during phase 0.

The reason for further subdivision of these drugs into classes Ia, Ib and Ic is that the earliest examples, **quinidine** and **procainamide** (class Ia), have different effects from many of the more recently developed drugs, even though all share the same basic mechanism of action. A partial explanation for these functional differences comes from electrophysiological studies of the characteristics of the Na⁺ channel block produced by the different types of class I drugs.

The central concept is that of *use-dependent channel block*. It is this characteristic that enables all class I drugs to block the high-frequency excitation of the myocardium that occurs in dysrhythmias, without preventing the heart from beating at normal frequencies. Sodium channels exist in three distinct functional states: *resting*, *open* and *refractory*. Channels switch rapidly from resting to open in response to depolarisation; this is known as activation. Maintained depolarisation, as in

Table 14.2 Summary of antidysrhythmic drugs (Vaughan Williams' classification)

Class	Examples	Mechanism	Cardiac effects*				
			MRD	APD	ERP	AV conduction	Contractility
Ia	Quinidine	Block of Na channels	↓↓	↑	↑	↓↓	↓
	Procainamide		↓↓	↑	↑	↓↓	↓
	Disopyramide		↓↓	↑	↑	↓↓	↓↓
Ib	Lignocaine	Block of Na channels (fast dissoc.)	↓	↓	↑↑	–	–
Ic	Flecainide	Block of Na channels (slow dissoc.)	↓↓↓	–	–	↓↓	↓↓
II	Propranolol	β-adrenoceptor antagonism	–	–	–	↓	↓↓
III	Amiodarone	Not known	–	↑↑↑	↑↑↑	↓	–
	Sotalol		–	↑↑↑	↑↑↑	↓	↓↓
IV	Verapamil	Ca-channel block	–	↓↓	–	↓↓	↓↓↓

* MRD = maximum rate of depolarisation; APD = action potential duration; ERP = effective refractory period

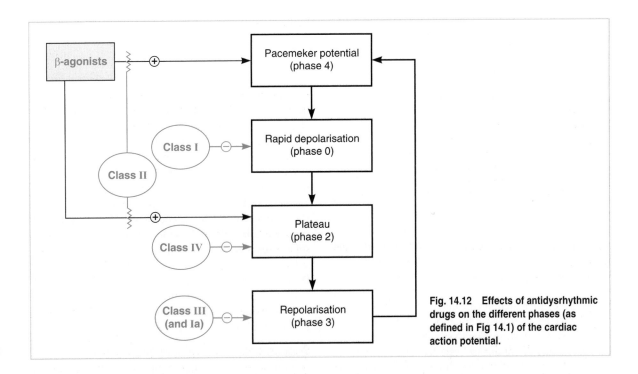

Fig. 14.12 **Effects of antidysrhythmic drugs on the different phases (as defined in Fig 14.1) of the cardiac action potential.**

ischaemic muscle, causes channels to change more slowly from open to refractory (inactivation) and the membrane must then be repolarised for a time to restore the channel to the resting state before it can be activated again. Class I drugs bind to channels most strongly when they are in either the open or refractory state, less strongly to channels in the resting state. Their action therefore shows the property of 'use-dependence' (i.e. the more frequently the channels are activated, the greater the degree of block produced).

Class Ib drugs, e.g. **lignocaine**, associate and dissociate rapidly within the time-frame of the normal heartbeat. Drug binds to open channels during phase 0 of the action potential (affecting the rate of rise very little, but leaving many of the channels blocked by the time the action potential reaches its peak). Dissociation occurs in time for the next action potential, provided the cardiac rhythm is normal. A premature beat, however, will be aborted because the channels are still blocked. Furthermore, class Ib drugs bind selectively to refractory channels, and thus block preferentially when the cells are depolarised, for example in ischaemia.

Class Ic drugs, such as **flecainide** and **encainide**, associate and dissociate much more slowly, thus reaching a steady-state level of block that does not vary appreciably during the cardiac cycle; they also show only a marginal preference for refractory channels, so are not specific for damaged myocardium. Therefore, they cause a rather general reduction in excitability, and do not discriminate particularly against occasional premature beats, as class Ib drugs do, but will suppress re-entrant rhythms that depend on unidirectional or intermittent conduction pathways operating at a low margin of safety (e.g. some forms of paroxysmal atrial fibrillation). They markedly inhibit conduction through the His–Purkinje system, thereby prolonging the QRS complex on the electrocardiogram.

Class Ia, the oldest group (e.g. **quinidine**, **procainamide**, **disopyramide**), lies midway in its properties between Ib and Ic, but in addition prolongs repolarisation, albeit less markedly than class III drugs (see below).

Class II drugs

Class II drugs comprise the β-adrenoceptor antagonists (e.g. **propranolol**).

Adrenaline can cause dysrhythmias by its effects on the pacemaker potential and on the slow inward calcium current (see above). Ventricular dysrhythmias following myocardial infarction are partly the result of increased sympathetic activity (see Fig. 14.7), providing a rationale for using β-adrenoceptor antagonists in this setting. AV conduction depends critically on sympathetic activity, and the refractory period of the AV node is increased by β-adrenoceptor-blocking drugs. β-adrenoceptor antagonists are also used as prophylaxis in patients with recurrent attacks of paroxysmal atrial fibrillation occurring in the setting of sympathetic activation.

Class III drugs

The class III category of antidysrhythmic action was originally based on the unusual behaviour of a single drug, **amiodarone** (see below), although others with similar properties (e.g. **sotalol**) have since been described. Both amiodarone and sotalol have more than one class of antidysrhythmic action. The special feature that defines them as class III drugs is that they substantially prolong the cardiac action potential. The mechanism of this effect is still not fully understood, but involves blocking some of the potassium channels involved in cardiac repolarisation including the outward (delayed) rectifier. Action potential prolongation is associated with an increased refractory period, accounting for powerful and varied antidysrhythmic activity, e.g. by interrupting re-entrant tachycardias and suppressing ectopic activity. However, all drugs that prolong the cardiac action potential (detected clinically as prolonged Q–T interval on the electrocardiogram) can paradoxically also have pro-arrhythmic effects, notably a polymorphic form of ventricular tachycardia called (somewhat whimsically) 'torsades de pointes' (because the appearance of the ECG trace is said to be reminiscent of this ballet sequence). This occurs particularly in patients taking other drugs that can prolong Q–T, such as the H_1-receptor antagonist **terfenadine** (Chs 5 and 48), class Ia drugs such as **disopyramide** and several antipsychotic drugs, in association with disturbances of those electrolytes involved in repolarisation (e.g. hypokalaemia, hypercalcaemia) or in individuals with hereditary prolonged Q–T (Ward–Romano syndrome).* The mechanism of pro-arrhythmia is not fully understood; possibilities include increased dispersion of repolarisation, and in-

creased Ca^{2+} entry during the prolonged action potential leading to increased after-depolarisation.

Class IV drugs

Class IV agents act by blocking voltage-sensitive calcium channels. Class IV drugs in therapeutic use as antidysrhythmic drugs (e.g. **verapamil**) all act on L-type channels. Class IV drugs slow conduction in the SA and AV nodes where action potential propagation depends on slow inward Ca^{2+} current, slowing the heart and terminating supraventricular tachycardias by causing partial AV block. They shorten the plateau phase of the action potential and reduce the force of contraction. Reduced calcium entry reduces the transient inward current and hence reduces after-depolarisation, and thus suppresses premature ectopic beats.

Details of individual drugs

Table 14.2 summarises the properties of important antidysrhythmic drugs. Clinical uses of Class I drugs are given in the clinical box (p. 269).

Quinidine, procainamide and disopyramide (class Ia)

Quinidine and **procainamide** are pharmacologically similar. They are now mainly of historical interest. **Disopyramide** resembles quinidine in its antidysrhythmic effects and uses, as well as its marked atropine-like effects which result in blurred vision, dry mouth, constipation and, in men, may cause urinary retention. It is more negatively inotropic than quinidine but is less likely to cause hypersensitivity reactions.

Lignocaine (class Ib)

Lignocaine remains the most clinically important class I drug, being given by intravenous infusion to treat and prevent ventricular arrhythmias in the immediate aftermath of myocardial infarction, although even in this setting its prophylactic use has not been proved to prolong life. It is almost completely extracted from the portal circulation by hepatic first-pass metabolism (Ch. 5), so cannot be administered orally. Its plasma half-life is normally about 2 hours, but its elimination is slowed if hepatic blood flow is reduced, for example by reduced cardiac output following myocardial infarction or by negative inotropes (e.g. β-adrenoceptor antagonists, also often used after myocardial infarction), and accumulation and toxicity may result if this is not anticipated and the rate of administration reduced accordingly.

The adverse effects of lignocaine are mainly manifestations of actions on the central nervous system, and include drowsiness, disorientation and convulsions. Because of its relatively short half-life, the plasma

---

*'A 3 year old girl began to have blackouts, which decreased in frequency with age. Her electrocardiogram showed a prolonged Q–T interval. When 18 years old she lost consciousness running for a bus. When she was 19, she became quite emotional as a participant in a live television audience and died suddenly.' The molecular basis of this rare inherited disorder is now known to be caused by a mutation in genes coding either for a particular K^+ channel—called *HERG*—or another gene *SCN5A* which codes for the Na^+ channel and disruption of which results in a loss of inactivation of the Na^+ current (see Welsh & Hoshi 1995, Nature 376: 640–641, for a commentary).

concentration can be adjusted fairly rapidly by varying the infusion rate.

Phenytoin (class Ib)

Phenytoin is used as an anticonvulsant (Ch. 36); it has antidysrhythmic actions on the heart, but its clinical use for this indication is obsolete.

Flecainide and encainide (class Ic)

Flecainide and encainide suppress ventricular ectopic beats. They are long-acting and are effective at reducing the frequency of ventricular ectopic beats when administered orally. However, they were found, in a well-controlled trial, actually to *increase* the incidence of sudden death associated with ventricular fibrillation after myocardial infarction, so they are no longer used in this setting. This study, together with the trials of phosphodiesterase inhibitors which improved haemodynamic indices while worsening mortality in patients with heart failure mentioned above, has had a profound impact on the way clinicians and drug regulators view the use of seemingly reasonable intermediate end-points (in this case reduction of frequency of ventricular ectopic beats) as evidence of efficacy in clinical trials.

β-adrenoceptor antagonists (class II)

The most important β-receptor antagonists are described in Chapter 8. Their clinical use for rhythm disorders is shown in the clinical box above. **Propranolol**, like several other drugs of this type, has some class

---

Clinical use of class I antidysrhythmic drugs

Class Ia
- Quinidine and procainamide are now seldom used, because of their side-effects. Disopyramide is similar to quinidine, and has marked atropine-like effects; it is sometimes used in patients with recurrent paroxysmal atrial fibrillation occurring in a setting of vagal overactivity.

Class Ib
- Lignocaine is used (intravenously) to treat ventricular tachycardia and prevent ventricular fibrillation during and immediately after myocardial infarction.
- Phenytoin has been used to treat digoxin-induced dysrhythmias, but this is obsolete.

Class Ic
- Flecainide reduces ventricular ectopics, but *increases* mortality after myocardial infarction. It is sometimes used for paroxysmal atrial fibrillation in patients with disabling symptoms, and for some patients with recurrent tachyarrhythmias associated with abnormal conducting pathways (e.g. Wolff–Parkinson–White syndrome).

Clinical use of Class II antidysrhythmic drugs
- Class II drugs (e.g. propranolol, timolol) *reduce mortality* in patients recovering from myocardial infarction, and should always be considered in this setting.
- Prophylaxis against recurrent tachyarrhythmias (e.g. paroxysmal atrial fibrillation) when these are provoked by increased sympathetic activity.

I action in addition to blocking β-receptors. This may contribute to its antidysrhythmic effects, though probably not very much since an isomer with little β-antagonist activity has little antidysrhythmic activity, despite similar activity as a class I agent.

Adverse effects are described in Chapter 8, the most important being bronchospasm in patients with asthma or other forms of obstructive airways disease, a negative inotropic effect and increased fatigue. It was hoped that the use of β₁-selective drugs (e.g. **metoprolol**, **atenolol**) would reduce the risk of bronchospasm, but their degree of selectivity is inadequate to achieve this goal in clinical practice, although their once-a-day convenience has led to their widespread use in patients without lung disease.

Amiodarone and sotalol (class III)

Amiodarone is highly effective at suppressing dysrhythmias (see clinical box, p. 270). Unfortunately, it has several peculiarities that complicate its use. It is extensively bound in tissues, has a long elimination half-life (10–100 days) and accumulates in the body during repeated dosing (see Ch. 4, p. 67), so its action normally takes days or weeks to develop. For this reason, a loading dose is used, and is given intravenously via a central vein (it causes phlebitis if given into a peripheral vessel) in treating life-threatening arrhythmias. Adverse effects are numerous and important; they include photosensitive skin rashes and a slate-grey/bluish discoloration of the skin, thyroid abnormalities (hypo- and hyper-, connected with its high iodine content), pulmonary fibrosis that is slow in onset but may be irreversible, corneal deposits, neurological and gastrointestinal disturbances.

Sotalol is a non-selective β-adrenoceptor antagonist, this activity residing in the L-isomer. Unlike other β-antagonists, it prolongs the cardiac action potential and the Q–T interval because of prolongation of the slow outward potassium current. This class III activity is present in both L- and D-isomers. Racemic sotalol (the form prescribed) appears to have similar efficacy to amiodarone in preventing chronic malignant ventricular tachyarrhythmias unassociated with acute myocardial

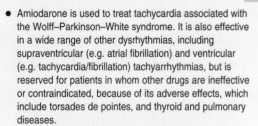

Clinical use of Class III antidysrhythmic drugs

- Amiodarone is used to treat tachycardia associated with the Wolff–Parkinson–White syndrome. It is also effective in a wide range of other dysrhythmias, including supraventricular (e.g. atrial fibrillation) and ventricular (e.g. tachycardia/fibrillation) tachyarrhythmias, but is reserved for patients in whom other drugs are ineffective or contraindicated, because of its adverse effects, which include torsades de pointes, and thyroid and pulmonary diseases.
- (Racemic) sotalol (i.e. the form available for prescription) combines class III with class II actions and adverse effects. It is used in paroxysmal supraventricular dysrhythmias, and suppresses ventricular ectopic beats and short runs of ventricular tachycardia. It can cause torsades de pointes, and is contraindicated in patients with asthma or other contraindications to β-blockade, but does not cause the idiosyncratic adverse effects associated with amiodarone.

infarction. It shares the ability of amiodarone to cause *torsades de pointes* but lacks its other adverse effects, and is valuable in patients in whom β-receptor antagonists are not contraindicated.

Verapamil and diltiazem (class IV)

Verapamil is given orally for its main indications (see clinical box, below). It is contraindicated in patients with Wolff–Parkinson–White syndrome. It has a plasma half-life of 6–8 hours and is subject to quite extensive first-pass metabolism, which is more marked for the isomer that is responsible for its cardiac effects. A slow-release preparation is available for once daily use, but

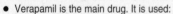

Clinical use of Class IV antidysrhythmic drugs

- Verapamil is the main drug. It is used:
  — to prevent recurrence of paroxysmal supraventricular tachycardia (SVT)
  — to reduce the ventricular rate in patients with atrial fibrillation (especially if inadequately controlled with digoxin). It is, however, contraindicated in patients with atrial fibrillation with Wolff–Parkinson–White or a related pre-excitation syndrome.
- Verapamil was previously given intravenously to terminate paroxysmal supraventricular tachycardia (SVT); it is now seldom used for this because adenosine is safer.
- They are ineffective and dangerous in ventricular dysrhythmias.

is less effective when used for prevention of arrhythmia than the regular preparation because the bioavailability of the cardioactive isomer is reduced by presenting a steady low concentration to the drug-metabolising enzymes in the liver.

Adverse effects and other actions of verapamil and diltiazem are described below in the section on Ca^{2+} channel antagonists. If verapamil is added to **digoxin** in patients with poorly controlled atrial fibrillation the dose of digoxin should be reduced and plasma digoxin concentration checked after a few days because verapamil both displaces digoxin from tissue-binding sites and reduces its renal elimination, hence predisposing to digoxin accumulation and toxicity (see Ch. 48). **Diltiazem** is similar to verapamil, but has relatively more smooth-muscle-relaxing effect, and produces less bradycardia.

Adenosine (unclassified in the Vaughan-Williams' classification)

Adenosine is produced endogenously and is an important chemical mediator (Ch. 9), with effects on breathing, cardiac muscle and afferent nerves and on platelets in addition to the effects on cardiac conducting tissue that underlie its therapeutic use. The A_1 receptor is responsible for its effect on the AV node. These receptors are linked to the same cardiac K^+ channel (termed K_{ACh}) that is activated by acetylcholine via M_2 muscarinic receptors, and adenosine hyperpolarises cardiac conducting tissue and slows the rate of rise of the pacemaker potential accordingly. It is used intravenously to terminate supraventricular tachycardia (SVT) if this rhythm persists despite manoeuvres such as carotid artery massage designed to increase vagal tone, and has largely replaced **verapamil** for this purpose because it is safer owing to its effect being short-lived. This is a consequence of its pharmacokinetics: it is taken up via a specific nucleoside transporter by red blood cells, and is also metabolised by enzymes on the lumenal surface of vascular endothelium. Consequently the effects of a bolus dose of adenosine last only 20–30 s. Once SVT has terminated the patient usually remains in sinus rhythm, even though adenosine is no longer present in plasma, but the unwanted effects resolve very rapidly. These include chest pain, shortness of breath, dizziness and nausea. **Theophylline** and other xanthine alkaloids block adenosine receptors and inhibit the actions of intravenous adenosine, whereas **dipyridamole** (a vasodilator and antiplatelet drug; see below and Ch. 17) blocks the nucleoside uptake mechanism, potentiating and prolonging its adverse effects. Both of these undesirable interactions are clinically important.

ANTIANGINAL DRUGS

The mechanism of anginal pain is discussed above (pp 258–259). Angina is managed by using drugs that either improve perfusion of the myocardium or reduce its metabolic demand, or both. Two of the main groups of drugs, *organic nitrates* and *calcium antagonists*, are vasodilators and produce both of these effects. The third group, the *β-adrenoceptor antagonists*, slow heart rate and hence reduce metabolic demand. Organic nitrates and calcium antagonists are described below, and β-adrenoceptor antagonists in Chapter 8.

The clinical box below summarises the clinical use of antianginal drugs.

Organic nitrates (see also Ch. 10)

The ability of organic nitrates to relieve anginal pain was discovered by Lauder Brunton, a distinguished British physician, in 1867. He had found that angina could be partly relieved by bleeding, and also knew that **amyl nitrite**, which had been synthesised 10 years earlier, caused flushing and tachycardia, with a fall in blood pressure, when its vapour was inhaled. He thought that the effect of bleeding resulted from hypotension, and

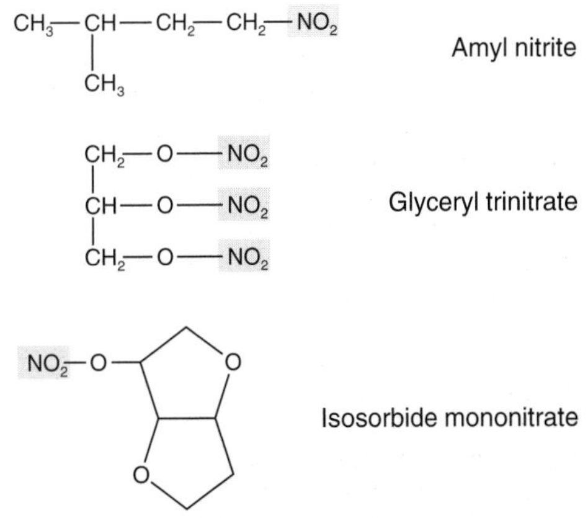

Fig. 14.13 Structures of some organic nitrates.

found that amyl nitrite inhalation worked much better. Amyl nitrite has now been replaced by **glyceryl trinitrate** (nitroglycerine).* Efforts to increase the duration of action of glyceryl trinitrate have led to the synthesis of several related organic nitrates, of which the most important is **isosorbide mononitrate** (Fig. 14.13).

Mechanism of action

Organic nitrates act by relaxing vascular smooth muscle. In common with other smooth muscle relaxants such as **nitroprusside** and natriuretic peptides (see above) they increase cGMP formation, and this is believed to be the basis of their cellular effects. The release of nitric oxide (NO) from organic nitrates at concentrations achieved during therapeutic use involves an enzymic step and possibly a reaction with tissue –SH groups. NO activates a soluble cytosolic form of guanylate cyclase in vascular smooth muscle by interacting with a haem group in the enzyme (see Ch. 11). cGMP formation is thereby increased, leading to changes in the degree of phosphorylation of various smooth muscle proteins and ultimately to *de*-phosphorylation of the myosin light chain, and hence relaxation.

Pharmacological effects

Organic nitrates cause marked venorelaxation, with a consequent reduction in central venous pressure (reduced pre-load). In healthy subjects, this reduces stroke volume. With small doses, there is little effect on arterioles, and

---

Antianginal therapy

- Unstable angina is caused by platelet–fibrin thrombus on coronary artery atheroma. The most important drug is aspirin (Ch. 17) because it reduces the incidence of myocardial infarction. Glyceryl trinitrate as an intravenous infusion is very effective in relieving pain in this setting.
- Stable angina is caused by fixed coronary artery narrowing due to atheroma. Drugs (especially statins) and diet (Ch. 16) are important long-term measures.
- Duration of pain in stable angina is usually only a few minutes on stopping exercise; this can be reduced by sublingual glyceryl trinitrate.
- The frequency of anginal attacks can be reduced by regular use of:
  — organic nitrates (e.g. isosorbide mononitrate given regularly by mouth or glyceryl trinitrate sublingually immediately before exertion)
  — β-adrenoceptor antagonists (e.g. atenolol, metoprolol)
  — calcium antagonists (e.g. diltiazem, amlodipine).
- Prinzmetal variant angina is uncommon; it is caused by coronary artery spasm often in an artery affected by atheromatous disease. The frequency and severity of attacks is reduced by coronary artery vasodilators including organic nitrates and calcium antagonists whereas β-adrenoceptor antagonists may increase vasospasm and worsen pain.

---

*Nobel discovered how to stabilise nitroglycerine with Kieselguhr, enabling him to exploit its explosive properties in dynamite, manufacture of which earned him the fortune with which he endowed the eponymous prizes.

the reduced stroke output is largely compensated by reflex tachycardia, so arterial pressure does not change. With larger doses, arterioles dilate, and arterial pressure falls. Venous pooling occurs when the subject stands up, and can cause postural hypotension and dizziness. Nevertheless, coronary flow is *increased* via coronary vasodilatation. Because both arterial pressure and cardiac output are decreased, myocardial oxygen consumption is reduced. This, and the increased coronary blood flow, cause a large increase in the oxygen content of coronary sinus blood.

If the coronary arteries are partially occluded by atheromatous disease, however, coronary flow is not increased by nitrates. In this situation, some benefit results from the reduction of myocardial oxygen consumption secondary to the lowering of arterial and central venous pressure. In addition, studies in experimental animals have shown that glyceryl trinitrate diverts blood from normal to ischaemic areas of myocardium. The mechanism involves *dilatation of collateral vessels* that bypass narrowed coronary artery segments (Fig. 14.14). It is interesting to compare this effect with that of other vasodilators (e.g. **dipyridamole**) which dilate arterioles but not collaterals. This drug is at least as effective as

nitrates in increasing coronary flow in normal subjects, but actually worsens angina. This is probably because arterioles in an ischaemic region are fully dilated by the ischaemia, and drug-induced dilatation of the arterioles in normal areas has the effect of diverting blood away from the ischaemic areas (Fig. 14.14), producing what is termed a vascular 'steal'. This effect is exploited in a pharmacological 'stress' test for coronary arterial disease in which dipyridamole is administered intravenously to patients in whom this diagnosis is suspected but who cannot exercise.

The direct relaxant action of nitrates on the coronary artery may be important in *variant angina*, which results from coronary spasm. Other vasodilators (e.g. Ca^{2+} antagonists) are also effective in this condition.

In summary, the antianginal action of nitrates involves:

- reduction of cardiac oxygen consumption, secondary to reduced arterial pressure and cardiac output
- redistribution of coronary flow towards ischaemic areas via collaterals
- relief of coronary spasm in variant angina.

Organic nitrates also relax non-vascular smooth muscle (e.g. in the oesophagus and biliary tract).

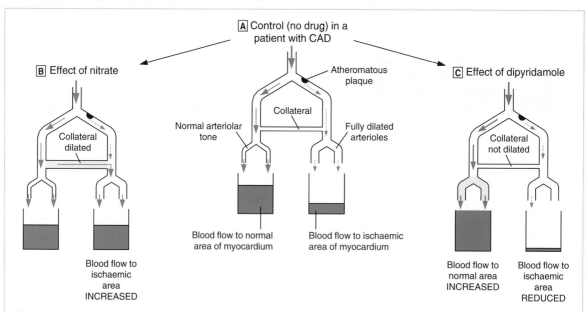

Fig. 14.14 Comparison of the effects of organic nitrates and an arteriolar vasodilator (dipyridamole) on the coronary circulation. A Control. B Nitrates dilate the collateral vessel, thus allowing more blood through to the under-perfused region (mostly by diversion from the adequately perfused area). C Dipyridamole dilates arterioles, increasing flow through the normal area at the expense of the ischaemic area (in which the arterioles are anyway fully dilated).

Tolerance and unwanted effects

Repeated administration of nitrates to smooth muscle preparations in vitro results in diminished relaxation, possibly partly because of *depletion of free –SH groups*, although attempts to prevent tolerance by agents that restore tissue –SH groups have not been clinically useful. Tolerance to the antianginal effect of nitrates does not occur to a clinically important extent with ordinary formulations of short-acting drugs (e.g. **glyceryl trinitrate**), but occurs with longer-acting drugs (e.g. **isosorbide mononitrate**) or when glyceryl trinitrate is administered by prolonged intravenous infusion or by frequent administration of slow-release transdermal patches (see below).

The main *adverse effects* of nitrates are a direct consequence of their main pharmacological actions and include postural hypotension and headache. This was the cause of 'Monday morning sickness' among workers in explosives factories. Tolerance to these effects develops quite quickly, but wears off after a brief nitrate-free interval (which is why the symptoms appeared on Mondays and not later in the week). Formation of *methaemoglobin*, an oxidation product of haemoglobin that is ineffective as an oxygen carrier, seldom occurs when nitrates are used clinically, but can be induced deliberately with amyl nitrate in the treatment of cyanide poisoning.

Pharmacokinetic and pharmaceutic aspects

Glyceryl trinitrate is rapidly inactivated by hepatic metabolism. It is well absorbed from the mouth, and is taken as a tablet under the tongue or as a sublingual spray, producing its effects within a few minutes. If swallowed, it is ineffective because of first-pass metabolism. Given sublingually, nitroglycerine is converted to di- and mono-nitrates, which have some activity and have half-lives of about 2 hours. Its effective duration of action is, however, only about 30 minutes. It is quite well absorbed through the skin, and a more sustained effect can be achieved by applying it as a *transdermal patch*. Once a bottle of the tablets has been opened its shelf life is quite short, because of evaporation of the volatile active substance; patients may be aware of this if their tablets no longer give them their usual headache. Patients who need only occasional treatment benefit from a *sublingual spray* from a metered sealed container, because, although more expensive than tablets, such sprays have an indefinite shelf life.

Isosorbide mononitrate (Fig. 14.13) is longer-acting than nitroglycerine (half-life approximately 4 hours) but has similar pharmacological actions. It is swallowed rather than taken sublingually and taken twice a day for prophylaxis (usually in the morning and at lunch, to allow a nitrate-free period during the night, when the patient is not exerting him/herself, to avoid tolerance). It is also available in slow-release form for once daily use.

Clinical use

The clinical use of organic nitrates is summarised below.

Potassium-channel activators

Nicorandil combines effects due to vascular smooth muscle K$^+$-channel activation (see Ch. 15) with effects as an NO donor. It has been used for angina in Japan for many years and was recently licensed for this indication

Organic nitrates

- Are powerful vasodilators, acting mainly on capacitance vessels to reduce pre-load.
- Act via NO, to which they are metabolised. NO stimulates cGMP formation, affecting both contractile proteins and calcium regulation.
- Tolerance occurs experimentally, and is important clinically with frequent use of long-acting drugs or sustained-release preparations.
- Effectiveness in angina is due partly to reduced cardiac load, partly to dilatation of collateral coronary vessels, causing more effective distribution of coronary flow. In variant angina, dilatation of constricted coronary vessels is beneficial.
- Important compounds are: glyceryl trinitrate, used sublingually for rapid antianginal effect; isosorbide mononitrate, used orally for prophylaxis and more sustained effect.
- No serious unwanted effects; headache and postural hypotension may occur initially. Overdose can, rarely, cause methaemoglobinaemia.

Clinical uses of organic nitrates

- Stable angina:
  — Prevention (e.g. regular isosorbide mononitrate; or glyceryl trinitrate sublingually immediately before exertion)
  — Treatment (sublingual glyceryl trinitrate)
- Unstable angina: intravenous glyceryl trinitrate (as supplement to aspirin, Ch. 17)
- To reduce cardiac pre-load in patients with heart failure, especially those unable to take angiotensin-converting enzyme inhibitors (see Ch. 15)
- Uses related to relaxation of other smooth muscles (e.g. uterine, biliary) are being investigated.

in the UK. It is both an arterial and a venous dilator and causes the expected unwanted effects of headache, flushing and dizziness. Its place in therapy remains to be established and at present it is usually reserved for patients who remain symptomatic despite optimal management with other drugs and/or surgery or angioplasty.

β-adrenoceptor antagonists

β-adrenoceptor antagonists (see Ch. 8) are important in prophylaxis of angina. They work by reducing cardiac oxygen consumption. Their effects on coronary vessels are of minor importance, although they are avoided in variant angina because of the theoretical risk that they will increase coronary spasm.

Calcium antagonists (calcium-entry blockers)

The term 'calcium antagonists' is often used for drugs that affect cellular entry of calcium rather than its intracellular actions, and are referred to by some authors as 'calcium-entry blockers' to make this distinction clear. There are several chemically distinct classes of such drugs (Fig. 14.15).

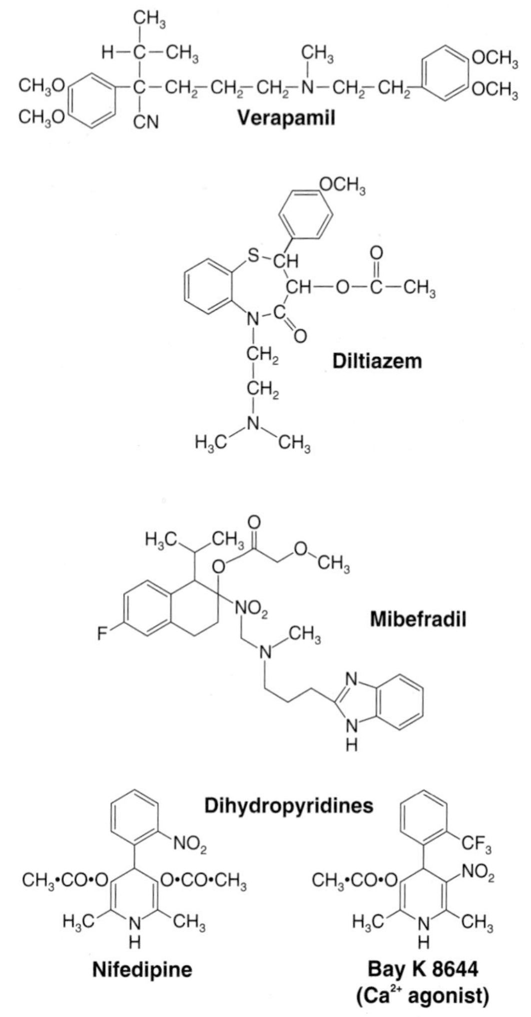

Mechanism of action: types of Ca²⁺ channel

The properties of voltage-gated calcium channels have been studied in great detail by voltage-clamp and patch-clamp techniques (see Ch. 2). Until recently all therapeutically important Ca^{2+} antagonists acted on L-type channels. L-type Ca^{2+} antagonists comprise three chemically distinct classes (Fig. 14.15): phenylalkylamines (e.g. **verapamil**), dihydropyridines, (e.g. **nifedipine, amlodipine**) and benzothiazepines (e.g. **diltiazem**). These each bind the α_1-subunit of the cardiac Ca^{2+} channel, but to distinct sites each of which interacts allosterically with each other and with the gating machinery of the channel, indirectly preventing diffusion of Ca^{2+} through its pore in the open channel. Many calcium antagonists show properties of use-dependence (i.e. they block more effectively in those cells in which the calcium channels are most active; see the discussion of class I anti-dysrhythmic drugs above). For the same reason, they also show voltage-dependent blocking actions, blocking more strongly when the membrane is depolarised causing calcium channel opening and inactivation.

Dihydropyridines affect Ca^{2+} channel function in a complex way, not simply by a physical plugging of the pore. This became clear when some dihydropyridines, exemplified by **Bay K 8644** (Fig. 14.15), were found to bind to the same site but to act in the converse way, that is, to promote the opening of voltage-gated calcium channels. Thus Bay K 8644 produces effects opposite

Fig. 14.15 Structures of calcium antagonists. Bay K 8644 (a calcium agonist) is included for comparison.

to those of the clinically used dihydropyridines, namely an increase in the force of cardiac contraction, and constriction of blood vessels; it is competitively antagonised by nifedipine. Studies on the response of single calcium channels to a step depolarisation of the membrane suggest that channels can exist in one of three distinct states (Fig. 14.16). When a channel is in mode 0 it does not open in response to depolarisation; in mode 1, depolarisation produces a low opening probability, and each opening is brief. In mode 2, depolarisation produces a very high opening probability, and single openings are prolonged. Under normal conditions, about 70% of

Mode	Mode 0	Mode 1	Mode 2	
	▲–Depolarizing–▲ step	▲–Depolarizing–▲ step	▲–Depolarizing–▲ step	------ Channel closed ------ Channel open
Opening probability	Zero	Low	High	
Favoured by	DHP antagonists		DHP agonists	
% of time normally spent in this mode	<1%	~70%	~30%	

Fig. 14.16   Mode behaviour of calcium channels. The traces shown in blue are patch-clamp recordings (see Ch. 2) of the opening of single Ca^{2+} channels (downward deflections) in a patch of membrane from a cardiac muscle cell. A depolarising step is imposed close to the start of each trace, causing an increase in the opening probability of the channel. When the channel is in mode 1 (centre), this causes a few brief openings to occur, in mode 2 (right) the channel stays open for most of the time during the depolarising step; in mode 0 (left) it fails to open at all. Under normal conditions the channel spends most of its time in modes 1 and 2, and only rarely enters mode 0.

Calcium antagonists

- Block Ca^{2+} entry by preventing opening of voltage-gated L-type and, recently, T-type Ca^{2+} channels.
- Three main L-type antagonists, typified by verapamil, diltiazem and dihydropyridines (e.g. nifedipine).
- Mainly affect heart and smooth muscle, inhibiting the Ca^{2+} entry caused by depolarisation in these tissues.
- Selectivity between heart and smooth muscle varies: verapamil is relatively cardioselective; nifedipine is relatively smooth-muscle selective and diltiazem is intermediate.
- Vasodilator effect (mainly dihydropyridines) is mainly on resistance vessels, causing reduced after-load. Calcium antagonists also dilate coronary vessels, which is important in variant angina.
- Effects on heart (verapamil, diltiazem): antidysrhythmic action (mainly atrial tachycardias) because of impaired AV conduction, and reduced contractility.
- Clinical uses include: antidysrhythmic therapy (mainly verapamil, especially atrial tachycardias), angina (by reducing cardiac work) and hypertension.
- Unwanted effects include headache, constipation (verapamil), and ankle oedema (dihydropyridines). There is a risk of causing cardiac failure or heart block, especially with verapamil and diltiazem.

the channels at any one moment exist in mode 1, with only 1% or less in mode 2; each channel switches randomly and quite slowly between the three modes. Dihydropyridines of the antagonist type bind selectively to channels in mode 0, thus favouring this non-opening state, whereas agonists bind selectively to channels in mode 2 (Fig. 14.16). This type of two-directional modulation resembles the phenomenon seen with the GABA/benzodiazepine interaction (Ch. 33), and invites speculation about possible endogenous dihydropyridine-like mediator(s) with a regulatory effect on calcium entry.

Mibefradil is distinctive in that it blocks T- as well as L-type channels at therapeutic concentrations but was withdrawn from therapeutic use because it caused adverse drug interactions by interfering with drug metabolism.

Pharmacological effects

The main effects of calcium antagonists, as used therapeutically, are confined to cardiac and smooth muscle. **Verapamil** mainly affects the heart, whereas most of the dihydropyridines (e.g. **nifedipine**) exert a greater effect on smooth muscle than on the heart. **Diltiazem** is intermediate in its actions.

Cardiac actions

The antidysrhythmic effects of **verapamil** and **diltiazem** have been discussed above. Ca^{2+} antagonists can cause AV block and cardiac slowing by their actions on conducting tissues, but this is offset by reflex increase in sympathetic activity secondary to their vasodilator action. Thus, **nifedipine**, for example, typically causes reflex tachycardia, **diltiazem** causes little or no change in heart rate and **verapamil** slows the heart rate. Ca^{2+} antagonists also have a negative inotropic effect, which results from the inhibition of the slow inward current during the action potential plateau. In spite of this the cardiac output usually stays constant or increases, because of the reduction in peripheral resistance. Again, there are clinically important differences between the different classes of drugs, with **verapamil** having the most marked negative inotropic action and therefore being contraindicated in heart failure, as are most other calcium antagonists. By contrast, in a recent trial in over 1000 patients with severe chronic heart failure treated for 6–33 months, **amlodipine** did not worsen cardiovascular morbidity or mortality.

Vascular smooth muscle

Ca^{2+} antagonists cause generalised arteriolar dilatation, but do not much affect the veins. They affect all vascular beds, though regional effects vary between different drugs to a considerable degree. Vasodilatation causes a fall in arterial pressure. They cause coronary vasodilatation in normal individuals and in patients with coronary artery spasm (variant angina). Other types of smooth muscle (e.g. biliary tract, urinary tract and uterus) are also relaxed by calcium antagonists, but these effects are less important than their actions on vascular smooth muscle, although they may contribute to adverse effects (see below).

Protection of ischaemic tissues

There are theoretical reasons (see Fig. 14.7) why calcium antagonists might exert a cytoprotective effect in ischaemic tissues, and thus be of clinical use in treating heart attack and stroke. Disappointingly, there is as yet little or no evidence from randomised clinical trials of beneficial (or harmful) effects of Ca^{2+} antagonists on cardiovascular morbidity or mortality in any patient group. The answers to these questions await the outcome of large ongoing trials that are due to report in the first decade of the next century. **Nimodipine** reduces the risk of cerebral vasospasm following subarachnoid haemorrhage, and has a distinct use in this relatively uncommon form of stroke.

Pharmacokinetics

Ca^{2+} antagonists in clinical use are all well absorbed from the gastrointestinal tract, and are given by mouth except for some special indications, such as following subarachnoid haemorrhage, for which intravenous preparations are available. They are extensively metabolised. Pharmacokinetic differences between different drugs and different pharmaceutical preparations are clinically important, because they determine the dose interval, and also the intensity of some of the unwanted effects such as headache and flushing (see below). **Amlodipine** has a long elimination half-life and is given once daily, whereas **nifedipine**, **diltiazem** and **verapamil** have shorter elimination half-lives and are either given more frequently or are formulated in various slow-release preparations to permit once daily dosing.

Unwanted effects

Several unwanted effects of Ca^{2+} antagonists are extensions of their main pharmacological actions. Short-acting dihydropyridines cause flushing and headache because of their vasodilator action, and in chronic use dihydropyridines not uncommonly cause ankle swelling, possibly because arteriolar dilatation increases capillary pressure, especially in the feet where venous pressure is greatest when standing. **Verapamil** commonly causes constipation, probably because of effects on Ca^{2+} channels in gastrointestinal nerves or smooth muscle. Effects on cardiac rhythm (e.g. heart block) and force of contraction (e.g. worsening heart failure) are discussed above.

Apart from these predictable effects, which cause tiresome but not usually very severe problems, it has been believed that the Ca^{2+} channel antagonists, as a class, are rather free from severe and unpredictable adverse effects. This view has been challenged recently on the basis of epidemiological data, but there is little evidence from randomised trials of harmful effects, and in the final analysis data from the ongoing randomised controlled trials of outcome referred to above will be needed to resolve these issues.

Clinical uses

The main clinical uses of calcium antagonists are summarised in the clinical box below.

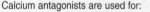

Clinical uses of calcium antagonists

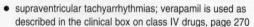

Calcium antagonists are used for:

- supraventricular tachyarrhythmias; verapamil is used as described in the clinical box on class IV drugs, page 270
- hypertension (see Ch. 15)
- reducing the frequency of attacks of angina.

REFERENCES AND FURTHER READING

Ad Hoc Subcommittee of the Liaison Committee of the World Health Organization and the International Society of Hypertension 1997 Effects of calcium antagonists on the risks of coronary heart disease, cancer and bleeding. J Hypertens 15: 105–115 *(Sober view: 'there is little or no reliable evidence from randomised trials of beneficial (or harmful) effects of calcium antagonists on major cardiovascular morbidity and mortality in any patient group.')*

Camm A J, Garratt C J 1991 Adenosine and supraventricular tachycardia. N Engl J Med 325: 1621–1628 *(Discusses its role as an endogenous mediator and its pharmacology and clinical use)*

Digitalis Investigation Group 1997 The effect of digoxin on mortality and morbidity in patients with heart failure. N Engl J Med 336: 525–533 *(Digoxin did not affect overall mortality, but reduced hospitalisations over an average follow-up of approximately 3 years)*

Ertel S I, Clozel J-P 1997 Mibefradil (Ro 40-5967): the first selective T-type Ca^{2+} channel blocker. Exp Opin Invest Drugs 6: 569–582 *(Tetralol derivative acting on L- and T-type Ca^{2+} channels, with 10-fold selectivity for T-type channels; reviews in vitro and in vivo pharmacology)*

Fine L G, Yellon D M (chairmen) 1993 Unstable angina. Report of a meeting of physicians and scientists, University College London Medical School. Lancet 341: 1323–1327 *(Discussion of myocardial 'stunning' and ischaemic preconditioning)*

Goto A, Yamada K, Yashioka M, Sugimoto T 1992 Physiology and pharmacology of endogenous digitalis-like factors. Pharmacol Rev 44: 377–399 *(Review, including ouabain-like substance)*

Hess P, Lansmann J B, Tsien R W 1984 Different modes of Ca-channel gating behaviour favoured by dihydropyridine Ca agonists and antagonists. Nature 311: 538–544 *(Evidence for three 'modes' of Ca^{2+} channels)*

ISIS-4 collaborative group 1995 ISIS-4: A randomised factorial trial assessing early oral captopril, oral mononitrate, and intravenous magnesium sulphate in 58,050 patients with suspected acute myocardial infarction. Lancet 345: 669–685 *(Impressive trial: disappointing results! Magnesium was ineffective; oral nitrate did not reduce 1-month mortality)*

Katz A M 1993 Cardiac ion channels. N Engl J Med 328: 1244–1251 *(Clear, readable synthesis of modern understanding of the cardiac action potential in terms of structural changes in the proteins that control ion fluxes across the plasma membrane)*

Katz A M 1996 Calcium channel diversity in the cardiovascular system. J Am Coll Cardiol 28: 522–528 *(Reviews the diverse Ca^{2+} channels that participate in signal transduction in the cardiovascular system)*

Liu G S, Thornton J, van Winkle D M, Stanly D W H, Olsson R A, Downey J M 1991 Protection against infarction afforded by preconditioning as mediated by A1 adenosine receptors in rabbit heart. Circulation 84: 350–356 *(Adenosine as mediator of cardiac protection)*

Murad F, Leitman D, Waldman S, Chang C-H, Hirata M, Kohse K 1988 Effects of nitrovasodilators, endothelium-dependent vasodilators and atrial peptides on cGMP. Cold Spring Harb Symp Quant Biol 53: 1005–1009 *(Cellular mechanisms)*

Prospective Randomized Amlodipine Survival Evaluation Study Group 1996 Effect of amlodipine on morbidity and mortality in severe chronic heart failure. N Engl J Med 335: 1107–1114 *(No adverse effect on survival in the group as a whole)*

Roques B P, Noble F, Daugée V, Fournie-Zaluski M-C, Beaumont A 1993 Neutral endopeptidase 24.11: structure, inhibition and experimental and clinical pharmacology. Pharmacol Rev 45: 87–146

Ruskin J N 1989 The cardiac arrhythmia suppression trial (CAST). N Engl J Med 321: 386–388 *(Showed increased mortality with active treatment despite suppression of arrhythmia)*

Ruskoaho H 1992 Atrial natriuretic peptide: synthesis, release and metabolism. Pharmacol Rev 44: 479–602

Smith T W 1988 Digitalis: mechanisms of action and clinical use. N Engl J Med 518: 358–365 *(Excellent review)*

Vaughan Williams E M 1989 Classification of antiarrhythmic actions. In: Vaughan Williams E M (ed) Antiarrhythmic drugs. Handbook of experimental pharmacology. Springer-Verlag, Berlin, vol 89 *(For a different approach see Circulation 1994, 84: 1848)*

Waldo A L, Wit A L 1993 Mechanisms of cardiac arrhythmias. Lancet 341: 1189–1193

Ward D E, Camm A J 1993 Dangerous ventricular arrhythmias— can we predict drug efficacy? N Engl J Med 329: 498–499 *(Commentary on the seemingly logical but problematic strategy of deliberately provoking arrhythmias in susceptible patients in order to select therapy individualised to their needs)*

The vascular system

This chapter is concerned mainly with the pharmacology of blood vessels. The walls of arteries, arterioles, venules and veins contain smooth muscle whose contractile state is controlled by mediators released locally from sympathetic nerve terminals and endothelial cells, and by circulating hormones. Parasympathetic nerves are not generally important in controlling vascular smooth muscle. Arterioles and small muscular arteries are the main resistance vessels in the circulation, while veins are capacity vessels. In terms of cardiac function, therefore, arteries and arterioles regulate the *after-load*, while veins and pulmonary vessels regulate the *pre-load* of the ventricles. Viscoelastic properties of large conduit arteries determine vascular compliance (i.e. the degree to which the volume of the arterial system increases as the pressure increases), an important factor in a circulatory system that is driven by an intermittent, rather than continuous, pump. Much of the blood that is ejected from the ventricle is accommodated, in the first instance, by distension of the arterial system, which absorbs the pulsations in cardiac output and delivers a relatively steady flow to the tissues. The greater the compliance of the system, the more effectively are fluctuations damped out,* and

the smaller the oscillations of arterial pressure with each heartbeat (known as the 'pulse pressure'). This is important because cardiac work (see Ch. 14) can be reduced by introducing additional compliance into the arterial system, even if the cardiac output and mean arterial pressure are unchanged, and indeed there is evidence that pulse pressure is an independent risk factor for cardiac disease.

Several important disorders affect large or small blood vessels (e.g. *atheroma* and *Raynaud's phenomenon* respectively). When atheroma involves peripheral arteries the commonest symptom is pain in the legs on walking ('claudication'), followed by pain at rest and, in severe cases, gangrene of the feet or legs. Treatment is often surgical (surgical reconstruction or amputation) or by angioplasty (disruption of atheroma by inflation of a balloon surrounding the tip of a catheter). Drug treatment (considered further in Chs 16 and 17) is often unsatisfactory. Vasodilator drugs (e.g. **oxypentifylline**) are popular in some countries; they increase blood flow at rest but controlled trials have not shown improvement in walking distance, reduction of rest pain or sustained increase in muscle blood flow during exercise. *Microvascular disease* can result from structural damage to capillary endothelium (e.g. in diabetes mellitus; Ch. 22) or from inappropriate vasoconstriction of arteries and arterioles. In the peripheral circulation this gives rise to Raynaud's phenomenon (blanching of the fingers during vasoconstriction, followed by blueness due to deoxygenation of the static blood and redness due to reactive hyperaemia following return of blood flow). This can be mild but if severe causes ulceration and gangrene of the fingers. It can occur in isolation ('Raynaud's disease') or in association with a number of other diseases including several so-called connective tissue diseases (e.g. systemic sclerosis, systemic lupus erythematosus). Treatment of Raynaud's phenomenon involves stopping smoking and avoiding the cold. Vasodilators (e.g. **nifedipine**) are of some benefit in severe cases.

---

*This cushioning action is called the 'Windkessel' effect, after a 19th century German toy which operated on this principle.

Actions of drugs on the vascular system can be broken down into effects on:

- total peripheral resistance (controlled mainly by the arterioles), which is one of the main determinants of arterial pressure and is relevant to the treatment of hypertension and shock
- the resistance of individual vascular beds, which determines the local distribution of blood flow to and within different organs; such effects are relevant to the drug treatment of angina (Ch. 14), migraine (Ch. 9), Raynaud's phenomenon and circulatory shock
- arterial compliance (controlled mainly by muscular arteries), which is relevant in the treatment of cardiac failure and angina
- venous capacity, which determines the central venous pressure and is relevant to the treatment of cardiac failure and angina
- atheroma (Ch. 16) and thrombosis (Ch. 17).

In this chapter we first consider the control of vascular smooth muscle tone, followed by the actions of vaso-constrictor and vasodilator drugs and clinical uses of vasodilators in the treatment of hypertension, shock and cardiac failure. The use of vasoactive drugs in treating angina is discussed in Chapter 14.

CONTROL OF VASCULAR SMOOTH MUSCLE TONE

Like other muscle cells, vascular smooth muscle contracts when the intracellular calcium concentration ($[Ca^{2+}]_i$) rises, but the coupling between $[Ca^{2+}]_i$ and contraction is less tight than in striated or cardiac muscle. Vasoconstrictors and vasodilators act by increasing or reducing $[Ca^{2+}]_i$, and/or by altering the sensitivity of the contractile machinery to $[Ca^{2+}]_i$. Figure 15.1 summarises cellular mechanisms that are involved in the control of smooth muscle contraction.

REGULATION OF $[Ca^{2+}]_i$

The regulation of $[Ca^{2+}]_i$ in vascular smooth muscle depends on the entry and exit of Ca^{2+} across the plasma membrane, and on sequestration of Ca^{2+} within the cell. Calcium entry occurs partly through voltage-gated Ca^{2+} channels, which open when the cell is depolarised, and partly through receptor-operated channels. To complicate matters, the opening probability of voltage-gated channels is influenced by second messengers produced in response to receptor occupation by agonists. However,

---

Vascular smooth muscle

- Vascular smooth muscle is controlled by mediators secreted by sympathetic nerves and vascular endothelium, and by circulating hormones.
- Smooth muscle cell contraction is initiated by a rise in $[Ca^{2+}]_i$ which activates myosin-light-chain kinase, causing phosphorylation of myosin or by sensitisation of the myofilaments to Ca^{2+} by inhibition of myosin phosphatase.
- Agents causing contraction may:
  — release intracellular Ca^{2+}, secondary to receptor-mediated IP_3 formation
  — depolarise the membrane and thus allow Ca^{2+} entry through voltage-gated Ca^{2+} channels
  — allow Ca^{2+} entry through receptor-operated Ca^{2+} channels.
- Agents causing relaxation may:
  — inhibit Ca^{2+} entry through voltage-gated Ca^{2+} channels either directly (e.g. nifedipine) or indirectly by hyperpolarising the membrane (K^+ activators, e.g. cromokalim)
  — increase intracellular cAMP or cGMP concentration; cAMP causes inactivation of myosin-light-chain kinase, and may facilitate Ca^{2+} efflux; cGMP opposes agonist-induced increases in $[Ca^{2+}]_i$.

---

many vasoconstrictors (e.g. noradrenaline) cause both a depolarisation by increasing the membrane perme-ability to cations (Na^+ and Ca^{2+}) and a further increase in Ca^{2+} uptake through distinct receptor-operated channels. This latter occurs even in preparations that are fully depolarised (by immersion in isotonic K^+ solution) and is unaffected by dihydropyridine-type calcium antagonists (which block voltage-gated Ca^{2+} channels). Ca^{2+} exit is mediated by Na^+/Ca^{2+}-ATPase and by Na^+/Ca^{2+} exchange.

Sequestration of intracellular Ca^{2+}

Intracellular Ca^{2+} in vascular smooth muscle is contained mainly in sarcoplasmic reticulum, which is the main storage site for *releasable* Ca^{2+}, and in mitochondria. Many vasoconstrictors activate membrane-bound phos-pholipase C (see Ch. 2), increasing IP_3. This acts on receptors on the sarcoplasmic reticulum to release Ca^{2+} into the cytoplasm. Recapture of the released Ca^{2+} occurs by an ATP-driven active transport system which is modulated by cAMP and cGMP.

Link between $[Ca^{2+}]_i$ and contraction

Smooth muscle differs from striated and cardiac muscle in that it contains no troponin. In smooth muscle, Ca^{2+}-calmodulin regulates *myosin-light-chain kinase* (MLCK)

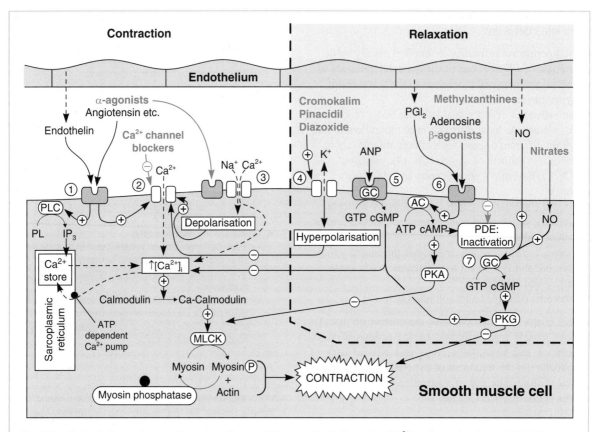

Fig. 15.1 Control of vascular smooth muscle. Agents elicit contraction by increasing $[Ca^{2+}]_i$, or increasing the sensitivity of myofilaments to Ca^{2+}. $[Ca^{2+}]_i$ is increased by: (1) Receptors coupled to phospholipase C (PLC), which lead to inositol trisphosphate (IP_3), production and the release of stored Ca^{2+}. (2) Voltage-gated Ca^{2+} channels, which open in response to depolarisation. (3) Receptor-operated channels, which allow Ca^{2+} entry and also cause depolarisation. (4) Decreased myosin phosphatase activity causes contraction via Ca^{2+} sensitisation. Agents that cause relaxation may work by reducing $[Ca^{2+}]_i$, or directly on the contractile machinery: (5) K^+ channels (sensitive to intracellular ATP) are opened by drugs such as diazoxide, causing hyperpolarisation, and thus preventing voltage-gated Ca^{2+} channels from opening. (6) Receptors (e.g. for PGI_2, adenosine) coupled to adenylate cyclase, activation of which cause increased cAMP production. This acts via protein kinase A (PKA) and myosin-light-chain kinase (MLCK) to inhibit contraction. Inhibitors of phosphodiesterase (PDE) protect cAMP or cGMP from degradation. (7) Stimulation of soluble guanylate cyclase by NO increases cGMP formation. (8) ANP occupies a receptor that is directly coupled to membrane-bound guanylate cyclase. (Enzymes: AC = adenylate cyclase; GC = guanylate cyclase; MLCK = myosin-light-chain kinase; PKA = cAMP-dependent protein kinase; PKG = cGMP-dependent protein kinase). Only the main pathways are shown in this diagram.

which phosphorylates myosin light chains, enabling myosin to interact with actin and thereby initiating contraction. Relaxation is usually initiated by a fall in $[Ca^{2+}]_i$ which leads to dephosphorylation of the myosin light chain via *myosin phosphatase*. The relatively indirect coupling between $[Ca^{2+}]_i$ and contraction in smooth muscle (as compared with striated muscle) allows for contraction to be regulated by mechanisms that increase or reduce the sensitivity of the contractile apparatus to $[Ca^{2+}]_i$. Decreased activity of myosin phosphatase or

increased activity of myosin-light-chain kinase results in Ca^{2+} sensitisation, while increased activity of myosin phosphatase or decreased activity of myosin-light-chain kinase causes Ca^{2+} desensitisation. One link between receptor activation and Ca^{2+} sensitisation is provided by a G-protein called RhoA which leads to inhibition of myosin phosphatase; it is of particular interest as a site of action of novel vasodilator drugs (see below). Many vasodilators work through either cAMP or cGMP, which activate protein kinases (PKA and PKG respectively;

see Ch. 2). PKA works by phosphorylating, and thereby inactivating, MLCK (see Fig. 15.1), and also by enhancing Ca^{2+} efflux. The special roles of MLCK and myosin phosphatase in smooth muscle explain the otherwise puzzling fact that mediators that increase cytoplasmic cAMP relax smooth muscle but increase cardiac contraction. The importance of IP_3-mediated Ca^{2+} release in smooth muscle is also relevant to this, since IP_3-mediated Ca^{2+} release is not affected by cAMP, whereas Ca^{2+} entry through voltage-gated channels is strongly increased by cAMP and is important for cardiac contraction. cGMP relaxes vascular smooth muscle through activation of PKG, and through sequestration of intracellular Ca^{2+}.

THE ROLE OF THE VASCULAR ENDOTHELIUM

A new chapter in our understanding of vascular control opened with the realisation that vascular endothelium acts not only as a passive barrier between plasma and extracellular fluid, but also as a source of numerous potent chemical mediators. These actively control the contraction of the underlying smooth muscle as well as influencing platelet and mononuclear cell function: the complex roles of the endothelium in haemostasis and thrombosis are discussed in Chapter 17. *Prostacyclin* (PGI$_2$; see Ch. 12), whose discovery by Bunting, Gryglewski, Moncada & Vane in 1976 ushered in this era, relaxes smooth muscle and inhibits platelet aggregation. Endothelial cells from microvessels synthesise prostaglandin (PG) E_2 which is a vasodilator and inhibits noradrenaline release from sympathetic nerve terminals, while lacking the effect of PGI$_2$ on platelets. Prostaglandin endoperoxide intermediates (PGG$_2$, PGH$_2$) are formed in endothelial cells, and act on thromboxane (TX) A_2 receptors which initiate effects opposite to those of PGI$_2$. The discovery of *endothelium-derived relaxing factor* (EDRF) by Furchgott & Zawadzki in 1980 and its subsequent identification as NO by the groups of Moncada and of Ignarro in 1988 enormously expanded the role of the endothelium (see Ch. 11). The endothelium also secretes several vasoactive peptides, including the vasodilators *C-natriuretic peptide* which is related to atrial natriuretic peptide and B-natriuretic peptide (Ch. 14) and *adrenomedulin* (a vasodilator peptide originally discovered in phaeochromocytoma tissue, but now known to be expressed in many tissues including vascular endothelium), and *endothelin*, a potent vasoconstrictor which we cover here.

Many endothelium-derived mediators are mutually antagonistic, conjuring an image of opposing rugby football players swaying back and forth in a never-ending scrimmage: in moments of exasperation one sometimes wonders whether all this makes sense or whether the designer simply could not make up his mind! An important distinction is whether a system is tonically active in resistance vessels under basal conditions as is the case with the noradrenergic nervous system (Ch. 8), EDRF/NO (Ch. 11) and, possibly, endothelin, or whether it only responds to injury, inflammation, etc. as with prostacyclin. Some of the latter may be functionally redundant, perhaps representing vestiges of mechanisms that were important to our evolutionary forebears, or they may simply be taking a breather on the touch-line and ready to rejoin the fray if called on by the occurrence of some vascular insult. In addition to producing an array of vasoactive mediators, the plasma membrane of endothelial cells contains several enzymes and transport mechanisms that act on circulating hormones and are important targets of drug action. *Angiotensin-converting enzyme* (ACE) is a particularly important example (see below).

The role of the endothelium in controlling vascular smooth muscle

- Endothelial cells release various vasoactive substances, including prostacyclin (vasodilator), nitric oxide (vasodilator) and endothelin (vasoconstrictor).
- Many vasodilator substances (e.g. acetylcholine and bradykinin) act via endothelial NO production. The NO derives from arginine, and is produced when $[Ca^{2+}]_i$ increases in the endothelial cell.
- NO causes smooth muscle relaxation by increasing cGMP formation.
- Endothelin is a potent and long-acting vasoconstrictor peptide, released from endothelial cells by many chemical and physical factors. It is not confined to blood vessels, and its physiological role is not yet clear.

Endothelin

Discovery, biosynthesis and secretion

Hickey et al. described a vasoconstrictor factor produced by cultured endothelial cells in 1985. This was identified as endothelin (ET), a 21-residue peptide, by Yanagisawa et al. (1988), who achieved the isolation, analysis and cloning of the gene for this peptide in a very short space of time. Three ET genes encode different sequences (ET-1, ET-2 and ET-3), each with a distinctive 'shepherd's crook' appearance due to two internal disulphide bonds (Fig. 15.2). The three isoforms are diversely and unevenly distributed (Table 15.1) suggesting that ET may have multiple functions that are not restricted to the cardiovascular system, and this is supported by observations

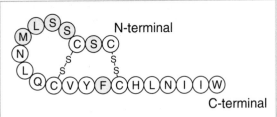

Fig. 15.2 Endothelins. The circles represent the sequence of amino acid residues in ET-1, labelled according to the single letter amino acid code. Solid circles show those residues that differ from ET-1 in ET-2 and/or ET-3.

Table 15.1 Distribution of endogenous ETs and subtypes of ET receptors in various tissues

Tissues	ET-1	ET-2	ET-3	ET_A	ET_B
Vascular tissue					
Endothelium	++++				+
Smooth muscle	+			++	
Brain	+++		+	+	+++
Kidney	++	++	+	+	++
Intestines	+	+	+++	+	+++
Adrenal gland	+		+++	+	++

++++ = highest; +++ = high; ++ = moderate; and + = low levels of expression of ETs or ET-receptor mRNA and/or immunoreactive ETs
Adapted from: Masaki (1993)

of mice in which the gene coding for ET-1 is disrupted (see below). ET-1 is the only ET present in endothelial cells and is also expressed in many other tissues. ET-2 is much less widely distributed but is present in kidney and intestine. ET-3 is present in brain, lung, intestine and adrenal gland. ET-1 is synthesised by transcription and translation of a 212-residue precursor molecule ('prepro ET') which is processed to 'big ET-1' and finally cleaved by an endothelin-converting enzyme to ET-1. Cleavage occurs not at the usual Lys–Arg or Arg–Arg position but at a Trp–Val pair implying a very atypical endopeptidase. The best candidate for the converting enzyme is a metalloprotease which is inhibited by **phosphoramidon**. Big ET-1 is converted to ET-1 intracellularly and also on the surface of endothelial and smooth muscle cells. Regulation of ET production occurs at the transcriptional level. Stimuli include activated platelets, endotoxin, thrombin, various cytokines and growth factors, angiotensin II, arginine vasopressin,

adrenaline, insulin, hypoxia and low shear stress. Inhibitors include NO, natriuretic peptides, prostaglandins E_2 and I_2, heparin and high shear stress. It was originally believed that ET-1 is generated de novo, and not stored intracellularly, but secretion of ET-1 can occur more rapidly than would be expected if it were always freshly synthesised (for example, in response to stretch), and there is evidence that preformed ET-1 can, in fact, be stored in endothelial cells although probably not in granules. Release mechanisms of such stored ET-1 are poorly understood.

Endothelin receptors and responses

There are at least two types of ET receptor, designated ET_A and ET_B (Table 15.2). Both belong to the superfamily of G-protein-coupled receptors (Ch. 2). ET_A-receptors are preferentially activated by ET-1. Messenger RNA for the ET_A-receptor is expressed in many human tissues including vascular smooth muscle, heart, lung and kidney. It is *not* expressed in endothelium. ET_A-mediated responses include vasoconstriction, bronchoconstriction and aldosterone secretion. ET_A-receptors are coupled to phospholipase C which initiates several effects including stimulation of Na^+/H^+ exchange, protein kinase C and mitogenesis as well as vasoconstriction. There are several selective ET_A-receptor antagonists including **BQ-123** (a cyclic pentapeptide) and several orally active non-peptide drugs (e.g. **BMS 182874**, a sulphonamide derivative). ET_B-receptors are activated to a similar extent by each of the three ET isoforms but **sarafotoxin S6c** (a 21-amino acid peptide which shares the shepherd's crook structure of the endothelins and was isolated from the venom of the burrowing asp) is a selective agonist and has proved useful as a pharmacological tool for studying the ET_B-receptor. Messenger RNA for the ET_B-receptor is mainly expressed in brain (especially cerebral cortex and cerebellum) with moderate expression in aorta, heart, lung,

Table 15.2 Subtypes of ET receptor

Receptor	Affinity	Pharmacological response
ET_A	ET-1 = ET-2 > Et-3	Vasoconstriction Bronchoconstriction Stimulation of aldosterone secretion
ET_B	ET-1 = ET-2 = ET-3	Vasodilatation Inhibition of ex vivo platelet aggregation

From: Masaki (1993)

kidney and adrenals. In contrast to the ET_A-receptor, it is *highly expressed* in endothelium, but it is also present in vascular smooth muscle like the ET_A-receptor. The receptor on endothelium has been called ET_{B1} while the vascular smooth muscle subtype is termed ET_{B2}, based on subtype-selective antagonists. Agonists acting on ET_{B1}-receptors cause vasodilatation by stimulating NO and PGI_2 production. They do this by increasing $[Ca^{2+}]_i$ in endothelium, NO synthase and phospholipase A_2 both being activated by Ca^{2+}-calmodulin. In contrast, ET_{B2}-mediated responses are vasoconstrictor, like responses mediated by ET_A.

Functions of endothelin

ET-1 is a paracrine mediator rather than a circulating hormone, although it stimulates the secretion of several hormones, including *atrial natriuretic peptide, aldosterone, adrenaline* and *hypothalamic* and *pituitary hormones*. The concentration of ET-1 in *thyroid follicles* is extremely high and it has been suggested that it may be involved in thyroglobulin synthesis. Administration of an ET_A-receptor antagonist into the brachial artery increases forearm blood flow, suggesting that ET-1 may be formed continuously in endothelial cells in resistance vessels in this vascular bed leading to tonic vasoconstriction via activation of ET_A-receptors on the underlying vascular smooth muscle. ET-1 is present in very high concentrations in amniotic fluid and has been implicated in the control of uteroplacental blood flow and in the genesis of *eclampsia*, a disease of the last trimester of pregnancy characterised by hypertension, oedema and seizures, and which is the leading cause of maternal and neonatal mortality in industrialised countries. Plasma concentrations of ET-1 are raised in several pathological conditions, especially those with a component of vasospasm, including acute myocardial infarction. ET may play a part in renal and cerebral vasospasm (see Fig. 15.3). The ET-1 gene has been disrupted experimentally in mouse embryo stem cells to produce mice deficient in ET-1 (see Ch. 3). Pharyngeal arch tissues develop abnormally in such mice and homozygotes die of respiratory failure at birth, implicating ET-1 in the development as well as the control of the cardiorespiratory systems.

THE ROLE OF THE RENIN–ANGIOTENSIN SYSTEM

The renin–angiotensin system acts synergistically with the sympathetic nervous system and stimulates aldosterone secretion; it plays a central role in the control of sodium excretion and fluid volume as well as of vascular tone.

Renin is a proteolytic enzyme that is secreted into the circulation by cells of the *juxtaglomerular apparatus* (see Fig. 20.2), an island of tissue lying at the point where the afferent arteriole is apposed to a specialised part of the distal tubule called the macula densa (see Ch. 20). The control of renin secretion is complex and only partly understood (see Fig. 15.4). It is secreted in response to various physiological stimuli, including a fall in sodium concentration of the fluid in the distal tubule to which the macula densa is exposed, and (independently) to a fall in renal perfusion pressure. Renal sympathetic nerve activity, β-adrenoceptor agonists and prostacyclin all stimulate renin secretion directly, whereas angiotensin II causes feedback inhibition. Atrial natriuretic peptide also inhibits renin secretion. The macula densa is rich in NO synthase, but the effect of NO on renin release is controversial, with conflicting claims that it either inhibits or stimulates this. Renin is cleared rapidly from plasma. It acts on *angiotensinogen* (a plasma globulin made in the liver) splitting off a decapeptide, *angiotensin I*, from the N-terminal end of the protein.

Angiotensin I has no appreciable activity *per se* but is converted by angiotensin-converting enzyme (ACE) to an octapeptide, *angiotensin II*, which is a potent vasoconstrictor. Angiotensin II can be broken down further by enzymes (aminopeptidase A and N) that remove single amino acids sequentially from the N-terminal end and giving rise respectively to angiotensin III and angiotensin IV (Fig. 15.5). These had been regarded as of little importance, but it is now known that angiotensin III stimulates aldosterone secretion and is involved in thirst. Angiotensin IV also has distinct actions, probably via its own receptor, including release of plasminogen activator inhibitor-I (PAI-I) from the endothelium (Ch. 17). Receptors for angiotensin IV have a distinctive distribution, including the hypothalamus.

ACE is a membrane-bound enzyme on the surface of endothelial cells, and is particularly abundant in the lung which has a vast surface area of vascular endothelium.* The common isoform of ACE is also present in other vascular tissues including heart, brain, striated muscle and kidney, and is not restricted to endothelial cells.** Consequently, local formation of angiotensin II can occur in different vascular beds, and provides local control independent of blood-borne angiotensin II. ACE inactivates bradykinin (see Ch. 13) and several other

---

*Approximately that of a football field.

**A different isoform of ACE is also present in testis, and male mice lacking ACE have markedly reduced fertility.

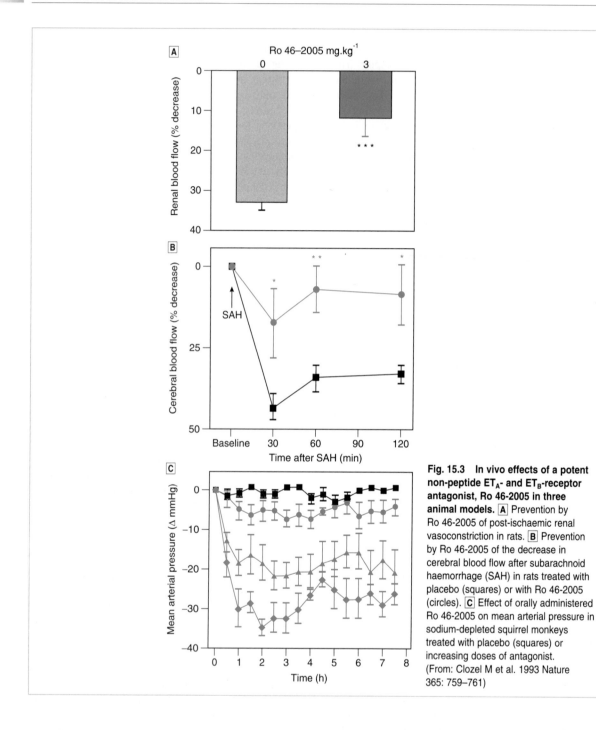

Fig. 15.3   In vivo effects of a potent non-peptide ET$_A$- and ET$_B$-receptor antagonist, Ro 46-2005 in three animal models. [A] Prevention by Ro 46-2005 of post-ischaemic renal vasoconstriction in rats. [B] Prevention by Ro 46-2005 of the decrease in cerebral blood flow after subarachnoid haemorrhage (SAH) in rats treated with placebo (squares) or with Ro 46-2005 (circles). [C] Effect of orally administered Ro 46-2005 on mean arterial pressure in sodium-depleted squirrel monkeys treated with placebo (squares) or increasing doses of antagonist. (From: Clozel M et al. 1993 Nature 365: 759–761)

vasodilator peptides. This may contribute to the pharmacological actions of ACE inhibitors (ACEI), as discussed below. The main actions of angiotensin II are mediated via a specific membrane-bound G-protein-coupled receptor called (somewhat confusingly) the angiotensin II subtype 1 receptor, or AT1 receptor. These actions include:

- generalised vasoconstriction, especially marked in efferent arterioles of the kidney

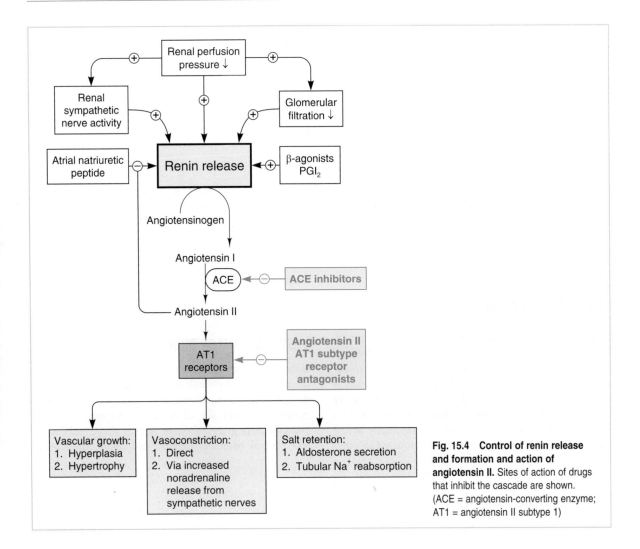

Fig. 15.4 Control of renin release and formation and action of angiotensin II. Sites of action of drugs that inhibit the cascade are shown. (ACE = angiotensin-converting enzyme; AT1 = angiotensin II subtype 1)

- increased release of noradrenaline from sympathetic nerve terminals, reinforcing vasoconstriction and increasing the rate and force of contraction of the heart
- stimulation of proximal tubular reabsorption of sodium ions
- secretion of aldosterone from the adrenal cortex (see Chs 20 and 24)
- cell growth in the cardiac left ventricle and in the arterial wall. These effects are initiated by the G-protein-coupled AT1 receptor acting via the same intracellular tyrosine phosphorylation pathways as are used by cytokines.*

An AT2 receptor has also been cloned and is expressed during foetal life and in distinct brain nuclei. Studies

of mice in which the AT2 receptor gene has been disrupted suggest that it may be involved in growth, development and exploratory behaviour. Cardiovascular effects of AT2 receptors (inhibition of cell growth and lowering of blood pressure) appear to be relatively subtle, and oppose those of AT1 receptors.

The renin–angiotensin pathway is important in the pathogenesis of heart failure, and several very important classes of therapeutic drugs act by inhibiting it at various points (see below).

*For example the 'Jak/Stat' pathway (see Ch. 2)—see Marrero M B et al. 1995 Direct stimulation of Jak/Stat pathway by the angiotensin II AT1 receptor. Nature 375: 247–250.

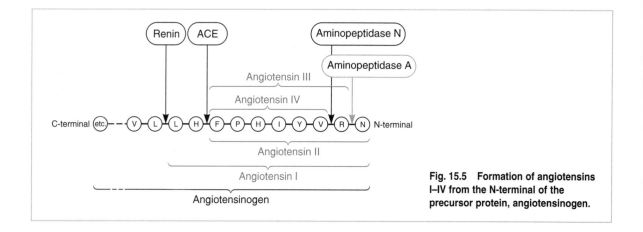

Fig. 15.5   Formation of angiotensins I–IV from the N-terminal of the precursor protein, angiotensinogen.

DRUGS THAT AFFECT VASCULAR SMOOTH MUSCLE CONTRACTION

Drugs can affect vascular smooth muscle either directly, by acting on the smooth muscle cells themselves, or indirectly, by acting on endothelial cells or on sympathetic nerve terminals. Another type of indirect action is exemplified by ACEI. Mechanisms of action of directly acting vasoconstrictors and vasodilators are summarised in Figure 15.1. Table 15.3 summarises indirectly acting vasoactive drugs, many of which are discussed in other

chapters. In this chapter we concentrate on agents that are not covered elsewhere, and discuss ways in which vasoactive drugs are used clinically.

VASOCONSTRICTOR DRUGS

α_1-adrenoceptor agonists and drugs that release noradrenaline from sympathetic nerve terminals or inhibit its reuptake ('sympathomimetic amines') cause vasoconstriction, and are discussed in Chapter 8. Some eicosanoids (e.g. thromboxane A_2; see above and Ch. 17) and several peptides, notably *endothelin*, *angiotensin*

Table 15.3   Classification of vasoactive drugs that act indirectly

Site	Mechanism	Examples	Further details
Vasoconstrictors			
Sympathetic nerve terminals	Noradrenaline release	Amphetamine, ephedrine, tyramine	Ch. 8
	Block of NA reuptake	Cocaine	Chs 8 and 38
Endothelium	Endothelin release from endothelial cells	Many agents, e.g.: thrombin, Ca^{2+} ionophore, TGF-β, PDGF, IL-1, TNF, angiotensin II, endotoxin, shear stress, etc.	Above
Vasodilators			
Sympathetic nerve terminals	Inhibition of NA release via presynaptic receptors	Many examples, e.g.: α_2-adrenoceptor agonists, muscarinic agonists, prostaglandins, etc.	Chs 7, 8 and 12
	Sympathetic-neuron-blocking drugs	Guanethidine, bethanidine	Ch. 8
Endothelium	Nitric oxide release	Many agents, e.g.: acetylcholine, bradykinin, substance P, Ca^{2+} ionophore, ATP, shear stress	
Central nervous system	Vasomotor inhibition	Anaesthetics	Ch. 32
		Clonidine, methyldopa	Ch. 78
Enzymes	ACE inhibition	Captopril, enalapril	Below
	Renin inhibition	Compounds in development (e.g. enalkiren)	

and *vasopressin* are also predominantly vasoconstrictor. **Sumatriptan** and ergot alkaloids acting through 5-HT$_2$- and 5-HT$_{1D}$-receptors also cause vasoconstriction (Ch. 9).

Angiotensin

The physiological role of the renin–angiotensin system in the control of the circulation is described above. Angiotensin II is an extremely powerful vasoconstrictor, being roughly 40 times as potent as noradrenaline in raising blood pressure. Its peripheral effects resemble those of α_1-receptor agonists, in that it mainly affects cutaneous, splanchnic and renal blood flow, with less effect on blood flow to brain and skeletal muscle. It has no routine clinical uses, its pharmacological importance lying in the fact that other drugs (e.g. **captopril** and **losartan**; see below) affect the cardiovascular system by altering its production or action.

Vasopressin (antidiuretic hormone)

Vasopressin is a posterior pituitary peptide hormone (Ch. 24). It is important mainly for its actions on the kidney (discussed in Ch. 20), but it is also a powerful vasoconstrictor. Its effects are initiated by two distinct types of receptor termed V$_1$ and V$_2$. Water retention is mediated through V$_2$-receptors, occurs at low plasma concentrations of vasopressin, and involves activation of adenylate cyclase and increased cAMP production in renal collecting ducts. Vasoconstriction is mediated through V$_1$-receptors, requires much higher concentrations of vasopressin and involves intracellular calcium mobilisation via IP$_3$ (see Ch. 2). Vasopressin causes generalised vasoconstriction, including the coeliac, mesenteric and coronary vessels. It also affects other (e.g. gastrointestinal and uterine) smooth muscle and causes abdominal cramps for this reason. It is sometimes used to treat patients with bleeding oesphageal varices and portal hypertension before more definitive treatment, although many gastroenterologists prefer to use **octreotide** (unlicensed indication; see Ch. 24) for this.

Endothelin

Endothelins are discussed above; as explained, they have both vasodilator and vasoconstrictor actions, but vaso-constriction predominates. Intravenous administration causes transient vasodilatation followed by profound and very long-lived vasoconstriction. The endothelins are more potent vasoconstrictors than angiotensin II. As yet they have no clinical uses and their pharmacological importance, like that of angiotensin II, will probably lie in drugs (not yet available for clinical use) that affect the cardiovascular system by altering their production or actions.

Vasoconstrictor substances

- The main groups are sympathomimetic amines (direct and indirect), certain eicosanoids (thromboxanes), peptides (angiotensin, vasopressin and endothelin) and a group of miscellaneous other drugs (e.g. ergot alkaloids).
- Clinical uses are limited mainly to local applications (e.g. nasal decongestion, co-administration with local anaesthetics). Usefulness in hypotensive states is not proven, apart from adrenaline in anaphylactic shock and in cardiac arrest. Vasopressin may be used to stop bleeding from oesophageal varices in patients with portal hypertension caused by liver disease.

VASODILATOR DRUGS

Many vasodilators are clinically important, being used in the treatment of common and chronic conditions including hypertension, cardiac failure and angina pectoris.

DIRECTLY ACTING VASODILATORS

There are several points at which drugs could act to cause relaxation of vascular smooth muscle. These include Ca^{2+} entry, either by blocking voltage-dependent Ca^{2+} channels or by causing hyperpolarisation, Ca^{2+} release from sarcoplasmic reticulum or reuptake into it, and enzymes that determine Ca^{2+} sensitivity. These mechanisms are exemplified by calcium antagonists, potassium channel activators and drugs that influence cytoplasmic concentrations of cyclic nucleotides. Recently, a pyridine drug (**Y27632**) has been described that causes vasorelaxation by inhibiting a Rho-associated protein kinase, thereby selectively inhibiting smooth muscle contraction by inhibiting Ca^{2+} sensitisation, so a whole new group of vasodilator drugs may be on the way!

Calcium antagonists

Calcium antagonists are discussed in detail in Chapter 14. They cause generalised vasodilatation, though individual agents differ in the regional distribution of this effect. Drugs of the **dihydropyridine** type act preferentially on vascular smooth muscle, whereas **verapamil** acts also on the heart; **diltiazem** is intermediate in specificity. The main difference that this makes is that dihydro-pyridines usually produce a transient reflex tachycardia as a result of lowering the blood-pressure. Verapamil and diltiazem do not, because although they also lower blood pressure they slow the cardiac pacemaker by their direct action on the heart.

Several calcium antagonists of the dihydropyridine type show special features:

- **Amlodipine** has a much longer elimination half-life leading to less variation in plasma concentration during chronic dosing and permitting once daily dosing.
- **Nimodipine** has some selectivity for *cerebral* vasculature and is used to prevent cerebral vasospasm following subarachnoid haemorrhage.

Drugs that activate K⁺ channels

Some drugs (e.g. **cromokalim**, **pinacidil**, **minoxidil** and **diazoxide**) relax smooth muscle by selectively increasing the membrane permeability to K^+. This hyperpolarises the membrane, switching off voltage-dependent Ca^{2+} channels and inhibiting action potential generation. Ion flux studies revealed that these drugs increase the efflux of radioactive rubidium (an ion that traverses K^+ channels). Patch-clamp recording (see Ch. 2) demonstrated that they open a high-conductance K^+ channel. This discovery coincided with studies demonstrating the existence of ATP-sensitive K^+ channels in various different cell types. In cardiac muscle and pancreatic islet insulin-secreting beta cells, for example, intracellular ATP was found to close these K^+ channels, thus causing the cell to depolarise.* Potassium channel activators work by antagonising the action of intracellular ATP on these channels (Fig. 15.6), thus opening them and causing relaxation when ATP would normally have kept them closed. **Diazoxide** belongs chemically to the same group as the thiazide diuretics (see Ch. 20) which have vasodilator properties as well as their renal actions. It causes hyperglycaemia (by inhibiting insulin secretion) which precludes its use in chronic therapy. It used to be given intravenously in the emergency treatment of hypertension, but has been superseded by other drugs which have fewer unwanted effects.

Minoxidil is a very potent and long-acting vasodilator, used as a drug of last resort in treating severe hypertension unresponsive to other drugs. It causes hirsutism which is unacceptable to most women, and its active metabolite is actually used as a rub-on cream to treat baldness. It causes marked salt and water retention and is usually prescribed with a loop diuretic (e.g. **frusemide**). It causes reflex tachycardia, and a β-adrenoceptor antagonist is used to prevent this. **Pinacidil**, **cromakalim** and

its active isomer **lemakalim** are more recently developed K^+ channel activators. Drugs of this type relax most kinds of smooth muscle, but have yet to establish a therapeutic niche.

Agents that act by increasing cyclic nucleotide concentration

Cyclase activation. Many drugs relax vascular smooth muscle by increasing the cellular concentration of either cGMP or cAMP. For example NO, nitrates and the natriuretic peptides act through cGMP (see Chs 11 and 14), while β₂-agonists, adenosine and prostacyclin act through cAMP (see Chs 8, 9 and 12). **Dopamine** has mixed vasodilator and vasoconstrictor actions, but is used therapeutically to dilate the renal vasculature where it increases cAMP by activating adenylate cyclase, and so is considered here. It is the precursor of noradrenaline in noradrenergic neurons (Ch. 8), and is also a transmitter in its own right in the brain (Ch. 28) and probably also in the periphery (Ch. 6). The proposal that dopamine might serve a role as a peripheral transmitter came from observations that stimulation of sympathetic nerves to the kidney causes vasodilatation that is not affected by adrenoceptor antagonists, but is prevented by dopamine-receptor antagonists such as **haloperidol** (see Ch. 28). Dopamine produces a mixture of cardiovascular effects resulting from its agonist actions on α- and β-adrenoceptors, as well as on dopamine receptors, when administered as an intravenous infusion. Blood pressure increases slightly, but the main effects are vasodilatation in the renal circulation and increased cardiac output. At low doses (e.g. 1–5 μg/kg body weight/min) it is relatively selective for dopamine receptors in the renal vasculature; at higher doses, effects on α- and β-adrenoceptors become progressively more evident. The main effects are:

- *vasodilatation*, particularly in the kidney but also in the mesenteric vascular bed, due to activation of dopamine receptors
- *vasoconstriction* in other vascular beds, caused by activation of α_1-adrenoceptors
- *increased force of contraction of the heart*, due to activation of β_1-adrenoceptors.

Dopamine is often used in intensive care units in patients in whom renal failure associated with decreased renal perfusion appears imminent; despite its beneficial effect on renal haemodynamics, it has not, however, been proved to improve survival in these circumstances.

Nitroprusside (nitroferricyanide) is a very powerful vasodilator with little effect outside the vascular system. It breaks down spontaneously under physiological

---

*This latter mechanism forms an important link between the metabolic state of the cell and membrane function, and sulphonylurea drugs cause insulin secretion by mimicking the action of ATP on these channels; see Chapter 22.

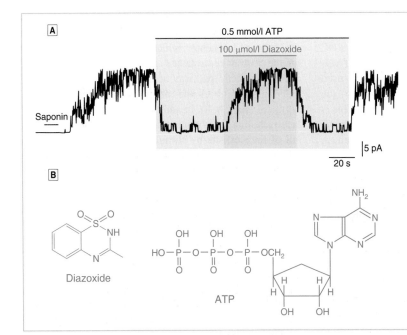

Fig. 15.6 Drugs that act at ATP-sensitive K⁺ channels. [A] K^+ channels opened by diazoxide. The records were obtained from insulin-secreting cells in culture by the patch-clamp technique (Ch. 2). Saponin caused permeabilisation of the cell, with loss of intracellular ATP, causing the channels to open (upward deflection) until they were inhibited by ATP. Addition of diazoxide, a vasodilator drug (which also inhibits insulin secretion; see text) causes opening of the channels. In an intact smooth muscle cell, this causes hyperpolarisation and relaxation. [B] Structure of diazoxide. (From: (A) Dunne et al. 1990 Br J Pharmacol 99: 169)

conditions to yield nitric oxide (NO) which activates soluble guanylate cyclase (Ch. 11). Unlike the organic nitrates which are enzymically converted to NO and preferentially dilate capacitance vessels, it acts equally on arterial and venous smooth muscle. Its clinical usefulness is limited because it must be given intravenously. In solution, particularly when exposed to light, nitroprusside is hydrolysed to cyanide. The intravenous solution has to be made up freshly from dry powder, and is protected from light by covering the container with foil. In the body, nitroprusside is rapidly converted to thiocyanate, its plasma half-life being only a few minutes, so it must be given as a continuous infusion with careful monitoring to avoid excessive hypotension. Continued use can lead to thiocyanate toxicity (weakness, nausea and inhibition of thyroid function) because thiocyanate is cleared only slowly from the bloodstream, so nitroprusside is only useful for short-term treatment (usually up to 72 hours maximum). It is used in intensive care units for hypertensive crises, to produce controlled hypotension during surgery, and to reduce cardiac work during the reversible cardiac dysfunction that occurs after cardiopulmonary bypass surgery.

Natriuretic peptides (ANP, BNP and CNP; see Ch. 14) also cause vasodilatation by activating guanylate cyclase, but act on the membrane-bound form of this enzyme which is directly linked with natriuretic peptide receptors. **Anaritide**, a 25-amino acid synthetic form of ANP which works by increasing cGMP (Ch. 14) and increases glomerular filtration rate by dilating afferent arterioles while constricting efferent arterioles, has been investigated in critically ill patients with acute renal failure: it did not improve the overall rate of dialysis-free survival, but appeared to be beneficial in the sub-group of patients who had oliguria (reduced urine formation) and harmful in those who did not, so it is currently undergoing further evaluation. Natriuretic peptides have not found a therapeutic use thus far; the alternative strategy of inhibiting their clearance or metabolism (e.g. with **candoxatril**, a neutral endopeptidase inhibitor) is still being evaluated.

Phosphodiesterase inhibition. Phosphodiesterase enzymes (PDE) are a growing family of potential drug targets, consisting currently of at least 14 genetically different isoenzymes. Existing therapeutic drugs, including methylxanthines (e.g. **theophylline**) and **papaverine**, are inhibitors of PDE though this is not their only action. Methylxanthines exert their main effects on non-vascular smooth muscle and on the central nervous system, and are discussed in Chapters 19 and 38. In addition to inhibiting PDE, some methylxanthines are also purine-receptor antagonists, which may partly account for their smooth muscle relaxant effects. They are not used clinically as vasodilators. Papaverine is closely related to **morphine** (see Ch. 37) and is also produced by the opium poppy. Pharmacologically, it is quite unlike morphine, however, its main action being to relax smooth muscle in blood vessels and elsewhere. Its mechanism is poorly understood, but seems to involve a combination of PDE inhibition (as with methylxanthines) and block of calcium channels. It (or **prostaglandin E₁**) have been used to treat erectile impotence by direct injection into the corpus cavernosum of the penis (Brindley 1986). This is highly effective and, although some readers may wince, has been much appreciated by many insulin-requiring diabetics who suffer from this complication of their disease and are no more needle-shy than the author of the above report whose paper describes the use of 17 drugs in one subject (himself). Many inhibitors of specific PDE isoenzymes are in development. PDE type III inhibitors are positive inotropes, but have not proved beneficial in treating heart failure, as explained in Ch. 14. *PDE type V inhibitors* (e.g. **sildenafil**) inhibit the breakdown of cGMP and are orally active in causing penile erection. They appear likely to revolutionise the treatment of impotence.

Vasodilators with unknown mechanism of action

Hydralazine

Hydralazine acts mainly on arteries and arterioles, causing a fall in blood pressure accompanied by reflex tachycardia and an increased cardiac output; it has little effect on the venous system. Its mechanism has not been determined in detail at the cellular level, although it appears to interfere with the action of IP_3 on calcium release from the sarcoplasmic reticulum. Its main clinical uses were in hypertension and in heart failure (see below) but its toxicity (especially an immune disorder resembling *systemic lupus erythematosus*) greatly limits its use and alternative agents are now usually preferred.

Ethanol

Ethanol (see Ch. 39) dilates cutaneous vessels, causing the familiar drunkard's flush. Several general anaesthetics (e.g. **propofol**) cause vasodilatation as an unwanted effect (Ch. 32).

INDIRECTLY ACTING VASODILATOR DRUGS

The two main groups of clinically important indirectly acting vasodilator drugs are:

- those that inhibit sympathetically mediated vasoconstriction
- those that inhibit the renin–angiotensin system.

The central control of sympathetically mediated vaso-

constriction is believed to involve not only catecholamine receptors, but also another class of receptor, termed the imidazoline I_1 receptor, which is present in the brainstem in the rostral ventrolateral medulla. Drugs can inhibit the sympathetic pathway at any point from the central nervous system to the peripheral sympathetic nerve terminal (see Ch. 8). In addition, many vasodilators (e.g. acetylcholine, bradykinin, substance P) exert some or all of their effects by stimulating biosynthesis of vasodilator prostaglandins or of NO (or of both) by vascular endothelium (see above and Ch. 11).

We concentrate here on the renin–angiotensin system which can be inhibited by drugs at four points:

- renin release: several drugs inhibit release (e.g. β-adrenoceptor antagonists) but only to a modest extent, and this is not generally an important mechanism.
- renin activity: renin inhibitors (e.g. **enalkiren**) have been developed, but are not used therapeutically.
- ACE: ACEI (e.g. **captopril**, **enalapril**) are very widely used therapeutically; see clinical box (p. 292) and Chapter 14.
- angiotensin II type 1 (AT1) receptors: AT1-receptor antagonists (e.g. **losartan**) have recently been introduced into clinical practice and are being used increasingly—see below.

All such drugs can increase plasma potassium ion concentration by reducing aldosterone secretion.

Renin inhibitors

Orally active renin inhibitors (e.g. **enalkiren**, **remikiren**) reduce plasma renin activity, but their effects on blood pressure in patients with hypertension have been disappointing.

Vasodilator drugs

- Vasodilators act:
  —to increase local tissue blood flow
  —to reduce arterial pressure
  —to reduce central venous pressure.
- Net effect is a reduction of cardiac pre-load (reduced filling pressure) and after-load (reduced vascular resistance), hence reduction of cardiac work.
- Main uses are:
  —antihypertensive therapy (e.g. ACEI, α_1-antagonists)
  —treatment of angina (e.g. Ca^{2+} antagonists)
  —treatment of cardiac failure (e.g. ACEI).

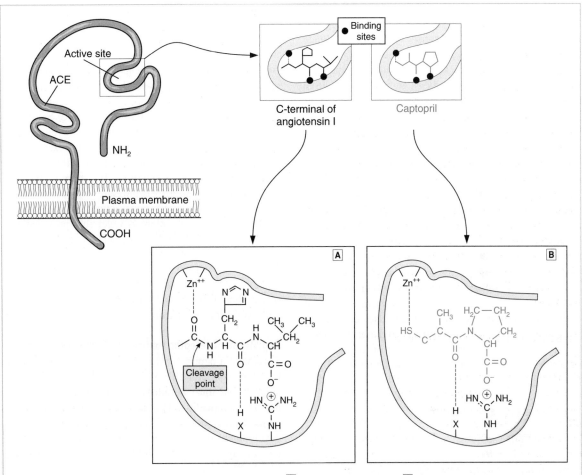

Fig. 15.7   The active site of angiotensin-converting enzyme. [A] Binding of angiotensin I. [B] Binding of the inhibitor, captopril, which is an analogue of the terminal dipeptide of angiotensin I.

Angiotensin-converting enzyme inhibitors (ACEI)

Several specific ACEI have been developed, the first of which was **captopril** (Fig. 15.7). ACE is a carboxypeptidase enzyme that cleaves the C-terminal pair of amino acids from peptide substrates. Its active site contains a zinc atom. The development of captopril was one of the first examples of successful drug design based on a chemical knowledge of the target molecule. Various small peptides had been found to be weak inhibitors of the enzyme,* but these were unsuitable as drugs because of their low potency and poor oral absorption. Captopril was designed to combine the steric properties of such

peptide antagonists in a non-peptide molecule, which contains a sulphydryl group appropriately placed to bind the zinc atom, coupled to a proline residue that binds the site on the enzyme that normally accommodates the terminal leucine of angiotensin I (Fig. 15.7). Several ACEI are now available, including **enalapril**, **lisinopril**, **ramipril**, **perindopril** and **trandolapril**. These differ in their durations of action, but share most of their pharmacological effects.

Pharmacological effects

Captopril is a powerful inhibitor of the effects of angiotensin I in the whole animal. It causes only a small fall in arterial pressure in normal animals or human subjects who are consuming the amount of salt contained in a usual western diet, but a much larger fall in hypertensive

---

*The lead compound was a nonapeptide derived from the venom of *Bothrops jacaraca*—a South American snake.

patients, particularly those in whom renin secretion is enhanced (e.g. in patients receiving diuretics). ACEI affect capacitance and resistance vessels, and reduce cardiac load as well as arterial pressure. They do not affect cardiac contractility, so cardiac output normally increases. They act preferentially on angiotensin-sensitive vascular beds, which include those of the kidney, heart and brain. This selectivity may be important in sustaining adequate perfusion of these vital organs in the face of reduced perfusion pressure. Critical renal artery stenosis represents an exception to this, where ACE inhibition results in a fall of glomerular filtration rate (see below).

Clinical uses

Clinical uses of ACEI are summarised in the box below.

Unwanted effects

Captopril was initially used in doses that, in retrospect, were excessive. In these large doses it caused rashes, taste disturbance, neutropenia, and heavy proteinuria. This pattern of adverse effects is also seen during treatment with **penicillamine** (Ch. 13) which also contains a sulphydryl group, and it has been argued that these effects are attributable to this chemical feature of the molecule rather than to ACE inhibition as such. Other ACEI that

---

Clinical uses of ACE inhibitors

- Hypertension
- Cardiac failure
- Following myocardial infarction (especially when there is ventricular dysfunction, even when this is mild)
- Diabetic nephropathy
- Progressive renal insufficiency

---

do not possess a sulphydryl group do not cause these effects. In contrast, adverse effects that are directly related to ACE inhibition are common to all drugs of this class. These include hypotension, especially after the first dose, and especially in patients with heart failure who have been treated with loop diuretics, in whom the renin–angiotensin system is highly activated. A dry cough, possibly the result of accumulation of bradykinin (Ch. 12) in the bronchial mucosa, is the commonest persistent adverse effect. Patients with bilateral renal artery stenosis predictably develop renal failure if treated with ACEI, because glomerular filtration in the face of low afferent arteriolar pressure is maintained by angiotensin II-mediated constriction of the efferent arteriole. Such renal failure is reversible provided it is recognised promptly and the ACEI stopped. If such renal failure occurs, *hyperkalaemia* may be severe owing to reduced aldosterone secretion, and potassium-sparing diuretics (e.g. **amiloride**; Ch. 20) or potassium supplements should not be used routinely in patients treated with ACEI for this reason.

Angiotensin II receptor subtype 1 (AT1) antagonists

Saralasin, a peptide analogue of angiotensin II, inhibits the vasoconstrictor effect of angiotensin II. It is a partial agonist, and must be administered parenterally so it is not used clinically. More recently, attention has again focused on angiotensin II receptor antagonists with the development of a number of non-peptide, orally active pure antagonists of the AT1 receptor (e.g. **losartan**; Fig. 15.8). ACE is not the only enzyme capable of forming angiotensin II, *chymase* (which is not inhibited by ACEI) providing an alternative route. It is not known if these alternative pathways of angiotensin II formation

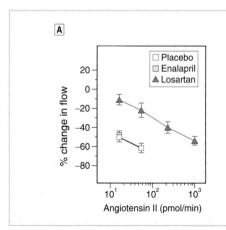

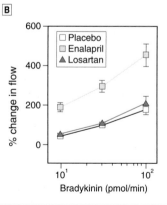

Fig. 15.8 Comparison of effects of angiotensin-converting enzyme inhibition and angiotensin-receptor blockade in the human forearm vasculature. [A] Effect of brachial artery infusion of angiotensin II on forearm blood flow after oral administration of placebo, enalapril (10 mg) or losartan (100 mg). [B] Effect of brachial artery infusion of bradykinin as in A. (From: Cockcroft J R et al. 1993 J Cardiovasc Pharmacol 22: 579–584)

are important under any clinically important conditions in vivo, but if so, then AT1-receptor antagonists could be more effective than ACEI in such situations. Losartan does not cause the dry cough that is sometimes caused by ACEI, consistent with the 'bradykinin accumulation' explanation of this side-effect mentioned above. It is useful in hypertensive patients who experience this side-effect with ACEI and find it unacceptable. Conversely, it is not known whether any of the beneficial effects of ACEI (e.g. reversal of left ventricular hypertrophy and improvement of endothelial dysfunction) are bradykinin/EDRF mediated, so it is unwise to assume that AT1-receptor antagonists will share all of the therapeutic properties of ACEI. Initial experience with losartan in elderly patients with heart failure has, however, been

---

Clinical uses of angiotensin II subtype 1 (AT1) receptor antagonists

- Experience with AT1 antagonists is more limited than with ACEI, and it cannot be assumed that they will prove to be therapeutically equivalent for all indications. Many clinicians therefore currently reserve them for patients with hypertension in whom an ACEI is indicated, but who are unable to tolerate this because of dry cough. (This side-effect is not caused by AT1 antagonists.)

Types of vasodilator drugs

- ACE inhibitors (e.g. captopril, enalapril): prevent conversion of angiotensin I to angiotensin II; therefore most effective when renin release is increased.
- Nitrates (e.g. glyceryl trinitrate, nitroprusside): act like endogenous NO, causing increased cGMP formation.
- Calcium antagonists (diltiazem, nifedipine and many other dihydropyridines): act by blocking Ca^{2+} entry in response to depolarisation; dilate both resistance and capacitance vessels.
- Drugs that interfere with sympathetic transmission (e.g. α_1-adrenoceptor antagonists).
- K^+ channel activators (e.g. diazoxide, cromokalim, pinacidil): open membrane K^+ channels, thus causing hyperpolarisation; thought to affect insulin-secreting cells and neurons, as well as smooth muscle, so produce various side-effects.
- Angiotensin II subtype 1 (AT1) receptor antagonists (e.g. losartan).
- Other agents include: β_2-adrenoceptor agonists; adenosine; methylxanthines (e.g. theophylline); various diuretics and numerous agents that stimulate endothelial NO production (Ch. 11).

---

encouraging so these drugs may come to have a place in the treatment of heart failure.

CLINICAL USES OF VASOACTIVE DRUGS

It is beyond the scope of this book to provide a detailed account of the clinical uses of vasoconstrictor and vasodilator drugs, but it is, nonetheless, useful to consider the various pharmacological approaches that are used in treating certain important clinical states. The conditions that will be briefly discussed are:

- hypertension
- cardiac failure
- shock.

HYPERTENSION

Hypertension is a common disorder, which, if not effectively treated, results in a greatly increased probability of coronary thrombosis, strokes and renal failure. Until about 1950, there was no effective treatment, and the development of antihypertensive drugs, which greatly increase life expectancy, has been a major, but largely unsung, therapeutic success story.

There are a few recognisable and surgically treatable causes of hypertension, such as phaeochromocytoma (Ch. 8), steroid-secreting tumours of the adrenal cortex, renal artery stenosis and so on, but the great majority of cases involve no obvious causative factor, and are grouped as *essential hypertension* (so called because it was originally thought that the raised blood pressure was essential to maintain adequate tissue perfusion). The pathophysiology is intimately related to the kidneys (as demonstrated by transplantation experiments in which kidneys are transplanted from or to animals with genetic hypertension, or to humans requiring renal transplants therapeutically: hypertension 'goes with' the kidney from a hypertensive donor and vice versa) and leads to narrowing of the lumen of systemic arterioles. The raised peripheral vascular resistance calls into play various physiological responses involving the cardiovascular system, nervous system and kidney. Certain vicious circles tend to become established, and these provide some of the targets for pharmacological attack.

Figure 15.9 summarises major physiological mechanisms that control arterial blood pressure, and shows the sites at which some antihypertensive drugs act. The main systems include the *sympathetic nervous system*, the *renin–angiotensin–aldosterone* system and *tonically active endothelium-derived autacoids* (NO and probably

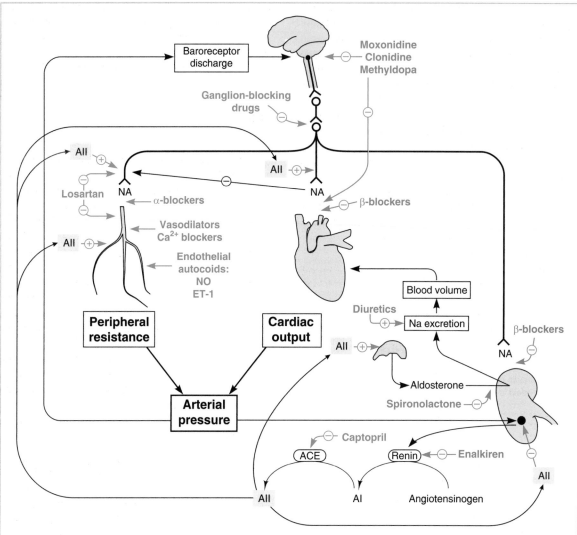

Fig. 15.9 Diagram showing the main mechanisms involved in arterial blood pressure regulation (black lines), and the sites of action of antihypertensive drugs (blue lines). NA = noradrenaline, AI = angiotensin I, AII = angiotensin II, ACE = angiotensin-converting enzyme.

endothelin 1; see above). One of the ways in which the primary process (which is unknown) leads to progressively worsening hypertension is that remodelling and hypertrophy, associated with proliferation of smooth muscle cells in the media of resistance arteries, occurs in response to the raised pressure, reducing the ratio of lumen diameter to wall thickness and increasing the peripheral vascular resistance. The role of cellular growth factors (including angiotensin II) and inhibitors of growth (e.g. NO) in the evolution of these structural changes

is currently of great interest to vascular biologists, and is potentially of importance to the therapeutic use of drugs such as ACEI.

Contrary to the earlier view that hypertension was 'essential' to sustain life, reducing arterial blood pressure greatly improves the prognosis of patients with hypertension (i.e. usual diastolic pressures >100 mmHg). The use of drugs to control mild hypertension (which is asymptomatic), without producing unacceptable side-effects, is therefore an important clinical need, and much effort has gone into devising satisfactory therapeutic regimes.* Treatment involves non-pharmacological measures (e.g. increased exercise, reduced dietary salt, weight and alcohol reduction) followed by the staged introduction of drugs, starting with those of proven benefit and least likely to produce side-effects. The preferred regimes have changed progressively as better drugs have become available. Centrally acting α_2-agonists (e.g. **clonidine**), or **methyldopa** (which is metabolised to α-methylnoradrenaline, an α_2-agonist that is released centrally as a false transmitter; Ch. 8) and drugs (e.g. **reserpine**) that deplete central neurotransmitter amines or block adrenergic neurons (e.g. **guanethidine**) or α_1-adrenoceptors (e.g. **prazosin**) all commonly have severe side-effects, respectively drowsiness, depression and postural hypotension. Diarrhoea and impotence are also common. Currently, *thiazide diuretics or β-adrenoceptor antagonists* are the usual starting point for patients who are otherwise healthy. They abolish the excess risk of stroke and reduce the excess risk of myocardial infarction conferred by a particular level of hypertension. They also have side-effects, though less severe than those of the other drugs mentioned above. In patients with moderate or severe hypertension it is often possible to control the pressure without causing side-effects by combining low doses of different drugs with complementary mechanisms of action (e.g. a diuretic, whose efficacy is limited by the increased plasma renin activity that it causes, with an ACEI that blocks the renin–angiotensin system), rather than increasing the dose of a single agent, the effectiveness of which is often limited by homeostatic mechanisms. High doses of antihypertensive drugs are thus often not very effective during chronic administration, and often cause side-effects.

ACEI and Ca^{2+} antagonists are used increasingly, mainly because of their relative lack of metabolic and other side-effects. α_1-adrenoceptor antagonists have also staged something of a comeback with longer-acting drugs such as **terazosin** and **doxazosin** that are well tolerated, used once daily and have theoretically desirable effects on plasma lipids (reduced LDL/HDL ratio; see Ch. 16). **Moxonidine** is a centrally acting antihypertensive drug that is an agonist at imidazoline I_1 receptors. It was licensed recently and clinical experience is relatively limited, but it causes less drowsiness than α_2-agonists and may come to have a place in treating some patients. Clinical trials to determine whether ACEI and Ca^{2+}

channel antagonists are as effective at reducing the risks of stroke and myocardial infarction as are diuretics and β-adrenoceptor antagonists are currently under way (and not before time!).

The main categories of antihypertensive drugs are summarised in Table 15.4.

CARDIAC FAILURE

The underlying abnormality in cardiac failure (see Ch. 14) is a cardiac output that is inadequate to meet the metabolic demands of the body during exercise (and ultimately also at rest). It may be caused by disease of the myocardium itself (most commonly ischaemic heart disease), or by circulatory factors such as volume overload (e.g. valvular incompetence, arteriovenous shunts caused by congenital defects)* or pressure overload (e.g. hypertension, valvular narrowing). When cardiac output decreases, an increase in fluid volume occurs, partly because increased venous pressure causes increased formation of tissue fluid, and partly because reduced renal blood flow activates the renin–angiotensin–aldosterone system, causing sodium and water retention. Irrespective of the cause, the outlook for adults with cardiac failure is grim: of those with the most severe grade 50% are dead in 6 months, and of those with 'mild/moderate' disease 50% are dead in 5 years.

A highly simplified diagram of the sequence of events is shown in Figure 15.10. Drugs can act to:

- *Increase the force of cardiac contraction.* Cardiac glycosides (see Ch. 14) are mainly used either in patients who also have chronic atrial fibrillation or in patients who remain symptomatic despite treatment with diuretic and ACEI. **Digoxin** does not reduce mortality in such patients, but does improve symptoms and reduce the need for hospital admission. **Dobutamine** (a β_1-selective adrenoceptor agonist; see Ch. 8) is used intravenously when a rapid response is needed in the short term, for example following open heart surgery.
- *Increase excretion of salt and water (natriuresis).* Diuretics (see Ch. 20) are essential, especially if there is pulmonary oedema.
- *Relax vascular smooth muscle.* **Glyceryl trinitrate** is used to treat acute cardiac failure, especially if there is associated ischaemic pain. Its venodilator effect

*The harsh realities of life on antihypertensive drugs are graphically described in an article entitled '80,000 pills: a personal history of hypertension' (Mills 1989 Br Med J 298: 445–448).

*So-called 'hole-in-the-heart' babies have a defect in the atrial or ventricular septum, leading to shunting of blood from high- to low-pressure parts of the circulation.

Table 15.4 Commonly used antihypertensive drugs

Mode of action	Drugs	Adverse effects			Special features
		Postural hypotension	Impotence	Other	
Reduction of blood Volume/indirect vasodilatation	Thiazide diuretics*	–	++	Urinary frequency, gout glucose intolerance, hypokalaemia, hyponatraemia, thrombocytopenia	Reduce stroke in clinical trials, inexpensive
Block of β-adrenoceptors[†]	Propranolol Atenolol Metoprolol	–	±	Fatigue, cold peripheries	Reduce stroke in clinical trials, inexpensive, additional benefit after MI. Contraindications: asthma, heart failure, heart block, peripheral vascular disease
ACE inhibition	Captopril Enalapril Lisinopril Trandolapril Ramipril	–	±	First dose hypotension, dry cough, reversible renal failure in patients with bilateral renal artery stenosis	Additional benefit in insulin-dependent diabetics with proteinuria, following MI, and in patients with heart failure; cause regression of left ventricular hypertrophy
Arteriolar vasodilatation	Ca^{2+} antagonists, e.g. nifedipine, amlodipine nicardipine	–	±	Flushing, headache, ankle oedema	
Block of α$_1$-adrenoceptors[†]	Prazosin Terazosin Doxazosin	+	±	First dose hypotension	Longer-acting drugs (e.g. terazosin, doxazosin) better tolerated than prazosin. Improve plasma lipids. Useful addition to other drugs when two drugs needed

MI = myocardial infarction; * see Chapter 20; [†] see Chapter 8.

reduces venous pressure, and its effect on arterial compliance reduces cardiac work. The combination of **hydralazine** (to reduce after-load) with an organic nitrate (to reduce pre-load) in patients with chronic heart failure improves survival, albeit less well than treatment with an ACEI. It is useful in patients in whom ACEI are contraindicated or are not tolerated.

• *Inhibit the renin–angiotensin system.* The renin–angiotensin system is inappropriately activated in patients with cardiac failure, especially when they are treated with diuretics. ACEI are now commonly used to counteract this. By blocking the formation of angiotensin II they reduce vascular resistance, thus improving tissue perfusion and reducing cardiac after-load, and cause natriuresis by inhibiting secretion of aldosterone and by reducing the direct stimulatory effect of angiotensin II on reabsorption of sodium bicarbonate in the early part of the proximal convoluted tubule. Most important of all, they prolong life. In one rather small trial in elderly patients with heart failure, **losartan** improved survival even more than ACEI, but this awaits confirmation.

• *β-adrenoceptor antagonists.* Heart failure is accompanied by potentially harmful activation of the sympathetic nervous system as well as of the renin–angiotensin system, providing a rationale for

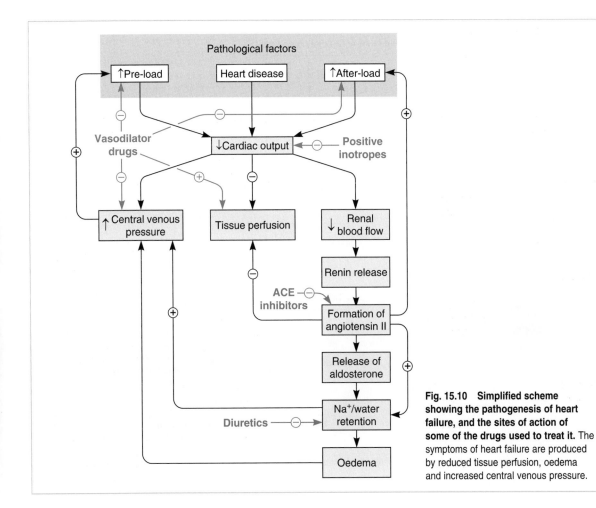

Pathological factors

↑Pre-load   Heart disease   ↑After-load

Vasodilator drugs

↓Cardiac output   Positive inotropes

↑Central venous pressure   Tissue perfusion   ↓Renal blood flow

Renin release

ACE inhibitors

Formation of angiotensin II

Release of aldosterone

Na⁺/water retention

Diuretics

Oedema

Fig. 15.10 Simplified scheme showing the pathogenesis of heart failure, and the sites of action of some of the drugs used to treat it. The symptoms of heart failure are produced by reduced tissue perfusion, oedema and increased central venous pressure.

using β-adrenoceptor antagonists for this disorder. Most clinicians have been very wary of this approach, because of the negative inotropic action of these drugs, but low doses have been shown to improve left ventricular ejection fraction and reduce hospitalisation. In one recent fairly small controlled trial, low-dose **carvedilol** reduced the risk of death when added to digoxin, diuretic and ACEI, and larger and hopefully definitive studies are due to report soon.

SHOCK AND HYPOTENSIVE STATES

Shock is a medical emergency characterised by inadequate perfusion of vital organs, usually because of a very low arterial blood pressure. This leads to anaerobic metabolism, and hence to increased lactate production. Mortality is extremely high, even with optimal treatment in an intensive care unit. Shock can be caused by various insults, including haemorrhage, burns, bacterial infections, anaphylaxis (Ch. 49) and myocardial infarction (Fig. 15.11). Reduced effective circulating blood volume (hypovolaemia) may be caused either directly by loss

---

Drugs commonly used in chronic heart failure

- Loop diuretics (e.g. frusemide; Ch. 20)
- ACE inhibitors (e.g. captopril, enalapril)
- Digoxin (see Ch. 14), especially for heart failure associated with established rapid atrial fibrillation. It is also indicated in patients who remain symptomatic despite treatment with loop diuretics and ACE inhibitors.
- Other vasodilators: organic nitrates (e.g. isosorbide mononitrate) reduce pre-load, and hydralazine reduces after-load. Used in combination, these prolong life, but less effectively than ACE inhibitors. They are used when ACE inhibitors are contraindicated or not tolerated.

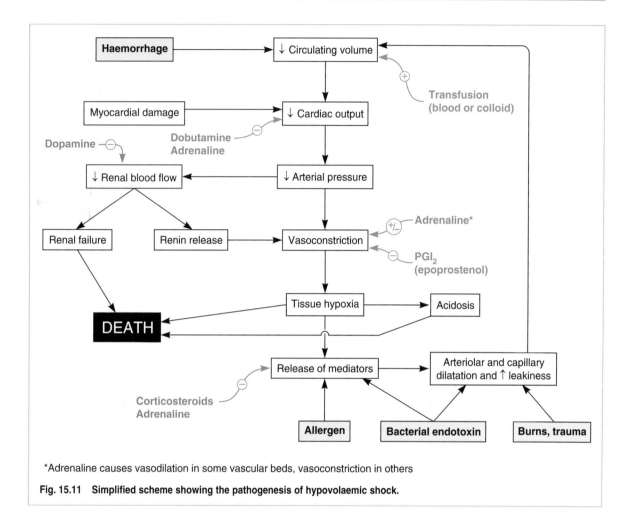

*Adrenaline causes vasodilation in some vascular beds, vasoconstriction in others

Fig. 15.11 Simplified scheme showing the pathogenesis of hypovolaemic shock.

of blood or by movement of fluid from the plasma to the tissues. The physiological (homeostatic) response to this is complex: vasodilatation in a vital organ (e.g. brain, heart or kidney) favours perfusion of that organ, but at the expense of a further reduction in blood pressure which leads to reduced perfusion of other organs. Ideally, there is a balance between vasoconstriction in non-essential vascular beds and vasodilatation in vital ones. The dividing line between the normal physiological response to blood loss and clinical shock is that, in the latter, tissue hypoxia produces secondary effects that tend to magnify rather than correct the primary disturbance. Thus, patients with established shock have profound and inappropriate vasodilatation in non-essential organs which is difficult to correct with vasoconstrictor drugs. The release of mediators (e.g. histamine, 5-hydroxytrypt-amine, bradykinin, prostaglandins, cytokines including

interleukins and TNF, NO and, undoubtedly, many more as yet unidentified substances) that cause capillary dilata-tion and leakiness, is the opposite of what is required to improve function in this setting.

Hypoperfusion leads to multiple organ failure, and intensive therapy specialists spend much effort trying to support the circulations of such patients with cocktails of vasoactive drugs (e.g. **adrenaline, dobutamine, dop-amine, prostacyclin**) designed to optimise flow to vital organs. In addition, there is great interest in antagonists of mediators that may be contributing to the hypotensive state. Clinical trials are in progress with drugs and macro-molecules (including monoclonal antibodies and soluble fragments of receptors) designed to block or neutralise endotoxin, interleukins, TNF and the inducible form of NO synthase among others. So far, these efforts have not yielded fruit: experimental work strongly suggests that dose will be critical since small amounts of mediators such as NO appear to be beneficial while larger amounts are harmful (Ch. 11). Clinical trials in this setting are extremely difficult because of the unique and distinctive haemodynamic features of each patient. Volume replacement is of proven benefit if there is hypovolaemia; antibiotics are essential if there is persistent infection;

adrenaline can be life-saving in anaphylaxis, corticosteroids suppress the formation of NO and of prostaglandins but are not of proven benefit once shock is established; vasoactive (dopamine, prostacyclin) and positively inotropic (adrenaline, dobutamine) drugs may help in individual patients but have not been proved to improve the ultimate clinical outcome.

REFERENCES AND FURTHER READING

Control of vascular smooth muscle tone

Gurney A M, Clapp L H 1994 Calcium channels and vasodilation. Adv Mol Cell Biol 8: 21–34 (*Reviews the properties of calcium channels in vascular smooth muscle*)

Nelson M T, Quayle J M 1995 Physiological roles and properties of potassium channels in arterial smooth muscle. Am J Physiol 268: C799–C822 (*Reviews four types of K^+ channel in regulation of membrane potential and vascular tone*)

Somlyo A P, Somlyo A V 1994 Signal transduction and regulation in smooth muscle Nature 372: 231–236 (*Smooth muscle contraction is regulated by $[Ca^{2+}]_i$ and by the Ca^{2+} sensitivity of the myofilaments*)

Vascular endothelium (see Ch 11 for further reading on NO)

Bunting S, Gryglewski R, Moncada S, Vane J R 1976 Arterial walls generate from prostaglandin endoperoxides a substance (prostaglandin X) which relaxes strips of mesenteric and coeliac arteries and inhibits platelet aggregation. Prostaglandins 12: 897–913

Furchgott R F, Zawadzki J V 1980. The obligatory role of endothelial cells in the relaxation of arterial smooth muscle by acetylcholine. Nature 288: 373–376

Furchgott R F, Vanhoutte P M 1989 Endothelium-derived relaxing and contracting factors. FASEB J 3: 2007–2018 (*Diversity of endothelium-derived mediators; references early work on endothelium-derived constricting factors which led to the discovery of endothelin*)

Hickey K A, Rubanyi G, Paul R J, Highsmith R F 1985 Characterization of a coronary vasoconstrictor produced by cultured endothelial cells. American Journal of Physiology 248(5 Pt 1): C550–C556

Karihara Y, Karihara H, Suzuki H et al. 1994 Elevated blood pressure and craniofacial abnormalities in mice deficient in endothelin-1. Nature 368: 703–710 (*Previously unsuspected role of endothelin-1 in development*)

Levin E R 1995 Endothelins. N Engl J Med 336: 356–363 (*Up-to-date review of cell biology, physiology, pathophysiology and central nervous system effects*)

Masaki T 1993 Endothelins: homeostatic and compensatory actions in the circulatory and endocrine systems. Endocr Rev 14: 256–268 (*Particularly useful on roles in endocrine—reproductive, neuroendocrine—systems*)

Vane J R, Anggard E E, Botting R M 1990 Regulatory functions of the vascular endothelium. N Engl J Med 323: 27–35 (*Superb review*)

Yanagisawa M, Kurihara H, Kimura S et al. 1988 A novel potent vasoconstrictor peptide produced by vascular endothelial cells. Nature 332: 411–415 (*Tour de force*)

Renin–angiotensin system

Dzau V J, Sasamura H, Hein L 1993 Heterogeneity of angiotensin

synthetic pathways and receptor subtypes: physiological and pharmacological implications. J Hypertens 11 (suppl 3): S13–S18 (*Explains why interrupting the renin–agiotensin system at different points in the pathway may have different effects*)

Goodfriend T L, Elliott M E, Catt K J 1996 Angiotensin receptors and their antagonists. N Engl J Med 334: 1649–1654 (*Succinct account*)

Hein L, Barsh G S, Pratt R E, Dzau V J, Kobilks B K 1995 Behavioural and cardiovascular effects of disrupting the angiotensin II type-2 receptor gene in mice. Nature 377: 744–747 ('*The AT2 receptor plays a role in the central nervous system and in cardiovascular functions that are mediated by the renin–angiotensin system.*' Pause for thought for clinicians inclined to prescribe ACEI and ATI-receptors antagonists interchangeably)

Ichiki T, Labosky P A, Shiota C et al. 1995 Effects on blood pressure and exploratory behaviour of mice lacking angiotensin II type-2 receptor Nature 377: 748–750 ('*Angiotensin II activates AT1 and AT2, which have mutually counteracting haemodynamic effects … AT2 regulates central nervous system functions, including behaviour.*')

Timmermans P B M W M, Wong P C, Chiu A T et al. 1993 Angiotensin II receptors and angiotensin II receptor antagonists. Pharmacol Rev 45: 205–251 (*Comprehensive review*)

Drugs (and clinical uses)

Allgren R A et al. for the Auriculin Anaritide Acute Renal Failure Study Group 1997 Anaritide in acute tubular necrosis. N Engl J Med 336: 828–834 (*A synthetic analogue of atrial natriuretic peptide may have improved survival in those patients with oliguria but worsened it in those with non-oliguric renal failure*)

Brindley G S 1986 Pilot experiments on the actions of drugs injected into the human corpus cavernosum penis. Br J Pharmacol 87: 495–500

Chertow G M et al. for the Auriculin Anaritide Acute Renal Failure Study Group 1996 Is the administration of dopamine associated with adverse or favourable outcomes in acute renal failure? Am J Med 101: 49–53 (*Low-dose dopamine did not improve survival in patients with acute renal failure*)

Cohen J N 1996 The management of chronic heart failure. N Engl J Med 335: 490–498 (*Excellent review including new approaches including β-adrenergic antagonists*)

Linz W, Scholkens B A 1992 A specific B_2-bradykinin receptor antagonist HOE140 abolishes the antihypertrophic effect of ramipril. Br J Pharmacol 105: 771–772 (*Some of the effects of angiotensin-converting enzyme inhibitors may be mediated by bradykinin*)

Maschio G et al. for the Angiotensin-converting-enzyme Inhibition in Progressive Renal Failure Study Group 1996

Effect of the angiotensin-converting-enzyme inhibitor benazepril on the progression of chronic renal insufficiency. N Engl J Med 334: 939–945 *(Benazepril protected against progression of renal insufficiency in patients with various renal diseases)*

Packer M et al. for the US Carvedilol Heart Failure Study Group 1996 The effect of carvedilol on morbidity and mortality in patients with chronic heart failure. N Engl J Med 334: 1349–1355 *(An accompanying editorial—Pfeffer M A, Stevenson L W 1996 β-adrenergic blockers and survival in heart failure. N Engl J Med 334: 1396–1397—comments in the context of other β-blocker trials in heart failure and concludes of the present study 'its promising results are not sufficient for us to conclude that they improve survival.')*

Uehata M, Ishizaki T, Satoh H et al. 1997 Calcium sensitization of smooth muscle mediated by a Rho-associated protein kinase in hypertension. Nature 389: 990–994 *(A pyridine derivative, Y-27632, selectively inhibits smooth muscle contraction by inhibiting calcium sensitisation via the Rho-associated protein kinase pathway, and lowers blood pressure in several experimental models of hypertension)*

Van Zwieten P A, Hamilton C A, Julius S, Prichard B N C (eds) 1996 The I_1-imidazoline receptor agonist moxonidine: a new antihypertensive, 2nd edn. The Royal Society of Medicine Press, London *(Succinct monograph on this recently licensed and novel centrally acting antihypertensive drug)*

16

Atherosclerosis and lipoprotein metabolism

LIPOPROTEINS AND OTHER RISK FACTORS FOR ATHEROSCLEROSIS

Lipoproteins (macromolecular complexes of lipid and protein) transport lipids and cholesterol through the bloodstream. Such a transport system is essential to life, but excessive concentrations in plasma of one important class of lipoprotein known as *low density lipoprotein* (LDL) increase the risk of ischaemic heart disease. Since this is the commonest cause of death in industrialised societies there is great interest in drugs that reduce the concentration of LDL in plasma.

Ischaemic heart disease is caused by plaques of atheroma in the coronary arteries which may rupture, exposing subendothelial material that acts as a focus for thrombosis, which causes myocardial infarction (see also Ch. 14, and Ch. 15 for comment on atheromatous disease in other vascular territories). One approach to the treatment and prevention of myocardial infarction is to use *fibrinolytic drugs* and *antiplatelet drugs*—notably **aspirin** (see Ch. 17). The other main approach to preventing myocardial infarction, described in the present chapter, is to attempt to inhibit atherogenesis by altering circulating lipoproteins. This has been mooted for many years, but remained intensely controversial until around 1994. The reason for the controversy was partly because the drugs available had only a small effect on LDL-cholesterol concentration. Furthermore, whereas it was generally accepted that there is a strong epidemiological association between raised LDL-cholesterol in plasma and risk of coronary artery disease, one camp held strongly to the view that *lowering* cholesterol pharmacologically might actually *increase* mortality from other causes such as cancer. HMG-CoA reductase inhibitors ('statins'—for example **simvastatin**, **pravastatin** and **lovastatin**) have greater effects on circulating cholesterol concentrations than the drugs that had been available previously and, more recently, several large clinical trials have demonstrated favourable effects on survival. This has led to a revolution in clinical practice. Statins are now very widely used, especially in the large numbers of patients with manifest coronary artery disease. This contrasts with the highly specialised treatment of patients with rare lipid disorders, often associated with pancreatitis and other clinical features, which were hitherto the main use for drugs that act on lipoprotein metabolism.

Epidemiological studies have identified numerous risk factors for atheromatous disease. Some of these cannot be altered (e.g. a family history of ischaemic heart disease) but others can (e.g. cigarette smoking, hypertension, hyperglycaemia, obesity, physical inactivity and increased plasma concentrations of total or LDL-cholesterol or reduced concentrations of high density lipoprotein—HDL). The present chapter describes drugs that affect lipoprotein metabolism. Other risk factors for atherosclerosis can also be favourably influenced by drugs, for example deficiency of oestrogen in postmenopausal women (see Ch. 26), increased concentrations in plasma of coagulation factors or of homocysteine, and serological evidence of chronic infection with *Chlamydia pneumoniae*. Much research is currently directed toward determining whether such drugs also prevent clinical manifestations of atherosclerotic disease.

Atherosclerosis is a *focal* disease of the intima of large and medium-sized arteries. Its pathogenesis evolves over many decades during most of which time the lesions are clinically silent, the occurrence of symptoms signalling advanced disease or supervening thrombosis. Until very recently there have been no good sub-primate models of advanced focal atherosclerotic disease, although transgenic animals deficient in specific key enzymes and receptors in lipoprotein metabolism (see Ch. 3) are now rapidly transforming this scene. Nevertheless, most of our understanding of atheroma comes from human pathology and from experimental studies in primates.

THE RELATIONSHIP BETWEEN ATHEROSCLEROSIS/THROMBOSIS AND LDL-CHOLESTEROL CONCENTRATION IN THE PLASMA

The pathogenesis of atherosclerosis is now beginning to be better understood, although some important details remain obscure. The role of chronic infection by organisms such as *Chlamydia pneumoniae* is particularly controversial, but potentially of great importance because of the therapeutic implications. Atherogenesis involves:

- Injury to endothelium encourages monocyte attachment, this process being markedly increased in hypercholesterolaemia. Turbulence may be responsible for the striking predilection of lesions for regions of disturbed flow such as the origin of vessels from the aorta. Chronic infections can initiate and perpetuate endothelial damage. Injury is initially undetectable morphologically but results in endothelial cell dysfunction with altered PGI_2 (Ch. 12) and NO (Ch. 11) biosynthesis.
- Endothelial cells bind LDL. When activated (e.g. by injury) these cells and attached monocytes/macrophages generate free radicals which oxidise LDL, resulting in lipid peroxidation and destruction of the receptor needed for normal receptor-mediated clearance of LDL.
- Modified LDL is taken up by macrophages via 'scavenger receptors'.
- Having taken up LDL, these macrophages (now *foam-cells*) migrate subendothelially. Subendothelial collections of foam-cells and T lymphocytes form the fatty streaks which presage atherosclerosis.
- Platelets, macrophages and endothelial cells release cytokines and growth factors. These cause proliferation of smooth muscle and deposition of connective tissue components. The excessive inflammatory fibroproliferative response leads to a dense fibrous cap of connective tissue overlying a core of lipid and necrotic debris.
- The plaque forms the substrate on which throm-

bosis develops subsequent to rupture (see Ch. 17, Fig. 17.10). Features of a plaque that make it liable to rupture include the presence of large numbers of macrophages, whereas vascular smooth muscle and matrix proteins may actually stabilise it.

One species of LDL, lipoprotein(a), that is strongly associated with atherosclerosis (and is localised in atherosclerotic lesions) contains a unique apoprotein, apo(a), which is similar in structure to plasminogen. Hence lipoprotein(a) competes with and inhibits the binding of plasminogen to its receptors on the endothelial cell. Plasminogen is normally the substrate for plasminogen activator which is secreted by and bound to endothelial cells, generating the fibrinolytic enzyme plasmin (see Fig. 17.10). The effect of the binding of lipoprotein(a) is that less plasmin is generated, fibrinolysis is inhibited and thrombosis promoted. LDL can also activate platelets, constituting a further thrombogenic effect of LDL.

Several steps in the atherogenic process are potential targets for pharmacological attack. Use of antioxidants is one such approach that is currently of particular interest, both because of evidence that this can improve endothelial function in patients with increased oxidant stress, and because of epidemiological evidence that a diet rich in antioxidants is associated with reduced risk of coronary artery disease. Results from clinical trials have so far been inconclusive, however. In contrast, drugs that lower plasma cholesterol are of proven benefit in preventing coronary artery disease. To understand how such drugs work it is necessary to know how lipids are handled in the body.

LIPOPROTEIN TRANSPORT IN THE BLOOD

Lipoproteins consist of a central core of hydrophobic lipid (triglycerides or cholesteryl esters) encased in a more hydrophilic coat of polar substances—phospholipids, free cholesterol and associated apolipoproteins. There are four main classes of lipoproteins, differing in the relative proportion of the core lipids and in the type of apoprotein. They also differ in size and density, and this latter property, as measured by ultracentrifugation, is the basis for their classification into:

- high density lipoproteins (HDL)
- low density lipoproteins (LDL)
- very low density lipoproteins (VLDL)
- chylomicrons.

Each of these lipoprotein classes has a specific role in

lipid transport in the circulation, and there are different 'pathways' for exogenous and for endogenous lipids. In the *exogenous pathway* (see Fig. 16.1), cholesterol and triglycerides derived from the gastrointestinal tract are transported in the lymph and then in the plasma as *chylomicrons* (diameter 100–1000 nm) to capillaries in muscle and adipose tissue. Here the core triglycerides are hydrolysed by a surface-bound lipoprotein lipase (which requires one of the apoproteins as a cofactor) and the resulting free fatty acids are taken up by the tissues.

The chylomicron remnants (diameter 30–50 nm), still containing their full complement of cholesteryl esters, pass to the liver, bind to apolipoprotein receptors on hepatocytes, and undergo endocytosis. Cholesterol is liberated within the liver cell and may be stored, or oxidised to bile acids, or secreted in the bile unaltered. Alternatively, it may enter the endogenous pathway of lipid transport in VLDL.

In the *endogenous pathway*, cholesterol and newly synthesised triglycerides are transported from the liver as

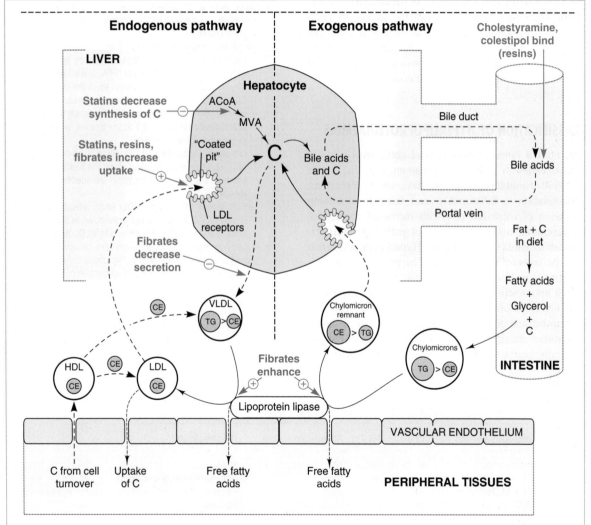

Fig. 16.1 Schematic diagram of cholesterol transport in the tissues, with sites of action of the main drugs affecting lipoprotein metabolism. (C = cholesterol; CE = cholesteryl ester; TG = triglyceride; MVA = mevalonate; HMG-CoA reductase = 3-hydroxy-3-methylglutaryl-CoA reductase; VLDL = very low density lipoprotein; LDL = low density lipoprotein; HDL = high density lipoprotein)

VLDL (diameter 30–80 nm) to muscle and adipose tissue where the triglycerides are hydrolysed and the resulting fatty acids enter the tissues as described above. During this process, the lipoprotein particles become smaller (diameter 20–30 nm), but still have a full complement of cholesteryl esters and ultimately become LDL which provides the source of cholesterol for incorporation into cell membranes and for synthesis of steroids (see Chs 24 and 26), and bile acids (Ch. 21). Cells take up LDL by endocytosis via LDL receptors that recognise LDL apolipoproteins. Some drugs (notably statins; see below) reduce the LDL concentration in the blood by stimulating the synthesis of these receptors in hepatocytes. Cholesterol can return to plasma from the tissues in HDL particles (diameter 7–20 nm). Cholesterol is esterified with long-chain fatty acid in HDL particles, and the resulting cholesteryl esters are subsequently transferred to VLDL or LDL particles by a transfer protein present in the plasma.

CLASSIFICATION OF HYPERLIPOPROTEINAEMIAS

The normal range of plasma total cholesterol concentration varies in different populations (e.g. in Britain 25–30% of middle-aged people have serum cholesterol concentrations > 6.5 mmol/l), and there is a smooth gradation of increased risk with increased cholesterol concentration, so the definition of pathological hypercholesterolaemia is arbitrary. Hyperlipoproteinaemia may be *primary* or *secondary*. The primary forms are genetically determined. They are classified, according to which lipoprotein particle is raised, into six phenotypes (the Frederickson classification; Table 16.1). This has prognostic and therapeutic implications, but is not a diagnostic classification. An especially great risk of ischaemic heart disease occurs in a subset of primary type

IIa hyperlipoproteinaemia due to a monogenic defect of LDL receptors called familial hypercholesterolaemia, in which the serum cholesterol concentration in adults is typically 9–11 mmol/l in heterozygotes. Study of this disorder enabled Brown & Goldstein (1986) to define the LDL-receptor pathway of cholesterol homeostasis.

Secondary forms of hyperlipoproteinaemia are a consequence of other conditions such as diabetes mellitus, alcoholism, nephrotic syndrome, chronic renal failure,

---

Lipoprotein metabolism and hyperlipoproteinaemia

- Lipids, such as cholesterol (C) and triglycerides (T), are transported in the plasma as lipoproteins, of which there are four classes:
  — chylomicrons which transport T and C from the GI tract to the tissues where they are split by lipoprotein lipase and the free fatty acids (FFA) are taken up. Chylomicron remnants are taken up in the liver, where C is stored, oxidised to bile acids, or released into:
  — very low density lipoproteins (VLDL), which transport C and newly synthesised T to the tissues, where T is removed as before, leaving:
  — low density lipoproteins (LDL) with a large component of C, some of which is taken up by the tissues and some by the liver, by endocytosis via specific LDL receptors
  — high density lipoproteins (HDL) which adsorb cholesterol derived from cell breakdown in tissues (including arteries) and transfer it to VLDL and LDL.
- Hyperlipoproteinaemias can be primary, or secondary to some generalised disease (e.g. hypothyroidism). They are classified according to which lipoprotein particle is raised, into six phenotypes (the Frederickson classification). The higher the plasma concentration of LDL-cholesterol, and the lower the concentration of HDL-cholesterol, the higher the risk of ischaemic heart disease.

Table 16.1 Frederickson/WHO classification of hyperlipoproteinaemia

Type	Lipoprotein elevated	Chol	TG	Atherosclerosis risk	Drug treatment
I	Chylomicrons	+	+++	NE	None
IIa	LDL	++	NE	High	HMG-CoA reductase ± resins
IIb	LDL + VLDL	++	++	High	Fibrates, HMG-CoA reductase inhibitor, nicotinic acid
III	βVLDL	++	++	Moderate	Fibrates
IV	VLDL	+	++	Moderate	Fibrates (± fish oil)
V	Chylomicrons + VLDL	+	++	NE	None (± fish oil)

Chol = cholesterol; TG = triglycerides; LDL = low density lipoprotein; VLDL = very low density lipoprotein; βVDL = a qualitatively abnormal form of VLDL identified by its pattern on electrophoresis; + = increased concentration; NE = not elevated

hypothyroidism, liver disease and administration of *drugs*, for example β-adrenoceptor antagonists (Ch. 8), thiazide diuretics (Chs 15 and 20), and **isotretinoin** (an isomer of vitamin A given by mouth as well as topically in the treatment of severe acne).

LIPID-LOWERING DRUGS

Several drugs are used to decrease plasma LDL-cholesterol. Drug therapy to lower plasma lipids is only one approach to treatment and is used in addition to dietary management and correction of other modifiable cardiovascular risk factors. The selection of patients to be treated with drugs remains controversial, not least for reasons of cost: the benefit is greatest for those who are at greatest risk, including those with symptomatic atherosclerotic disease and with many cardiovascular risk factors as well as those with the highest plasma concentrations of cholesterol.

The main classes of drugs used clinically are:

- HMG-CoA reductase inhibitors ('statins')
- bile acid binding resins
- fibrates.

Other drugs include **nicotinic acid** (or one of its derivatives) and **probucol**. Fish oil can be used in severe hypertriglyceridaemia, but can increase plasma cholesterol. D-thyroxine and neomycin are obsolete.

HMG-CoA REDUCTASE INHIBITORS (STATINS)

The rate-limiting enzyme in cholesterol synthesis is HMG-CoA reductase which catalyses the conversion of HMG-CoA* to mevalonic acid (MVA) (see Fig. 16.1). Several fungal metabolites are potent inhibitors of this enzyme (Fig. 16.2). **Simvastatin** and **pravastatin** have been extensively investigated and are specific, reversible, competitive inhibitors with K_i values of approximately 1 nmol/l. The resulting decrease in hepatic cholesterol synthesis leads to *increased synthesis of LDL receptors* and thus *increased clearance of LDL* and reduced concentration of LDL-cholesterol in plasma. They also cause a small reduction in plasma triglycerides and a small increase in HDL-cholesterol. Several large randomised placebo-controlled clinical trials to determine the effects of HMG-CoA reductase inhibitors on morbidity and mortality have been positive. These include:

*HMG-CoA = 3-hydroxy-3-methylglutaryl-coenzyme A.

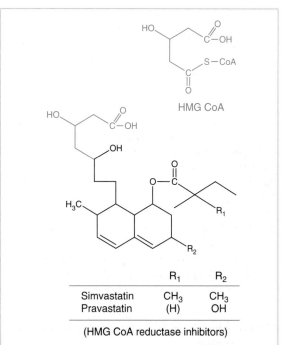

	R₁	R₂
Simvastatin	CH₃	CH₃
Pravastatin	(H)	OH

(HMG CoA reductase inhibitors)

Fig. 16.2 Structure of HMG-CoA and two inhibitors of HMG-CoA reductase.

- The Scandinavian Simvastatin Survival Study ('4S')—see Figure 16.3—of 4444 patients with angina or who had recovered from a heart attack and whose plasma cholesterol was 5.5–8.0 mmol/l; serum LDL-cholesterol was lowered by simvastatin by 35%. Treatment continued for a median 5.4 years and produced a 30% reduction in risk of death, accounted for by a 42% reduction in death from coronary disease.
- The West of Scotland Coronary Prevention Study ('WOSCOPS') involved randomisation of over 6500 45- to 64-year-old healthy men to placebo or pravastatin, which reduced LDL-cholesterol by 26%, overall mortality by 22% and the risk of heart attack or death from coronary disease by 31%.
- Cholesterol and Recurrent Events ('CARE') trial in which over 4000 patients who had recovered from myocardial infarction and in whom plasma cholesterol concentration was less than 6.2 mmol/l were allocated to treatment with placebo or pravastatin. Pravastatin lowered LDL-cholesterol by 28% and the risk of either death from coronary disease or recurrent myocardial infarction by 24% and the risk of stroke by 31%.

Atorvastatin causes long-lasting inhibition of HMG-CoA reductase, and lowers triglycerides as well as

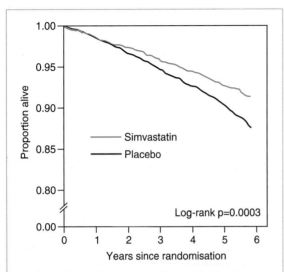

Fig 16.3   Survival in patients with coronary heart disease and serum cholesterol 5.5–8.0 mmol/l treated either with placebo or with simvastatin. The relative risk of death in the simvastatin group was 0.70 (95% confidence intervals 0.58–0.85). (Based on: 4S study 1994 Lancet 344: 1383–1389)

Clinical use of HMG-CoA reductase inhibitors ('statins')

- **Simvastatin** and **pravastatin** reduce mortality as well as morbidity in appropriately selected individuals.
- Such drugs are indicated in patients who have symptomatic atherosclerotic disease, and in patients who are at increased risk of coronary heart disease because of elevated serum cholesterol concentration, especially if there are other risk factors for atherosclerosis. Tables are available to help target treatment to those at greatest risk.
- In contrast to their usefulness in patients with heterozygous familial hypercholesterolaemia, most statins are ineffective in those rare patients with the *homozygous* form of this disease who cannot make LDL receptors (**atorvastatin** is an exception, having some useful effect on serum cholesterol in such patients).
- Main unwanted effect is myositis, which is rare but can be severe
- Statins are used with caution (or not at all) in patients with liver disease. They are contraindicated in pregnancy. Itraconazole and cyclosporin increase the risk of myositis.

cholesterol. Its effect on coronary events and survival has not been reported.

Pharmacokinetics

HMG-CoA reductase inhibitors are given by mouth last thing before going to bed at night. They are well absorbed and extracted by the liver, their site of action, and are subject to extensive presystemic metabolism. **Simvastatin** is an inactive lactone pro-drug which is metabolised in the liver to its active form, the corresponding β-hydroxy fatty acid.

Adverse effects

HMG-CoA reductase inhibitors are well tolerated: mild and infrequent unwanted effects include gastrointestinal disturbance, insomnia and rash. More serious adverse effects are rare but include severe myositis ('rhabdomyolysis'), hepatitis and angio-oedema.

Clinical uses

See the clinical box on this page.

BILE ACID BINDING RESINS

Cholestyramine and **colestipol** are anion exchange resins. When taken by mouth, they sequester bile acids in the intestine and prevent their reabsorption and entero-

hepatic recirculation (Fig. 16.1). The result is decreased absorption of exogenous cholesterol and increased metabolism of endogenous cholesterol into bile acids in the liver. This leads to increased expression of LDL receptors on liver cells, and hence to increased removal of LDL from the blood and a reduced concentration of LDL-cholesterol in plasma. The concentration of HDL-cholesterol is unchanged and there may be an unwanted increase in triglycerides. The American Lipid Research Clinics' trial of middle-aged men with primary hypercholesterolaemia showed that addition of a resin to dietary treatment caused a mean 13% fall in plasma cholesterol and a 20–25% fall in coronary heart disease over 7 years.

Unwanted effects

Since resins are not absorbed, systemic toxicity is low, but gastrointestinal symptoms of nausea, abdominal bloating, constipation or diarrhoea are common and dose-related. Resins are bulky and unappetising, although this can be minimised by suspending them in fruit juice. They interfere with the absorption of fat-soluble vitamins, and of drugs such as **chlorothiazide**, **digoxin** and **warfarin**, which should therefore be taken at least 1 hour before or 4–6 hours after the resin.

Clinical use

See the clinical box on page 307.

FIBRATES

Several fibric acid derivatives ('**fibrates**') are available including **bezafibrate**, **ciprofibrate**, **gemfibrozil**, **feno-fibrate** and **clofibrate**. These cause a marked reduction in circulating VLDL, and hence triglyceride, with a modest (approximately 10%) reduction in LDL and an approximately 10% increase in HDL. **Gemfibrozil** reduced coronary heart disease by approximately one-third compared with placebo in middle-aged men with primary hyperlipoproteinaemia in one study, but did not improve overall survival.

The mechanism of action of fibrates (see Fig. 16.1) is incompletely understood, but they stimulate lipoprotein lipase, hence increasing hydrolysis of triglyceride in chylomicron and VLDL particles as these traverse capillaries and liberating free fatty acid for storage in fat or metabolism in striated muscle. They also probably reduce hepatic VLDL production and increase hepatic LDL uptake. In addition to these effects on lipoproteins, fibrates also reduce plasma fibrinogen and improve glucose tolerance, although it is unknown if these potentially advantageous effects are clinically important.

Adverse effects

Myositis is unusual but can be severe ('rhabdomyolysis'), when it can cause myoglobinuria and acute renal failure. It occurs particularly in patients with renal impairment, because of reduced protein binding and impaired elimination of the drug. Fibrates should be avoided in such patients and also in alcoholics who are predisposed to hypertriglyceridaemia and are at risk of rhabdomyolysis.* Myositis can also be caused (rarely) by

---

*For several reasons, including a tendency to lie immobile for prolonged periods in gutters followed by generalised convulsions—'rum fits'—and *delirium tremens*.

Statins (see above) and the combined use of fibrates with this class of drugs is therefore generally inadvisable. Fibrates can cause a variety of mild gastrointestinal symptoms. **Clofibrate** predisposes to *gallstones* and its use is therefore limited to patients who have had a cholecystectomy.

Clinical use

See the clinical box below.

OTHER LIPID-LOWERING DRUGS

Nicotinic acid

Nicotinic acid is a vitamin which has been used in gram quantities as a lipid-lowering agent. **Acipimox** is a derivative of nicotinic acid which is used in lower dose and may have less marked adverse effects, although it is unclear whether the recommended dose is as effective as are standard doses of nicotinic acid. These drugs inhibit hepatic triglyceride production and VLDL secretion (see Fig. 16.1), which leads indirectly to a modest reduction in LDL and increase in HDL. Long-term administration is associated with reduced mortality, but its clinical use is limited by its *unwanted effects*, especially as there are now more effective and better tolerated drugs available in the form of the statins. Adverse effects include flushing, palpitations and gastrointestinal disturbances. Flushing is associated with production of *prostaglandin D_2* (Ch. 12) and is reduced by taking the dose half an hour after a dose of **aspirin**. High doses can cause disorders of liver function, impair glucose tolerance and precipitate gout.

Probucol

Probucol lowers the concentration in the plasma of both LDL and HDL. Its place in therapy has not been defined—it has distinctive properties that could be either desirable (e.g. antioxidant properties) or the reverse (e.g. lowering HDL and prolonging the cardiac action potential). A large clinical trial of its quantitative effects on atheroma in the femoral arteries ('PQRST') did not show any significant improvement in vessel narrowing. Its mechanism of action is not understood. Probucol has unusual pharmacokinetic properties: it is markedly lipophilic, and most of the circulating drug is associated with LDL. It remains in body fat for several months after chronic administration is discontinued. Its peak effect on plasma cholesterol occurs only after 1–3 months' administration. Gastrointestinal disturbances occur in 10% of patients. Probucol should be avoided in patients with a long Q–T interval on the electrocardiogram (see Ch. 14). Drugs that influence cardiac repolarisation such as **amiodarone**, **sotalol** and **terfenadine** should be avoided if possible in patients who have received probucol within the past few months because of the possibility of precipitating a form of ventricular tachycardia known as 'torsades de pointes' (Ch. 14).

Fish oil

ω-3 marine triglycerides reduce plasma triglyceride concentrations but increase cholesterol. Plasma triglyceride concentrations are less strongly associated with coronary artery disease than is cholesterol, and an effect of fish oil on cardiac morbidity or mortality is unproven, although there is epidemiological evidence that eating fish regularly does reduce ischaemic heart disease. The mechanism of action of fish oil on plasma triglyceride concentrations is unknown. Fish oil is rich in highly unsaturated fatty acids including *eicosapentaenoic* and *docosahexaenoic* acids and has other potentially important effects including inhibition of platelet function, prolongation of bleeding time, anti-inflammatory effects and reduction of plasma fibrinogen. Eicosapentaenoic acid substitutes for arachidonic acid in cell membranes and gives rise to 3-series prostaglandins and thromboxanes (that is, prostanoids with three double bonds in their side-chains rather than the usual two), and 5-series leukotrienes. This probably accounts for their effects on haemostasis since thromboxane A_3 is much less active as a platelet-aggregating agent than is thromboxane A_2, whereas prostaglandin I_3 is similar in potency as an inhibitor of platelet function to prostaglandin I_2 (prostacyclin). The alteration in leukotriene biosynthesis probably underlies the anti-inflammatory effects of fish oil. Fish oil is contraindicated in patients with type IIa hyperlipoproteinaemia because of the increase in LDL-cholesterol that it causes.

REFERENCES AND FURTHER READING

Anonymous 1996 Management of hyperlipidaemia. Drug Ther Bull 34: 89–93 *(Modern approach to management, based on succinct summary and analysis of clinical trial data)*

Brown M S, Goldstein J L 1986 A receptor-mediated pathway for cholesterol homeostasis. Science 232: 34–47 *(Classic from these Nobel Prize winners: read with Goldstein & Brown, see below)*

Canner P L, Berge K G, Wenger J et al. 1986 Fifteen year mortality in coronary drug project patients: long-term benefit with niacin. J Am Coll Cardiol 8: 1245–1255 *(Mortality benefit from niacin)*

Davies M J, Woolf N 1993 Atherosclerosis: what is it and why does it occur? Br Heart J 69: S3–S11 *(Reviews the pathology/pathogenesis)*

Dart A et al. 1997 A multi-center, double-blind, one-year, study comparing safety and efficacy of atorvastatin versus simvastatin in patients with hypercholesterolemia. Am J Cardiol 80: 39–44

Durrington P N 1989 Hyperlipidaemia: diagnosis and management. Wright, London *(Extremely readable, authoritative book; for a more recent review of lipid and lipoprotein disorders by the same author see Weatherall D J, Ledingham G G, Warrel D A (eds) 1996 Oxford textbook of medicine, 3rd edn. Oxford University Press, Oxford, vol 2, pp 1399–1415)*

Goldstein J L, Brown M S 1990 Regulation of the mevalonate pathway. Nature 343: 425–430

Gupta G, Leatham E W, Carrington D, Mendall M A, Kaski J C, Camm A J 1997 Elevated *Chlamydia pneumoniae* antibodies, cardiovascular events, and azithromycin in male survivors of myocardial infarction. Circulation 96: 404–407 *(A short course of azithromycin may lower risk of MI. If confirmed, prevention would be dynamite. What would we do with all the unemployed interventional cardiologists?)*

Hajjar K A, Gavish D, Breslow J L, Nachman R 1989 Lipoprotein(a) modulation of endothelial cell surface fibrinolysis and its potential role in atherosclerosis. Nature 339: 303–305

McCully K S 1996 Homocysteine and vascular disease. Nature Med 2: 386–389 *(Commentary on this recently recognised risk factor for atherosclerosis; discusses therapeutic promise of increased dietary folate and vitamin B_6)*

McLean J W, Tomlinson J E, Kuang W-J et al. 1987 cDNA sequence of human apolipoprotein(a) is homologous to plasminogen. Nature 300: 132–137

Miles L A, Fless G M, Levin E G, Scann A M, Plow E F 1989 A potential basis for the thrombotic risks associated with lipoprotein(a). Nature 339: 301–303 *(See also comment: Scott J 1989 Thrombogenesis linked to atherogenesis at last? Nature 341: 22–33)*

Nathan L, Chaudhuri G 1997 Estrogens and atherosclerosis. Annu Rev Pharmacol Toxicol 37: 477–515 *(Actions include effects on endothelium and vascular smooth muscle)*

Ramsay L E, Haq I U, Jackson P R, Yeo W W, Pickin D M, Payne J N 1996 Targeting lipid-lowering drug therapy for primary prevention of coronary disease: an updated Sheffield table. Lancet 348: 387–388 *(Controversial/influential tables based on targeting treatment to individuals with a coronary heart disease event rate of 3% per year or greater)*

Ridker P M, Cushman M, Stampfer M J, Tracy R P, Hennekens C H 1997 Inflammation, aspirin, and the risk of cardiovascular disease in apparently healthy men. N Engl J Med 336: 973–979 *(See also accompanying editorial by Attilio Maseri: 'Inflammation, atherosclerosis, and ischemic events—exploring the hidden side of the moon' N Engl J Med 336: 1014–1015)*

Ross R 1993 The pathogenesis of atherosclerosis: a perspective for the 1990s. Nature 362: 801–809 *(Enormously influential review)*

Scandinavian Simvastatin Survival Study Group 1994 Randomised trial of cholesterol lowering in 4444 patients with coronary heart disease: the Scandinavian Simvastatin Survival Study (4S). Lancet 344: 1383–1389 *(Demonstrated major effect of drug treatment not only on cholesterol but on clinical end-points including mortality)*

Steinberg D, Parthasarathy S, Carew T E, Khoo J C, Witztum J L 1989 Beyond cholesterol: modifications of low-density lipoprotein that increase its atherogenicity. N Engl J Med 320: 915–924 *(The oxidised LDL hypothesis)*

Treasure C B et al. 1995 Beneficial effects of cholesterol-lowering therapy on the coronary endothelium in patients with coronary artery disease N Engl J Med 332: 481–487 *(See also a review by Levine G N, Keaney J F & Vita J A in the same issue of the journal, pp 512–519: discusses studies of plaque rupture and endothelial function)*

Walldius G, Erikson U, Olsson A G et al. 1994 The effect of probucol on femoral atherosclerosis: the Probucol Quantitative Regression Swedish Trial. Am J Cardiol 74: 875–883 *(Failed to detect a beneficial effect of this antioxidant lipid-lowering drug. The acronym PQRST brings to mind the electrocardiogram: perhaps a salutary reminder in view of the pro-arrhythmic effect of probucol!)*

17

Haemostasis and thrombosis

Haemostasis is the arrest of blood loss from damaged blood vessels and is essential to life. A wound causes vasoconstriction, accompanied by:

- adhesion and activation of platelets
- fibrin formation.

Platelet activation leads to the formation of a haemostatic plug that stops the bleeding, and is subsequently reinforced by fibrin. The relative importance of each process depends on the type of vessel (arterial, venous or capillary) that has been injured.

Thrombosis is the pathological formation of a 'haemostatic' plug within the vasculature in the absence of bleeding. Over a century ago, Rudolph Virchow defined three predisposing factors still known as 'Virchow's triad'. This comprises: *injury to the vessel wall*—for example when an atheromatous plaque ruptures; *altered blood flow*—for example in the left atrial appendage of the heart during atrial fibrillation or in the veins of the legs while sitting cramped up on a long journey; and *abnormal coagulability of the blood*—as occurs, for example, in the later stages of pregnancy or during treatment with certain oral contraceptives (see Ch. 26).

Increased coagulability of the blood can be inherited, and is referred to as 'thrombophilia'. A *thrombus*, which forms in vivo, should be distinguished from a *blood clot*, which forms in static blood in vitro. Clots are amorphous, consisting of a diffuse fibrin meshwork in which all the cells of the blood are trapped. By contrast, arterial and venous thrombi each have a distinct structure.

Arterial thrombus (see Fig. 17.1) is composed of so-called 'white thrombus' consisting mainly of platelets and leukocytes in a fibrin mesh. It is usually associated with *atherosclerosis*. It interrupts blood flow, causing ischaemia or death (infarction) of the tissue beyond. *Venous thrombus* is composed of 'red thrombus' and consists of a small white head and a large jelly-like red tail, similar in composition to a blood clot, which streams away in the flow. Thrombus can break away forming an *embolus* which lodges in the lungs or, if it comes from the left heart or a carotid artery, in the brain or other organs, causing death or other disaster.

Drug therapy to promote haemostasis is rarely necessary, being required only when this essential process

---

Haemostasis and thrombosis

- Haemostasis is the arrest of blood loss from damaged vessels and is essential to life. The main phenomena are:
  - platelet adhesion and activation
  - blood coagulation (fibrin formation).
- Thrombosis is a pathological condition resulting from inappropriate activation of haemostatic mechanisms.
  - Venous thrombosis is usually associated with stasis of blood; a venous thrombus has a small platelet component and a large component of fibrin.
  - Arterial thrombosis is usually associated with atherosclerosis, and the thrombus has a large platelet component.
- A portion of a thrombus may break away, travel as an embolus and lodge downstream, causing ischaemia and infarction.

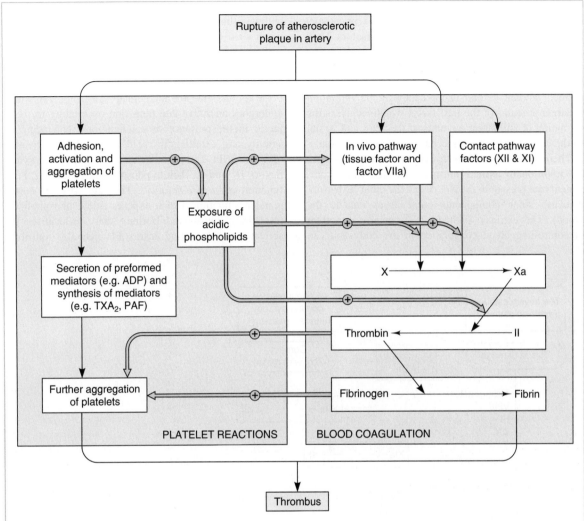

Fig. 17.1 The main events in the formation of an arterial thrombus. (A similar series of events occurs when there is vascular damage, leading to haemostasis.) The exposure of the acidic phospholipids of the platelets also provides the surface on which are localised the interactions of factors IXa and VIIa with factor X, and of factor Xa with factor II, as illustrated in more detail in Figure 17.4. Activation of factor XII also initiates the fibrinolytic pathway, which is shown in Figure 17.10.

is defective (e.g. coagulation factors in haemophilia or following excessive anticoagulant therapy) or when it proves difficult to staunch haemorrhage following surgery or for menorrhagia (e.g. antifibrinolytic and haemostatic drugs; see below). Drug therapy to treat or prevent thrombosis or thromboembolism, on the other hand, is extensively used because such diseases are common as well as serious. Drugs affect haemostasis and thrombosis in three distinct ways:

- by modifying blood coagulation (fibrin formation)
- by modifying platelet function
- by affecting fibrin removal (fibrinolysis).

BLOOD COAGULATION

COAGULATION CASCADE

Blood coagulation means the conversion of fluid blood to a solid gel or clot. The main event is the conversion of soluble fibrinogen to insoluble strands of fibrin, the last step in a complex enzyme cascade. The components ('factors') are present in blood as inactive precursors ('zymogens') of proteolytic enzymes and cofactors. They are activated by proteolysis, the active forms being designated by the suffix 'a'. Factors XIIa, XIa, IXa, Xa, and thrombin (IIa) are all serine proteases. Activation of a small amount of one factor catalyses the formation of larger amounts of the next factor which catalyses the formation of still larger amounts of the next, and so on, so the cascade provides a mechanism of amplification.

There are two main pathways of fibrin formation, one traditionally termed 'intrinsic' (because all the components are present in the blood) and the other 'extrinsic' (because some components come from outside the blood). The extrinsic pathway is especially important in controlling blood coagulation in the body and can

accurately be called the *in vivo* pathway. The intrinsic pathway (better called the contact pathway) is activated when shed blood comes into contact with an artificial surface such as glass.

The cascade is outlined in Figure 17.2. The *in vivo* (extrinsic) *pathway* is initiated by 'tissue factor', which is the cellular receptor and cofactor for factor VII, which undergoes an active site transition on binding to tissue factor in the presence of calcium ions, enhancing its activity and resulting in rapid autocatalytic activation of VII to VIIa. The tissue factor–VIIa complex activates factors IX and X. Acidic phospholipids (see Fig. 17.2) function as *surface catalysts*. They are provided during platelet activation, which exposes acidic phospholipids (especially phosphatidylserine) that co-localise and activate various clotting factors. Platelets also contribute

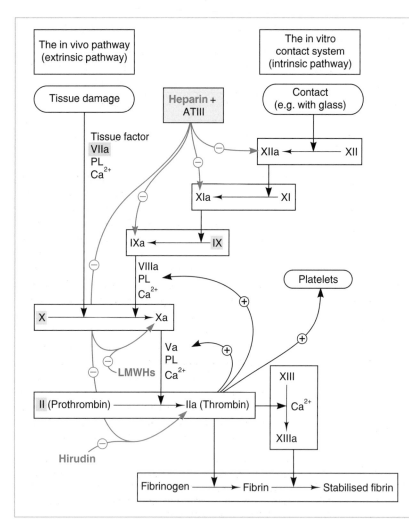

Fig. 17.2 The blood coagulation cascade with the sites of action of the anticoagulant drugs. Tissue factor also activates factor IX. Oral anticoagulants interfere with the essential post-translational γ-carboxylation of factors II, VII, IX and X (shown in light blue boxes). See Figure 17.4 for this latter action. Heparin and other antithrombin agents inactivate the enzymic forms of the coagulation factors. Coagulation of 100 ml of blood requires 0.2 mg of factor VIII, 2 mg of factor X, 15 mg of prothrombin and 250 mg of fibrinogen. (PL = a negatively charged phospholipid (supplied by activated platelets); AT III = antithrombin III; LMWHs = low-molecular-weight heparins)

by secreting coagulation factors, including factor Va and fibrinogen. Coagulation is sustained by further generation of factor Xa by IXa–VIIIa–calcium–phospholipid complex. This is needed because the tissue factor–VIIa complex is rapidly inactivated in plasma by tissue factor pathway inhibitor and by antithrombin III. Factor Xa, in the presence of calcium, phospholipid and factor Va, activates prothrombin to *thrombin*, the main enzyme of the cascade.

The role of thrombin. Thrombin (factor IIa) cleaves fibrinogen, producing fragments that polymerise to form fibrin. It also activates factor XIII, a fibrinoligase, which strengthens fibrin-to-fibrin links thereby stabilising the coagulum. In addition to its coagulant action, thrombin also causes platelet aggregation, stimulates cell proliferation and modulates smooth muscle contraction. Paradoxically, it can inhibit as well as promote coagulation (see below). Effects of thrombin on platelets and smooth muscle are initiated by interaction with specific thrombin receptors, which belong to the superfamily of G-protein-coupled receptors. The signal transduction mechanism is unusual: receptor activation requires proteolysis by thrombin of the extracellular N-terminal domain of the receptor, revealing a new N-terminal sequence that acts as a 'tethered agonist' (see Fig. 2.8, p. 32).

The *contact* (intrinsic) *pathway* commences when factor XII ('Hageman factor') adheres to a negatively charged surface, and converges with the in vivo pathway at the stage of factor X activation (see Fig. 17.2). The proximal part of this pathway is not crucial for blood coagulation in vivo. The two pathways are not entirely separate even before they converge, and various positive feedbacks promote coagulation.

As might be expected, this accelerating enzyme cascade has to be controlled by inhibitors, since otherwise all the blood in the body would solidify within minutes of the initiation of haemostasis. One of the most important inhibitors is an α_2-globulin, *antithrombin III*, which neutralises all the serine proteases in the cascade. Another, heparin cofactor II, inhibits only thrombin. Vascular endothelium also actively limits thrombus extension (see below).

VASCULAR ENDOTHELIUM IN HAEMOSTASIS AND THROMBOSIS

Vascular endothelium, the container of the circulating blood, plays a dual role in preserving the integrity of the circulation: it can change from a non-thrombogenic to a thrombogenic structure in response to different

---

Blood coagulation (fibrin formation)

The clotting system consists of a cascade of proteolytic enzymes and cofactors.

- Inactive precursors are activated in series, each giving rise to more of the next.
- The last enzyme, thrombin, derived from prothrombin (II), converts soluble fibrinogen (I) to an insoluble meshwork of fibrin in which blood cells are trapped, forming the clot.
- There are two pathways in the cascade:
  — the extrinsic pathway which operates in vivo
  — the intrinsic or contact pathway which operates in vitro.
- Both pathways result in activation of factor X, which then converts prothrombin to thrombin.
- Calcium and a negatively charged phospholipid (PL) are essential for three steps, namely the actions of:
  — factor IXa on X
  — factor VIIa on X
  — factor Xa on II.
- PL is provided by activated platelets adhering to the damaged vessel.
- Some factors promote coagulation by *binding* to PL and a serine protease factor, e.g. factor Va in the activation of II by Xa; VIIIa in the activation of X by IXa.
- Blood coagulation is controlled by:
  — enzyme inhibitors, e.g. antithrombin III
  — fibrinolysis.

---

demands. Normally, it provides a non-thrombogenic surface by virtue of surface *heparan sulphate*, a glycosaminoglycan related to **heparin**, which is, like heparin, a cofactor for antithrombin III. Endothelium thus plays an essential role in preventing intravascular platelet activation and coagulation. However, it also plays an active part in haemostasis, synthesising and storing several key haemostatic components: von Willebrand factor*, tissue factor and plasminogen activator inhibitor 1 ('PAI-1') are particularly important. PAI-1 is secreted in response to *angiotensin IV*, receptors for which are present on endothelial cells, providing a link between the renin–angiotensin system and thrombosis (see Ch. 15). These *prothrombotic factors* are involved, respectively, in platelet adhesion and in coagulation and clot stabilisation. However, the endothelium is also implicated in *thrombus limitation*. Thus it generates *prostacyclin* (Ch. 12) and *nitric oxide* (Ch. 11), converts the platelet

---

*Von Willebrand factor is a glycoprotein of 10^6 daltons, which is missing in a hereditary haemorrhagic disorder called von Willebrand's disease. It is synthesised by vascular endothelial cells and is also present in platelets.

agonist ADP to *adenosine* which inhibits platelet function (Ch. 9), synthesises *tissue plasminogen activator* (see below) and expresses *thrombomodulin*, a receptor for thrombin. After combination with thrombomodulin, thrombin activates *protein C*, a vitamin K-dependent anticoagulant. Activated protein C, helped by its cofactor protein S, inactivates factors Va and VIIa. This is known to be physiologically important, because a naturally occurring mutation of the gene coding for factor V ('factor V Leiden') that confers resistance to activated protein C, results in the commonest recognised form of inherited thrombophilia.

Endotoxin and cytokines, including tumour necrosis factor, tilt the balance of prothrombotic and antithrombotic endothelial functions toward thrombosis by causing loss of heparan and expression of tissue factor. If other mechanisms limiting coagulation are also faulty or become exhausted, *disseminated intravascular coagulation* can result. This is a serious complication of sepsis and of certain malignancies, and the main treatment is to correct the underlying disease.

DRUGS THAT ACT ON THE COAGULATION CASCADE

Drugs are used to modify the cascade either when there is a *defect in coagulation* or when there is *unwanted coagulation*.

COAGULATION DEFECTS

Genetically determined deficiencies of clotting factors are rare. Examples are *classical haemophilia*, caused by lack of factor VIII, and an even rarer form of haemophilia (haemophilia B or Christmas disease) caused by lack of factor IX (also called Christmas factor). Missing factors can be supplied by giving fresh plasma or concentrated preparations of factor VIII or factor IX. In the past these have transmitted viral infections including HIV and hepatitis B (Ch. 44). Pure forms of several human factors are now available, synthesised by recombinant technology, but are difficult to manufacture because of the need for post-translational modification in mammalian cells and are expensive.*

---

*The first publicly announced cloned sheep with a human transgene—Polly—contains the gene for human factor IX; if, as confidently expected, she and her clones secrete this in their milk, production costs will be dramatically reduced!

Some *acquired* clotting defects are more common than hereditary ones. These include liver disease, vitamin K deficiency (universal in neonates) and excessive oral anticoagulant therapy, each of which may require treatment with vitamin K.

VITAMIN K

Vitamin K (for 'Koagulation' in German) is a fat-soluble vitamin occurring naturally in two forms—as vitamin K_1 (*phytomenadione*; Fig. 17.3) in plants, and as vitamin K_2 which is synthesised by bacteria in the gastrointestinal tract. Vitamin K_2 is not a single compound but a series of substances with side-chains of varying lengths.

Vitamin K is essential for the formation of clotting factors II, VII, IX and X. These are all glycoproteins with several γ-*carboxyglutamic acid* (Gla) residues clustered at the N-terminal end of the peptide chain. The γ-carboxylation occurs *after* the synthesis of the chain and the carboxylase requires vitamin K as a cofactor. The role of the vitamin is clarified by considering the interaction of factors Xa and prothrombin (factor II) with calcium and phospholipid as shown in Figure 17.4. Binding does not occur in the absence of γ-carboxylation.

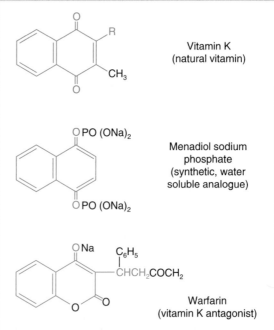

Fig. 17.3 Vitamin K, its congeners and warfarin. Warfarin, a vitamin K antagonist, is used as an oral anticoagulant drug.

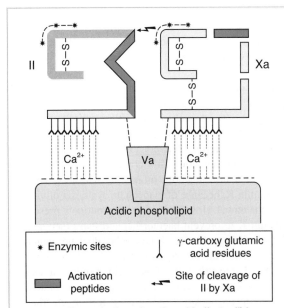

Fig. 17.4 The activation of prothrombin (factor II) by factor Xa. The peptide chains of both factors are very similar and are indicated schematically. The complex of factor Va with a negatively charged phospholipid surface (both partly supplied by aggregated platelets) forms a binding site for factor Xa and prothrombin. Platelets thus serve as a localising focus. Calcium ions are essential for the binding of the factors. When X is activated, with the removal of an activation peptide, it activates prothrombin (again with the removal of an activation peptide) liberating enzymic thrombin (shown in grey). Factor Xa is held at the surface by intrachain sulphydryl bonds, but thrombin is released. Factor V has to be converted from a non-functional to a functional binding protein (Va)—possibly by thrombin, which is thus autocatalytic. (Modified from: Jackson C M 1978 Br J Haematol 39: 1)

Reduced vitamin K is an essential cofactor in the carboxylation of glutamate residues (Fig. 17.5). Similar considerations apply to the proteolytic activation of factor X by IXa and by VIIa (see Fig. 17.2).

There are several other vitamin K-dependent Gla-proteins, including proteins C and S (see above) and osteocalcin in bone. The effect of the vitamin on osteoporosis is under investigation.

Administration and pharmacokinetic aspects

Natural vitamin K (phytomenadione) may be given orally or by intramuscular or intravenous injection. If given by mouth, it requires bile salts for absorption and this occurs by a saturable energy-requiring process in the

---

> **Clinical use of vitamin K**
>
> The treatment and/or prevention of:
>
> - bleeding due to oral anticoagulant drugs (e.g. warfarin)
> - haemorrhagic disease of the newborn
> - vitamin K deficiencies:
>   —sprue, coeliac disease, steatorrhoea
>   —lack of bile (e.g. with obstructive jaundice).

top part of the small intestine. A synthetic preparation, **menadiol** sodium phosphate (Fig. 17.3) is also available. It is water-soluble and thus does not require bile salts for its absorption. This synthetic compound takes longer to act than phytomenadione. There is very little storage of vitamin K in the body. It is metabolised to more polar substances that are excreted in the urine and the bile.

Clinical uses of vitamin K are summarised in the clinical box above.

THROMBOSIS

Thrombotic and thromboembolic disease is common and has severe consequences including myocardial infarction, stroke, deep vein thrombosis and pulmonary embolus. The main drugs used for platelet-rich 'white' thrombi are the antiplatelet drugs (notably **aspirin**) and fibrinolytic drugs, which are considered below. The main drugs used to prevent or treat red thrombus are:

- oral anticoagulants (**warfarin** and related compounds)
- injectable anticoagulants (**heparin** and newer thrombin inhibitors).

ORAL ANTICOAGULANTS

Oral anticoagulants became available as an indirect result of a change in agricultural policy in North America in the 1920s. Sweet clover was substituted for corn in cattle-feed, and an epidemic of deaths of cattle from haemorrhage ensued. This turned out to be due to *bis-hydroxycoumarin* in spoiled sweet clover. One of the first uses to which this observation was put was the development of such compounds as rat poison. Related compounds were developed for clinical use. **Warfarin** (Fig. 17.3) is the most important of these; other oral anticoagulants, e.g. **phenindione**, are now used only in rare patients who experience idiosyncratic adverse reactions to warfarin.

Mechanism

Oral anticoagulants act only in vivo and have no effect on clotting if added to blood in vitro. They interfere with the post-translational γ-carboxylation of glutamic acid residues in clotting factors II, VII, IX and X (see Fig. 17.5). They do this by *preventing the reduction of vitamin K*. The structural similarity of warfarin to vitamin K is illustrated in Figure 17.3. Their effect takes several days to develop because of the time taken for degradation of carboxylated factors. Their onset of action thus depends on the elimination half-lives of the relevant factors. Factor VII, with a half-life of 6 hours, is affected first, then IX, X and II with half-lives of 24, 40 and 60 hours respectively.

Administration and pharmacokinetic aspects

Warfarin is given orally and is absorbed quickly and totally from the gastrointestinal tract. It has a small distribution volume, being strongly bound to plasma albumin (see Ch. 4). The peak concentration in the blood occurs within an hour of ingestion, but because of the mechanism of action this does not coincide with the peak pharmacological effect, which occurs about 48 hours later. The effect of a single dose does not start for 12–16 hours, and lasts 4–5 days. Warfarin is metabolised by the hepatic mixed function oxidase P450 system and its half-life is very variable, being of the order of 40 hours in many individuals.

Oral anticoagulants cross the placenta and are not given in the first months of pregnancy because they are teratogenic (6–14 weeks is the critical period), nor in the later stages because they cause intracranial haemorrhage in the baby during delivery. They also appear in the milk during lactation. This could theoretically be important because newborn infants are naturally deficient in vitamin K, because of inadequate synthesis of vitamin K in the bowel. However, infants are routinely prescribed vitamin K to prevent haemorrhagic disease (see above), and warfarin treatment of the mother does not generally pose a risk to the breast-fed infant.

The therapeutic use of warfarin requires a careful balance between giving too little, leaving unwanted co-agulation unchecked, and giving too much thereby causing haemorrhage. Therapy is complicated not only because the effect of a particular dose is only seen 2 days after giving it, but also because of numerous conditions

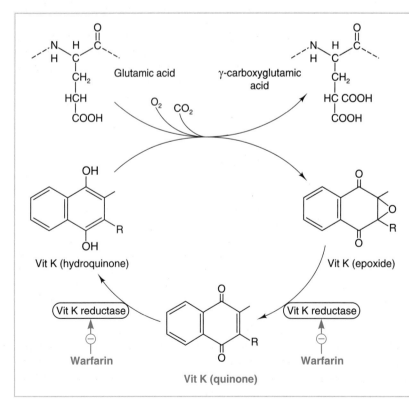

Fig. 17.5 The probable mechanism of action of vitamin K and the site of action of oral anticoagulants. After the peptide chains in clotting factors II, VII, IX and X have been synthesised, reduced vitamin K (the hydroquinone) acts as a cofactor in the conversion of glutamic acid (glu) to γ-carboxyglutamic acid (gla). During this reaction, the reduced form of vitamin K is converted to the epoxide, which in turn is reduced to the quinone and then the hydroquinone.

that modify sensitivity to warfarin, including interactions with other drugs. The effect is monitored by measuring the prothrombin time, which is expressed as an International Normalised Ratio (INR).* Dosage is usually adjusted to give an INR of 2–4, the precise target depending on the clinical situation. The duration of treatment also varies, but for several indications (e.g. to prevent thromboembolism in chronic atrial fibrillation) treatment is long-term.

Factors that potentiate oral anticoagulants

Various diseases and drugs potentiate warfarin, increasing the risk of haemorrhage:

Disease

Liver disease interferes with the synthesis of clotting factors; conditions in which there is a high metabolic rate, such as *fever* and *thyrotoxicosis*, increase the effect of anticoagulants by increasing degradation of clotting factors.

Drugs (see also Chs 5 and 48)

Many drugs potentiate warfarin, including:

- *Agents that inhibit hepatic drug metabolism.* Examples include **cimetidine**, **imipramine**, **co-trimoxazole**, **chloramphenicol**, **ciprofloxacin**, **metronidazole**, **amiodarone** and many antifungal **azoles**. Stereoselective effects (warfarin is a racemate, and its isomers are metabolised differently from one another) are described in Chapter 48.
- *Drugs that inhibit platelet function*, for example nonsteroidal anti-inflammatory drugs, **moxalactam**, **carbenicillin**. **Aspirin** increases the risk of bleeding if given during warfarin therapy, although this combination can be used safely with careful monitoring.
- *Drugs that displace warfarin from binding sites* on plasma albumin result in a transient increase in the concentration of free warfarin in plasma. Examples include some of the non-steroidal anti-inflammatory drugs, and **chloral hydrate**. This mechanism is

---

*The *prothrombin time* (PT) is the time taken for clotting of citrated plasma after the addition of calcium and standardised reference thromboplastin, and expressed as the ratio (PT ratio) of the PT of the patient to the PT of a pool of plasma from healthy subjects on no medication. The INR is a common scale designed to take account of differences between laboratories: the sensitivity of the local method is expressed as an index, the international sensitivity index (ISI) which is the slope of a logarithmic plot of PT obtained using the primary international reference preparation of thromboplastin against PT obtained with the local standard. INR is calculated as (PT ratio)[ISI].

seldom important, unless accompanied by an additional effect on warfarin metabolism (Ch. 48).

- *Drugs that inhibit reduction of vitamin K*, for example **cephalosporins**.
- *Drugs that decrease the availability of vitamin K.* Broad-spectrum antibiotics and some sulphonamides (see Ch. 43) depress the intestinal flora which normally synthesises vitamin K_2, but this has little effect unless there is a concurrent dietary deficiency.

Factors that lessen the effect of oral anticoagulants

Physiological state/disease

There is a decreased response to warfarin in conditions (e.g. *pregnancy*) where there is increased coagulation factor synthesis. Similarly, the effect of oral anticoagulants is lessened in *hypothyroidism*, which is associated with reduced degradation of coagulation factors.

Drugs (see also Chs 5 and 48)

Several drugs reduce the effectiveness of warfarin; this leads to increased doses being used to achieve the target INR. If the dose of warfarin is not reduced when the interacting drug is discontinued, this can result in over-anticoagulation and haemorrhage.

- *Vitamin K* is present in some parenteral feeds and vitamin preparations.
- *Drugs that induce hepatic P450 enzymes* increase the degradation of warfarin (e.g. **rifampicin**, **carbomazepine**, **barbiturates**, **griseofulvin**). Induction may wane only slowly after the inducing drug is discontinued, making it difficult to adjust the dose appropriately.
- *Drugs that reduce absorption*, for example **cholestyramine**.

Unwanted effects

Haemorrhage (especially into the bowel or the brain) is the main hazard. Depending on the urgency of the situation, treatment may consist of withholding warfarin (for minor problems), administration of vitamin K or fresh plasma or coagulation factor concentrates (for life-threatening bleeding). Oral anticoagulants are teratogenic. Hepatotoxicity is uncommon. Necrosis of soft tissues (for example breast or buttock) due to thrombosis in venules, occurs rarely shortly after starting treatment and is attributed to inhibition of biosynthesis of protein C, which has a shorter elimination half-life than do the vitamin K-dependent coagulation factors; this results in a procoagulant state soon after starting treatment. Treatment with heparin is usually started before warfarin, avoiding this problem.

Procoagulant drugs: vitamin K
- The reduced form of vitamin K is a cofactor in the post-translational γ-carboxylation of a cluster of glutamic acid (glu) residues in each of factors II, VII, IX and X; vitamin K is oxidised during the reaction. The γ-carboxylated glutamic acid (gla) residues are essential for the interaction of these factors with Ca^{2+} and negatively charged phospholipid.

Oral anticoagulants, e.g. warfarin
- These inhibit the reduction of vitamin K, thus inhibiting the γ-carboxylation of glu in II, VII, IX and X.
- They act only in vivo and the effect is delayed.
- Many factors modify their action; drug interactions are especially important.
- There is wide variation in response; their effect is monitored by measuring the INR and the dose individualised accordingly.

Injectable anticoagulants, e.g. heparin, low-molecular-weight heparins (LMWHs)
- These increase the rate of action of antithrombin III (AT III), a natural inhibitor which inactivates Xa and thrombin.
- They act both in vivo and in vitro.
- Anticoagulant activity is due to a unique pentasaccharide sequence with high affinity for AT III.
- The effect of heparin is monitored by the APTT and the dose individualised.
- LMWHs have the same effect on factor X as heparin but less effect on thrombin; they have equivalent anticoagulant effect to heparin but less action on platelet function.
- They are given subcutaneously or i.v. and the onset of action is rapid. A standard dose (per kg body weight) is given without the need for monitoring or individual dose adjustment. Patients can administer them at home.

INJECTABLE ANTICOAGULANTS

Heparin and low-molecular-weight heparins

Heparin was discovered in 1916 by a second-year medical student at Johns Hopkins Hospital. During a vacation project in which he was attempting to extract thromboplastic (i.e. coagulant) substances from various tissues, he found instead a powerful anticoagulant activity. This was named 'heparin' because it was first extracted from liver.

Heparin is not a single substance but a family of sulphated glycosaminoglycans (mucopolysaccharides) with a range of molecular weights up to 40 000. It is present (in the form of large polymers of MW 750 000) together with histamine in the granules of mast cells. It is extracted from beef lung or hog intestine and, since preparations differ in potency, assayed biologically against an agreed international standard: doses are specified in units of activity rather than of mass.

Heparin fragments, referred to as low-molecular-weight heparins (LMWHs), are used increasingly in place of unfractionated heparin. The molecular weights of different preparations vary from 4000 to 15 000.

Mechanism

Heparin inhibits coagulation both in vivo and in vitro, by activating antithrombin III (see above). Antithrombin III inhibits thrombin and other serine proteases by binding to the active serine site. Heparin modifies this interaction by binding, via a unique pentasaccharide sequence (Fig. 17.6), to antithrombin III, changing its conformation and accelerating its rate of action.

Thrombin is considerably more sensitive to the inhibitory effect of the heparin–antithrombin III complex than is factor X. To inhibit thrombin, it is necessary for heparin to bind to the enzyme as well as to antithrombin III; to inhibit factor X it is only necessary for heparin

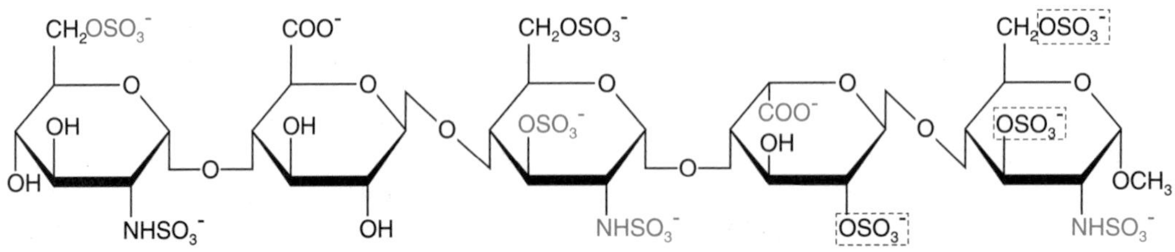

Fig. 17.6 **The pentasaccharide sequence in heparin which is the binding site for antithrombin III.** The groups in blue are critical for high-affinity binding; the groups in dotted boxes increase AT III binding but are not essential for it.

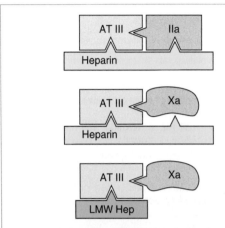

Fig. 17.7 Schematic diagram of the interaction of heparin, antithrombin III (AT III) and clotting factors. To increase the rate of inactivation of thrombin (IIa) by AT III, heparin needs to interact with both substances, but to speed up its effect on factor Xa it need only interact with AT III. The small, low-molecular-weight heparins (LMW Hep) can increase action of AT III on factor Xa, but cannot increase the action of AT III on thrombin because they cannot bind both simultaneously. (Modified from: Hirsh J & Levine M 1992 Blood 79: 1–17)

to bind to antithrombin III (see Fig. 17.7). Antithrombin III deficiency is a very rare cause of resistance to heparin therapy.

Low-molecular-weight heparins increase the action of antithrombin III on factor Xa but not its action on thrombin, since the molecules are too small to bind to both enzyme and inhibitor, essential for inhibition of thrombin but not of factor Xa (Fig. 17.7).

The anticoagulant action of heparin is modified by platelets, fibrin and plasma proteins. Not only do platelets release a heparin-neutralising protein, platelet factor 4, but factor Xa, when newly generated on the platelet surface (Fig. 17.4), is protected from the action of the heparin–antithrombin III complex. Thrombin when bound to fibrin is likewise protected from the action of the complex.

Administration and pharmacokinetic aspects

Heparin is not absorbed from the gut because of its charge and large size, and is therefore given intravenously or subcutaneously (intramuscular injections would cause haematomas). After intravenous injection of a bolus dose there is a phase of rapid elimination followed by a more gradual disappearance due both to saturable processes (involving binding to sites on endothelial cells and macrophages) and slower first-order processes

including renal excretion. As a result, once the dose exceeds the saturating concentration, a greater proportion is dealt with by these slower processes and the apparent half-life increases with increasing dose ('saturation kinetics'; see Ch. 5). Heparin acts immediately following intravenous administration, but the onset is delayed by up to 60 minutes when it is given subcutaneously. The elimination half-life is approximately 40–90 minutes. In urgent situations it is therefore usual to start treatment with a bolus intravenous dose, followed by a constant-rate infusion. The activated partial thromboplastin time (APTT), or some other in vitro clotting test, is measured and the dose of unfractionated heparin adjusted to achieve a value within a target range (e.g. 1.5–2.5 times control).

LMWHs are given subcutaneously. They have a longer elimination half-life than unfractionated heparin and this is independent of dose (first-order kinetics), so the effects are more predictable and dosing less frequent (once or twice a day). LMWHs do not prolong the APTT; their quality is consistent and, unlike unfractionated heparin, the effect of a standard dose (per kg body weight) is sufficiently predictable that monitoring is not required routinely. They are not neutralised by platelet factor 4 and are eliminated mainly by renal excretion. They are at least as safe and effective as unfractionated heparin, and are more convenient to use, since patients can be taught to inject themselves at home and there is generally no need for blood tests and dose adjustment.

Unwanted effects

The main hazard is haemorrhage which is treated by stopping therapy and, if necessary, giving **protamine** sulphate. This heparin antagonist is a strongly basic protein that forms an inactive complex with heparin and is given intravenously. The dose is estimated from the dose of heparin that has been administered recently, and it is important not to give too much as this can itself cause bleeding. If necessary, an in vitro neutralisation test is performed on a sample of blood from the patient to provide a more precise indication of the required dose.

Thrombosis is an uncommon but serious adverse effect of heparin and, as with warfarin necrosis (see above), may be misattributed to the natural history of the disease for which heparin is being administered. Paradoxically, it is associated with thrombocytopenia. A transitory early decrease in platelet numbers is not uncommon and is not clinically important. More serious thrombocytopenia occurring 2–14 days after the start of therapy is rarer, and is caused by IgM or IgG antibodies against complexes of heparin and platelet factor 4. Circulating immune complexes bind to Fc receptors (see Ch. 12) on circulating platelets, thereby activating them and releasing more platelet factor 4 and causing thrombocytopenia. Antibody also binds to platelet factor 4 complexed with glycosaminoglycans on the surface of endothelial cells, leading to immune injury of the vessel wall, thrombosis and disseminated intravascular coagulation. LMWHs are less liable than standard heparin to activate platelets to release platelet factor 4, and bind less avidly to platelet factor 4. Consequently, LMWHs are less likely than unfractionated heparin to cause thrombocytopenia and thrombosis. If antibodies to heparin–platelet factor 4 complexes have formed, however, it is to be expected that LMWHs could trigger these related immunologically mediated adverse effects.

Osteoporosis with spontaneous fractures has been reported with long-term (6 months or more) treatment with heparin (usually during pregnancy). Its explanation is unknown. *Hypoaldosteronism* (with consequent hyperkalaemia) has also been described, but is extremely rare.

Hypersensitivity reactions to heparin are rare, but are more common with protamine.

Newer thrombin-related agents

Dermatan sulphate is a glycosaminoglycan related to heparin. It potentiates heparin cofactor II, which inhibits thrombin selectively; so it is hoped that it may cause less bleeding than heparin. Its safety and efficacy has yet to be compared with LMWHs.

Antithrombin-III-independent anticoagulants

Several direct inhibitors of thrombin are under investigation, including **hirudin**, **hirugen**, **argatroban** and a tripeptide chloromethyl ketone inhibitor, **PPACK**.

Hirudin, the anticoagulant from the medicinal leech, has been synthesised by recombinant DNA techniques. Clinical trials, including GUSTO-2 and TIMI-9, have been somewhat disappointing. Hirugen is a synthetic dodecapeptide derived from hirudin. Argatroban, an arginine-based compound, is a weak competitive inhibitor of thrombin. PPACK alkylates the active site in thrombin, inhibiting it irreversibly. The latter three compounds can reach and inactivate thrombin that is bound to fibrin, but it is unknown whether this will prove clinically advantageous. These drugs may have a niche in the treatment of patients who have developed immune thrombocytopenia/thrombosis during treatment with heparin, from which they are immunologically quite distinct.

Various other approaches are being explored. These include several naturally occurring anticoagulants (tissue factor pathway inhibitor, thrombomodulin and protein C)

> **Clinical use of anticoagulants**
>
> Uses relate mainly to venous thrombosis, and include:
>
> - prevention of deep vein thrombosis (e.g. perioperatively)
> - preventing extension of established deep vein thrombosis or recurrence of pulmonary embolus
> - preventing thrombosis and embolisation in patients with atrial fibrillation (see Ch. 14)
> - preventing thrombosis on prosthetic heart valves
> - prevention of clotting in extracorporeal circulations (e.g. during haemodialysis or bypass surgery).
> - In addition, heparin is also used in unstable angina.
>
> Heparin (often as LMWH) is used acutely for short-term action and warfarin for prolonged therapy.

synthesised by recombinant technology. A particularly ingenious approach is the development of thrombin *agonists* that are selective for the anticoagulant properties of thrombin. One such modified thrombin, differing by a single amino acid substitution, is selective for the anticoagulant substrate protein C. It produces anticoagulation in monkeys without prolonging bleeding times, suggesting a reduced potential for bleeding complications in comparison with standard anticoagulation.

The clinical use of anticoagulants is summarised in the box above.

PLATELET ADHESION AND ACTIVATION

Platelets maintain the integrity of the circulation: a low platelet count results in *thrombocytopenic purpura*.* When activated, they undergo a complex sequence of reactions that is essential for haemostasis, important for the healing of damaged blood vessels and plays a part in inflammation (see Ch. 12). These reactions, several of which are redundant (in the sense that if one pathway of activation is blocked another is available) and several are autocatalytic, include:

- *adhesion* following vascular damage (via von Willebrand factor bridging between subendothelial macromolecules and glycoprotein Ib receptors on the platelet surface)**

---

*'Purpura' means a purple rash caused by spontaneous bleeding in the skin. Bleeding can occur into other organs including the gut and brain.

**Various platelet membrane glycoproteins are receptors or binding sites for adhesive proteins such as von Willebrand factor or fibrinogen.

- *shape change* (from smooth discs to spiny spheres with protruding pseudopodia)
- centralisation of dense granules and α-granules followed by *secretion* of the granule contents (including platelet agonists, such as ADP and 5-HT, and coagulation factors and growth factors such as platelet-derived growth factor) into a canalicular system that leads to the extracellular space
- *biosynthesis of labile mediators* such as platelet-activating factor and thromboxane (TX) A_2 (see Fig. 12.7)
- *aggregation* (i.e. platelets sticking to one another via fibrinogen bridging between glycoprotein IIb/IIIa receptors expressed on their surfaces during activation)
- *exposure of acidic phospholipid* on their outer surface promoting thrombin formation (and hence further platelet activation via thrombin receptors and fibrin formation via cleavage of fibrinogen; see above).

These processes are essential for haemostasis but may be inappropriately triggered if the vessel wall is diseased, most commonly with atherosclerosis, resulting in thrombosis (Figs 17.1 and 17.10).

ANTIPLATELET DRUGS

Since platelets play such a critical role in thromboembolic disease, antiplatelet drugs are potentially of immense therapeutic value. Advances in this area, particularly clinical trials of **aspirin**, have radically altered clinical practice. Sites of action of antiplatelet drugs are shown in Figure 17.8.

Aspirin (see Ch. 13) alters the balance between TXA_2 which promotes aggregation and prostacyclin (PGI_2) which inhibits it. Aspirin inactivates cyclo-oxygenase—acting mainly on the constitutive enzyme, COX-1—by irreversibly acetylating a serine residue in its active site. This reduces both TXA_2 synthesis in platelets and prostacyclin synthesis in endothelium. Vascular endothelial cells, however, can synthesise new enzyme whereas platelets cannot. After administration of aspirin, TXA_2 synthesis does not recover until the affected cohort of platelets is replaced in 7–10 days. Furthermore, higher doses of aspirin are needed to inhibit cyclo-oxygenase in vascular endothelium than in platelets, especially when administered by mouth. This is because platelets are exposed to aspirin in the portal blood, whereas systemic vasculature is partly protected by presystemic metabolism of aspirin to salicylate by

esterases in the liver. Thus low doses of aspirin given intermittently decrease the synthesis of thromboxane A_2 without drastically reducing prostacyclin synthesis. Clinical trials have demonstrated the efficacy of aspirin in several clinical settings (see p. 324). Treatment of acute myocardial infarction involves fibrinolytic drugs as well (see Fig. 17.9 and below).

The value of **dipyridamole**—a phosphodiesterase inhibitor—remains uncertain, but has been somewhat clarified by a European stroke prevention trial (ESPS-2) in patients with a history of ischaemic stroke or transient cerebral ischaemic attack. This showed that a modified release form of dipyridamole reduced the risk of stroke and death in such patients by around 15%—a similar effect to that of aspirin (25 mg twice daily).* The beneficial effects of aspirin and dipyridamole were additive. Headache was the commonest adverse effect of dipyridamole; unlike aspirin it caused no excess risk of bleeding.

The effectiveness of aspirin is limited by the fact that there are alternative pathways to platelet activation independent of TXA_2. Prostacyclin, in contrast, inhibits all pathways of platelet activation. It is available for clinical use (as **epoprostenol**) but, because of its very short half-life and the need for parenteral administration, its place in therapy is very limited. Stable analogues (e.g. **iloprost**) could extend these applications, but cause vasodilatation (and consequently flushing and headache) as well as inhibiting platelet function.

Ticlopidine, a thienopyridine derivative, inhibits ADP-dependent activation of the GPIIb/IIIa receptor (Fig. 17.9). Its action is slow in onset, taking 3–7 days to reach maximal effect, and it works through an active metabolite. Its efficacy in reducing stroke is similar to that of aspirin but unwanted effects, especially neutropenia, have limited its long-term use. Short-term (1 month) use has, however, recently increased substantially, in the context of a procedure in which an expansile device is positioned in a diseased coronary artery in an attempt to maintain its patency following balloon angioplasty ('stenting'). This stems from a clinical trial in which treatment for 1 month with a combination of ticlopidine plus aspirin was compared with conventional treatment with aspirin, heparin and oral anticoagulant. Ticlopidine with aspirin substantially reduced cardiac events and haemorrhagic and vascular complications compared with the conventional treatment. **Clopidogrel**

---

*This dose of aspirin is unconventional, being somewhat lower than the 75 mg per day that is the lowest dose commonly used in thromboprophylaxis.

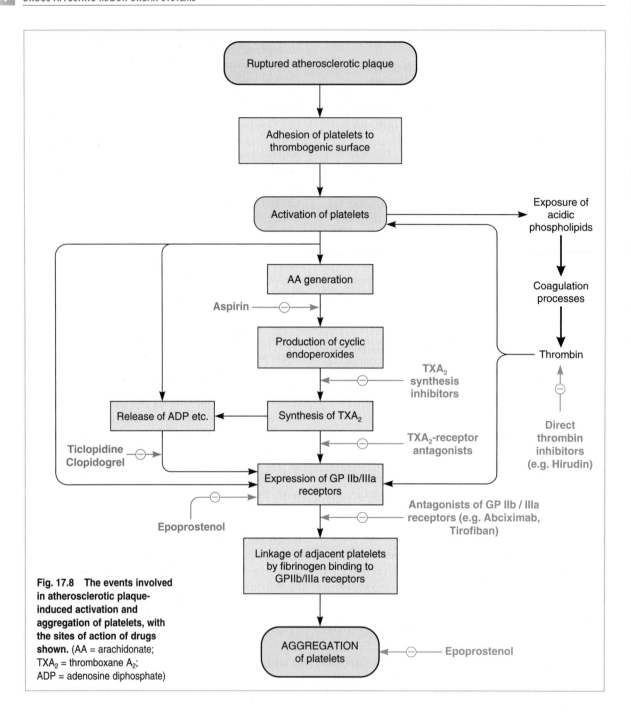

Fig. 17.8 The events involved in atherosclerotic plaque-induced activation and aggregation of platelets, with the sites of action of drugs shown. (AA = arachidonate; TXA_2 = thromboxane A_2; ADP = adenosine diphosphate)

is structurally related to ticlopidine, and has a similar but more potent action. Like ticlopidine it can cause rash or diarrhoea, but neutropenia is no more common than with aspirin. Clopidogrel was marginally more effective than aspirin (in the unconventionally large dose of 325 mg/

day) in reducing a composite outcome of ischaemic stroke, myocardial infarction or vascular death in a large recent trial. Its safety profile was similar to that of aspirin.

Antagonists of the GPIIb/IIIa receptor have the attrac-

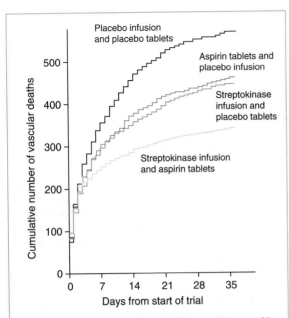

Fig. 17.9 Cumulative vascular mortality in patients with myocardial infarction treated either with placebo, aspirin alone, streptokinase alone or a combined aspirin–streptokinase regime. The figures indicate the number of deaths in the number of patients given a particular treatment, with, in brackets, the % mortality after 35 days. (ISIS-2 trial 1988 Lancet ii: 350–360)

tion that they inhibit all pathways of platelet activation. A hybrid murine/human monoclonal antibody Fab fragment directed against the GPIIb/IIIa receptor, which rejoices in the catchy little name of '**abciximab**', is licensed for use in high-risk patients undergoing coronary angioplasty as an adjunct to heparin and aspirin. It reduces the risk of restenosis at the expense of an increased risk of bleeding. Immunogenicity limits its use to a single administration. Cyclic peptides based on the Arg–Gly–Asp ('RGD') sequence that is common to ligands for IIa/IIIa receptors (e.g. **tirofiban**, **lamifiban**) are in development.

Because thrombin is a powerful stimulant of platelet activation and aggregation, drugs that inhibit its action could be regarded as antiplatelet agents and are therefore included in Figure 17.8.

Antiplatelet drugs in development. *TXA₂-receptor antagonists* (e.g. **GR32191**) have been investigated. These are unlikely to be more effective than low-dose aspirin, but could have less adverse effects. They are much more expensive than aspirin. *TXA₂-synthesis inhibitors* (e.g. **dazoxiben**, an analogue of imidazole)

increase prostacyclin synthesis, as a consequence of diversion of endoperoxide intermediates from TXA_2 synthesis to prostacyclin synthesis, as well as reducing TXA_2 production. However, they only weakly inhibit platelet function in vitro, probably because prostaglandin endoperoxides (e.g. PGH_2) are agonists at thromboxane receptors. Compounds which have both TXA_2 synthetase inhibition as well as TXA_2-receptor blocking activity offer a better possibility of selectively inhibiting thromboxane synthesis while increasing prostacyclin synthesis, and drugs with this combination of activities (e.g. **ridogrel**) are in development.

The clinical use of antiplatelet drugs is summarised on page 324.

Platelets and antiplatelet drugs

Platelets
- Healthy vascular endothelium prevents platelet adhesion.
- Platelets adhere to diseased or damaged areas and become activated, i.e. they change shape, exposing negatively charged phospholipids and GPIIb/IIIa receptors, and synthesise and release various mediators, e.g. TXA_2, ADP, which stimulate other platelets to aggregate.
- Aggregation entails links formed by fibrinogen binding to the GPIIb/IIIa receptors on adjacent platelets.
- The activated platelets constitute the localising focus for fibrin formation.
- Chemotactic factors and growth factors necessary for repair, but also implicated in atherogenesis, are released.

Antiplatelet drugs, e.g. aspirin
- Aspirin inhibits cyclo-oxygenase irreversibly. The balance between prostacyclin (an inhibitor of aggregation generated by vascular endothelium) and TXA_2 (a stimulant of aggregation generated by platelets) is thus altered, since the endothelium can synthesise more enzyme but platelets cannot. TXA_2 synthesis only recovers when new platelets are formed.
- Other clinically available antiplatelet drugs include: epoprostenol (synthetic prostacyclin), ticlopidine and clopidogrel (which inhibit expression of GPIIb/IIIa receptors in response to ADP) and a monoclonal antibody against the GPIIb/IIIa receptor (abciximab). Drugs being tested include agents that either inhibit TXA_2 synthesis or block TXA_2 receptors or have both actions.

FIBRINOLYSIS (THROMBOLYSIS)

When the intrinsic coagulation system is activated, the fibrinolytic system is also set in motion via several endo-

---

Clinical use of antiplatelet drugs

The main drug is aspirin. Uses mainly relate to arterial thrombosis, and include:

- acute myocardial infarction
- high risk of myocardial infarction, including:
  — patients who have recovered from myocardial infarction
  — patients with symptoms from atherosclerosis, including angina, transient cerebral ischaemic attacks, intermittent claudication
- following coronary artery bypass grafting
- following coronary artery angioplasty and stenting; (either ticlopidine or abciximab are used in some patients in addition to aspirin)
- acute thrombotic stroke
- atrial fibrillation in patients who have a contraindication to oral anticoagulation.

Other antiplatelet drugs (e.g. epoprostenol, dipyridamole) have limited clinical applications.

---

genous *plasminogen activators*, including tissue-type plasminogen activator (tPA), urokinase-type plasminogen activator (uPA), kallikrein and neutrophil elastase. In addition, there are several exogenous activators of fibrinolysis, including **streptokinase**. tPA is believed to be inhibited by a structurally related lipoprotein, lipoprotein(a), increased concentrations of which constitute a strong independent risk factor for myocardial infarction (Ch. 16).

Some tPA is derived from endothelium and phagocytic cells, and some by the action of factor XIIa on pro-activators in plasma or tissues (Fig. 17.10). *Plasminogen*, a serum β-globulin of MW 143 000, is deposited on the fibrin strands within a thrombus. Plasminogen activators are serine proteases and are unstable in circulating blood. They diffuse into thrombus and cleave plasminogen to release plasmin (see Fig. 17.10). Plasmin is trypsin-like, acting on Arg–Lys bonds, and thus digests not only fibrin but fibrinogen, factors II, V, and VIII and many other proteins. It is formed locally and acts on the fibrin meshwork, generating fibrin degradation products and lysing the clot. Its action is localised to the clot because plasminogen activators are effective mainly on plasminogen adsorbed to fibrin; any plasmin that escapes into the circulation is inactivated by plasmin inhibitors, including PAI-1 (see above), which protect us from digesting ourselves from within.

Drugs affect this system by increasing or inhibiting fibrinolysis (*fibrinolytic* and *antifibrinolytic drugs* respectively).

FIBRINOLYTIC DRUGS

Figure 17.10 summarises the interaction of the fibrinolytic system with the coagulation cascade and platelet activation, and the action of drugs that modify this. Several fibrinolytic (thrombolytic) drugs are used clinically, principally to reopen the occluded coronary artery in patients with acute myocardial infarction.

Streptokinase is a non-enzymic protein with a molecular weight of 47 000 daltons. It is extracted from cultures of β-haemolytic streptococci and is biologically assayed and standardised. It binds plasminogen, exposing active-site serine and causing plasmin activity. Infused intravenously, it reduces mortality in acute myocardial infarction and this beneficial effect is additive with aspirin (Fig. 17.9). Its action is blocked by antistreptococcal antibodies, which appear about 4 days or more after the initial dose. At least 1 year must elapse before it is used again.

Anistreplase (APSAC) is a complex of human lysplasminogen and streptokinase which has been rendered inactive by introducing a para (p) anisoyl group at its catalytic centre. The anisoyl group is removed in vivo, so anistreplase is a pro-drug of streptokinase. The half-life of activation is about 2 hours, both in blood and in thrombus. Anistreplase is given intravenously over 4–5 minutes, and fibrinolytic activity is sustained for 4–6 hours.

Alteplase and **duteplase** are recombinant tPA, the first being single-chain, the second double-chain. Their activity is enhanced in the presence of fibrin, i.e. they are more active on fibrin-bound plasminogen than on plasma plasminogen and are thus said to be 'clot selective'. tPA is not antigenic and can be used in patients likely to have antibodies to streptokinase. Because of their short half-lives, they must be give as intravenous infusions. **Reteplase** is similar, but has a longer elimination half-life than tPA, allowing for bolus administration and making for simplicity of administration. It is available for clinical use in myocardial infarction.

Urokinase (u-PA) is prepared from cultures of human embryonic kidney cells and is biologically assayed and standardised. It acts directly as a plasminogen activator, but its effectiveness in myocardial infarction has not been established, and its clinical use is limited.

Unwanted effects and contraindications

The main hazard of all fibrinolytic agents is bleeding, including gastrointestinal haemorrhage and stroke. If serious, bleeding may be treated with **tranexamic acid** (see below), fresh plasma or coagulation factors. Streptokinase and anistreplase can cause allergic reactions

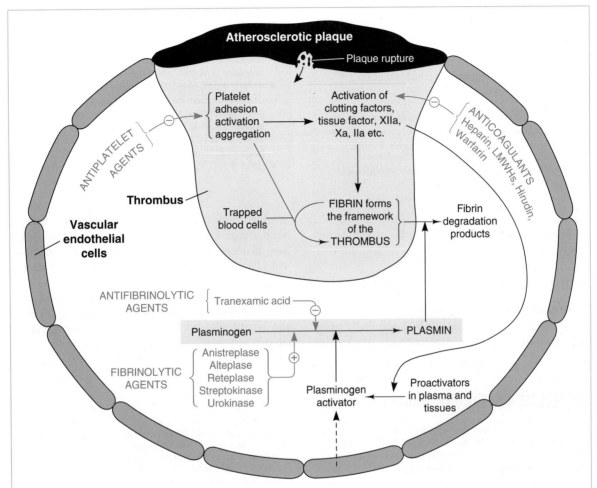

Fig. 17.10 Schematic diagram of thrombus formation showing the interaction of the fibrinolytic (thrombolytic) system with the coagulation cascade and the platelet-activation system, and the action of drugs which modify these systems. LMHs = low-molecular-weight heparins. For more detail of platelet activation and the coagulation cascade refer to Figures 17.1 and 17.2.

and the former produces low-grade fever in about 25% of patients. Streptokinase causes a burst of plasmin formation, generating kinins (see Ch. 12) and causing hypotension.

Contraindications to the use of these agents are active internal bleeding, haemorrhagic cerebrovascular disease, bleeding diatheses, pregnancy, uncontrolled hypertension, invasive procedures in which haemostasis is important and recent trauma—including vigorous cardiopulmonary resuscitation.

Which fibrinolytic agent is best?

Several large placebo-controlled studies in patients with myocardial infarction have shown convincingly

that fibrinolytic drugs reduce mortality if given within 12 hours from the onset of symptoms. Much has been written as to which drug is best. This has considerable commercial implications (doubtless the motivation behind much of the verbiage), but a recent authoritative review (Collins et al. 1997) concluded that: 'the choice of fibrinolytic drug makes little difference to the overall probability of stroke-free survival, because the regimens that dissolve coronary thrombi more rapidly produce greater risks of cerebral haemorrhage. ... It is ... important that any uncertainties about which fibrinolytic regimen or dose of aspirin to use do not engender uncertainty about whether to use fibrinolytic and antiplatelet therapies routinely.'

Clinical use of fibrinolytic drugs

The main drugs are streptokinase and tissue plasminogen activators (tPA). The main use is:

- acute myocardial infarction, within 12 hours of onset

Other uses include:

- acute thrombotic stroke within 3 hours of onset (tPA), in selected patients
- deep vein thrombosis, pulmonary embolus, clearing thrombosed shunts and cannulae, acute arterial thromboembolism and (urokinase) local thrombolysis in the anterior chamber of the eye.

Fibrinolysis and drugs modifying fibrinolysis

- A fibrinolytic cascade is initiated concomitantly with the coagulation cascade, resulting in the formation within the coagulum of plasmin, which digests fibrin.
- Various agents promote the formation of plasmin from its precursor plasminogen, e.g. streptokinase and its pro-drug anistreplase (APSAC), and tissue plasminogen activators such as alteplase, duteplase and reteplase. Most have to be infused; anistreplase and reteplase can be given as bolus injections.
- Some drugs (e.g. tranexamic acid) inhibit fibrinolysis.

The clinical use of fibrinolytic agents is summarised above.

ANTIFIBRINOLYTIC AND HAEMOSTATIC DRUGS

Tranexamic acid inhibits plasminogen activation and thus prevents fibrinolysis. It can be given orally or by intravenous injection. It is used to treat various conditions in which there is bleeding or risk of bleeding, such as haemorrhage following prostatectomy or dental extraction, in menorrhagia (excessive menstrual blood loss) and following thrombolytic overdose. It is also used in patients with the rare disorder of hereditary angioedema.

Aprotinin inhibits proteolytic enzymes, and is used for hyperplasminaemia caused by fibrinolytic drug overdose and in patients at risk of major blood loss during cardiac surgery.

REFERENCES AND FURTHER READING

Antiplatelet Trialists' Collaboration 1994 Collaborative overview of randomised trials of antiplatelet therapy I, II, III. Br Med J 308: 81–105, 159–168, 235–246 (*Overview of large number of randomised trials, leaves no room for doubt—well hardly any: 2p < 0.00001 in many comparisons*)

Aster R H 1995 Heparin-induced thrombocytopenia and thrombosis. N Engl J Med 332: 1374–1376 (*Succinct and lucid editorial; see also accompanying paper, pp 1330–1335*)

Biggs R, Rizza C R 1984 Human blood coagulation, haemostasis and thrombosis, 3rd edn. Blackwell Scientific Publications, Oxford (*Authoritative source reference; especially useful for methodology*)

CAPRIE Steering Committee 1996 A randomised, blinded trial of clopidogrel versus aspirin in patients at risk of ischaemic events (CAPRIE). Lancet 348: 1329–1339 (*19 185 patients randomised. Clopidogrel was marginally more effective than aspirin with an overall safety profile at least as good as that of aspirin*)

Clouse L H, Comp P C 1987 The regulation of hemostasis: the protein C system. N Engl J Med 314: 1298–1304

Collins R, Peto R, Baigent C, Sleight P 1997 Aspirin, heparin and thrombolytic therapy in suspected acute myocardial infarction. N Engl J Med 336: 847–860 (*Unbiased and authoritative overview. Includes a section on 'general problems of unduly selective emphasis'—fighting stuff!*)

Diener H, Cunha L, Forbes C, Sivenius J, Smets P, Lowenthal A 1996 European stroke prevention study 2. Dipyridamole and acetylsalicylic acid in the secondary prevention of stroke. J Neurol Sci 143: 1–14 (*Slow-release dipyridamole 200 mg twice daily was as effective as aspirin 25 mg twice daily, and the effects of aspirin and dipyridamole were additive*)

EPIC Investigators 1994 Use of a monoclonal antibody directed against the platelet glycoprotein IIb/IIIa receptor in high-risk coronary angioplasty. N Engl J Med 330: 956–961 (*Ischaemic complications were reduced by 35% at the cost of increased bleeding*)

Fears R 1990 Biochemical pharmacology and therapeutic aspects of thrombolytic agents. Pharmacol Rev 42: 201–224

Furie B, Furie B C 1992 Molecular and cellular biology of blood coagulation. N Engl J Med 326: 800–806

Gibbs C S 1995 Conversion of thrombin into an anticoagulant by protein engineering. Nature 387: 413–416 (*A single amino acid substitution shifts thrombin's specificity in favour of the anticoagulant protein C. See also accompanying editorial 'The thrombin paradox' by J H Griffin, pp 337–338*)

Gresele P, Deckmyn H 1991 Thromboxane synthase inhibitors, thromboxane receptor antagonists and dual blockers in thrombotic disorders. Trends Pharmacol Sci 12: 158–163 (*Rationale for the approach of simultaneous blockade of thromboxane receptors and inhibition of thromboxane synthesis*)

Hirsh J 1991 Heparin. N Engl J Med 324: 1565–1574

Hirsh J 1991 Oral anticoagulant drugs. N Engl J Med 324: 1865–1873 (*See also subsequent editorial by the same author on the optimal duration of anticoagulant therapy for venous thrombosis in N Engl J Med 1995; 332: 1710–1711*)

International Joint Efficacy Comparison of Thrombolytics 1995 Randomised, double-blind comparison of reteplase double-bolus administration with streptokinase in acute myocardial infarction (INJECT): trial to investigate equivalence. Lancet

346: 329–335 (*Reteplase is a safe, effective and convenient to administer alternative to streptokinase*)

Levine M 1995 A comparison of low-molecular-weight heparin administered primarily at home with unfractionated heparin administered in the hospital for proximal deep vein thrombosis. N Engl J Med 334: 677–681 (*Concludes that LMWH can be used safely and effectively at home. This has potentially very important implications for patient care*)

Longenecker G L (ed) 1985 The platelets: physiology and pharmacology. Academic Press, London

Mannuccio M 1998 Hemostatic drugs. N Engl J Med 333: 245–253

Nichols A J, Ruffolo R R et al. 1992 Development of GPIIb/IIIa antagonists as antithrombotic drugs. Trends Pharmacol Sci 13: 413–417

Patrono C 1994 Aspirin as an antiplatelet drug. N Engl J Med 330: 1287–1294

Salzman E W 1992 Low-molecular-weight heparin and other new antithrombotic drugs. N Engl J Med 326: 1017–1019 (*Review*)

Schömig A 1996 A randomized comparison of antiplatelet and anticoagulant therapy after the placement of coronary-artery stents. N Engl J Med 334: 1084–1089 (*Combined therapy with aspirin and ticlopidine was safer and more effective than conventional treatment with aspirin plus anticoagulant*)

Suttie J W 1980 Vitamin K-dependent carboxylation. Trends Biochem Sci 5: 302–304

Special Writing Group of the Stroke Council of the American Health Association 1996 Guidelines for thrombolytic therapy for acute stroke: a supplement to the guidelines for the management of patients with acute ischemic stroke. Stroke 27: 1711–1718 (*Recommends using tPA in selected patients within the first 3 hours of ischaemic stroke. Highly contentious—see for example editorial comment by Dorman & Sandercock in Lancet 1996; 348: 1600–1601*)

Turpie A G G 1993 A comparison of aspirin with placebo in patients treated with warfarin after heart-valve replacement. N Engl J Med 329: 524–529 (*Considerable benefit of combined treatment with aspirin and warfarin. Meticulous monitoring mandatory!*)

Vane J 1994 Towards a better aspirin. Nature 367: 215–216

Vermeer C, Hamulyak K 1991 Pathophysiology of vitamin K-deficiency and oral anticoagulants. Thromb Haemost 66: 153–159

Ware J A, Heisted D D 1993 Platelet–endothelium interactions. N Engl J Med 328: 628–635

Weitz J I, Hirsh J 1992 Antithrombins: their potential as antithrombotic agents. Annu Rev Med 43: 9–16

18

The haemopoietic system

The main components of the haemopoietic system are the bone marrow and the blood, with the spleen and the liver as important accessory organs. The spleen acts as a graveyard for time-expired red blood cells. The liver stores **vitamin B$_{12}$**—which is essential for erythrocyte generation—and is involved in the process of breakdown of the haemoglobin liberated when the red blood cells are destroyed. The kidney manufactures **erythropoietin**—a growth factor which stimulates red cell production. Cells from various other organs, synthesise and release haemopoietic growth factors—termed **colony-stimulating factors**—which regulate the production of leukocytes and platelets. The function of platelets is discussed in Chapter 17 and that of leukocytes in Chapter 12.

The term 'erythron' is used to describe the circulating red blood cells and their precursors. In a healthy adult the erythron is in a steady state, cell loss being precisely balanced by new production of cells.

The main function of the red cells is to carry oxygen, and their oxygen-carrying power depends on their haemoglobin content. About 3.3 mg of iron is contained in 1 g of haemoglobin, and the production of haemoglobin depends on the supply of iron.

Types of anaemia

Anaemia is defined as a reduced concentration of haemoglobin in the blood. It may give rise to symptoms of fatigue but, especially if it is chronic, is often surprisingly asymptomatic. The commonest cause is blood loss related to menstruation and child bearing, but there are several different types of anaemia, and several different diagnostic levels. Microscopical examination of a stained blood smear of blood allows characterisation into:

- hypochromic, microcytic anaemia (small red cells with low haemoglobin, due to iron deficiency)
- macrocytic anaemia (large red cells, few in number)
- normochromic normocytic anaemia (fewer normal-sized red cells with normal haemoglobin)
- mixed pictures.

Further evaluation may include examination of smears of bone marrow, determination of folic acid in the red cells and serum analysis. These lead to more precise diagnostic groupings of anaemias into:

- Deficiency of nutrients necessary for haemopoiesis, most importantly:
  —iron
  —folic acid and vitamin B$_{12}$
  —pyridoxine, vitamin C.
- Depression of the bone marrow, due to:
  —toxins (e.g. the drugs used in chemotherapy)
  —radiation therapy
  —diseases of the bone marrow of unknown origin (e.g. aplastic anaemia, leukaemias)
  —reduced production of, or responsiveness to erythropoietin (e.g. chronic renal failure, rheumatoid arthritis, AIDS).
- Excessive destruction of red blood cells, i.e. haemolytic anaemia. This can have many causes including adverse reactions to drugs and inappropriate immune reactions.

The commonest anaemias are due to deficiencies of nutrients and this chapter deals mainly with the widely prescribed haematinics: iron, folic acid and vitamin B$_{12}$. The use of agents which stimulate the proliferation and maturation of the red and white blood cells and platelets will also be covered.

It is important to note that the use of haematinics is

often only an adjunct to treatment of the underlying cause of the anaemia—for example removal of the colon for colon cancer (a common cause of iron deficiency) or anthelminthic drugs for patients with hookworm (a frequent cause of anaemia in parts of Africa and Asia; Ch. 47). Sometimes treatment consists of stopping the offending drug, e.g. a non-steroidal anti-inflammatory drug that causes blood loss from the stomach (Ch. 13, p. 233).

IRON

Iron is a transition metal with two important properties relevant to its biological role:

- the ability to exist in several oxidation states
- the tendency to form stable coordination complexes.

The body of a 70-kg man contains about 4 g of iron, 65% of which circulates in the blood as the oxygen-transporting molecule, haemoglobin. About one-half of the remainder is stored in the liver, spleen and bone marrow, chiefly as *ferritin* and *haemosiderin*. The iron in these molecules is available for fresh haemoglobin synthesis. The rest, which is not available for haemoglobin synthesis, is present in myoglobin, cytochromes and various enzymes.

The distribution of iron in an average normal adult male is shown in Table 18.1. The values for an average female would be about 55% of these. Since most of the iron in the body is either part of—or destined to be

Table 18.1 The distribution of iron in the body of a normal 70-kg male

Protein	Tissue	Iron content (mg)
Haemoglobin	Erythrocytes	2600
Myoglobin	Muscle	400
Enzymes (cytochromes, catalase, etc.)	Liver and other tissues	25
Transferrin	Plasma and extracellular fluid	8
Ferritin and haemosiderin	Liver	410
	Spleen	48
	Bone marrow	300

Data from: Jacobs A, Worwood M 1982 In: Hardisty R M, Weatherall D J (eds) Blood and its disorders. Blackwell Scientific Publications, Oxford, ch 5

part of—the haemoglobin in red cells, the most obvious clinical result of iron deficiency is anaemia, and the only indication for therapy with iron is to provide material for haemoglobin synthesis.

Haemoglobin is made up of four protein chain subunits (globins), each of which contains one *haem* moiety. Haem consists of a tetrapyrrole porphyrin ring containing ferrous (Fe^{2+}) iron. Each haem group can carry one O_2 molecule, which is bound reversibly to the Fe^{2+} and to a histidine residue in the particular globin chain to which the haem is linked. This reversible binding is the basis of O_2 transport.

Iron turnover and balance

Both the normal physiological turnover of iron and *pharmacokinetic factors* affecting iron when it is given therapeutically will be dealt with here.

The normal daily requirement for iron is approximately 5 mg for men, and 15 mg for growing children and for women during the reproductive period. A pregnant woman needs between two and ten times this amount because of the demands of the foetus and the increased requirements of the mother.*

The average diet in Western Europe provides 15–20 mg of iron daily, mostly in meat. Iron in meat is generally present as haem and about 20–40% of haem iron is available for absorption. The human body appears to be specifically adapted to absorb iron in the form of haem. It is thought that one reason why modern man has problems in maintaining iron balance (there are an estimated 500 million people with iron deficiency in the world) is that the change from hunting to grain cultivation 10 000 years ago led to cereals, which have a relatively small amount of utilisable iron, constituting a significant proportion of the diet.

Non-haem iron in food is mainly in the ferric state and this needs to be converted to ferrous iron for absorption. Ferric iron, and to a lesser extent ferrous iron, has low solubility at the neutral pH of the intestine; but in the stomach, iron dissolves and binds to mucoprotein which functions as a carrier, transporting the iron to the intestine. In the presence of ascorbic acid, fructose and various amino acids, iron is detached from the carrier, forming soluble low-molecular-weight complexes which enable it to remain in soluble form in the intestine. Ascorbic acid stimulates iron absorption partly by

*Each pregnancy 'costs' the mother 680 mg of iron, equivalent to 1300 ml of blood, owing to the demands of the foetus, plus an extra 450 mg to meet the requirements of the expanded blood volume.

forming soluble iron–ascorbate chelates and partly by reducing ferric iron to the more soluble ferrous form.

Tetracycline forms an insoluble iron chelate resulting in impaired uptake of both substances.

The amount of iron in the diet and the various factors affecting its availability are thus important determinants in absorption, but the *regulation* of iron absorption is a function of the intestinal mucosa, influenced by the body's iron stores. Because there is no mechanism whereby iron excretion is regulated, the absorptive mechanism holds a central role in iron balance since it is the sole mechanism by which body iron can be controlled.

The site of iron absorption is the duodenum and upper jejunum, and absorption is a two-stage process involving firstly a rapid uptake across the brush border and then transfer from the interior of the cell into the plasma. The second stage, which is rate-limiting, is energy dependent. Haem iron, as explained above, is absorbed as intact haem and the iron is released in the mucosal cell by the action of haem oxidase. Non-haem iron is absorbed in the ferrous state. Within the cell, ferrous iron is oxidised to ferric iron which is bound to an intracellular carrier, a transferrin-like protein; the iron is then either held in storage in the mucosal cell as *ferritin* (if body stores of iron are high) or passed on to the plasma (if iron stores are low).

Iron is carried in the plasma bound to *transferrin*—a β-globulin with two binding sites for ferric iron—which is normally only 30% saturated. Plasma contains 4 mg of iron at any one time, but the daily turnover is about 30 mg (Fig. 18.1). Most of the iron which enters the plasma is derived from the mononuclear phagocyte system, following the degradation of time-expired erythrocytes. Intestinal absorption and mobilisation of iron from storage depots contribute only small amounts. Most of the iron which leaves the plasma daily is used for haemoglobin synthesis by red cell precursors. These cells have receptors which bind transferrin molecules, releasing them after the iron has been taken up.

Iron is stored in two forms—soluble ferritin and insoluble haemosiderin. *Ferritin* is found in all cells, the mononuclear phagocytes of liver, spleen and bone marrow containing especially high concentrations. It is also present in plasma. The precursor of ferritin, *apoferritin*, is a large protein of molecular weight 450 000, composed of 24 identical polypeptide subunits which enclose a cavity in which up to 4500 iron molecules can be stored. Apoferritin takes up ferrous iron, oxidises it and deposits the ferric iron in its core. In this form it constitutes ferritin, the primary storage form of iron, from which the iron is most readily available. The life span of this iron-laden protein is only a few days. *Haemosiderin*

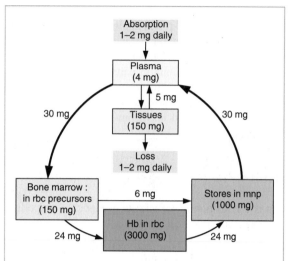

Fig. 18.1 Schematic illustration of the distribution of iron in the body, with an indication of the daily intake, movement between compartments, and loss. The intensity of colour indicates concentration of iron and the thickness of the arrows, the amount transferred between compartments. (Hb = haemoglobin; rbc = red blood cells; mnp = mononuclear phagocytes)

is a degraded form of ferritin in which the iron cores of several ferritin molecules have aggregated, following partial disintegration of the outer protein shells.

The ferritin in plasma has virtually no iron associated with it. It is in equilibrium with the storage ferritin in cells and its concentration in the plasma provides an estimate of total body iron stores.

The body has no means of actively excreting iron. Small amounts leave the body through the peeling off of mucosal cells containing ferritin, and even smaller amounts leave in the bile, the sweat and the urine. A total of about 1 mg is lost daily. The iron balance is therefore critically dependent on the active absorption mechanism in the intestinal mucosa. This absorption is influenced by the iron stores in the body, but the precise mechanism of this control is still a matter of debate. It is suggested that the amount of ferritin in the intestinal mucosa may be important in regulating absorption, as may the balance between ferritin and the transferrin-like carrier molecule in these cells. The daily movement of iron in the body is illustrated in Figure 18.1.

The clinical use of iron is given on page 331.

Administration

Iron is usually given orally but may be given parenterally in special circumstances.

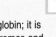

Clinical use of iron

Iron deficiency anaemia, which can be due to:

- chronic blood loss (e.g. with menorrhagia)
- increased demand (e.g. in pregnancy and early infancy)
- inadequate dietary intake or absorption (uncommon in developed countries).

Iron

- Iron is important for the synthesis of haemoglobin; it is also present in myoglobin, and in the cytochromes and other enzymes.
- Ferric iron (Fe^{3+}) must be converted to ferrous iron (Fe^{2+}) for absorption in the GIT.
- Absorption involves active transport into mucosal cells, whence it can be transported into the plasma and/or stored intracellularly as ferritin; in iron deficiency, the former route predominates.
- Iron loss occurs mainly by sloughing of ferritin-containing mucosal cells; iron is not excreted in the urine.
- Iron in plasma is bound to transferrin, and most is used for erythropoiesis. Some is stored as ferritin in other tissues. Iron from time-expired erythrocytes enters the plasma for re-use.
- Preparation: ferrous sulphate.
- Unwanted effects: GI tract disturbances. Severe toxic effects occur if large doses are ingested; these can be countered by desferrioxamine, an iron chelator.

Several different preparations of ferrous iron salts are available for oral administration. The main one is **ferrous sulphate**, which has an elemental iron content of 200 µg per mg. Others are ferrous succinate, ferrous gluconate, and ferrous fumarate, with elemental iron concentrations of 350 µg, 120 µg and 330 µg per mg respectively. These are all absorbed to a comparable extent.

Parenteral iron is rarely given but may be necessary in individuals who are not able to absorb oral iron because of malabsorption syndromes or as a result of surgical procedures or inflammatory conditions involving the gastrointestinal tract. The preparations used are **iron dextran** or **iron-sorbitol**, both given by deep intramuscular injection. Iron-dextran (but not iron-sorbitol) can be given by slow intravenous infusion, but this method of administration should only be used if absolutely necessary because of the risk of anaphylactoid reactions.

Unwanted effects

The unwanted effects of oral iron administration are dose-related and include nausea, abdominal cramps and diarrhoea.

Acute iron toxicity, usually seen in young children who have swallowed attractively coloured iron tablets in mistake for sweets, occurs after ingestion of large quantities of iron salts. This can result in severe necrotising gastritis with vomiting, haemorrhage and diarrhoea, followed by circulatory collapse.

Chronic iron toxicity or iron overload is virtually always due to causes other than ingestion of iron salts, the commonest being the giving of repeated blood transfusions. Patients on chronic transfusion programmes need regular therapy with desferrioxamine (see below).

The treatment of acute and chronic iron toxicity involves the use of iron chelators, such as **desferrioxamine**, which is given both intragastrically (to bind iron in the bowel lumen and prevent its absorption following acute overdose) and intramuscularly and, if necessary, intravenously. In severe poisoning it is given by slow intravenous infusion. Desferrioxamine forms a complex with ferric iron which is excreted in the urine.

A new, oral iron chelator, L1, is under test.

FOLIC ACID AND VITAMIN B₁₂

Vitamin B_{12} and folic acid are necessary constituents of man's diet, being essential for DNA synthesis and cell proliferation. Deficiency of either vitamin B_{12} or folate affects principally those tissues with a rapid cell turnover, particularly bone marrow and the gastrointestinal tract. The main manifestation of such deficiency is *megaloblastic haemopoiesis* in which there is a marked disorder of erythroblast (pronormoblast) proliferation and defective erythropoiesis. There are increased numbers of large abnormal erythrocyte precursors in the bone marrow, each with a high RNA : DNA ratio due to decreased DNA synthesis during the cell cycle (see Fig. 42.3). The circulating erythrocytes are large fragile cells, distorted in shape, but with normal cytoplasm and haemoglobin. Some degree of leukopenia and thrombocytopenia usually accompanies the anaemia.

The principal cause of vitamin B_{12} deficiency is decreased absorption of the vitamin due either to a lack of *intrinsic factor* (see below) or to conditions which interfere with its absorption in the ileum.

Intrinsic factor is a protein secreted by the stomach and is essential for B_{12} absorption. It is lacking in patients with *pernicious anaemia* and in individuals who have had total gastrectomies. In pernicious anaemia there is atrophic gastritis, thought to be due to a genetically influenced, local autoimmune reaction. There is often a concurrent neurological disorder—*subacute combined degeneration of the spinal cord*, caused by the deficiency of B_{12}. The anaemia was originally termed 'pernicious' because it seemed to be untreatable, but in 1926 Minot & Murphy showed that there was a remarkable response to the feeding of raw liver. Castle and his associates subsequently established that liver contained an **extrinsic factor** (later defined as **vitamin B_{12}**), and that this, together with an 'intrinsic factor' present in normal gastric juice, was necessary for normal maturation of red cells.

Other conditions resulting in B_{12} deficiency include disorders of the terminal ileum and various inflammatory conditions of the bowel.

Part of the reason that Minot & Murphy obtained a response with raw liver in pernicious anaemia was the presence in this tissue of **folic acid**.*

FOLIC ACID

Folic acid (pteroylglutamic acid) consists of a pteridine ring, para-aminobenzoic acid and glutamic acid (Fig. 18.2). It probably does not occur in nature as such, but can be regarded as the parent compound of a group of naturally occurring folates. These differ from folic acid in several respects. Different states of reduction of the pteridine ring may occur, several one-carbon units may be attached to N^5 or N^{10} or both, and additional glutamic acid residues may be attached to the glutamate moiety by unusual γ-peptide bonds, giving folate polyglutamates. (Some aspects of folate structure and metabolism are dealt with in Ch. 42.)

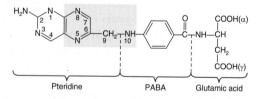

Fig. 18.2 Folic acid (pteroylglutamic acid). Folates may also contain: (1) extra hydrogens at positions 7 and 8 (dihydrofolate) or at 5, 6, 7 and 8 (tetrahydrofolate); (2) one-carbon units such as a methyl group ($-CH_3$) at N^5, a formyl group ($-CHO$) at N^5 or N^{10}, a methylene ($-CH_2-$) or a methenyl ($=CH-$) group between N^5 and N^{10}; (3) additional glutamic acid residues attached to the γ-carboxyl of the glutamate moiety. The area in the grey box is the part of the molecule involved in one-carbon transfers in purine and pyrimidine synthesis.

*In the 1930s, 'Marmite' was shown to have anti-anaemia action, said at the time to be due to an unknown 'Marmite factor' dubbed 'vitamin M'—later shown to be folic acid.

The average daily diet in Western Europe and the USA contains about 600 mg of folate, of which about 100 mg is absorbed. The folates in food are in the form of polyglutamates. These are converted to the monoglutamate before absorption, and are transported in the blood in this form. The folates in tissues are mostly polyglutamates.

Actions

Folates are essential for DNA synthesis in that they are cofactors in the synthesis of purines and pyrimidines. They are also necessary for reactions involved in amino acid metabolism. In all reactions, the polyglutamates are considerably more active than the monoglutamates. For activity, folate must be in the tetrahydro form, in which it is maintained by the enzyme dihydrofolate reductase. This enzyme reduces dietary folic acid to tetrahydrofolate (FH_4) in a two-step reaction, and also reduces the dihydrofolate (FH_2) produced from FH_4 during thymidylate synthesis (see Figs 18.3 and 42.11). Folate antagonists act by inhibiting dihydrofolate reductase (see also Chs 41, 42 and 46).

Folates are especially important for the conversion of deoxyuridylate monophosphate (DUMP) to deoxythymidylate monophosphate (DTMP). This is catalysed by thymidylate synthetase and folate acts as a $-CH_3$ donor (Fig. 18.4). During this reaction, tetrahydrofolate (FH_4) is oxidised to dihydrofolate (FH_2) (see Figs 18.4 and 42.11) and must be reduced before it can act again. The thymidylate synthetase reaction is rate-limiting in mammalian DNA synthesis.

The clinical use of folic acid is given on page 334.

Pharmacokinetic aspects

Folic acid is usually given orally, but preparations for parenteral use are available. In the intestine, folic acid is absorbed unchanged. Folates are taken up into the

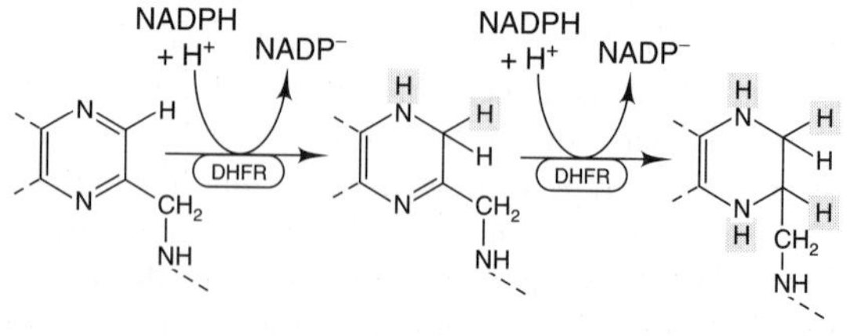

Fig. 18.3 The reduction of folic acid to dihydrofolate (FH_2) then to tetrahydrofolate (FH_4) by the enzyme dihydrofolate reductase (DHFR). Only a portion of the pteridine moiety of the folate molecule is included (that portion shown in the grey box in Fig. 18.2). The grey boxes indicate the hydrogen atoms added to FH_2 and FH_4.

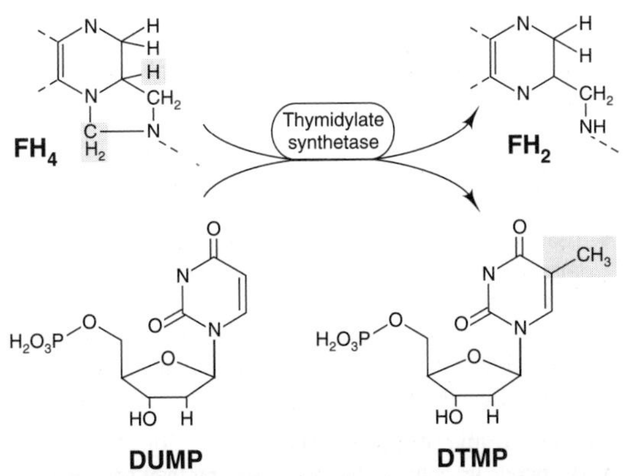

Fig. 18.4 The synthesis of 2-deoxythymidylate (DTMP).
DTMP is synthesised by the transfer of a methyl group from
N^5N^{10}-methylene tetrahydrofolate (FH$_4$) to 2-deoxyuridylate
(DUMP), the FH$_4$ being oxidised to dihydrofolate (FH$_2$) in the
process. Only a portion of the pteridine moiety of the folates
is included in the diagram—that portion shown in the grey
box in Figure 18.2.

liver and into bone marrow cells by active transport,
there being separate carrier mechanisms for folic acid
and reduced folates (see also Ch. 42). Reduced folates are
taken up more readily than folic acid.

Within the cells, folic acid is reduced and methylated
or formylated before being converted to the polyglutamate form. **Folinic acid**, a synthetic tetrahydrofolic acid,
is converted much more rapidly to the polyglutamate
form. Recent studies suggest that methyltetrahydrofolate
is a poor substrate for polyglutamate formation, unlike
dihydrofolate, tetrahydrofolate and formyltetrahydrofolate. (This has relevance for the effect of vitamin B$_{12}$
deficiency on folate metabolism, as is explained below.)

Unwanted effects

Unwanted effects do not occur even with large doses
of folic acid—except possibly in the presence of B$_{12}$
deficiency, because if vitamin B$_{12}$ deficiency is treated
with folic acid, the blood picture may improve and give
the appearance of cure while the neurological lesions
get worse. It is therefore important to determine whether
a megaloblastic anaemia is due to a folate or a vitamin
B$_{12}$ deficiency.

VITAMIN B$_{12}$

Vitamin B$_{12}$ is a complex cobalamin compound. The
vitamin B$_{12}$ used medically is **hydroxocobalamin**. In

the diet, the principal sources of vitamin B$_{12}$ are
meat (particularly liver), eggs and dairy products. All
cobalamins, dietary and therapeutic, must be converted to
methyl-cobalamin (methyl-B$_{12}$) or *5′-deoxyadenosyl-
cobalamin* (ado-B$_{12}$) for activity in the body.

The average daily diet in Western Europe contains
5–25 µg of B$_{12}$ and the daily requirement is 2–3 µg.
Absorption requires intrinsic factor (p. 331) which forms
a one-to-one complex with B$_{12}$. The stomach secretes
a huge excess of intrinsic factor—what limits absorption
is the amount the ileum is capable of absorbing. B$_{12}$
is taken up by active transport, intrinsic factor being
removed on the way.

B$_{12}$ is carried in the plasma by B$_{12}$-binding proteins
called *transcobalamins* (TCs). The vitamin is stored
mainly in the liver, the total amount in the body being
about 4 mg.

The daily requirement is so low that, if B$_{12}$ absorption
is stopped suddenly—as after a total gastrectomy—it takes
2–4 years for evidence of deficiency to become manifest.

Actions

Vitamin B$_{12}$ is required for two main biochemical
reactions in man:

- the conversion of methyl-FH$_4$ to FH$_4$
- isomerisation of methylmalonyl-CoA to succinyl-
CoA.

The conversion of methyl-FH$_4$ to FH$_4$

The reaction involves both conversion of 5-methyl-
tetrahydrofolate (methyl-FH$_4$) to FH$_4$ and homocysteine
to methionine, and the enzyme which accomplishes
this is homocysteine–methionine methyl-transferase; the
reaction requires B$_{12}$ as cofactor and 5-methyltetra-
hydrofolate as the methyl donor. It is thought that the
5-methyltetra-hydrofolate donates the methyl group to
B$_{12}$, the cofactor. The methyl group is then transferred
to homocysteine to form methionine (Fig. 18.5). This
vitamin-B$_{12}$-dependent reaction thus has a significant
role in the generation of the tetrahydrofolate from
methyltetrahydrofolate.

Methyltetrahydrofolate (the form in which folates are
usually carried in blood and in which they enter cells)
is a functionally inactive form of folate. Vitamin B$_{12}$
deficiency results in the 'trapping' of folate in the inactive methyltetrahydrofolate form and the consequent
depletion of all intracellular folate polyglutamate co-
enzymes (which are necessary for early stages of DNA
synthesis), since methyltetrahydrofolate is not converted
to the polyglutamate form, which is the active form of the
coenzyme (see above, p. 332).

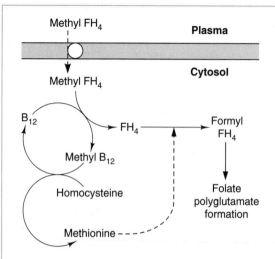

Fig. 18.5   The role of vitamin B$_{12}$ in the synthesis of folate polyglutamate co-enzymes. 5-methyltetrahydrofolate monoglutamate (methyl-FH$_4$) enters the cells by active transport. The methyl group is transferred to homocysteine to form methionine via vitamin B$_{12}$, which is bound to the apoenzyme, homocysteine–methionine methyltransferase. (Vitamin B$_{12}$ is shown as 'B$_{12}$' and as 'methyl B$_{12}$', but the enzyme is not shown.) Methionine is important in the donation of formate (shown by dashed line) for the conversion of tetrahydrofolate (FH$_4$) to formyl tetrahydrofolate (formyl-FH$_4$) which is the preferred substrate for the formation of folate polyglutamates.

B$_{12}$-dependent methionine synthesis may also affect the synthesis of folate polyglutamate coenzymes by an additional mechanism. There is evidence that the preferred substrate for polyglutamate synthesis is formyl-tetrahydrofolate, and the conversion of tetrahydrofolate to formyltetrahydrofolate requires a formate donor such as methionine.

The proposed role of vitamin B$_{12}$ in folate coenzyme synthesis is indicated in Figure 18.5.

It is through the events described above and shown in Figure 18.5 that the metabolic activities of vitamin B$_{12}$ and folic acid are linked and implicated in the synthesis of DNA.

Isomerisation of methylmalonyl-CoA to succinyl-CoA

The isomerisation reaction is part of a route by which propionate is converted to succinate. Through this pathway, cholesterol, odd-chain fatty acids, some amino acids and thymine may be used for energy production via the tricarboxylic acid cycle, or for gluconeogenesis. Vitamin B$_{12}$, in the form of deoxyadenosyl cobalamin (ado-B$_{12}$) is a cofactor in the reaction. In vitamin B$_{12}$ deficiency

Vitamin B$_{12}$ and folic acid

Both vitamin B$_{12}$ and folic acid are needed for DNA synthesis. Deficiencies affect mainly erythropoiesis.

Folic acid
- Folic acid consists of a pteridine ring, *p*-aminobenzoic acid and a glutamate residue.
- There is active uptake into cells and reduction to tetrahydrofolate (FH$_4$) by dihydrofolate reductase; extra glutamates are then added.
- Folate polyglutamate is a cofactor (a carrier of one-carbon units) in the synthesis of purines and pyrimidines (especially thymidylate).

Vitamin B$_{12}$ (hydroxocobalamin)
- B$_{12}$ needs an 'intrinsic factor' (a glycoprotein) secreted by gastric parietal cells for absorption.
- It is required for:
  — conversion of methyl-FH$_4$ (inactive form of FH$_4$) to active formyl-FH$_4$ which, after polyglutamation, is a cofactor in the synthesis of purines and pyrimidines (see above)
  — isomerisation of methylmalonyl-CoA to succinyl-CoA.
- B$_{12}$ is given by injection.

states, the reaction cannot occur and methylmalonyl-CoA accumulates. This can cause fatty acid synthesis in neural tissue to be distorted, and may be the basis of the neuropathy which occurs in these states.

The clinical use of vitamin B$_{12}$ is summarised in the clinical box above.

Administration and pharmacokinetic aspects

When vitamin B$_{12}$ is used therapeutically (as hydroxocobalamin), it is almost always given by intramuscular injection, since B$_{12}$ deficiency is virtually always due to malabsorption of the vitamin. Plasma transport and distribution of therapeutically administered B$_{12}$ have been described above.

Patients with pernicious anaemia require lifelong therapy. Unwanted effects do not occur.

HAEMOPOIETIC GROWTH FACTORS

Every 60 seconds, a human being must generate about 120 million granulocytes and 150 million erythrocytes, as well as numerous mononuclear cells and platelets. The cells responsible for this remarkable productivity are derived from a relatively small number of self-renewing, pluripotent stem cells laid down during embryogenesis. Maintenance of haemopoiesis necessitates a balance between self-renewal on the one hand, and differentiation into the various types of blood cell on the other. The factors involved in controlling this balance are the *haemopoietic growth factors*, which direct the division and maturation of the progeny of these cells down eight possible lines of development (Fig. 18.6). These cytokine growth factors are glycoproteins with high biological activity, acting at concentrations of 10^{-12}–10^{-10} mol/l. They are normally present at very low concentrations in the plasma, but the levels can increase very rapidly by 1000-fold within hours—in response to stimulation. **Erythropoietin** is the factor which regulates the red cell line and the signal for its production is blood loss and/or low tissue O_2 tension. The **colony-stimulating factors** regulate the myeloid divisions of the white cell line, and the main stimulus for their production is infection. See also Chapter 12.

The genes for several haemopoietic factors have been cloned, and recombinant erythropoietin, recombinant granulocyte-colony-stimulating factor, recombinant granulocyte-macrophage-colony-stimulating factor and recombinant thrombopoietin are being used clinically. Some of the other haemopoietic growth factors (e.g.

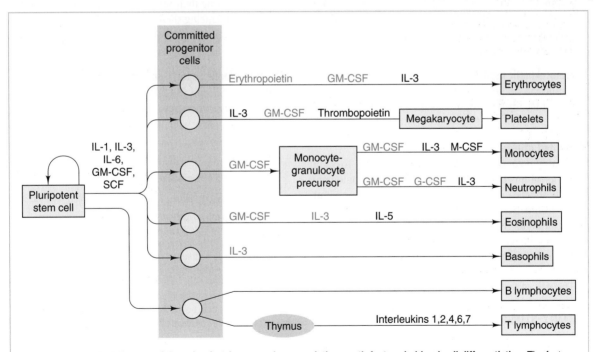

Fig. 18.6 Simplified diagram of the role of endogenous haemopoietic growth factors in blood cell differentiation. The factors shown in blue are in clinical use under different names (see text). Most T cells generated in the thymus die by apoptosis; those that emerge are either CD4+ or CD8+. (CSF = colony-stimulating factor; GM-CSF = granulocyte-macrophage-CSF; G-CSF = granulocyte-CSF; M-CSF = macrophage-CSF; IL-3 = interleukin-3, or multi-CSF; IL-1 = interleukin-1; SCF = stem cell factor) (See also Ch. 12, p. 224, and Fig. 12.3.)

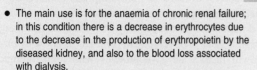

Clinical use of epoietin

- The main use is for the anaemia of chronic renal failure; in this condition there is a decrease in erythrocytes due to the decrease in the production of erythropoietin by the diseased kidney, and also to the blood loss associated with dialysis.
- Other potential future uses are: the anaemia of AIDS (which is exacerbated by zidovudine treatment); the anaemia of chronic inflammatory conditions such as rheumatoid arthritis; the anaemia of cancer; the anaemia which occurs in premature infants.

interleukin-1, interleukin-2 and various cytokines) are covered in Chapter 12.

ERYTHROPOIETIN

Erythropoietin is produced in juxtatubular cells in the kidney and also in macrophages, and its action is to stimulate committed erythroid progenitor cells to proliferate and generate erythrocytes (Fig. 18.6). Two forms of recombinant human erythropoietin, **epoietin alpha** and **epoietin beta** are now available. These are clinically indistinguishable and will be referred to here as simply as 'epoietin'.

The clinical use of epoietin is given above.

Pharmacokinetic aspects

Epoietin can be given intravenously, subcutaneously or intraperitoneally, the response being greatest after subcutaneous injection and fastest after intravenous injection.

Unwanted effects

Flu-like symptoms, which are transient, are likely to occur. Hypertension is common and can cause encephalopathy with headache, disorientation and sometimes convulsions. Iron deficiency can be induced because more iron is required for the enhanced erythropoiesis and there can be an increase in blood viscosity since the plasma volume does not increase commensurately with the increase in red cell mass.

The risk of thrombosis during dialysis is increased.

COLONY-STIMULATING FACTORS (CSFs)

The colony-stimulating factors are so called because they were found to stimulate the formation of maturing colonies of leukocytes in semi-solid medium in vitro. CSFs not only stimulate particular committed progenitor cells to proliferate (Fig. 18.6), but cause irreversible differentiation. The responding precursor cells have

membrane receptors to CSFs and may express receptors for more than one factor, thus permitting collaborative interactions between factors. The CSFs are classified as 'cytokines' (see Ch. 12. p. 224).

Granulocyte-macrophage-colony-stimulating factor (GM-CSF) is produced by many cell types and is important in the control of at least five of the eight lines of blood cell development. Granulocyte-colony-stimulating factor (G-CSF) is produced mainly by monocytes, fibroblasts and endothelial cells, and controls primarily the development of neutrophils. Recombinant G-CSF is available as **filgrastim** and **lenograstim**, and recombinant GM-CSF as **molgramostim**, and **sargramostim**.

Actions

GM-CSF stimulates the development of the progenitors of neutrophils, monocytes, eosinophils, and (under some circumstances) megakaryocytes and erythrocytes (Fig. 18.6). It also enhances the functional activity and survival of the mature cells. GM-CSF may increase the production of other cytokines.

G-CSF acts only on the neutrophil line (Fig. 18.6)—increasing the proliferation and maturation of neutrophils, stimulating their release from bone marrow storage pools and enhancing their function.

The clinical use of colony-stimulating factors is given below.

Pharmacokinetic aspects and unwanted effects

Both GM-CSF and G-CSF can be given either subcutaneously or by intravenous infusion.

Both CSFs are well tolerated. Bone pain occurs in 10–20% of patients.

Clinical uses of the CSFs

CSFs are used in specialist cancer chemotherapy centres:

- to reduce the severity and duration of the neutropenia induced by cytotoxic drugs during:
  — conventional anticancer chemotherapy
  — intensive courses of chemotherapy which damage the haemopoietic tissue necessitating autologous bone marrow rescue
- to stimulate release into the circulation of progenitor cells which can then be harvested and infused with, or instead of, bone marrow cells after high-dose, intensive chemotherapy
- to expand the number of harvested progenitor cells ex vivo before re-infusing them.

Other possible roles: in aplastic anaemia; for myelodysplasia; for the anaemia which occurs in AIDS and is exacerbated by zidovudine.

GM-CSF frequently produces fever and can cause skin rashes, muscle pain and lethargy. There may be pain and reddening at the site of the injection. With intravenous infusion, a syndrome of flushing, hypotension, tachycardia, breathlessness, nausea and vomiting and arterial oxygen desaturation has occurred; this is reversed by giving oxygen and intravenous fluids. At high doses (> 20 mg/kg per day) pleural and pericardial effusions, venous thrombosis and pulmonary embolism, have been reported.

G-CSF has produced mild dysuria (rare) and reversible abnormalities in liver function tests. Vasculitis has been reported with long-term use.

Thrombopoietin

Thrombopoietin stimulates proliferation of the progenitor cells of the platelet lineage and strikingly increases platelet production. Recombinant thrombopoietin is being tested clinically.

Haemopoietic growth factors

Erythropoietin
- Regulates red cell production
- Is given intravenously, subcutaneously, intraperitoneally
- Can cause transient flu-like symptoms, hypertension, iron deficiency and increased blood viscosity
- Is available as epoietin

Granulocyte colony-stimulating factor (G-CSF)
- Stimulates neutrophil progenitors
- Is available as filgrastim; given intravenously, subcutaneously

Granulocyte-macrophage colony-stimulating factor (GM-CSF)
- Stimulates development of many types of progenitor cells
- Is available as molgramostim; given intravenously, subcutaneously
- Can cause fever, rashes, bone pain, hypotension, GIT symptoms and arterial oxygen desaturation

---

REFERENCES AND FURTHER READING

Dale D C 1995 Where now for colony-stimulating factors? Lancet 346: 135–136

Erslev A J 1991 Erythropoietin. N Engl J Med 324: 1339–1344

Finch C A, Hueber S H 1982 Perspectives in iron metabolism. N Engl J Med 306: 1520–1528 (*Good background article on iron*)

Frewin R, Henson A, Provan D 1997 ABC of clinical haematology: iron deficiency anaemia. Br Med J 314: 360–363

Goodenough L T, Monk T G, Andriole G L 1997 Erythropoietin therapy. N Engl J Med 336: 933–938 (*A useful 'Current Concepts' article*)

Hoelzer D 1997 Haemopoietic growth factors—not whether, but when and where. N Engl J Med 336: 1822–1824 (*An edifying editorial comment*)

Levin J 1997 Thrombopoietin—clinically realised? N Engl J Med 336: 434–436 (*A useful editorial*)

Lieschke G J, Burges A W 1992 Granulocyte colony-stimulating factor and granulocyte-macrophage colony-stimulating factor. N Engl J Med 327: 1–35, 99–106 (*Worthwhile, comprehensive reviews*)

Nimer S D 1997 Platelet stimulating agents—off the launch pad. Nature Med 3: 154–155 (*Thrombopoietic growth factors prove useful in clinical trials*)

Petros W P, Peters W P 1996 Colony-stimulating factors. In: Chabner B A, Longo D L (eds) Cancer chemotherapy and biotherapy, 2nd edn. Lippincott-Raven, Philadelphia, pp 639–654 (*Covers mechanism of action, biological effects and clinical pharmacology*)

Spivak J L 1993 Recombinant erythropoietin. Annu Rev Med 44: 243–253

Steinberg S E 1984 Mechanisms of folate homeostasis. Amer J Physiol 246: G319–324 (*Good background article on folate*)

Toh B-H, van Driel I R, Gleeson P A 1997 Pernicious anaemia. N Engl J Med 337: 1441–1448 (*Immunopathogenesis of pernicious anaemia; excellent figures*)

Wald N J, Bower C 1994 Folic acid, pernicious anaemia, and prevention of neural tube defects. Lancet 343: 307

19

The respiratory system

The chief functions of respiration are to supply oxygen to the body and to remove carbon dioxide. In addition, the evaporation of water in the respiratory passages assists in regulating the temperature of the body.

THE REGULATION OF RESPIRATION

Respiration is controlled by spontaneous rhythmic discharges from the respiratory centre in the medulla, modulated by input from pontine and higher CNS centres and vagal afferents from the lungs. Various chemical factors affect the respiratory centre including the blood P_{CO_2} (by an action on medullary chemoreceptors) and the blood P_{O_2} (by an action on the chemoreceptors in the aortic and carotid bodies).

A moderate degree of voluntary control can be superimposed on the automatic regulation of breathing, and this implies connections between the cortex and the motor neurons innervating the muscles of respiration. Bulbar poliomyelitis and certain lesions in the brainstem result in loss of the automatic regulation of respiration without loss of voluntary regulation. (This has been referred to as 'Ondine's curse'. Ondine was a water nymph who fell in love with a mortal. When he was unfaithful to her, the king of the water nymphs put a curse on him—that he must stay awake in order to breathe. When exhaustion finally supervened and he fell asleep, he died.)

THE REGULATION OF THE MUSCULATURE, BLOOD VESSELS AND GLANDS OF THE AIRWAYS

In the normal neurohumoral control of the airways, the *efferent pathways* are the acetylcholine-releasing parasympathetic nerves, the noradrenaline-releasing sympathetic nerves, circulating adrenaline and the non-noradrenergic, non-cholinergic (NANC) inhibitory neurons. The *afferent pathways* include three different types of sensory receptor, described below.

In pathological conditions such as asthma and bronchitis, other mediators—the inflammatory mediators (see Ch. 12) and, possibly, the NANC contractile mediators—have a significant role.

The signal transduction mechanisms for the various receptors mediating contraction and relaxation of bronchiolar muscle are discussed by Dale & Hirst (1993).

The tone of the bronchial muscle affects the airways resistance, and in asthma and bronchitis the state of the mucosa and the activity of the glands also contribute. The airways resistance can be measured indirectly by instruments which record the volume or flow of forced expiration. FEV_1 is the 'forced expiratory volume in 1 second'. The 'peak expiratory flow rate' (PEFR) is the maximal flow (l/min) after a full inhalation.

Efferent pathways

Parasympathetic innervation
Parasympathetic ganglia are embedded in the walls of the bronchi and bronchioles, and the post-ganglionic fibres innervate airway smooth muscle, vascular smooth muscle and glands. There are three types of muscarinic (M) receptors present (see Ch. 7, Table 7.1). M_1-receptors are localised in ganglia, on the postsynaptic cells, and their

stimulation facilitates neurotransmission mediated by acetylcholine acting on the nicotinic receptors. M_2-receptors are 'autoreceptors' mediating negative feedback effects of acetylcholine on cholinergic nerves. M_3-receptors are found on bronchial smooth muscle and glands and mediate contraction of the former and secretion from the latter. Stimulation of the vagus causes broncho-constriction—mainly in the larger airways. The possible clinical relevance of the heterogeneity of muscarinic receptors in the airways is discussed below on page 346.

Sympathetic innervation and catecholamines
Sympathetic nerves innervate blood vessels and glands, the released noradrenaline causing constriction of the former and inhibiting secretion by the latter (Ch. 8). Contrary to general belief there is no sympathetic inner-vation of the bronchial smooth muscle; there is good experimental evidence that all 'sympathetic' effects are due to circulating catecholamines.

Autoradiography shows that β-adrenoceptors occur in the smooth muscle, the epithelium and glands, and also, in very large numbers, in the alveoli (though what they are doing in this last site is anybody's guess). They are also found on mast cells. In humans, virtually all the β-receptors in the airways are β_2; those in the alveoli are both β_1 and β_2. In contrast with the muscarinic receptors, the density of β-receptors increases from trachea to bronchioles.

Stimulation of the airway β-receptors with drugs results in relaxation of smooth muscle, inhibition of mediator release from mast cells, and increased mucoci-liary clearance.

α-adrenoceptor agonists have no effect on normal airways but cause contraction if the airways are diseased.

Non-noradrenergic, non-cholinergic (NANC) mediators
There is evidence that airway function is influenced by neuronal mediators other than acetylcholine and nor-adrenaline; these are referred to as NANC mediators (see Ch. 6, p. 104).

The inhibitory NANC mediator—the *main* neuro-transmitter relaxant in the airways—is now believed to be nitric oxide (see Ch. 11 and Barnes 1996). Inducible nitric oxide synthase (NOS) and both forms of con-stitutive NOS are present in human airways, and the inducible form is implicated in asthma and other types of airway inflammation.

The stimulant NANC mediators are thought to be excitatory neuropeptides* (see Chs 10 and 12) that are

---

*These peptides are considered to be the mediators of neurogenic inflammation, which may also be a contributing factor in various inflammatory conditions (Ch. 12, p. 223).

released from sensory C fibres when stimulated by inflammatory mediators and irritant chemicals. The main neuropeptides are substance P (which increases vascular permeability and induces mucus secretion), and neuro-kinin A (a potent spasmogen).

The inflammatory mediators are dealt with below.

Sensory receptors and afferent pathways
The receptors involved in the central regulation of respir-ation by the respiratory centre are the *slowly adapting stretch receptors*. In addition, there are *unmyelinated sensory C fibres* and *rapidly adapting irritant receptors* associated with myelinated vagal fibres.

Chemical stimuli, acting on irritant receptors on myelinated fibres in the upper airways and/or C-fibre receptors in the lower airways, cause coughing, broncho-constriction and an increase in mucus secretion. The stimuli that produce these effects include both exogenous agents, such as ammonia, sulphur dioxide, cigarette smoke and the experimental tool, capsaicin as well as endogenous stimuli such as the inflammatory mediators.

Regulation of airway muscle, blood vessels and glands

Afferent pathways
- Irritant receptors and C-fibres respond to exogenous chemicals, inflammatory mediators and physical stimuli (e.g. cold air) causing bronchoconstriction and mucus secretion through acetylcholine release in the upper airway and release of excitatory neuropeptides in the lower.

Efferent pathways
- The parasympathetic nerves mediate bronchial constriction and mucus secretion through an action on muscarinic M_3-receptors.
- Sympathetic nerves innervate blood vessels (causing constriction) and glands (inhibiting secretion), but not airway smooth muscle.
- Circulating adrenaline acts on β_2-receptors to relax airway smooth muscle.
- The main neurotransmitter causing relaxation of airway smooth muscle is the NANC inhibitory transmitter, thought to be nitric oxide.
- NANC excitatory transmitters are peptides released from sensory neurons.

DRUGS WHICH AFFECT RESPIRATION

Drugs may produce an effect on respiration inadvertently (e.g. the unwanted effects of some CNS depressants) or because they are intended to (e.g. respiratory stimulants).

RESPIRATORY STIMULANTS

Respiratory stimulants are used only in certain specific conditions (e.g. postoperative respiratory depression, acute respiratory failure) and then only under expert supervision in hospital. The main drug used is **doxapram** which stimulates both carotid chemoreceptors and the respiratory centre. It should not be used in severe acute asthma (*status asthmaticus*), or in respiratory depression which is caused by drug overdose (see below).

DRUGS CAUSING RESPIRATORY DEPRESSION

Many drugs which have a depressant action on the central nervous system cause a greater or lesser degree of respiratory depression. These include the **narcotic analgesics**, **barbiturates**, many **H_1 histamine-receptor antagonists**, some **antidepressants** and **ethanol**. Most of these agents generally depress respiration to a significant degree only in excessive dosage, but the **opiates** cause some degree of respiratory depression in the therapeutic dose range. The respiratory depression caused by the majority of the above agents can prove fatal; however, this is less likely to occur with the benzodiazepines. These hazards are discussed in more detail in the chapters devoted to each of these agents.

Opiate analgesics and barbiturates (and possibly other CNS depressant drugs) first affect the sensitivity of respiration to increased P_{CO_2} and only later, in larger doses, do they affect the hypoxic drive.

Drugs which affect respiration

- Depression of respiration can be produced by excessive doses of most drugs that have depressant actions on the CNS.
- Benzodiazepines cause relatively little depression (but may do so to a dangerous degree if combined with alcohol).
- Narcotic analgesics cause some degree of depression in therapeutic doses.
- Doxapram is occasionally used as a respiratory stimulant in emergencies.

DISORDERS OF RESPIRATORY FUNCTION

Two of the main disorders of the respiratory system are bronchial asthma and cough. Others, less susceptible to treatment, are chronic bronchitis with resultant chronic obstructive airway disease, and the adult respiratory distress syndrome.

BRONCHIAL ASTHMA

Asthma may be loosely defined as a syndrome in which there is recurrent 'reversible' obstruction of the airways in response to stimuli which are not in themselves noxious and which do not affect non-asthmatic subjects. The asthmatic subject has intermittent attacks* of dyspnoea (disorder of breathing), wheezing, and cough, the dyspnoea consisting of difficulty in breathing *out*. It contrasts with the obstructive airway disease mentioned above, which is not reversible. But note that the term 'reversible' as applied to asthma needs to be qualified since it is only the acute attack of dyspnoea that is reversible—the underlying pathological change may not be reversible and indeed can progress. In *acute severe asthma* (also known as *status asthmaticus*) the airway obstruction causing the dyspnoea can take days to reverse, and in some cases is not reversible at all and proves to be fatal.

Asthma affects over 5–10% of the population in industrialised countries. Most authorities agree that it is increasing in prevalence and severity. Some chest physicians consider that the increase in morbidity may be the result of the currently available therapy not being used optimally; if this is indeed so, it may stem from the fact that recent advances in the understanding of the pathogenesis of asthma have not been universally appreciated.

10 years or so ago, asthma was thought to be purely a type I hypersensitivity reaction (Ch. 12, p. 209), the actual attack occurring in a sensitised individual when allergen interacted with IgE antibodies on mast cells, leading to release of histamine and other mediators, which caused a simple bronchoconstriction. That view is now known to be an oversimplification—not all asthma is due to allergy and, even in allergic asthma, numerous elements other than the interaction of allergen with mast-cell-fixed IgE are involved.** This has relevance for the use of drugs in treatment.

It is currently recognised that the characteristic features of most cases of asthma are *inflammatory changes in the airways* associated with *bronchial hyper-*

---

*The term 'chronic asthma' is sometimes used; it is employed rather indiscriminately to mean the propensity for repeated attacks and/or a state of semi-continuous low-grade asthma.

**The NSAIDs, especially aspirin, can precipitate asthma in sensitive individuals.

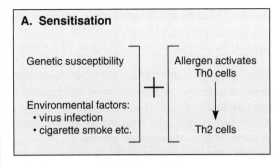

A. Sensitisation

Genetic susceptibility

Environmental factors:
• virus infection
• cigarette smoke etc.

+

Allergen activates
Th0 cells

↓

Th2 cells

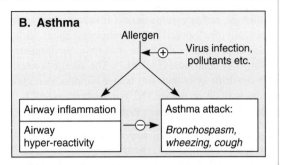

B. Asthma

Allergen

Virus infection,
pollutants etc.

Airway inflammation

Airway
hyper-reactivity

Asthma attack:

*Bronchospasm,
wheezing, cough*

Fig. 19.1 Simplified outline of the development of allergic asthma. Sensitisation: allergen interacts with dendritic cells and Th0 helper lymphocytes giving rise to Th2 cells which generate cytokines whose actions result in differentiation and activation of eosinophils, the production of IgE and the expression of IgE receptors on mast cells and eosinophils. Re-exposure to allergen triggers an asthma attack and initiates a process of airway inflammation and hyper-reactivity, which predispose to further attacks. Once hyper-reactivity has been established, an asthma attack can be set off by exercise, cold air, SO_2, etc. For details of the cells and mediators involved in the airway inflammation, and the action of anti-asthma drugs, see Figure 19.3.

reactivity;* in allergic asthma, these are related to, and follow from, prior sensitisation (Fig. 19.1).

Inflammatory changes are present even in patients with very mild asthma and in some individuals these may even precede the development of overt asthma. But note that the episodic asthma associated with viral infections can occur without underlying chronic inflammation.

The term bronchial hyper-reactivity (or hyper-responsiveness) refers to abnormal sensitivity to a wide range of stimuli such as irritant chemicals, cold air, stimulant drugs, etc., all of which can result in broncho-constriction. Stimuli which cause the actual asthma attacks are many and varied, and include allergens (in sensitised individuals), exercise (in which the stimulus may be cold air), respiratory infections and atmospheric pollutants such as sulphur dioxide.

The development of asthma probably involves both genetic and environmental factors, and the asthmatic attack itself consists, in many subjects, of two main phases—the immediate phase and the late (or delayed) phase. These phases can be demonstrated by tests of FEV_1 (Fig. 19.2).

This division into two phases is fairly arbitrary—indeed, in some subjects, only one of the phases may be obvious—but it provides a useful basis for discussing the physiopathological changes in the bronchi as well as the locus of action and the effects of drugs used in treatment.

Fig. 19.2 The two phases of asthma as demonstrated by the changes in the forced expiratory volume in 1 second (FEV_1) after inhalation of grass pollen in an allergic subject. (From: Cockcroft D W 1983 Lancet 1: 253)

The full details of the complex events involved are still a matter of debate, with various authors championing their particular inflammatory cell or mediator as being the principal agent in the development of asthma. In the following paragraphs we give a simplified version of asthma pathogenesis (see Holgate 1993; and for a comprehensive coverage by numerous authors in 33 chapters, see Weiss & Stein 1993). We emphasise that an understanding of this topic is necessary for rational use of current (and future) drugs in the treatment of asthma.**

---

*But note that only during the latter part of the 20th century has a simplistic interpretation of asthma pathogenesis held sway. Several aspects of the current view of asthma as an inflammatory disease date back to astute observations made during the 19th century—and subsequently overlooked (see Persson 1997).

**We write this bearing in mind the words of one aspiring general practitioner in 1989: 'Asthma is easy to understand and simple to treat. It's just histamine-induced bronchospasm—all you need to do is prescribe a good bronchodilator'.

The development of allergic asthma

In allergic asthma, sensitisation involves exposure of genetically predisposed individuals to allergens such as pollen or proteins of the house dust mite; environmental factors may contribute (Fig. 19.1). The allergens interact with dendritic cells and Th0 helper lymphocytes giving rise to a clone of helper Th2 lymphocytes (see Ch. 12, p. 204 and Fig. 12.3) which then:

- generate various B-cell-activating cytokines, leading to IgE production and release
- generate cytokines such as interleukin-5 (IL-5) that promote differentiation and activation of eosinophils
- generate various cytokines (e.g. IL-4)* that induce expression of IgE receptors, mainly on mast cells but also on eosinophils; IL-4 also induces endothelium to express receptors that specifically attract eosinophils.

The system thus becomes primed so that subsequent re-exposure to the relevant allergen will cause an asthmatic attack (Fig. 19.1).

The immediate phase of the asthmatic attack

In allergic asthma, the immediate phase, i.e. the initial response to allergen provocation, occurs abruptly and is due mainly to *spasm of the bronchial smooth muscle*. Allergen interaction with mast cell-fixed IgE releases histamine, but this is not the only or even the main spasmogen—LTC_4 and LTD_4 (Ch. 12, p. 218) are now known to be more important, and other mediators (e.g. PDG_2, neurokinin A) may also contribute. Various chemotaxins (e.g. LTB_4) and chemokines (see Ch. 12, p. 224) attract leukocytes—particularly eosinophils and mononuclear cells—into the area, setting the stage for the delayed phase.

Most exercise-induced asthma appears to involve mainly the phenomena of this first phase.

The late phase

The second, late phase or delayed response (see Fig. 19.2), occurs at a variable time after exposure to the eliciting stimulus and may be nocturnal. This phase is in essence a progressing *inflammatory reaction*, initiation of which occurred during the first phase, the influx of Th2 lymphocytes being of particular importance. The inflammation is different from that seen, for example, in bronchitis. It has special characteristics in that there is infiltration not only by the usual inflammatory cells (Ch. 12, p. 201),

---

*The genes for both IL-4 and IL-4 receptors have been shown to be linked to asthma.

but also, and more specifically, by activated cytokine-releasing Th2 cells and by eosinophils, whose products cause damage and loss of epithelium—with the repercussions outlined in Figures 19.1, 19.2 and 19.3 (reviewed by Corrigan & Kay 1992). The epithelial loss means that irritant receptors and C fibres are more accessible to irritant stimuli; this is thought to be the basis of the hyper-reactivity.

Other factors that have been put forward as putative mediators of the inflammatory process in the delayed phase are adenosine (acting on the A_1 receptor), induced nitric oxide (see Ch. 11, Ch. 12, p. 223), and the neuropeptides (see Ch. 12, pp. 217–219).

Growth factors released from inflammatory cells act on smooth muscle cells, causing hypertrophy and hyperplasia, and the smooth muscle can itself release pro-inflammatory mediators and autocrine growth factors (Ch. 12).

There are two categories of anti-asthma drugs—**bronchodilators** and **anti-inflammatory agents**. Bronchodilators are effective in reversing the bronchospasm of the immediate phase, anti-inflammatory agents in inhibiting or preventing the inflammatory components of both phases (Fig. 19.3). But note that these two categories are not mutually exclusive—some drugs classified as bronchodilators may also act on inflammatory cells.

Many authorities now consider that progression of the condition, with increase in the severity of the asthmatic attacks, is due to a gradual increase in the mucosal inflammation. Over-reliance on bronchodilators, which overcome the acute attacks of bronchospasm without significantly modifying the underlying inflammation, could well contribute to this.

The problem of how to use the above two categories of drugs in the clinical treatment of asthma is complex. A recent set of guidelines (see British Thoracic Society et al. 1997) specifies five therapeutic steps—the first involving only a short-acting β-agonist, progressing, if this type of agent is needed more than once daily, to subsequent steps involving both bronchodilators and anti-inflammatory drugs. There is now general agreement on the need to implement early anti-inflammatory treatment in many cases, rather than relying on symptomatic treatment with bronchodilators alone.

DRUGS USED TO TREAT ASTHMA—BRONCHODILATORS

Drugs used as bronchodilators include the $β_2$-adrenoceptor agonists, the xanthines and the muscarinic-receptor antagonists.

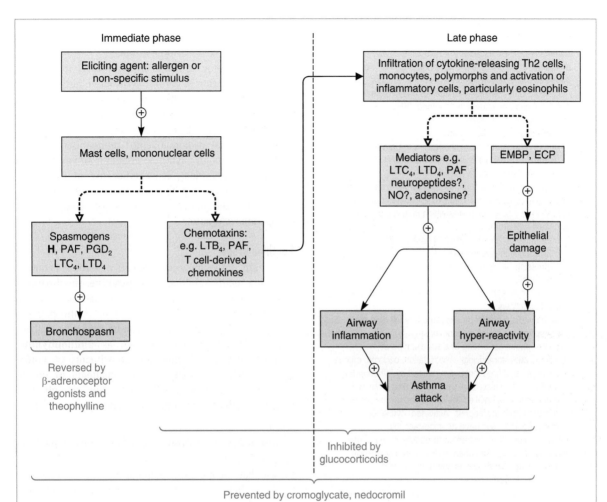

Fig. 19.3   Outline of the reactions thought to occur in asthma, with the actions of the main drugs. (H = histamine; PAF = platelet-activating factor; LTB_4, LTC_4 and LTD_4 = leukotrienes B_4, C_4 and D_4; EMBP = eosinophil major basic protein; ECP = eosinophil cationic protein; NO = nitric oxide.) For more detail of the Th2-derived cytokines and chemokines, see Chapter 12, pages 223–224 and Figure 12.3. Note that not all asthmatic subjects respond to cromoglycate or nedocromil, and that theophylline is only a second-line drug.

β_2-adrenoceptor agonists

β_2-adrenoceptor agonists are dealt with in detail in Chapter 8.

Their primary effect in asthma is to dilate the bronchi by a direct action on the β_2-adrenoceptors on the smooth muscle. Being physiological antagonists (see Ch. 1, pp. 14, 15), they relax the bronchial muscle whatever the spasmogens involved. They also inhibit mediator release from mast cells and the release from monocytes of one of the primary mediators of inflammation (see Ch. 12, p. 224)—tumour necrosis factor (TNF-α). In addition, they may increase mucus clearance by an action on cilia.

These drugs are usually given by inhalation of aerosol, powder or nebulised solution, but some may be given orally or by injection. A metered-dose inhaler is used for aerosol preparations; if patients (e.g. children, the elderly) have problems using these, 'spacer' devices can be used instead.

Two categories of β_2-adrenoceptor agonists are used in asthma:

- Short-acting agents—**salbutamol** and **terbutaline**; given by inhalation, the maximum effect is within 30 minutes and the duration 4–6 hours; they are usually used on an 'as needed' basis to control symptoms.

- Asthma is defined as recurrent reversible airway obstruction. The asthmatic attack comprises wheezing, cough and difficulty in breathing out; the airways resistance is increased—manifest as a decrease in the 'forced expiratory volume in 1 second' (FEV$_1$). Severe attacks are life-threatening.
- Two characteristic features are:
  — underlying inflammatory changes in the airways
  — underlying bronchial hyper-responsiveness, i.e. abnormal sensitivity to stimuli.
- The development of allergic asthma involves exposure of genetically sensitive individuals to allergens; these cause activation of Th2 lymphocytes which in turn generate cytokines that promote:
  — differentiation and activation of eosinophils
  — IgE production and release
  — expression of IgE receptors on mast cells and eosinophils.
- In many subjects the asthmatic attack consists of two phases as follows:
  — an immediate phase on exposure to eliciting agent consisting mainly of bronchospasm
  — a later phase consisting of a special type of inflammation comprising: vasodilatation, oedema, mucus secretion and bronchospasm caused by inflammatory mediators released from eosinophils and other cells; damage to bronchial epithelium is caused by proteins released from eosinophils. Activated, cytokine-releasing Th2 cells have an important role.
- Important mediators: histamine (probably in first phase only), LTC$_4$, LTD$_4$, (and possibly PgD$_2$, neuropeptides and nitric oxide) and various chemotaxins and chemokines in both phases.
- In acute severe asthma (status asthmaticus) the airway obstruction can be fatal.
- Anti-asthmatic drugs include:
  — bronchodilators
  — anti-inflammatory agents.

- Longer-acting agents—**salmeterol**; given by inhalation, the duration is 12 hours; They are not used 'as needed' but are given regularly, twice daily, as adjunctive therapy in patients whose asthma is inadequately controlled by glucocorticoids.

Others are **rimeterol** (with shorter duration of action than salbutamol), **pirbuterol** and **reprotelol**. Bambuterol, a pro-drug of terbutaline, is also now available.

The unwanted effects of β$_2$-adrenoceptor agonists result from systemic absorption and are given in Chapter 8. In the context of their use in asthma, the commonest adverse effect is tremor. There is some evidence that β-agonist tolerance can occur in asthmatic airways (see

Cockroft et al. 1993) and that steroids can reduce the possibility of the development of tolerance because they inhibit β-receptor down-regulation.

β$_2$-adrenoceptor agonists are also used to improve respiratory function in chronic obstructive lung disease.

It should be stressed that non-selective β-adrenoceptor agonists, such as adrenaline and isoprenaline, which act on both β$_1$- and β$_2$-receptors, are no longer used in asthma and that β$_2$-adrenoceptor *antagonists*, such as propranolol, though having no effect on airway function in normal individuals, cause wheezing in asthmatics and can precipitate a potentially serious acute asthmatic attack—by abrogating the effect of compensatory endogenous adrenaline.

Xanthine drugs

There are three pharmacologically active, naturally occurring methylxanthines, **theophylline**, **theobromine** and **caffeine** (see also Chs 14 and 38). The xanthine usually employed in clinical medicine is theophylline (1,3-dimethylxanthine), which can be used also as theophylline-ethylene-diamine, known as **aminophylline**. Caffeine and theophylline are constituents of coffee and tea, and theobromine is a constituent of cocoa. Theophylline has bronchodilator action, though it is rather less effective than the β$_2$-adrenoceptor agonists.

Actions

Anti-asthmatic actions. Xanthines have long been used as bronchodilators.* Several clinical studies have shown that theophylline preparations can be effective both in relieving the acute attack and in the treatment of chronic asthma. Actions in addition to bronchodilatation seem to be involved since there is some evidence that theophylline can inhibit the late phase, as shown by measurement of FEV$_1$ after bronchial allergen challenge (Pauwels 1989); but it does not appear to prevent bronchial hyper-responsiveness. Analogues currently under test have more specific and more potent effects on the underlying mechanisms of the late phase of asthma (see below).

Actions on the central nervous system. The methylxanthines have a stimulant effect on the CNS, causing increased alertness (see Ch. 38). They can cause tremor and nervousness and can interfere with sleep and have a stimulant action on respiration.

Actions on the cardiovascular system. All the xan-

---

*Over 200 years ago, William Withering recommended 'coffee made very strong' as a remedy for asthma, belief in its efficacy was reinforced by Salter in 1859.

thines stimulate the heart (see Ch. 14), having positive chronotropic and inotropic actions. They cause vaso-dilatation in most blood vessels, though some can cause constriction in some vascular beds, more particularly cerebral blood vessels.

Actions on kidney. Methylxanthines have a weak diuretic effect, involving both an increased glomerular filtration rate and reduced reabsorption in the tubules.

Mechanisms of action

The way in which these drugs produce effects in asthma is still unclear.

The relaxant effect on smooth muscle has been attributed to inhibition of phosphodiesterase (PDE) with resultant increase in cyclic AMP (see Fig. 15.1). An increase in cyclic AMP could also attenuate the actions of inflammatory cells and explain the effect of theophylline in the late phase. However, the concentrations necessary to inhibit the isolated enzyme greatly exceed the therapeutic range.

There is some evidence that the smooth muscle relaxation could be related to an effect on a cyclic *GMP* phosphodiesterase.

Recent work has shown that subtypes of the PDE enzyme exist, including one (type 5) that is selective for cyclic GMP. This raises the possibility that inhibitors with selective action could be of value, and a plethora of new compounds that inhibit these more specifically are under test (see below). These may well replace theophylline in the near future.

One proposed mode of action has been competitive antagonism of adenosine at adenosine receptors, but the PDE inhibitor enprofylline, which is a more potent bronchodilator, is not an adenosine antagonist.

Unwanted effects

When theophylline is used in asthma, most of its other effects, such as those on the CNS, cardiovascular system and gastrointestinal tract, are unwanted side-effects. Furthermore, the plasma concentration range for an optimum therapeutic effect is 30–100 µmol/l, and adverse effects are likely to occur with concentrations greater than 110 µmol/l. Measurements of the plasma concentration are necessary when the drug is given intravenously for treatment of *status asthmaticus*, and are advisable to optimise therapy at high oral doses.

Gastrointestinal symptoms (anorexia, nausea and vomiting) and nervousness and tremor are sometimes seen with concentrations only slightly higher than the clinically effective levels. Serious cardiovascular and CNS effects can occur when the plasma concentration exceeds 200 µmol/l. The most serious cardiovascular effect is arrhythmia, which can be fatal. In children, seizures can occur with theophylline concentrations at or slightly above the upper limit of the therapeutic range. Seizures can be fatal in patients with respiratory compromise due to severe asthma.

Pharmacokinetic aspects

Xanthine drugs are given orally in sustained-release preparations; it is not feasible to give them by inhalation. Aminophylline can also be given by *slow* intravenous injection of a loading dose followed by intravenous infusion, in the treatment of *status asthmaticus*.

Theophylline is well absorbed from the gastrointestinal tract. It is metabolised in the liver and the plasma half-life is about 8 hours in adults but varies widely in different subjects.

The half-life of theophylline is *increased* in liver disease, cardiac failure, and viral infections and is *decreased* in heavy cigarette smokers and drinkers. Theophylline is implicated as a culprit in many unwanted drug interactions. Its plasma concentration is decreased by drugs that increase P450 enzymes such as **rifampicin**, **phenobarbital**, **phenytoin** and **carbamazepine**; its serum concentration is increased by drugs that inhibit P450 enzymes such as **oral contraceptives**, **erythromycin**, **ciprofloxacin**, **calcium-channel blockers**, **fluconazole** and **cimetidine** (but not **ranitidine**). These factors should be borne in mind in view of the narrowness of the range of safe and effective therapeutic concentrations.

The clinical use of theophylline is summarised below.

Histamine H₁-receptor antagonists

Although mast cell mediators are thought to play a part in the immediate phase of allergic asthma (Fig. 19.3) and in some types of exercise-induced asthma, histamine H_1-receptor antagonists have had no place in therapy. Recently, clinical trials have shown that some newer, non-sedating antihistamines, such as **loratidine** (see p. 241) are moderately effective in mild atopic asthma.

Clinical use of theophylline

- As a second-line drug in asthma therapy, i.e. as an alternative, or in addition, to steroids and other anti-asthmatic agents in patients whose asthma does not respond adequately to β₂-adrenoceptor agonists.
- To reduce symptoms of chronic obstructive pulmonary disease.

Muscarinic-receptor antagonists

Muscarinic-receptor antagonists are dealt with in detail in Chapter 7. The main compound used specifically as an anti-asthmatic is **ipratropium**. Oxitropium is also available. Ipratropium relaxes bronchial constriction caused by parasympathetic stimulation; this occurs particularly in asthma produced by irritant stimuli (see p. 340) and can occur in allergic asthma.

Ipratropium is a quaternary derivative of N-isopropyl-atropine. It does not discriminate between muscarinic receptor subtypes (see Ch. 7), and it is possible that its blockade of M_2-autoreceptors on the cholinergic nerves increases acetylcholine release and reduces the effectiveness of its antagonism at the M_3-receptors on the smooth muscle. It is not particularly effective against allergen challenge but it inhibits the augmentation of mucus secretion which occurs in asthma and may increase the mucociliary clearance of bronchial secre-

---

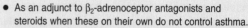

Clinical use of ipratropium bromide

- As an adjunct to β_2-adrenoceptor antagonists and steroids when these on their own do not control asthma.
- As a bronchodilator in some cases of chronic bronchitis, and in bronchospasm precipitated by β_2-adrenoceptor antagonists.

---

tions. It has no effect on the late inflammatory phase of asthma.

It is given by aerosol inhalation. It is not well absorbed into the circulation and thus does not have much action at muscarinic receptors other than those in the bronchi. The maximum effect occurs after 30 minutes or so, but then lasts for 3–5 hours. It has few unwanted effects and is, in general, safe and well tolerated. It can be used with β_2-adrenoceptor agonists.

DRUGS USED TO TREAT ASTHMA—ANTI-INFLAMMATORY AGENTS

Glucocorticoids

Glucocorticoids are dealt with in detail in Chapter 24 (p. 418). They are not bronchodilators and are not effective in the treatment of the immediate response to the eliciting agent. In the management of chronic asthma, in which there is a predominant inflammatory component, their efficacy is unequivocal.*

The basis of their anti-inflammatory action is discussed on page 419. An important action, of relevance for asthma, is that they decrease formation of cytokines (Fig. 12.3), in particular the Th2 cytokines that recruit and activate eosinophils and are responsible for promoting the production of IgE and the expression of IgE receptors (p. 342 above and Ch. 12). Glucocorticoids also inhibit the generation of the vasodilators, PGE_2 and PGI_2 by inhibiting of induction of cyclo-oxygenase-2 (Fig. 12.4). In addition, by virtue of inducing lipocortin, they may inhibit production of the spasmogens, LTC_4 and LTD_4, and decrease synthesis of the leukocyte chemotaxins, LTB_4 and PAF, thus reducing recruitment and activation of inflammatory cells (Fig. 12.4). Broncho-alveolar lavage studies have shown that they

---

Anti-asthma drugs—bronchodilators

- β_2-adrenoceptor agonists (e.g. salbutamol) are first-line drugs (for details see Ch. 8).
  - They act as physiological antagonists of the spasmogenic mediators, but have little or no effect on the bronchial hyper-reactivity.
  - Salbutamol is given by inhalation; its effects start immediately and last 3–5 h; it can also be given by intravenous infusion in status asthmaticus.
  - Salmeterol is given by inhalation; its duration of action is 12 h.
- Theophylline is a second-line drug.
  - It is a xanthine compound; the mechanism of action is uncertain but may be by inhibition of cyclic GMP- or cyclic AMP-phosphodiesterase.
  - It has a narrow therapeutic window; unwanted effects include chronotropic and inotropic effects on the heart, CNS stimulation and gastrointestinal disturbances.
  - It is given intravenously (by slow infusion) for status asthmaticus, or orally (as a sustained-release preparation) as a second-line treatment.
  - It is metabolised in the liver, and liver dysfunction and viral infections increase its plasma concentration and $t_{1/2}$ (normally 12 h with sustained-release preparation).
  - Drug interactions with theophylline are important, some (e.g. some antibiotics) increase the $t_{1/2}$, others (e.g. antiepileptic drugs) decrease it.
- Muscarinic-receptor antagonists (e.g. ipratropium bromide) are second-line drugs (see Ch. 7 for details).
  - Ipratropium bromide binds to all muscarinic receptor subtypes (M_1, M_2 and M_3); it inhibits acetylcholine-mediated bronchospasm. It is given by aerosol inhalation.

---

*In 1900, Solis-Cohen reported that dried bovine adrenals had anti-asthma action. He noted that the extract did not serve acutely 'to cut short the paroxysm' but was 'useful in averting recurrence of paroxysms'. Mistaken for the first report on the effect of adrenaline, his astute observation was probably the first on the efficacy of steroids in asthma (see Persson 1997).

inhibit the allergen-induced influx of eosinophils into the lung. Glucocorticoids can up-regulate β_2-adreno-ceptors, decrease microvascular permeability and reduce mediator release from eosinophils. The reduction in the synthesis of IL-3 (the cytokine that regulates mast cell production) may explain why *long-term* steroid treatment eventually reduces the early-phase response to allergens and prevents exercise-induced asthma.

The main compounds used are **beclomethasone**, **budesonide**, and **fluticasone** which are given by inhalation with a metered-dose inhaler, the full effect being attained only after several days of therapy.

For chronic asthma and severe or rapidly deteriorating asthma, a short course of an *oral* glucocorticoid (e.g. **prednisolone**) is indicated, combined with an inhaled steroid to reduce the oral dose required. In *status asthmaticus*, **hydrocortisone** is given intravenously followed by oral prednisolone.

Unwanted effects are uncommon with inhaled steroids. Oropharyngeal candidiasis, i.e. thrush (Ch. 45), can occur, as can dysphonia (voice problems), but these are less likely to occur if 'spacing' devices are used which decrease oropharyngeal deposition of the drug and increase airway deposition. Regular large doses can produce adrenal suppression, particularly in children, and necessitate the carrying of a 'steroid card'. The unwanted effects of oral glucocorticoids are given in Chapter 24, p. 423; these can sometimes occur with inhaled steroids if part of an inhaled dose is ingested. This is less likely with fluticasone as it has limited absorption from the gastrointestinal tract and undergoes almost complete first-pass metabolism.

Sodium cromoglycate

Sodium cromoglycate is unique in that it was first tested—and its efficacy demonstrated—in allergic asthma in humans, without prior testing in animals.

Actions and mechanisms of action

Sodium cromoglycate and the related drug, **nedocromil sodium**, are not bronchodilators; they do not have any direct effects on smooth muscle, nor do they inhibit the actions of any of the known smooth muscle stimulants. If given prophylactically they can reduce both the immediate and the late-phase asthmatic responses and reduce bronchial hyper-reactivity. They are effective in antigen-induced, exercise-induced and irritant-induced asthma, though not all asthmatic subjects respond, and it is not possible to predict which patients will benefit. Children are more likely to respond than adults.

The mechanism of action is not fully understood.

Cromoglycate was originally thought to act as a 'mast cell stabiliser', preventing histamine release from mast cells. However, although it has this effect it is clearly not the basis of its action in asthma because many other compounds have been produced which are equally or more potent than cromoglycate at inhibiting mast cell histamine release but none has proved to have any anti-asthmatic effect at all in humans.

There is evidence that cromoglycate depresses the exaggerated neuronal reflexes that are triggered by stimulation of the 'irritant receptors'; it suppresses the response of sensory C fibres to the irritant, capsaicin, and *may* inhibit the release of preformed T cell cytokines. Various other effects on the inflammatory cells and mediators involved in asthma have been described. (See review by Garland 1991.)

Pharmacokinetic aspects

Cromoglycate is extremely poorly absorbed from the gastrointestinal tract. It is given by inhalation as an aerosol, as a nebulised solution or in powder form; about 10% is absorbed into the circulation when it is given in this way. It is excreted unchanged—50% in the bile and 50% in the urine. Its half-life in the plasma is 90 minutes.

Nedocromil is also given by inhalation and is rather better absorbed.

Unwanted effects

Unwanted effects are few and consist mostly of the effects of irritation in the upper respiratory tract. Hypersensitivity reactions have been reported (urticaria, anaphylaxis), but are rare.

SEVERE ACUTE ASTHMA (STATUS ASTHMATICUS)

Severe acute asthma is a medical emergency requiring hospitalisation. Treatment includes oxygen, inhalation of **salbutamol** in oxygen given by nebuliser, and intravenous **hydrocortisone** followed by a course of oral **prednisolone**. Additional measures include nebulised **ipratropium**, **intravenous salbutamol** or **aminophylline** and **antibiotics** (if bacterial infection is present).

POSSIBLE FUTURE STRATEGIES FOR ASTHMA THERAPY

Of the currently used anti-asthmatic drugs, none is ideal in that none actually 'cures' all patients by eliminating the underlying inflammation and bronchial hyper-reactivity. The glucocorticoids are the most active in this regard but they have potentially serious unwanted effects. Ideally what are required are new anti-inflammatory

---

Anti-asthma drugs—anti-inflammatory agents

Glucocorticoids (for details see Ch. 24)

- These reduce the inflammatory component in chronic asthma and are life-saving in *status asthmaticus* (acute severe asthma).
- They are not effective in the treatment of the immediate response to the eliciting agent.
- The mechanism of action involves decreased formation of cytokines, particularly those generated by Th2 lymphocytes (see Key Points Box on p. 423), decreased activation of eosinophils and other inflammatory cells, and decreased formation of prostaglandins and possibly of PAF, LTC$_4$ and LTD$_4$ (see Fig. 12.4).
- They are given by inhalation (e.g. beclomethasone); systemic unwanted effects are rare, but oral thrush and voice problems can occur. In deteriorating asthma, an oral glucocorticoid (e.g. prednisolone) or intravenous hydrocortisone is also given.

Sodium cromoglycate

- Given prophylactically this can prevent both phases of asthma and reduce bronchial hyper-responsiveness in many but not all patients. Children are more likely to respond than adults.
- The mechanism of action is uncertain. Depression of release of neuropeptides, antagonism of tachykinin receptors, inhibition of cytokine release and inhibition of PAF interaction with platelets and eosinophils may be important; mast cell stabilisation is not.
- It is given by inhalation and acts locally. 10% is absorbed; it is excreted unchanged.
- Unwanted effects are minor respiratory tract irritation and (rarely) hypersensitivity.

---

agents that are active by the oral route and that do not have the drawbacks of steroid drugs.

Several potentially useful compounds are in development.

New bronchodilators

Cysteinyl leukotriene (CystLT)-receptor antagonists. Note that LTC$_4$, LTD$_4$ and LTE$_4$ act on the same CystLT-receptor (see Chs 12 and 13). Several CystLT-receptor antagonists are in clinical trial; these may prove to be one of the most effective anti-asthmatic treatments yet. **Zafirlukast** (who thinks up these names?) has received FDA approval in the USA and **pranlucast** has been approved for treatment of asthma in Japan, both drugs being orally active. Others in clinical trial are **cinalukast** and **montelucast**.*

Zafirlukast is a potent competitive antagonist at the LTD$_4$-receptor. It prevents aspirin-sensitive asthma as

---

*The full montelukast?

well as antigen-induced and exercise-induced bronchospasm. It relaxes the airways in mild asthma, its bronchodilator activity being one-third that of salbutamol. Its effects are additive with β_2-adrenoceptor agonists and its eventual role may be in combination therapy with these drugs, particularly in aspirin-sensitive asthmatic subjects.

5-lipoxygenase inhibitors. Several 5-lipoxygenase inhibitors are in clinical trial. These agents prevent the production of not only the spasmogenic leukotrienes LTC$_4$ and LTD$_4$, but also LTB$_4$, a chemotaxin that recruits leukocytes into the bronchial mucosa and then activates them (see Ch. 12). **Zileutin** is the prototype compound. It blocks antigen- and exercise-induced bronchospasm and may inhibit or reduce late phase inflammation. It is given orally but has low potency and is short-lived, necessitating large doses three to four times daily. Other similar compounds which are more potent and longer-acting are in the pipeline. Also under investigation are agents with 5-lipoxygenase inhibitory activity by virtue of an action on FLAP—the **f**ive **l**ipoxygenase **a**ctivating **p**rotein—a membrane protein with which the enzyme needs to be associated in order to act on arachidonate (see Ch. 12).

New cyclic nucleotide phosphodiesterase inhibitors. An increase in intracellular cyclic AMP reduces not only smooth muscle contraction but the activation of inflammatory and immune cells. Agents that specifically inhibit the phosphodiesterase (PDE) isoenzymes that convert cyclic AMP to 5'AMP could be potent anti-asthmatic drugs. There are seven families of PDE isoenzymes, PDE4 being of particular importance in neutrophils, eosinophils, mast cells and basophils, and PDE3 in monocytes/macrophages and lymphocytes. Theophylline is a non-selective inhibitor of the PDE enzymes. A prodigious amount of experimental work is currently underway to develop selective PDE4 inhibitors as anti-asthma agents. At least two are in phase II clinical trial and one is in phase III trial. See Texeira et al. 1997.

It has recently become clear that there are at least six subtypes of PDE4 selectively regulated and expressed in different cell types and that chronic activation of inflammatory cells is associated with modulation of the number and activity of these subtypes.

DRUGS USED FOR COUGH

Cough is a protective reflex mechanism that removes foreign material and secretions from the bronchi and bronchioles. It can be inappropriately stimulated by inflammation in the respiratory tract or neoplasia. In these cases *antitussive* (or cough suppressant) drugs are sometimes used, for example for the dry painful cough associated with bronchial carcinoma or with inflammation of the pleura. It should be understood that these drugs merely suppress the symptom without influencing the underlying condition. In cough associated with bronchiectasis (suppurating bronchial inflammation) or chronic bronchitis, antitussive drugs can cause harmful sputum thickening and retention. They should not be used for the cough associated with asthma.

Antitussive drugs act by an ill-defined effect in the brainstem, depressing an even more poorly defined 'cough centre'. The **narcotic analgesics** (see Ch. 37) have effective antitussive action in doses below those required for pain relief, and various isomers of these agents, that are neither analgesic nor addictive, are also effective against cough. New opioid analogues, that suppress cough by inhibiting release of excitatory neuropeptides through an action on μ-receptors (see Table 37.2) on sensory nerves in the bronchi, are being assessed.

Codeine

Codeine, or methylmorphine, is an opiate (see Ch. 37) that has considerably less addiction liability than the main opioid analgesics and is an effective cough suppressant. However, it also decreases secretions in the bronchioles, which thickens sputum, and inhibits ciliary activity, which reduces clearance of the thickened sputum. Constipation also occurs because of the well-known action of opiates on the gastrointestinal tract (see Chs 21 and 37).

Dextromethorphan

Dextromethorphan is related to levorphanol, a synthetic narcotic analgesic. Its antitussive potency is equivalent to that of codeine and it produces only marginally less constipation and inhibition of mucociliary clearance.

Pholcodine, which is a non-analgesic opiate of the same chemical class as papaverine, is also used as a cough suppressant.

ADULT RESPIRATORY DISTRESS SYNDROME

The adult respiratory distress syndrome is a serious disease of the lungs which has a 60% mortality. It affects 150 000 individuals in the USA each year. It is characterised by pulmonary arterial hypertension with vasoconstriction. There is extensive injury and occlusion of the pulmonary microvasculature resulting in oedema and progressive hypoxia. Multi-organ dysfunction follows. Its causes are many and varied: direct injury to the lungs (pneumonia, aspiration of gastric contents, inhalation of toxic chemicals) or systemic disorders (sepsis, drug reactions). A variety of inflammatory mediators are involved in the microvascular damage and neutrophils are known to play a significant part through the generation of toxic oxygen radicals and the release of elastase. There is a pool of marginated neutrophils in the lung which may be of relevance here. Early clinical studies suggest that inhalation of **nitric oxide** could be beneficial (see p. 196).

REFERENCES AND FURTHER READING

Anderson G P, Coyle A J 1994 T_H2 and 'T_H2-like' cells in asthma: pharmacological perspectives. Trends Pharmacol Sci 15: 324–331

Barnes P J 1996 NO or no NO in asthma? Thorax 51: 218–220 (*The possible role of nitric oxide in asthma*)

Bertrand C, Geppetti P 1998 Tachykinin and kinin receptor antagonists: therapeutic perspectives in allergic airway disease. Trends Pharmacol Sci 17: 255–259 (*New approach to asthma pathophysiology*)

British Thoracic Society et al. 1997 The British guidelines on asthma management. Thorax 52 (suppl): S1–S21 (*Important precepts for asthma treatment*)

Chauhan A J, Krishna M T, Holgate S 1996 Aetiology of asthma. Mol Med Today (May): 192–197 (*Valuable analysis of asthma aetiology*)

Cockroft D W, McParland C P et al. 1993 Regular inhaled salbutamol and airway responsiveness to allergen. Lancet 342: 833–837

Corrigan C J, Kay A B 1992 T cells and eosinophils in the pathogenesis of asthma. Immunol Today 13: 501–507 (*Initiation of inflammation by activated T cells; and the role of eosinophils*)

Dale M M, Hirst S J 1993 Advances in receptor biochemistry. In: Weiss E B, Stein M S 1993 (eds) Bronchial asthma: mechanisms and therapeutics, 3rd edn. Little Brown, Boston, ch 16, pp 203–216 (*Covers signal-transduction mechanisms in smooth muscle*)

Drazen J M, Gaston B, Shore S A 1995 Chemical regulation of airway tone. Annu Rev Physiol 57: 151–170 (*Review covering cysteinyl leukotrienes, neuropeptides and nitrogen oxides*)

Garland L G 1991 Pharmacology of prophylactic anti-asthma drugs. In: Page C P, Barnes P J (eds) Handbook of experimental pharmacology. Springer-Verlag, Berlin, vol 98, ch 9, pp 261–290 (*Commendable review*)

Hall I P 1997 The future of asthma. Br Med J 314: 45–49 (*Thought-provoking article on future developments in therapy*)

Hamid Q, Sprongall D R et al. 1993 Induction of nitric oxide synthase in asthma. Lancet 342: 1510–1513

Hay D P, Torphy T J, Undem B J 1995 Cysteinyl leukotrienes in asthma: old mediators up to new tricks. Trends Pharmacol Sci 16: 304–309 (*Discusses role in asthma and lists potential new compounds*)

Holgate S 1993 Mediator and cytokine mechanisms in asthma. Thorax 48: 103–109

Johnson S R, Knox A J 1997 Synthetic functions of smooth muscle in asthma. Trends Pharmacol Sci 18: 288–292

Kollef M H, Schuster D P 1995 The acute respiratory distress syndrome. N Engl J Med 332: 27–37

McFadden E R, Gilbert I A 1994 Exercise-induced asthma. N Engl J Med 330: 1362–1366 *(Effective coverage)*

McGill K A, Busse W W 1996 Zileutin. Lancet 348: 519–523 *(Drug profile)*

Nelson H S 1995 β-adrenergic bronchodilators. N Engl J Med 333: 499–506 *(Worthwhile)*

Nicholson C D, Shahid M 1994 Inhibitors of cyclic nucleotide phosphodiesterase isoenzymes—their potential utility in the therapy of asthma. Pulmonary Pharmacol 7: 1–17 *(Edifying, comprehensive)*

Page C 1994 Sodium cromoglycate, a tachykinin antagonist? Lancet 343: 70

Pauwels R A 1989 New aspects of the therapeutic potential of theophylline in asthma. J Allergy Clin Immunol 83: 548–553

Persson C G A 1997 Centenial notions of asthma as an eosinophilic, desquamative, exudative, and steroid-sensitive disease. Lancet 349: 1021–1024

Richardson P J 1997 Asthma: blocking adenosine with antisense. Nature 385: 684–685 *(Possible new approach to therapy)*

Rosenwasser L J 1997 Interleukin-4 and the genetics of atopy. N Engl J Med 337: 1766–1767 *(Editorial comment)*

Salmon J A, Garland L G 1991 Leukotriene antagonists and inhibitors of leukotriene biosynthesis as potential therapeutic agents. Prog Drug Res 37: 10–80

Spina D, Landells L J, Page C P 1998 The role of phosphodiesterase enzymes in allergy and asthma. Adv in Pharmacol volume 44 *(Excellent, up-to-date review)*

Texeira M M, Gristwood R W et al. 1997 Phosphodiesterase (PDE)4 inhibitors: anti-inflammatory drugs of the future. Trends Pharmacol Sci 18: 164–170 *(Thought-provoking review)*

Venables K M, Chan-Yeung M 1997 Occupational asthma. Lancet 349: 1465–1468 *(Succinct coverage)*

Weinberger M E, Hendeles L 1996 Theophylline in asthma. N Engl J Med 334: 1380–1388 *(Addresses the possible role of theophylline in asthma therapy)*

Weiss E B, Stein M S 1993 (eds) Bronchial asthma: mechanisms and therapeutics, 3rd edn. Little Brown, Boston, pp 1256 *(Substantial coverage; 95 chapters by different authors working on asthma)*

20

The kidney

The main function of the kidney is the excretion of waste products such as urea, uric acid and creatinine. In the course of this activity it fulfils another function, crucially important in homeostasis—the regulation of the salt and electrolyte content and the volume of the extracellular fluid. It also plays a part in acid–base balance.

The kidneys receive about a quarter of the cardiac output. From the several hundred litres of plasma which flow through them each day, they filter an amount equivalent to about 15 times the extracellular fluid volume. This filtrate is similar in composition to plasma, the main difference being that it has very little protein or protein-bound substances. As it passes through the renal tubule, about 99% of it is reabsorbed while some substances are secreted, and eventually about 1.5 litres of the filtered fluid are voided as urine (Table 20.1).

The most important group of drugs employed for their effect on the kidney are the **diuretics**. In essence, these drugs increase the excretion of salt and water. They are employed mainly in the therapy of heart failure and other causes of salt and water retention (often manifested clinically as oedema, a condition in which there is an accumulation of extracellular fluid); but have another important use in the treatment of hypertension (see Ch. 15).

Drugs may also be used to alter the pH of the urine and to modify the excretion of some organic compounds such as uric acid.

Table 20.1   Reabsorption of fluid and solute in the kidney*

	Filtered/day	Excreted/day[†]	% reabsorbed
Na^+ (mEq)	25 000	150	99+
K^+ (mEq)	600	90	93+
Cl^- (mEq)	18 000	150	99+
HCO_3^- (mEq)	4900	0	100
Total solute (mosm)	54 000	700	87
H_2O (litres)	180	~1.5	99+

Renal blood flow = 1200 ml/min (20–25% of cardiac output); renal plasma flow = 660 ml/min; glomerular filtration rate = 125 ml/min[‡]

*Adapted from: Ganong W F 1993 Review of medical physiology, 16th edn. Prentice-Hall, London, p 774
†These are typical figures for an individual eating a western diet. The kidney excretes more or less of each of these substances to maintain the constancy of the internal milieu, so on a low-sodium diet (for instance) NaCl excretion may be reduced to as low as 20 mmol/day.
‡Typical values for a healthy young adult

In structure, each kidney consists of an outer cortex, an inner medulla and a hollow pelvis which empties into the ureter. The functional unit is the nephron, of which there are about 1.3×10^6 in each kidney.

THE STRUCTURE AND FUNCTION OF THE NEPHRON

The nephron consists of a glomerulus, proximal convoluted tubule, loop of Henle, distal tubule and collecting duct (Fig. 20.1). The glomerulus comprises a tuft of capillaries projecting into a dilated end of the renal tubule. Most nephrons lie largely or entirely in the cortex. The remaining 12%, called the juxtamedullary nephrons, have their glomeruli and convoluted tubules next to the junction of the medulla and cortex, and their loops of Henle pass deep into the medulla.

The blood supply to the nephron

The nephron possesses the special characteristic of having two capillary beds in series with each other (see Fig. 20.1). For those nephrons which lie entirely in the cortex, the afferent arterioles branch to form the capillaries of the glomerulus; these empty into the efferent arterioles which in turn branch to form a second capillary network in the cortex, around the convoluted tubules and loops of Henle, before emptying into the veins. In the case of the juxtamedullary nephrons, some of the branches of the afferent arterioles bypass the convoluted tubules, and instead form bundles of vessels which pass deep into the medulla with the thin loops of Henle. These loops of vessels are called *vasa recta* and they have a role in counter-current exchange (see p. 357).

The juxtaglomerular apparatus

A conjunction of afferent arteriole, efferent arteriole and distal convoluted tubule near the glomerulus comprises the *juxtaglomerular apparatus* (Fig. 20.2). At this site there are specialised cells in both the afferent arteriole and in the tubule. The latter, termed *macula densa* cells, respond to changes in the rate of flow and the composition of tubule fluid, and control renin release from the specialised granular renin-containing cells in the afferent arteriole (Ch. 15). The juxtaglomerular apparatus is important in controlling the blood flow to the nephron and the glomerular filtration rate. Factors extrinsic to the kidney can influence these processes through circulating hormones and through noradrenergic sympathetic fibres which supply the afferent and efferent arterioles and the specialised cells. They will thus influence the generation of angiotensin I and II. The role of the juxtaglomerular

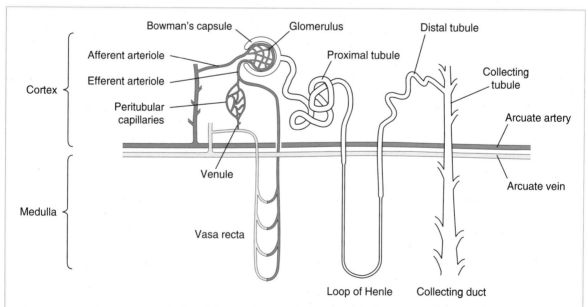

Fig. 20.1 Simplified diagram of a juxtamedullary nephron and its blood supply. The tubules and the blood vessels are shown separately for clarity. In the kidney the peritubular capillary network surrounds the convoluted tubules, and the distal convoluted tubule passes close to the glomerulus, between the afferent and efferent arterioles. (This last is shown in more detail in Fig. 20.2.)

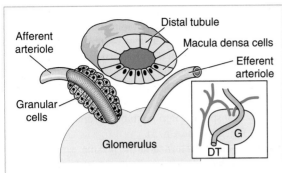

Fig. 20.2 The juxtaglomerular apparatus. The cutaway sections show the granular renin-containing cells round the afferent arteriole, and the *macula densa* cells in the distal convoluted tubule. The inset shows the general relationships between the structures. (G = glomerulus; DT = distal tubule) (Modified from: Sullivan & Grantham 1982)

apparatus in the control of sodium balance is dealt with below, and its role in cardiovascular dynamics is considered in Chapter 15.

Glomerular filtration

Fluid is driven from the capillaries into the tubular capsule (Bowman's capsule) by hydrodynamic force. It crosses three layers: the capillary endothelium, the basement membrane, and the epithelial cell layer of the capsule. These form a complex filter which excludes large molecules. Normally, all constituents in the plasma, except the plasma proteins, appear in the filtrate, and the blood which passes on through the efferent arteriole to the peritubular capillaries has a higher concentration of plasma proteins and thus a higher oncotic pressure than normal. (The term 'oncotic pressure' refers to osmotic pressure contributed by large molecules such as the plasma proteins.)

TUBULAR FUNCTION

In the epithelium of the tubules, as in all epithelia, the apex or luminal surface of each cell is surrounded by a *zonula occludens*, a specialised region of membrane which forms a tight junction between it and neighbouring cells, and which separates the intercellular space from the lumen (see Fig. 20.10). The movement of ions and water across the epithelium can occur both through the cells (the transcellular pathway) and between the cells through the *zonulae occludentes* (the paracellular pathway). The *zonulae* in different parts of the nephron vary in their degree of functional tightness, i.e. their relative

permeability to ions. The tightness or leakiness of the epithelium of various portions of the nephron is an important factor in their function (see Taylor & Palmer 1982). Tight epithelium is found in the distal portion of the nephron, which is the site of action of the major hormones involved in the control of salt and water excretion.

Normally, 70–75% of the volume of the filtrate is absorbed back into the blood in the proximal convoluted tubule, with virtually no change in the sodium concentration or the osmotic pressure of the remaining tubular fluid. In the rest of the renal tubule the electrolyte concentrations and osmotic pressure of the filtrate vary a great deal owing to differential absorption of salt and water and the effects of the antidiuretic hormone (ADH), mineralocorticoids and the counter-current system in the medulla.

A detailed account of the renal handling of sodium, chloride, water, amino acids and glucose is given by Burg (1985).

The proximal convoluted tubule

The apical (luminal) surface of the cells of this part of the tubule is extensively increased by numerous microvilli, forming a brush border, and the surface area is further increased by numerous ridges and folds (Fig. 20.3). The epithelium is 'leaky', i.e. the *zonula occludens* is permeable to ions and water and permits passive flows in either direction. This prevents the build-up of significant ionic or osmotic gradients; separate regulation of the movements of ions and water occurs mainly in the distal part of the tubule.

Some of the transport processes in the proximal tubule are shown in Figure 20.4 and below in Figure 20.14.

About 60–70% of the sodium in the filtrate is reabsorbed in the proximal tubule. It enters the cells passively through the sodium-permeable apical membrane, and is

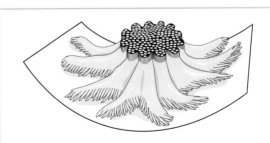

Fig. 20.3 Simplified three-dimensional reconstruction of a cell in the proximal convoluted tubule. (Modified from: Sullivan & Grantham 1982)

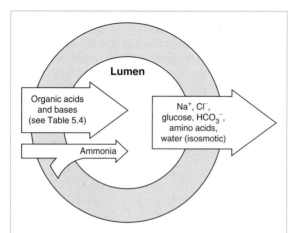

Fig. 20.4 The main transport processes in the proximal convoluted tubule. The main driving force for the absorption of solutes and water from the lumen is the Na^+/K^+-ATPase in the basolateral membrane of the tubule cells. Many drugs are secreted into the proximal tubule (see Ch. 5). (Redrawn from: Burg 1985)

transported out by *the primary active transport mechanism in the nephron*—the Na^+/K^+-ATPase (the sodium pump) in the basolateral membrane. Some sodium enters in exchange for hydrogen ions.

Water is reabsorbed as a result of the osmotic force generated by this solute reabsorption, the increased oncotic pressure in the peritubular capillaries contributing to this effect.

The movement of sodium into the cell is coupled to that of other solutes by various *symport* systems.* *Glucose* enters the cell with sodium by such a symport process, the co-transport being driven by the electrochemical gradient for sodium across the apical membrane. There are similar symport processes for various *amino acids* with sodium. It is assumed that in these symport systems there is a two-site carrier in the membrane with one site for sodium and one for glucose or an amino acid. On the luminal side, where the concentration of sodium is high, sodium combines with its specific site and this increases the affinity of the other site for the other solute. Re-orientation of the binding sites to the inner side of the membrane, where the sodium

---

*In a symport or co-transport system, the transport of one substance is coupled to that of another, both being transported across a membrane in the same direction, as opposed to an antiport system in which two substances are exchanged with each other across a membrane.

concentration is low, favours dissociation of the sodium and consequently of the other solute.

Atrial natriuretic peptide (Ch. 14) reduces reabsorption of sodium and water in the proximal tubule.

Chloride absorption is largely passive. Some diffuses through the *zonula occludens*.

Many organic acids and bases are actively secreted by specific transporters into the tubule from the blood (see below, Fig. 20.4 and Ch. 5).

Bicarbonate is returned to the plasma—mainly in the proximal tubule—by an indirect method involving the action of carbonic anhydrase (for detail see Fig. 20.14). Drugs, such as acetazolamide, which inhibit carbonic anhydrase, increase the volume of urine flow (i.e. are diuretic) by preventing bicarbonate reabsorption (Figs 20.5 and 20.14). They also result in a depletion of extracellular bicarbonate.

After passage through the proximal tubule, the remaining 25–30% of the filtrate, which is still isosmotic with plasma, passes on to the loop of Henle.

The loop of Henle

The loop of Henle plays an important part in regulating the osmolarity of the urine, and hence in regulating the osmotic balance of the body as a whole. Its function is summarised in Figure 20.6. The loop consists of a descending and an ascending portion (Figs 20.1 and 20.6), the ascending portion having both thick and thin segments.

The *descending* limb is highly permeable to water, which moves out passively under the influence of osmotic forces. These forces arise because the interstitial fluid of the medulla is hypertonic (see below and p. 357). In juxtamedullary nephrons with long loops, there is extensive movement of water out of the tubule (and also movement of urea in) so that the fluid eventually reaching the tip of the loop has a high osmolarity—up to 1500 mosmol/l under conditions of dehydration.

The *ascending* limb has very low permeability to water. In the thick segment of this limb, there is active reabsorption of sodium chloride, not accompanied by water, which reduces the osmolarity of the tubular fluid and makes the interstitial fluid of the medulla hypertonic (Figs 20.5 and 20.6). Sodium and chloride move into the cell by a co-transport system involving $Na^+/K^+/2Cl^-$, this process being driven by the electrochemical gradient for sodium produced by the Na^+/K^+-ATPase in the basolateral membrane. **Loop diuretics** inhibit this process as shown in Figures 20.5 and 20.10. Chloride then passes out of the cell into the circulation, partly by diffusion through chloride channels and partly by a symport

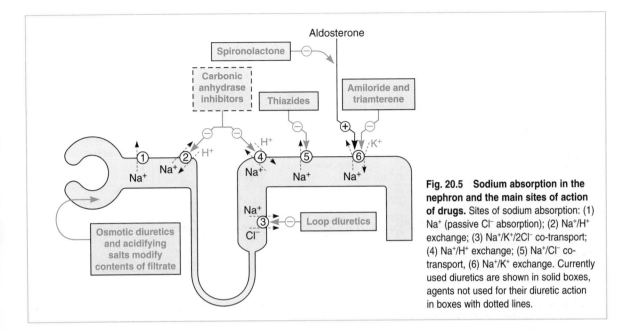

Fig. 20.5 Sodium absorption in the nephron and the main sites of action of drugs. Sites of sodium absorption: (1) Na^+ (passive Cl^- absorption); (2) Na^+/H^+ exchange; (3) $Na^+/K^+/2Cl^-$ co-transport; (4) Na^+/H^+ exchange; (5) Na^+/Cl^- co-transport, (6) Na^+/K^+ exchange. Currently used diuretics are shown in solid boxes, agents not used for their diuretic action in boxes with dotted lines.

mechanism with potassium (see Fig. 20.10). Most of the potassium taken into the cell by the co-transport system cycles back to the lumen but some potassium is reabsorbed along with magnesium and calcium.

The tubular fluid, after passage through the loop of Henle, has been reduced in volume by a further 5% and, because of the absorption of salt, it is hypotonic with respect to plasma as it enters the distal convoluted tubule. The thick ascending limb of the loop of Henle is sometimes referred to as the 'diluting segment' because the absorption of salt with very little water results in this marked dilution of the filtrate.

The early distal tubule

In the early distal tubule, active salt transport, coupled with impermeability of the *zonula occludens*, continues to dilute the tubular fluid and the osmolarity falls further below that of plasma. Potassium and hydrogen ions are added to the filtrate. The transport is driven by the sodium–potassium pump in the basolateral membrane, sodium entering the cell from the lumen, accompanied by chloride by means of an electroneutral Na^+/Cl^- carrier (Fig. 20.12). **Thiazide diuretics** act by inhibiting this carrier.

This part of the nephron is where calcium excretion is regulated. Parathyroid hormone and calcitriol both increase calcium reabsorption (see Ch. 27).

The collecting tubule and the collecting duct

Several distal tubules empty into each collecting tubule and the collecting tubules join to form collecting ducts (see Fig. 20.1). The collecting tubule has two different cell types: the principal cells that reabsorb sodium and secrete potassium and the intercalated cells that are involved mainly in hydrogen ion secretion. The principal cells have sodium and potassium *channels*, not co-transporters, in the luminal membrane.

This portion of the nephron has 'tight' junctions between the cells, i.e. the *zona occludens* has low permeability to both ions and water. Because of this property, the movement of ions and water can be dissociated and individual regulation of each can be influenced by hormones. The absorption of salt is under the control of the mineralocorticoid, **aldosterone**, and the absorption of water is under the control of the **antidiuretic hormone** (ADH), also termed **vasopressin** (see Chs 15 and 24).

Aldosterone enhances sodium reabsorption and promotes potassium excretion. It has a threefold action on sodium reabsorption. Firstly, according to recent work, it has a rapid effect through stimulation of the Na^+/H^+ exchanger by an action on membrane aldosterone receptors.* Secondly, it has a delayed effect by binding

---

*A mechanism distinct from regulation of gene transcription which is the normal transduction mechanism for steroid hormones.

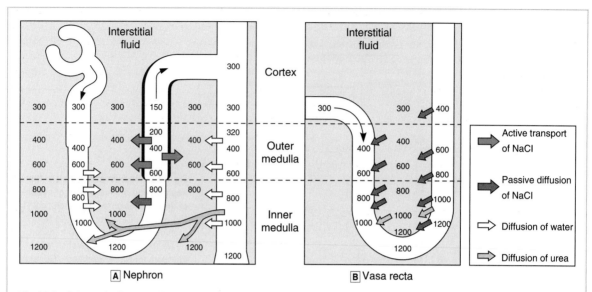

Fig. 20.6 Schematic diagram of the counter-current mechanisms for concentrating the urine. (The figures are in milliosmoles per litre.) A Renal tubules. B Vasa recta.
The main factors are:

- A counter-current multiplier mechanism involving the tubules and a counter-current exchange mechanism involving the vasa recta.
- A source of energy, which is supplied by the sodium pump and the active transport of sodium chloride in the ascending loop of Henle. (Loop diuretics act by inhibiting this active transport, thus interfering with the counter-current concentrating mechanism.)
- Differences in permeability between tubules carrying fluid in opposite directions. The thickened outline of the ascending limb of Henle's loop indicates decreased permeability to water in contrast to the water-permeable descending loop.
- Diffusion of salt into the vessels taking blood down into the medulla, and out of vessels passing back up to the cortex, maintaining hypertonicity in the medulla.

The absorption of water in the collecting ducts is controlled by the antidiuretic hormone. Additional active reabsorption of sodium chloride occurs in the distal tubule and is controlled by aldosterone.

to receptors within the cell (see Chs 2 and 24) and directing the synthesis of a specific mediator protein that activates sodium channels in the apical membrane which allow transcellular passage of sodium. **Amiloride** and **triamterene** inhibit these channels as shown in Figures 20.5 and 20.13. Thirdly it exerts long-term effects by increasing the number of basolateral sodium pumps.

Aldosterone secretion is controlled indirectly by the juxtaglomerular apparatus (see Fig. 20.2) which is sensitive to the composition of the fluid in the distal tubule. A decrease in the sodium chloride concentration of the filtrate is sensed by the *macula densa* cells of the distal tubule, which stimulate renin release. This leads to the formation of angiotensin I and, subsequently, angiotensin II (see Ch. 15), which in turn stimulates the synthesis and release of aldosterone by the adrenal cortex. The renin–angiotensin system and the mechanism of action of aldosterone are considered in more detail in Chapters 15 (p. 290) and 24 (p. 425). **Spironolactone** exerts a

diuretic effect by antagonising the action of aldosterone in this part of the nephron; shown in Figures 20.5 and 20.13.

Antidiuretic hormone (ADH) produces a sustained increase in the permeability to water in this part of the nephron, allowing its passive reabsorption. This hormone is secreted by the posterior pituitary gland (Ch. 24) and binds to receptors in the basolateral membrane. These receptors, which are different from those involved in vascular responses (p. 287), are termed V_2-receptors.

The eventual result of stimulation of the V_2-receptors is an increase in the number of aquaporins (water channels) in the apical membrane.*

An inhibition of the action of ADH occurs as a

*Six aquaporins have been identified in mammalian cells. The channel in the apical membrane that allows water into the cell is aquaporin 2; aquaporins 3 and 4 are located in the basolateral membrane.

side-effect of some drugs—**lithium carbonate** (used in psychiatric disorders; see Ch. 35), **demeclocycline** (an antibiotic; see Ch. 43) and agents which affect the microtubules, such as **colchicine** (Ch. 13) and the **vinca alkaloids** (see Ch. 42).

Urea is reabsorbed from the medullary section of the collecting tubule, and passes into the interstitial tissue where it plays a part in increasing the osmolarity of this area (see Fig. 20.6).

The main site at which the urine is concentrated is in the collecting tubule as it passes into the medulla where there is passive reabsorption of water due to the increasing osmolarity of the interstitial fluid. This absorption depends on ADH, and in its absence, the low water permeability of the collecting ducts means that the hypo-osmolarity of the distal tubular fluid is maintained as the fluid traverses the collecting ducts, and a large volume of hypotonic urine is excreted.

Natriuretic peptides

Endogenous natriuretic peptides are involved in the regulation of sodium excretion in the distal nephron. The atrial natriuretic peptide (see Ch. 14) is released when the arterial pressure is high. It causes solute and water diuresis, thus decreasing blood volume and therefore reducing atrial pressure. This peptide also inhibits the biosynthesis of renin, aldosterone and ADH (reviewed by Cogan 1990). Another peptide, similar to atriopeptin and termed urodilatin, is now thought to be produced in the distal tubule and is believed to promote sodium excretion and produce diuresis by action on receptors on the luminal side of the collecting duct cells.

The counter-current multiplier and exchange system in the medulla

The loops of Henle function as counter-current multipliers and the *vasa recta* as counter-current exchangers. In the ascending limb, salt is actively absorbed in the thick part and passively absorbed in the thin part. *This results in hypertonicity of the interstitial tissue.* In the descending limb, water moves out of the tubule and the fluid becomes more concentrated as it reaches the bend. There is thus an osmotic gradient in the medulla which ranges from isotonicity (300 mosmol/l) at the cortical boundary to 1200–1500 mosmol/l or more in the innermost area (see Fig. 20.6). Urea contributes to this gradient because it is more slowly reabsorbed than water throughout most of the nephron (it may be *added* to the fluid in the descending limb; Fig. 20.6) and so its concentration rises until it reaches the collecting tubules in the medulla where it diffuses out into the interstitia. It is thus 'trapped' in the inner medulla.

These differences in salt concentration are the basis of the counter-current multiplier system, the main principle being that a small horizontal osmotic gradient is multiplied vertically (see Fig. 20.6). The primary generating force is the active reabsorption of salt in the ascending limb of the loop of Henle.

The osmotic gradient would be dissipated if all the excess salt in the medulla were carried away by the blood vessels. This does not happen because the vasa recta function as counter-current exchangers in that salt diffuses passively out of the vessels which take blood to the cortex and into those which descend into the medulla (Fig. 20.6), while water diffuses out of the descending and into the ascending vessels.

> **Renal tubular function**
>
> - All the constituents of the plasma, other than proteins, are filtered into the tubules.
> - Transport of sodium out of the tubules by the Na^+/K^+-ATPase in the basolateral membrane is the main primary active transport process throughout the tubules.
> - In the proximal tubules, 75% of the filtrate is reabsorbed isosmotically and organic acids and bases are secreted into the tubular lumen.
> - In the descending limb of Henle's loop, water is reabsorbed owing to hypertonicity in the medulla; fluid of high osmolarity therefore reaches the thick ascending limb.
> - The thick ascending limb is impermeable to water, and within it there is active, marked reabsorption of NaCl (the major factor in producing hypertonicity in the medulla). The ions are transported by a $Na^+/2Cl^-/K^+$ carrier (inhibited by loop diuretics). The filtrate is diluted.
> - Counter-current mechanisms maintain hypertonicity in the medulla.
> - In the distal convoluted tubule there is moderate absorption of Na^+ and Cl^- by an electroneutral carrier (inhibited by thiazides). K^+ is secreted into the tubule.
> - The collecting tubules and ducts have low permeability to salts and water. Na^+ is absorbed through Na^+ channels, which are stimulated by the aldosterone mediator (and inhibited by amiloride). Aldosterone also increases the number of basolateral sodium pumps. Water absorption through water channels is stimulated by antidiuretic hormone. K^+ and H^+ are secreted into the tubule.

ACID–BASE BALANCE

The kidneys participate in the regulation of the hydrogen ion concentration of the body fluids. Though either an acid or alkaline urine can be excreted according to need, the usual requirement is the formation of an acid urine to compensate for the tendency to a decrease in body pH consequent on the metabolic production of CO_2. The compensating renal mechanism is the secretion of hydrogen ions into the tubular fluid and the conservation of bicarbonate. This depends on the carbonic-anhydrase-catalysed reactions illustrated in Figure 20.14.

POTASSIUM BALANCE

The extracellular potassium concentration is controlled rapidly and within narrow limits through regulation of potassium excretion by the kidney. This regulation is very important because small changes in extracellular [K^+] affect the function of many excitable tissues, particularly the heart, brain and skeletal muscle. Urinary potassium excretion is normally about 50–100 mEq in 24 hours, but can be as low as 5 mEq or as high as 1000 mEq. The amount which normally appears in the urine represents mainly potassium secreted into the filtrate in the collecting tubule, as much of the filtered potassium is reabsorbed in the proximal tubule and loop of Henle. Some diuretics cause significant potassium loss (see below). This may be particularly important if such potassium-losing agents are administered at the same time as cardiac glycosides or class II antidysrhythmic drugs (whose toxicity is increased by low plasma potassium; see Ch. 14).

In the collecting duct, potassium is transported into the cell from the blood and the interstitial fluid by the Na^+/K^+-ATPase in the basolateral membrane; it then leaks into the tubule through a selective ion channel. This potassium secretory flux is regulated by the extent to which sodium is re-absorbed, because the influx of sodium into the cell through sodium channels down the electrochemical gradient created by the basolateral sodium pump results in depolarisation of the luminal but not the basolateral membrane. This generates a lumen-negative potential difference across the cell and this increases the driving force for potassium secretion.

It follows that potassium loss will be *increased* in the following circumstances:

- When more sodium reaches the collecting duct—as occurs with the **thiazide** and **loop diuretics**, which decrease sodium absorption in earlier parts of the nephron and therefore increase its delivery to the collecting ducts (see pp. 363 and 361). (The high

flow rate of filtrate produced by these diuretics will also favour potassium excretion by continually flushing it away, increasing the gradient from cell to lumen.)
- When sodium reabsorption in the collecting ducts is markedly increased—as occurs in hyperaldosteronism. Aldosterone indirectly increases potassium excretion because of its stimulant effect on sodium uptake (see above). Aldosterone may also directly increase luminal membrane potassium permeability.

Potassium loss will be *reduced* in the following circumstances:

- When sodium reabsorption in the collecting ducts is decreased—as occurs with **amiloride** and **triamterene**, which block the sodium channel in this part of the nephron (see p. 365) and with **spironolactone**, which blocks the action of aldosterone (see p. 365).

Recent work suggests that the kidney has a previously unsuspected mechanism for primary, active potassium absorption in the collecting duct, possibly by a luminal membrane H^+/K^+-ATPase similar to that on gastric parietal cells.

EXCRETION OF ORGANIC MOLECULES

There are different mechanisms for the excretion of organic anions and organic cations (see Ch. 5) but both involve active transport, the power being derived from the action of the basolateral Na^+/K^+-ATPase in the basolateral membrane.

Organic anions bound to plasma albumin do not pass into the glomerular filtrate, but when the blood from the glomerulus passes into the peritubular capillary plexus they may be secreted into the proximal convoluted tubule. They are exchanged with α-ketoglutarate by an antiport in the basolateral membrane and diffuse passively into the tubular lumen (Fig. 20.4). Among the drugs excreted in this way are the **thiazides**, **ethacrynic acid**, **frusemide**, **salicylates** and most **penicillins** and **cephalosporins**.

Organic cations are thought to diffuse into the cell from the interstitia and are then actively transported into the tubular lumen in exchange for H^+. Some diuretics (**triamterene**, **amiloride**) are added to the tubular fluid in this way and many drugs are eliminated by this route, including **atropine**, **morphine** and **quinine**.

This topic is dealt with in more detail in Chapter 5 (see Table 5.4, p. 85).

ARACHIDONIC ACID METABOLITES AND RENAL FUNCTION

The metabolites of arachidonic acid, the eicosanoids, which are generated in the kidney, modulate its haemo-dynamics and excretory functions. Details of the eicosanoids are given in Chapter 12.

Prostanoids, the products of the cyclo-oxygenase pathway, are synthesised in all parts of the kidney, the predominant products being PGE_2 in the medulla and PGI_2 in the glomeruli. Factors which stimulate their synthesis include ischaemia, mechanical trauma, circulating angiotensin II, catecholamines, antidiuretic hormone and bradykinin.

Influence on haemodynamics

Under basal conditions, prostaglandins probably do not have much effect. However, in circumstances in which vasoconstrictor agents (angiotensin II, noradrenaline) are generated and released, the vasodilator prostaglandins, PGE_2 and PGI_2, modulate the effects of these agents in the kidney by causing compensatory vasodilatation. This action is relevant to the unwanted renal effects of some NSAIDs (see Ch. 13, p. 233, and Ch. 49; reviewed by de Broe & Elseviers 1998). Prostaglandins play a part in the control of renin release under basal conditions, and also in conditions of intravascular volume depletion.

Influence on the renal control of salt and water

The overall effect of the renal prostaglandins is to increase renal blood flow and cause natriuresis. This can, in some circumstances, be an important consideration when NSAIDs, whose action is inhibition of prosta-glandin production (see Ch. 13), are used in therapy. Thus, NSAIDs can cause renal failure in several clinical conditions in which renal blood flow depends on vaso-dilator prostaglandins, for example cirrhosis of the liver, heart failure, nephrotic syndrome and glomerulo-nephritis. They exacerbate salt and water retention in patients with heart failure.

DRUGS ACTING ON THE KIDNEY

DIURETICS

Diuretics are drugs which increase the excretion of sodium and water from the body by an action on the kidney. Their primary effect is to decrease the reabsorp-tion of sodium and chloride from the filtrate, increased

water loss being secondary to the increased excretion of salt. This can be achieved by:

- a direct action on the cells of the nephron
- indirectly modifying the content of the filtrate.

Since a very large proportion of the salt and water which passes into the tubule in the glomerulus is reabsorbed (Table 20.1), a small decrease in reabsorption can result in a marked increase in excretion. A summary diagram of the mechanisms and sites of action of various diuretics is given in Figure 20.5.

Note that the diuretics which have a direct action on the cells of the nephron (with the exception of spirono-lactone) act from within the tubular lumen and reach their sites of action by being secreted into the proximal tubule.

THE DEVELOPMENT OF DIURETIC DRUGS

The diuretics used prior to 1920 were **xanthines** (e.g. theophylline and caffeine) and **osmotic diuretics** (e.g. urea). The next group of compounds introduced were the **carbonic-anhydrase inhibitors**. These were developed from the sulphonamides, following on the observation that sulphanilamide (Ch. 43) caused, as a side-effect, a mild diuresis.

As a result of further modifications of the original structure, **acetazolamide** (Fig. 20.7) was introduced in 1950. Further molecular modifications, in which diuretic activity was sought rather than carbonic-anhydrase inhibition, resulted in studies of metadisulphonamides (Fig. 20.7) and gave rise eventually to **chlorothiazide** and **hydrochlorothiazide**, then **bendrofluazide**, the series showing increasing potency in promoting sodium excretion, not accompanied by equivalent potency on potassium excretion (Fig. 20.7). Numerous other similar compounds have been produced.* A by-product of the research on thiazides was the development of diazoxide, an antihypertensive agent; see page 288.

Further molecular modifications led in the early 1960s to the compounds **frusemide**, **bumetanide** and later **piretanide** and **torasemide**. These agents, though also sulphonamide derivatives, have very few chemical features in common with the thiazides (Fig. 20.8). Their

---

*It would be apposite to mention, in this context, that molecular modification of a derivative of sulphanilamide gave rise to the oral antidiabetic agents (see Ch. 22), the sulphonylureas, and that investigation of the goitrogenic action of sulphaguanidine led to the development of the antithyroid drugs, thiouracil, propylthiouracil and methimazole (see Ch. 25).

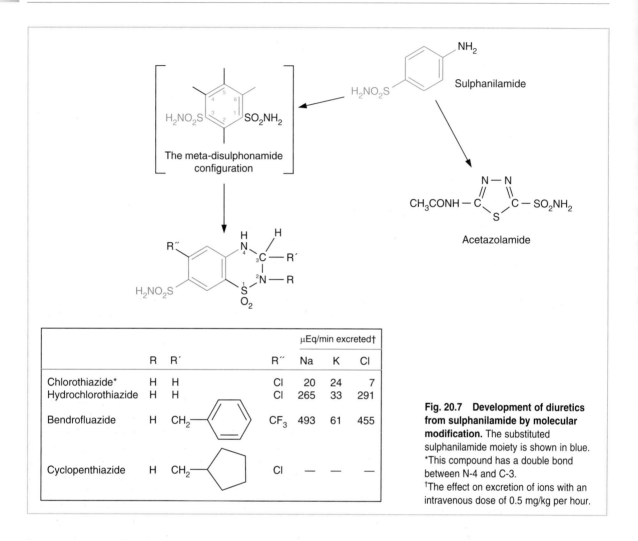

Fig. 20.7 Development of diuretics from sulphanilamide by molecular modification. The substituted sulphanilamide moiety is shown in blue. *This compound has a double bond between N-4 and C-3. †The effect on excretion of ions with an intravenous dose of 0.5 mg/kg per hour.

	R	R′		R″	Na	K	Cl
					μEq/min excreted†		
Chlorothiazide*	H	H		Cl	20	24	7
Hydrochlorothiazide	H	H		Cl	265	33	291
Bendrofluazide	H	CH₂—		CF₃	493	61	455
Cyclopenthiazide	H	CH₂—		Cl	—	—	—

mechanism of action is also different from that of the thiazides. They are *loop diuretics* with a 'ceiling' of diuresis much higher than that of the thiazides; their action is similar to that of **ethacrynic acid** (Fig. 20.8), a compound which was developed in a quite different research programme.

Although all these compounds proved to be very effective in promoting sodium excretion, they all caused potassium loss, and this prompted the search for potassium-sparing diuretics. Aldosterone antagonists such as **spironolactone**, introduced in 1962, partially satisfied this requirement, but they had several drawbacks. Numerous compounds were screened and eventually **amiloride** and **triamterene** emerged. These two drugs were developed from two different research programmes, but they have rather similar sites of action.

Another development in this area is the attempt to develop uricosuric diuretics to overcome the problem that most currently used diuretics tend to produce an increase in the plasma uric acid concentration. So far this has been unsuccessful.

DIURETICS ACTING DIRECTLY ON THE CELLS OF THE NEPHRON

Drugs which cause salt loss by an action on cells must obviously affect those parts of the nephron where most of the *active* and *selective* solute reabsorption occurs:

- the ascending loop of Henle
- the early distal tubule
- the collecting tubules and ducts.

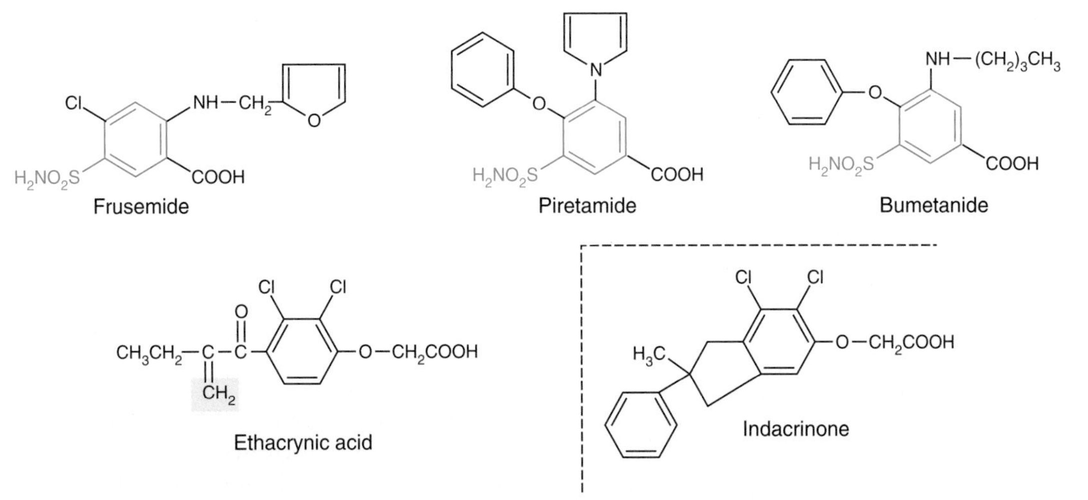

Fig. 20.8 Loop diuretics. The boxed methylene group of ethacrynic acid forms an adduct with cysteine in vivo and this adduct is thought to be the pharmacologically active form of the drug. The substituted sulphanilamide moiety is shown in blue. Indacrinone has uricosuric activity.

Diuretics

- Diuretics are drugs which increase the excretion of salt (NaCl, NaHCO$_3$) and water. Normally (i.e. in the absence of diuretics), less than 1% of filtered sodium is excreted. The main diuretics are the loop diuretics and the thiazides.
- Loop diuretics (e.g. frusemide) cause up to 15–20% of filtered Na$^+$ to be excreted, with copious urine production. They act by inhibiting the Na$^+$/K$^+$/2Cl$^-$ co-transporter in the thick ascending loop. They increase K$^+$ and Ca^{2+} loss. Main unwanted effects: hypokalaemia, metabolic alkalosis and hypovolaemia.
- Thiazides (e.g. bendrofluazide) are less potent. They act by inhibiting the Na$^+$/Cl$^-$ co-transporter in the distal convoluted tubule. They increase K$^+$ loss and reduce Ca^{2+} loss. Main unwanted effects: hypokalaemia and metabolic alkalosis.
- Potassium-sparing diuretics:
  — These act in the collecting tubules and are very weak diuretics.
  — Amiloride and triamterene act by blocking the Na$^+$ channels controlled by aldosterone's protein mediator.
  — Spironolactone is an antagonist at the aldosterone receptor.

Loop diuretics

Loop diuretics are the most powerful of all diuretics, capable of causing 15–25% of the sodium in the filtrate to be excreted (see Fig. 20.9 for comparison with a thiazide). They are termed 'high ceiling' diuretics and their action is often described—in a phrase that conjures up a rather uncomfortable picture—as causing 'torrential urine flow'. The main example is **frusemide**; others are **bumetanide, piretanide, torasemide** and **ethacrynic acid**. These drugs act primarily on the thick segment of the ascending loop of Henle, inhibiting the transport of sodium chloride out of the tubule into the interstitial tissue by inhibiting the Na$^+$/K$^+$/2Cl$^-$ carrier in the luminal membrane (see Figs 20.5 and 20.10). **Frusemide, bumetanide, torasemide** and **piretanide** have a direct inhibiting effect on the carrier, acting on the chloride-binding site. **Ethacrynic acid** forms a complex with cysteine, the complex being the active form of the drug.

As has been explained above, the reabsorption of solute at this site is the basis for the ability of the kidney to concentrate the urine by creating a hypertonic interstitial area in the medulla, which provides the osmotic force by which water is reabsorbed from the collecting tubules under the influence of the antidiuretic hormone. The action of the loop diuretics has the additional effect that more solute is delivered to the distal portions of the nephron where its osmotic pressure further reduces water reabsorption. Essentially, some of the solute which normally passes into the medullary interstitium and draws water out of the collecting ducts,

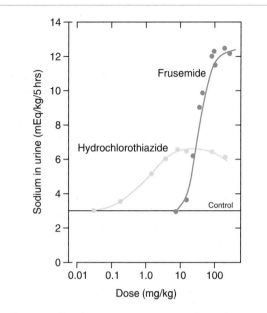

Fig. 20.9 **The dose–response curves for frusemide and hydrochlorothiazide, showing differences in potency and 'ceiling'.** Note that these doses are not used clinically. (Adapted from: Timmerman R J et al. 1964 Curr Ther Res 6: 88)

now remains in the tubular fluid and holds water with it. As much as 25% of the glomerular filtrate may pass out of the nephron (compared with the normal loss of about 1%), resulting in a profuse diuresis.

Loop diuretics appear to have a venodilator action, directly and/or indirectly through the release of a renal factor. After intravenous administration to patients with acute heart failure (see Ch. 14), a therapeutically useful vascular effect is seen *before* the onset of the diuretic effect. **Piretanide**, in particular, has general vasodilator actions.

The increased sodium concentration that reaches the distal tubule results in increased loss of H^+ and potassium (see above, p. 383). Loop diuretics may thus produce a metabolic alkalosis.

There is an increase in the excretion of calcium and magnesium and a decreased excretion of uric acid. The effect on calcium is made use of in the treatment of hypercalcaemia. **Torasemide** causes less loss of potassium and calcium.

Pharmacokinetic aspects

The loop diuretics are readily absorbed from the gastro-intestinal tract and may also be given by injection. They are strongly bound to plasma protein and so do not

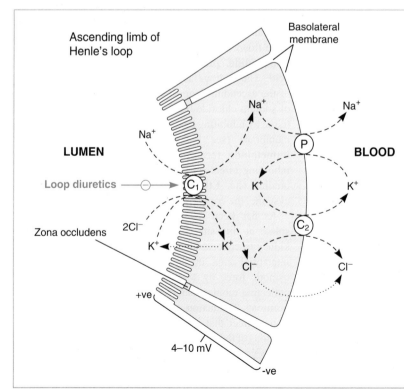

Fig. 20.10 **Ion transport in the cells of the thick ascending limb of Henle's loop, showing the site of action of loop diuretics.** The sodium pump (P) is the main primary active transport mechanism. Na^+, K^+ and Cl^- enter by a co-transport system (C_1). Chloride leaves the cell both by passive diffusion (dotted lines) and by an electroneutral K^+/Cl^- co-transport system (C_2). Some sodium is absorbed paracellularly, through the zonula occludens, and some potassium leaves the cell by passive diffusion (not shown). Note that the diagram is simplified and thus the stoichiometry is not accurate; e.g. each time the sodium pump works, it exchanges 3 Na^+ for 2 K^+. (Based on Greger 1998, and Hendry & Ellory 1988)

Clinical use of loop diuretics

- In patients with salt and water overload due to:
  - — acute pulmonary oedema
  - — chronic heart failure
  - — hepatic cirrhosis complicated by ascites
  - — nephrotic syndrome
  - — renal failure.
- In hypertension, especially if accompanied by renal impairment.
- In acute treatment of hypercalcaemia.

pass into the glomerular filtrate to any marked degree. They reach their site of action—the luminal membrane of the cells of the thick ascending loop—by being secreted in the proximal convoluted tubule by the organic acid transport mechanism; the fraction thus secreted will pass out in the urine. The fraction not secreted is metabolised in the liver—**bumetanide** and **torasemide** being metabolised by cytochrome P450 pathways and **frusemide** being glucuronidated. Given orally, they act within 1 hour; given intravenously, they produce a peak effect within 30 minutes. The half-lives are about 90 minutes (longer in renal failure) and the duration of action 3–6 hours, except in the case of **torasemide** which has a longer half-life and longer duration of action and can therefore be given once a day. The clinical use of loop diuretics is given above.

Unwanted effects

Some unwanted effects are common with loop diuretics, and are directly related to their renal actions. *Potassium loss* (see p. 362), resulting in low plasma potassium (hypokalaemia), and *metabolic alkalosis* due to hydrogen ion excretion are both very likely to occur. Hypokalaemia can be averted or treated by concomitant use of potassium-sparing diuretics (see below) or by potassium supplements. *Depletion of magnesium and calcium* is common, and in elderly patients, *hypovolaemia* and *hypotension*, with collapse due to sudden loss of extracellular fluid volume, can follow the profuse diuresis produced by these agents.

Unwanted effects which are not related to the renal actions of the drugs are rare. They include nausea, allergic reactions (more common in those agents related to sulphonamides) and, infrequently, deafness (compounded by concomitant use of an aminoglycoside antibiotic). Ethacrynic acid is more likely to cause gastrointestinal disturbances and deafness and is consequently less widely used.

Diuretics acting on the early distal tubule

The diuretics acting at this site—sometimes referred to as the distal convoluted tubule—include the **thiazides** and related drugs.

The development of these agents is outlined above. The main thiazide is **bendrofluazide**. Others are **hydrochlorothiazide**, and **cyclopenthiazide**, but many similar drugs are available (Fig. 20.11). Drugs with similar actions include **chlorthalidone**, and newer ones such as **indapamide**, **xipamide** and **metolazone**.

This group of drugs has a moderately powerful diuretic action (see comparison with loop diuretics in Fig. 20.9). They decrease active reabsorption of sodium and accompanying chloride by binding to the chloride site of the electroneutral Na^+/Cl^- co-transport system and inhibiting its action (Figs 20.5 and 20.12). They do not have any action on the thick ascending loop of Henle. Potassium loss with these drugs is significant (by mechanisms explained on p. 358) and can be serious. Excretion of uric acid and calcium is decreased; that of magnesium is increased.

Hypochloraemic alkalosis can occur.

Thiazide diuretics have a paradoxical effect in diabetes insipidus where they *reduce* the volume of urine.

They have some extrarenal actions—they produce vasodilatation and can cause hyperglycaemia. When used in the treatment of hypertension (Ch. 15), the initial

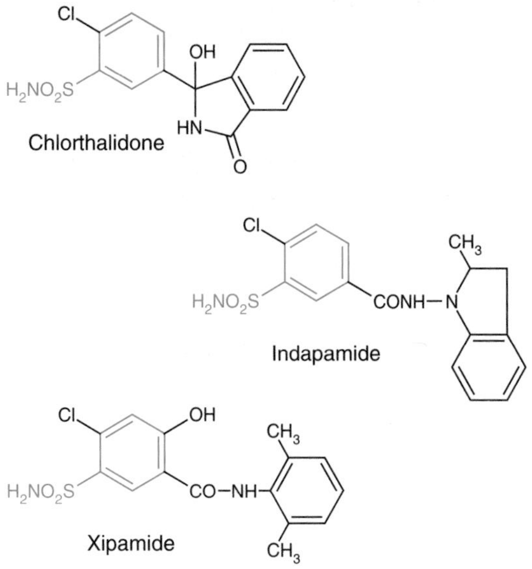

Fig. 20.11 Some diuretics related to the thiazide compounds. The substituted sulphanilamide moiety is shown in blue.

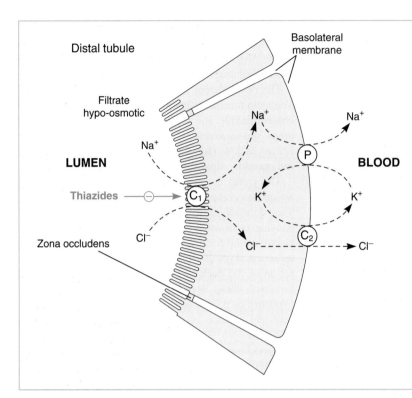

Fig. 20.12 Salt transport in the distal convoluted tubule showing the proposed site of action of thiazide diuretics. The sodium pump (P) in the basolateral membrane is the primary active transport mechanism. Na^+ and Cl^- enter by an electroneutral co-transport carrier (C_1). Some K^+ is transported out of the cell by the co-transport carrier (C_2), and some by passive diffusion (not shown). Note that the diagram is simplified and thus the stoichiometry is not accurate; e.g. each time the sodium pump works, it exchanges 3 Na^+ for 2 K^+. (Adapted from: Greger 1988, Hendry & Ellory 1988)

fall in blood pressure is due to decreased blood volume resulting from diuresis, but the later phase seems to be due to a direct action on the blood vessels. Note that **diazoxide**, a non-diuretic thiazide, has powerful vasodilator effects (see Ch. 15). and also increases the blood sugar (but is now seldom used). Both actions are due to the same mechanism, namely the opening of membrane K^+ channels (see Ch. 15). **Indapamide** is said to lower blood pressure at sub-diuretic doses with less metabolic disturbance.

Pharmacokinetic aspects

The thiazides and related drugs are all effective orally, being well absorbed from the gastrointestinal tract. All are excreted in the urine mainly by tubular secretion (see p. 358). Their tendency to increase plasma uric acid is due to competition with uric acid for tubular secretion mechanisms. With the shorter-acting drugs such as **bendrofluazide**, **hydrochlorothiazide**, **chlorothiazide** and **cyclopenthiazide**, onset of action is within 12 hours, maximum effect at about 4–6 hours and duration between 8 and 12 hours. The longer-acting drugs such as **chlor-thalidone** have a similar onset but a longer duration of action and can be given on alternate days. The clinical use of thiazide diuretics is given in the Clinical Box on this page.

Clinical use of thiazide diuretics

- In hypertension.
- In mild heart failure.
- In severe resistant oedema (metolazone, especially, is used, together with loop diuretics).
- To prevent recurrent stone formation in idiopathic hypercalciuria.
- In nephrogenic diabetes insipidus.

Unwanted effects

These agents have a fairly large therapeutic index and serious unwanted effects are relatively rare. The main unwanted effects of thiazides are the result of some of the renal actions; a *decreased plasma potassium* is particularly significant. Others are *metabolic alkalosis*, *increased plasma uric acid* (with the possibility of gout) and *hyperglycaemia* (which could exacerbate diabetes mellitus). **Indapamide** has little obvious effect on potassium, uric acid and glucose excretion.

Unwanted effects not related to the main renal actions of the thiazides include increased plasma cholesterol (with long-term use), male impotence (reversible on stopping the drug) and, infrequently, hypersensitivity reactions (skin rashes, blood dyscrasias and, more rarely still, pancreatitis, acute pulmonary oedema). In cases of hepatic failure, thiazides can precipitate encephalopathy. An unusual but potentially serious unwanted effect is hyponatraemia.

Spironolactone

Spironolactone has a limited diuretic action. It is an antagonist of aldosterone, a mineralo corticoid (p. 425) competing for intracellular aldosterone receptors in the cells of the distal tubule (see Ch. 24). The spironolactone–receptor complex does not apparently attach to the DNA, and the subsequent processes of transcription, translation and production of mediator protein(s)—see page 426 and Figure 20.13—do not occur. The result is an inhibition of the sodium-retaining action of aldosterone (see Fig. 20.5), and a concomitant decrease in its potassium-secreting effect. Spironolactone has subsidiary actions in decreasing hydrogen ion secretion and also uric acid excretion.

Potassium canrenoate (see below) has effects similar to spironolactone.

Pharmacokinetic aspects

Spironolactone is well absorbed from the gastrointestinal tract. Its plasma half-life is only 10 minutes but its active metabolite, canrenone, has a plasma half-life of 16 hours. The action of spironolactone is believed to be largely but not entirely due to canrenone. The onset of action is very slow, taking several days to develop.

Potassium canrenoate is given parenterally. The clinical use of spironolactone is given in the Clinical Box on page 366.

Unwanted effects

Gastrointestinal upsets occur fairly frequently. If spironolactone is used on its own it will cause hyperkalaemia and possibly metabolic acidosis. Actions on steroid receptors in tissues other than the kidney can result in gynaecomastia, menstrual disorders and testicular atrophy. Peptic ulceration has been reported.

Triamterene and amiloride

Like spironolactone, triamterene and amiloride have a limited diuretic efficacy. They act on the collecting tubules and collecting ducts, inhibiting sodium reabsorption and decreasing potassium excretion (see Figs 20.5 and 20.13). Amiloride blocks the luminal sodium channels by which aldosterone produces its main effect, making less sodium available for transport across the basolateral membrane. Triamterene probably has a similar action.

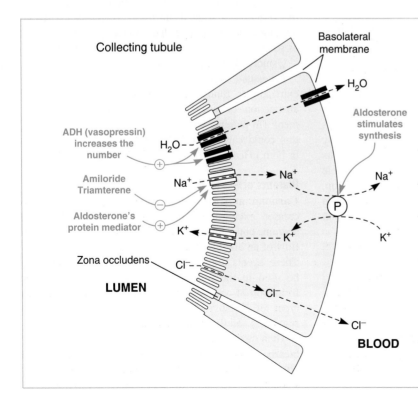

Fig. 20.13 Simplified diagram of the action of hormones and drugs on the principal cells of the collecting tubule. The cells are normally impermeable to water in the absence of antidiuretic hormone (ADH), and to sodium in the absence of aldosterone. Salt and water reabsorption in this part of the tubule are controlled physiologically by these two hormones, through their respective effects on the water channels and sodium channels. Aldosterone acts within the tubule (see p. 355). Spironolactone antagonises aldosterone action. The Na⁺ pump (P) in the basolateral membrane is the main source of energy for ion movement. Note that the diagram is simplified and thus the stoichiometry is not accurate; e.g. each time the sodium pump works, it exchanges 3 Na⁺ for 2 K⁺. (Adapted from: Hendry & Ellory 1988)

Both are mildly uricosuric, i.e. they promote the excretion of uric acid.

The main importance of these diuretics lies in their *potassium-sparing ability*. They can be given with potassium-losing diuretics like the thiazides in order to maintain potassium balance.

Pharmacokinetic aspects

Triamterene is well absorbed in the gastrointestinal tract. Its onset of action is within 2 hours and its duration of action 12–16 hours. It is partly metabolised in the liver and partly excreted unchanged in the urine. Amiloride is poorly absorbed and has a slower onset, with a peak action at 6 hours and a duration of action of about 24 hours. Most of the drug is excreted unchanged in the urine. The clinical use of triamterene and amiloride is given on this page.

Unwanted effects

The main unwanted effect is related to the pharmacological action of the drugs—hyperkalaemia, which can be dangerous. Metabolic acidosis can occur, as can skin rashes. Gastrointestinal disturbances have been reported but are infrequent.

DIURETICS WHICH ACT INDIRECTLY BY MODIFYING THE CONTENT OF THE FILTRATE

Diuretics which act indirectly by modifying the content of the filtrate do so by increasing either the osmolarity or the sodium load.

Osmotic diuretics

Osmotic diuretics are pharmacologically inert substances (e.g. **mannitol**) which are filtered in the glomerulus but incompletely reabsorbed or not reabsorbed at all by the nephron (see Fig. 20.5). They can be given in amounts sufficiently large for them to constitute an appreciable fraction of the plasma osmolarity. Within the nephron, their main effect is exerted on those parts of the nephron which are freely permeable to water—the proximal tubule, descending limb of the loop and the collecting tubules. Passive water reabsorption is reduced by the presence of the non-reabsorbable solute within the tubule; consequently a larger volume of fluid remains within the proximal tubule. This has the secondary effect of reducing sodium reabsorption, since the sodium concentration within the proximal tubule is lower than it otherwise would be, and this alters the electrochemical gradient for reabsorption.

Therefore, the main effect of osmotic diuretics is to increase the amount of water excreted, with a relatively smaller increase in sodium excretion. Hence, they are not useful in treating conditions associated with sodium retention, but have much more limited therapeutic applications. These include *acutely raised intracranial or intraocular pressure* and *prevention of acute renal failure*. In this latter condition, the glomerular filtration rate is reduced, and absorption of salt and water in the proximal tubule becomes almost complete, so that more distal parts of the nephron virtually dry up, and urine flow ceases. Retention of fluid within the proximal tubule by administration of an osmotic diuretic limits these effects.

The treatment of acutely raised intracranial pressure (cerebral oedema) and raised intraocular pressure (glaucoma) relies on the increase in plasma osmolarity by solutes that do not enter the brain or eye; this results in extraction of water from these compartments. It has nothing to do with the kidney; indeed the effect is lost as soon as the osmotic diuretic appears in the urine.

Osmotic diuretics are usually given intravenously.

Unwanted effects include transient expansion of the extracellular fluid volume and hyponatraemia due to abstraction of water from the intracellular compartment. (In patients who are totally unable to form urine, this could cause cardiac failure or pulmonary oedema or both.) Headache, nausea and vomiting can occur.

Diuretics acting on the proximal tubule

Carbonic anhydrase inhibitors (Fig. 20.14) cause increased excretion of bicarbonate with accompanying sodium, potassium and water, resulting in an increased flow of an alkaline urine and a mild metabolic acidosis. These agents, though not now used as diuretics, may be used in the treatment of glaucoma to reduce the formation of aqueous humor, and also in some unusual types of epilepsy. Examples are **acetazolamide** (see Fig. 20.7) and **dichlorphenamide**.

Their action results in a depletion of extracellular bicarbonate and their effect is self-limiting as the blood bicarbonate falls.

Their mechanism of action is shown in Figure 20.14.

> **Clinical use of the potassium-sparing diuretics**
>
> - With potassium-losing diuretics to prevent potassium loss (spironolactone is used less frequently than amiloride or triamterene because it is poorly tolerated).
> - Spironolactone is used:
>   — in primary hyperaldosteronism (Conn's syndrome), which is rare
>   — in secondary hyperaldosteronism due to hepatic cirrhosis complicated by ascites.

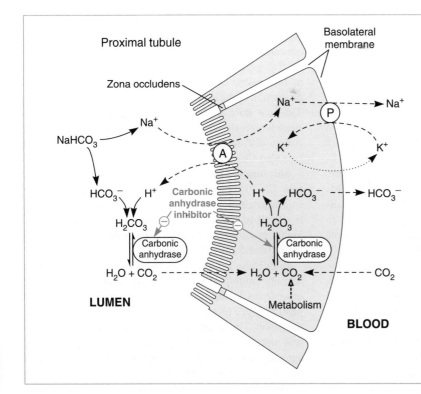

Fig. 20.14 **Renal mechanisms for conserving base showing the action of carbonic anhydrase inhibitors.** Sodium is absorbed and hydrogen ions secreted at the luminal surface by an antiport mechanism (A). Most bicarbonate in the filtrate is 'reabsorbed' in this way in the proximal tubule. In the distal tubule, bicarbonate is added to the plasma, and monobasic phosphate or ammonium chloride is added to the urine (not shown). The primary active transport mechanism is the sodium pump (P). Dashed lines with K^+ indicate passive diffusion. (Amiloride inhibits the Na^+/H^+ exchange or antiport, but this is not a major factor in its diuretic action.) Note that the diagram is simplified and thus the stoichiometry is not accurate; e.g. each time the sodium pump works, it exchanges 3 Na^+ for 2 K^+. (Adapted from Hendry & Ellory 1988)

DRUGS WHICH ALTER THE pH OF THE URINE

In various conditions it is of advantage to alter the pH of the urine, and it is possible to produce urinary pH values ranging from 5–8.5.

Agents which increase the urinary pH

Sodium or **potassium citrate** or other salts (acetate, lactate) are metabolised and the cations are excreted with bicarbonate to give an alkaline urine. This may have some antibacterial effects, as well as decreasing irritation or inflammation in the urinary tract. Alkalinisation is important in preventing certain drugs, such as some sulphonamides, from crystallising out in the urine; it also decreases the formation of uric acid and cystine stones.

It is possible to increase the excretion of drugs which are weak acids (e.g. **salicylates** and some **barbiturates**) by alkalinising the urine (see Ch. 5). **Sodium bicarbonate** given intravenously is used in patients with salicylate overdose.

Note that sodium overload can be dangerous in cardiac failure, and that overload with either sodium or potassium can be harmful in renal insufficiency.

Agents which decrease urinary pH

A decrease in urinary pH can be produced with **ammonium chloride** but this is now rarely if ever used clinically except in a specialised test for renal tubular acidosis.

The ammonia is metabolised to urea in the liver, leaving chloride and hydrogen ion. The chloride displaces bicarbonate (which is dissipated by conversion to carbonic acid then to CO_2 and H_2O) so that a hyperchloraemic acidosis results. The chloride, with accompanying sodium, appears in the glomerular filtrate and passes out in the urine with an osmotic equivalent of water, causing a mild diuresis. Then the base-conserving mechanisms come into play, the tubules secrete hydrogen ions in exchange for sodium, ammonia is generated and an acid urine (containing ammonium chloride) is excreted.

DRUGS WHICH ALTER THE EXCRETION OF ORGANIC MOLECULES

The main organic molecules to be considered are **uric acid** and **penicillin**. Uric acid metabolism and excretion is relevant in the treatment of gout and a few points about its excretion are made here.

Uric acid is derived from the catabolism of the purine bases and is present in plasma mainly as ionised urate. In man it passes freely into the glomerular filtrate, and most is then reabsorbed in the proximal convoluted tubule while a small amount is simultaneously secreted into the tubule by the anion-secreting mechanisms (see p. 358). The net result is excretion of approximately 8–12% of the filtered urate. Under physiological conditions, a rise in the level of urate in the plasma results in increased secretion into the proximal tubule. This process regulates urate concentrations but in some individuals these concentrations are high, predisposing to gout. In this disorder, urate crystals are deposited in joints and soft tissues, resulting in the arthritis and chalky tophi characteristic of this condition. Drugs which *increase* the elimination of urate (uricosuric agents) may be useful in such cases, although these have largely been supplanted by allopurinol which inhibits urate synthesis (Ch. 13, p. 239).

Some uricosuric agents *decrease* the secretion of penicillin and may also be used for this purpose. The two main uricosuric agents are probenecid and sulphinpyrazone.

Probenecid is a lipid-soluble derivative of benzoic acid, which inhibits the reabsorption of urate in the proximal convoluted tubule and thus increases its excretion. It has the opposite effect on penicillin, inhibiting its secretion into the tubules and raising its plasma concentration. Given orally, probenecid is well absorbed in the gastrointestinal tract, maximal concentrations in the plasma occurring in about 3 hours. The greater proportion of the drug (90%) is bound to plasma albumin. The free drug passes into the glomerular filtrate, but more is actively secreted into the proximal tubule whence it may diffuse back because of its high lipid solubility (see also Ch. 5).

Sulphinpyrazone is a congener of phenylbutazone (see Ch. 13) with powerful inhibitory effects on uric acid reabsorption in the proximal convoluted tubule. It is absorbed from the gastrointestinal tract, becomes highly protein-bound in the plasma and is secreted into the proximal convoluted tubule.

Both these agents, if given in sub-therapeutic doses, actually *inhibit* secretion of urate. **Salicylates**, on the other hand, inhibit secretion in doses within their therapeutic range, producing an increase in urate levels in the blood. They may thus exacerbate gouty arthritis and will antagonise the effects of more powerful uricosuric agents. But note that salicylates become uricosuric themselves at very high doses.

Most diuretics cause an increase in plasma uric acid. Current research is aimed at developing diuretics with uricosuric properties; **indacrinone** is one such agent.

REFERENCES AND FURTHER READING

Barter D C 1983 Pharmacodynamic considerations in the use of diuretics. Annu Rev Pharmacol 123: 45–62

Berger B E, Warnock D G 1985 Clinical uses and mechanisms of action of diuretic agents. In: Brenner B M, Rector F C (eds) The kidney, 3rd edn. W B Saunders, Philadelphia, pp 433–455

Brater D C 1998 Diuretic therapy. N Eng J Med 339: 387–395 (*Pharmacodynamics, clinical pharmacology and adverse effects of loop diuretics*)

Breyer J, Jacobson H R 1990 Molecular mechanism of diuretic agents. Annu Rev Med 41: 265–275 (*Succinct review, useful diagrams*)

Burg M B 1985 Renal handling of sodium, chloride, water, amino acids and glucose. In: Brenner B M, Rector F C (eds) The kidney, 3rd edn. W B Saunders, Philadelphia, pp 145–175

Cogan M G 1990 Renal effects of atrial natriuretic factor. Annu Rev Physiol 52: 699–708

Connolly D L, Shanahan C M, Weissberg P L 1996 Water channels in health and disease. Lancet 347: 210–211

Cragoe E J (ed) 1983 Diuretics: chemistry, pharmacology and medicine. John Wiley, New York

De Broe M E, Elseviers M M 1998 Current concepts: analgesic nephropathy. N Engl J Med 338: 446–452

Friedel H A, Buckley M M 1991 Torasemide. A review of its pharmacological properties and therapeutic potential. Drugs 41: 81–83

Funder J W 1993 Aldosterone action. Annu Rev Physiol 55: 115–130 (*Covers biosynthesis, receptors and physiology*)

Gennari F J 1998 Hypokalemia. N Eng J Med 339: 451–458 (*Regulation of potassium balance, with nice diagram; drug-induced alterations of balance*)

Greger R 1985 Ion transport mechanisms in thick ascending limb of Henle's loop of mammalian nephron. Physiol Rev 65: 760–797 (*Comprehensive in-depth review*)

Greger R 1988 Chloride transport in thick ascending limb, distal convolution and collecting duct. Annu Rev Physiol 50: 111–122 (*Seminal review on chloride transport*)

Greven J 1987 The pharmacological basis of the action of loop diuretics. In: Puschett J B, Greenberg A (eds) Diuretics II: chemistry pharmacology and clinical implications. Elsevier, Amsterdam, pp 173–181

Halperin M L, Kamel K S 1998 Potassium. Lancet 352: 135–140. (*Good review of potassium homeostasis; useful diagrams*)

Hendry B M, Ellory J C 1988 Molecular sites for diuretic action. Trends Pharmacol Sci 9: 416–421

Houston M C 1991 Nonsteroidal anti-inflammatory drugs and antihypertensives. Am J Med 90: 42(S)–47(S)

Jamison R, Maffly R H 1976 The urinary concentrating mechanism. N Engl J Med 295: 1059–1067

Kaplan M R, Mount D B et al. 1996 Molecular mechanisms of NaCl cotransport. Annu Rev Physiol 58: 649–668

King L S, Agre P 1996 Pathophysiology of the aquaporin water channels. Annu Rev Physiol 58: 619–648 (Detailed review; covers structure, function and pathophysiology)

Koga H, Sat H, Dan T, Aoki B 1991 Studies on uricosuric diuretics. J Med Chem 34: 2702–2708

Kumar S, Berl T 1998 Sodium. The Lancet 352: 220–228 (Sodium homeostasis, its disorders and treatments)

Levenson D J, Simmons C E, Brenner B M 1982 Arachidonic acid metabolism, prostaglandins and the kidney. Am J Med 72: 354–374

Orme M 1990 Thiazides in the 1990s. Br Med J 300: 1668–1669

Pritchaed J B, Miller D S 1993 Mechanisms mediating renal secretion of organic anions and cations. Physiol Rev 73: 765–796

Reeves W B, Andreoli T E 1992 Renal epithelial chloride channels. Annu Rev Physiol 54: 29–50

Rose B D 1991 Diuretics. Kidney Int 39: 336–352 (Useful, detailed introductory paper to a Nephrology forum)

Schafer J A, Hawk C T 1992 Regulation of Na^+ channels in the cortical collecting duct by AVP and mineralocorticoids. Kidney Int 41: 255–268 (Editorial review)

Schuster V L 1993 Function and regulation of collecting duct intercalated cells. Annu Rev Physiol 55: 267–288

Sullivan L P, Grantham J J 1982 The physiology of the kidney, 2nd edn. Lea & Febiger, Philadelphia

Taylor A, Palmer L G 1982 Hormonal regulation of sodium chloride and water transport in epithelia. In: Goldberger R F, Yamamoto K R (eds) Biological regulation and development. Plenum Press, New York, vol 3A, pp 253–298

Wasnick R, Davis J, Ross P, Vogel J 1990 Effect of thiazides on rates of bone mineral loss: a longitudinal study. Br Med J 301: 1303–1305

Wehling M, Christ M, Gerzer R 1993 Aldosterone-specific membrane receptors and related rapid, non-genomic effects. Trends Pharmacol Sci 14: 1–4

Wingo C S, Cain B D 1993 The renal ATP-ase: physiological significance and role in potassium homeostasis. Annu Rev Physiol 55: 323–347

21

The gastrointestinal tract

In addition to its main function of digestion and absorption of food, the gastrointestinal tract is one of the major endocrine systems in the body. It also has its own integrative neuronal network, the enteric nervous system (see Ch. 6, p. 96), which contains about the same number of neurons as the spinal cord; the topic is reviewed by Del Valle & Yamada (1990) and Goyal & Hirano (1996).

THE INNERVATION AND THE HORMONES OF THE GASTROINTESTINAL TRACT

The elements under neuronal and hormonal control are the smooth muscle, the blood vessels and the glands (exocrine, endocrine and paracrine).

Neuronal control

There are two principal intramural plexuses in the tract—the *myenteric plexus* (*Auerbach's plexus*) between the outer, longitudinal and the middle, circular muscle layers, and *Meissner's plexus*, or *submucous plexus*, on the luminal side of the circular muscle layer. The plexuses are interconnected and their ganglion cells receive preganglionic *parasympathetic fibres* from the vagus which are mostly cholinergic and mostly excitatory, though some are inhibitory. Incoming *sympathetic fibres* are largely postganglionic and these, in addition to innervating blood vessels, smooth muscle and some glandular cells directly, may have endings in the plexuses where they inhibit acetylcholine secretion (see Ch. 6).

The neurons within the plexuses constitute the enteric nervous system and secrete not only acetylcholine and noradrenaline but 5-HT, purines, nitric oxide and a variety of pharmacologically active peptides. The enteric plexus contains sensory neurons which respond to mechanical and chemical stimuli.

Hormonal control

The hormones of the gastrointestinal tract include both *endocrine* secretions and *paracrine* secretions. The endocrine secretions (i.e. substances released into the bloodstream) are mainly peptides synthesised by endocrine cells in the mucosa, and the most important is **gastrin**. The paracrine secretions, or local hormones, many of them regulatory peptides, are released from special cells found throughout the wall of the tract. These hormones act on nearby cells, and in the stomach the most important of these is **histamine**. Some of these paracrine secretions also function as neurotransmitters. Histamine, gastrin and acetylcholine are considered below in the context of the local control of acid secretion.

The *main functions* of the gastrointestinal tract that are important from a pharmacological point of view are:

- gastric secretion
- vomiting (emesis)

- the motility of the bowel and the expulsion of the faeces
- the formation and excretion of bile.

GASTRIC SECRETION

The stomach secretes about 2.5 litres of gastric juice daily. The principal exocrine secretions are pepsinogens, from the *chief* or *peptic cells*, and hydrochloric acid and intrinsic factor (see Ch. 18) from the *parietal* or *oxyntic cells*. Mucus is secreted by mucus-secreting cells found amongst the surface cells throughout the gastric mucosa. Bicarbonate ions are also secreted and are trapped in the mucus, creating a gradient of pH from 1–2 in the lumen to 6–7 at the mucosal surface. The mucus and bicarbonate form an unstirred gel-like layer protecting the mucosa from the gastric juice. Alcohol and bile can disrupt this layer. Locally-produced prostaglandins stimulate the secretion of both mucus and bicarbonate.

Disturbances in the above secretory functions are thought to be involved in the pathogenesis of peptic ulcer, and the therapy of this condition involves drugs which modify each of these factors.

THE REGULATION OF ACID SECRETION BY PARIETAL CELLS

The regulation of acid secretion by parietal cells is especially important in peptic ulcer and constitutes a particular target for drug action. The secretion of the parietal cells is an isotonic solution of HCl (150 mmol/l) with a pH less than 1, the concentration of hydrogen ion being more than a million times higher than that of the plasma.

The Cl^- is actively transported into canaliculi in the cells which communicate with the lumen of the gastric glands and thus with the lumen of the stomach. K^+ accompanies the Cl^- and is then exchanged for H^+ from within the cell by a K^+/H^+-ATPase (Fig. 21.1). H_2CO_3, formed from CO_2 and H_2O, dissociates in a reaction catalysed by carbonic anhydrase to form H^+ and HCO_3^-. The HCO_3^- exchanges across the basal membrane for Cl^-. Three main stimuli act on the parietal cells:

- **gastrin** (a hormone)
- **acetylcholine** (a neurotransmitter)
- **histamine** (a local hormone).

Prostaglandins E_2 and **I_2** inhibit acid secretion. Figure 21.2 summarises the actions of these chemical mediators.

Gastrin

Gastrin is a peptide hormone synthesised in endocrine cells of the mucosa of the gastric antrum and duodenum,

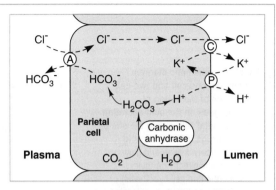

Fig. 21.1 A schematic illustration of the secretion of hydrochloric acid by the gastric parietal cell. Secretion involves a proton pump (P) which is a H^+/K^+-ATPase, a symport carrier (C) for K^+ and Cl^-, and an antiport (A) which exchanges Cl^- and HCO_3^-. A Na^+/H^+ antiport at the interface with the plasma may also have a role (not shown).

and secreted into the portal blood. Its main action is stimulation of the secretion of acid by the parietal cells, but there is controversy as to the mechanism of action (discussed below). Gastrin receptors on the parietal cells have been demonstrated with radioactively labelled gastrin. The receptors are blocked by **proglumide** (Fig. 21.2)—a drug used only as an experimental tool.

Gastrin also indirectly increases pepsinogen secretion and stimulates blood flow and gastric motility.

Control of gastrin release involves both neuronal transmitters and blood-borne mediators, and the direct effects of the stomach contents. Within the stomach, the important stimuli are amino acids and small peptides, which act directly on the gastrin-secreting cells. Milk and solutions of calcium salts are also effective stimulants, so it is inappropriate to use calcium-containing salts as antacids.

Gastrin secretion is inhibited when the pH of the gastric contents falls to 2.5 or lower.

An excessive secretion of gastrin resulting in excessive secretion of acid is seen with rare tumours of gastrin-secreting cells, gastrinomas—the complex of signs and symptoms constituting the Zollinger–Ellison syndrome.

Acetylcholine

Acetylcholine is released from neurons and stimulates specific muscarinic receptors on the surface of the parietal cells and on the surface of histamine-containing cells, as determined by studies with competitive antagonists (see Ch. 7).

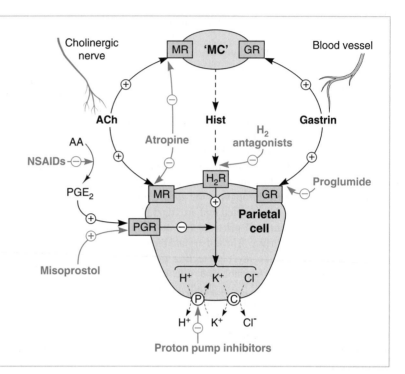

Fig. 21.2 Schematic diagram showing the one-cell and two-cell hypotheses of the action of secretagogues on the acid-secreting gastric parietal cell, giving the site of action of drugs influencing acid secretion. Acetylcholine and gastrin may act mainly directly on their receptors (the one-cell hypothesis) or partly directly, and partly by releasing histamine (the two-cell hypothesis). ('MC' = mast-cell-like, histamine-secreting cell; Hist = histamine; ACh = acetylcholine; MR = muscarinic receptor; H_2R = histamine H_2-receptor; GR = gastrin receptor; PGR = prostaglandin E_2 (PGE_2) receptor; AA = arachidonic acid; NSAIDs = non-steroidal anti-inflammatory drugs; P = proton pump (H^+/K^+-ATPase); C = symport carrier for K^+ and Cl^-).

Histamine

Histamine is discussed in Chapter 12. Only those aspects of its pharmacology relevant to gastric secretion will be dealt with here.

Considerable clarification of the role of histamine followed from the development of the histamine H_2-receptor antagonists (see below). The parietal cells are stimulated by histamine acting on H_2-receptors. They respond to amounts that are below the threshold concentration that acts on H_2-receptors in blood vessels. The histamine is derived from mast cells (or histamine-containing cells similar to mast cells) that lie close to the parietal cell. There is a steady basal release of histamine which is increased by gastrin and acetylcholine.

The role of acetylcholine, histamine and gastrin in acid secretion

The exact mechanism of action of the three secretagogues on the parietal cell is not entirely clear. A general scheme is given in Figure 21.2 which summarises the two main theories—the *single-cell* hypothesis and the *two-cell* hypothesis.

According to the *single-cell* hypothesis, the parietal cell has H_2-receptors for histamine, muscarinic M_2-receptors for acetylcholine, and also gastrin receptors.

Stimulation of the H_2-receptors increases cAMP, and stimulation of the M_2- and gastrin receptors increases cytosolic calcium; these intracellular messengers synergise to produce acid secretion. In this scheme, all three secretagogues act directly on the parietal cell. Evidence for independent action of all three secretagogues comes from experiments with isolated canine parietal cells. However, the situation in vivo is more complicated, in that **cimetidine**, (an H_2-receptor antagonist) and atropine (a muscarinic receptor antagonist) can block gastrin

---

Secretion of gastric acid, mucus and bicarbonate

- Acid is secreted from gastric parietal cells by a proton-pump (K^+/H^+-ATPase).
- The three endogenous secretagogues for acid are histamine, acetylcholine and gastrin.
- PGE_2 and PGI_2 inhibit acid and stimulate mucus and bicarbonate secretion.
- The genesis of peptic ulcers involves:
  — infection of the gastric mucosa with *H. pylori* plus
  — other factors such as an imbalance between the mucosal-damaging mechanisms (acid, pepsin), and the mucosal-protecting mechanisms (mucus, bicarbonate, local synthesis of PGE_2 and PGI_2).

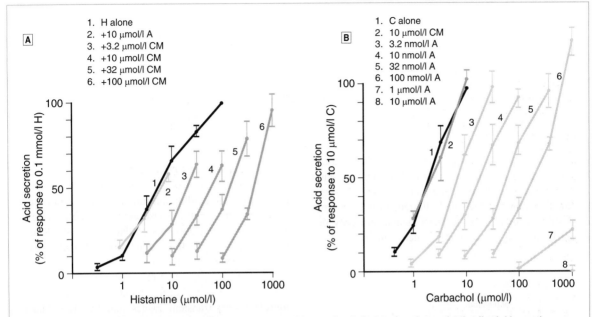

Fig. 21.3 **The effect of antisecretory agents on stimulated acid secretion in isolated canine parietal cells.** Acid secretion was measured by the accumulation of a radiolabelled weak base, aminopyrine, in the secretory channels of the parietal cell. [A] Parallel displacement of the histamine dose–response curve by cimetidine (CM) but not by atropine (A). (The pA₂ value for cimetidine calculated from such data was 6.) [B] Parallel displacement of the carbachol dose–response curve by atropine but not cimetidine. (See Ch. 1 for discussion of parallel displacement of dose–response curves.) (Adapted from: Soll A H 1980 Am J Physiol 238: G366–375)

action. The concentration–response effects of histamine and of carbachol (each with and without cimetidine and atropine) on isolated parietal cells is shown in Figure 21.3.

According to the *two-cell* hypothesis, gastrin and acetylcholine act either only by releasing histamine, or partly by releasing histamine and partly by direct action on their respective receptors on the parietal cell. This is discussed by Black & Shankley (1987), Soll & Berglindh (1987) and Sandvik & Waldrum (1991).

DRUGS USED TO INHIBIT OR NEUTRALISE GASTRIC ACID SECRETION

The principal pathological conditions in which it is useful to reduce acid secretion are **peptic ulceration** (both duodenal and gastric), **reflux oesophagitis** (in which gastric juice causes damage to the oesophagus) and the **Zollinger–Ellison syndrome** (a rare condition which is due to a gastrin-producing tumour).

The reason why peptic ulcers develop is not fully understood. Infection of the stomach mucosa with *Helicobacter pylori**—a Gram-negative bacillus that causes chronic gastritis—is now generally considered to

be a major cause, especially of duodenal ulcer; but there are still some sceptics (see Graham 1995). Treatment of *H. pylori* infection is discussed below. However, the presence of this organism does not invariably result in peptic ulcer; other factors may be involved such as a shift in the balance between mucosal-damaging mechanisms (the secretion and action of acid and pepsin) and mucosal-protecting mechanisms (the secretion and action of mucus and bicarbonate).

The mucosal-protecting mechanisms can be abrogated by NSAIDs (Ch. 13), which decrease the synthesis of prostaglandins. (Prostaglandins normally stimulate mucus and bicarbonate secretion, decrease acid secretion and cause vasodilatation, thereby increasing the elimination of acid that has diffused into the sub-mucosa.)

Antisecretory therapy of peptic ulcer and reflux oesophagitis involves decreasing the secretion of acid with **H₂-receptor antagonists** or **proton-pump inhibitors**, and/or neutralising secreted acid with **antacids** (see

---

*H. pylori infection in the stomach is an important risk factor for gastric cancer. *H. pylori* has been classified as a class 1 (definite) carcinogen for this type of malignancy.

Colin-Jones 1990). But treatment of peptic ulcer should include eradication of *H. pylori*.

H₂-RECEPTOR ANTAGONISTS

The introduction of the H₂-receptor antagonists in the mid 1970s by Black and his colleagues constituted a major breakthrough in drug treatment of peptic ulcer.

H₂-receptor antagonists competitively inhibit histamine actions at all H₂-receptors, but their main clinical use is as inhibitors of gastric acid secretion. They inhibit histamine-stimulated and gastrin-stimulated acid secretion and decrease acetylcholine-stimulated acid secretion; pepsin secretion also falls with the reduction in volume of gastric juice (Fig. 21.4). These agents not only decrease both basal and food-stimulated acid secretion by

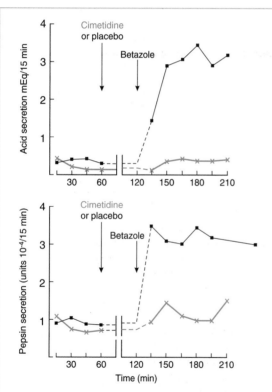

Fig. 21.4 The effect of cimetidine on betazole-stimulated gastric acid and pepsin secretion in man.
Either cimetidine (×) or a placebo (■) was given orally 60 minutes prior to injecting betazole (1.5 mg/kg) subcutaneously. (Betazole, an isomer of histamine which is a relatively specific H₂-receptor agonist, stimulates gastric acid secretion.) (Modified from: Binder H J, Donaldson R M 1978 Gastroenterology 74: 371–375)

90% or more, but promote healing of duodenal ulcers, as shown by numerous clinical trials. Relapses are likely to follow when treatment with H₂-receptor antagonists is stopped.

The drugs used are **cimetidine** (see Table 12.1b) and **ranitidine**. Newer H₂ antagonists, such as **nizatidine** and **famotidine**, are also available. The results of experiments with cimetidine on gastric secretion in humans are given in Figure 21.4. The clinical use of H₂-receptor antagonists is given in the clinical box on page 375.

Pharmacokinetic aspects and unwanted effects

The drugs are given orally and are well absorbed. Preparations of cimetidine and ranitidine for intramuscular and intravenous use are also available. With these two preparations, oral doses twice daily, even single doses nocturnally, are effective. Famotidine and nizatidine need only be given once a day.

Unwanted effects are rare and are usually readily reversed on withdrawal of treatment. Diarrhoea, dizziness, muscle pains, transient rashes and hypergastrinaemia have been reported. Cimetidine sometimes causes gynaecomastia in men and, rarely, decrease in sexual function. This is probably due to a modest affinity for androgen receptors. Cimetidine also inhibits cytochrome P450 and can retard the metabolism (and thus potentiate the action) of drugs such as the **oral anticoagulants**, **phenytoin**, **carbamazepine**, **quinidine**, **nifedipine**, **theophylline** and the **tricyclic antidepressants**. It can also cause confusion in the elderly. Ranitidine has less effect on androgen receptors and the P450 system. Both cimetidine and ranitidine reduce renal tubular secretion of basic drugs.

PROTON-PUMP INHIBITORS

The first proton-pump inhibitor was the substituted benzimidazole, **omeprazole**. It acts by irreversible inhibition of the H⁺/K⁺-ATPase (the proton pump), the terminal step in the acid secretory pathway (see Figs 21.1 and 21.2). It markedly inhibits both basal and stimulated gastric acid secretion (Fig. 21.5). It is inactive at neutral pH, but, being a weak base, accumulates in the acid environment of the canaliculi of the stimulated parietal cell where it is activated. This preferential accumulation in areas of very low pH, such as occur uniquely in the secretory canaliculi of gastric parietal cells, means that it has a specific effect on these cells. Other proton-pump inhibitors now licensed are **lansoprazole** and **pantoprazole**.

The clinical use of proton-pump inhibitors is given in the clinical box on page 375.

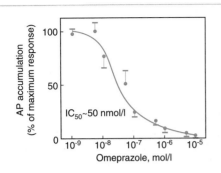

Fig. 21.5   The inhibitory action of omeprazole on acid secretion from isolated human gastric glands stimulated by 50 μmol/l histamine. Mean and standard error for tissue from eight patients. Acid secretion was measured by the accumulation of a radiolabelled weak base, aminopyrine (AP), in the secretory channels. (Adapted from: Lindberg P et al. 1987 Trends Pharmacol Sci 8: 399–402)

Pharmacokinetic aspects and unwanted effects

Omeprazole is given orally but as it degrades rapidly at low pH it is administered as capsules containing enteric-coated granules. It is absorbed and from the blood passes into the parietal cells and then into the canaliculi. Increased doses give disproportionately higher increases in plasma concentration (possibly because its inhibitory effect on acid secretion improves its own relative bio-availability). It is eliminated rapidly and completely by metabolism to inactive products. Although its half-life is about 1 hour, a single daily dose affects acid secretion for 2–3 days because it accumulates in the canaliculi. With daily dosage there is an increasing antisecretory effect for up to 5 days, after which a plateau is reached.

Unwanted effects are not common. They include headache, diarrhoea (both sometimes severe) and rashes. Dizziness, somnolence, mental confusion, impotence, gynaecomastia, and pain in muscles and joints have been reported.

ANTACIDS

Antacids act by neutralising gastric acid and thus raising the gastric pH. This has the effect of inhibiting peptic activity, which practically ceases at pH 5. Given in sufficient quantity for long enough they can produce healing of duodenal ulcers but are less effective for gastric ulcers.

The antacids in common use are salts of magnesium and aluminium. Magnesium salts cause diarrhoea and aluminium salts constipation, so mixtures of these two can, happily, be used to preserve normal bowel function.

Some preparations of these substances (e.g. magnesium trisilicate mixture and some proprietary aluminium preparations) contain high concentrations of sodium and should not be given to patients on a sodium-restricted diet.

Numerous antacid preparations are available; a few of the main ones are given below.

Magnesium hydroxide is an insoluble powder that forms magnesium chloride in the stomach. It does not produce systemic alkalosis since magnesium ion is poorly absorbed from the gut.

Magnesium trisilicate is an insoluble powder which reacts slowly with the gastric juice forming magnesium chloride and colloidal silica. This agent has a prolonged antacid effect, and it also adsorbs pepsin.

Aluminium hydroxide gel forms aluminium chloride in the stomach; when this reaches the intestine the chloride is released and is reabsorbed. Aluminium hydroxide raises the pH of the gastric juice to about 4; it also adsorbs pepsin. It acts gradually and its effect continues for several hours.* Colloidal aluminium hydroxide combines with phosphates in the gastrointestinal tract and the increased excretion of phosphate in the faeces which occurs results in decreased excretion of phosphate via the kidney. This is important in the management of patients with chronic renal failure.

Sodium bicarbonate acts rapidly and is said to raise the pH of gastric juice to about 7.4. Carbon dioxide is

---

Clinical use of agents affecting gastric secretion

- H$_2$-receptor antagonists, e.g. ranitidine:
  — peptic ulcer
  — reflux oesophagitis.
- Proton-pump inhibitors, e.g. omeprazole:
  — peptic ulcers resistant to H$_2$-receptor antagonists
  — reflux oesophagitis.
  — as one component of therapy for *Helicobacter* infection
  — Zollinger–Ellison syndrome (a rare condition) (drugs of choice).
- Antacids, e.g. magnesium trisilicate, aluminium hydroxide:
  — dyspepsia
  — symptomatic relief in peptic ulcer.
- Bismuth chelate:
  — as one component of therapy for *Helicobacter* infection.

---

*There was a suggestion—no longer widely believed—that aluminium, if absorbed, could be involved in the pathogenesis of Alzheimer's disease. In fact, aluminium is said not to be absorbed to any significant extent during administration of aluminium hydroxide, but some perhaps overly cautious practitioners may prefer to use other antacids.

liberated and this causes belching. The CO_2 stimulates gastrin secretion and can result in a secondary rise in acid secretion. Since some sodium bicarbonate is absorbed in the intestine, large doses or frequent administration of this antacid can cause alkalosis, the onset of which can be insidious. This agent should therefore not be prescribed for long-term treatment; nor should it be given to patients who are on a sodium-restricted diet.

Alginates are sometimes combined with antacids for use in reflux oesophagitis, because they are believed to increase adherence of mucus to the oesophageal mucosa.

The clinical use of antacids is given on page 375.

TREATMENT OF *H. PYLORI* INFECTION

As specified above, *H. pylori* is implicated in the production of gastric and, more particularly, duodenal ulcers and is a risk factor for gastric cancer.*

Combination therapy with three drugs is employed to eradicate *H. pylori* using omeprazole, amoxycillin and metronidazole.

Other combinations used are omeprazole, clarythromycin, and amoxycillin *or* tetracycline, metronidazole and bismuth chelates.

The antibiotics are all covered in Chapter 43 and bismuth chelates are considered below.

Elimination of the bacillus can produce long-term remission of ulcers but reinfection with the organism can occur.

DRUGS WHICH PROTECT THE MUCOSA

Some agents, termed 'cytoprotective', are said to enhance the mucosal protection mechanisms (see above) and/or provide a physical barrier over the surface of the ulcer.

Bismuth chelate

Bismuth chelate (colloidal bismuth subcitrate, tripotassium dicitratobismuthate) is used in combination regimes to treat *H. pylori* involvement in peptic ulcer. It has toxic effects on the bacillus and may also prevent its adherence to the mucosa or inhibit its proteolytic enzymes. It is also believed to have other mucosal-protecting actions—coating the ulcer base, adsorbing pepsin, enhancing local prostaglandin synthesis and stimulating bicarbonate secretion.

---

*Some authorities have proposed that *H. pylori*-induced gastroduodenitis should be considered as a disease in its own right, with peptic ulcer and gastric cancer as its important complications.

The small amount of bismuth which is absorbed is excreted in the urine. If renal excretion is impaired, the raised plasma concentrations of bismuth can result in encephalopathy.

Unwanted effects include nausea and vomiting, and blackening of the tongue and faeces.

Sucralfate

Sucralfate is a complex of aluminium hydroxide and sulphated sucrose, which, in the presence of acid, releases aluminium, acquires a strong negative charge and binds to positively charged groups in proteins, glycoproteins, etc. It can form complex gels with mucus, an action which is thought to decrease the degradation of mucus by pepsin and to limit the diffusion of hydrogen ions. In vitro studies indicate that it can inhibit the action of pepsin. It also stimulates the mucosal-protecting mechanisms—mucus and bicarbonate secretion and prostaglandin production.

It is given orally and in the acid environment of the stomach the polymerised product forms a viscous paste; about 30% is still present in the stomach 3 hours after administration. A small amount is absorbed into the systemic circulation and 1–2% of the drug given appears in the urine. It reduces the absorption of a number of other drugs, including **fluoroquinolone antibiotics**, **theophylline**, **tetracycline**, **digoxin** and **amitriptyline**. Since it requires an acid environment for activation, **antacids** given concurrently or prior to its administration will reduce its efficacy.

Unwanted effects are few, the most common being constipation which occurs in 0–15% of patients treated. Less common are dry mouth, nausea, vomiting, headache and rashes.

Misoprostol

Prostaglandins (PGs) are synthesised in large amounts by the gastric and intestinal mucosa and the E and I series can protect the deeper mucosal cells from experimental necrotic damage. A deficiency in prostaglandin production may contribute to ulcer formation. **Misoprostol** is a stable analogue of PGE_1. It inhibits gastric acid secretion, both basal and that occurring in response to food, histamine, pentagastrin and caffeine by a direct action on the parietal cell (Fig. 21.2). It maintains or increases mucosal blood flow and increases the secretion of mucus and bicarbonate.

It is given orally and is used to prevent the gastric damage that can occur with chronic use of **non-steroidal anti-inflammatory drugs** (NSAIDs).

Unwanted effects are diarrhoea and abdominal cramps;

uterine contractions can also occur (see Ch. 26). Prosta-glandins and NSAIDs are discussed in Chapters 12 and 13.

VOMITING

The act of vomiting is a complicated one necessitating coordinated activity of the somatic respiratory and abdominal muscles, and the involuntary muscles of the gastrointestinal tract.

THE REFLEX MECHANISM OF VOMITING

Borison & Wang (1953) showed that the central neural regulation of vomiting is vested in two separate units in the medulla:

- *the vomiting centre*, which controls the interrelated movements of the relevant smooth muscle and striated muscle
- *the chemoreceptor trigger zone* in the *area postrema* on the floor of the fourth ventricle, close to the vagal nuclei.

The chemoreceptor trigger zone (CTZ) is sensitive to chemical stimuli and is the site of action of drugs such as **apomorphine**, **morphine** and the **cardiac glycosides**, and of emetogenic substances released by cytotoxic cancer chemotherapy drugs. These agents reach the CTZ through the bloodstream and an action on the CTZ is probably the mechanism by which endogenous substances produced in uraemia, radiation sickness and various clinical disorders, stimulate vomiting. The CTZ is also concerned in the mediation of motion sickness.

The blood–brain barrier is relatively permeable in the neighbourhood of the CTZ, allowing circulating mediators to act on it directly.

Motion sickness—a reflex whose ability to incapacitate and cause extreme misery to those afflicted seems quite out of proportion to any conceivable biological function that it may serve—is caused by certain kinds of movement, and the origin of the stimuli is primarily the vestibular apparatus. There is at least one primary afferent relay, in the vestibular nucleus, and the cerebellum may function as a secondary relay. However, it is not clear how the vestibular apparatus relays to the CTZ, since the cells of the CTZ do not appear to receive synaptic inputs, but respond only to substances in the blood and cerebrospinal fluid. A neurohumoral factor in the cerebrospinal fluid may be implicated.

Impulses from the CTZ pass to those areas of the brainstem—known collectively as the vomiting centre—

which control and integrate the visceral and somatic functions involved in vomiting. An outline of the suggested interrelationships is given in Figure 21.6.

Vomiting can be triggered by a variety of stimuli. Some examples are given in Figure 21.6.

The main neurotransmitters considered to be involved in the control of vomiting are acetylcholine, histamine, 5-hydroxytryptamine and dopamine.* Receptors for these transmitters have been demonstrated in the relevant areas and are illustrated in Figure 21.6.

EMETIC DRUGS

In some circumstances, such as when a toxic substance has been swallowed, it may be necessary to stimulate vomiting. This should never be attempted if the patient is not fully conscious or if the substance is corrosive. The drug usually used to produce vomiting is **ipecacuanha**, which acts locally in the stomach, its irritant action being due to the presence of two alkaloids *emetine* and *cephaeline*.

Ipecacuanha is also used in a human model of emesis employed in phase I studies of anti-emetic drugs—the 'vomiting medical student'** (an advance on the 'vomiting ferret' model).

Emetine has also been used in the treatment of amoebiasis (see Ch. 46).

ANTI-EMETIC DRUGS

Different anti-emetic agents are used for different conditions, though there may be some overlap. Anti-emetic drugs are of particular importance as an adjunct to cancer chemotherapy to combat the nausea and vomiting produced by many cytotoxic drugs (see Ch. 42). These agents can cause almost unendurable nausea and vomiting.***

In using drugs to treat the morning sickness of pregnancy, the problem of potential damage to the foetus has to be borne in mind. In general, all drugs should

---

*It has been hypothesised that enkephalins (see Ch. 10) are implicated in the mediation of vomiting, acting possibly at δ-receptors in the CTZ and at μ-receptors in the vomiting centre, and that cytotoxic drugs which cause emesis may act by inhibiting the metabolising enzymes which break down the enkephalins in the CTZ.

**Voluntary! Voluntary!

***It is reported that a young medically qualified patient being treated by combination chemotherapy for sarcoma stated that 'the severity of the nausea and vomiting at times made the thought of death seem like a welcome relief'.

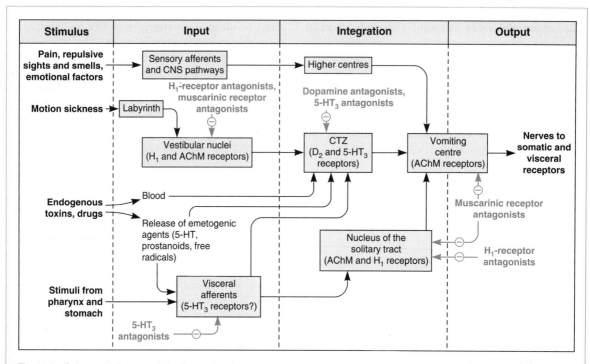

Fig. 21.6 **Schematic diagram of the factors involved in the control of vomiting, with the probable sites of action of anti-emetic drugs.** The cerebellum may function as a second relay or gating mechanism in the link between labyrinth and CTZ (not shown). (CTZ = chemoreceptor trigger zone; H_1 = histamine H_1; M = muscarinic; D_2 = dopamine D_2; 5-HT_3 = 5-hydroxytryptamine$_3$) (Based partly on a diagram from Borison H L et al. 1981 J Clin Pharmacol 21: 235–295)

be avoided, if possible, during the first three months of pregnancy.

Details of the main categories of agents are given below and a summary of the main clinical uses of anti-emetic drugs is given on page 379.

H_1-receptor antagonists

H_1-receptor antagonists are dealt with in Chapter 13. They have little or no activity against vomiting produced by substances acting directly on the CTZ but are effective in motion sickness and against vomiting caused by substances which act locally in the stomach. Examples are **cinnarizine**, **cyclizine**, **dimenhydrinate** and **promethazine**. It is possible that the component of anti-muscarinic activity in some H_1-receptor antagonists plays a part in their effects. Promethazine is effective in the morning sickness of pregnancy, but see proviso above.

H_1-receptor antagonists are most effective if given before the onset of nausea and vomiting but may have some action in controlling it when established. Their peak anti-emetic effect occurs about 4 hours after ingestion and can last 24 hours.

Muscarinic-receptor antagonists

Drugs which antagonise acetylcholine at muscarinic receptors are dealt with in Chapter 7. **Hyoscine** is active against nausea and vomiting of labyrinthine origin and against vomiting due to local stimuli in the stomach but is ineffective against substances which act directly on the CTZ.

Hyoscine is the most potent agent available for the prevention of motion sickness, though it is less useful once sickness occurs. Its anti-emetic action peaks 1–2 hours after ingestion. The main unwanted actions are drowsiness and dry mouth; other side-effects (e.g. blurring of vision and retention of urine) do not usually occur with the doses employed for anti-emetic effect. A transdermal preparation of hyoscine is available, often applied fetchingly behind the ear.

5-hydroxytryptamine (5-HT) antagonists

5-hydroxytryptamine (see Ch. 9), released in either CNS or gut, is an important transmitter in emesis. Selective 5-HT_3-receptor antagonists, for example **ondansetron**, are proving to be of particular value in preventing and treating vomiting caused by cytotoxic drugs.

Ondansetron is given orally and/or by slow intravenous injection or infusion and its $t_{1/2}$ is 5 hours. Unwanted effects include headache and gastrointestinal upsets.

Other 5-HT$_3$ antagonists, with similar action, are **granisetron** and **tropisetron**.

Phenothiazines

Phenothiazines are dealt with in Chapter 34; only those aspects relevant to the control of vomiting will be considered here.

Antipsychotic phenothiazines, such as **chlorpromazine**, **prochlorperazine** and **trifluoperazine** are effective anti-emetics, while some phenothiazines, such as **thiethylperazine**, are employed only as anti-emetic drugs. They are active against agents which directly stimulate the CTZ but most are not active against emetic stimuli in the gut. They are thought to act mainly as antagonists of the dopamine D$_2$-receptors in the chemoreceptor trigger zone (see Fig. 21.6). However, they also have some degree of blocking action at histamine and muscarinic receptors and may have other sites of action.

Halogenation of the R$_1$ side-chain, as in trifluoperazine and prochlorperazine, increases anti-emetic activity and extrapyramidal effects (see Ch. 34), and decreases the occurrence of sedation and hypotension.

The main unwanted effects are dealt with in Chapter 34.

Phenothiazines can be given orally, rectally or parenterally, which means that unlike some anti-emetics they can be given after a patient starts to vomit.

Metoclopramide

Metoclopramide is a dopamine-receptor antagonist (Fig. 21.6) and acts in the CTZ*. Like the phenothiazines, its unwanted effects are related to its blockade of other CNS dopamine receptors (see Ch. 34) but they differ qualitatively from the adverse effects of the phenothiazines. Disorders of movement occur and are more common in children and young adults. Many patients feel drowsy and fatigued but some experience motor restlessness, spasmodic torticollis (involuntary twisting of the neck) and occulogyric crises (rapid involuntary eye movements). Metoclopramide stimulates prolactin release (see Ch. 24) and can cause galactorrhoea and disorders of menstruation; diarrhoea can result from its action on gut motility (see below, p. 381). It is given orally, has a plasma $t_{1/2}$ of 4 hours and is excreted in the urine.

Metoclopramide also has peripheral actions, increasing the motility of the stomach and intestine, which add to

*In high doses, it may cause some 5-HT$_3$-receptor antagonism.

its anti-emetic effect and which may be used in therapy of gastrointestinal disorders (see p. 381).

Cannabinoids

A synthetic cannabinol derivative, **nabilone**, decreases vomiting due to agents which stimulate the CTZ. Its anti-emetic effect is antagonised by **naloxone** which implies that opioid receptors may be important in the action of this drug.

Nabilone is given orally, is well absorbed from the gastrointestinal tract and is metabolised in many tissues. Its plasma half-life is approximately 120 minutes, and its metabolites are excreted in the urine and faeces.

Unwanted effects are common, especially drowsiness, dizziness and dry mouth. Mood changes and postural hypotension are also fairly frequent. Some patients experience hallucinations and psychotic reactions, resembling the effect of other cannabinoids (see Ch. 39).

Steroids

High-dose glucocorticoids (**dexamethasone** and **methylprednisolone**; see Ch. 24) can have anti-emetic action the mechanism of which is unknown. They can be used alone or in combination with a phenothiazine or with ondansetron. They synergise with **ondansetron**.

Other anti-emetic agents

Other anti-emetic agents include the non-phenothiazine antipsychotic drugs **haloperidol** and **droperidol** (Ch. 34)

The reflex mechanism of vomiting

- Emetic stimuli:
  — chemicals in blood
  — neuronal input from GI tract, labyrinth and CNS.
- Impulses from chemoreceptor trigger zone, and various CNS centres relay to the vomiting centre.
- Chemical transmitters: histamine, acetylcholine, dopamine, 5-hydroxytryptamine acting on H$_1$, muscarinic, D$_2$ and 5-HT$_3$-receptors respectively.
- Anti-emetic drugs:
  — H$_1$-receptor antagonists (e.g. cyclizine)
  — muscarinic antagonists (e.g. hyoscine)
  — 5-HT$_3$-receptor antagonists (e.g. ondansetron)
  — D$_2$-receptor antagonists (e.g. thiethylperazine, metoclopramide)
  — cannabinoids (e.g. nabilone).
- Main side-effects of principal anti-emetics:
  — drowsiness and antiparasympathetic effects (hyoscine, nabilone > cinnarizine)
  — dystonic reactions (thiethylperazine > metoclopramide)
  — general CNS disturbances (nabilone)
  — headache, GIT upsets (ondansetron).

which have given good results against strongly emetic cytotoxic drugs (e.g. cisplatin). **Domperidone**, a dopamine D$_2$-receptor antagonist (see Ch. 15 and below) is also used as an anti-emetic in postoperative vomiting and against moderately emetogenic anticancer drugs.

THE MOTILITY OF THE GASTROINTESTINAL TRACT

Drugs which increase movements include the *purgatives*, which accelerate the passage of food through the intestine, and *agents which increase the motility* of the gastrointestinal smooth muscle without causing purgation. The main agents decreasing movements are the *antidiarrhoeal* drugs and the *antispasmodics*. These four groups of agents are dealt with below.

PURGATIVES

The transit of food through the intestine may be hastened by several different methods:

- by increasing the volume of non-absorbable solid residue with *bulk laxatives*
- by increasing the water content with *osmotic laxatives*
- by altering the consistency of the faeces with *faecal softeners*
- by increasing motility and secretion (*stimulant purgatives*).

Good, comparative clinical studies of laxatives are not available; folk-lore and old wives' tales abound.

Bulk laxatives

The bulk laxatives include **methylcellulose** and certain plant gums, for example **sterculia**, **agar**, **bran** and **ispaghula husk**. These agents are polysaccharide polymers which are not broken down by the normal processes of digestion in the upper part of the gastrointestinal tract. They act by virtue of their capacity to retain water in the gut lumen and so promote peristalsis. They take several days to work but have no serious unwanted effects.

Osmotic laxatives

Osmotic laxatives consist of poorly absorbed solutes—the **saline purgatives** and **lactulose**. These maintain an increased volume of fluid in the lumen of the bowel by osmosis, which accelerates the transfer of the gut contents through the small intestine and results in an abnormally large volume entering the colon. This causes distension which leads to purgation about an hour later. Abdominal cramps can occur. Isotonic or hypotonic solutions of saline purgatives cause purgation, hypertonic solutions can cause vomiting.

The main salts in use are **magnesium sulphate** and **magnesium hydroxide**. These are virtually insoluble; they remain in the lumen and retain water, increasing the volume of the faeces. The amount of magnesium absorbed after an oral dose is usually too small to have adverse systemic effects but these salts should be avoided in small children and in patients with poor renal function, in whom they can cause heart block, neuromuscular block or CNS depression.

Lactulose is a semisynthetic disaccharide of fructose and galactose. In the colon, bacteria convert it to its two component sugars which are poorly absorbed; when these are fermented, the lactic and acetic acid formed function as osmotic laxatives. It takes 2–3 days to act. Unwanted effects, with high doses, are flatulence, cramps, diarrhoea and electrolyte disturbance. Tolerance can develop.

Faecal softeners

Docusate sodium is a surface-active compound which acts in the gastrointestinal tract in a manner similar to a detergent, and produces softer faeces. It is also a weak stimulant laxative.

Stimulant purgatives

These drugs act mainly by increasing water and electrolyte secretion by the mucosa and also by increasing peristalsis—possibly by stimulating enteric nerves. The following are the more important purgatives in this group:

- bisacodyl
- sodium picosulphate
- preparations of senna.

These agents sometimes cause abdominal cramps; prolonged use can lead to deterioration of intestinal function, and can result in atonic colon.

Senna has laxative activity because it contains derivatives of anthracene (e.g. emodin) combined with sugars to form glycosides. The drug passes unchanged into the colon where bacteria hydrolyse the glycoside bond, releasing the free anthracene derivatives which are absorbed and have a direct stimulant effect on the myenteric plexus, resulting in smooth muscle activity and thus defaecation. Some emodin is excreted in the urine and some may appear in the milk of women who are breast feeding.

A single dose usually produces a laxative action within 8 hours, which may be accompanied by griping.

Bisacodyl can be given orally but is usually administered as a suppository, causing stimulation of the rectal mucosa which results in peristaltic action and defaecation in 15–30 minutes. **Sodium picosulphate** has a similar action; it is given orally and is often used in preparation for intestinal surgery.

DRUGS WHICH INCREASE GASTROINTESTINAL MOTILITY

Some agents increase gut motility. The main drugs used are:

- domperidone
- metoclopramide
- cisapride.

Domperidone

Domperidone is primarily a dopamine-receptor antagonist acting at D_2-receptors, and is used as an anti-emetic as described above. It is also effective in increasing gastrointestinal motility, by an unknown mechanism. Clinically, it increases lower oesophageal sphincter pressure (thus inhibiting gastro-oesophageal reflux), increases gastric emptying and enhances duodenal peristalsis. It does not stimulate gastric acid secretion. It is useful in disorders of gastric emptying and in chronic gastric reflux.

Its main unwanted effect is hyperprolactinaemia, consistent with its action on dopamine receptors (see Chs 26 and 28).

Metoclopramide

In addition to its central effects as an anti-emetic (see above), metoclopramide exerts a significant local stimulant effect on gastric motility, causing a marked acceleration of gastric emptying with no concomitant stimulation of gastric acid secretion. Metoclopramide is useful in gastro-oesophageal reflux and in disorders of gastric emptying, but is ineffective in paralytic ileus.

Cisapride

Cisapride stimulates acetylcholine release in the myenteric plexus in the upper gastrointestinal tract. This raises oesophageal sphincter pressure and increases gut motility. It is used in reflux oesophagitis and in disorders of gastric emptying. It has no anti-emetic action.

Unwanted effects, which are rare, include diarrhoea, abdominal cramps and tachycardia.

ANTIDIARRHOEAL AGENTS

Diarrhoea is the frequent passage of liquid faeces. There are numerous causes including infectious agents, toxins, anxiety, drugs, etc. The repercussions will depend not only on the cause, but also on the state of nutrition and health of the patient. They can range from discomfort and inconvenience in a healthy well-nourished adult, to a medical emergency requiring hospitalisation and parenteral fluid and electrolyte therapy. On a world-wide basis, acute diarrhoeal disease is one of the principal causes of death in malnourished infants; this is particularly important in developing countries.

Diarrhoea involves both an increase in the motility of the gastrointestinal tract, along with increased secretion and decreased absorption of fluid, and thus a loss of electrolytes (particularly sodium) and water. Details of electrolyte transport in diarrhoea are given by Field et al. (1989). Cholera toxins and some other bacterial toxins produce not only loss of gut contents but a profound increase in secretion through their effect on the guanine nucleotide regulatory proteins which couple the surface receptors of the mucosal cells to adenylate cyclase (see Ch. 2).

There are three approaches to the treatment of severe acute diarrhoea:

- maintenance of fluid and electrolyte balance
- use of anti-infective agents
- use of non-antimicrobial antidiarrhoeal agents.

The maintenance of fluid and electrolyte balance by means of oral rehydration is the first priority and wider appreciation of this could save the lives of many infants in the developing world. Many cases require no other treatment. In the ileum, as in parts of the nephron, there is co-transport of sodium and glucose across the epithelial cell and, therefore, glucose enhances sodium absorption and thus water uptake; amino acids have a similar effect. Preparations of sodium chloride and glucose for oral use are available in powder form, ready to be dissolved in water before use.

The use of anti-infective agents is usually not necessary in simple gastroenteritis since most infections are usually viral in origin, and those that are bacterial generally resolve without antibacterial therapy. *Campylobacter* is the commonest bacterial organism causing gastroenteritis in the UK, and severe cases may require **erythromycin** or **ciprofloxacin** (Ch. 43). Chemotherapy may be necessary in some types of enteritis (e.g. typhoid, amoebic dysentery and cholera).

The use of non-antimicrobial antidiarrhoeal agents is dealt with below, and these include antimotility agents, adsorbents and agents which modify fluid and electrolyte transport.

Traveller's diarrhoea. More than 3 000 000 people cross international borders each year. Many travel hopefully but come back ill, having encountered enterotoxin-producing *Escherichia coli* or other organisms. Most infections are self-limiting and require only oral replacement of fluid and salt as detailed above. General principles for the treatment of traveller's diarrhoea are detailed by DuPont & Ericsson (1993) and Gorbach (1987), who makes the pertinent remark 'travel broadens the mind and loosens the bowels'.

Antimotility agents

The main pharmacological agents which decrease motility are **opiates** (details in Ch. 37) and **muscarinic receptor antagonists** (details in Ch. 7). Agents in this latter group are seldom employed as primary therapy for diarrhoea because of their actions on other systems; but small doses of atropine are used combined with diphenoxylate (see below).

The action of **morphine**, the archetypal opiate, on the alimentary tract is complex; it increases the tone and rhythmic contractions of the intestine but diminishes propulsive activity. Its overall effect is constipating. The pyloric, ileocolic and anal sphincters are contracted and the tone of the large intestine is markedly increased.

The main opiates used in diarrhoea are **codeine** (a morphine congener), **diphenoxylate** and **loperamide** (both pethidine congeners which do not readily penetrate the blood–brain barrier, and are used only for their actions in the gut). All have unwanted effects which

occur mainly with chronic use and include constipation, abdominal cramps, drowsiness and dizziness. Paralytic ileus can also occur. They should not be used in young children.

Loperamide has a relatively selective action on the gastrointestinal tract and undergoes significant enterohepatic cycling. It has low solubility in water which discourages abuse by injection. In traveller's diarrhoea loperamide reduces the frequency of passage of faeces and the duration of the illness.

Diphenoxylate, given once in the therapeutic dose suitable for diarrhoea, does not have morphine-like activity in the CNS, though large doses (25-fold higher) produce typical opioid effects. However, its salts are, for practical purposes, insoluble in water and thus the drug does not have potential for abuse by injection. Preparations of diphenoxylate usually contain atropine as well.

Codeine and loperamide have antisecretory actions in addition to their effects on intestinal motility.

Bismuth subsalicylate, which is used for traveller's diarrhoea, is said to be safe in healthy young adults and is reported to prevent up to 65% of cases of diarrhoea in areas of high risk. It decreases fluid secretion in the bowel and may work largely by virtue of its salicylate component.

Bismuth subsalicylate can cause tinnitus and blackening of the faeces and may have as yet unknown unwanted effects.

Adsorbents

Adsorbent agents are used extensively in the treatment of diarrhoea, although properly controlled trials proving adequacy have not been carried out.

The main preparations used are **kaolin**, **pectin**, **chalk**,

---

Drugs and GI tract motility

- Purgatives:
  - bulk laxatives, e.g. ispaghula husk (first choice for slow action)
  - osmotic laxatives, e.g. lactulose
  - faecal softeners, e.g. docusate sodium
  - stimulant purgatives, e.g. senna.
- Drugs which increase motility without purgation:
  - domperidone, used in disorders of gastric emptying.
- Drugs used to treat diarrhoea:
  - oral rehydration with isotonic solutions of NaCl plus glucose or starch-based cereal (important in infants)
  - antimotility agents, e.g. loperamide (unwanted effects: drowsiness and nausea)
  - adsorbents, e.g. magnesium aluminium silicate.

charcoal, **methyl cellulose** and **activated attapulgite** (magnesium aluminium silicate).

It has been suggested that these agents may act by adsorbing microorganisms or toxins, by altering the intestinal flora or by coating and protecting the intestinal mucosa but there is no hard evidence for this.

ANTISPASMODIC AGENTS

Drugs which reduce spasm in the gut are of value in irritable bowel syndrome and diverticular disease.

Muscarinic receptor antagonists are dealt with in Chapter 7. They decrease spasm by inhibiting parasympathetic activity. Agents available include **propantheline** and **dicyclomine**. The last named is thought to have some additional direct relaxant action on smooth muscle. Unwanted effects—dry mouth, blurred vision, dry skin, tachycardia, difficulty with urination—are due to parasympathetic inhibition in other tissues; they are less marked and less common with dicyclomine.

Mebeverine, a derivative of reserpine, has a direct relaxant action on gastrointestinal smooth muscle. Unwanted effects are few.

DRUGS FOR CHRONIC INFLAMMATORY BOWEL DISEASE

Chronic inflammatory bowel disease comprises ulcerative colitis and Crohn's disease (a granulomatous condition affecting especially the terminal ileum and the colon), both of uncertain aetiology. The following agents are used.

Glucocorticoids—these anti-inflammatory agents are dealt with in Chapter 24. See also Figure 12.4. Prednisolone is given locally in the bowel by suppository or enema.

Sulphasalazine is a combination of the sulphonamide, sulphapyridine, with 5-aminosalicylic acid. The latter is the active moiety; it is released in the colon and is not absorbed. Its mechanism of action is not known. It may act by scavenging free radicals, inhibiting prostaglandin and leukotriene production and/or by decreasing neutrophil chemotaxis and superoxide generation. Its unwanted effects are diarrhoea, salicylate sensitivity and interstitial nephritis. The sulphapyridine moiety is absorbed and its unwanted effects are those associated with the sulphonamides (see Ch. 43). Sulphasalazine is not useful for the actual attack of inflammatory bowel

disease, but is valuable in preventing recurrence in patients who are in remission.

Newer compounds are **mesalazine** (5-amino-salicylic acid itself) and **olsalazine** (two molecules of 5-amino-salicylic acid linked by a diazo bond, which is broken by colonic bacteria).

The immunosuppressant, **azathioprine** (see Ch. 13), is used in patients with severe disease.

DRUGS AFFECTING THE BILIARY SYSTEM

Drugs used to treat cholesterol cholelithiasis

The commonest pathological condition of the biliary tract is cholesterol cholelithiasis, i.e. the formation of cholesterol gallstones. Drugs which dissolve non-calcified cholesterol gallstones are **chenodeoxycholic acid** (CDCA) and **ursodeoxycholic acid** (UDCA). CDCA is one of the two primary bile acids. UDCA, the 7 β-hydroxy epimer of CDCA, occurs in small amounts in human bile and is the main bile acid in the bear (hence 'urso'). UDCA and CDCA are interconvertible during enterohepatic cycling in humans. Given orally, UDCA and CDCA are handled by the body in the same way as endogenous bile acids; both agents decrease hepatic synthesis and secretion of cholesterol. Diarrhoea is the main unwanted effect.

The clinical use of these agents is appropriate only in selected patients with gallstones as surgery is the preferred treatment in most cases when active intervention is indicated.

Drugs affecting biliary spasm

The pain produced by the passage of gallstones down the bile duct (biliary colic) can be very intense, and immediate relief may be required. **Morphine** relieves the pain, owing to its central narcotic analgesic action, but it may have an undesirable local effect since it constricts the sphincter of Oddi and raises the pressure in the bile duct. **Buprenorphine** may be preferable. **Pethidine** has similar actions, although it relaxes other smooth muscle, for example that of the ureter. **Atropine** is commonly employed to relieve biliary spasm since it has antispasmodic action. It may be used in conjunction with morphine.

The **nitrates** (see Ch. 14) can produce a marked fall of intrabiliary pressure and may relieve biliary spasm.

REFERENCES AND FURTHER READING

Innervation and hormones of the gastrointestinal tract

Del Valle J, Yamada T 1990 The gut as an endocrine organ. Annu Rev Med 41: 447–455

Goyal R K, Hirano I 1996 The enteric nervous system. N Engl J Med 334: 1106–1115

Walsh J H 1988 Peptides as regulators of gastric acid secretion. Annu Rev Physiol 50: 41–63

Gastric secretion

Allen A, Garnet A 1980 Mucus and bicarbonate secretion in the stomach and their possible role in mucosal protection. Gut 21: 249–262

Angus J A, Black J W 1982 The interaction of choline esters, vagal stimulation and H_2-receptor blockade on acid secretion in vitro. Eur J Pharmacol 80: 217–224

Black J W, Shankley N P 1987 How does gastrin act to stimulate oxyntic cell secretion? Trends Pharmacol Sci 8: 486–490

Black J W, Duncan W A M, Durant C J, Ganellin C R, Parsons E M 1972 Definition and antagonism of histamine H_2-receptors. Nature 236: 385–390 *(Seminal paper)*

Blaser M J 1998 *Helicobacter pylori* and gastric disease. Br Med J 316: 1507–1510 *(Succinct review, emphasis on future developments)*

Graham J R 1995 *Helicobacter pylori*: human pathogen or simply an opportunist? Lancet 345: 1095–1097

Sachs G, Shin J M et al. 1995 The pharmacology of the gastric acid pump: the $H^+,K^+ATPase$. Annu Rev Pharmacol Toxicol 35: 277–305 *(Comprehensive review)*

Sandvik A K, Waldrum H L 1991 Gastrin is a potent stimulant of the parietal cell—maybe. Am J Physiol 260: G925–G928

Soll A H, Berglindh T 1987 Physiology of isolated gastric glands and parietal cells: receptors and effectors regulating function. In: Johnson L R (ed) Physiology of the gastrointestinal tract, 2nd edn. Raven Press, New York, pp 883–908

Drugs in gastric disorders

Alper J 1993 Ulcers as an infectious disease. Science 260: 159–160

Axon A, Forman D 1997 Helicobacter gastroduodenitis: a serious infectious disease. Br Med J 314: 1430–1431 *(Editorial comment)*

Bateman D N 1997 Proton-pump inhibitors: three of a kind? Lancet 349: 1637–1638 *(Editorial commentary)*

Blaser M J 1996 The bacteria behind ulcers. Scientific American (Feb): 92–97 *(Simple coverage, very good diagrams)*

Colin-Jones D G 1990 Acid suppression: how much is needed. Br Med J 301: 564–565

Feldman M, Burton M E 1990 Histamine H_2-receptor antagonists: standard therapy for acid-peptic disease. N Engl J Med 323: 1672–1680, 1749–1755

McCarthy D M 1991 Sucralfate. N Engl J Med 325: 1017–1025

Marks I N, Schmassmann A et al. 1992 Antacid therapy today. Eur J Gastroenterol Hepatol 4: 977–983

Rauws E A J, van der Hulst R W M 1998 The management of *H. pylori* infection. Br Med J 316: 162–163 *(Editorial commentary)*

Walsh J H, Peterson W L 1995 The treatment of *Helicobacter pylori* infection in the management of peptic ulcer disease. N Engl J Med 333: 984–991 *(Useful coverage)*

Walt R P 1992 Misoprostol for the treatment of peptic ulcer and anti-inflammatory-drug-induced gastroduodenal ulceration. N Engl J Med 327: 1575–1580

Yeomans N D, Tulassy Z et al. 1998 A comparison of omeprazole with ranitidine for ulcers associated with nonsteroidal antiinflammatory drugs. N Engl J Med 338: 719–726 *(Results: omeprazole healed and prevented ulcers more effectively than ranitidine)*

Vomiting

Borison H L, Wang S C 1953 Physiology and pharmacology of vomiting. Pharmacol Rev 5: 193–230

Bunce K, Tyers M, Beranek P 1991 Clinical evaluation of $5-HT_3$ receptor antagonists as anti-emetics. Trends Pharmacol Sci 12: 46–48

Tramèr M R, Moore R et al. 1997 A quantitative systematic review of ondansetron in treatment of established postoperative nausea and vomiting. Br Med J 314: 1088–1092

Motility of the gastrointestinal tract

Avery M E, Snyder J D 1990 Oral therapy for acute diarrhoea. N Engl J Med 323: 891–894

Bateman D N, Smith J M 1989 A policy for laxatives. Br Med J 298: 1420–1421

Costello A M de L, Bhutta T I 1992 Antidiarrhoeal drugs for acute diarrhoea in children: none work, and many may be dangerous. Br Med J 304: 1–2

DuPont H L, Ericsson C D 1993 Prevention and treatment of travellers diarrhoea. N Engl J Med 328: 1281–1287

Farthing M J G 1993 Travellers diarrhoea: mostly due to bacteria and difficult to prevent. Br Med J 306: 1425–1426

Field M, Rao M C, Chang E B 1989 Intestinal electrolyte transport and diarrhoeal disease. N Engl J Med 321: 800–806, 879–883

Gorbach S L 1987 Bacterial diarrhoea and its treatment. Lancet 2: 1378–1382

Huizinga J D, Thuneberg L et al., 1997 Interstitial cells of Cajal as targets for pharmacological intervention in gastrointestinal motor disorders. Trends Pharmacol Sci 18: 393–403

Spiller R 1990 Management of constipation. Part 2: When fibre fails. In: Controversies in therapeutics. Br Med J 300: 1064–1065

The biliary system

Bateson M C 1997 Bile acid research and applications. Lancet 349: 5–6

Editorial 1992 Bile acid therapy in the 1990s. Lancet 340: 1260–1261

Johnston D E, Kaplan M M 1993 Pathogenesis and treatment of gallstones. N Engl J Med 328: 412–421

Inflammatory bowel disease

Kamm M A, Senapati A 1992 Drug management of ulcerative colitis. Br Med J 305: 35–38

22

The endocrine pancreas and the control of blood glucose

PANCREATIC ISLET HORMONES

The endocrine portion of the pancreas, namely the islets of Langerhans, contains four main cell types: B-cells that secrete *insulin*, A-cells that secrete glucagon, D-cells that secrete somatostatin and PP cells that secrete pancreatic polypeptide (the function of which is unknown). The core of each islet contains mainly the predominant B-cells surrounded by a mantle of A-cells with D-cells or, in the posterior part of the head of the pancreas, PP cells (see Fig. 22.1). The B-cells secrete, as well as insulin, a peptide known as *islet amyloid polypeptide* (or amylin). Amylin opposes the action of insulin by stimulating breakdown of glycogen in striated muscle and delays gastric emptying thereby inhibiting insulin secretion, although the biological importance of these effects is controversial (see below). Insulin controls the metabolism of carbohydrate, fat and protein and normally determines blood glucose concentration. Diseases in which there is deficient or excessive insulin production (*diabetes mellitus* or functioning B-cell tumours known as *insulinomas*, respectively) are characterised by profound metabolic disturbances. Glucagon increases blood glucose; decreased glucagon secretion is not known to cause disease; excessive secretion (from functioning tumours of A-cells, known as *glucagonomas*) causes only moderate hyperglycaemia but profound catabolic effects on muscle protein. Somatostatin has an indirect paracrine role in that it inhibits secretion of insulin and of glucagon. Somatostatin is widely distributed outside the pancreas and is also released from the hypothalamus, thereby inhibiting the release of growth hormone from the pituitary (p. 411).

INSULIN

Insulin was the first protein whose amino acid sequence was determined (by Brown and his co-workers in 1955). It consists of two peptide chains (A and B, of 21 and 30 amino acid residues respectively) connected by two disulphide bridges.

Synthesis and secretion

Like other islet hormones, insulin is synthesised as a precursor (preproinsulin) in the rough endoplasmic reticulum. Preproinsulin is transported to the Golgi apparatus where it undergoes post-translational modification in the form of successive proteolytic cleavage to proinsulin and then to insulin and C-peptide. These are stored in granules in the B-cells and are normally cosecreted by exocytosis in equimolar amounts together with smaller and variable amounts of proinsulin. This relationship is altered in diabetes mellitus. Secretion normally occurs in pulses every 15–30 minutes. The main factor controlling the synthesis and secretion of insulin is the *blood glucose* concentration (Fig. 22.1). The B-cell responds to both the absolute glucose concentration and also to the *rate of change* of blood glucose. There is a steady basal release of insulin and also a response to a rise in blood glucose. This response has two phases—an initial rapid phase reflecting release of stored hormone, and a slower, delayed phase reflecting both continued release of stored hormone and new synthesis (Fig. 22.2). The response is abnormal in diabetes mellitus, as discussed later.

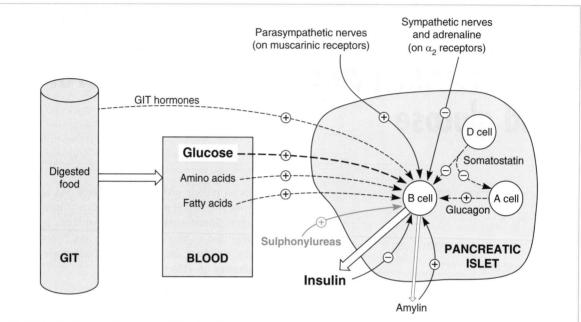

Fig. 22.1 **Endogenous factors regulating insulin secretion by B-cells of the islets of Langerhans.** Blood glucose is the most important factor. Drugs used to stimulate insulin secretion are shown in blue. Glucagon potentiates insulin release but opposes some of its peripheral actions and increases blood glucose; see Table 22.2. (GIT = gastrointestinal tract)

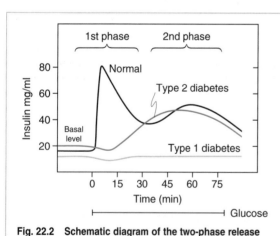

Fig. 22.2 **Schematic diagram of the two-phase release of insulin in response to a constant glucose infusion.** The first phase is missing in type 2 (non-insulin-dependent) diabetes mellitus and both are missing in type 1 (insulin-dependent) diabetes mellitus. The first phase is also produced by amino acids, sulphonylureas, glucagon and GIT hormones. (Data from: Pfeifer et al. 1981 Am J Med 70: 579–588)

ATP-sensitive K^+ channels determine the resting membrane potential in B-cells. Glucose enters B-cells via a membrane transporter called Glut-2, and its subsequent

metabolism via *glucokinase* (the rate-limiting enzyme that acts as the 'glucose sensor' linking insulin secretion to extracellular glucose) and glycolysis increases the intracellular concentration of ATP, which blocks the ATP-sensitive K^+ channels, causing membrane depolarisation. This opens voltage-dependent Ca^{2+} channels, leading to Ca^{2+} influx. There is evidence that the Ca^{2+} signal caused by glucose in the B-cell induces insulin secretion only in the presence of amplifying intracellular messengers including diacylglycerol (DAG), non-esterified arachidonic acid (which facilitates further Ca^{2+} entry) and 12-lipoxygenase products of arachidonic acid (mainly 12-S-HETE; see Ch. 12). Most phospholipases are activated by Ca^{2+} but free arachidonic acid is liberated in B-cells by an ATP-sensitive Ca^{2+}-insensitive ('ASCI') phospholipase A_2. Thus, both Ca^{2+} entry and arachidonic acid production are driven by ATP in the B-cell.

Other stimuli to insulin release (besides glucose) include amino acids (particularly arginine and leucine), fatty acids, the *parasympathetic nervous system*, glucagon and various hormones from the gastrointestinal tract and the *sulphonylurea drugs* (see below). These elicit only the first phase of insulin release. Gastrointestinal hormones that stimulate insulin secretion, including *gastrin, secretin, cholecystokinin, gastric inhibitory poly-peptide* (GIP) and enteroglucagon-related peptides such as *glucagon-like peptide* (GLP) and GLP_1 (the amide of a fragment of GLP), are released by eating. This explains why oral glucose causes greater insulin release than does intravenous glucose. Such GIT hormones (in particular GIP and GLP_1) provide an anticipatory signal from the GIT to the islets.

Insulin release is inhibited by several peptide hormones including somatostatin, galanin (an endogenous ATP-sensitive K^+ channel activator) and amylin and by the *sympathetic nervous system* (Fig. 22.1). Adrenaline increases blood glucose by inhibiting insulin release from the islets (via α_2-receptors) and by promoting glycogenolysis via β_2-receptors in striated muscle and liver. These activate adenylate cyclase, leading to conversion of glycogen phosphorylase from the inactive to the active form (see Ch. 2).

About one-fifth of the insulin stored in the pancreas of the human adult (approximately 5 mg) is secreted daily, and the mean plasma concentration after an overnight fast is 20–50 pmol/l. Insulin is secreted into the portal circulation and in the fasted state its concentration in the portal vein is approximately threefold higher than in the rest of the circulation, reflecting hepatic clearance. This differential may rise to a ratio of 10 : 1 after the islets have been stimulated by glucose.

Circulating insulin can be measured by radioimmunoassay, but this may give an overestimate because many insulin antibodies cross-react with proinsulin. Plasma insulin concentration is reduced in patients with type 1 ('insulin-dependent') diabetes mellitus (see below) and markedly increased in patients with insulinomas, as is C-peptide with which it is co-released.*

Actions

Insulin is the main hormone controlling intermediary metabolism, having actions on liver, muscle and fat (Table 22.1). Its overall effect is to conserve fuel by facilitating the uptake, utilisation and storage of glucose, amino acids and fats after a meal. Acutely, it *reduces blood sugar.* Conversely, a fall in plasma insulin reduces

---

*Insulin for injection does *not* contain C-peptide, which therefore provides a means of distinguishing endogenous from exogenous insulin. This is used to differentiate insulinoma (an insulin-secreting tumour causing high circulating insulin with high C-peptide) from surreptitious injection of insulin (high insulin, normal or low C-peptide). Deliberate induction of hypoglycaemia by self-injection with insulin is a well-recognised, if unusual, manifestation of psychiatric disorder, especially in health professionals—it has also been used in murder.

cellular glucose uptake and mobilises endogenous sources of fuel. The biochemical pathways through which insulin exerts its effects are summarised in Figure 22.3 and molecular aspects of its mechanism are discussed below.

Effect of insulin on carbohydrate metabolism

Insulin influences glucose metabolism in all tissues, especially the *liver* where it inhibits glycogenolysis (glycogen breakdown) and gluconeogenesis (synthesis of glucose from non-carbohydrate sources) while stimulating glycogen synthesis. It also increases glucose utilisation (glycolysis), but the overall effect is to increase hepatic glycogen stores.

In *muscle*, unlike liver, uptake of glucose is slow and is the rate-limiting step in carbohydrate metabolism. The main effect of insulin is to increase facilitated transport of glucose via a transporter called Glut-4, and to stimulate glycogen synthesis and glycolysis.

Insulin increases glucose uptake by Glut-4 in *adipose tissue* as well as in muscle, enhancing glucose metabolism. One of the main end-products of glucose metabolism in adipose tissue is glycerol, which is esterified with fatty acids to form triglycerides, thereby affecting fat metabolism (see below and Table 22.1).

Effect of insulin on fat metabolism

Insulin increases fatty acid synthesis and triglyceride formation in *adipose tissue*, while inhibiting lipolysis, partly via dephosphorylation (and hence inactivation) of lipases (Table 22.1). It also inhibits the lipolytic actions of adrenaline, growth hormone and glucagon by opposing their actions on adenylate cyclase. Insulin also causes lipogenesis in the *liver*.

Effect of insulin on protein metabolism

Insulin stimulates the uptake of amino acids into *muscle* and increases protein synthesis. It also decreases protein catabolism and inhibits the oxidation of amino acids in the *liver*.

Other metabolic effects of insulin

Other metabolic effects of insulin include transport into cells of K^+,* Ca^{2+}, nucleosides and inorganic phosphate.

Long-term effects of insulin

In addition to its immediate effects on metabolism, insulin has longer-term actions by increasing or decreasing enzyme synthesis. It is an important anabolic hormone, especially during foetal development. It

---

*This action is used in the emergency treatment of hyperkalaemia by intravenous glucose with insulin.

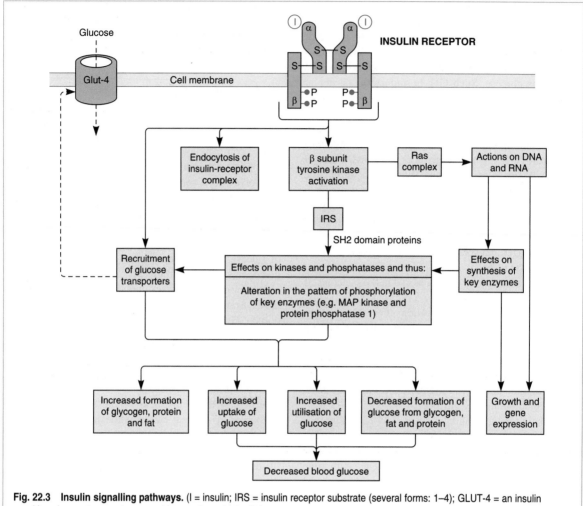

Fig. 22.3   Insulin signalling pathways. (I = insulin; IRS = insulin receptor substrate (several forms: 1–4); GLUT-4 = an insulin sensitive glucose transporter present in muscle and fat cells)

Table 22.1   Summary of the effects of insulin on carbohydrate, fat and protein metabolism in liver, muscle and adipose tissue

Type of metabolism	Liver cells	Fat cell	Muscle
Carbohydrate metabolism	↓ gluconeogenesis ↓ glycogenolysis ↑ glycolysis ↑ glycogenesis	↑ glucose intake ↑ glycerol synthesis	↑ glucose uptake ↑ glycolysis ↑ glycogenesis
Fat metabolism	↑ lipogenesis ↓ lipolysis	↑ synthesis of triglycerides ↑ fatty acid synthesis ↓ lipolysis	–
Protein metabolism	↓ protein breakdown	–	↑ amino acid uptake ↑ protein synthesis

stimulates cell proliferation and is implicated in somatic and visceral growth and development.

Mechanism of action

Insulin binds to a specific receptor on the surface of its target cells. The receptor is a large (approximately 400 kDa) transmembrane glycoprotein complex consisting of two α- and two β-subunits linked by disulphide bridges (Fig. 22.3). The α-subunits are entirely extracellular and each carries an insulin-binding site, whereas the β-subunits are transmembrane proteins with tyrosine kinase activity. This activity is suppressed by the α-subunits, but insulin binding causes a conformational change that derepresses (activates) the tyrosine kinase activity of the β-subunits (see Fig. 22.3 and Ch. 2), which act on each other (autophosphorylation) as well as on other target proteins (such as IRS proteins; see below). Binding data for insulin and its receptors are not linear when displayed on a Scatchard plot (cf. Fig. 1.8), probably because of 'negative cooperativity' (i.e. binding of insulin to the binding site on one α-subunit reduces the affinity for insulin of the site on the neighbouring α-subunit).

At concentrations of insulin that produce maximum effects, less than 10% of the receptors are occupied. On interaction with insulin, they aggregate into clusters and the insulin–receptor complexes are subsequently internalised in vesicles, resulting in down-regulation. Internalised insulin is degraded in lysosomes, but receptors are recycled to the plasma membrane. The signal transduction mechanisms that link receptor-binding to the biological effects of insulin are complex. The immediate *metabolic actions* are mediated largely through alteration of the state of key enzymes via activation of a cascade of kinases and phosphatases, initiated by tyrosine kinase activity of the β-subunit of the receptor. Insulin receptor substrate (IRS) proteins undergo rapid tyrosine phosphorylation in response to insulin and insulin-like growth factor-1 (IGF-1) but not to other growth factors that act through receptor tyrosine kinases. The best characterised of these is IRS-I, which contains 22 tyrosine residues as potential phosphorylation sites which interact with proteins that contain a so-called SH2 domain (see Ch. 2), thereby passing on the insulin signal. Knockout mice lacking IRS-1 are hyporesponsive to insulin ('insulin resistant'), but do not become diabetic because of robust B-cell compensation with increased insulin secretion. By contrast, mice lacking IRS-2 fail to compensate and develop overt diabetes, implicating IRS-2 as a candidate gene for human type 2 diabetes. Activation of phosphatidylinositol 3-kinase by interaction of its SH2 domain with phosphorylated IRS has several important effects including recruitment of insulin-sensitive glucose transporters (GLUT-4) from the Golgi apparatus to the plasma membrane in muscle and fat cells.

The *longer-term actions* of insulin entail effects on DNA and RNA, mediated partly at least by the Ras signalling complex. Ras is a protein that regulates cell growth and cycles between an active GTP-bound form and an inactive GDP-bound form (see Chs 2 and 42). Insulin shifts the equilibrium in favour of the active form and initiates a phosphorylation cascade that results in activation of mitogen-activated protein kinase (MAP kinase) which in turn activates several nuclear transcription factors leading to the expression of genes that are involved both with cell growth and with intermediary metabolism. Regulation of the rate of specific messenger RNA transcription by insulin provides an important means of modulating enzyme activity. Insulin-like growth factor (IGF) can also bind to and activate insulin receptors.

> **Endocrine pancreas and blood glucose**
>
> - Islets of Langerhans secrete insulin (and amylin) from B-cells, glucagon from A-cells, and somatostatin from D-cells.
> - Many factors stimulate insulin secretion, but the main one is blood glucose.
> - Insulin has essential metabolic actions as a fuel-storage hormone, and also affects cell growth and differentiation. It decreases blood glucose by:
>   — increasing glucose uptake into muscle and fat via Glut-4
>   — increasing glycogen synthesis
>   — decreasing gluconeogenesis
>   — decreasing glycogen breakdown.
> - Glucagon is a fuel-mobilising hormone, stimulating gluconeogenesis and glycogenolysis, also lipolysis and proteolysis. It increases blood sugar and also increases the force of contraction of the heart.
> - Diabetes mellitus is a chronic metabolic disorder in which there is hyperglycaemia. There are two main forms:
>   — type 1 (insulin-dependent) diabetes, with an absolute deficiency of insulin
>   — type 2 (non-insulin-dependent) diabetes, with a relative deficiency of insulin associated with reduced sensitivity to its action ('insulin resistance').

GLUCAGON

Glucagon is a single chain polypeptide of 21 amino acid residues.

Synthesis and secretion

Glucagon is synthesised mainly in the A-cell of the islets, but also in the stomach. It has considerable structural homology with other gastrointestinal tract hormones including *secretin*, *vasoactive intestinal peptide* and *gastric inhibitory peptide* (see Ch. 10).

One of the main physiological stimuli to glucagon secretion is the concentration of amino acids, in particular arginine, in plasma. Thus an increase in secretion follows ingestion of a high protein meal, but in contrast to insulin, which fluctuates markedly, there is rather little change in plasma glucagon concentrations throughout the day. Glucagon secretion is stimulated by low, and inhibited by high concentrations of glucose and fatty acids in the plasma. Sympathetic nerve activity and circulating adrenaline stimulate glucagon release via β-adrenoceptors. Parasympathetic nerve activity also increases secretion, whereas somatostatin, released from D-cells adjacent to the glucagon-secreting A-cells in the periphery of the islets, inhibits glucagon release.*

Actions

Glucagon acts on specific receptors that are coupled by stimulatory G-proteins to adenylate cyclase, and its actions are somewhat similar to β-adrenoceptor-mediated actions of adrenaline. Unlike adrenaline, however, its metabolic effects are more pronounced than its cardiovascular actions. As regards metabolic actions, glucagon is proportionately more active on liver, while adrenaline is more active on muscle and fat. Glucagon acts on the liver to *stimulate* glycogen breakdown and gluconeogenesis, and to *inhibit* glycogen synthesis and glucose oxidation. Consequently, it increases blood glucose. It causes lipolysis in liver and fat cells (the fatty acids so produced further increase gluconeogenesis), and catabolism of protein in muscle. Its actions on target tissues are thus the opposite of those of insulin. Paradoxically, glucagon increases insulin release (Figs 22.1 and 22.2).

Glucagon increases the rate and force of contraction of the heart, though less markedly than adrenaline.

Clinical uses are specialised and are summarised in the box on this page.

SOMATOSTATIN

Somatostatin is secreted by the D-cells of the islets. It is also the growth hormone release-inhibiting factor generated in the hypothalamus (see Ch. 24). It provides

---

*Octreotide, a somatostatin analogue (see p. 411), is used to treat the rare syndrome caused by functional glucagonomas.

> **Clinical uses of glucagon**
>
> Glucagon can be administered intramuscularly or subcutaneously as well as intravenously:
>
> - to treat hypoglycaemia in unconscious patients (who cannot drink), or if there is difficulty in obtaining intravenous access. In contrast to intravenous glucose it can be administered by non-medical personnel (e.g. spouses and ambulance crew).
> - to increase the force of contraction of the heart (positive inotropic action) in acute cardiac failure precipitated by injudicious use of β-adrenoceptor antagonists.

local, paracrine, inhibitory regulation of insulin and glucagon release within the islet. **Octreotide** is a long-acting octapeptide analogue of somatostatin. It inhibits release of a number of hormones and is used clinically to relieve symptoms from several uncommon gastroentero-pancreatic endocrine tumours, and for treatment of the endocrine disorder caused by a functioning tumour of cells that secrete growth hormone from the anterior pituitary (see Ch. 24) and known as *acromegaly*. (It is used either short term before surgery on the pituitary tumour, or while waiting for radiotherapy of the tumour to take effect, or if other treatments have been ineffective.)

AMYLIN (ISLET AMYLOID POLYPEPTIDE)

Amyloid is an amorphous protein that is deposited in different tissues in a variety of diseases. Amyloid deposits occur in the pancreas of patients with diabetes mellitus, although it is not known if this is functionally important or a secondary phenomenon. In 1987 the major structural component of pancreatic amyloid was identified as a 37-amino-acid peptide now known as *islet amyloid polypeptide* or *amylin*. This is stored with insulin in secretory granules in B-cells and cosecreted with insulin in response to glucose and other stimuli. The molar ratio of secreted amylin to insulin varies, increasing during prolonged stimulation by elevated glucose. Fasting amylin concentrations in plasma of healthy humans are around 1–10 pmol/l, postprandial concentrations rising to 5–20 pmol/l (i.e. approximately one-tenth of plasma insulin concentrations). Amylin delays gastric emptying. Supraphysiological concentrations stimulate the breakdown of glycogen to lactate in striated muscle, with an increase in plasma lactate concentration and subsequent rise in glucose concentration that may reflect gluconeogenesis from lactate in liver. Amylin also inhibits insulin secretion (Fig. 22.1).

It is structurally related to *calcitonin* and has weak calcitonin-like actions on calcium metabolism and osteoclast activity in patients with Paget's disease (a metabolic disorder of bone characterised by focal areas of increased bone turnover; see Ch. 27). It is also about 50% identical with *calcitonin gene-related peptide* (CGRP; see Ch. 10) and large intravenous doses cause vasodilatation via activation of adenylate cyclase, presumably by an action on CGRP receptors. Circulating concentrations of amylin are reduced to the detection limit of current assays in patients with type 1 diabetes, and increased in patients with type 2 (non-insulin-dependent) diabetes mellitus (see below). Whether amylin has a significant role in the physiological control of glucose metabolism is controversial, but there is interest in the therapeutic potential of amylin agonists (such as **pramlintide**, an analogue with three proline substitutions introduced into the amylin molecule to reduce its tendency to aggregate into insoluble fibrils) as a supplement to insulin therapy in type 1 diabetes mellitus. A recent multicentre trial (Thompson et al. 1997) showed that pramlintide lowers mean and postprandial glucose concentrations in such patients.

CONTROL OF BLOOD GLUCOSE

The control of blood glucose (Table 22.2) must be seen in the context of the necessity of maintaining adequate fuel supplies (glucose is the obligatory source of meta-bolic energy for the brain, in particular) in the face of intermittent food intake and variable metabolic demand (e.g. with exercise). More fuel is made available by feeding than is immediately required, excess calories being stored as glycogen or fat. During fasting, these energy stores need to be mobilised in a regulated manner.

The blood glucose concentration is controlled by a feedback system between liver, muscle and fat and the pancreatic islets—the main regulatory hormone being insulin, and the overall pattern of control of blood glucose differing in basal (i.e. fasting) and fed states.

DIABETES MELLITUS

Diabetes mellitus is a chronic metabolic disorder characterised by a *high blood glucose concentration—hyperglycaemia* (fasting plasma glucose > 7.0 mmol/l, or plasma glucose > 10 mmol/l, 2 hours after a meal) due to insulin deficiency and/or insulin resistance. Hyperglycaemia occurs because of uncontrolled hepatic glucose output and reduced uptake of glucose by skeletal muscle with reduced glycogen synthesis. When the renal threshold for glucose reabsorption is exceeded, glucose spills over into the urine (*glycosuria*) and causes an osmotic diuresis (*polyuria*) which in turn results in dehydration, thirst and increased drinking (*polydipsia*). Insulin deficiency causes wasting due to increased breakdown and reduced synthesis of proteins. Ketosis occurs in the absence of insulin because there is accel-

Table 22.2 The effect of hormones on the control of blood glucose

Hormone	Main actions	Main stimulus for secretion	Main effect
Main regulatory hormone			
Insulin	↑ glucose uptake ↑ glycogen synthesis ↓ glycogenolysis ↓ gluconeogenesis	Moment-to-moment fluctuations in blood glucose	↓ blood glucose
Main counter-regulatory hormones			
Glucagon	↑ glycogenolysis ↑ gluconeogenesis		
Catecholamines	↑ glycogenolysis ↓ glucose uptake	Hypoglycaemia, i.e. blood glucose less than 3 mM (e.g. with exercise, stress, high protein meals, etc.)	↑ blood glucose
Glucocorticoids	↑ gluconeogenesis ↓ glucose uptake and utilisation		
Growth hormone	↓ glucose uptake		

erated fat breakdown to acetyl CoA. In the absence of aerobic carbohydrate metabolism, acetyl CoA is converted anaerobically to acetoacetate, β-hydroxybutyrate and acetone.

As a consequence of the metabolic derangements in diabetes, various complications develop, often over many years. Many of these are due to disease of blood vessels, either large (*macrovascular disease*) or small (*micro-angiopathy*). Dysfunction of the vascular endothelium (see Ch. 15), and abnormalities of endothelium-derived mediators, appear to be early and possibly critical events. Oxygen-derived free radicals, protein kinase C and non-enzymatic products of glucose and albumin (called *advanced glycosylation end-products*, or 'AGE') have been implicated in these changes. Macrovascular disease is due to accelerated atheroma which is much more common and severe in diabetic patients. Micro-angiopathy is a distinctive feature of diabetes mellitus and particularly affects retina, kidney and peripheral nerves. Coexistent *hypertension* promotes progressive renal damage, and treatment of hypertension slows the progression of diabetic nephropathy, which can be detected by the excretion of small amounts of albumin in the urine ('microalbuminuria'). Treatment of hypertension with *angiotensin-converting enzyme inhibitors* (ACEI; Ch. 15) appears to be more effective in preventing diabetic nephropathy than treatment with other antihypertensive drugs. Trials are in progress to determine whether ACEI are also of benefit in diabetic patients with normal blood pressures.

Diabetic neuropathy is associated with accumulation of poorly metabolised osmotically active metabolites of glucose such as sorbitol, produced by the action of aldose reductase. This underpinned hopes that aldose reductase inhibitors would be effective in preventing diabetic complications. Results to date have not, however, been encouraging, and the first such drug to have been marketed (**tolrestat**) has been withdrawn because of lack of efficacy.

There are two main forms of diabetes mellitus:

- type 1 diabetes (also known as insulin-dependent diabetes mellitus—IDDM—or juvenile onset diabetes)
- type 2 diabetes (also known as non-insulin-dependent diabetes mellitus—NIDDM—or maturity onset diabetes).

In type 1 diabetes there is an absolute deficiency of insulin resulting from autoimmune destruction of B-cells, and unless insulin treatment is provided the patient will die with diabetic ketoacidosis. Such patients are usually young (children or adolescents) and not obese when they first develop symptoms. There is an inherited predisposition, with a 10-fold increased incidence in first-degree relatives of an index case, and strong associations with particular histocompatibility antigens (HLA types). Studies of identical twins have shown that genetically predisposed individuals must additionally be exposed to an environmental factor such as viral infection (e.g. with Coxsackie or Echo virus). Viral infection may damage pancreatic B-cells and expose antigens that initiate a self-perpetuating autoallergic process. The patient becomes overtly diabetic only when more than 90% of the B-cells have been destroyed. This natural history provides a tantalising prospect of intervening in the prediabetic stage, and a variety of strategies have been mooted including *immunosuppression* with **cyclosporin** or **azathioprine**, dietary modifications, antioxidants, tumour necrosis factor and many others. Studies from New Zealand suggest that pharmacological doses of **nicotinamide** induce remission in patients with newly diagnosed type 1 diabetes, and delay onset of diabetes in prediabetic children with antibodies against islet cells. It is suggested that it may work by influencing DNA repair. A controlled study is currently in progress.

In type 2 diabetes there is both insulin resistance (which precedes overt disease) and impaired regulation of insulin secretion. Such patients are usually obese and usually present in adult life, the incidence rising progressively with age as B-cell function declines. Treatment is initially dietary although supplementary oral hypoglycaemic drugs or insulin often become necessary.

The alterations in insulin secretion in the two main forms of diabetes are shown schematically in Figure 22.2 and are contrasted with the normal response. In a healthy individual there is a basal level of insulin secretion and the response to an intravenous infusion of glucose (equivalent to what might happen after a meal) has two phases. The first phase is rapid and short-lived and the second is prolonged. In type 2 diabetes there is hyperglycaemia and a normal or slightly raised basal insulin concentration. The first phase of the insulin-secretory response to glucose is virtually absent, but the delayed response is present. The response to non-glucose secret-agogues (e.g. amino acids, sulphonylureas, glucagon and GI tract hormones) is nearly normal (not shown). In type 1 diabetic patients there is severe B-cell dysfunction. Basal insulin secretion is extremely low and there is virtually no response to glucose, or to any other stimulus, leading to hyperglycaemia, proteolysis, lipolysis and ketosis.

There are many other less common forms of diabetes

mellitus in addition to the two main ones described above, and hyperglycaemia can also be a clinically important adverse effect of several drugs, including glucocorticoids (Ch. 24), thiazide diuretics (Ch. 20) and several of the protease inhibitors used to treat HIV infection (Ch. 44).

TREATMENT OF DIABETES MELLITUS

Insulin is essential to treat type 1 diabetes. For many years it was assumed, as an act of faith, that normalising plasma glucose would prevent diabetic complications. The Diabetes Control and Complications Trial (American Diabetes Association 1993) showed that this faith was well placed: type 1 diabetic patients were randomly allocated to intensive or conventional management. Mean blood glucose concentration was 2.8 mmol/l lower in the intensively managed group, who had a substantial reduction in the occurrence and progression of retinopathy, nephropathy and neuropathy over a period of 4–9 years. These benefits outweighed a threefold increase in severe hypoglycaemic attacks and modest excess weight gain.

Realistic goals in type 2 diabetic patients (especially in older obese patients) are likely to be less ambitious than in younger type 1 patients. Diet is the cornerstone (albeit one with a tendency to crumble) often combined with oral agents (e.g. **metformin** or **acarbose** and sulphonylureas) and/or **insulin**. Dietary advice to prevent atheromatous disease (Ch. 16) is extremely important, since macrovascular disease causes much of the excess mortality and morbidity of both forms of diabetes mellitus. Details of dietary management are beyond the scope of this book, as is laser treatment of microvascular complications in the retina.

INSULIN TREATMENT

The effects of insulin and its mechanism of action have been described above. It is destroyed in the gastrointestinal tract, and must be given parenterally—usually subcutaneously, but intravenously or occasionally intramuscularly in emergencies.

Insulin is assayed biologically against an international standard and its dosage expressed in 'units'. Insulin for clinical use was once either porcine or bovine, but is now almost entirely human (made by recombinant DNA technology). No major advantage of human insulin emerged during clinical trials, but manufacturing advantages over animal insulins are substantial.

One of the main problems in using insulin is to avoid wide fluctuations in plasma concentration and thus in blood glucose. To address this, various formulations of insulin are available, varying in their peak effect and duration of action. Early preparations were acidic and tended to precipitate in the tissues or when mixed with other insulin formulations. To counter this, acetate-buffered neutral solutions were introduced. This type of insulin (soluble insulin) produces a rapid and short-lived effect, and can be given intravenously. Longer-acting preparations are made by precipitating insulin with protamine or zinc, thus forming finely divided amorphous solid or relatively insoluble crystals, which are injected as a suspension from which insulin is slowly absorbed. These include **isophane insulin**, a suspension of insulin (porcine, bovine or human) in the form of a complex with protamine; **amorphous insulin zinc suspension**, and **crystalline insulin zinc suspension**. Mixtures of different forms in fixed proportions are available and are widely used. **Insulin lispro** is a recently introduced insulin analogue in which a lysine and a proline residue

---

Drugs in diabetes

Insulin can be extracted from porcine or bovine pancreas. Increasingly, 'human' insulin is used, usually made by recombinant DNA technology. For routine use it is given subcutaneously (by intravenous infusion in emergencies).

- Different formulations of insulin differ in their duration of action:
  - Fast- and short-acting soluble insulin. Peak action after s.c. dose 2–4 hours; duration 6–8 hours. It can be given i.v.
  - Intermediate-acting, e.g. isophane insulin. It can be mixed with soluble insulin.
  - Long-acting, e.g. insulin zinc suspension.
- The main unwanted effect is hypoglycaemia.

Oral hypoglycaemic drugs: used in type 2 diabetes
- Biguanides (e.g. metformin):
  - have complex peripheral actions in the presence of residual insulin, increasing glucose uptake in striated muscle and inhibiting hepatic glucose output and intestinal glucose absorption
  - cause anorexia and assist in weight loss
  - are used with sulphonylureas when these have ceased to work adequately.
- Sulphonylureas (e.g. tolbutamide, glibenclamide, glipizide, gliclazide):
  - stimulate insulin secretion
  - can cause hypoglycaemia (which stimulates appetite and leads to weight gain)
  - are only effective if B-cells are functional
  - block ATP-sensitive K^+ channels in B-cells.

are 'switched'. It acts more rapidly but for a shorter time than natural insulin, a feature that enables patients to inject themselves soon before the start of a meal.

Pharmacokinetic aspects

Various regimes of insulin administration may be used. A common one for type 1 patients involves injecting a combination of short- and intermediate-acting insulins twice daily, before breakfast and before the evening meal. Intensified regimes may be used to improve control of blood glucose; these involve multiple daily injections or continuous subcutaneous infusion of soluble insulin through a pump. The most sophisticated forms of pump regulate the dose by means of a sensor which continuously measures blood glucose, but these are not routinely available. Intravenous and intraperitoneal infusions are also used. *Intravenous* infusion of soluble insulin is used routinely in emergency treatment of diabetic keto-acidosis, in conjunction with large volumes of isotonic saline and potassium chloride to replace Na^+, K^+ and Cl^- depletion. *Intraperitoneal* insulin can be used in diabetic patients with end-stage renal failure treated by *ambulatory peritoneal dialysis*.

Intranasal and inhalation routes of administration are being investigated. Other new techniques include incorporation of insulin into biodegradable polymer microspheres, and its encapsulation with a lectin in a glucose-permeable membrane. This latter technique could be self-regulatory, because there is competitive binding of glucose and glycosylated insulin to the lectin.

Once in the blood, insulin has a $t_{1/2}$ of about 10 minutes. It is inactivated enzymically in the liver and kidney, and 10% is excreted in the urine. Renal impairment reduces insulin requirement.

Unwanted effects

The main undesirable effect of insulin is *hypoglycaemia*. This is common, and can cause brain damage. Intensive insulin therapy results in a threefold increase in severe hypoglycaemia. The treatment of hypoglycaemia is to take a sweet drink or snack, or, if the patient is unconscious, to give intravenous glucose (50% w/v solution) or intramuscular glucagon (see above). *Rebound hyperglycaemia* ('*Somogyi effect*') can follow excessive insulin administration. This results from the release of the insulin-opposing or counter-regulatory hormones in response to insulin-induced hypoglycaemia. This can cause hyperglycaemia before breakfast following an unrecognised hypoglycaemic attack during sleep in the early hours of the morning. It is essential to recognise

this possibility to avoid the mistake of *increasing* (rather than reducing) the dose of insulin in this situation.

Allergy to insulin is unusual but may take the form of local or systemic reactions. Severe insulin resistance as a consequence of antibody formation is rare. A high titre of circulating anti-insulin antibodies is more likely to occur with bovine than with porcine insulin. Note, however, that virtually all patients treated with animal insulin have antibodies against the hormone, albeit usually of low titre. 'Human' insulin is less immunogenic than animal insulin but may still evoke an antibody response, since the source of the hormone is not the only determinant of immunogenicity; insulins undergo physical changes before and after injection which can increase their potential for provoking an immune response.

Clinical uses of insulin are summarised below.

ORAL HYPOGLYCAEMIC AGENTS

The main groups of oral agents that lower blood sugar (see box on p. 393) are the *biguanides* and the *sulphonylureas* and related compounds. In addition, **acarbose** (an α-glucosidase inhibitor) is available, and several other classes of drugs are in development (see below).

Biguanides

These are orally active hypoglycaemic agents that do not require functioning B-cells. Their action is complex and incompletely understood. They increase glucose uptake in skeletal muscle, and have effects on glucose absorption and hepatic glucose production. **Metformin**, the only drug of this class presently available in the UK, has additional metabolic actions in that it reduces plasma concentrations of low density lipoprotein and very low density lipoprotein, effects that could theo-

---

Clinical uses of insulin

- Patients with type 1 diabetes require long-term maintenance treatment with insulin.
- Many patients with type 2 diabetes ultimately require chronic insulin treatment.
- Short-term treatment with insulin may be needed in patients with type 2 diabetes or impaired glucose tolerance during intercurrent events (e.g. infections, myocardial infarction, pregnancy, during major operations).
- An entirely separate use is in emergency treatment of hyperkalaemia, when insulin is given with glucose to lower extracellular K^+ via redistribution into cells.

retically be useful in reducing atheroma (see Ch. 16). It has a half-life of about 3 hours, and is excreted unchanged in the urine.

Metformin does not stimulate appetite (rather the reverse!), and is consequently useful in the majority of type 2 patients who are obese and who fail treatment with diet alone. It can be combined with sulphonylurea drugs. The main unwanted effect is transient gastro-intestinal disturbance. A rare but potentially fatal toxic effect is lactic acidosis and metformin should never be given to patients with renal disease or severe pulmonary or cardiac disease, who are predisposed to this adverse effect because of reduced drug elimination or increased anaerobic metabolism respectively. Metformin does not cause hypoglycaemia and does not result in weight gain. Long-term use may interfere with absorption of vitamin B_{12}.

Sulphonylureas

The sulphonylurea group of drugs was developed as a result of the chance observation that a sulphonamide derivative (used to treat typhoid) resulted in a marked lowering of blood glucose. These drugs act by stimulating insulin release (see below) and thus require functional islet cells.

There are now numerous sulphonylureas available. The first used therapeutically were **tolbutamide** and **chlorpropamide**. Chlorpropamide has a long duration of action and a substantial fraction is excreted in the urine. Consequently it can cause severe hypoglycaemia in elderly patients in whom there is a progressive decline in glomerular filtration rate (Ch. 5). It causes flushing after alcohol because of a **disulfiram**-like effect (Ch. 39) and has an action like that of antidiuretic hormone on the distal nephron giving rise to hyponatraemia and water intoxication. Williams (1994) comments that 'time honoured but idiosyncratic chlorpropamide should now be laid to rest'—a sentiment with which we concur. Tolbutamide, however, remains widely used. So-called second-generation sulphonylureas (e.g. **glibenclamide**, **glipizide**, and **gliclazide**; see Fig. 22.4 and Table 22.3) are more potent (on a milligram basis), but their maximum hypoglycaemic effect is no greater and failure of treatment to control blood sugar is just as common as with tolbutamide. They all contain the sulphonylurea moiety, but different substitutions result in differences in pharmacokinetics and hence in duration of action (see Table 22.3). Glibenclamide is best avoided in the elderly and in patients with even mild renal impairment because of the risk of hypoglycaemia since several of its metabolites are excreted in urine and are moderately active.

Mechanism of action

The principal action of the sulphonylureas is on the B-cells of the islets (Fig. 22.1), stimulating insulin secre-

---

Table 22.3 Oral hypoglycaemic sulphonylurea drugs

Drug	Relative potency*	Duration of action and (half-life) in hours	Pharmacokinetic aspects	General comments
Tolbutamide	1	6–12 (4)	Some converted in liver to weakly active hydroxytolbutamide. Some carboxylated to inactive compound. Renal excretion	A safe drug. Least likely to cause hypoglycaemia. May decrease iodide uptake by thyroid. Contraindicated in liver failure
Glibenclamide†	150	18–24 (10)	Some is oxidised in the liver to moderately active products and is excreted in urine; 50% is excreted unchanged in the faeces	May cause hypoglycaemia. The active metabolite accumulates in renal failure
Glipizide	100	16–24 (7)	Peak plasma levels in 1 hour. Most is metabolised in the liver to inactive products which are excreted in urine. 12% is excreted in faeces	May cause hypoglycaemia. Has diuretic action. Only inactive products accumulate in renal failure

*Relative to tolbutamide
†Termed 'gliburide' in USA
All are largely protein-bound (90–95%).

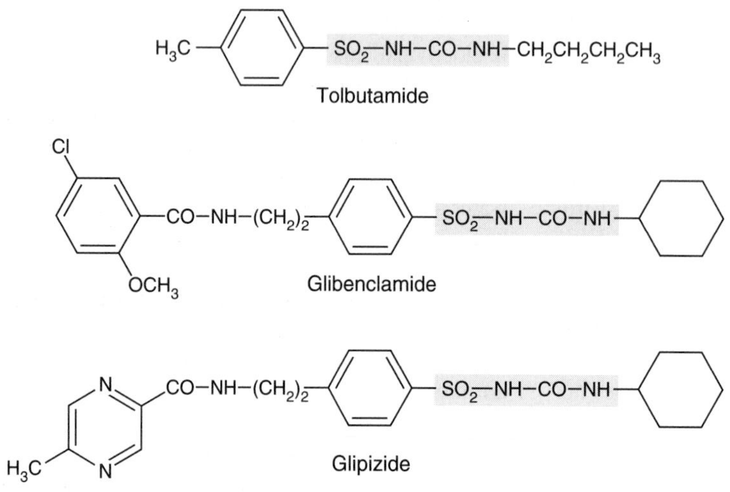

H_3C—⟨benzene⟩—SO_2—NH—CO—NH—$CH_2CH_2CH_2CH_3$
Tolbutamide

Cl / OCH$_3$ ⟨benzene⟩—CO—NH—$(CH_2)_2$—⟨benzene⟩—SO_2—NH—CO—NH—⟨cyclohexane⟩
Glibenclamide

H_3C—⟨pyrazine, N⟩—CO—NH—$(CH_2)_2$—⟨benzene⟩—SO_2—NH—CO—NH—⟨cyclohexane⟩
Glipizide

Fig. 22.4 Structures of some oral hypoglycaemic drugs. The sulphonylurea moiety is shown within the light blue box.

tion (the equivalent of phase I in Fig. 22.2) and thus reducing plasma glucose concentration.

High-affinity receptors for sulphonylureas are present on the ATP-sensitive K^+ channels in B-cell plasma membranes, and the binding of various sulphonylureas parallels their potency in stimulating insulin release. The drugs reduce the potassium permeability of B-cells by blocking the ATP-sensitive potassium channels (see p. 288), causing depolarisation, Ca^{2+} entry and hence insulin secretion.

Basal insulin secretion and the secretory response to various stimuli are enhanced in the first few days of treatment with sulphonylurea drugs. With longer treatment, insulin secretion continues to be augmented, and tissue sensitivity to insulin also improves, by an unknown mechanism.

Pharmacokinetic aspects

Sulphonylureas are well absorbed after oral administration and most reach peak plasma concentrations within 2–4 hours. The duration of action varies (Table 22.3). All bind strongly to plasma albumin, and are implicated in interactions with other drugs (e.g. salicylates and sulphonamides) that compete for these binding sites (see below and Ch. 48). Most sulphonylureas (or their active metabolites) are excreted in the urine, so their action is increased in elderly patients or in those with renal disease.

Sulphonylureas cross the placenta and stimulate foetal B-cells to release insulin causing severe hypoglycaemia at birth; as a result, their use is contraindicated in preg-

nancy, and gestational diabetes is managed with diet supplemented if necessary with insulin.

Unwanted effects

The sulphonylureas are usually well tolerated. Side-effects are specified in Table 22.3. In addition, as with insulin, sulphonylurea drugs *stimulate appetite* and often cause *weight gain*. This is a major concern in obese diabetic patients. *Hypoglycaemia*, which can be severe, may occur. Its incidence is related to the potency and duration of action, the highest incidence occurs with chlorpropamide and glibenclamide and the lowest with tolbutamide. Such hypoglycaemia can be prolonged, and this can be serious in elderly patients and in patients with impaired renal function. About 3% of patients experience *gastrointestinal upsets. Allergic skin rashes* can occur, and *bone marrow damage* (Ch. 49), though very rare, can be severe.

A vexing question is whether prolonged therapy with oral hypoglycaemic drugs has *adverse effects on the cardiovascular system*. A study in the USA in 1970 found that after 4–5 years of treatment there appeared to be an *increase* in cardiovascular-related deaths in the group treated with oral drugs as compared with the groups treated with insulin or placebo. Blockade of ATP-sensitive K^+ channels in heart and vascular tissue could have adverse effects, and more selective drugs are under investigation. However, in the US study there was no statistically significant increase in total mortality in the sulphonylurea group as compared with the others and a reappraisal of the data does not support the view

> **Oral hypoglycaemic drugs**
>
> Oral hypoglycaemic drugs are only of use in the treatment of type 2 diabetes and only as a supplement to diet. They include:
>
> - metformin (a biguanide)
> - sulphonylureas (e.g. tolbutamide, glibenclamide, glipizide, gliclazide)
> - acarbose (an α-glucosidase inhibitor).

that sulphonylurea therapy is necessarily harmful. Conversely, there is no evidence that oral hypoglycaemic drugs reduce the cardiovascular complications of diabetes.

Drug interactions

Several compounds *augment* the hypoglycaemic effect of the sulphonylureas and several such interactions are potentially clinically important. Non-steroidal anti-inflammatory drugs (including **azapropazone**, **phenylbutazone** and salicylates), coumarins, some uricosuric drugs (e.g. **sulphinpyrazone**), alcohol, monoamine oxidase inhibitors, some antibacterials (including sulphonamides, **trimethoprim** and **chloramphenicol**), some antifungal drugs (including **miconazole** and possibly **fluconazole**) have all been reported to produce severe hypoglycaemia when given with the sulphonylureas. The probable basis of the interaction is competition for the metabolising enzymes, but interference with plasma protein binding or with excretion may play a part.

Agents that *decrease* the action of the sulphonylureas

include diuretics (thiazides and loop diuretics) and corticosteroids.

α-glucosidase inhibitors

Acarbose, an inhibitor of intestinal α-glucosidase, is used in type 2 patients inadequately controlled by diet with or without other agents. It delays carbohydrate absorption, reducing the postprandial increase in blood glucose. The commonest adverse effects are related to its main action and consist of flatulence, loose stools or diarrhoea and abdominal pain and bloating. Its precise place in treatment has still to be established, but like **metformin** it may be particularly helpful in obese type 2 patients.

Potential new antidiabetic drugs

Several agents are currently being studied including α_2-antagonists, inhibitors of fatty acid oxidation and agents that enhance the response of tissues to insulin, notably the *thiazolidinediones*. The first such drug to be marketed in the UK was **troglitazone**, which is mildly vasodilatory and lowers blood pressure as well as reducing insulin resistance. It was withdrawn because of hepatotoxicity. It is not known whether such toxicity is a class effect of the thiazolidinediones or is unique to troglitazone. Lipolysis in fat cells is controlled by adrenoceptors of the β_3-subtype (see Ch. 8). The possibility of using selective β_3-agonists, currently in development, in the treatment of obese patients with type 2 diabetes is being investigated (see Ch. 23).

REFERENCES AND FURTHER READING

Several of the references below are to specific chapters of particular relevance in Pickup J C, Williams J (eds) 1997 Textbook of diabetes, 2nd edn. Blackwell Science, Oxford. This superbly illustrated and extremely readable textbook offers an excellent 'way in' to all aspects of the original literature.

American Diabetes Association 1993 Implications of the diabetes control and complications trial. Diabetes 42: 1555–1558 *(Landmark clinical trial)*

Barnett A H, Owens D R 1997 Insulin analogues. Lancet 349: 47–51 *(Reviews the potential impact of modification of amino acid structure to produce 'designer insulins')*

Bishop A, Polak J M 1997 The anatomy, organization and ultrastructure of the islets of Langerhans. In: Pickup J C, Williams J (eds) Textbook of diabetes, 2nd edn Blackwell Science, Oxford

Brown H, Sanger F, Kitai R 1955 The structure of pig and sheep insulin. Biochemical Journal 60: 356–365

Cohen R A 1993 Dysfunction of vascular endothelium in diabetes mellitus. Circulation 87 (suppl V): V-67–V-76 *(Endothelial*

dysfunction may underlie vascular disease in diabetes mellitus)

deFronzo R A, Goodman A M 1995 Efficacy of metformin in patients with non-insulin-dependent diabetes mellitus. N Engl J Med 333: 541–549 *(See also accompanying editorial on metformin by O B Crofford, pp 588–589)*

Dunn M J 1997 Familial persistent hyperinsulinemic hypoglycemia of infancy and mutations in the sulfonylurea receptor. N Engl J Med 336: 703–706 *(A rare disease resulting from disorder of potassium channels as a result of mutation in the sulphonylurea receptor)*

Flatt P R 1997 The hormonal and neural control of endocrine pancreatic function. In: Pickup J C, Williams J (eds) Textbook of diabetes, 2nd edn Blackwell Science, Oxford

Gerich J E 1989 Oral hypoglycemic agents. N Engl J Med 321: 1231–1245

Howell S L 1997 The biosynthesis and secretion of insulin. In: Pickup J C, Williams J (eds) Textbook of diabetes, 2nd edn Blackwell Science, Oxford

Klip A, Leiter L A 1990 Cellular mechanism of action of metformin. Diabetes Care 13: 696–704

Maratos-Flier E, Goldstein B J, Kahn C R 1997 The insulin receptor and postreceptor mechanisms. In: Pickup J C, Williams J (eds) Textbook of diabetes, 2nd edn Blackwell Science, Oxford

Myers M G Jr, White M F 1993 Perspectives in diabetes. The new elements of insulin signaling. Insulin receptor substrate-1 and proteins with SH2 domains. Diabetes 42: 643–650 *(Signal transduction following occupation of the insulin receptor)*

Pociot F, Reimers J I, Anderson H U 1993 Nicotinamide— biological actions and therapeutic potential in diabetes prevention. Diabetologia 34: 362–365

Thompson R G, Peterson J, Gottlieb A, Mullane J 1997 Effects of pramlintide, an analog of human amylin, on plasma glucose profiles in patients with IDDM: results of a multicenter trial. Diabetes 46: 632–636 *(This amylin analogue lowered blood glucose when added to patients' usual insulin)*

Turk J, Gross R W, Ramanadham S 1993 Perspectives in diabetes. Amplification of insulin secretion by lipid messengers. Diabetes 42: 367–374 *(Amplifying intracellular messengers include diacylglycerol (DAG), non-esterified arachidonic acid 12-S-HETE)*

Williams G 1994 Management of non-insulin-dependent diabetes mellitus. Lancet 343: 95–100

Withers D J, Gutierrez J S, Towery H et al. 1998 Disruption of IRS-2 causes type 2 diabetes in mice. Nature 391: 900–904 *(Dysfunction of IRS-2 may 'contribute to the pathophysiology of human type 2 diabetes'; see also accompanying commentary on pp 846–847 by J Avruch 'A signal for β-cell failure')*

23

Obesity

The survival of an animal species requires a continuous supply of energy for physiological functioning even though the supply of food is intermittent. This requirement has been met by the evolution of a mechanism for storing energy in fuels, mainly the triglycerides of fat, from which it can be quickly mobilised. The mechanism, controlled by the so-called thrifty genes, was an obvious asset to our hunter-gatherer ancestors. But, in affluent societies that combine sedentary lifestyles with an ample supply of calorie-rich foods, it is the cause of an increasing medical problem—obesity.

BACKGROUND

It had long been thought that the body had a homeostatic system for controlling body fat and that the CNS was involved. At the beginning of this century it was observed that patients with damage to the hypothalamus tended to get fat. In the 1940s, it was shown that discrete lesions in the hypothalamus of rodents caused them to become obese. In 1953, Kennedy proposed, on the basis of experiments on rats, that the suggested homeostatic mechanism did in fact exist and that it involved a hormone from the adipose tissue acting on the hypothalamus. Hervey (1958) provided further evidence by showing that ablation of the ventromedial nucleus of the hypothalamus in one member of a parabiotic pair led to death by starvation in the unlesioned animal.* He suggested that in the lesioned animal (in which the normal feedback loop with the hypothalamus was disrupted) the fatty tissue released excessive amounts of a 'satiety' factor that led to the parabiont eating less. The details of this homeostatic system are only now becoming clear and are leading to an understanding of the problem of obesity.

DEFINITION OF OBESITY

Obesity has been variously defined as 'an excess of body fat' or 'body weight that is 20% over the ideal'. These phrases leave us with the problem of defining what is meant by 'excess' or 'ideal'. The nutritionists achieved more precision, if not more understanding, by defining a new unit: the 'body mass index' or BMI. The BMI is body mass (kg) divided by the square of the height (metres); it is highly correlated with body fat. 'Healthy' people have a BMI of 20–25, those with a BMI of 25–30 are deemed to be 'overweight' and those with a BMI of >30 are said to be obese.

The level of BMI is obviously an integral part of the energy balance equation. An operational definition

---

*Parabiosis is the joining of the circulations of two animals.

of obesity therefore, would be that it is a multifactorial disorder of energy balance in which chronic calorie intake has been greater than energy output resulting in an excessively large BMI.

We will cover first the current understanding of the homeostatic mechanisms that control energy balance and BMI—derived from experimental studies in mice. We will go on to consider the main health aspects of obesity, then its pathophysiology and then the possible pharmacological agents that might be used in therapy.

THE HOMEOSTATIC MECHANISMS CONTROLLING ENERGY BALANCE

Energy balance depends on food intake, energy storage in fat and energy expenditure. An effective system for the regulation of energy balance would require:

- mechanisms for sensing the level of energy stores in body fat and …
- relaying the information to controlling sites in the hypothalamus where …
- it could be integrated and in turn …
- determine energy balance through control of food intake and energy expenditure.

Many reviews of energy balance control contain spaghetti* diagrams of interacting factors—endocrines (glucocorticoids, oestrogens, etc.), autonomic mediators, gastrointestinal peptides, CNS transmitters, etc., all impinging on the hypothalamus which in turn releases mediators that act on CNS, autonomic and endocrine systems—which then affect food intake and energy balance. Phew!

In this chapter, we will have to confine ourselves to the main strips of pasta.

MECHANISM FOR SENSING THE LEVEL OF ENERGY STORES IN BODY FAT

A mechanism for sensing the level of energy stores in body fat would involve the generation of a factor by the adipose tissue, as proposed by Kennedy in 1953. Does such a factor exist? There has been phenomenal progress in research in this area in recent years.

The unravelling of the story started with a study of fat rodents. For many years it had been known that mice can become obese due to mutations of certain genes, at least five of which have been identified—including the

ob (obesity) gene and the db (diabetes) gene.** Mice that are homozygous for mutant forms of these genes—ob/ob mice and db/db mice—eat excessively and have low energy expenditure; they become grossly fat and have numerous metabolic and other abnormalities including hyperglycaemia, hyperinsulinaemia, hypothermia, decreased thyroid hormone levels and reduced reproductive function. Weight gain in an ob/ob mouse is suppressed if its circulation is linked to that of a normal mouse, implying that the obesity is due to lack of a blood-borne factor.

In 1994, Friedman and his colleagues (see Zhang et al. 1994) cloned the ob gene and identified its protein product—leptin. (The word 'leptin' is derived from the Greek 'leptos' meaning thin. Some authorities prefer to term the normal gene that codes for leptin, 'lep', and reserve the term ob for the mutated gene). Leptin is found in the blood of normal mice but not of genetically obese ob/ob mice, and when recombinant leptin is given intraperitoneally to ob/ob mice, it strikingly reduces body weight, food intake (Fig. 23.1), body fat and the levels of glucose and insulin in the blood. It also normalises body temperature, increases the level of activity in the recipient mice and restores reproductive function. If directly injected into the lateral or the third ventricle of ob/ob mice, it reduces food intake and weight gain, implying that it acts on the neural networks of the brain that control food intake and energy balance. If large doses are injected into normal rodents, leptin causes both weight loss and the neuroendocrine responses specified above, and significantly, the neuroendocrine responses occur at lower doses than the weight loss.

Leptin mRNA is expressed only in fat cells. Synthesis of leptin can be detected in all adipose tissue depots, but the intracellular messengers involved are not yet known. The concentration of leptin in the circulation is proportional to fat stores and BMI in normal subjects (Fig. 23.2); and leptin concentrations in the plasma are pulsatile and inversely related to hydrocortisone levels. The generation of leptin in fatty tissue is increased by glucocorticoids, oestrogens and possibly insulin and is reduced by β-adrenoceptor agonists.

So leptin, it would seem, fulfils the role of signalling the level of fat; and it has become evident that, as Flier (1995) has put it, the fat cell is not only a storage depot for fat, it is a node on the energy information highway.

But note that other factors derived from adipose tissue

---

*Somehow images of food keep intruding.

**The other genes are termed agouti yellow, and (named with geneticist tongue in cheek as usual) tubby, and fat. Versions of all five genes occur in humans.

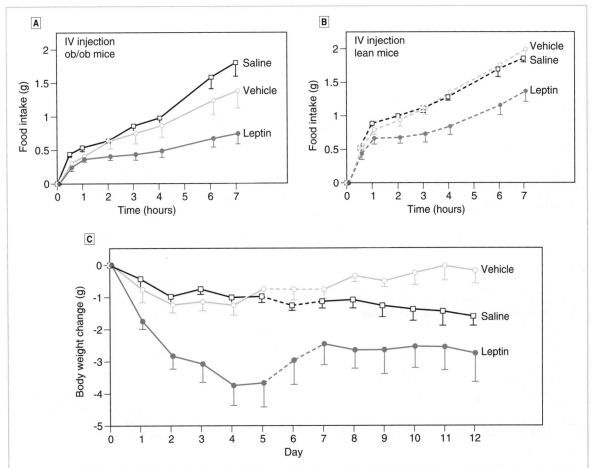

Fig. 23.1 The effect of recombinant leptin on food intake and body weight in mice. *Ob/ob* mice are genetically obese mice with a mutation in the gene coding for leptin. **A** and **B** The effect of a single i.v. injection on food intake in *ob/ob* and lean mice. **C** The effect on body weight in *ob/ob* mice, of two daily intraperitoneal injections for two 5-day periods, separated by a 2-day interval. (Data from Campfield et al. 1995)

(e.g. tumour necrosis factor-α) may be part of the traffic on the highway.

RELAY OF INFORMATION FROM FAT DEPOTS TO THE HYPOTHALAMUS

On reaching the brain, leptin enters by saturable transport (though the concentration of leptin in the CSF in humans is only 5% of that in the circulation). The next question is—how does leptin act in the hypothalamus? Is there a specific receptor? Studies on *db/db* mice provide a clue. Weight gain in a *db/db* mouse is not suppressed by parabiosis with a lean mouse or by leptin injections— suggesting that *db/db* mice are defective in the *response* to leptin, possibly owing to a mutation in the leptin

receptor. The leptin receptor, OB-R, has recently been identified by genetic mapping and shown to be a product of the *db* gene. (Some refer to the normal gene for the leptin receptor as Lepr, and confine the term *db* to the mutated gene). Leptin receptors are found not only in the CNS, but also the lungs, kidney, muscle and adipose tissue. The leptin receptor gene is complex and it has become clear that the receptors form a subfamily of the superfamily of cytokine receptors (see Chs 2 and 12). One member of the family is responsible for intracellular signalling, some bind and transport leptin in the circulation, and one variant is a carrier protein that transports leptin across membranes (possibly across the blood–CSF barrier in the choroid plexus).

The signal transduction mechanisms following leptin

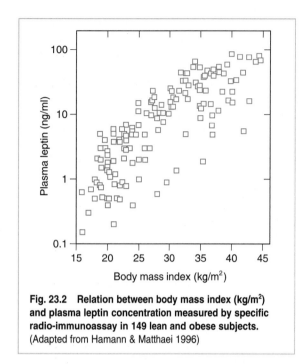

Fig. 23.2 Relation between body mass index (kg/m²) and plasma leptin concentration measured by specific radio-immunoassay in 149 lean and obese subjects. (Adapted from Hamann & Matthaei 1996)

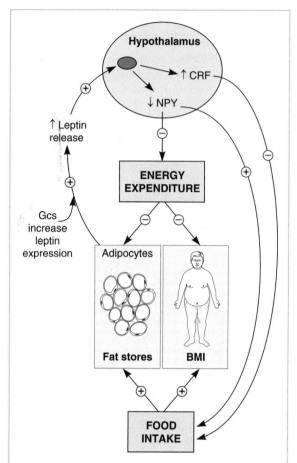

Fig. 23.3 Simplified outline of the homeostatic regulation of energy balance. Energy balance depends on food intake, energy storage in fat—which is correlated with body mass index (kg/m²)—and energy expenditure. Factors involved in energy expenditure include increased sympathetic activity, decreased thermogenesis and increased metabolic energy utilisation. (NPY = neuropeptide Y; CRF = corticotrophin-releasing factor; Gcs = glucocorticoids)

receptor activation are not yet known but are thought to involve the Jak/Stat pathway (Ch. 2).

INTEGRATION OF INFORMATION AND EFFECT ON ENERGY BALANCE

The integration of the information on fat stores with other information and the subsequent effect on factors determining energy balance is obviously very complex since both involve the basic processes of metabolism and the systems controlling it; leptin is only one part of the jigsaw.

An important target of leptin is the group of neurons that release neuropeptide Y (NPY). It acts on these neurons to *reduce* NPY production (Fig. 23.3). NPY is found mainly in the paraventricular nucleus, having been synthesised in the arcuate nucleus. Food deprivation increases hypothalamic production of NPY. Its action is to stimulate food intake and decrease sympathetic outflow, thus lowering energy expenditure. It also promotes the synthesis and storage of fat by an action on the lipoprotein lipase in adipose tissue. However, there is redundancy in this system, since although NPY is an important component of the response, other mechanisms can compensate if it is missing.

NPY neurons are not the only targets on which leptin acts. Injected into the third ventricle in rats, leptin in-

creases gene expression of corticotrophin-releasing factor (CRF) in the hypothalamus. CRF is known to reduce food intake (Fig. 23.3). The action of melanocyte-stimulating hormone (MSH) may also be required for the response to leptin (see Friedman 1997). Other neurotransmitter peptides, e.g. orexins, produced in the hypothalamus are also thought to function as mediators in the central feedback mechanism regulating feeding behaviour.

The interaction of insulin, glucocorticoids and leptin in the CNS is not fully understood and their interrelationship with other peptides that affect food intake (e.g. galanin, cholecystokinin, corticotrophin-releasing factor and enterostatin) is not yet clear; but it seems that leptin, generated in adipose tissue when fat cells increase in size and number, may function in the hypothalamus as a coordinator of various neuronal and hormonal actions that regulate food intake and energy balance.

Some of the existing information on energy balance and the control of body weight and fat depots has been put together in Figure 23.3.

Energy balance

Energy balance depends on food intake, energy storage in fat, and energy expenditure. Control of energy balance involves:

- Mechanisms that signal the level of fat stores, e.g. leptin. Plasma leptin concentrations are proportional to fat stores; variations in leptin concentration occur as follows:
  — with increased food intake and/or reduced energy expenditure, fat cells increase in size and number and
  — their *ob* genes are activated and increase the basal levels of leptin synthesis and release.
- The relay of the information on fat stores to centres in the hypothalamus (e.g. neurons with leptin receptors).
- The integration of the signal with other systems, e.g. NPY- and CRF-containing neurons and subsequent effects on systems that affect food intake and/or energy expenditure.

SYSTEMS FOR REGULATION OF ENERGY EXPENDITURE AND FOOD INTAKE

Energy expenditure

Energy is expended in metabolism, physical activity and thermogenesis (heat production). The metabolic aspects of energy expenditure include, amongst other things, cardiorespiratory work, the maintenance of ion gradients and the actions of a multitude of enzymes. Physical activity increases all these as well as increasing energy expenditure by the skeletal muscles. The sympathetic nervous system plays a significant part in the regulation of energy expenditure not only as regards effects on cardiovascular and skeletal muscle function during physical activity but in thermogenesis (see below).

Fat cells, both white and brown, but particularly brown, have a major role in thermogenesis. Brown fat cells contain abundant mitochondria and are remarkable heat generators, producing more heat and less ATP than white fat cells. The basis for this, as determined in mice, is the presence of a special mitochondrial protein, UCP1, that uncouples oxidative phosphorylation, i.e. it uncouples combustion from ATP synthesis. Another uncoupling protein, UCP2, occurs in both white and brown fat and is up-regulated if mice are fed a high-fat diet. The genes that code for these proteins are known and human fat cells have a gene similar to the mouse gene for UP2.

Brown fat cells, more abundant in infants and children than adults, have an extensive sympathetic innervation. Noradrenaline, acting on β-adrenoceptors (mainly β_3) in brown fat, increases lipolysis and fatty acid oxidation, increasing heat production. The expression of β_3-adrenoceptors is decreased in genetically obese mice.

Food intake

Food intake is modified by a multitude of factors (hormones, paracrine mediators, neuropeptides, etc.) too numerous to cover adequately here. We confine ourselves to two that are particularly relevant to the present topic—cholecystokinin and insulin.

Cholecystokinin is a peptide secreted by the duodenum in the presence of food; it acts on cholecystokinin A receptors in the gastrointestinal tract to decrease food intake. Circulating cholecystokinin does not cross the blood–brain barrier but the peptide is synthesised in the brain and acts on cholecystokinin B receptors to function as a satiety factor.

Insulin is secreted by pancreatic beta cells and its concentration in the blood is proportional to the fat mass in the body. It stimulates leptin release from fat cells and also enters the CNS where it may decrease food intake by affecting the actions of cholecystokinin and NPY. However, the main effect of insulin on food intake is to *increase* it, presumably indirectly, by an effect on blood glucose. Thus non-insulin-dependent diabetes mellitus (NIDDM) patients usually gain weight on insulin or sulphonylureas—an effect that is clinically very important (see Ch. 22).

IS THERE A 'SET POINT' FOR BODY WEIGHT IN THE HYPOTHALAMUS?

The body clearly has a complex homeostatic system for regulating fat stores and controlling energy balance. Some authorities talk of the hypothalamus having a leptin-controlled 'lipostat' for regulating the extent of fat stores. Some talk of a 'set-point' for energy balance, meaning that central hypothalamic mechanisms continuously adjust the systems of energy intake (factors controlling appetite, satiety, etc.) and energy expenditure to maintain a particular balance that is expressed as a target weight. Others consider that the control is more complex and refer to a 'settling point'. By 'settling point' it is meant that maintenance of energy balance (and thus of weight) depends on numerous metabolic feedback loops—tuned by an individual's particular susceptibility genes (see below)—'*settling* into a happy* equilibrium with the individual's environment'. (See summary by Gibbs 1996.) These questions have yet to be settled.

OBESITY AS A HEALTH PROBLEM

Obesity is a growing and costly health problem in many of the richest nations of the world. Approximately 33% of adults in the USA are said to be obese and the incidence in other developed nations is increasing. In Europe, 15–20% of the middle-aged population is obese (Björntorp 1997).

With a BMI above 30 there is a 3–4 times increase in the risk of non-insulin-dependent diabetes mellitus (NIDDM), hypertension, hypertriglyceridaemia, and ischaemic heart disease. (The relationship between NIDDM, increased BMI and insulin-resistance, is discussed in Ch. 22; see also O'Rahilly 1997.) Obese subjects have an increased risk of colon, breast, prostate, gall bladder, ovary and uterine cancer; and numerous other disorders are associated with excess body weight, including osteoarthritis, gall bladder disease, hyperuricaemia and male hypogonadism. Gross obesity (BMI over 40) is associated with a 12-fold increase in mortality in the age group 25–35 compared with those in this age group with a BMI of 20–25.

The distribution of the adipose tissue is also important: a central distribution of fat—visceral fat—is associated with a higher morbidity and mortality than a peripheral distribution. A simple clinical measure of visceral fat is the waist circumference divided by the hip circumference—the waist : hip ratio or WHR. The WHR should not be greater than 1.0 in men and 0.85 in women.

THE PATHOPHYSIOLOGY OF OBESITY

As specified above, energy balance depends on food intake, energy storage in fat and energy expenditure, energy being expended in metabolism, physical activity and thermogenesis. In most adult subjects, body fat and body weight remain more or less constant over many years, even decades, in the face of very large variations in food intake and energy expenditure—amounting to about a million calories per year. As has been stressed,

the steady-state body weight and BMI of an individual is the result of the integration of multiple interacting factors; and perturbations—either in the direction of increase or decrease—are resisted by homeostatic mechanisms. How, then, does obesity occur? How is it that some individuals can eat as much as they like without putting on weight while others, with similar food intake, get fat? Why is it so difficult for the obese to lose weight and maintain the lower weight?

Since many factors influence energy balance and they interact at many levels, determining the pathophysiology of obesity is difficult. The main determinant is manifestly a disturbance of the homeostatic mechanisms that control energy balance, but genetic endowment underlies this disturbance. Other factors such as food intake, and lack of physical activity contribute and there are, of course, social, cultural and psychological aspects. We will deal below with imbalance of homeostatic mechanisms and genetic endowment and then briefly mention the role of food intake and physical activity.

OBESITY AS A DISORDER OF THE HOMEOSTATIC CONTROL OF ENERGY BALANCE

Although it is clear that a disturbance of the homeostatic mechanisms that control energy balance causes obesity, it is less clear *how* the balance is disturbed, since the mechanisms are extremely complex and involve most of the systems in the body.

When the leptin story unfolded, it was thought that alterations in leptin kinetics might provide a simple explanation of how the energy balance was disturbed in obese subjects, and that increasing the leptin concentrations in obese subjects might be therapeutically useful. But most of the information on leptin has been derived from experiments with rodents. What is the situation in humans?

Plasma leptin is higher in obese individuals, compared with non-obese subjects, not lower as might be expected (Fig. 23.2), and the concentration increases with increasing body fat; in fact leptin concentrations are proportional to body fat mass in both lean and obese subjects (Table 23.1). Thus, obesity is not due to a deficient concentration of circulating leptin. Factors and conditions influencing leptin concentration in the serum are listed in Table 23.1.

The data suggest that disturbances in plasma leptin concentration *per se* are not the cause of obesity. However, leptin or congeners might nevertheless be useful in treatment by tipping the energy balance towards increased basal energy expenditure. Some groups are

---

*Happy? A questionable concept in relation to gross obesity, some would say.

Table 23.1 Factors and conditions affecting plasma concentrations of leptin in human subjects*

Factors	Effects on leptin concentration
Leanness or obesity	Leptin concentration proportional to fat mass in both. Rate of leptin production per unit of adipose mass and rate of leptin clearance from the circulation similar in both
Weight loss on low-calorie diet with subsequent regain of weight	Decreases with weight loss, then increases with weight regain
Weight loss on low-calorie diet, the loss being subsequently maintained	Sustained reduction
Weight loss on low calorie diet maintained by diet and exercise program	Sustained reduction
Acute (i.e. short-term) caloric restriction	No change
Fasting for 24 h followed by food intake	Decrease during fast; recovery after feeding
Variation in the fat content of isocaloric diets	No change
Insulin-induced reduction of hyperglycaemia in NIDDM† patients	Increase as compared to NIDDM patients not given insulin
Circadian variation	Stable during day, increases at night

*Adapted from: Campfield et al. 1996
†Non-insulin-dependent diabetes

optimistic that this may be so and clinical trials are under way.

Resistance to leptin might be a factor in the development of obesity. Such resistance could involve a defect in the carriage of leptin in the circulation or in its transport into the CNS; and indeed there is preliminary evidence that less leptin is transferred from plasma to CSF in obese subjects than in lean individuals. Other possible disorders of the leptin system include defects in the leptin receptor (as occurs in *db/db* mice) or in the transducing systems, e.g. overexpression of NPY or decreased expression of CRF. (Data on the leptin receptor gene are given below.)

Dysfunction of mediators other than leptin could be implicated in obesity. Tumour necrosis factor-α, another cytokine that relays information from fat to brain, is increased in the adipose tissue of insulin-resistant obese individuals.

It has been suggested that one of the proteins that uncouple oxidative phosphorylation in fat cells, UP2, is dysfunctional in obese individuals. A further suggestion is that alteration of function of the PPAR* transcription factors α, β and γ, may have a role in obesity. These transcription factors regulate gene expression of enzymes associated with lipid and glucose homeostasis, and

*PPAR = peroxisome proliferation-activated receptor.

also promote the genesis of adipose tissue. PPARγ is expressed preferentially in fat cells and synergises with another transcription factor, C/EBPα, to convert precursor cells to fat cells (see Spiegelman & Flier 1996). The gene for UCP (see above) in white fat cells has regulatory sites for PPARα and C/EBPα. A new class of agents, the thiazoladinediones, bind to and activate PPARγ (see Ch. 25). One of these, troglitazone, is licensed in the UK for treatment of NIDDM.

Reduced function of β₃-adrenoceptors in brown adipose tissue (see above) could also be implicated in the development of obesity.

In addition, the pathophysiology of obesity could involve disturbance(s) in any of the multitude of other factors involved in energy balance. Further research is needed to solve these problems.

GENETIC FACTORS AND OBESITY

Studies in twins and in adoptees and their families indicate that from 40% to as much as 80% of the variance of BMI can be attributed to genetic factors. It is estimated that heritability is as high as 30–40% for factors relevant to energy balance such as body fat distribution, resting metabolic rate, energy expenditure after overeating, lipoprotein lipase activity and basal rates of lipolysis. It appears that modern populations have a genetic propensity, more manifest in some individuals than others, to increase their fat depots—as a result of the 'thrifty genes' developed during evolution by our forebears to code for proteins that promote fat storage at feasts to sustain them during famine.

There are some rare diseases in which obesity is the consequence of a single gene disorder, but in most cases it is believed that a limited number of genes interact with other factors to produce obesity.

Genes thought to be involved in energy balance are being studied: particularly the leptin and leptin receptor genes. As the information on leptin in rodents burgeoned, it was thought that the cause of obesity in humans would prove to be mutations in these genes; however, most obese subjects so far studied have not had any abnormalities in either the leptin or the leptin receptor genes.

Linkage of human obesity to genes for other factors relevant to energy balance have been reported. Some are specified below.

- The β_3-adrenoceptor, decreased function of which could be associated with impairment of lipolysis in white fat or with thermogenesis in brown fat. A mutation of the β_3-adrenoceptor gene has been found to be associated with abdominal obesity, insulin resistance and early onset NIDDM in some subjects and an increased propensity to gain weight in a separate group of morbidly obese subjects.
- The glucocorticoid receptor, which could be associated with obesity through the permissive effect of glucocorticoids on several aspects of fat metabolism and energy balance.

FOOD INTAKE AND OBESITY

As Spiegelman & Flier (1996) point out 'one need not be a rocket scientist to notice that increased food intake tends to be associated with obesity'. A typical obese subject will usually have put on 20 kg over 10 years. This means that there has been a daily excess of energy input over output of 30–40 kcal initially, increasing gradually to maintain the increased body weight.

The type of food eaten can play a part in upsetting the energy balance. Fat has more calories per gram and it may be that the mechanisms regulating appetite react rapidly to carbohydrate and protein but slowly to fat—too slowly to stop an individual consuming too much high-fat food before the satiety systems come into play.

Obese individuals diet to lose weight. However, when a subject reduces calorie intake, shifts into negative energy balance and loses weight, the resting metabolic rate decreases, and there is a concomitant reduction in energy expenditure. This could be said to be due to homeostatic mechanisms trying to return the body weight to the 'set-point'. Thus, an individual who was previously obese and is now of normal weight, generally needs fewer calories to maintain that weight than an individual who has never been obese. The decrease in energy expenditure appears to be largely due to an alteration in the conversion efficiency of chemical energy to mechanical work in the skeletal muscles. This adaptation to the caloric reduction contributes to the difficulty of *maintaining* weight loss by diet.

PHYSICAL EXERCISE AND OBESITY

It used to be said that the only exercise effective in combating obesity was pushing one's chair back from the table. It is now recognised that physical activity—i.e. increased energy expenditure—has a more positive role in reducing fat storage and adjusting energy balance in the obese, particularly if associated with modification of the diet. An inadvertent, natural population study provides an example. Many years ago, a tribe of Pima Indians split into two groups. One group settled in Mexico and continued to live simply at subsistence level, eating frugally and spending most of the week in hard physical labour. They are generally lean and have a low incidence of non-insulin-dependent diabetes (NIDDM). The other group moved to the USA—an environment with easy access to calorie-rich food and less need for hard physical work. They are on average 57 pounds heavier than the Mexican group and have a high incidence of early-onset NIDDM.

PHARMACOLOGICAL APPROACHES TO THE PROBLEM OF OBESITY

At present, there are no effective agents that alter the central regulation of body weight; dietary regimes and planned exercise programs are the mainstay of treatment for obesity. The surgical measures sometimes used for gross obesity are beyond the remit of this book.

Pharmacological approaches to the problem can be considered under three headings: drugs currently used; drugs under development; and potential leads to future drug development.

Drugs currently used to treat obesity

Drug treatment is advised only for subjects with a BMI of >30 and thus at medical risk from obesity and, if given

Obesity

- Obesity is a multifactorial disorder of energy balance in which chronic calorie intake is greater that energy output.
- It is characterised by an excessive body mass index (BMI) which is the weight in kg divided by the height in metres^2.
- A subject with a BMI less than 20 is considered as having a healthy body weight, one with a BMI of 20–30 as overweight, and one with a BMI >30 as obese.
- Obesity is a growing problem in most rich nations; the incidence—at present 30% in the USA and 15–20% in Europe—is increasing.
- A BMI over 30 increases by three- to fourfold the risk of non-insulin-dependent diabetes, hypercholesterolaemia, ischaemic heart disease; the risk of various cancers is also increased.
- Obesity is primarily an energy balance disorder, the details of which are not clear but may include the following:
  — deficiencies in the genesis of, and/or the response to leptin or other fat depot sensors
  — defects in the hypothalamic neuronal systems responding to leptin, e.g. NPY (normally reduced by increased leptin), CRF (normally increased by increased leptin)
  — defects in the systems controlling energy expenditure, e.g. reduced sympathetic activity; decreased metabolic expenditure of energy; decreased thermogenesis in adipocytes due to reduction of β_3-adrenoceptor-mediated action on lipid metabolism and/or dysfunction of the proteins that uncouple oxidative phosphorylation.
- The disturbance of energy balance underlying obesity could be due to a genetic propensity, developed during evolution, to store fat at feasts for sustenance during famine.
- The rapid advance of knowledge of the factors controlling energy balance and BMI may well lead to new drugs for obesity in the near future.

Drugs under development for obesity therapy

Agents acting in the CNS

The following are in clinical trial: *leptin*, several *neuropeptide Y inhibitors* and *sibutramine*, (which acts as a sympathomimetic and as an agonist on 5-HT receptors).

The following agents are under investigation: *cholecystokinin promoters*; these increase the A type receptors for cholecystokinin, a transmitter that reduces appetite.

Agents acting on fat

Troglitazone, an analogue of an intracellular messenger in adipocytes that activates the transcription factor PPARγ (thus increasing lipolysis, decreasing glycolysis, promoting adipogenesis and reducing insulin resistance) has been licensed in some countries for NIDDM and is in phase III clinical trial in others. It or its congeners may be of value in obesity.

β_3-adrenoceptor agonists acting on fat cells are under investigation.

Agents acting in the gastrointestinal tract (GIT)

The following are in clinical trial:

- A *pancreatic lipase inhibitor*, orlistat, that reduces lipid breakdown in the intestine allowing a proportion of ingested fat to be excreted.
- A synthetic version of a *glucagon-like peptide*, insulotropin, that slows emptying of the stomach and increases insulin levels; it is destined for use mainly in NIDDM.
- *Butabindide*, an inhibitor of an enzyme that degrades cholecystokinin in the GIT.

Potential leads to future drug development

Because of the possible role of the PPAR transcription factors α, β, and γ, in the pathophysiology of obesity (see above, p. 405), it has been suggested that it might be worth exploring synthetic libraries of the ligands that affect these transcription factors. Agents that modify this system might inhibit formation of white fat cells or increase that of brown.

Further investigation of the proteins that uncouple oxidative phosphorylation specifically in fat cells might also be profitable.

To sum up. There are, at present, no totally effective, safe drugs for the treatment of obesity, but the understanding of the possible basis of obesity is progressing rapidly. Pharmacology is almost certain to come to the aid of the obese eventually, but for the present, all one can usefully say to obese patients is 'stick to the diet and keep jogging'.

at all, should be used only as an adjunct to dietary and exercise regimes.

Inhibitors of 5-hydroxytryptamine uptake, fenfluramine and dexfenfluramine, were licensed for obesity therapy but proved to cause pulmonary hypertension and heart valve defects and have been withdrawn from the market. Fluoxetine, a 5-HT uptake inhibitor used mainly as an antidepressant (Ch. 35), promotes weight loss for several months after the start of therapy.

Phentermine, a sympathomimetic, causes weight loss, when used with fenfluramine, but its use is restricted to 12 weeks, after which there is rebound weight gain, so there is little advantage in giving the drug.

REFERENCES AND FURTHER READING

Andersson L B 1996 Genes and obesity. Editorial. Ann Med 28: 5–7

Arner P 1995 The β_3-adrenergic receptor—a cause and cure of obesity. N Engl J Med 333: 382–383 *(Editorial commentary)*

Auwerx J, Staels B 1998 Leptin. Lancet 351: 737–742 *(Valuable short review covering signalling pathways in CNS and periphery, intracellular transduction mechanisms and relationship to body weight)*

Bennett W I 1995 Beyond overeating. N Engl J Med 332: 673–674 *(Editorial commentary)*

Björntorp P 1997 Obesity. Lancet 350: 423–426

Bray G 1998 Obesity: a time bomb to be defused. The Lancet 352: 160–161 *(Editorial: includes mention of the pancreatic lipase inhibitor, orlistat)*

Campfield et al. 1995 Recombinant mouse OB protein: evidence for a peripheral signal linking adiposity and central neural networks. Science 269: 546–549

Campfield L A, Smith F J, Burn P 1996 The OB protein (leptin) pathway—a link between adipose tissue and central neural networks. Horm Metab Res 28: 619-632 *(Valuable review)*

Caro J, Sinha M K et al. 1996 Leptin: the tale of an obesity gene. Diabetes 45: 1455–1462

Finer N (ed) 1997 Obesity. Br Med Bull 53(2): 450

Flier J S 1995 The adipocyte: storage depot or node on the information highway. Cell 80: 15–18

Flier J S, Flier E M 1998 Obesity and the hypothalamus: novel peptides for new pathways. Cell 92: 437–440 *(Excellent minireview)*

Friedman J M 1997 The alphabet of weight control. Nature 385: 119–120 *(Melanocyte-stimulating hormone has opposite action to NPY in weight control)*

Gibbs W W 1996 Gaining on fat. Scientific American (August): 70–76 *(Simple, well-written analysis)*

Hamann A, Matthaei S 1996 Regulation of energy balance by leptin Exp Clin Endocrinol Diabetes 104: 293–300

Hervey G R 1958 The effect of lesions in the hypothalamus in parabiotic rats. J Physiol 145: 336–352

Hirsch J 1997 Obesity. Some heat but not enough light. Nature 387: 27–28

Kaiyala K J, Woods S C, Schwartz M W 1995 New model for the regulation of energy balance and adiposity by the central nervous system. Am J Clin Nutr 62 (suppl): 1123S–1134S

Kennedy G C 1953 The role of depot fat in the hypothalamic control of food intake in the rat. Proc R Soc 140: 578–592

Licinio J et al. 1997 Human leptin levels are pulsatile and inversely related to pituitary–adrenal function. Nature Med 3: 575–579

Lindpainter K 1995 Clinical implications of basic research: Finding an obesity gene—a tale of mice and man. N Engl J Med 332: 679–680

Lönnqvist F 1996 The obese (*Ob*) gene and its product leptin—a new route toward obesity treatment in man. Q J Med 89: 327–332

National Taskforce on the Prevention and Treatment of Obesity 1996 Long-term pharmacotherapy in the management of obesity. JAMA 276: 1907–1915

O'Rahilly S 1997 Non-insulin dependent diabetes mellitus: the gathering storm. Br Med J 314: 955-960 *(Clinical review)*

Pi-Sunyer F X 1996 Obesity: advances in understanding and treatment. A round up of IBC's 2nd annual international symposium on obesity. Molec Med Today (Oct): 410–411

Rosenbaum M, Liebel R L, Hirsch J 1997 Obesity. N Engl J Med 337: 396–407 *(General review of the regulation of energy storage, intake and expenditure)*

Sakurai T, Amemiya A et al. 1998 Orexins and orexin receptors: a family of hypothalamic neuropeptides and G protein-coupled receptors that regulate feeding behaviour. Cell 92: 573–585

Schwartz M W 1998 Orexins and appetite: the big picture of energy homeostasis gets a little bigger. Nature Med 4: 385–386 *(Short article on new appetite-stimulating mediator(s))*

Schwartz M W, Seeley R J 1997 Neuroendocrine responses to starvation and weight loss. N Engl J Med 336: 1802–1811

Serhan C N 1996 Signalling the fat controller. Nature 384: 23–24

Sørensen T I, Echwald S, Holm J-C 1996 Leptin in obesity: Tells the brain how much fat there is, but in obese people the message may not get through. Br Med J 313: 953–954

Spiegelman B M, Flier J S 1996 Adipogenesis and obesity: rounding out the big picture. Cell 87: 377–389 *(Excellent review)*

Strossberg A D 1997 Association of β_3-adrenoceptor polymorphism with obesity and diabetes current status. Trends Pharmacol Sci 18: 449–454

White D W, Tartaglia L A 1996 Lepti and OB-R: Body weight regulation by a cytokine. Cytokine and Growth Factor Rev 7: 303–309 *(Minireview of leptin receptor)*

Zhang Y, Proenca R et al. 1994 Positional cloning of the mouse obese gene and its human homologue. Nature 372: 425–432

24

The pituitary and adrenal cortex

The pituitary and adrenal glands release 'hormones'. This word, as introduced by Bayliss & Starling, referred to chemicals secreted without benefit of duct into the bloodstream, for action on a distant tissue. As pointed out in Chapter 12, the concept of 'hormones' as distinct from 'neurotransmitters' has become increasingly elastic. There appears to be, instead, a spectrum of agents, with substances that are predominantly neurotransmitters, acting at very short range (e.g. acetylcholine) at one end and substances that are predominantly hormones, in the classical sense, acting at long range, (e.g. sex steroids) at the other, with a range of substances acting more or less locally lying in between. In this chapter we consider substances that are mainly hormones in the classical Bayliss & Starling sense.

THE PITUITARY

The pituitary gland is composed of three sections arising from two different embryological sites. The *anterior* *pituitary* is derived from the endoderm of the buccal cavity, as is the *intermediate lobe* (which can thus be considered for practical purposes as part of the anterior pituitary), while the *posterior pituitary* is derived from neural ectoderm. Both main parts of the gland have an intimate functional relationship with the hypothalamus, the neurons of which contribute to two quite distinct systems influencing the anterior and posterior pituitary respectively.

ANTERIOR PITUITARY (ADENOHYPOPHYSIS)

The anterior pituitary secretes a number of different hormones vital for normal physiological function, some of which are involved in the regulation of other endocrine glands (Table 24.1). The cells of the anterior pituitary can be classified into corticotrophs, lactotrophs (mammotrophs), somatotrophs, thyrotrophs and gonadotrophs, according to the substances they secrete.

Secretion from the anterior pituitary is largely regulated by factors (hormones) derived from the hypothalamus, which reach the pituitary through the bloodstream. Blood vessels to the hypothalamus divide in its tissue to form a meshwork of capillaries—the primary plexus (Fig. 24.1), which drains into the hypophyseal portal vessels. These pass through the pituitary stalk to feed a secondary plexus of capillaries in the anterior pituitary. (Some portal veins which drain into these capillaries originate from a different primary plexus in the *posterior* pituitary.) Peptidergic neurons in the hypothalamus secrete a variety of releasing or release-inhibiting factors or hormones directly into the capillaries of the primary plexus (Table 24.1 and Fig. 24.1). Most of these regulate the secretion of hormones from the anterior lobe. The melanocyte-stimulating hormones are secreted mainly from the intermediate lobe.

There is a balance—involving various negative feed-back pathways—between the hypothalamic factors, the anterior pituitary hormones whose release they regulate

Table 24.1 Hormones secreted by the hypothalamus and the anterior pituitary

Hypothalamic factor/ hormone (and related drugs)	Hormone affected in anteror pituitary (and related drugs)	Main effects of anterior pituitary hormone
Corticotrophin-releasing factor (CRF)	Corticotrophin (ACTH; tetracosactrin)	Stmulates secretion of adrenal cortical hormones (mainly glucocorticoids). Maintains integrity of adrenal cortex
Thyrotrophin-releasing hormone (TRH; protirelin)	Thyrotrophin	Stimulates synthesis and secretion of thyroid hormones, T_3 and T_4. Maintains integrity of thyroid gland
Growth hormone-releasing factor (GHRF) Growth hormone-release inhibiting factor (GHRIF; somatostatin, octreotide)	Growth hormone (GH; somatotropin, somatropin, somatrem)	Regulates growth, partly directly, partly through evoking the release of somatomedins from the liver and elsewhere. Increases protein synthesis, increases blood glucose, stimulates lipolysis
Gonadotrophin-releasing hormone (GnRH; somatorelin, sermorelin)	Follicle-stimulating hormone (FSH). See Chapter 26	Stimulates the growth of the ovum and the Graafian follicle in the female and gametogenesis in the male. With LH, stmulates the secretion of oestrogen throughout the menstrual cycle and progesterone in the second half
	Luteinising hormone (LH) or interstitial-cell-stimulating hormone (ICSH). See Chapter 26	Stimulates ovulation and the development of the corpus luteum. With FSH, stmulates secretion of oestrogen throughout the menstrual cycle, and progesterone in the second half. In male, regulates testosterone secretion
Prolactin release-inhibiting factor (PRIF). Probably dopamine Prolactin-releasing factor (PRF)	Prolactin	Together with other hormones, prolactin promotes development of mammary tissue during pregnancy. Stimulates milk production in the postpartum period
Melanocyte-stimulating hormone releasing factor (MSH-RF) MSH release-inhibiting factor (MSH-RIF)	α-, β- and γ-melanocyte-stmulating hormones	Darken the skin in amphibia and fish. Function in humans not known

and the secretions of the peripheral endocrine glands. In general, the long negative feedback pathways, in which the mediators are the hormones that are secreted from the peripheral glands, affect both the hypothalamus and the anterior pituitary. The mediators of the short negative feedback pathways are anterior pituitary hormones that act on the hypothalamus.

The peptidergic neurons in the hypothalamus are themselves influenced by higher centres in the CNS. This action is mediated through dopamine, noradrenaline, 5-hydroxytryptamine and the opioid peptides, the latter being found in very high concentration in the hypothalamus (see Ch. 10).

Another means of hypothalamic control of the anterior pituitary is exerted through the tuberohypophyseal dopaminergic pathway, the neurons of which lie in close apposition to the primary capillary plexus (see Ch. 28). Dopamine can be secreted directly into the hypophyseal portal circulation and thus reach the anterior pituitary.

HYPOTHALAMIC HORMONES

There are at least six sets of hormones (also referred to as 'factors') which originate in the hypothalamus and which regulate the secretion of anterior pituitary hormones. These are listed in Table 24.1 and are described in more detail below. Some are used clinically for diagnosis or treatment; some are used as research tools. Many of these hormones also function as neurotransmitters or neuromodulators elsewhere in the central nervous system (Ch. 28), but their concentrations are highest and their functions best understood, in the hypothalamus.

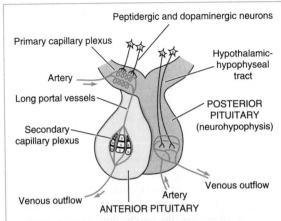

Fig. 24.1 Schematic diagram of vascular and neuronal relationships between the hypothalamus, the posterior pituitary and the anterior pituitary. The main portal vessels to the anterior pituitary lie in the pituitary stalk and arise from the primary plexus in the hypothalamus, but some (the short portal vessels) arise from the vascular bed in the posterior pituitary (not shown).

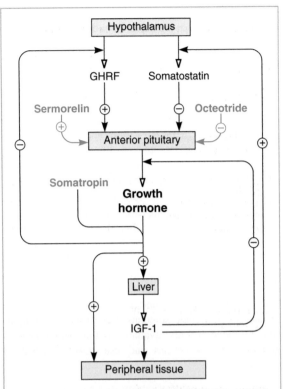

Fig. 24.2   Control of growth hormone secretion and its actions. Drugs are shown in blue. (GHRF = growth hormone-releasing factor; ILG-1 = insulin-like growth factor-1)

GROWTH HORMONE-RELEASING FACTOR (GHRF; SOMATORELIN)

GHRF is a peptide with 40–44 amino acid residues, active at a concentration of 10^{-15} mol/l. An analogue, **sermorelin**, has been introduced as a diagnostic test for growth hormone secretion.

The main action of GHRF is summarised in Figure 24.2. Given intravenously, subcutaneously or intranasally, it causes secretion of growth hormone within minutes and peak concentrations in 60 minutes. The action is selective for the somatotrophs in the anterior pituitary, no other pituitary hormones being released. Unwanted effects are rare.

SOMATOSTATIN

Somatostatin is a peptide of 14 amino acid residues. Somatostatin inhibits the release of growth hormone and thyrotrophin from the anterior pituitary (Figs 24.2 and 25.4), and insulin and glucagon from the pancreas, and decreases the release of most gastrointestinal hormones. It also reduces gastric acid and pancreatic secretion.

Octreotide is a long-acting analogue of somatostatin. It is used for the treatment of tumours secreting vasoactive intestinal peptide (Ch. 10), carcinoid tumours (Ch. 9), glucagonomas and various pituitary adenomas. It has a place in the therapy of acromegaly (a condition in which there is oversecretion of growth hormone in an adult) and of bleeding oesophageal varices.

It is given subcutaneously, the peak action is at 2 hours and the suppressant effect lasts for up to 8 hours.

Unwanted effects include pain at the injection site and gastrointestinal disturbances. Gallstones and post-prandial hyperglycaemia have also been reported and acute hepatitis has occurred in a few cases.

THYROTROPHIN-RELEASING HORMONE (TRH; PROTIRELIN)

TRH from the hypothalamus releases thyrotrophin (thyroid-stimulating hormone, TSH), from the anterior pituitary. **Protirelin** is a synthetic TSH; it is used for the diagnosis of mild thyroid disorders (see Fig. 25.4, p. 430). Given intravenously in normal subjects it elicits an increase in plasma thyrotrophin concentration, whereas in cases of hyperthyroidism, there is a blunted response to protirelin because the raised blood thyroxine concentration has a negative feedback effect on the anterior pituitary. The opposite occurs with hypothyroidism, in which the defect is in the thyroid itself.

CORTICOTROPHIN-RELEASING FACTOR (CRF)

CRF is a peptide which releases corticotrophin and β-endorphin from the anterior pituitary. Synthetic preparations are available. CRF acts synergistically with arginine vasopressin, and both its action and its release are inhibited by **glucocorticoids** (see Fig. 24.5).

Its main use is in diagnostic tests: to assess the ability of the pituitary to secrete corticotrophin; to assess whether a deficiency of corticotrophin is due to a pituitary or a hypothalamic defect; and to evaluate hypothalamic pituitary function after therapy for Cushing's syndrome (see Fig. 24.8).

GONADOTROPHIN-RELEASING HORMONE (GnRH)

Gonadotrophin-releasing hormone is a decapeptide which releases both follicle-stimulating hormone and luteinising hormone. It is also available as a preparation called **gonadorelin**. Its actions and uses are described in Chapter 26.

ANTERIOR PITUITARY HORMONES

The main hormones of the anterior pituitary are listed in Table 24.1. The gonadotrophins are dealt with in Chapter 26 and thyrotrophin in Chapter 25. The others are dealt with below.

GROWTH HORMONE (GH; SOMATOTROPIN)

Growth hormone is derived from the somatotroph cells and is found in the anterior pituitary in larger quantities than any other pituitary hormone. Secretion of growth hormone is high in the newborn, decreasing at 4 years to an intermediate level, which is then maintained until after puberty when there is a further decline.

A preparation of growth hormone, **somatropin**, produced by recombinant DNA technology and identical to growth hormone, is available for clinical use.

Regulation of secretion

Secretion of GH is regulated by the action of hypothalamic growth hormone-releasing factor (GHRF) modulated by somatostatin as described above and outlined in Figure 24.2.

One of the mediators of growth hormone action, *insulin-like growth factor 1* (*IGF-1*) which is released from the liver (see below) has an inhibitory effect on growth hormone secretion by stimulating somatostatin release from the hypothalamus (Fig. 24.2).

Growth hormone release, like that of other anterior pituitary secretions, is pulsatile, and its plasma concentration fluctuates 10- to 100-fold. These surges occur repeatedly during the day and night and reflect changes in hypothalamic control. Deep sleep is a potent stimulus to growth hormone secretion, particularly in children.

Actions

The main effect of growth hormone and its analogues is to stimulate normal growth and, in doing this, it affects many tissues, acting in conjunction with other hormones secreted from the thyroid, the gonads and the adrenal cortex. It stimulates the production, mainly from the liver, of several polypeptide mediators, the insulin-like growth factors (IGFs)—also termed somatomedins—which are responsible for most of its anabolic actions (see Fig. 24.2). IGF-1 is the main mediator of growth hormone action. Receptors for IGF-1 exist on many cell types, including liver cells and fat cells.

Protein synthesis is stimulated by growth hormone, and the uptake of amino acids into cells is increased, especially in skeletal muscle. IGF-1 mediates many of these anabolic effects, acting on skeletal muscle and also on the cartilage at the epiphyses of long bones, thus influencing bone growth.

The effects on *carbohydrate metabolism* are complex. At high concentrations, an early 'insulin-like' effect is produced, but at physiological concentrations this does not occur.

The main action on *fat metabolism* is to act in concert with glucocorticoids to cause lipolysis.

Growth hormone also has prolactin-like effects (see below).

Disorders of production and clinical use

Deficiency of growth hormone results in pituitary dwarfism. In this condition, which can be produced by lack of GHRF or a failure of IGF generation or action, the normal proportions of the body are maintained.

The only established clinical use is in patients with growth hormone deficiency and in short stature due to Turner's syndrome. Satisfactory linear growth can be achieved by giving **somatropin**.* It is given subcutaneously, six to seven times per week, and therapy is most successful when started early.

---

*Growth hormone extracted from cadaver pituitaries has caused Creutzfeldt–Jakob disease, a severe neurodegenerative disease (see Ch. 31) and its use has been discontinued.

The availability of the synthetic peptide has opened up the possibility of many other uses based on the anabolic and central effects.

An excessive production of growth hormone in children results in gigantism. An excessive production in adults, which is usually the result of a benign pituitary tumour, results in acromegaly—a condition in which there is enlargement mainly of facial structures and of the hands and feet.* The dopamine agonist **bromocriptine** (see Ch. 9 and below) and **octreotide** (see Ch. 42) may ameliorate the condition, but effective treatment consists of removal or irradiation of the tumour.

PROLACTIN

Prolactin is secreted by mammotroph (lactotroph) cells which are abundant in the anterior pituitary and which increase in number during pregnancy, probably under the influence of oestrogen.

Regulation of secretion

Prolactin is unusual in that its secretion is under *tonic inhibitory* control by the hypothalamus (Fig. 24.3 and Table 24.1). The inhibitory influence is exerted through the dopaminergic tuberohypophyseal pathway (see Ch. 30); the *prolactin release-inhibiting factor* (PRIF) secreted by the hypothalamus is generally held to be dopamine itself.

The main stimulus for prolactin release is suckling. Neural reflexes from the breast may stimulate the secretion from the hypothalamus of a *prolactin-releasing factor* (PRF) (and/or TRH—there are receptors for TRH on the mammotrophs). Oestrogens increase both prolactin secretion and the proliferation of lactotrophs through release, from a subset of lactotrophs, of the neuropeptide, galanin.

Dopamine antagonists (used mainly as antipsychotic drugs; see Ch. 34) are potent stimulants of prolactin release.

Dopamine agonists such as **bromocriptine** (see below) suppress prolactin release. Bromocriptine is also used in parkinsonism (Ch. 31).

Actions

The main function of prolactin in females is the control of milk production; one can only speculate as to what its function is in males. At parturition, when the blood level of oestrogen falls, the prolactin concentration rises and lactation is initiated. Maintenance of lactation depends on suckling, which stimulates a reflex secretion

*'Acral' means distal.

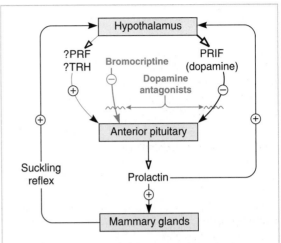

Fig. 24.3 Control of prolactin secretion and the drugs which modify it. (TRH = thyrotrophin-releasing hormone; PRF = prolactin-releasing factor; PRIF = prolactin release-inhibiting factor)

of prolactin by neural pathways, causing a 10- to 100-fold increase within 30 minutes.

Prolactin, along with other hormones, is responsible for the proliferation and differentiation of mammary tissue during pregnancy. It inhibits gonadotrophin release and/or the response of the ovaries to these trophic hormones. This is one of the reasons why ovulation does not usually occur during breast feeding, and it is believed to constitute a natural contraceptive mechanism.

According to one rather appealing hypothesis, the high post-delivery concentration of prolactin reflects its biological function of 'parental' hormone. Certainly broodiness and nest-building activity can be induced in birds by prolactin injections, and equivalent 'parental' behaviour can be induced in mice and rabbits. It is rather attractive to think that it might have a similar action in humans, but this is conjectural.

Modification of prolactin secretion

Prolactin itself is not used clinically; in the context of prolactin physiology, the main clinical need is to *decrease* its secretion, and the agent used for this purpose is **bromocriptine**.

Bromocriptine is well absorbed orally, and peak concentrations occur after 2 hours. It is metabolised in the liver and excreted in the bile. Unwanted reactions include nausea and vomiting, which may be ameliorated by taking the drug with meals. Dizziness, constipation and postural hypotension may also occur.

Clinical use of bromocriptine

- To prevent lactation without causing pain or engorgement of the breast, as well as to suppress established lactation; it is more effective than oestrogens in this latter action.
- To treat galactorrhoea, i.e. non-puerperal lactation due to excessive prolactin secretion.
- To treat prolactin-secreting pituitary tumours (prolactinomas).
- In the treatment of parkinsonism (Ch. 31) and of acromegaly.

CORTICOTROPHIN

Corticotrophin (also termed adrenocorticotrophic hormone or ACTH) is the adenohypophyseal endocrine secretion which controls the synthesis and release of the glucocorticoids of the adrenal cortex (see Table 24.1 and p. 418). It is a polypeptide hormone (prepared from animal pituitary glands) with 39 amino acid residues. It is rarely used in therapy because its action is less predictable than that of the corticosteroids and it provokes antibody formation. **Tetracosactrin**, a synthetic polypeptide that consists of the first 24 N-terminal amino acids of human ACTH, is less immunogenic than corticotrophin because the immunogenicity resides mainly in the 15 amino acids at the C-terminal end.

(Detail of the regulation of corticotrophin secretion is given on p. 418 and shown in Fig. 24.5.)

The concentration of corticotrophin in the blood is reduced by glucocorticoids, forming the basis of the dexamethasone suppression test (see p. 424).

Actions

Corticotrophin and tetracosactrin have two actions on the adrenal cortex:

- Stimulation of the synthesis and release of glucocorticoids from the adrenal cortex. There is also a slight release of aldosterone and weakly androgenic steroids. The main effect is to increase the concentration of the starting substrate for steroid synthesis, cholesterol (Fig. 24.5). The action is very rapid—a release of glucocorticoids occurs within minutes of injection and the main biological actions are those of the steroids released.
- A trophic action on adrenal cortical cells, and regulation of the levels of key mitochondrial steroidogenic enzymes. The loss of this effect accounts for the adrenal atrophy that results from chronic gluco-

corticoid administration (see p. 423) which suppresses ACTH secretion.

The main use of tetracosactrin is in the diagnosis of adrenal cortical insufficiency. The drug is given intramuscularly, and then the concentration of hydrocortisone in the plasma is measured by radioimmunoassay (see Ch. 3).

Anterior pituitary and hypothalamus

- The anterior pituitary secretes hormones which regulate:
  - the release of glucocorticoids from adrenal cortex
  - the release of thyroid hormones
  - ovulation in the female and spermatogenesis in the male, and the release of sex hormones (Ch. 26)
  - growth
  - mammary gland structure and function.
- Each anterior pituitary hormone is regulated by a specific hypothalamic releasing factor. Feedback mechanisms influence the release of these factors.
- Substances available for clinical use are:
  - growth hormone-releasing factor (sermorelin) and analogues of growth hormone (GH, somatrem, somatropin)
  - thyrotrophin-releasing factor (protirelin) and thyrotrophin (used to test thyroid function)
  - octreotide, an analogue of somatostatin, which inhibits GH release
  - corticotrophin-releasing factor, used in diagnosis
  - gonadotrophin-releasing factor (see Ch. 26).

POSTERIOR PITUITARY (NEUROHYPOPHYSIS)

The posterior pituitary gland consists largely of the terminals of nerve cells which lie in the supraoptic and paraventricular nuclei of the hypothalamus. Their axons form the hypothalamic–hypophyseal tract, and the fibres terminate in dilated nerve endings in close association with capillaries in the posterior pituitary gland (Fig. 24.1). Peptides, synthesised in the hypothalamic nuclei, pass down the axons into the posterior pituitary where they are stored and eventually secreted into the bloodstream. See also Chapter 10.

The two main hormones of the posterior pituitary are **oxytocin** (which contracts the smooth muscle of the uterus; see Ch. 26) and the **antidiuretic hormone** (also called **vasopressin**; see Chs 15 and 20). The structure of these hormones is given in Figure 24.4.

Several similar peptides have been synthesised which vary in their antidiuretic, vasopressor and oxytocic (uterine stimulant) properties.

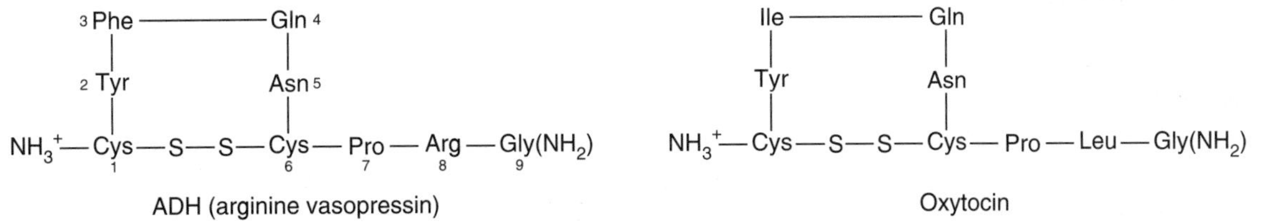

Fig. 24.4 **The structures of the two posterior pituitary peptides.**

Posterior pituitary

- The posterior pituitary secretes:
  — oxytocin (see Ch. 26)
  — the antidiuretic hormone (vasopressin) which acts on V_2-receptors in the distal kidney tubule to increase water reabsorption, and, in higher concentrations, on V_1-receptors to cause vasoconstriction. (It also participates in the control of ACTH secretion.)
- Substances available for clinical use are vasopressin, and the analogues, desmopressin, lypressin, terlipressin.

ANTIDIURETIC HORMONE (ADH; VASOPRESSIN)

Regulation of secretion and physiological role

ADH released from the posterior pituitary has a crucial role in the control of the water content of the body through its action on the cells of the distal part of the nephron and the collecting tubules in the kidney (see Ch. 20). Specific nuclei in the hypothalamus which control water metabolism lie close to the nuclei which synthesise and secrete ADH.

One of the main stimuli to ADH release is an *increase in plasma osmolality* (which produces a sensation of thirst). A *decrease in circulating blood volume* (hypo-volaemia) is another major factor causing secretion of ADH, the stimuli arising from baroreceptors in the cardiovascular system. Angiotensin also releases ADH.

The main disorder of ADH secretion is *diabetes insipidus*, a condition in which there is continuous pro-duction of copious amounts of hypotonic urine. It results from either reduced circulating ADH, termed *neuro-hypophyseal diabetes insipidus*, or an impaired response of the nephron to normal ADH levels, termed *nephro-genic diabetes insipidus*. This latter is due in many cases to defective V_2-receptors (see below).

The receptors for ADH

There are two classes of receptors for ADH (vaso-pressin)—V_1 and V_2. The V_2-receptors, which mediate its main physiological actions on the kidney, are coupled to adenylate cyclase; and the V_1-receptors, of which there are two types—V_{1a} and V_{1b}—are coupled to the phospholipase C/IP_3 system.

Actions

Renal actions

ADH binds to V_2-receptors in the basolateral membrane of the cells of the distal tubule and collecting ducts of the nephron. Its main effect in the collecting duct is to increase the rate of insertion of water channels into the lumenal membrane, thus increasing the permeability of the membrane to water. (Details of this action are given in Ch. 20.) It also activates urea transporters and transiently increases sodium absorption, particularly in the distal tubule.

Several drugs affect the action of ADH. **NSAIDs** and **carbamazepine** increase ADH effects; **lithium**, **colchicine** and **vinca alkaloids** decrease it, the latter two agents by virtue of their action on microtubules—organelles required for the movement of the water channels. **Demeclocycline** counteracts the action of ADH and can be used to treat patients with hyponatraemia (and thus water retention) due to excessive secretion of ADH.

Non-renal actions

ADH causes contraction of *smooth muscle*, particularly in the cardiovascular system, by acting on V_{1a}-receptors (see Ch. 15). The affinity of these receptors for ADH is lower than that of the V_2-receptors, and smooth muscle effects are only seen with doses larger than those affecting the kidney.

In the CNS, ADH acts as a neuromodulator and neurotransmitter, and released into the pituitary 'portal circulation' it promotes the release of corticotrophin from the anterior pituitary by an action on V_{1b}-receptors (Fig. 24.5). It tends to increase the concentration of factor VIII in the blood.

Preparations used and pharmacokinetic aspects

Various analogues of vasopressin have been developed for clinical use, the aims being (a) to increase the duration of action and (b) to shift the potency between V_1- and V_2-receptors. The main analogues are:

- Vasopressin (ADH) itself, the prototype; this has short duration of action, weak selectivity for V_2-receptors and is usually given by subcutaneous or intramuscular injection, or by intravenous infusion. It has 0.8 times the diuretic action of ADH and 60% of its vasopressor potency.
- Desmopressin (1-deamino-DArg8-vasopressin); this has increased duration of action, is V_2-selective and is usually given as a nasal spray. It has 12 times the diuretic action of ADH and 0.4% of its vasopressor potency.
- Lypressin (Lys^8-vasopressin); this is similar in potency to vasopressin but is given as a nasal spray.
- Terlipressin (triglyceryl-Lys^8-vasopressin); this has increased duration of action, is V_1-selective and is given intravenously. It has low but protracted vasopressor action and minimal antidiuretic properties.
- Felypressin (Phe^2-Lys^8-vasopressin); this has a short duration of action and is V_1-selective. Its vasoconstrictor effect is used with local anaesthetics to prolong their action.

Vasopressin and lypressin are rapidly eliminated, both having a plasma half-life of 10 minutes and a short duration of action. Metabolism is by tissue peptidases, and 33% of vasopressin is removed by the kidney. Desmopressin is less subject to degradation by peptidases, and its plasma half-life is 75 minutes.

Various synthetic peptide and non-peptide agonists and antagonists of vasopressin have been synthesised and are used as experimental tools.

The clinical uses of vasopressin and analogues are given on this page.

Unwanted effects

There are few unwanted effects if the antidiuretic peptides are used intranasally in therapeutic doses. Nausea and abdominal cramps, and hypersensitivity reactions have been reported. Intravenous vasopressin may cause spasm of the coronary arteries with resultant angina, and it frequently causes abdominal and uterine cramps.

OXYTOCIN

Oxytocin is discussed in Chapter 26.

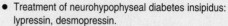

> **Clinical use of vasopressin and analogues**
>
> - Treatment of neurohypophyseal diabetes insipidus: lypressin, desmopressin.
> - The initial treatment of bleeding oesophageal varices: vasopressin, terlipressin, lypressin. (Octreotide is also used but sclerotherapy is the main treatment.)
> - As prophylactic therapy (e.g. before tooth extraction) in haemophilia: vasopressin, desmopressin (by increasing the concentration of factor VIII; somatostatin is also effective).
> - Felypressin is used as a vasoconstrictor with local anaesthetics (see Ch. 40).
> - Desmopressin is used in older children and adults with persistent enuresis.

ADRENAL STEROIDS

The steroids secreted by the adrenal cortex have two main actions:

- those seen primarily in the resting state and which are 'permissive' in nature, i.e. they permit or facilitate the actions of other hormones
- those which occur in response to a threatening environment.

These latter actions are crucial for survival, an animal deprived of its adrenal cortex being able to survive only in rigorously controlled conditions.

The principal adrenal steroids are those with *mineralocorticoid* and *glucocorticoid* activity, but some *sex steroids*—mainly androgens—are also secreted. The mineralocorticoids affect water and electrolyte balance and the main endogenous hormone is **aldosterone**. The glucocorticoids affect carbohydrate and protein metabolism and the main endogenous hormones are **hydrocortisone** and **corticosterone**. The two actions are not completely separated in naturally occurring steroids, some glucocorticoids having quite substantial effects on water and electrolyte balance.* In addition to their metabolic effects, glucocorticoids also have anti-inflammatory and immunosuppressive activity, and it is for these actions that they are most commonly used therapeutically. When they are used as anti-inflammatory

---

*In fact hydrocortisone and aldosterone are equiactive on mineralocorticoid receptors; but, in mineralocorticoid-sensitive tissues such as the kidney, the action of 11b-hydroxysteroid dehydrogenase converts hydrocortisone to receptor-inactive cortisone.

and immunosuppressive agents, all of their other actions are unwanted side-effects.

Synthetic steroids have been developed in which it has been possible to separate the glucocorticoid from the mineralocorticoid actions (see Table 24.2), but it has not been possible to separate the anti-inflammatory actions from the other actions of the glucocorticoids.

A deficiency in corticosteroid production, *Addison's disease*, is characterised by muscular weakness, low blood pressure, depression, anorexia, loss of weight and hypoglycaemia. Addison's disease may have an auto-immune aetiology, or may be due to destruction of the gland by chronic inflammatory conditions such as tuberculosis. A decreased production of *endogenous* corticoids

Table 24.2 Comparison of the main corticosteroid agents (using hydrocortisone as a standard)

Compound	Relative affinity for glucocorticoid receptors*	Approx. relative potency in clinical use:		Duration of action after oral dose	Comments
		Anti-inflam.	Sodium-retaining		
Hydrocortisone (cortisol)	1	1	1	S	Drug of choice for replacement and emergencies
Cortisone	0.01	0.8	0.8	S	Cheap. Inactive until converted to hydrocortisone. Not used as anti-inflammatory because of mineralocorticoid effects
Corticosterone	0.85	0.3	15	S	–
Prednisolone	2.2	4	0.8	I	Drug of choice for systemic anti-inflammatory and immunosuppressive effects
Prednisone	0.05	4	0.8	I	Inactive until converted to prednisolone. Anti-inflammatory and immunosuppressive
Methylprednisolone	11.9	5	Minimal	I	Anti-inflammatory and immunosuppressive
Triamcinolone	1.9	5	None	I	Relatively more toxic than others. Anti-inflammatory and immunosuppressive
Dexamethasone	7.1	30	Minimal	L	Anti-inflammatory and immunosuppressive, used especially where water retention is undesirable, e.g. cerebral oedema. Drug of choice for suppression of ACTH production
Betamethasone	5.4	30	Negligible	L	Anti-inflammatory and immunosuppressive, used especially where water retention is undesirable. Used for suppression of ACTH production
Beclomethasone		+	–	–	Anti-inflammatory and immunosuppressive. Used topically and as an aerosol
Budesonide		+	–	–	
Deoxycortone	0.19	Negligible	50	–	
Fludrocortisone	3.5	15	150	S	Drug of choice for mineralocorticoid effects
Aldosterone	0.38	none	500	–	Endogenous mineralocorticoid

*Human foetal lung cells
Duration of action: S: $t_{1/2}$ = 8–12 h; I: $t_{1/2}$ = 12–36 h; L: $t_{1/2}$ = 36–72 h
Data for relative affinity obtained from: Baxter & Rousseau 1979

also occurs when glucocorticoids are given therapeutically for prolonged periods; this can result in deficiency eventually, when treatment is discontinued.

When corticosteroids are produced in excess, the clinical picture depends on which of the steroids predominate. Excessive glucocorticoid activity results in *Cushing's syndrome*, the manifestations of which are outlined in Figure 24.8. This can be caused by hypersecretion from the adrenal glands or by prolonged administration of glucocorticoids. An excessive production of mineralocorticoids results in disturbances of sodium and potassium balance. This may occur with hyperactivity of the adrenals or tumours of the glands (*primary hyperaldosteronism*, or Conn's syndrome, an uncommon but important cause of hypertension; see Ch. 15), or with excessive renin–angiotensin action such as occurs in kidney disease, cirrhosis of the liver or congestive cardiac failure (*secondary hyperaldosteronism*). Excessive production of adrenal androgens results in *adrenal virilism*.

The glucocorticoids are dealt with below and the mineralocorticoids on page 425.

Corticotrophin and the adrenal steroids

- Corticotrophin (ACTH) stimulates synthesis and release of glucocorticoids (e.g. hydrocortisone) from adrenal cortex (also some androgens).
- Corticotrophin-releasing factor (CRF) from the hypothalamus regulates corticotrophin release and is in turn regulated by neural factors and negative feedback effects of plasma glucocorticoids.
- Mineralocorticoid (e.g. aldosterone) release from the adrenal cortex is controlled by the renin–angiotensin system.

GLUCOCORTICOIDS

Synthesis and release

Adrenal steroids are not stored preformed; they are synthesised and released as needed, and the main physiological stimulus for synthesis and release of the glucocorticoids is *corticotrophin* (adrenocorticotrophic hormone, or ACTH) secreted from the anterior pituitary gland (see p. 414 and Fig. 24.5). Corticotrophin secretion is regulated partly by *corticotrophin-releasing factor* (CRF) derived from the hypothalamus (see Table 24.1 and Fig. 24.5) and partly by the level of glucocorticoids in the blood. (Antidiuretic hormone, which may reach the pituitary through short portal vessels from the posterior

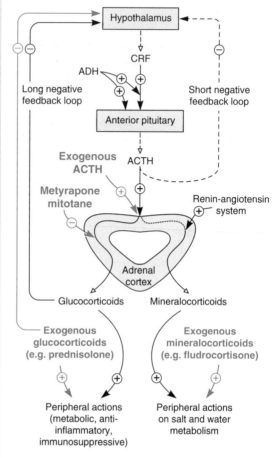

Fig. 24.5   Regulation of synthesis and secretion of adrenal corticosteroids. The long negative feedback loop is more important than the short one (dashed line). ACTH has only a minimal effect on mineralocorticoid production (indicated by dotted line). (ACTH = adrenocorticotrophic hormone (corticotrophin); ADH = antidiuretic hormone (vasopressin); CRF = corticotrophin-releasing factor)

pituitary, also stimulates ACTH release and may have a physiological role.) The release of CRF in turn is inhibited by the level of glucocorticoids and, to a lesser extent, of corticotrophin in the blood, and is influenced by input from the central nervous system. There is a basal release of glucocorticoids. Opioid peptides normally exercise a tonic inhibitory control on the secretion of CRF. Psychological factors can affect the release of CRF, as can stimuli such as excessive heat or cold, injury or infections; this is the mechanism, in fact, by which the pituitary adrenal system is activated in response to a threatening environment.

The interrelationship of these factors is outlined in Figure 24.5.*

For a discussion of the interaction of CNS transmitters with the hypothalamic–pituitary–adrenal axis in stress (see Chrousos 1995).

The concentration of endogenous corticosteroids in the blood is high in the morning, at 8 a.m. and low at midnight.

The starting substance for synthesis of glucocorticoids is *cholesterol* (Fig. 24.6) which is obtained mostly from the plasma and is present in the lipid granules of the cells of the middle layer of the adrenal cortex. The first step, the conversion of cholesterol to *pregnenolone* is the rate-limiting step and is regulated by ACTH. Some of the reactions in the synthesis can be inhibited by drugs.

Metyrapone prevents the β-hydroxylation at C_{11} and thus the formation of hydrocortisone and corticosterone (Fig. 24.6). Synthesis is stopped at the 11-deoxycorticosteroid stage and, as these substances have no negative feedback effects on the hypothalamus and pituitary, there is a marked increase in ACTH in the blood. Metyrapone can therefore be used to test ACTH production and may also be used in some cases of Cushing's syndrome. **Trilostane** (of use in Cushing's syndrome and primary hyperaldosteronism) blocks an earlier step in the pathway—the 3β-dehydrogenase.

Aminoglutethimide inhibits an earlier stage in the synthetic pathway and has the same effect as metyrapone (Fig. 24.6). **Ketoconazole**, an antifungal agent (Ch. 45), used in higher doses, inhibits steroidogenesis and can be of value in Cushing's syndrome.

Actions

The pharmacological actions of the glucocorticoids may be considered under three main headings:

- general effects on metabolism, water and electrolyte balance and organ systems
- negative feedback effects on the anterior pituitary and hypothalamus (lipocortin-1 is involved; see below)
- anti-inflammatory and immunosuppressive effects.

General metabolic and systemic effects

The main metabolic effects are on carbohydrate and protein metabolism. The hormones cause both a decrease in the uptake and utilisation of glucose and an increase in gluconeogenesis, resulting in a tendency to hyperglycaemia (see Ch. 22). There is a concomitant increase in glycogen storage which may be due to insulin secretion in response to the increase in blood sugar. There is decreased protein synthesis and increased protein breakdown, particularly in muscle. Glucocorticoids have a 'permissive' effect on the lipolytic response to catecholamines and other hormones, which act by increasing intracellular cAMP concentration (see Ch. 2). Such hormones cause lipase activation through a cAMP-dependent kinase, the synthesis of which requires the presence of glucocorticoids (see below). Large doses of glucocorticoids given over a long period result in the redistribution of fat characteristic of Cushing's syndrome (see Fig. 24.8).

The glucocorticoids, in non-physiological concentrations, have some mineralocorticoid actions (see below), causing sodium retention and potassium loss—possibly by occupying mineralocorticoid receptors.

Glucocorticoids tend to produce a negative calcium balance by decreasing calcium absorption in the gastrointestinal tract and increasing its excretion by the kidney. This can result in osteoporosis (see below).

Negative feedback effects on the anterior pituitary and hypothalamus

Both endogenous and exogenous glucocorticoids have a negative feedback effect on the secretion of CRF and ACTH (see Fig. 24.5). Administration of exogenous glucocorticoids depresses the secretion of CRF and ACTH thus inhibiting the secretion of endogenous glucocorticoids and causing atrophy of the adrenal cortex. If therapy is prolonged, it may take many months to return to normal function when the drugs are stopped.

Anti-inflammatory and immunosuppressive effects

When given therapeutically, glucocorticoids have powerful anti-inflammatory and immunosuppressive effects. They inhibit both the early and the late manifestations of inflammation, i.e. not only the initial redness, heat, pain and swelling (p. 199), but also the later stages of wound healing and repair and the proliferative reactions seen in chronic inflammation (p. 210). They affect *all* types of inflammatory reactions whether caused by invading pathogens, by chemical or physical stimuli or by inappropriately deployed immune responses such as are seen in hypersensitivity or autoimmune disease (pp 209–210). When used clinically to suppress graft rejection, glucocorticoids suppress the initiation and generation of a 'new' immune response more efficiently than a response that is already established and in which clonal proliferation has already occurred.

---

*When released, the corticosteroids pass first through the adrenal medulla because both the medulla and cortex of the adrenal gland have a common blood supply. Glucocorticoids play a part in controlling the conversion of noradrenaline to adrenaline, through a stimulant action on the relevant methyltransferase (see Ch. 8).

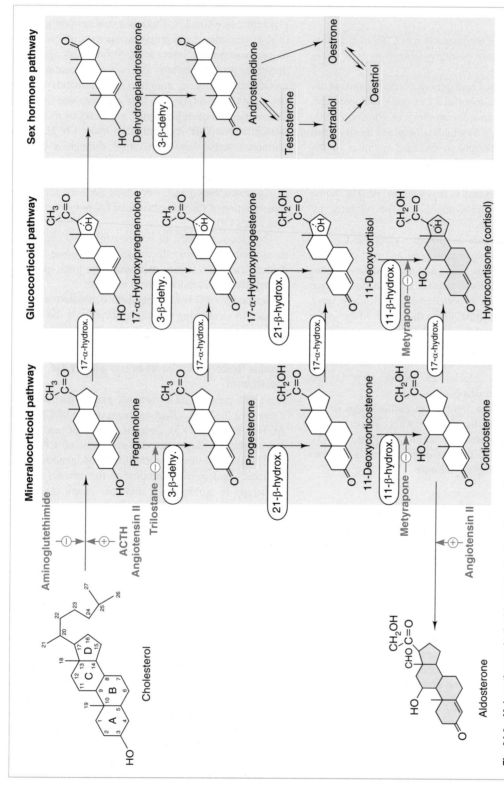

Fig. 24.6 Main pathways in the biosynthesis of corticosteroids and adrenal androgens with sites of action of drugs indicated. Note that the drugs have selective actions on different cortical cell types. Glucocorticoids are produced by cells of the zona fasciculata and their synthesis is stimulated by ACTH; aldosterone is produced by cells of the zona glomerulosa and its synthesis is stimulated by angiotensin II. Metyrapone inhibits glucocorticoid synthesis, aminoglutethimide inhibits both glucocorticoid and sex hormone synthesis, and trilostane blocks synthesis of all three types of adrenal steroid. (Further details of sex steroid biosynthesis are given in Fig. 26.3.) (3-β-dhy. = 3-β-dehydrogenase; 17-α-hydrox. = 17-α-hydroxylase; 21-β-hydrox. = 21-β-hydroxylase; 11-β-hydrox. = 11-β-hydroxylase)

Actions on inflammatory cells:

- Decreased egress of neutrophils from blood vessels and reduced activity of neutrophils and macrophages due to decreased transcription of the genes for cell adhesion factors and the relevant cytokines (see below).
- Decreased action of T helper cells and reduced clonal proliferation of T cells, mainly through decreased transcription of the genes for IL-2 and the IL-2 receptor. (See below and Fig. 12.3.)
- Decreased fibroblast function and therefore less production of collagen and glycosaminoglycans; the contribution of these events to chronic inflammation is reduced but so also is healing and repair.
- Reduced function of osteoblasts and increased activity of osteoclasts—and thus a tendency to develop osteoporosis (see below).

Action on the mediators of inflammatory and immune responses:

- Decreased production of prostanoids due to decreased expression of COX-2 (see Fig. 12.4).
- Decreased generation of cytokines—IL-1, IL-2, IL-3, IL-4, IL-5, IL-6, IL-8, TNF-γ and cell adhesion factors (see Ch. 12), GM-CSF (see Ch. 18, p. 336)—due to inhibition of transcription of the relevant genes (see below).
- Reduction in the concentration of complement components in the plasma (see p. 200).
- Decreased generation of induced nitric oxide (see below).
- Decreased histamine release from basophils.
- Decreased IgG production.

These anti-inflammatory and immunosuppressive actions of the glucocorticoids have generally been considered to be 'pharmacological' actions only, i.e. to be qualitatively different from the physiological effects (namely the metabolic and regulatory actions) of endogenously produced glucocorticoids. It is now understood that the anti-inflammatory and immunosuppressive actions *do* have a physiological role in that they prevent 'overshoot' of the body's powerful defence reactions, that might otherwise themselves threaten homeostasis (see Munck et al 1984).

The consequence of these powerful actions of the glucocorticoids is that they can be of great value when used to treat certain conditions in which there is hypersensitivity and unwanted inflammation, but they carry the hazard that they can suppress the necessary protective responses to infection and can decrease essential healing processes.

Glucocorticoids

Drugs used: hydrocortisone, prednisolone and dexamethasone.

Metabolic actions
- On carbohydrates: decreased uptake and utilisation of glucose, and increased gluconeogenesis; this causes a tendency to hyperglycaemia.
- On proteins: increased catabolism, reduced anabolism.
- On fat: a permissive effect on lipolytic hormones, and a redistribution of fat, as in Cushing's syndrome.

Regulatory actions
- On hypothalamus and anterior pituitary: a negative feedback action resulting in reduced release of endogenous glucocorticoids.
- On vascular events: reduced vasodilatation, decreased fluid exudation.
- On cellular events:
  — in areas of acute inflammation: decreased influx and activity of leukocytes
  — in areas of chronic inflammation: decreased activity of mononuclear cells, decreased proliferation of blood vessels, less fibrosis
  — in lymphoid areas: decreased clonal expansion of T and B cells and decreased action of cytokine-secreting T cells.
- On inflammatory and immune mediators:
  — decreased production and action of cytokines including many interleukins, TNFγ, GM-CSF
  — reduced generation of eicosanoids
  — decreased generation of IgG
  — decrease in complement components in the blood.
- Overall effects: reduction in chronic inflammation and autoimmune reactions but also decreased healing and diminution in the protective aspects of the inflammatory response.

Mechanism of action

Glucocorticoid effects involve interactions between the steroids and intracellular receptors that belong to the superfamily of receptors that control gene transcription (see Ch. 2).This superfamily also includes the receptors for mineralocorticoids, the sex steroids, thyroid hormones, vitamin D_3 and retinoic acid. There are believed to be 10–100 steroid-responsive genes in each cell.

The glucocorticoids, after entering cells, bind to specific receptors in the cytoplasm (Fig. 24.7A). These receptors, which have a high affinity for glucocorticoids, are found in virtually all tissues—about 3000 to 10 000 per cell, the number varying in different tissues. After interaction with the steroid, the receptor becomes 'activated', i.e. it undergoes a conformational change which exposes a DNA-binding domain (see Figs 24.7B, 2.2

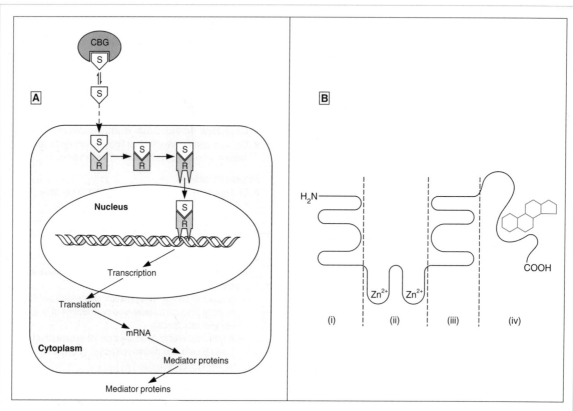

Fig. 24.7 **Mechanism of action of glucocorticoids at the cellular level and the functional domains of the glucocorticoid receptor.** [A] Diagram showing glucocorticoid-mediated induction (initiation of transcription). Note that the glucocorticoids can also *repress* induction by inhibiting transcription factors such as AP-1 and NF-κB. (S = steroid; R = receptor; CBG = corticosteroid-binding globulin). After the binding of steroid to receptor and before interaction with DNA, there is dimer formation, i.e. the linking of two steroid–receptor complexes (not shown). [B] Diagram of the glucocorticoid receptor domains with the main functions associated with each domain. Note that three domains are involved in transcription and three in dimer formation. (i) Regulatory domain: activates gene-specific transcription, and can bind other protein factors. (ii) The DNA-binding domain: determines which genes will be influenced by the receptor (it contains two 'zinc fingers' which wrap around the DNA helix), controls transcriptional activation (i.e. positive as opposed to negative genomic events) and is involved in dimer formation. (iii) Hinge domain: is involved in nuclear localisation, transcription and dimer formation. (iv) Steroid-binding domain: binds steroid and is involved in nuclear localisation and dimer formation. (Modified from: Landers & Spelsberg 1992)

and 2.3). The steroid–receptor complexes form dimers (pairs), then move to the nucleus and bind to steroid-response elements in the DNA. The effect is either to repress (prevent transcription of) or induce (i.e. initiate transcription of) particular genes.

Repression is brought about in part by inhibition of the action of various transcription factors* such as AP-1** and NF-κB*** (see Marx 1995). These transcription factors normally switch on the genes for COX-2, various cytokines, and the inducible form of nitric oxide synthase (see above and Ch. 14). Basal and induced transcription of the genes for collagenase are modified and vitamin

D_3 induction of the ostecalcin gene in osteoblasts is inhibited. (See Funder 1997, Krane 1993, Landers & Spelsberg 1992, Marx 1995.)

---

*These factors bind to the DNA upstream from the start site of transcription and act as enhancers of transcription.

**AP-1 is a heterodimer of Fos and Jun proteins which are the products of Fos and Jun proto-oncogenes. See Figure 42.3.

***Glucocorticoids *induce* the transcription of the inhibitory factor-κBa gene, and the resultant protein binds nuclear factor-κB transcription factor in the cytosol, preventing its translocation to the nucleus.

Induction involves the formation of specific messenger RNAs, which direct the synthesis of specific proteins. In addition to the enzymes involved in their metabolic action (e.g. the cyclic AMP-dependent kinase), the glucocorticoids induce the formation of lipocortin-1, a member of the family of calcium-regulated phospholipid-binding proteins termed 'annexins'. Lipocortin-1 is important in the negative feedback action of glucocorticoids on the hypothalamus and anterior pituitary and has anti-inflammatory actions (possibly by inhibiting phospholipase A_2).

Much is now known about the anti-inflammatory and immunosuppressive actions of the glucocorticoids, but their *metabolic actions* are less well understood. Several relevant enzymes can be shown, in vitro, to be induced by glucocorticoids (e.g. the cAMP-dependent kinase), but these do not as yet explain all of the metabolic actions seen in vivo.

Mechanism of action of the glucocorticoids

Glucocorticoids interact with intracellular receptors; the resulting steroid–receptor complexes dimerise (form pairs) then interact with DNA to modify gene transcription—inducing synthesis of some proteins and inhibiting synthesis of others.

- For metabolic actions, most mediator proteins are enzymes, e.g. cAMP-dependent kinase, but not all actions on genes are known.
- For anti-inflammatory and immunosuppressive actions, some actions at the level of the genes are known:
  — inhibition of transcription of the genes for COX-2, cytokines (e.g. the interleukins), cell adhesion molecules and the inducible form of nitric oxide synthase
  — block of vitamin D_3-mediated induction of the osteocalcin gene in osteoblasts and modification of transcription of the collagenase genes
  — increased synthesis of lipocortin 1, which is important in negative feedback on hypothalamus and anterior pituitary and may have anti-inflammatory actions.

Unwanted effects

Unwanted effects are likely to occur with large doses or prolonged administration but should not occur with replacement therapy. These effects are inherent in the three categories of pharmacological actions associated with the drugs:

- *Suppression of the response to infection or injury.* An intercurrent infection can be potentially very serious unless recognised and treated with antimicrobial agents along with an increase in the dose of steroid.* Wound healing may be impaired, but peptic ulceration is probably not the problem it has been considered to be in the past, the incidence being only slightly higher in patients treated with steroids than in controls. However, patients on concurrent high doses of **aspirin** (e.g. in rheumatoid arthritis) are more at hazard from peptic ulceration.
- *Suppression of the patients' capacity to synthesise corticosteroids.* Sudden withdrawal of the drugs after prolonged therapy may result in acute adrenal insufficiency.** Careful procedures for phased withdrawal should be followed. Recovery of full adrenal function usually takes about 2 months, though it can take 18 months or more.
- *Metabolic effects.* When the drugs are used in anti-inflammatory and immunosuppressive therapy, the metabolic actions and the effects on water and electrolyte balance and organ systems are unwanted side-effects, and iatrogenic Cushing's syndrome may occur (see Fig. 24.8).

Osteoporosis, with the attendant hazard of fractures, is probably one of the main limitations to long-term glucocorticoid therapy. Glucocorticoids influence bone by regulation of calcium and phosphate metabolism and through effects on collagen synthesis by osteoblasts and collagen degradation by collagenase. Glucocorticoids modify transcription of the collagenase genes and inhibit vitamin D_3-mediated induction of genes in osteoblasts (see above). Given long-term, glucocorticoids reduce the function of osteoblasts (which lay down bone matrix) and increase the activity of osteoclasts (which digest bone matrix). The effect on osteoclasts is indirect—through decreasing the intestinal absorption of calcium, resulting in increased parathormone secretion, which in turn stimulates these cells. Therapy with biphosphonates can limit glucocorticoid-induced osteoporosis.

The tendency to hyperglycaemia which occurs with exogenous glucocorticoids may develop into actual diabetes.

---

*This is because the exogenous glucocorticoids will have suppressed the necessary general hypothalamo–pituitary–adrenal response to the stress of illness or trauma.

It is advisable that a patient on long-continued glucocorticoid therapy should carry a card stating: 'I am a patient on STEROID TREATMENT which **must not be stopped abruptly and in the case of intercurrent illness may need to be increased'. This is because the exogenous glucocorticoids will have suppressed the necessary general hypothalamo–pituitary–adrenal response to the stress of illness or trauma.

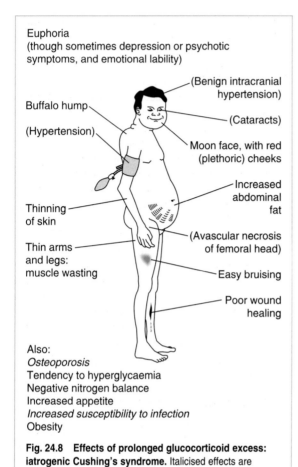

Euphoria
(though sometimes depression or psychotic symptoms, and emotional lability)

(Benign intracranial hypertension)

Buffalo hump

(Cataracts)

(Hypertension)

Moon face, with red (plethoric) cheeks

Increased abdominal fat

Thinning of skin

(Avascular necrosis of femoral head)

Thin arms and legs: muscle wasting

Easy bruising

Poor wound healing

Also:
Osteoporosis
Tendency to hyperglycaemia
Negative nitrogen balance
Increased appetite
Increased susceptibility to infection
Obesity

Fig. 24.8   Effects of prolonged glucocorticoid excess: iatrogenic Cushing's syndrome. Italicised effects are particularly common. Less frequent effects, related to dose and duration of therapy, are shown in brackets. (Adapted from: Baxter & Rousseau 1979)

Another limitation is the development of muscle wasting and weakness.

In children, the metabolic effects (particularly those on protein metabolism) may result in inhibition of growth, even with fairly low doses, though this is not likely to occur unless treatment is continued for more than 6 months. A depressant effect on DNA synthesis and cell division in some tissues may also be implicated in this effect.

There is often euphoria, but some patients may become depressed or develop psychotic symptoms.

An effect on the blood supply to bone can result in avascular necrosis of the head of the femur.

The incidence of cataracts is higher after prolonged administration of the glucocorticoids in patients with rheumatoid arthritis, and cataracts have occurred in children as well.

Other toxic effects that have been reported are glaucoma, raised intracranial pressure, hypercoagulability of the blood, fever and disorders of menstruation. Oral thrush (a fungal infection; see Ch. 45) frequently occurs when glucocorticoids are taken by inhalation.

Pharmacokinetic aspects

Glucocorticoids may be given by a variety of routes. Most are active when given orally. All can be given systemically, either intramuscularly or intravenously. They may also be given topically—injected intra-articularly, given by aerosol into the respiratory tract, administered as drops into the eye or the nose, or applied in creams or ointments to the skin. There is much less likelihood of systemic toxic effects after topical administration unless large quantities are used. When prolonged use of systemic glucocorticoids is necessary, alternate-day therapy may decrease the unwanted effects.

The endogenous glucocorticoids are carried in the plasma, bound to corticosteroid-binding globulin (CBG) and to albumin. CBG has high affinity for naturally occurring glucocorticoids. It is present in plasma in very low concentration and accounts for about 77% of hydro-cortisone bound. CBG does not bind synthetic steroids. Albumin has a lower affinity for hydrocortisone; it binds both natural and synthetic steroids. Both CBG-bound and albumin-bound steroids are biologically inactive.

Steroids, being small lipophilic molecules, enter their target cells by simple diffusion.

Hydrocortisone has a plasma half-life of 90 minutes, though its main biological effects occur only after 2–8 hours. The main step in inactivation is the reduction of the double bond between C_4 and C_5. This occurs in liver cells and elsewhere. The ketone at C_3 is reduced in the liver, and most compounds are then linked enzymically to sulphate or glucuronic acid at the C_3 hydroxyl, and finally excreted in the urine. Hydrocortisone may under-go an oxidation at C_{17} to give a 17-ketosteroid along with a two-carbon fragment. Virtually all of the metabolites are excreted within 72 hours. Metabolism is slowed if there is a double bond between carbon atoms 1 and 2 (methylprednisolone and prednisolone) and if there is a fluorine atom at C_9 (dexamethasone, betamethasone). Cortisone and prednisone are inactive until converted in vivo to hydrocortisone and prednisolone respectively.

The clinical use of the glucocorticoids is given on page 425.

Dexamethasone can be used to test hypothalamic–pituitary–adrenocortical function in the 'dexamethasone suppression test'. A low dose, usually given at night, should suppress the hypothalamus and pituitary, and result in reduced corticotrophin secretion and hydro-cortisone output, the hydrocortisone being measured in the plasma about 9 hours later. Failure of suppression

implies hypersecretion of corticotrophin or of gluco-corticoids (Cushing's syndrome).

Pharmacokinetics and unwanted actions of the glucocorticoids

- Administration: oral, topical and parenteral; the drugs are bound to corticosteroid-binding globulin in the blood and enter cells by diffusion; metabolised in the liver.
- Unwanted effects are seen mainly with prolonged systemic use as anti-inflammatory or immunosuppressive agents (in which case all the metabolic actions are unwanted), but not usually with replacement therapy. The most important are:
  — suppression of response to infection
  — suppression of endogenous glucocorticoid synthesis
  — metabolic actions (see above)
  — osteoporosis
  — iatrogenic Cushing's syndrome (see Fig. 24.8).

Clinical use of glucocorticoids

- Replacement therapy for patients with adrenal failure (e.g. Addison's disease). All the actions of the corticosteroids are required, and a mineralocorticoid will need to be given along with a glucocorticoid.
- Anti-inflammatory/immunosuppressive therapy (see also Ch. 13):
  — in asthma (by inhalation or, in severe cases, systemically; see Ch. 19)
  — topically in various inflammatory conditions of skin, eye, ear or nose (e.g. eczema, allergic conjunctivitis or rhinitis)
  — in hypersensitivity states (e.g. severe allergic reactions to drugs or insect venom)
  — in miscellaneous diseases with autoimmune and inflammatory components (e.g. rheumatoid arthritis and other 'connective tissue' diseases, inflammatory bowel diseases, some forms of haemolytic anaemia, idiopathic thrombocytopenic purpura)
  — to prevent graft-versus-host disease following organ or bone marrow transplantation.
- In neoplastic disease (see also Ch. 42):
  — in combination with cytotoxic drugs in treatment of specific malignancies (e.g. Hodgkin's disease, acute lymphocytic leukaemia)
  — to reduce cerebral oedema in patients with metastatic or primary brain tumours (dexamethasone is the drug used)
  — as a component of anti-emetic treatment in conjunction with chemotherapy (see Ch. 21).

When they are used as anti-inflammatory and immunosuppressive agents, all of their metabolic actions are unwanted side-effects.

MINERALOCORTICOIDS

The main endogenous mineralocorticoid is **aldosterone**, which is produced in the outermost of the three zones of the adrenal medulla, the *zona glomerulosa*. Its main action is to increase sodium reabsorption by an action on the distal tubules in the kidney, with concomitant increased excretion of potassium and hydrogen ions (see Ch. 20). An excessive secretion of mineralocorticoids, as in Conn's syndrome, causes marked sodium and water retention with resultant increase in the volume of extra-cellular fluid, hypokalaemia, alkalosis and hypertension. A decreased secretion, as in Addison's disease, causes increased sodium loss which is relatively more pro-nounced than water loss. The osmotic pressure of the extracellular fluid is thus reduced, resulting in a shift of fluid into the intracellular compartment and a marked decrease in extracellular fluid volume. There is a con-comitant decrease in the excretion of potassium ions resulting in hyperkalaemia, and also a moderate decrease in plasma bicarbonate.

Regulation of aldosterone synthesis and release

The control of the synthesis and release of aldosterone is complex. Control depends mainly on the electrolyte composition of the plasma and on the angiotensin II system (Fig. 24.5 and Chs 15 and 20). Low plasma sodium or high plasma potassium concentrations affect the *zona glomerulosa* cells of the adrenal directly, stimulating aldosterone release. A depletion in body sodium also activates the *renin–angiotensin system* (see Fig. 15.4). One of the effects of angiotensin II is to increase the synthesis and release of aldosterone.

Mechanism of action

Aldosterone, like other steroids, binds to specific intra-cellular receptors. Unlike the glucocorticoid-binding receptors which occur in most tissues, aldosterone receptors occur in only a few target tissues such as the kidney, and in the transporting epithelia of the colon and bladder. Cells containing mineralocorticoid receptors also contain 11-β–hydroxysteroid dehydrogenase.* This enzyme converts glucocorticoids, but not mineralocorticoids, to

---

*This enzyme is inhibited by carbenoxolone (used to treat ulcers; see Ch. 21) and liquorice; marked inhibition causes a syndrome of mineralocorticoid excess similar to Conn's syndrome (primary hyperaldosteronism).

metabolites that have only low affinity for the mineralo-corticoid receptors, thus ensuring that the cells are affected only by bona fide mineralocorticoids.

As with the glucocorticoids, the interaction of ligand with receptor initiates DNA transcription of specific proteins resulting in:

- an early increase in the number of sodium channels in the apical membrane of the cell, mainly by the activation of previously quiescent channels; the protein mediator that activates these channels has not been identified
- a later phase of increase in the number of Na^+/K^+-ATPase molecules in the basolateral membrane (see Ch. 20, Fig. 20.13).

The increased K^+ excretion into the tubule produced by aldosterone results from the influx of K^+ into the cell through the action of the basal Na^+/K^+-ATPase, coupled with an increased efflux of K^+ through apical K^+ channels.

In addition to the effects mediated through DNA, there is evidence for a rapid non-genomic effect of aldosterone on Na^+ influx, through an action on the Na^+/H^+ exchanger in the apical membrane.

Spironolactone is a competitive antagonist of aldosterone, and it also prevents the mineralocorticoid effects of other adrenal steroids on the renal tubule (Ch. 20).

Clinical use of mineralocorticoids

The main clinical use of mineralocorticoids is in replacement therapy (Table 24.2). The most commonly used drug is **fludrocortisone** (Table 24.2 and Fig. 24.5) which can be taken orally.

Mineralocorticoids

- Fludrocortisone is given orally to produce a mineralocorticoid effect. This agent:
  - increases Na^+ reabsorption in distal tubules and increases K^+ and H^+ efflux into the tubules
  - acts, like most steroids, on intracellular receptors that modulate DNA transcription causing synthesis of protein mediators
  - is used with a glucocorticoid in replacement therapy.

REFERENCES AND FURTHER READING

The hypothalamus and pituitary

Clark R G, Robinson I C A F 1996 Up and down the growth hormone cascade. Cytokine and Growth Factor Rev 1: 65–80 (*A review covering the cascade that controls the primary regulators of growth and metabolism, namely growth hormone and the insulin-like growth factors*)

Jørgensen J O L, Christiansen J S 1993 Growth hormone therapy. Lancet 341: 1247–1248

Lamberts S W J, van der Lely A-J, et al. 1996 Octreotide N Engl J Med 334: 246–254 (*A review covering somatostatin receptors, somatostatin analogues, treatment of tumours expressing somatostatin receptors with octreotide*)

Lamberts, S W J, Bruining H A, De Jong F S 1997 Corticosteroid therapy in severe illness. N Engl J Med 337: 1285–1292 (*Review with succinct coverage of normal response of adrenal to illness, followed by more detail on clinical therapy*)

László F A, László F, De Wied D 1991 Pharmacology and clinical perspectives of vasopressin antagonists. Pharmacol Rev 43: 73–104 (*Detailed review covering structure/activity relationships, the physiological and pathological roles of V_1 and V_2 antagonists and their clinical significance*)

Lightman S L 1993 Molecular insights into diabetes insipidus. N Engl J Med 328: 1562–1563

Manger J A 1990 Thyroid-stimulating hormone: biosynthesis, cell biology, and bioactivity. Endocr Rev 11: 354–385 (*Detailed review of synthesis of thyroid-stimulating hormone and its actions*)

Orlander P R, Nader S 1996 Youthful hormones. Lancet 348: (suppl II): 6 (*End of year review of key 1996 references on growth hormone and insulin-like growth factors*)

Owens M J, Nemeroff C B 1991 Physiology and pharmacology of corticotropin-releasing factor. Pharmacol Rev 43: 425–464 (*Detailed review of corticotrophin-releasing factor (CRF)-containing neurons and receptors and CRF regulation of neuroendocrine function*)

Page R B 1982 Pituitary blood flow. Am J Physiol 243: E427–442

Vance M L 1994 Hypopituitarism. N Engl J Med 330: 1651–1662 (*Review of causes, clinical features and hormone-replacement therapy of hypopituitarism*)

Wass J A H 1993 Acromegaly: treatment after 100 years. Br Med J 307: 1505–1506 (*Short editorial on surgical and pharmacological treatment of acromegaly*)

ACTH and the adrenal corticosteroids

Barnes P J, Adcock I 1993 Anti-inflammatory actions of steroids: molecular mechanisms. Trends Pharmacol Sci 14: 436–441 (*Clear review covering the binding of glucocorticoid receptor to heat shock protein 90, and AP-1-mediated transcription of genes for inflammatory mediators; useful diagrams*)

Bastl C, Hayslett J P 1992 The cellular action of aldosterone in target epithelia. Kidney Int 42: 250–264 (*A detailed review covering the aldosterone receptor and regulation of gene expression, aldosterone action on electrogenic and electroneutral sodium transport, and on potassium and proton secretion*)

Baxter J D, Rousseau G G (eds) 1979 Glucocorticoid hormone action. Monographs on endocrinology. Springer-Verlag, Berlin, vol 12 (*Early review of glucocorticoid action with memorable diagram of Cushing's syndrome*)

Buckingham J C, Flower R J 1997 Lipocortin 1: a second messenger of glucocorticoid action in the hypothalamic–pituitary–adrenocortical axis. Mol Med Today 3:

296–302 (*Outline of HPA axis function, glucocorticoid action and the possible role of lipocortin 1 in both*)

Chrousos G 1995 The hypothalamic–pituitary–adrenal axis and immune-mediated inflammation. N Engl J Med 332: 1351–1362 (*Review covering the interaction between the CNS/autonomic transmitters, inflammatory mediators and the HPA axis in stress*)

Funder J W 1997 Glucocorticoid and mineralocorticoid receptors: biology and clinical relevance. Annu Rev Med 48: 231–240 (*Succinct review of glucocorticoid (GR) and mineralocorticoid (MR) receptors, differences in GR- and MR-mediated transcription and responses, and steroid resistance*)

Krane S M 1993 Some molecular mechanisms of glucocorticoid action. Br J Rheumatol 32: 3–5 (*Briefly covers inhibition by glucocorticoids of AP-1 induction of collagenase and interleukin-1*)

Landers J P, Spelsberg T C 1992 New concepts in steroid hormone action: transcription factors, proto-oncogenes, and the cascade model of gene expression. Crit Rev Eukaryotic Gene Expression 2: 19–63 (*Excellent, detailed review on topics in the title, with useful diagrams*)

Marx J 1995 How the glucocorticoids suppress immunity. Science 270: 232–233 (*Clear, succinct coverage of recent information on glucocorticoid inhibition of gene transcription*)

Munck A, Guyre P M, Holbrook N J 1984 Physiological functions of glucocorticoids in stress and their relation to pharmacological actions. Endocr Rev 5: 25–44 (*Review suggesting that the anti-inflammatory/immunosuppressive actions of the glucocorticoids have a physiological function*)

Ramirerz V D 1996 How do steroids act? Lancet 347: 630–631 (*Short discussion of the non-genomic actions of steroids, with particular reference to aldosterone*)

Rhodes D, Klug A 1993 Zinc fingers. Scientific American (Feb): 32–39 (*Clear discussion of the role of zinc fingers in regulating gene transcription; excellent diagrams, of course*)

Tsai M-J, O'Malley B W 1994 Molecular mechanisms of action of steroid/thyroid receptor superfamily members. Annu Rev Biochem 63: 451–486 (*Detailed review of molecular biology of these receptors, including gene activation and gene silencing*)

Wilckens T 1995 Glucocorticoids and immune dysfunction: physiological relevance and pathogenic potential of hormonal dysfunction. Trends Pharmacol Sci 16: 193–197 (*Covers glucocorticoid (Gc) interaction with Gc receptors, heat shock protein 90, and AP-1 and NF-κB transcription factors; clear diagram*)

25

The thyroid

The thyroid is essential for many physiological processes. It secretes three main hormones: **thyroxine (T_4)**, **triiodothyronine (T_3)** and **calcitonin**. T_4 was isolated from thyroid tissue in crystalline form by Kendall in 1914 and subsequently synthesised by Harington & Barger in 1927. The presence in the thyroid of T_3, which is three- to fivefold more active than thyroxine, was shown by Gross & Pitt-Rivers in 1952.

T_4 and T_3 are critically important for normal growth and development and for energy metabolism. Calcitonin is involved in the control of plasma calcium and is dealt with in Chapter 27. The term 'thyroid hormone' will be used here to refer to T_4 and T_3.

SYNTHESIS, STORAGE AND SECRETION OF THYROID HORMONE

The functional unit of the thyroid is the follicle or acinus. Each follicle consists of a single layer of epithelial cells around a cavity, the follicle lumen, which is filled with a thick colloid containing *thyroglobulin*. Thyroglobulin is a large glycoprotein, each molecule of which contains about 115 tyrosine residues. It is synthesised, glycosylated and then secreted into the lumen of the follicle where iodination of the tyrosine residues occurs. Surrounding the follicles is a rich capillary network, and the rate of blood flow through the gland is very high in comparison with other tissues. The main steps in the synthesis, storage and secretion of thyroid hormone (Fig. 25.1), are as follows:

- uptake of plasma iodide by the follicle cells
- oxidation of iodide and iodination of tyrosine residues in the thyroglobulin of the colloid
- secretion of thyroid hormone.

The uptake of plasma iodide by the follicle cells
This is an energy-dependent transport process occurring against a gradient, which is normally about 25 : 1.

The oxidation of iodide and iodination of tyrosine residues
This is brought about by an enzyme, thyroperoxidase, at the inner, apical surface of the cell at the interface with the colloid. It is very rapid—labelled iodide (^{125}I) can be found in the lumen within 40 seconds of intravenous injection—and requires H_2O_2 as an oxidising agent. Iodination (referred to as 'organification' of iodine) occurs *after* the tyrosine has been incorporated into thyroglobulin. The process believed to occur is shown in Figure 25.2.

Tyrosine is iodinated first at position 3 on the ring and then, in some molecules, on position 5 as well, forming *monoiodotyrosine* (MIT) in the first case, and *diiodotyrosine* (DIT) in the second. Two of these molecules are then coupled—either MIT with a DIT to form T_3 or two DIT molecules to form T_4 (Fig. 25.3). The mechanism for coupling is believed to involve a peroxidase system similar to that involved in iodination. About one-fifth of the tyrosine residues in thyroglobulin are iodinated.

The iodinated thyroglobulin of the thyroid forms a large store of thyroid hormone and, as is explained below, there is a relatively slow turnover of hormone in the tissues. This is in contrast to other endocrine secretions, such as growth hormone secreted by the anterior pituitary or the hormones of the adrenal cortex, which are synthesised on demand.

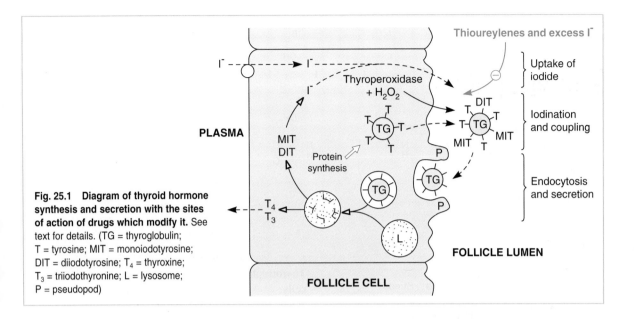

Fig. 25.1 Diagram of thyroid hormone synthesis and secretion with the sites of action of drugs which modify it. See text for details. (TG = thyroglobulin; T = tyrosine; MIT = monoiodotyrosine; DIT = diiodotyrosine; T_4 = thyroxine; T_3 = triiodothyronine; L = lysosome; P = pseudopod)

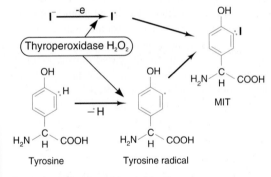

Fig. 25.2 Iodination of tyrosyl by the thyroperoxidase–H_2O_2 complex. This probably involves two sites on the enzyme, one of which removes an electron from iodide to give the free radical, I˙, and another removes a monohydrogen (monoelectron) from tyrosine to give the tyrosine radical (shown by the blue dot). Formation of monoiodotyrosine (MIT) results from addition of the two radicals.

Secretion of thyroid hormone

The thyroglobulin molecule is taken up into the follicle cell by endocytosis of some of the colloid in the lumen (see Fig. 25.1). The endocytotic vesicles then fuse with lysosomes, proteolytic enzymes act on thyroglobulin, and T_4 and T_3 are released and secreted into the plasma. The MIT and DIT which are released at the same time are normally metabolised within the cell, the iodide being removed enzymically and re-used.

REGULATION OF THYROID FUNCTION

Thyrotrophin-releasing hormone (TRH) from the hypothalamus releases thyrotrophin (thyroid-stimulating hormone, TSH) from the anterior pituitary (see Fig. 25.4 and Fig. 24.2), as does **protirelin**, a synthetic tripeptide (pyroglutamyl-histidyl-proline amide). The actions and uses of protirelin are considered on page 411. Somatostatin (see p. 411) reduces basal thyrotrophin release.

The production of thyrotrophin is also influenced by a negative feedback effect of thyroid hormones, T_3 being more active than T_4.

The control of the secretion of thyrotrophin thus depends on a balance between the actions of T_4 and TRH, and probably also somatostatin, on the pituitary, but even high concentrations of thyroid hormone do not *completely* inhibit thyrotrophin secretion.

Thyrotrophin acts on receptors on the membrane of thyroid follicle cells and its main second messenger is cAMP. It controls all aspects of thyroid hormone synthesis:

- the uptake of iodide by follicle cells, by an action on the synthesis of the transport proteins; *this is the main mechanism by which it regulates thyroid function*
- the synthesis and secretion of thyroglobulin
- the generation of hydrogen peroxide and the iodination of tyrosine

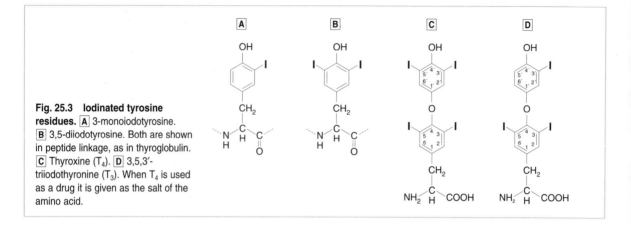

Fig. 25.3   Iodinated tyrosine residues. A 3-monoiodotyrosine. B 3,5-diiodotyrosine. Both are shown in peptide linkage, as in thyroglobulin. C Thyroxine (T_4). D 3,5,3'-triiodothyronine (T_3). When T_4 is used as a drug it is given as the salt of the amino acid.

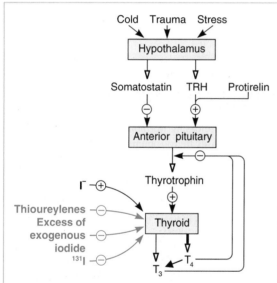

Fig. 25.4   Regulation of thyroid hormone secretion. Agents used clinically are shown in blue. For the endogenous substances (shown in black) the thickness of the lines indicates the relative importance of each factor. Iodide (I^-) is essential for thyroid hormone synthesis, but excess of exogenous iodide ($30 \times$ the daily requirement of iodine) inhibits the increased thyroid hormone production which occurs in thyrotoxicosis. (TRH = thyrotrophin-releasing hormone)

- endocytosis and proteolysis of thyroglobulin
- secretion of T_3 and T_4
- the blood flow through the gland
- the transcription of the thyroperoxidase and thyroglobulin genes.

Thyrotrophin also has a trophic action on the thyroid cells.

The other main factor influencing thyroid function is the plasma iodide concentration. About 100 nmol of T_4 is synthesised daily, necessitating the gland taking up approximately 500 nmol of iodide each day (equivalent to about 70 mg of iodine). A reduced iodine intake with reduced plasma iodide concentration will result in a decrease of hormone production and an increase in thyrotrophin secretion. An increased plasma iodide has the opposite effect, though this may be modified by other factors (see below). The overall feedback mechanism responds to changes of iodide only slowly—over fairly long periods, days or weeks, since there is a large reserve capacity for the binding and uptake of iodide in the thyroid. The size and vascularity of the thyroid are reduced by an increase in plasma iodide. A prolonged decrease of iodine in the diet results in a continuous excessive secretion of thyrotrophin and eventually in an increase in vascularity, and hypertrophy of the gland.

ACTIONS OF THE THYROID HORMONES

The physiological actions of the thyroid hormones fall into two categories:

- those affecting metabolism
- those affecting growth and development.

Effects on metabolism

The hormones are regulators of metabolism in most tissues, T_3 being three to five times more active than T_4 (Fig. 25.5). They produce a general increase in the metabolism of carbohydrates, fats and proteins. Most of

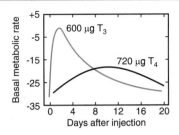

Fig. 25.5   Schematic diagram of the effect of single equimolar doses of T$_3$ and T$_4$ on basal metabolic rate in a hypothyroid subject. Note that this figure is meant only to illustrate differences in potency; thyroxine is not given clinically in a single bolus dose but in regular daily doses so that the effect builds up to a plateau. (From: Blackburn C M et al. 1954 J Clin Invest 33: 819)

these effects involve modulation of the actions of other hormones such as insulin, glucagon, the glucocorticoids and the catecholamines, although the thyroid hormones also control, directly, the activity of some of the enzymes of carbohydrate metabolism. There is an increase in O$_2$ consumption and heat production which is manifested as an increase in basal metabolic rate. This reflects action on some tissues, such as heart, kidney, liver and muscle, but not others, such as the gonads, brain and spleen. The calorigenic action is important as part of the response to a cold environment. Administration of thyroid hormone results in augmented cardiac rate and output and increased tendency to dysrhythmias such as atrial fibrillation.

Effects on growth and development

The thyroid hormones have a critical effect on growth, partly by a direct action on cells and partly indirectly by influencing growth hormone production and potentiating its effects. The hormones are important for a normal response to parathormone and calcitonin, and for skeletal development; they are particularly necessary for normal growth and maturation of the CNS.

Mechanism of action

The hormones act by a mechanism rather similar to that of the steroids (Ch. 24 p. 421 and Fig. 24.7). After they enter the cell, T$_4$ is converted to T$_3$ which binds with high affinity to specific receptors associated with DNA in the nucleus. (T$_4$ can be regarded mainly as a *prohormone*.) Without bound ligand, the receptors *repress* basal transcription ('gene silencing'); when T$_3$ is bound the receptors change conformation and *activate* transcription, resulting in generation of mRNA and protein synthesis.

TRANSPORT AND METABOLISM

The normal plasma concentrations of the hormones, which can be measured by radioimmunoassay, are 10^{-7} M for T$_4$ and 2×10^{-9} M for T$_3$. Both hormones are bound mainly to thyroxine-binding globulin (TBG).

The thyroid hormones are eventually degraded by deiodination, deamination and conjugation with glucuronic and sulphuric acids. This occurs mainly in the liver, and the free and conjugated forms are excreted partly in the bile and partly in the urine. The metabolic clearance of T$_3$ is 20 times faster than that of T$_4$ (which is about 6 days).

In summary:

- There is a large pool of T$_4$ in the body; it has a low turnover rate and is found mainly in the circulation.
- There is a small pool of T$_3$ in the body; it has a fast turnover rate and is found mainly intracellularly.

ABNORMALITIES OF THYROID FUNCTION

Hyperthyroidism (thyrotoxicosis)

In thyrotoxicosis there is excessive activity of the thyroid hormones resulting in a high metabolic rate, an increase in temperature and sweating and a marked sensitivity to heat. Nervousness, tremor, tachycardia, fatiguability and increased appetite associated with loss of weight occur. There are several types of hyperthyroidism but only two are common: *diffuse toxic goitre* (also called Graves' disease or exophthalmic goitre) and *toxic nodular goitre*.

Diffuse toxic goitre is an organ-specific autoimmune disease caused by thyroid-stimulating immunoglobulins directed at the thyrotrophin receptor. Constitutively active mutations of the thyrotrophin-releasing hormone receptor (see Ch. 2) may be involved. (As is indicated by the name, patients with exophthalmic goitre have protrusion of the eyeballs; the pathogenesis of this condition is not fully understood.) There is also increased sensitivity to catecholamines.

Toxic nodular goitre is due to a benign neoplasm or adenoma and may develop in patients with long-standing simple goitre (see below). This condition does not usually have concomitant exophthalmos.

The antidysrhythmic drug, **amiodarone** (Ch. 14), is rich in iodine and has a propensity to cause either hyperthyroidism or hypothyroidism.

Hypothyroidism

A decreased activity of the thyroid results in hypothyroidism, and in severe cases *myxoedema*. It is immunological in origin and the manifestations are low metabolic rate, slow speech, deep hoarse voice, lethargy, bradycardia, sensitivity to cold and mental impairment. Patients also develop a characteristic thickening of the skin which gives myxoedema its name. *Hashimoto's thyroiditis*, a chronic autoimmune disease in which there is an immune reaction against thyroglobulin or some other component of thyroid tissue, can lead to hypothyroidism and myxoedema. Therapy of thyroid tumours with **radioiodine** (see below) is another cause of hypothyroidism.

Thyroid deficiency during development, caused by congenital absence or incomplete development of the thyroid, causes *cretinism* which is characterised by gross retardation of growth and mental deficiency.

Simple, non-toxic goitre

A dietary deficiency of iodine, if prolonged, causes a rise in plasma thyrotrophic hormone and eventually an increase in the size of the gland. This condition is known as *simple* or *non-toxic goitre*. Another cause is ingestion of goitrogens (e.g. from cassava root). The enlarged thyroid usually manages to produce normal amounts of thyroid hormone, though if the iodine deficiency is very severe, hypothyroidism may supervene.

DRUGS USED IN DISEASES OF THE THYROID

Drugs are used to treat both hyperthyroidism and hypothyroidism.

DRUGS USED IN HYPERTHYROIDISM

Hyperthyroidism may be treated pharmacologically or surgically. In general, surgery is only used when there are mechanical problems due to compression of the trachea.

Although the condition of hyperthyroidism can be controlled with antithyroid drugs, the disease is not 'cured' since the drugs do not alter the underlying autoimmune mechanisms. Furthermore, there is little evidence that these drugs affect the course of the exophthalmos associated with Graves' disease.

Radioiodine

Radioiodine is a first-line treatment for hyperthyroidism (particularly in the USA). The isotope used is ^{131}I. Given orally, it is taken up and processed by the thyroid in the same way as the stable form of iodide, eventually becoming incorporated into thyroglobulin. It emits both β-particles and γ-rays. The γ-rays pass through the tissue, but the β-radiation has a very short range and exerts a cytotoxic action virtually restricted to the cells of the thyroid follicles—resulting in significant destruction. ^{131}I has a half-life of 8 days; by 2 months its radioactivity has effectively disappeared. It is used in one single dose, but its cytotoxic effect on the gland is delayed for 1–2 months and does not reach its maximum for a further 2 months.

Hypothyroidism will eventually occur after treatment with radioiodine, particularly in patients with Graves' disease, but is easily managed by replacement therapy with thyroxine. Radioiodine is best avoided in children and also in pregnant patients because of potential damage to the foetus

The uptake of ^{131}I and other isotopes of iodine may be used as a test of thyroid function. A tracer dose of the isotope is given orally or intravenously and the amount accumulated by the thyroid is measured by a gamma scintillation counter placed over the gland.

Thioureylenes

The thioureylenes used are **carbimazole**, **methimazole** and **propylthiouracil**. They are related to thiourea,

---

> **Thyroid**
>
> - Thyroid hormones are synthesised by iodination of tyrosine residues on thyroglobulin within the lumen of the thyroid follicle.
> - The thyroglobulin is endocytosed and thyroxine (T_4) and triiodothyronine (T_3) are secreted.
> - Synthesis and secretion of T_3 and T_4 are regulated by thyrotrophin, and influenced by plasma iodide.
> - T_3 and T_4 actions are:
>   — to stimulate metabolism generally, causing increased O_2 consumption and increased metabolic rate
>   — to influence growth and development.
> - Within cells, the T_4 is converted to T_3 which interacts with a nuclear receptor; the receptor represses basal transcription when not bound to T_3, and activates transcription when bound.
> - There is a large pool of T_4 in the body; it has a low turnover rate and is found mainly in the circulation.
> - There is a small pool of T_3 in the body; it has a fast turnover rate and is found mainly intracellularly.
> - Abnormalities of thyroid function include:
>   — hyperthyroidism (thyrotoxicosis), either diffuse toxic goitre or toxic nodular goitre
>   — hypothyroidism; in adults this causes myxoedema, in infants, cretinism
>   — simple non-toxic goitre, due to dietary iodine deficiency, usually with normal thyroid function.

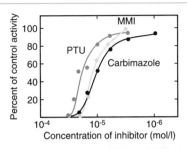

Fig. 25.6 Dose–response curves for inhibition of thyroperoxidase-catalysed iodination of thyroglobulin. The IC^{50} for carbimazole: 10.5 µmol/l; for methimazole (MMI): 11.5 µmol/l; and for propylthiouracil (PTU): 18.5 µmol/l. (Modified from: Taurog A 1976 Endocrinology 98: 1031)

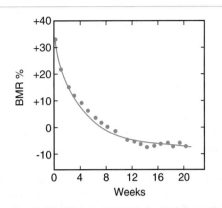

Fig. 25.7 Average time-course of fall of basal metabolic rate (BMR) during treatment with an antithyroid drug, carbimazole. The curve is exponential, corresponding to a daily decrease in BMR of 3.4%. (From: Furth E O et al. 1963 J Clin Endocrinol Metab 23: 1130)

the thiocarbamide group (S–C–N) being essential for antithyroid activity.

Action

Thioureylenes decrease the output of thyroid hormones from the gland and cause a gradual reduction in the signs and symptoms of thyrotoxicosis, the basal metabolic rate and pulse rate returning to normal over a period of 3–4 weeks. Their mode of action is not completely understood, but there is evidence that they inhibit the iodination of tyrosyl residues in thyroglobulin (see Figs 25.1, 25.2 and 25.6). It is thought that they inhibit the thyroperoxidase-catalysed oxidation reactions by acting as substrates for the postulated peroxidase–iodinium complex, thus competitively inhibiting the interaction with tyrosine. Propylthiouracil has the additional effect of reducing the de-iodination of T$_4$ to T$_3$ in peripheral tissues.

Pharmacokinetic aspects

Thioureylenes are given orally. Carbimazole is rapidly converted to methimazole which is the active compound. Methimazole is distributed throughout the body water and has a plasma half-life of 6–15 hours. An average dose of carbimazole produces more than 90% inhibition of thyroid organification of iodine within 12 hours. The clinical response to this and other antithyroid drugs, however, may take several weeks (Fig. 25.7). This is not only because thyroxine has a long half-life but also because the thyroid may have large stores of hormone which need to be depleted before the drug's action can be manifest. Propylthiouracil may act somewhat more rapidly because of its effect in inhibiting peripheral conversion of T$_4$ to T$_3$.

Both methimazole and propylthiouracil cross the placenta and also appear in the milk, but this effect is less pronounced with propylthiouracil because it is more strongly bound to plasma protein. After degradation, the metabolites are excreted in the urine, propylthiouracil being excreted more rapidly than methimazole. The thioureylenes are not concentrated in the thyroid.

Unwanted effects

The most important unwanted effect is granulocytopenia (see Ch. 49), which, fortunately, is relatively rare, having an incidence of 0.1–1.2% and being reversible if the drug is stopped. Rashes are more common (2–25%), and other symptoms such as headaches, nausea, jaundice and pain in the joints can occur.

Iodine/iodide

Iodine is converted in vivo to iodide (I$^-$) which temporarily inhibits the release of thyroid hormones. When high doses of iodine are given to thyrotoxic patients, the symptoms subside within 1–2 days. There is inhibition of the secretion of thyroid hormones and, over a period of 10–14 days, a marked reduction in vascularity of the gland, which becomes smaller and firmer. Iodine solution in potassium iodide ('Lugol's iodine') is given orally. With continuous administration its effect reaches maximum within 10–15 days and then decreases.

The mechanism of action is not entirely clear; it may inhibit iodination of thyroglobulin, possibly by inhibiting the H$_2$O$_2$ generation which is necessary for this process.

The main uses are for the preparation of hyperthyroid subjects for surgery and as part of the treatment of severe thyrotoxic crisis (thyroid storm).

Allergic reactions can occur—these include angio-oedema, rashes, drug fever, lacrimation, conjunctivitis, pain in the salivary glands and a cold-like syndrome.

Other drugs used

β-adrenoceptor antagonists, for example propranolol (Ch. 8), are not in fact antithyroid agents, but they are useful for decreasing many of the signs and symptoms of hyperthyroidism—the tachycardia, dysrhythmias, tremor and agitation. They are used in preparation for surgery, for the initial treatment of most hyperthyroid patients while the thioureylenes or radioiodine are taking effect, and as part of the treatment of thyroid storm.

Guanethidine, a noradrenergic blocking agent (Ch. 7), is used in eye drops to ameliorate the exophthalmos of hyperthyroidism (which is not relieved by antithyroid drugs); it acts by relaxing the sympathetically innervated smooth muscle that causes eyelid retraction.

Glucocorticoids (e.g. prednisolone) or surgical decompression may be needed for the exophthalmia of Graves' disease.

DRUGS USED IN HYPOTHYROIDISM

There are no drugs that specifically augment the synthesis or release of thyroid hormones. The only effective treatment of hypothyroidism, unless it is due to iodine deficiency (which is treated with iodide; see above), is to administer the thyroid hormones themselves—used as replacement therapy. **Thyroxine** and **triiodothyronine** (**liothyronine**) are available and are given orally. Thyroxine is the drug of choice, liothyronine being reserved for the rare condition of myxoedema coma when its more rapid action is required for emergency treatment.

The actions and mechanisms of action of T_4 and T_3 are detailed on page 430.

Unwanted effects may occur with overdose, and in addition to the signs and symptoms of hyperthyroidism there is a risk of precipitating angina pectoris, cardiac dysrhythmias or cardiac failure. The effects of less severe overdose are more insidious; the patient feels well but bone resorption is increased leasing to osteoporosis.

The clinical use of drugs acting on the thyroid is given on this page.

Drugs in thyroid disease

Drugs for hyperthyroidism
- Radioiodine, given orally, is selectively taken up by thyroid and damages cells; it emits short-range β-radiation which affects only thyroid follicle cells. Hypothyroidism will eventually occur.
- Thioureylenes (e.g. propylthiouracil) decrease the synthesis of thyroid hormones; the mechanism is through inhibition of thyroperoxidase thus reducing iodination of thyroglobulin. Given orally.
- Iodine, given orally in high doses, transiently reduces thyroid hormone secretion and decreases vascularity of the gland.

Drugs for hypothyroidism
- Thyroxine has all the actions of endogenous T_4, (see box on p. 432); given orally
- Liothyronine (T_3) has all the actions of endogenous T_3 (see box on p. 432); given intravenously.

Clinical use of drugs acting on the thyroid

Radioiodine is used:
- as first-line treatment for hyperthyroidism (particularly in the USA); recurrence is rare provided the dose is adequate
- for treatment of relapse of hyperthyroidism after thioureylene therapy or surgery.

The **thioureylenes** are used:
- for hyperthyroidism (diffuse toxic goitre), at least 1 year of treatment being necessary; recurrence occurs eventually in over half the patients but can be managed by a repeat course of treatment
- as a preliminary to surgery for toxic goitre
- as part of the treatment of thyroid storm (very severe hyperthyroidism); propylthiouracil is preferred because of its action in decreasing the conversion of T_4 to T_3 in the tissues.

Thyroid hormones
- Thyroxine is the standard replacement therapy for hypothyroidism.
- Liothyronine is the treatment of choice for myxoedema coma.

REFERENCES AND FURTHER READING

Brent G A 1994 The molecular basis of thyroid hormone action. N Engl J Med 331: 847–854 (*A review covering receptor subtypes; T_3 regulation of genes in liver, adipocytes, cardiac and skeletal muscle; resistance to thyroid hormone*)

Franklin J A 1995 The management of hyperthyroidism. N Engl J Med 330: 1731–1738 (*An excellent review of the drug treatment of hyperthyroidism*)

Franklin J F, Sheppard M 1992 Radioiodine for hyperthyroidism: perhaps the best option. Br Med J 305: 728–729 (*An editorial commenting on the role of radioiodine in the treatment of thyrotoxicosis*)

Hermus A R, Huysmans D A 1998 Treatment of benign nodular thyroid disease. N Engl J Med 338: 1438–1447

Lazarus J H 1997 Hyperthyroidism. Lancet 349: 339–343 (*A 'seminar' covering aetiology, clinical features, pathophysiology, diagnosis and treatment*)

Lindsay R S 1997 Hypothyroidism. Lancet 349: 413–417 (*A 'seminar' emphasising the management of hypothyroidism*)

Oppenheimer J H, Schwartz H L et al. 1987 Advances in our understanding of thyroid hormone action at the cellular level. Endocr Rev 8: 288–308 (*Early, general review of the molecular basis of thyroid hormone action at the nuclear level*)

Paschke R, Ludgate M 1997 The thyrotropin receptor and its diseases. N Engl J Med 337: 1675–1679 (*Up-to-date review on aspects of molecular biology*)

Perlmann T, Vennstrom B 1995 Nuclear receptors: the sound of silence. Nature 377: 387–388 (*A simple commentary on two articles which provide evidence that thyroid hormone silences basal transcription*)

Surks M I, Sievert R 1995 Drugs and thyroid function. N Engl J Med 333: 1688–1694 (*Review covering drugs affecting secretion of TSH, secretion of thyroid hormone, T_4 absorption, the transport of T_4 and T_3 in blood, and the metabolism of T_3 and T_4*)

Tsai M-J, O'Malley B W 1994 Molecular mechanisms of action of steroid/thyroid receptor superfamily members. Annu Rev Biochem 63: 451–486 (*Detailed review of molecular biology of these receptors, including gene activation and gene silencing*)

Wagner R L, Apriletti J W et al. 1995 A structural role for hormone in the thyroid hormone receptor. Nature 378: 690–697 (*The molecular biology of ligand–receptor interaction*)

26

The reproductive system

ENDOCRINE ASPECTS

Hormonal control of the reproductive system in both the male and female involves *sex steroids* from the gonads, the *hypothalamic peptides* and the *glycoprotein gonadotrophins* from the anterior pituitary.

NEUROHORMONAL CONTROL OF THE FEMALE REPRODUCTIVE SYSTEM

At puberty an increased output of the hormones of the hypothalamus and anterior pituitary stimulates secretion of oestrogenic sex steroids. These are responsible for the maturation of the reproductive organs and the development of the secondary sexual characteristics, and also for a phase of accelerated growth followed by closure of the epiphyses of the long bones. Sex steroids are there-

after involved in the regulation of the cyclic changes expressed in the menstrual cycle and are important in pregnancy. A simplified outline of the interrelationship of these substances in the physiological control of the menstrual cycle is given in Figures 26.1 and 26.2.

The menstrual cycle is taken as beginning with the start of menstruation. This lasts for 3–6 days, during which the superficial layer of the endometrium of the uterus is shed. When the menstrual flow stops, the endometrium regenerates.

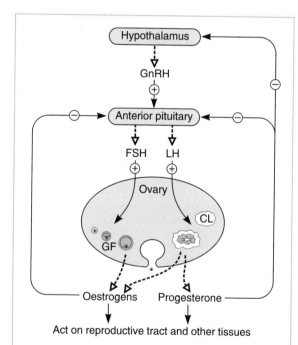

Fig. 26.1 Hormonal interrelationship in the control of the female reproductive system. The Graafian follicle (GF) is shown developing on the left, then involuting to form the corpus luteum (CL) on the right, after the ovum (●) has been released. (LH = luteinising hormone; FSH = follicle-stimulating hormone; GnRH = gonadotrophin-releasing hormone)

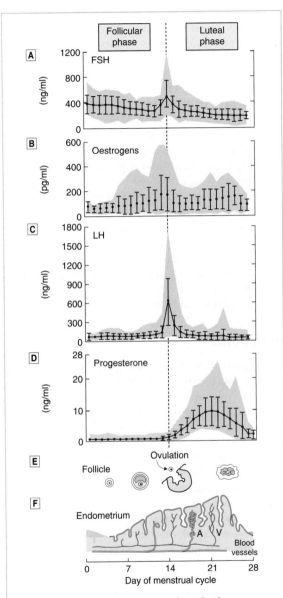

Fig. 26.2 Plasma concentrations of ovarian hormones and gonadotrophins in women during normal menstrual cycles. Values are the mean ± standard deviation of 40 women. The shaded areas indicate the entire range of observations. Day 1 is the onset of menstruation. E and F show diagrammatically the changes in the ovarian follicle and the endometrium during the cycle. Ovulation on day 14 of the menstrual cycle occurs with the midcycle peak of LH, represented by the dashed line. (After: Van de Wiele R L, Dyrenfurth I 1974 Pharmacol Rev 25: 189–217)

A releasing factor, the gonadotrophin-releasing hormone (**GnRH**), is secreted from peptidergic neurons in the hypothalamus in a pulsatile fashion, the frequency being about 1 discharge per hour. The GnRH stimulates the anterior pituitary to release gonadotrophic hormones (Fig. 26.1)—the follicle-stimulating hormone (**FSH**) and the luteinising hormone (**LH**). In the first phase of the cycle—the follicular phase—these gonadotrophins act on the ovaries (Fig. 26.2A), promoting the development of small groups of follicles, each of which contains an ovum. One of these develops faster than the others and forms the *Graafian follicle* (Figs 26.1 and 26.2E), and the rest degenerate.

The ripening Graafian follicle has a fluid-filled centre surrounded by granulosa cells within which lies the ovum, and surrounding these is a layer of thecal cells. **Oestrogens** are produced by the granulosa cells stimulated by FSH, from androgen precursor molecules derived from thecal cells stimulated by LH. The oestrogens (Fig. 26.2B), are responsible for the *early, proliferative* phase of endometrial regeneration which occurs from day 5 or 6 until midcycle (see Fig. 26.2F). During this phase the endometrium increases in thickness and vascularity, and at the peak of oestrogen secretion there is a prolific cervical secretion of mucus of pH 8–9, rich in protein and carbohydrate, which is thought to make the passage of the spermatozoa easier. The secreted oestrogens have a negative feedback effect on the anterior pituitary, decreasing gonadotrophin release (Fig. 26.1). The high oestrogen secretion just before midcycle sensitises LH-releasing cells of the pituitary to the action of the GnRH and thus is instrumental in determining the midcycle surge of LH secretion (Fig. 26.2C), which causes rapid swelling and rupture of the main follicle, resulting in ovulation (Fig. 26.2E). If fertilisation occurs, the fertilised ovum passes down the fallopian tubes to the uterus, starting to divide as it goes.

An important action of the oestrogens is to promote the formation of progesterone receptors in target tissues. They also have mild anabolic effects and tend to increase retention of salt and water.

Under the influence of LH, the cells of the ruptured follicle proliferate and the follicle develops into the *corpus luteum* which secretes **progesterone** (Fig. 26.2C, D and E). During the second part of the menstrual cycle, this hormone acts on the oestrogen-primed endometrium, stimulating the *secretory* phase of its regeneration which renders the endometrium suitable for the implantation of a fertilised ovum (Fig. 26.2F). At this stage the cervical mucus becomes more viscid, less alkaline, less copious and in general less welcoming for the sperm.

Progesterone has a negative feedback effect on hypothalamus and pituitary, decreasing the release of LH. It also has a *thermogenic* effect, causing a rise in body temperature of about 0.5°C which commences at ovulation and is maintained until the end of the cycle. If implantation of the ovum has not occurred, progesterone secretion stops, and its sudden cessation is one of the main triggers for the onset of menstruation.

If implantation does occur and pregnancy results, the *corpus luteum* continues to secrete progesterone, which, by its effect on hypothalamus and anterior pituitary, prevents further ovulation.

As pregnancy proceeds, the placenta develops hormonal functions and secretes **gonadotrophins**, **progesterone** and **oestrogens**. Progesterone secreted during pregnancy controls the development of the secretory alveoli in the mammary gland, while oestrogen stimulates the lactiferous ducts. After parturition, oestrogens, along with **prolactin** (see Ch. 24, p. 413), are responsible for stimulating and maintaining lactation, though high doses of exogenous oestrogen will inhibit it.

Oestrogens are dealt with below, progestogens (progesterone-like drugs) on page 442, androgens on page 444, and the gonadotrophins on page 447.

Hormonal control of the female reproductive system

- The menstrual cycle starts with menstruation.
- Hypothalamic GnRH acts on the anterior pituitary to release the gonadotrophins, FSH and LH, which act on the ovary.
- The gonadotrophins stimulate follicle development. FSH is the main hormone stimulating oestrogen release. LH stimulates ovulation at midcycle and is the main hormone controlling subsequent progesterone secretion from the corpus luteum.
- Oestrogen controls the proliferative phase of the endometrium and has negative feedback effects on the anterior pituitary. Progesterone controls the later secretory phase and has negative feedback effects on both hypothalamus and anterior pituitary.
- If a fertilised ovum is implanted, the corpus luteum continues to secrete progesterone during the pregnancy.

THE BEHAVIOURAL EFFECTS OF SEX HORMONES

As well as exerting a cyclical control over the menstrual cycle, sex steroids affect sexual behaviour. Two types of control are recognised, namely *organisational* and *activational*. The former refers to the fact that sexual differentiation of the brain can be permanently altered by the presence or absence of sex steroids at a key stage in development.

In rats, administration of androgens to females within a few days of birth results in virilisation of behaviour. Conversely, neonatal castration of male rats causes them to develop behaviourally as females. It is believed that brain development in the absence of sex steroids follows female lines, but that it can be switched to the male pattern by exposure of the hypothalamic cells to androgen at a key stage of development. In primates, similar but less complete behavioural virilisation of female offspring has been demonstrated following androgen administration or hypersecretion in pregnant mothers. This probably happens in humans also, if pregnant women secrete, or are treated with, androgens.

The *activational* effect of sex steroids refers to their ability to modify sexual behaviour after brain development is complete. In general, oestrogens and androgens increase sexual activity in the appropriate sex. Recent animal experiments have shown that oxytocin, known to be important during parturition, has a role in mating, pair bonding and parenting behaviours, its action in the CNS being regulated by oestrogen.

OESTROGENS

Oestrogens are synthesised mainly by the ovary but also in fairly large amounts by the placenta, and in small amounts by the testis in males and by the adrenal cortex in both sexes. Some other tissues, such as liver, muscle, fat and hair follicles, can also convert steroid precursors into oestrogens.

The starting substance for oestrogen synthesis is cholesterol (see Fig. 24.6). The immediate precursors to the oestrogens are androgenic substances—androstenedione or testosterone (Fig. 26.3).

There are three main endogenous oestrogens in humans—**oestradiol, oestrone** and **oestriol** (Fig. 26.3). Oestradiol is the most potent and is the principal oestrogen secreted by the ovary. At the beginning of the menstrual cycle, the plasma concentration is 0.2 nmol/l rising to ~2.2 nmol/l in midcycle (see Fig. 26.2). In the liver, oestradiol is converted to oestrone (Fig. 26.3) which may be converted to oestriol, a shorter-acting compound. Oestradiol and oestrone are the two main endogenous oestrogens and are readily interconvertible.

Actions

The effects of oestrogens given as drugs depend on the age at which they are administered. Given at age 11–13 (with progestogens) for primary hypogonadism, oestro-

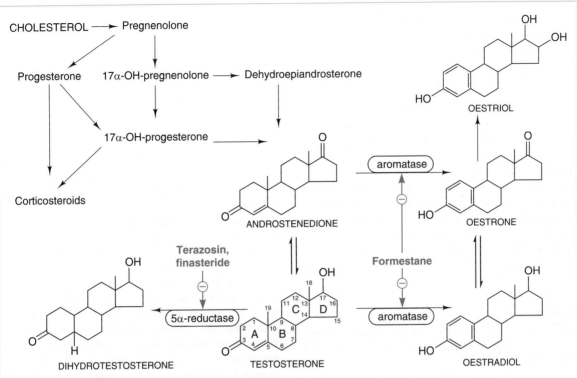

Fig. 26.3 The biosynthetic pathway for the androgens and oestrogens with sites of drug action. (See also Fig. 24.6.) Finasteride is used in benign prostatic hyperplasia and formestane to treat breast cancer in postmenopausal women.

gens stimulate the development of the secondary sexual characteristics and the phase of accelerated growth. In the adult with primary amenorrhoea, oestrogens, given cyclically with a progestogen, will induce an artificial cycle. Their main use in adult women, however, is for oral contraception and in postmenopausal hormone replacement therapy (HRT), and their pharmacological actions when thus used are described on pages 447 and 443 respectively.

Oestrogens have several metabolic actions which may become manifest when they are used as drugs. They cause some degree of retention of salt and water (as occurs with endogenous oestrogens in the latter half of the menstrual cycle) and they have mild anabolic actions. The concentration of serum triglycerides and of high density lipoproteins is raised, whereas that of low density lipoproteins is decreased (these effects may contribute to the relatively low risk of atheromatous disease in premenopausal women).

They affect bone in that they decrease resorption (Fig. 27.1) and can maintain bone mass in post-menopausal women; this effect may be indirect.

An impairment in glucose tolerance can occur in some individuals.

Oestrogens increase the coagulability of the blood. This increase in coagulability is the basis for the increased risk of thromboembolism which occurred with contraceptive pills containing a high oestrogen content. The low doses of oestrogens now used in contraceptive pills and in hormone replacement therapy do not themselves produce significant change in clotting mechanisms.

Mechanism of action

As with most other steroids, the action of oestrogen involves binding to receptors in the nucleus.* Binding is followed by interaction of the resultant complexes with nuclear sites and subsequent genomic effects—either gene transcription (i.e. DNA-directed RNA and protein synthesis) or gene repression (inhibition of transcription).

---

*Corticosteroids are an exception in that they bind to receptors in the cytoplasm.

More details are given in Chapters 2 and 24; see especially Figure 24.7.

Oestrogen receptors occur mainly in the cells of its principal target tissues: the reproductive system (uterus, vagina, mammary glands) and the anterior pituitary. These tissues contain about 15 000 to 21 000 high-affinity oestrogen-binding sites per cell, but smaller numbers of sites also occur in the liver, kidney, adrenal and ovary. One of the principal effects of the oestrogens on DNA is the induction of synthesis of progesterone receptors in target tissues such as uterus, vagina, anterior pituitary and hypothalamus.

Progesterone decreases oestrogen receptor expression in the reproductive tract even in the presence of continuously high plasma oestrogen concentrations, by interfering with the de novo synthesis of the receptors. **Prolactin** (see Ch. 24, p. 413) increases the numbers of oestrogen receptors in the mammary gland and liver but has no effect on those in the uterus.

Preparations

Many preparations of oestrogens are available.* Some of the more commonly used ones are listed in Table 26.1

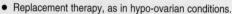

Clinical use of oestrogens

- Replacement therapy, as in hypo-ovarian conditions.
- Treatment of menopausal symptoms or for postmenopausal replacement therapy.
- Contraception.
- Vaginitis (topical oestrogen preparations are used).
- Therapy of prostatic cancer and for some cases of breast cancer (these uses have largely been superseded by other hormonal manipulations; see Ch. 42).

Very different doses are used for these different indications; see footnote on this page.

and some chemical structures are given in Figures 26.3 and 26.4.

The clinical use of oestrogens is given above.

Pharmacokinetic aspects

Both the natural and synthetic oestrogens used in therapy are well absorbed in the gastrointestinal tract, but after absorption, the natural oestrogens are rapidly metabolised in the liver, whereas the synthetic oestrogens and non-steroidal oestrogen-like compounds are less rapidly degraded. There is a variable amount of enterohepatic cycling. Most oestrogens are readily absorbed from skin and mucous membranes and can be given by transdermal patches. They may be given topically in the vagina as creams or pessaries for local effect (some may be absorbed). In the plasma, natural oestrogens are bound to albumin and to a sex-steroid-binding globulin. Natural oestrogens are excreted in the urine as glucuronides and sulphates.

Unwanted effects

In general, the unwanted effects of oestrogens are tenderness in the breasts, nausea, vomiting, anorexia, retention of salt and water with resultant oedema, and increased risk of thromboembolism and of alteration of carbohydrate metabolism (see below). More details of the unwanted effects which can occur with oral contraceptives are given on page 418.

Used for postmenopausal replacement therapy, oestrogens frequently cause menstruation-like bleeding, and can produce endometrial hyperplasia unless given cyclically with a progestogen. When administered to males, oestrogens result in feminisation.

Oestrogen administration to pregnant women carries the hazard of potential non-malignant genital abnormality in the offspring, whether male or female.

There is evidence that carcinoma of the vagina and the cervix is more common in young women whose

Table 26.1	Oestrogens
Drug	Comment
Oestradiol	A natural oestrogen. Usually given i.m. Long-acting preparations are available. Oestradiol valerate is active by mouth. Patch preparations for transdermal use have proved effective
Oestriol	A natural oestrogen. Can be given orally
Oestrone	Given orally as piperazone oestrone sulphate. Oestrone sulphate is the main ingredient of conjugated oestrogens
Ethinyl oestradiol	Semi-synthetic. Given orally. Effective and cheap. The drug of choice. Used in many contraceptive preparations
Mestranol	Synthetic. Converted to oestradiol in the body
Dienoestrol	Used topically in the vagina

*Note that very different doses of oestrogens are used for different conditions, for example ethinyloestradiol is used in a dose of 10–20 µg/day for postmenopausal hormone replacement therapy, 20–50 µg/day in the combined contraceptive pill, 1–3 mg/day for breast cancer.

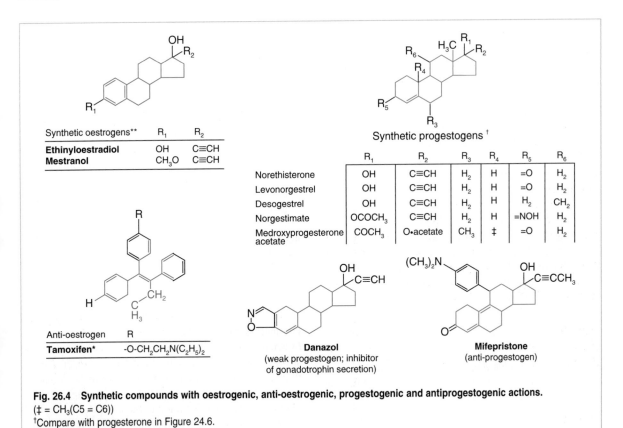

Synthetic oestrogens**

Synthetic oestrogens**	R_1	R_2
Ethinyloestradiol	OH	C≡CH
Mestranol	CH₃O	C≡CH

Synthetic progestogens [†]

	R_1	R_2	R_3	R_4	R_5	R_6
Norethisterone	OH	C≡CH	H₂	H	=O	H₂
Levonorgestrel	OH	C≡CH	H₂	H	=O	H₂
Desogestrel	OH	C≡CH	H₂	H	H₂	CH₂
Norgestimate	OCOCH₃	C≡CH	H₂	H	=NOH	H₂
Medroxyprogesterone acetate	COCH₃	O•acetate	CH₃	‡	=O	H₂

Anti-oestrogen	R
Tamoxifen*	-O-CH₂CH₂N(C₂H₅)₂

Danazol
(weak progestogen; inhibitor of gonadotrophin secretion)

Mifepristone
(anti-progestogen)

Fig. 26.4 Synthetic compounds with oestrogenic, anti-oestrogenic, progestogenic and antiprogestogenic actions.
(‡ = CH₃(C5 = C6))
[†]Compare with progesterone in Figure 24.6.
*See Wiseman (1994), Figure 3.
**Compare with oestrogen in Figure 26.3.

mothers were given the synthetic oestrogen preparation, stilboestrol, in early pregnancy (see Ch. 49).

ANTI-OESTROGENS

Anti-oestrogens (Fig. 26.4) are inactive or weakly active themselves, but compete with natural oestrogens for receptors in target organs.

Tamoxifen is a non-steroidal compound with anti-oestrogenic action on mammary tissue but oestrogenic action on plasma lipids, endometrium and bone. It produces the same side-effects as the oestrogens themselves, but they are less marked. This drug binds to the oestrogen receptor in the nucleus, but there is little or no stimulation of transcription, possibly because the complex binds to a different nuclear acceptor site. Moreover, the complex does not readily dissociate, so there is interference with the recycling of receptors.

Tamoxifen up-regulates the cytokine, transforming growth factor-β (TGF-β), decreased function of which is associated with the progression of malignancy; this may play a part in the anticancer action of drug. The anti-osteoporotic action of tamoxifen may also be due to up-regulation of TGF-β since this cytokine has a role in controlling the balance between bone-producing osteoblasts and bone-resorbing osteoclasts. See also Chapter 42, p. 677.

Newer analogues are in clinical trial, **doloxifene** for mammary cancer, **raloxifene** (selective estrogen receptor modulator, SERM) for osteoporosis.

Tamoxifen is discussed in Chapter 42.

Clomiphene (see Fig. 26.6) and **cyclofenil** inhibit oestrogen binding in the anterior pituitary, so preventing the normal modulation by negative feedback and causing increased secretion of GnRH and gonadotrophins. This results in a marked stimulation and enlargement of the ovaries and increased oestrogen secretion. The main effect of their anti-oestrogen action in the pituitary is that they *induce ovulation*. These compounds are used in treating infertility due to lack of ovulation. Multiple pregnancies commonly occur.

PROGESTOGENS

The natural progestational hormone or progestogen is *progesterone* (see Figs 24.6 and 26.3) which is secreted mainly by the *corpus luteum* in the second part of the menstrual cycle. Small amounts are also secreted by the testis in the male and the adrenal cortex in both sexes, and large amounts are secreted by the placenta.

Mechanism of action

Progestogens act by the same mechanism as other steroids (see Ch. 24, p. 421 and Fig. 24.7). The presence of adequate numbers of progesterone receptors depends on the prior action of oestrogens (see above).

Preparations

There are two main groups of progestogens:

- *The naturally occurring hormone and its derivatives* (see Fig. 24.6). **Progesterone** itself is virtually inactive orally because after absorption it is metabolised in the liver. Preparations are available for intramuscular injection and for topical use in the vagina and rectum. Hydroxyprogesterone is an intermediate in the pathway of synthesis of hydrocortisone and

testosterone (see Fig. 24.6), and has progesterone-like activity. It is given by intramuscular injection as **hydroxyprogesterone hexanoate**—the esterification at C_{17} inhibiting its further enzymic conversion. Medroxyprogesterone can be given orally or by injection, dyhydrogesterone orally.

- *Testosterone derivatives.* **Norethisterone** (see Fig. 26.4), norgestrel, and ethynodiol are all derivatives of testosterone with progesterone-like activity, and all can be given orally. The first two have some androgenic activity and are metabolised to give oestrogenic products. Newer progestogens used in contraception are given on page 447.

Actions

The pharmacological actions of the progestogens are in essence the same as the physiological actions described above. Specific effects relevant to contraception are detailed on page 448.

Pharmacokinetic aspects

Injected progesterone is bound to albumin, not to the sex-steroid-binding globulin. Some is stored in adipose tissue. It is metabolised in the liver, and the products, pregnanolone and pregnanediol, are conjugated with glucuronic acid and excreted in the urine.

The main *clinical use* of progestogens is in contraception (see below). They have an ill-defined place in the therapy of various gynaecological conditions such as menstrual disorders, endometriosis and dysmenorrhoea. They are also used in the treatment of endometrial carcinoma, and, in conjunction with oestrogen, for hormone replacement therapy.

Unwanted effects include weak androgenic actions of some of the progestogens derived from testosterone. Other unwanted effects are considered under 'Drugs used for contraception' on pages 448–449.

ANTIPROGESTOGENS

Mifepristone (Fig. 26.4) is a partial agonist at progesterone receptors; thus it has some inherent progestogen agonist properties but inhibits progesterone action. It sensitises the uterus to the action of prostaglandins. It is given orally and has a plasma half-life of 21 hours.

Mifepristone is used as a medical alternative to surgical termination of pregnancy (see p. 452). Given within 49 days of the last menstrual period, mifepristone, in a single oral dose, followed 48 hours later by the prostaglandin analogue, **gemeprost**, given as an intravaginal pessary (see p. 452), results in complete abortion in 95% of cases. There is evidence that mifepristone combined with oral prostaglandin analogue, e.g. **misoprostol**,* is also effective.

If given in the late follicular phase of the menstrual cycle, mifepristone inhibits ovulation and hence has potential as a postcoital contraceptive agent. Mifepristone also has a significant antagonist action at the glucocorticoid receptor, though in higher concentration.

Progestogens and antiprogestogens

- The endogenous hormone is progesterone. Examples of exogenous hormones are the progesterone derivative, medroxyprogesterone, and the testosterone derivative, norethisterone.
- Mechanism of action: as for oestrogens. Prior oestrogen action is required for the synthesis of progesterone receptors.
- Main pharmacological use: in oral contraception regimes.
- The antiprogestogen, mifepristone, in combination with prostaglandin analogues, is an effective medical alternative to surgical termination of early pregnancy.

POSTMENOPAUSAL HORMONE REPLACEMENT THERAPY (HRT)

At the menopause, either natural or surgically induced, ovarian function decreases and oestrogen levels fall but gonadotrophin secretion continues and is increased because of loss of negative feedback. Exogenous oestrogens, the main hormones used for HRT, have clear-cut beneficial effects:

- Reduction in the menopausal symptoms associated with the decline in oestrogen production, namely the hot flushes, inappropriate sweating, paraesthesias, palpitations, atrophic vaginitis, mood changes, etc.
- A reduction in the risk of coronary heart disease (the commonest cause of death in postmenopausal women); epidemiological studies suggest that there is a 50% reduction. Recent evidence indicates that addition of progestogens to the HRT regime, (necessary for women with an intact uterus) does not attenuate this cardioprotective effect (Grodstein et al. 1996).
- Reduction of osteoporotic change and the concomitant risk of fracture.
- Observational studies indicate that women on HRT have a reduced incidence and/or a delayed onset of Alzheimer's disease.

*For use in protection against NSAID-induced gastric damage; see page 233.

The use of oestrogen in HRT has some drawbacks, as follows:

- An increase in the risk of endometrial cancer. This risk can be reduced if progestogens are given for 10 days each month.
- A possible increase in the risk of breast cancer—said to be a 20% increase up to the age of 60 and a 70% increase after 60 (this is controversial).
- Uterine bleeding; this occurs if cyclical progestogens are included in the HRT regime.
- Minor gastrointestinal symptoms and mood changes (the latter mainly due to the progestogen component).
- A small increase in the risk of venous thromboembolism and pulmonary embolism; there are about 19 and 6 extra cases per 100 000 HRT-taking women per year respectively.

Oestrogens used in HRT can be given orally (conjugated oestrogens, oestradiol, oestriol), vaginally (oestriol), by transdermal patch (oestradiol) or by subcutaneous implant (oestradiol). A steroid marketed specifically for the treatment of postmenopausal vasomotor and vaginal symptoms is **tibolone**, which has weak oestrogenic, progestogenic and androgenic properties.

There is still some controversy about the use of HRT (see Toozs-Hobson & Cardozo 1996 versus Jacobs 1996; **Khaw K-T 1988**) but many authorities consider that the benefits outweigh the risks. A recent 20-year retrospective study using data from 34 000 women showed a 20% reduction in overall mortality for HRT users, the reduction being greater for women with a higher risk of coronary disease. Survival benefit decreases with longer duration of use (see Brinton & Schairer 1997).

Raloxifene, a newer analogue, is in clinical trial for prevention of osteoporosis (see Ch. 27).

NEUROHORMONAL CONTROL OF THE MALE REPRODUCTIVE SYSTEM

As in the female, endocrine secretions from the hypothalamus, anterior pituitary and gonads control the male reproductive system. A simplified outline of the interrelationship of these factors is given in Figure 26.5. The gonadotrophin-releasing hormone (**GnRH**) controls the secretion of gonadotrophins by the anterior pituitary. This secretion is not cyclical as in the menstruating female; in both sexes it is pulsatile (see below). **FSH** is responsible for the integrity of the seminiferous tubules and, after puberty, is important in gametogenesis through an action on the Sertoli cells which nourish and support the developing spermatozoa. **LH**, which in the male is

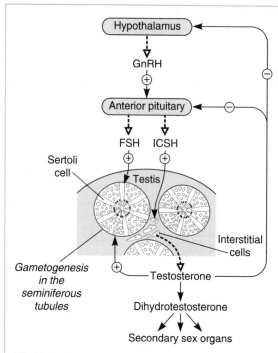

Fig. 26.5 **Hormonal interrelationships in the control of the male reproductive system.** (GnRH = gonadotrophin-releasing hormone; FSH = follicle-stimulating hormone; ICSH = interstitial-cell-stimulating hormone (equivalent to luteinising hormone in the female))

also called *interstitial cell stimulating hormone* (**ICSH**), stimulates the interstitial cells (Leydig cells) to secrete androgens—in particular **testosterone**. The secretion of LH begins at puberty, and the testosterone secreted is responsible for the maturation of the reproductive organs and the development of the secondary sexual characteristics. Thereafter, the primary function of testosterone is the maintenance of spermatogenesis and hence fertility—an action mediated by the Sertoli cells. This steroid is also important in the maturation of the spermatozoa as they pass through the epididymis and vas deferens. A further action is a feedback effect on the anterior pituitary, modulating its sensitivity to GnRH and thus influencing the concentration of ICSH in the circulation. In addition it has marked anabolic effects in puberty causing development of the musculature and increased bone growth resulting in a rapid increase in height. This is followed by closure of the epiphyses of the long bones.

Though the secretion of testosterone is controlled largely by ICSH, FSH may also play a part, possibly

by inducing the release from the Sertoli cells (which are its primary target) of a factor similar to GnRH. The interstitial cells which synthesise testosterone also have receptors for **prolactin**, and this substance may influence testosterone production by increasing the number of receptors for ICSH.

ANDROGENS

Testosterone is the main natural androgen, and it is synthesised not only by the interstitial cells of the testis in males, but in small amounts by the ovary in females and the adrenal cortex in both sexes. Adrenal production of androgens is under the control of corticotrophin. Cholesterol is the starting substance (see Figs 24.6 and 26.3), and precursor substances are dehydroepiandro-sterone and androstenedione, which may be released from the gonads and the adrenal cortex in both sexes and subsequently converted to testosterone in the liver (see Fig. 26.3).

Actions

In general the effects of exogenous androgens are the same as those of the endogenous hormones and will depend on the age of the patient to whom they are given.

If administered to males at the age of puberty, there is rapid development of the secondary sexual characteristics, maturation of the reproductive organs and a marked increase in muscular strength. Height increases more gradually. The anabolic effects can be accompanied by retention of salt and water. The skin becomes thickened and sometimes darkens, and the sebaceous glands become more active (which can result in acne). There is growth of hair on the pubic and axillary regions and on the face. The vocal cords hypertrophy resulting in a lower pitch to the voice. Androgens cause a feeling of well-being and an increase in physical vigour and may increase libido. Whether they are responsible for sexual behaviour as such is controversial, as is their contribution to aggressive behaviour.

If given to prepubertal males, the individuals concerned do not reach their full height because of premature closure of the epiphyses of the long bones.

Administration to women results in masculinisation changes similar to those seen in the pubertal male. With long-continued administration many of the effects are irreversible.

Mechanism of action

Testosterone is converted to dihydrotestosterone in most target cells by a 5α-reductase, though it is testosterone itself which is involved in virilisation of the genital tract in the male embryo and in the regulation of ICSH production. Both testosterone and dihydrotestosterone modify gene transcription by the same mechanisms as other steroids (see p. 421).

Preparations

Testosterone itself can be given by subcutaneous implantation. **Testosterone enanthate** and **testosterone proprionate** are given by intramuscular depot injection. **Testosterone undecanoate** and **mesterolone** can be given orally.

The clinical use of androgens is given in the box on page 446.

Pharmacokinetic aspects

Testosterone is rapidly metabolised in the liver if given orally, though this does not happen if it is absorbed from the buccal mucosa or from rectal suppositories. Virtually all testosterone in the circulation is bound to plasma protein—mainly to the sex-steroid-binding globulin. The half-life of free testosterone is 10–21 minutes. It is inactivated in the liver by conversion to androstenedione (see Fig. 26.3) which has weak androgenic activity, and 90% of its metabolites are excreted in the urine. Synthetic androgens are less rapidly metabolised and some are excreted in the urine unchanged.

Unwanted effects

Unwanted effects of treatment with testosterone include eventual decrease of gonadotrophin release with resultant infertility, and salt and water retention leading to oedema. Adenocarcinoma of the liver has been reported. In children, the androgens cause disturbances in growth and in females, acne and masculinisation.

Alprostadil (synthetic prostaglandin E_1), injected into the corpus cavernosum, can be effective in men with erectile dysfunction.

Androgens and the hormonal control of the male reproductive system

- GnRH from the hypothalamus acts on the anterior pituitary to release both FSH, which stimulates gametogenesis, and LH (also called interstitial-cell-stimulating hormone) which stimulates androgen secretion.
- The endogenous hormone is testosterone; an exogenous preparation is mesterolone.
- Mechanism of action: as for oestrogens.

ANABOLIC STEROIDS

It is possible to modify the structure of androgens so as to enhance the anabolic effects and decrease other effects. Many have been produced; examples are **nandrolone** and **stanozolol**. They are believed to increase protein synthesis and enhance muscle development, resulting in weight gain. These agents are used to decrease the itching of chronic biliary obstruction and in the therapy of some aplastic anaemias. They may have a place in the treatment of debilitating and wasting conditions and in terminal disease, in which they can improve appetite and promote a welcome feeling of well-being. They are used in some cases of hormone-dependent metastatic mammary cancer. Unwanted effects can occur, in particular cholestatic jaundice.

Anabolic steroids are used by some athletes in the expectation that they will increase strength and athletic performance. When combined with strength training, a short course of weekly 600 mg doses of testosterone (a dose six times higher than that used for replacement therapy) increased fat-free mass and muscle size. As anabolic steroid abusers may take up to 26 times the therapeutic dose, serious unwanted effects can occur—not only those specified above under 'androgens', but numerous others including testicular atrophy, sterility and gynaecomastia in men, and inhibition of ovulation, hirsutism, deepening of the voice, alopecia and acne in women.

Increased aggressiveness and psychotic symptoms have been described. In both sexes there is increased risk of coronary heart disease, and there have been instances of sudden death in young athletes in which there was a strong suspicion that anabolic steroid use had been contributory.

ANTI-ANDROGENS

Both oestrogens and progestogens have anti-androgen activity, oestrogens mainly by inhibiting gonadotrophin secretion and progestogens by competing with androgens in target organs. **Cyproterone** is a derivative of progesterone and has weak progestational activity. It is a partial agonist at androgen receptors, competing with dihydrotestosterone for receptors in androgen-sensitive target tissues. Through its effect in the hypothalamus it depresses the synthesis of gonadotrophins. It is used as an adjunct in the treatment of prostatic cancer during initiation of GnRH treatment (see below). It is also used in the therapy of precocious puberty in males, and of masculinisation and acne in women. It seems also to have an effect in the central nervous system, decreasing libido. It has been proposed for use in the treatment of severe hypersexuality in male sexual offenders.*

Flutamide is a non-steroidal anti-androgen used with GnRH in the treatment of prostate cancer.

Drugs can have anti-androgen action by inhibiting the enzymes which give rise to the active steroids. **Finasteride** inhibits the enzyme 5α-reductase that converts testosterone to dihydrotestosterone (Fig. 26.3) which has greater affinity for androgen receptors. It is well absorbed after oral administration, has a half-life of about 7 hours and is excreted in the urine and faeces. It is used to treat benign prostatic hyperplasia though the α_1-adrenoceptor antagonist, **terazosin**, is more effective. There is now a selective α_{1A}-adrenoceptor antagonist, **tamsulosin**, that blocks the receptors in prostatic smooth muscle but not in the vasculature; there is thus less postural hypertension than with **terazosin**. Surgery is the preferred option (especially by surgeons).

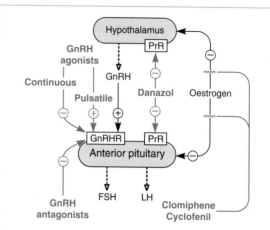

Fig. 26.6 The regulation of gonadotrophin release from the anterior pituitary by endogenous gonadotrophin-releasing hormone (GnRH) and drugs. (GnRHR = GnRH receptor; PrR = progestogen receptor; FSH = follicle-stimulating hormone; LH = luteinising hormone)

Clinical use of androgens and anti-androgens

- Androgens (testosterone preparations) are used for replacement therapy in testicular failure and as anabolic agents.
- Anti-androgens (e.g. flutamide, cyproterone) are used as part of the treatment of prostatic cancer.

GONADOTROPHIN-RELEASING HORMONE: AGONISTS AND ANTAGONISTS

Gonadotrophin-releasing hormone (GnRH) controls the secretion by the anterior pituitary of both FSH and LH.

The secretion of GnRH is controlled by neural input from other parts of the brain and, in the female particularly, through negative feedback by the sex steroids (Figs 26.1 and 26.6). Exogenous androgens, oestrogens and progestogens all inhibit the secretion of the peptide, but only the progestogens, when given on their own, seem to have this effect without having marked hormonal actions on peripheral tissues. This is presumably because in the absence of oestrogen there is less induction of progesterone receptors in the reproductive tract.

Synthetic GnRH is termed **gonadorelin**. Numerous analogues of GnRH, both agonists and antagonists, have

been synthesised. Analogues with agonist activity are **buserelin, leuprorelin, goserelin** and **nafarelin**, the last being 200 times more potent than endogenous GnRH.

An agent which inhibits the release of both GnRH and the gonadotrophins is **danazol** (see below). **Clomiphene** and **cyclofenil** stimulate gonadotrophin release by inhibiting the negative feedback effects of endogenous oestrogen (see above and Fig. 26.6).

Administration of the antagonists results in a decrease not in total FSH per se but in biologically active FSH, because greater amounts of the deglycosylated FSH isoforms with antagonist action are released.

Pharmacokinetics and clinical use

GnRH antagonists were synthesised because it was thought they might constitute a new non-steroidal method of contraception. This approach has so far been less rewarding than expected, but is still being explored.

GnRH agonists, given subcutaneously in pulsatile fashion by a miniaturised pump, can stimulate gonadotrophin release (Fig. 26.6) and have been used successfully to induce ovulation. Continuous use has, paradoxically, the opposite effect—desensitising the pituitary and *inhibiting gonadotrophin generation* (Fig. 26.6). For this inhibitory action on gonadotrophin production, GnRH analogues are given by subcutaneous injection, by nasal spray or as depot preparations. GnRH analogues given in this fashion are used in various conditions in which gonadal suppression is desirable, such as endometriosis

---

*As with the oestrogens, very different doses are used for these different conditions, for example 2 mg/day for acne, 100 mg/day for hypersexuality, 300 mg/day for prostatic cancer.

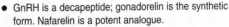

(endometrial tissue outside the uterine cavity), precocious puberty, sex-hormone-dependent cancers (particularly advanced prostatic cancer), and hirsutism due to the polycystic ovary syndrome. Continuous, non-pulsatile administration will also lead to inhibition of spermatogenesis and ovulation. This latter effect has been used to permit timed follicular recruitment by exogenous FSH for the harvesting of oocytes for in vitro fertilisation. Intranasal administration is being considered for use in contraception.

The *unwanted effects* of the GnRH agonists are hypo-oestrogenism, which is associated with hot flushes, decreased libido and headache. With prolonged use, osteoporosis may be a problem.

DANAZOL

Danazol inhibits the output of gonadotrophins (Fig. 26.6), affecting particularly the midcycle surge in the female and inhibiting steroid synthesis in the ovary. It is also active in males, reducing androgen synthesis and spermatogenesis. It has weak androgenic activity.

It is used in various conditions in which decreased sex hormone production would be beneficial, more particularly endometriosis, but also menorrhagia (excessive menstruation) and other menstrual disorders as well as gynaecomastia in men. Unwanted effects are common and include gastrointestinal disturbances, weight gain, fluid retention, dizziness, muscle cramps and headache. It has a virilising action in females.

Gestrinone has similar actions to danazol and is also used in endometriosis.

GONADOTROPHINS AND ANALOGUES

Follicle-stimulating hormone (FSH) and luteinising hormone (LH) are produced in moderate amounts by the anterior pituitary (see Ch. 24 and Table 24.1) in both males and females, and in large amounts by the placenta during pregnancy in the female. These hormones are glycoproteins with two different subunits, designated α and β; biological specificity depends on the β-subunit.

Preparations

Substances with gonadotrophin activity are extracted from biological material—**chorionic gonadotrophin** (mostly LH) from the urine of pregnant women and menotrophin (LH and FSH) and urofollitrophin (FSH) from the urine of postmenopausal women. A preparation of recombinant FSH (follitrophin) is also now available.

The gonadotrophin preparations have to be given by

> **Gonadotrophin-releasing hormone (GnRH) and gonadotrophins**
>
> - GnRH is a decapeptide; gonadorelin is the synthetic form. Nafarelin is a potent analogue.
> - Given in pulsatile fashion they stimulate gonadotrophin release; given continuously they inhibit it.
> - The gonadotrophins, FSH and LH, are glycoproteins.
> - Preparations of gonadotrophins (e.g. chorionic gonadotrophin, extracted from the urine of pregnant women) are used to treat infertility due to lack of ovulation.
> - Danazol is a modified progestogen which inhibits gonadotrophin production by an action on the hypothalamus and anterior pituitary.

injection. They are used primarily to treat infertility due to lack of ovulation.

DRUGS USED FOR CONTRACEPTION

ORAL CONTRACEPTIVES

There are two main types of oral* contraceptives:

- combinations of an oestrogen with a progestogen (the combined pill)
- progestogen alone (the progestogen-only pill).

(For review, see Baird & Glasier 1993.)

The combined pill

The oestrogen in most combined preparations (second-generation pills)** is **ethinyloestradiol**, though a few preparations contain **mestranol** instead. The progestogen may be **norethisterone**, **levonorgestrel**, **ethynodiol**, or—in third-generation pills—the newer compounds, **desogestrel** or **gestodene**, which are more potent, have less androgenic action and cause less change in lipoprotein metabolism. The oestrogen content of the pill should be no more than 50 μg of ethinyl-oestradiol or its equivalent, and the progestogen content should also

---

*For oral contraceptives to be effective, they must of course be absorbed. Gastrointestinal disturbances with vomiting and diarrhoea may impair absorption. A bout of traveller's diarrhoea, for example, could have unexpected consequences.

**The first-generation pills, containing more than 50 μg oestrogen, were shown, in the 1970s, to be associated with increased coagulability of the blood and an increased risk of deep vein thrombosis and, in some cases, pulmonary embolism.

be low. This combined pill is taken for 21 consecutive days followed by 7 pill-free days. The mode of action is thought to be as follows:

- The oestrogen inhibits the release of FSH and thus suppresses the development of the ovarian follicle.
- The progestogen inhibits the release of LH and thus prevents ovulation, and it also makes the cervical mucus less suitable for the passage of sperm.
- Together they alter the endometrium in such a way as to discourage implantation.

They may also interfere with the coordinated contractions of cervix, uterus and fallopian tubes which are thought to be necessary for successful fertilisation and implantation. When administration ceases after 21 days, it is the withdrawal of the progestogen which precipitates menstruation.

The progestogen-only pill

The drugs used include **norethisterone**, **levonorgestrel** or **ethynodiol**. The pill is taken daily without interruption. The mode of action is primarily on the cervical mucus which is made inhospitable to sperm. The progestogen probably also hinders implantation through its effect on the endometrium and on the motility and secretions of the fallopian tubes (described above).

Potential unwanted and beneficial effects of the combined pill

The experience of the last 30 years or more indicates that the combined pill constitutes a safe and effective method of contraception. There are distinct health benefits from taking the pill (see below) but serious adverse effects are rare. However, minor unwanted effects constitute possible drawbacks to its use and several important questions need to be considered.

Possible drawbacks

- There can be a gain in weight, due to fluid retention or an anabolic effect or both.
- General symptoms, such as nausea, flushing, dizziness, depression or irritability occur in some individuals.
- Skin changes, such as acne and/or an increase in pigmentation are occasionally reported.
- Amenorrhoea of variable duration on cessation of taking the pill is sometimes seen. Permanent loss of fertility is rare and normal cycles of menstruation usually commence fairly soon.

Questions that need to be considered

Is there an increased risk of cardiovascular disease (venous thromboembolism, myocardial infarction,

stroke)? With second-generation pills (oestrogen content less than 50 μg), the risk of thromboembolism is small and is confined to specific subgroups in whom other factors contribute, such as smoking (which can increase the risk substantially) and long-continued use of the pill, especially in women over 35 years old. On the other hand, the oestrogens in these pills are thought to *reduce* the risk of cardiovascular disease by protecting the arterial walls against atheromatous change.

With third-generation pills, and to a lesser extent with second-generation pills that contain **gestodene** or **desogestrel**, there is a small increase in risk of thromboembolic disease because these progestogens induce resistance to the blood's natural anticoagulation system. See Rosing et al. (1997); Vandenbroucke & Rosendaal (1997). However, the consensus seems to be that in healthy women, the greatest risk to health comes from smoking while taking the pill rather than from the type of pill.

Is there an increase in the risk of cancer? A study of more than 150 000 women has shown that there is a small increase in the risk of breast cancer, the risk being 0.5 excess cancers per 10 000 women aged 16–19, and 4.7 excess cancers per 10 000 women at age 25–29. The cancers were less advanced in pill users and thus potentially more treatable (see Hemminki 1996). Evidence suggests that oral contraceptives *decrease* the incidence of ovarian and endometrial cancer and do not cause cervical cancer. An association between liver cancer and oral contraceptive use has been reported; but this cancer is very rare in Europe and the USA and the possibility of a confounding role of hepatitis B in these cancers must be taken into account.

Does the pill increase the risk of hypertension? Some degree of hypertension occurs in about 4–5% of women who take the combined pill, and pre-existing hypertension can be increased. The effect is usually reversible.

Is there an impairment in glucose tolerance? Older progestogen preparations could impair glucose tolerance; the newer compounds are thought not to have this effect.

Beneficial effects

The use of the combined pill markedly decreases the incidence of amenorrhoea, irregular periods and intermenstrual bleeding. The incidence of iron deficiency anaemia and of premenstrual tension is reduced, as is the incidence of benign breast disease, uterine fibroids and functional cysts of the ovaries. There is less risk of thyroid disease. Amongst the beneficial effects should be included the fact that unwanted pregnancy has been avoided, in the light of the further fact that pregnancy carries an overall maternal mortality ranging from 1 in 10 000 in developed countries to 1 in 150 in Africa.

In general, as stated by Baird & Glasier (1993), 'the evidence suggests (but not proves conclusively) that after risk factors (e.g. smoking, hypertension, and obesity) have been identified, combined oral contraceptives are safe for most women for most of their reproductive lives'.

Potential beneficial and unwanted effects of the progestogen-only pill

Inhibition of ovulation with the progestogen-only pill is variable and inconsistent. The contraceptive effect is less reliable than that of the combination pill, and missing a dose may result in conception. Disturbances of menstruation are common; in particular there is liable to be irregular bleeding. Only a small proportion of women use this form of contraception and information on the long-term risks is not available.

An advantage is that the progestogen-only pill can be taken after parturition as, unlike oestrogen-containing pills, it does not interfere with lactation.

Oral contraceptives

The combined pill

- The combined pill contains an oestrogen and a progestogen. It is taken for 21 consecutive days out of 28.
- Mode of action: the oestrogen inhibits FSH release and therefore follicle development; the progestogen inhibits LH release and therefore ovulation, and makes cervical mucus inhospitable for sperm; together they render the endometrium unsuitable for implantation.
- Drawbacks: weight gain, nausea, mood changes and skin pigmentation can occur.
- Serious unwanted effects are rare. A small proportion of women develop reversible hypertension; there is evidence both for and against an increased risk of breast cancer; there is a small increased risk of thromboembolism with third-generation pills.
- There are several beneficial effects, not least the avoidance of unwanted pregnancy which itself carries a not insignificant risk.

The progestogen-only pill

- The progestogen-only pill is taken continuously. It differs from the combined pill in that the contraceptive effect is less reliable and is mainly due to the alteration of cervical mucus. Irregular bleeding is likely to occur. It does not interfere with lactation.

OTHER DRUG REGIMES USED FOR CONTRACEPTION

Postcoital oral contraceptives

Oral administration of oestrogen (100 µg) with levonorgestrel (250 µg) within 72 hours of unprotected intercourse, followed by further administration of these doses 12 hours later, has been effective for contraception. Nausea and vomiting are likely to occur (and the pills may then be lost).

A single dose of **mifepristone** is also reported to be effective.

Long-acting progestogen-only contraception

Medroxyprogesterone can be given intramuscularly as a contraceptive. This is effective and safe. However, menstrual irregularities are common, and infertility may persist for many months after cessation of treatment.

Levonorgestrel implanted subcutaneously in nonbiodegradable capsules is being used by ~3 million women world-wide. This route of administration bypasses the liver, thus avoiding first-pass metabolism. The tubes slowly release their progestogen content over 5 years. Common unwanted effects are irregular bleeding and headache.

A **levonorgestrel-impregnated intrauterine device** has contraceptive action for 3–5 years.

Contraceptives for males

Oral contraceptives for males are still in the experimental stage.

THE UTERUS

The physiological and pharmacological responses of the uterus vary at different stages of the menstrual cycle and pregnancy.

The motility of the uterus

Uterine muscle contracts rhythmically both in vitro and in vivo. the contractions originating in the muscle itself. Myometrial cells in the fundus act as pacemakers and give rise to conducted action potentials, the electrophysiological activity of these pacemaker cells being regulated by the sex hormones.

The non-pregnant human uterus shows weak spontaneous contractions during the first part of the cycle and stronger, more coordinated contractions in the latter part and during menstruation. In early pregnancy, uterine movements are depressed, but towards the end of the

9-month period, contractions start to occur; these increase in force and become fully coordinated during parturition. Administration of **oestrogen** hyperpolarises myometrial cells, suppressing spontaneous activity, and subsequent administration of **progesterone** increases this effect. During pregnancy, a condition of electrical and mechanical quiescence and relative inexcitability is produced by endogenous progesterone.

Innervation of the uterus and the action of sympathomimetic amines

The nerve supply to the uterus includes both excitatory and inhibitory sympathetic fibres.

In both pregnant and non-pregnant women, **adrenaline**, acting on β-adrenoceptors inhibits uterine contractions and **noradrenaline**, acting on α-adrenoceptors, stimulates them. Selective β$_2$-adrenoceptor agonists, such as **ritodrine**, **salbutamol** and **terbutaline**, inhibit both the spontaneous and oxytocin-induced contractions of the pregnant uterus. These uterine relaxants are used in selected patients to prevent premature labour. Pulmonary oedema can occur.

Posterior pituitary hormones and uterine function

As explained in Chapter 24, the neurohypophyseal hormones are important in the regulation of myometrial activity. **Oxytocin** release can be stimulated by certain peripheral stimuli such as suckling. Cervical dilatation can also cause its release. The non-pregnant human uterus and the uterus in early pregnancy have greater sensitivity to **vasopressin** than to oxytocin.

DRUGS CAUSING CONTRACTION OF THE UTERUS

Agents which stimulate the pregnant uterus and are of importance in obstetrics are: oxytocin, ergometrine and the E and F type prostaglandins.

Oxytocin

Oxytocin for clinical use is prepared synthetically. Its chemical structure is given in Figure 24.4. The S–S bond of cystine is crucial for its activity.

Actions

On the uterus. Oxytocin contracts the uterus. At parturition, the uterus has an oestrogen-induced increase in oxytocin receptors and is highly sensitive to oxytocin.

Oxytocin, given by slow intravenous infusion at term, causes regular coordinated contractions which travel from fundus to cervix, and both the amplitude and the frequency of the contractions are related to dose, the uterus relaxing completely between contractions. Large doses cause an increase in the frequency of the contractions such that there is incomplete relaxation between them. Very high doses cause sustained contractions which interfere with blood flow through the placenta and lead to foetal distress or death.

*Other actions.** Oxytocin causes contraction of the myoepithelial cells of the mammary gland, which leads to 'milk let-down'—the expression of milk from the alveoli and ducts. When given by intravenous injection, it also has a vasodilator action. A weak vasopressin-like antidiuretic action, which can result in water retention, occurs if large doses are infused; this may constitute an unwanted effect if oxytocin is used in patients with cardiac or renal disease, or pre-eclampsia.**

The clinical use of oxytocin is given in the box on page 451.

Pharmacokinetic aspects

Oxytocin can be given by intravenous injection or intramuscularly, but is most often given by intravenous infusion. It is inactivated in the liver and kidneys and by circulating placental oxytocinase.

Unwanted effects with large doses include transient but serious hypotension with associated tachycardia. If oxytocin is given by rapid intravenous injection, ECG abnormalities can occur, as can water retention in both mother and foetus.

An analogue of oxytocin that competitively inhibits the effect of oxytocin and could suppress preterm labour is being investigated.

Ergometrine

Ergot (*Claviceps purpurea*) is a fungus which grows on rye and on certain grasses and contains a surprising variety of pharmacologically active substances (see Ch. 9). Ergot poisoning, which occurred frequently in Europe in the past, was often associated with abortion and it was clear that ergot contained an active principle which had powerful effects on the uterus. In 1935, **ergometrine** was isolated and was recognised as the oxytocic principle in ergot.

Actions

Ergometrine has a rapid stimulant effect on the postpartum human uterus in vivo. Its action depends partly

---

*Oxytocin receptors are found not only in the uterus but in the brain, particularly in the limbic system. Animal experiments have shown that oxytocin is important in mating and parenting behaviour.

**Eclampsia is a pathological condition (involving, among other things, high blood pressure) which can occur in pregnant women.

on the state of the organ, thus on a normally contracting uterus, ergometrine has little effect, but if the uterus is quiescent, it initiates a prolonged series of strong contractions.

Ergometrine has a moderate degree of vasoconstrictor action.

The mechanism of action of ergometrine on smooth muscle is not understood. It is possible that it acts on α-adrenoceptors, like the related alkaloid ergotamine, which is a partial agonist on these receptors (see Ch. 8), though it may produce effects through stimulation of 5-HT receptors.

The clinical use of ergometrine is given in the box on this page.

Pharmacokinetic aspects and unwanted effects

Ergometrine can be given orally, intramuscularly or intravenously. It has a very rapid onset of action and its effect lasts for 3–6 hours.

Ergometrine can produce vomiting, probably by an effect on dopamine D_2-receptors in the chemoreceptor trigger zone (see Fig. 21.6). Vasoconstriction with an increase in blood pressure associated with nausea, blurred vision and headache can occur, as can vasospasm of the coronary arteries resulting in anginal pain.

Prostaglandins

Endogenous prostaglandins

The endometrium and the myometrium of the uterus have significant prostaglandin-synthesising capacity, particularly in the second, proliferative phase of the menstrual cycle. The vasoconstrictor prostaglandin, **PGF$_{2\alpha}$**, is generated in particularly large amounts and is thought by some to be implicated in the ischaemic necrosis of the endometrium which precedes menstruation (though it is said by others to have little vasoconstrictor action on human blood vessels). The vasodilator prostaglandins, **PGE$_2$** and **prostacyclin**, are also generated by the uterus. (Prostaglandins are discussed in detail in Ch. 12.)

In addition to their vasoactive properties, the E- and F-type prostaglandins cause contractions of both the non-pregnant and the pregnant uterus. The sensitivity of the uterine muscle to prostaglandins increases during gestation.

Prostaglandins play a significant role in two of the main disorders of menstruation, **dysmenorrhoea** (painful menstruation) and **menorrhagia** (excessive blood loss).

Menorrhagia, in the absence of uterine pathology, appears to be due to a combination of increased vasodilatation and reduced haemostasis, the increased vasodilatation being associated with an increased production of PGE_2 and PGI_2 as compared with $PGF_{2\alpha}$. Haemostasis depends on both platelet aggregation and fibrin formation, the former providing a surface for the latter (Fig. 17.1) There are fewer platelets in menstrual blood than in normal blood, and they have a reduced capacity to aggregate and to synthesise thromboxane A_2. Increased generation by the uterus of prostacyclin (which inhibits platelet aggregation) will clearly impair haemostasis as well as causing vasodilatation.

Dysmenorrhoea of the spasmodic type is now known to be associated with increased production of the spasmogenic prostaglandins, PGE_2 and $PGF_{2\alpha}$.

Non-steroidal anti-inflammatory drugs (see Ch. 13) can be used with success to treat spasmodic dysmenorrhoea. Taken for a few days immediately before and during the marked blood loss, they can also be of value in menorrhagia, though 20% of patients with this condition do not respond at all.

Exogenous prostaglandins

On the pregnant uterus, prostaglandins of the E and F series promote a series of coordinated contractions of the body of the organ, along with relaxation of the cervix; they also, in contrast to oxytocin, tend to increase uterine tone. In early and middle pregnancy, oxytocin generally cannot cause expulsion of the uterine contents (since,

Clinical uses of drugs acting on the uterus

Myometrial stimulants (oxytocics)
- Oxytocin is used to induce or augment labour when the uterine muscle is not functioning adequately. It can also be used to treat postpartum haemorrhage.
- Ergometrine can be used to treat postpartum haemorrhage.
- A preparation containing both oxytocin and ergometrine is used for the management of the third stage of labour; the two agents together can also be used, prior to surgery, to control bleeding due to incomplete abortion.
- Dinoprostone given by the extra-amniotic route is used for late (second trimester) therapeutic abortion; given as vaginal gel, it is used for cervical ripening and induction of labour.
- Gemeprost, given as vaginal pessary, following mifepristone, is used as a medical alternative to surgical termination of pregnancy (up to 63 days' gestation).
- Carboprost can be used to treat postpartum haemorrhage in patients who do not respond to oxytocin or ergometrine.

Myometrial relaxants
- β-adrenoceptor agonists (e.g. ritodrine) are used to prevent preterm labour.

at this time, the myometrial cells are not very sensitive to its action), whereas the prostaglandins can, and are therefore abortifacient.

The prostaglandins used in obstetrics are **dinoprostone** (PGE$_2$), **carboprost** (15-methyl PGF$_{2\alpha}$) and **gemeprost** (a PGE$_1$ analogue). Dinoprostone can be given intravaginally as a gel or as tablets or by the extra-amniotic route as a solution. Carboprost is given by deep intramuscular injection. Gemeprost is given intravaginally by pessary.

The clinical use of prostaglandin analogues is given on page 451.

Unwanted effects include uterine pain, nausea and vomiting, which are reported to occur in about 50% of patients when the drugs are used as abortifacients. Dinoprost may cause cardiovascular collapse if it escapes into the circulation after intra-amniotic injection. Phlebitis at the site of intravenous infusion has occurred. Systemic side-effects are also likely to occur when prostaglandins are given as abortifacients, by intravaginal

pessary. When combined with **mifepristone**, a progestogen antagonist (see p. 442), which sensitises the uterus to prostaglandins, lower doses of the prostaglandins (e.g. misoprostol; see p. 443) can be used for termination of pregnancy, and the incidence and severity of side-effects are correspondingly reduced.

Drugs acting on the uterus

- At parturition, oxytocin causes regular coordinated uterine contractions, each followed by relaxation; ergometrine, an ergot alkaloid, causes uterine contractions with an increase in basal tone.
- Prostaglandin analogues, e.g. dinoprostone (PGE$_2$) and dinoprost (PGF$_{2\alpha}$), cause increased tone and contractions of the body of the pregnant uterus but relaxation of the cervix.
- β_2-adrenoceptor analogues (e.g. ritodrine) inhibit both spontaneous and oxytocin-induced contractions of the pregnant uterus.

REFERENCES AND FURTHER READING

Endocrine aspects

Bagatelle C J, Bremner W J 1996 Androgens in men—uses and abuses. N Engl J Med 334: 707–714 (*A review of the biology, pharmacology and use of androgens*)

Baird D T, Glasier A F 1993 Editorial: hormonal contraception. N Engl J Med 328: 1543–1549 (*A careful review of the pros and cons of hormonal contraception*)

Brinton L A, Schairer C 1997 Postmenopausal hormone replacement therapy—time for a reappraisal? N Engl J Med 336: 1821–1822 (*Editorial comment on 20-year retrospective study of 34 000 women*)

Davidson N E 1995 Breast versus heart versus bone. N Engl J Med 332: 1638–1639

Eastell R 1998 Treatment of postmenopausal osteoporosis. N Engl J Med 338: 736–746 (*Excellent, comprehensive review of pathophysiology and drug treatment of postmenopausal osteoporosis, with review of clinical trials of drugs used, and future therapies*)

Fuleihan G E-H 1997 Tissue-specific estrogens—the promise for the future. N Engl J Med 337: 1686–1687 (*Editorial on potential use of 'designer oestrogens'*)

Ginsberg J (ed) 1996 Drug therapy in reproductive endocrinology. Arnold, London, p 372 (*An excellent, up-to-date, multi-author textbook on the reproductive system, covering pathophysiology, pharmacology and clinical aspects*)

Grainger D J, Metcalf J C 1996 Tamoxifen: teaching an old drug new tricks. Nature Med 2: 381–385 (*An outline of the actions and mechanisms of action of tamoxifen, namely the anticancer, anti-osteoporotic effects, etc.*)

Grodstein F et al. 1996 Postmenopausal estrogen and progestin use and the risk of cardiovascular disease. N Engl J Med 335: 453–460 (*A retrospective study of data on 59 337 women that provides evidence that progestin does not decrease cardioprotection when added to HRT regimes*)

Guillebaud J 1998 Time for emergency contraception with levonorgestrol alone. Lancet 352: 46 (*A commentary that expands on the title*)

Hemminki E 1996 Oral contraceptives and breast cancer. Br Med J 313: 63–64 (*An editorial summarising the results of a study that analysed the data from 150 000 women*)

Hotchkiss J, Knobil E 1994 The menstrual cycle and its control. In Knobil E, Neil J D (eds) The physiology of reproduction. Raven Press, New York, ch 48, pp 711–749

Jacobs J 1996 Not for everybody. Br Med J 313: 351–352 (*One side of a debate on the desirability of prescribing HRT, the opposite point of view being given by Toozs-Hobson P, Cardozo L 1996*)

Khaw K-T 1998 Hormone replacement therapy again: Risk-benefit relation differs between population and individuals. Brit Med J 316: 1842–1843 (*Emphasises concerns over the risk-benefit balance of long-term use of HRT in healthy women*).

LaCroix A Z, Burke W 1997 Breast cancer and hormone replacement therapy. Lancet 350: 1042–1043

Landers J P, Spelsberg T C 1992 New concepts in steroid hormone expression: transcription factors, proto-oncogenes, and the cascade model for steroid regulation of gene expression. Crit Rev Eukaryotic Gene Expression 2: 19–63 (*The molecular biology of steroid hormones*)

McCarthy M, Altemus M 1997 Central nervous system actions of oxytocin and modulation of behaviour in humans. Mol Med Today 3: 269–275 (*A review of recent work*)

McPherson K 1996 Third generation oral contraception and venous thromboembolism. Br Med J 312: 68–69 (*Editorial analysing the problem in the title and quoting three other papers on the subject in the same issue*)

Mascarenhas L 1994 Long-acting methods of contraception: much to offer. Br Med J 308: 991–992 (*Editorial*)

Neven P, De Muylder X 1995 Hormonal interventions and cancer risk. Lancet 346 (suppl): 8 *(A short analysis of the 1995 key references on this topic)*

Pedersen A T, Lidegaard Ø et al. 1997 Hormone replacement therapy and risk of non-fatal stroke. Lancet 350: 1277–1283

Pritchard K I 1998 Is tamoxifen effective in prevention of breast cancer? Lancet 352: 80–81 *(A large trial in 13,388 women has shown 45% reduction in breast cancer; two smaller trials had not. This is discussed)*

Rosing J, Tans G, et al. 1997 Oral contraceptives and venous thromboembolism: different sensitivities to activated protein C in women using second- and third-generation oral contraceptives. Br J Haematol 97: 233–238 *(A proposed explanation for the thrombogenic potential of third-generation pills)*

Toozs-Hobson P, Cardozo L 1996 Hormone replacement therapy for all? Universal prescription is desirable. Br Med J 313: 350–351 *(One side of a debate on the desirability of prescribing HRT, the opposite point of view being given by Jacobs J 1996)*

Utiger R D 1998 A pill for impotence. N Engl J Med *(Editorial comment)*

Vandenbroucke J P, Rosendaal F R 1997 End of the line for 'third generation-pill' controversy? *(A short article quoting evidence for the mechanisms whereby newer progestogens increase the risk of thromboembolism)*

WHO Collaborative study of cardiovascular disease and steroid hormone contraception. Results of international multicentre case-control studies on: (1) Ischaemic stroke and combined oral contraceptives. Lancet 1996 348: 498–510; (2) Acute myocardial infarction and combined oral contraceptives Lancet 1997 349: 1202–1209

Wise J 1997 Hormone replacement therapy increases the risk of breast cancer. Br Med J 315: 969

Wiseman H 1994 Tamoxifen: new membrane-mediated mechanisms of action and therapeutic advances. Trends Pharmacol Sci 15: 83–89

Uterus

Huzar G, Roberts J M 1982 Biochemistry and pharmacology of the myometrium and labor: regulation at the cellular and molecular levels. Am J Obstet Gynecol 142: 225–236 *(A review on uterine muscle)*

Wray S 1993 Uterine contraction and physiological mechanisms of modulation. Am J Physiol 264 (Cell Physiol 33): C1–C18 *(A review on uterine function)*

27

Bone metabolism

BONE STRUCTURE AND COMPOSITION

The human skeleton consists of 80% cortical bone and 20% trabecular bone. Cortical bone is the dense, compact outer part and trabecular bone the inner meshwork. The former predominates in the shafts of long bones, the latter in the vertebrae, the epiphyses of long bones and the iliac crest. Trabecular bone, having a large surface area, is metabolically more active and more affected by factors that lead to bone loss (see below).

The main minerals in bone are calcium and phosphates. More than 99% of the calcium in the body is in the skeleton, mostly as crystalline hydroxyapatite (see above) but some as non-crystalline phosphates and carbonates; together, these make up half the bone mass. Phosphates are also a major constituent of bone and are important in modifying the calcium concentration in bone and other tissues, in part by an effect on the synthesis of calcitriol (outlined in Fig. 27.4).

The organic matrix of bone is osteoid, the principal component of which is collagen; but there are also other components such as osteocalcin (a vitamin-K-dependent protein that binds calcium by virtue of γ-carboxyglutamic

acid residues; see Ch. 17, pp. 314–315) and various phosphoproteins, one of which, osteonectin, binds to both calcium and collagen and thus links these two major constituents of bone matrix. Calcium phosphate crystals in the form of hydroxyapatite $[Ca_{10}(PO_4)_6(OH)_2]$ are deposited in the osteoid, converting it into hard bone matrix.

BONE REMODELLING

Bone mass is continuously being remodelled—some bone being resorbed and new bone being laid down—so that gradually all the bone in the body will turn over during an average lifetime and adult humans wind up with a skeleton completely different from the one they started out with.

Remodelling involves the following:

- cells—osteoblasts that secrete new bone matrix and osteoclasts that break it down
- the actions of cytokines such as the bone morphogenic proteins (also termed osteogenic proteins), interleukin-6 (IL-6) and insulin-like growth factor-1 (IGF-1)
- the turnover of bone minerals—particularly calcium and phosphate
- the action of hormones: parathyroid hormone, the vitamin D family and calcitonin.

Diet, drugs and physical factors (exercise, loading) also affect remodelling. Formation of new bone predominates in the young, bone loss in the old. Bone loss—of 0.5–1% per year—starts in the 35–40 age group in both sexes. The rate accelerates by as much as 10-fold during the menopause in women (or with castration in men) and then gradually settles at 1–3% per year. The loss during the menopause is due to *increased osteoclast activity* (see below) and affects mainly trabecular bone; the later loss in both sexes with increasing age, is due to *decreased osteoblast numbers* (see below) and affects mainly cortical bone.

We discuss first the factors involved in bone re-modelling, then bone disorders and then the drugs used to modify bone remodelling and treat bone disorders.

FACTORS INVOLVED IN BONE REMODELLING

CELLS AND CYTOKINES

A cycle of remodelling starts with recruitment of osteo-clasts, by cytokines, e.g. IL-6. The osteoclasts adhere to an area of trabecular bone and move along it digging a pit by secreting hydrogen ions and proteolytic enzymes; this gradually liberates factors such as IGF-1 that are embedded in the osteoid (Fig. 27.1). These factors recruit and activate successive teams of osteoblasts that have been stimulated to develop from precursor cells by para-thyroid hormone and calcitriol, and are awaiting the call to duty (see Fig. 27.1 and below). The osteoblasts

invade the site, synthesising and secreting the organic matrix of bone, the osteoid. The osteoblasts and their precursors, stimulated as described above, secrete IGF-1 (which becomes embedded in the osteoid; see above), and eventually other cytokines such as IL-6 and IL-11, which in turn recruit osteoclasts—and we are back to the beginning of the cycle. (See Alper 1994, Manolagas & Jilka 1995, Whitfield & Morley 1995.)

Other important cytokines involved in bone re-modelling are the bone morphogenic proteins.

Bone morphogenic proteins

Bone morphogenic proteins (BMPs)—also known as osteogenic proteins (OPs)—are a family of cytokines related to the transforming growth factor-β superfamily. Fifteen BMPs have been recognised and they have wide-ranging actions, affecting the growth and differentiation of many tissues including bone, kidney, teeth, eyes, skin

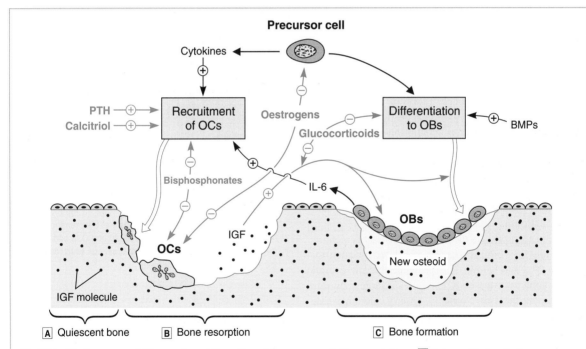

Fig 27.1 The bone-remodelling cycle and the action of hormones, cytokines and drugs. [A] Quiescent trabecular bone. Cytokines such as insulin-like growth factor (IGF), shown as dots, embedded in the bone matrix. [B] Bone resorption. Mobile multinuclear osteoclasts (OCs) move towards the quiescent area, resorbing bone and releasing the embedded cytokines. [C] Bone formation. The released cytokines recruit osteoblasts (OBs) which lay down osteoid and embed cytokines in it, and release interleukin-6 (IL-6), which recruits osteoclasts. The osteoid then becomes mineralised and lining cells cover the area (not shown). (PTH = parathyroid hormone; BMPs = bone morphogenic proteins. Oestrogens cause apoptosis (programmed cell death) of osteoclasts through transforming growth factor-β. Note that pharmacological concentrations of glucocorticoids have the effects specified above, but physiological concentrations are *required* for osteoblast differentiation; also that under some circumstances, parathyroid hormone can inhibit osteoblast proliferation.

and heart. BMP-2 and BMP-7 (the latter also known as OP-1) are the members of the family important in bone remodelling; in particular, they stimulate the differentiation of bone marrow stem cells into osteoblasts and may stimulate local mesenchymal cells to differentiate into chondrocytes (which secrete collagen). Bone itself contains BMPs and the main production site of BMP-7 is the kidney—which also generates another important morphogen, erythropoietin (see Ch. 18). BMP-2 and BMP-7 are being tested in multicentre trials for their ability to facilitate union of fractures and promote healing of bone defects.

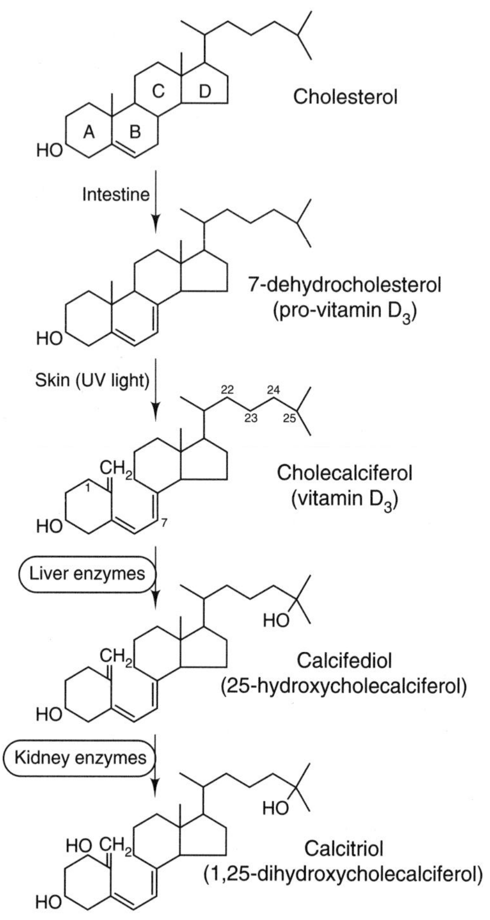

THE TURNOVER OF BONE MINERALS

The main bone minerals are calcium and phosphates.

Calcium metabolism

The daily turnover of bone minerals during remodelling involves about 700 mg of calcium. Calcium has numerous roles in physiological functioning. Intracellular calcium constitutes only a small proportion of body calcium, but it has a major role in cellular function (see Ch. 2). An influx of calcium with increase of calcium in the cytosol is part of the signal transduction mechanism of many cells; thus the concentration of calcium in the extracellular fluid and the plasma needs to be controlled with great precision. The concentration of calcium in the cytoplasm of cells is about 100 nmol/l, whereas in the plasma it is about 2.5 mmol/l. As described below, the normal plasma calcium concentration is regulated by complex interactions between **parathyroid hormone** and various forms of **vitamin D** (Figs 27.2, 27.3 and 27.4). **Calcitonin** also plays a part.

Calcium absorption in the intestine involves a calcium-binding protein whose synthesis is regulated by calcitriol (see Fig. 27.3 and below). It is probable that the overall calcium content of the body is regulated largely by this absorption mechanism. Normally, urinary calcium excretion remains more or less constant. However, with high blood calcium concentrations, urinary excretion increases, and with low blood concentrations, urinary excretion can be reduced by parathyroid hormone and calcitriol, both of which enhance calcium reabsorption in the renal tubules (Fig. 27.3).

Phosphate metabolism

Phosphates are not only an important constituent of bone they are critically important in the structure and function of all the cells of the body. They play a significant part

Fig. 27.2 The basic structures of the members of the vitamin D3 system. The B ring of the precursor 7-dehydrocholesterol is cleaved by UV irradiation. Both vitamin D2 (calciferol) and its precursor, ergosterol (neither shown here), have a double bond between C22 and C23 and a methyl group at C24. Hydroxylation at various sites results in the active vitamin D metabolites.

in enzymic reactions in the cell; they have roles as intracellular buffers and in the excretion of hydrogen ions in the kidney.

Phosphate absorption is an energy-requiring process regulated by calcitriol (see below). Phosphate deposition in bone, as hydroxyapatite, depends on the plasma concentration of parathyroid hormone, which, with calcitriol, tends to mobilise both calcium and phosphate from the bone matrix. Phosphate is excreted by the kidney; here parathyroid hormone inhibits reabsorption and thus increases excretion.

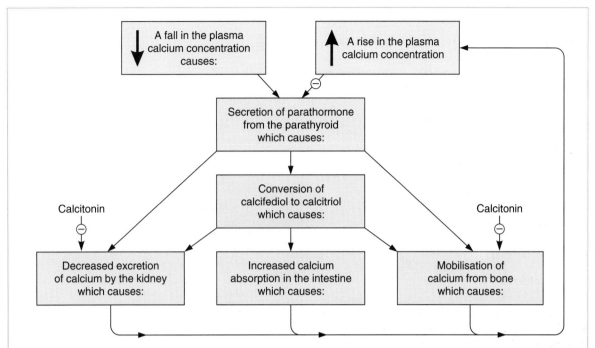

Fig. 27.3 **The main factors involved in maintaining the concentration of calcium in the plasma.** Calcifediol and calcitriol are metabolites of vitamin D_3 and constitute the 'hormones' 25-hydroxy-vitamin D_3 and 1,25-dihydroxy-vitamin D_3 respectively. (Calcitonin, secreted by the thyroid, inhibits calcium mobilisation from bone and decreases its resorption in the kidney, thus reducing blood calcium.)

HORMONES INVOLVED IN BONE METABOLISM AND REMODELLING

The main hormones involved in bone metabolism and remodelling are parathyroid hormone, the vitamin D family and calcitonin. Glucocorticoids also affect bone.

Parathyroid hormone (PTH)

Parathyroid hormone is an important regulator of calcium metabolism. It maintains the plasma calcium concentration by mobilising calcium from bone, by promoting its reabsorption by the kidney and, in particular, by stimulating the synthesis of calcitriol which in turn increases calcium absorption from the intestine and synergises with PTH in mobilising bone calcium (Figs 27.3 and 27.4). PTH promotes phosphate excretion, and thus its net effect is to increase the concentration of calcium in the plasma and lower that of phosphate.

The mobilisation of calcium from bone by PTH is mediated, at least in part, by stimulation of the recruitment and activation of osteoclasts. In some circumstances, osteoblast activity is also inhibited (not shown in Fig. 27.1).

PTH-related agents—fragments of PTH—paradoxically *stimulate* osteoblast activity and enhance bone formation.

PTH is synthesised in the cells of the parathyroid glands and stored in vesicles. The principal factor controlling secretion is the concentration of ionised calcium in the plasma, low plasma calcium stimulating secretion. The parathyroid cell has a calcium sensor in its membrane and calcium binding leads to inhibition of parathyroid hormone secretion.

Vitamin D

Vitamin D is a prehormone which is converted in the body into a number of biologically active metabolites. These function as true hormones, circulating in the blood and regulating the activities of various cell types (see Reichel et al 1989). The main action is the maintenance of plasma calcium by increasing calcium absorption in the intestine, mobilising calcium from bone and decreasing its renal excretion (see Fig. 27.3). Vitamin D itself is really a family of sterol derivatives. In humans, there are two sources of vitamin D:

- dietary ergocalciferol (D_2), derived from ergosterol in plants

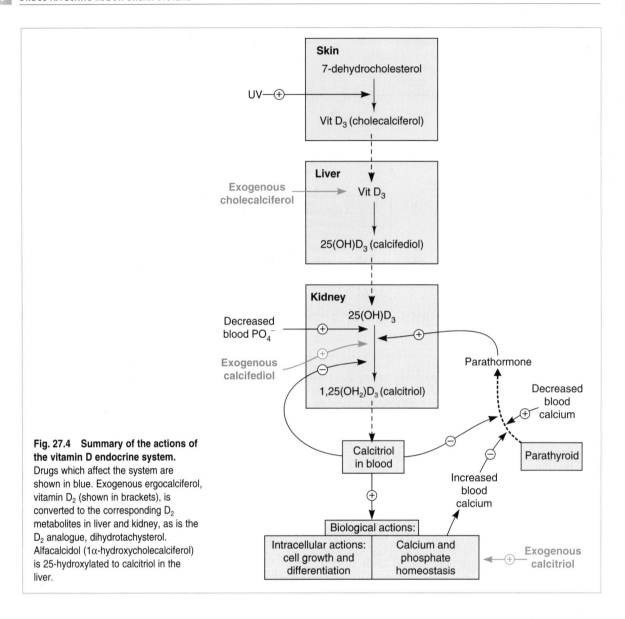

Fig. 27.4 Summary of the actions of the vitamin D endocrine system.
Drugs which affect the system are shown in blue. Exogenous ergocalciferol, vitamin D_2 (shown in brackets), is converted to the corresponding D_2 metabolites in liver and kidney, as is the D_2 analogue, dihydrotachysterol. Alfacalcidol (1α-hydroxycholecalciferol) is 25-hydroxylated to calcitriol in the liver.

- cholecalciferol (D_3) generated in the skin from 7-dehydrocholesterol by the action of ultraviolet irradiation, the 7-dehydrocholesterol having been formed from cholesterol in the wall of the intestine (Table 27.1).

Cholecalciferol (vitamin D_3) is a secosteroid, i.e. a steroid in which one of the rings has undergone fission, in this case ring B. The basic structure is outlined in Figure 27.2. It is converted to 25-hydroxy-vitamin D_3 (*calcifediol*) in the liver, and this is converted to a series of other metabolites of varying activity in the kidney, the most

potent of which is 1,25-dihydroxy-vitamin D_3 (*calcitriol*) (see Figs 27.2 and 27.4).

Calcifediol is the main vitamin D metabolite in the circulation. The synthesis of calcitriol from calcifediol is regulated by parathyroid hormone, and is also influenced by the phosphate concentration in the plasma and by the calcitriol concentration itself through a negative feedback mechanism (Fig. 27.4). Receptors for calcitriol have been identified in virtually every tissue except liver and it is now considered that calcitriol may be important in the functioning of many cell types, possibly participating in the regulation of intracellular calcium and in the

Table 27.1 Vitamin D and its main derivatives

Compound	Alternative name	Comments
Vitamin D_3	Cholecalciferol*	Formed in skin from dehydrocholesterol by ultraviolet radiation
Vitamin D_2	Ergocalciferol* (calciferol)*	Formed in plants by ultraviolet radiation
25-hydroxy-vitamin D_3	Calcifediol	Formed in liver from cholecalciferol or ergosterol. Main 'storage' form of vitamin D. Thought to be important in reabsorbing calcium in the renal tubules and regulating calcium flux in muscle
1,25-hydroxy-vitamin D_3	Calcitriol*	Formed from cacifediol in kidney. Most potent metabolite in regulating plasma [Ca^{2+}]
Analogue of vitamin D_3	Dihydrotachysterol*	A crystalline compound prepared by reduction of vitamin D_2. Activated by 25-hydroxylation in the liver
1α-hydroxycholecalciferol	Alfacalcidol	A synthetic 1α-hydroxylated derivative of vitamin D_3. Undergoes hepatic 25-hydroxylation to calcitriol

*Compounds available for clinical use

control of cell differentiation and growth—particularly in bone marrow. (The vitamin D endocrine system is reviewed by Reichel et al. 1989.)

The main actions of calcitriol are the stimulation of absorption of calcium and phosphate in the intestine and the mobilisation of calcium from bone, but it also increases calcium reabsorption in the kidney tubules (Fig. 27.3).

Its effect on bone involves promotion of maturation of osteoclasts and indirect stimulation of their activity (Figs 27.1 and 27.3). It decreases collagen synthesis by osteoblasts, and its effect on these cells is by the classical steroid pathway, involving intracellular receptors and an effect on the DNA. However, the effect on bone is complex, and is clearly not confined to mobilising calcium, since in clinical vitamin D deficiency (see below), in which the mineralisation of bone is impaired, administration of vitamin D restores bone formation. One explanation may lie in the fact that calcitriol stimulates synthesis of osteocalcin, the vitamin-K-dependent, calcium-binding protein of bone matrix.

Oestrogens

During reproductive life in the female, oestrogens have an important role in maintenance of bone integrity. They inhibit the cytokines that recruit osteoclasts and oppose the bone-resorbing, calcium-mobilising action of PTH.

Calcitonin

Calcitonin is a hormone secreted by the specialised 'C' cells found in the thyroid follicles.

The main action of calcitonin is on bone; it inhibits calcium resorption by binding to a specific receptor on osteoclasts inhibiting their action. In the kidney it decreases the reabsorption of both calcium and phosphate in the proximal tubules. Its overall effect is to decrease the plasma calcium concentration.

Secretion is determined mainly by the plasma calcium concentration.

Glucocorticoids

Physiological concentrations of glucocorticoids are required for osteoblast differentiation. Excessive pharmacological concentrations inhibit bone formation by inhibiting osteoblast differentiation and activity (see Fig. 27.1). This latter effect is also evident when pathological concentrations of endogenous glucocorticoids are present as in Cushing's syndrome (see Fig. 24.8).

Bone remodelling

- Bone is continuously remodelled throughout life. The events of the remodelling cycle are as follows:
  - osteoclasts dig pits in trabecular bone into which osteoblasts secrete osteoid (bone matrix) that consists mainly of collagen, but also contains osteocalcin, osteonectin and phosphoproteins
  - the osteoid is then mineralised, i.e. complex calcium phosphate crystals (hydroxyapatites) are deposited.
- Bone metabolism and mineralisation involves the action of parathyroid hormone, the vitamin D family, cytokines (e.g. bone morphogenic proteins) and calcitonin.

DISORDERS OF BONE

Disorders of the structure of bone

The reduction of bone mass with distortion of the microarchitecture is termed 'osteoporosis'; a reduction in the mineral content is termed 'osteopenia'. Osteoporotic bone can fracture easily after minimal trauma—and frequently does. The commonest causes of osteoporosis are postmenopausal deficiency of oestrogen and age-related deterioration in bone homeostasis, but it can also result from other factors such as excessive glucocorticoid or thyroxine administration. Since life expectancy has increased significantly, osteoporosis has become an important public health problem and drugs that prevent its development are being sought actively. Other diseases of bone requiring drug therapy are *osteomalacia* and *rickets* (the juvenile form of osteomalacia) in which there are defects in bone mineralisation due to vitamin D deficiency, and *Paget's disease* in which there is distortion of the processes of bone resorption and remodelling.

Disorders of bone mineral metabolism

Hypocalcaemia occurs with hypoparathyroidism, vitamin D deficiencies, congenital rickets and some kidney diseases; *hypercalcaemia* with hyperparathyroidism and some malignancies.

Phosphate deficiency and *hypophosphataemia* can occur in nutritional deficiency states (e.g. in alcoholics and patients receiving parenteral nutrition).

Hyperphosphataemia is a common problem in patients with renal failure and is treated with calcium- or aluminium-containing antacids (Ch. 21) that bind phosphate and prevent its absorption from the gut.

DRUGS USED IN BONE DISORDERS

BISPHOSPHONATES

Bisphosphonates (also termed diphosphonates) are enzyme-resistant analogues of pyrophosphate—which normally inhibits mineralisation in bone. In bisphosphonates, the P–O–P structure of pyrophosphate is replaced by P–C–P. They reduce the turnover of bone in a dose-dependent manner—mainly by inhibiting recruitment and promoting apoptosis (cell suicide) of osteoclasts (Fig. 27.1). They also indirectly stimulate osteoblast activity.

The efficacy of bisphosphonates in retarding bone loss in the elderly, and reducing the incidence of fractures, has been confirmed in long-term trials.

The main bisphosphonates available for clinical use are **disodium etidronate** and **alendronate**. Others are **disodium pamidronate** and **sodium clodronate**.

Bisphosphonates are given orally and are poorly absorbed. About 50% of a dose accumulates at sites of bone mineralisation, where it remains, potentially for months or years, until the bone is resorbed. The free drug is excreted unchanged by the kidney.

Absorption is impaired by food, particularly milk, so the drugs must be taken on an empty stomach, which can cause gastric pain and oesophagitis. More potent drugs now in development may overcome these problems.

Unwanted effects. These include gastrointestinal upsets and occasionally bone pain. Alendronate can cause oesophagitis.

Disodium etidronate can *increase* the risk of fractures due to reduced calcification of bone; this is less likely if it is given cyclically.

Clinical use of bisphosphonates

- To treat Paget's disease of bone.
- To treat malignant hypercalcaemia.
- As an alternative to, or in addition to oestrogens for postmenopausal osteoporosis.
- For treating glucocorticoid-induced osteoporosis.

They are under investigation for the treatment of cancer metastases in bone.

OESTROGENS AND ANTI-OESTROGENS

Oestrogens have an important place in the prevention of postmenopausal osteoporosis (discussed in Ch. 26).

Anti-oestrogens (e.g. **tamoxifen**) have anti-oestrogenic action on mammary tissue but oestrogenic action on bone, plasma lipids, and endometrium. Their anti-osteoporotic effect in bone is thought to be due to up-regulating transforming growth factor-β which has a role in controlling the balance between osteoblasts and osteoclasts (see Grainger & Metcalf 1996). A newer anti-oestrogen—a member of a new class of agents, the selective oestrogen receptor modulators—**raloxifene**, is currently in clinical trial.

VITAMIN D AND PARATHYROID HORMONE (PTH)

There is little or no clinical use for PTH as such; but, as mentioned above, fragments of PTH paradoxically stimulate osteoblast activity and enhance bone formation;

they are in clinical trial for the treatment of osteoporosis (see Whitfield & Morley 1995).

Hypoparathyroidism is treated by vitamin D—acute hypoparathyroidism necessitating the use of intravenous calcium and injectable vitamin D preparations.

The main vitamin D preparation used clinically is **ergocalciferol**; also available for clinical use are **alfacalcidol** and **calcitriol** (Table 27.1). All can be given orally and are well absorbed from the intestine. Vitamin D preparations are fat-soluble and bile salts are necessary for absorption. Injectable forms of calciferol are available.

Pharmacokinetic aspects

Given orally, vitamin D is bound to a specific α-globulin in the blood. The plasma half-life is about 22 hours but vitamin D can be found in the fat for many months. The main route of elimination is in the faeces.

The clinical use of vitamin D preparations is given in the box below.

Unwanted effects

Excessive intake of vitamin D causes hypercalcaemia, the manifestations of which include constipation, depression, weakness and fatigue. Renal effects include a reduced ability to concentrate the urine, resulting in polyuria and polydipsia. If hypercalcaemia persists, calcium salts are deposited in the kidney and urine causing renal failure and kidney stones.

Some anticonvulsant drugs (e.g. phenytoin; see Ch. 36) increase the requirement for vitamin D.

Clinical use of vitamin D preparations

- To prevent and to treat various forms of rickets, osteomalacia and vitamin D deficiency due to malabsorption and liver disease (ergocalciferol).
- To treat the hypocalcaemia associated with hypoparathyroidism (ergocalciferol).
- To treat the osteodystrophy of chronic renal failure, which is due to decreased calcitriol generation (calcitriol or alphacalcidol).

Plasma calcium levels should be routinely monitored (usually weekly) during therapy with vitamin D.

CALCITONIN

The preparations available for clinical use (see the clinical box on this page) are porcine (natural) **calcitonin** and **salcatonin** (synthetic salmon calcitonin). Synthetic

human calcitonin is now also available. Porcine calcitonin may contain traces of thyroid hormones and can lead to the production of antibodies. Calcitonin is given by subcutaneous or intramuscular injection, and there may be a local inflammatory action at the injection site. It can also be given intranasally. Its plasma half-life is 4–12 minutes, but its action lasts for several hours.

Unwanted effects include nausea and vomiting. Facial flushing may occur, as may a tingling sensation in the hands and an unpleasant taste in the mouth.

Clinical use of calcitonin/salcatonin

- To lower the plasma calcium in hypercalcaemia—for example that associated with neoplasia.
- To treat Paget's disease of bone (it relieves the pain and reduces some of the neurological complications).
- As part of the therapy of postmenopausal and corticosteroid-induced osteoporosis.

CALCIUM SALTS

Calcium salts used therapeutically include **calcium gluconate** and **calcium lactate**, given orally. Calcium gluconate is also used for intravenous injection; intramuscular injection is not used because it causes local necrosis. An oral preparation of **hydroxyapatite** is available.

The clinical use of the calcium salts is given in the box on this page.

Unwanted effects. Oral calcium salts can cause gastrointestinal disturbance. Intravenous administration requires care, especially in patients on cardiac glycosides (see Ch. 14).

Clinical use of calcium salts

- In dietary deficiencies and for chronic hypocalcaemia due to hypoparathyroidism or malabsorption (given orally).
- Hypocalcaemic tetany (given i.v.).
- Osteoporosis:
  - with oestrogen and calcitonin in postmenopausal osteoporosis; regimes involving calcium with vitamin D preparations and/or etidronate and/or calcitriol are also used
  - with calcitriol and calcitonin for corticosteroid-induced osteoporosis (see below).
- Cardiac dysrhythmias caused by severe hyperkalaemia (given i.v.).

GLUCOCORTICOIDS

These tend to cause osteoporosis as an unwanted effect. This is due partly to decreased intestinal absorption of calcium and phosphate associated with increased renal excretion, and partly to an inhibition of bone formation. This latter action is due mainly to inhibition of osteoblast differentiation and activity (see Fig. 27.1). These effects can be made use of in the therapy of some types of hypercalcaemia, particularly that associated with sarcoidosis.

Parathyroid, vitamin D and bone mineral homeostasis

- The vitamin D family are true hormones; precursors are converted to calcifediol in the liver, then to the main hormone, calcitriol, in kidney.
- Calcitriol increases plasma calcium by mobilising it from bone, increasing its absorption in the intestine and decreasing its excretion by the kidney.
- Parathyroid hormone (PTH) increases blood calcium by increasing calcitriol synthesis, mobilising calcium from bone and reducing renal calcium excretion.
- Calcitonin (secreted from the thyroid) reduces calcium resorption from bone by inhibiting osteoclast activity.

- Truncated PTH analogues, possibly formed from PTH in vivo, may paradoxically enhance bone formation
- Drugs affecting this system are:
  - the vitamin D preparations: ergocalciferol, calcitriol; given orally
  - the bisphosphonates which reduce bone turnover: disodium etidronate; given orally or by i.v. infusion
  - salcatonin (synthetic salmon calcitonin); given subcutaneously or intranasally
  - oestrogens and anti-oestrogens which control bone density by preventing its resorption; given orally

---

REFERENCES AND FURTHER READING

Alper J 1994 Boning up: newly isolated proteins heal bad breaks. Science 263: 323–324 (*Succinct article on osteogenic proteins*)
Barnes D 1987 Close encounters with an osteoclast. Science 236: 914–916
Bouillon R 1998 The many faces of rickets. N Engl J Med 338: 681–682 (*Editorial: A succinct account of recent information about the metabolic activation of the vitamin D family and its relation to rickets*)
Bushinskey D A, Monk R D 1998 Calcium. The Lancet 352: 306–311 (*Calcium homeostasis, its disorders and the treatment thereof*)
Davidson N E 1995 Breast versus heart versus bone. N Engl J Med 332: 1638–1639
Delmas P D 1996 Editorial: Bisphosphonates in the treatment of bone diseases. N Engl J Med 335: 1836–1837 (*Editorial commentary*)
Eastell R 1998 Treatment of postmenopausal osteoporosis. N Engl J Med 338: 736–746 (*Excellent, comprehensive review of pathophysiology and drug treatment of postmenopausal osteoporosis, with review of clinical trials of drugs used, and future therapies*)
Fraser D R 1995 Vitamin D. Lancet 345: 104–108
Fuleihan G E-H 1997 Tissue-specific estrogens—the promise for the future. N Engl J Med 337: 1686–1687 (*Editorial commentary*)
Grainger D J, Metcalf J C 1996 Tamoxifen: teaching an old drug new tricks Nature Med 2: 381–385
Gustafsson J-Å 1998 Raloxifene: magic bullet for heart and bone. Nature Med 4: 152–153

Horowitz M C 1993 Cytokines and estrogen in bone: anti-osteoporotic effects Science 260: 626–627
Manolagas S C, Jilka R L 1995 Bone marrow, cytokines, and bone remodeling. N Engl J Med 332: 305–311
Raisz L G 1996 Estrogen and bone: new pieces to the puzzle. Nature Med 2: 1077–1078
Ralston S H 1997 Osteoporosis. Br Med J 315: 496–472 (*Good article; covers genetics and osteoporosis, cellular basis of bone remodelling. Good diagrams*)
Reddi A H 1997 BMPs: actions in flesh and bone. Nature Med 3: 837–839
Reichel H, Koeftler H P, Norman A W 1989 The role of the vitamin D endocrine system in health and disease. N Engl J Med 320: 980–991 (*Comprehensive review*)
Reid I R 1997 Editorial: Preventing glucocorticoid-induced osteoporosis. N Engl J Med 337: 420–421
Riggs B L, Melton L J 1992 The prevention and treatment of osteoporosis. N Engl J Med 327: 620–627 (*Valuable review*)
Sambrook P N 1995 Editorial: The treatment of postmenopausal osteoporosis. N Engl J Med 333: 1495-1496 (*Editorial commentary*)
Silverberg S S, Bone H G et al. 1997 Short-term inhibition of parathyroid hormone secretion by a calcium-receptor agonist in patients with primary hyperparathyroidism. N Engl J Med 337: 1506–1510
Whitfield J M, Morley P 1995 Small bone-building fragments of parathyroid hormone: new therapeutic agents for osteoporosis. Trends Pharmacol Sci 16: 382–385 (*Useful review, cheerful diagram of bone remodelling*)

THE CENTRAL NERVOUS SYSTEM

28

Chemical transmission and drug action in the central nervous system

INTRODUCTION

There are two reasons why understanding the action of drugs on the CNS presents a particularly challenging problem. The first is that centrally acting drugs are of special significance to mankind. Not only are they of major clinical and therapeutic importance,* but they are also the drugs that humans most commonly administer to themselves without the intervention of the medical profession (e.g. alcohol, tea and coffee, cannabis, nicotine, opiates, amphetamines and so on). The second reason is that the CNS is functionally far more complex than any other system in the body, and this makes the understanding of drug effects very much more difficult. The relationship between the behaviour of individual cells and that of the organ as a whole is far less direct in the brain than, for example, in the heart or kidney. In these latter organs, a detailed understanding of how a drug affects the cells gives us a fairly clear idea of what effect it will produce on the organ (and on the animal) as a whole. In the brain, this is simply not true. Thus, we may know that a drug mimics the action of 5-HT in its effect on nerve cells, and we know empirically that this type of action is often associated with drugs that cause halluci-

---

*A 1977 study of general practitioners prescribing in the UK showed that one person in six was given a prescription for a centrally acting drug in 1 year. In women aged 45–59 the figure was one in three.

nations, but the link between these two events remains wholly mysterious. In spite of sustained progress in understanding the cellular and biochemical effects produced by centrally acting drugs, the gulf between the description of drug action at this level and the description of drug action at the functional and behavioural level remains, for the most part, very wide. Attempts to bridge it seem, at times, like throwing candy floss into the Grand Canyon.

A few bridgeheads have none the less been established, some more firmly than others. Thus the relationship between dopaminergic pathways in the extrapyramidal system and the effects of drugs in alleviating or exacerbating the symptoms of parkinsonism (see Ch. 31) is clear cut. Also reasonably firm is the link between the functions of noradrenaline and 5-HT in certain parts of the brain and the symptoms of depression (see Ch. 35). Less well established is the connection between hyperactivity in dopaminergic pathways and schizophrenia (see Ch. 34). At the other end of the spectrum attempts to relate the condition of epilepsy to an identifiable cellular disturbance (see Ch. 36) have been very disappointing, even though the abnormal neuronal discharge pattern in epilepsy seems, on the face of it, a much simpler kind of disturbance than, for example, the altered mood of a depressed patient. In this chapter, we outline the general principles governing the action of drugs on the central nervous system. Most neuroactive drugs work by interfering with the chemical signals that underlie brain function, and the next two chapters discuss the major CNS transmitter systems, and the ways in which drugs affect them. In Chapter 31 we focus on neurodegenerative diseases, and the remaining chapters in this section deal with the main classes of neuroactive drugs that are currently in use.

Background information will be found in neurobiology textbooks such as Kandel et al. (1993), Levitan & Kaczmarek (1997) and in texts on neuropharmacology such as Carvey (1998), Cooper et al. (1996). For exhaustive coverage, see Bloom & Kupfer (1995).

CHEMICAL SIGNALLING IN THE NERVOUS SYSTEM

The brain (like every other organ in the body!) is basically a chemical machine, able to control the main functions of a higher animal across timescales ranging from milliseconds (e.g. returning a 100 mph tennis serve) to years (e.g. remembering how to ride a bicycle).* The chemical signalling mechanisms cover a correspondingly wide dynamic range, as summarised, in a very general way, in Figure 28.1. Currently, we understand much about drug effects on events at the fast end of the spectrum—synaptic transmission and neuromodulation—but much less about long-term adaptive processes, though it is quite evident that the latter are of great importance for the neurological and psychiatric disorders that are susceptible to drug treatment.

The original concept of neurotransmission envisaged a substance released by one neuron and acting rapidly, briefly, and at short range on the membrane of an adjacent neuron, producing a change in conductance which either increased or decreased the excitability of the postsynaptic cell. The biology of synaptic transmission, which applies to the central as well as the peripheral nervous system, is described in Chapter 6. It is now clear that chemical mediators within the brain can produce slow and long-lasting effects; that they can act rather diffusely, at a considerable distance from their site of release; and they can produce diverse effects, for example on transmitter synthesis and on the expression of neurotransmitter receptors, in addition to affecting the ionic conductance of the postsynaptic cells. The term '*neuromodulator*' was coined to denote a neuronally released mediator, the actions of which do not conform to the original neurotransmitter concept. The term is not clearly defined, and it covers not only the diffusely acting neuropeptide mediators, but also mediators such as nitric oxide and arachidonic acid metabolites, which are not stored and released like conventional neurotransmitters, and may come from non-neuronal cells as well as neurons. In general, neuromodulation relates to *synaptic plasticity*, including short-term events, such as the regulation of pre-synaptic transmitter release or postsynaptic excitability, and longer-term events such as neuronal gene regulation.

Neurotrophic factors act over even longer timescales to regulate the growth and morphology of neurons, as well as their functional properties.

TARGETS FOR DRUG ACTION

To recapitulate what was discussed in Chapters 1 and 2, most drugs act on one of four types of target proteins, namely *ion channels*, *receptors*, *enzymes* and *transport proteins*; receptors can in turn be divided into four main types, namely *channel-linked receptors*, *G-protein-coupled receptors*, *kinase-linked receptors* and *receptors linked to gene transcription*. All of these can serve as targets for neuroactive drugs, but the most important in relation to drugs in current use are *receptors*, *transporters* and *ion channels*.

In the last two decades, knowledge about these targets in the CNS has accumulated rapidly, particularly as follows:

- The number of putative transmitters has jumped from about 10 'classical' transmitters (mainly small mono-amines and amino acids) to 40 or more, with the discovery of a host of neuropeptides (see Ch. 10). At the same time, the importance of other 'non-classical' mediators—NO, eicosanoids, growth factors, etc.—has become apparent.
- Cloning of genes for a wide variety of receptors, ion channels, and other functional proteins has revealed a remarkable diversity. All of the known receptor molecules appear to be expressed in at least three or four (often more) subtypes, with quite characteristic distributions in different brain areas. Ion channels, including ligand-gated channels, are multimeric proteins comprising four or five subunits surrounding the central pore (Fig. 2.4). The monomers (termed α, β, γ, etc.) in this complex differ from each other, and each can be expressed in different isoforms (often including splice variants),** so the possible diversity within what had hitherto been regarded as a single physiological or pharmacological entity, is enormous. In some cases (e.g. dopamine receptor subtypes, Ch. 30) we are beginning to understand what the diversity means at a functional level, but in many cases (e.g. NMDA receptors, Ch. 29; sodium channels, Ch. 40), we have no real idea. From the pharmacological standpoint, the molecular diversity of such targets raises the possi-bility that drugs with improved selectivity of action—blocking one kind of sodium channel without affecting

---

**RNA splicing is the process by which sections of the sequence of the primary RNA transcript are excised to form messenger RNA. Variations can occur in the extent of the deleted sections, allowing 'splice variant' forms of mRNA (and hence variant forms of the protein) to be produced from the same gene.

---

*Memory of the basic facts of pharmacology seems to come some-where in the middle of this range (skewed towards the short end).

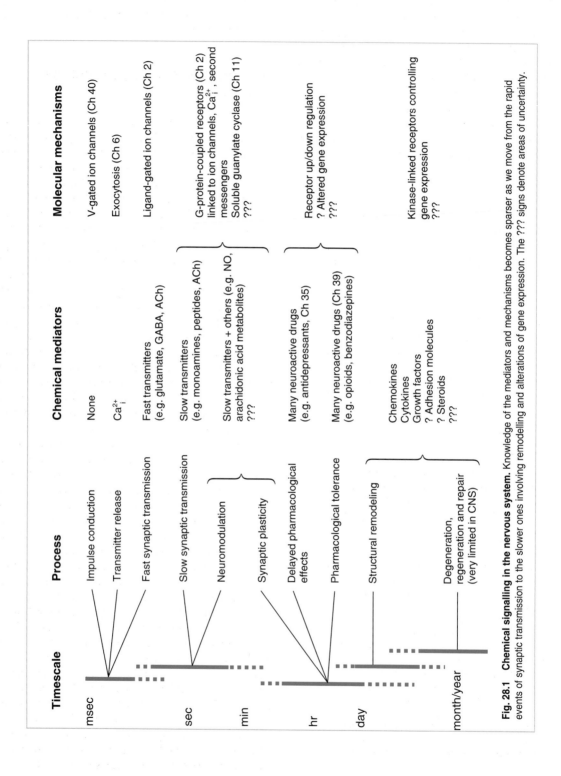

Fig. 28.1 Chemical signalling in the nervous system. Knowledge of the mediators and mechanisms becomes sparser as we move from the rapid events of synaptic transmission to the slower ones involving remodelling and alterations of gene expression. The ??? signs denote areas of uncertainty.

others, for example—may be discovered, and these may provide tools with which to study the functional importance of the different isoforms. Other approaches to elucidating the function of novel isoforms include the use of transgenic animals, which either lack or overexpress specific isoforms (see Ch. 3), or the use of antisense oligonucleotides (Ch. 50) to block expression in a specific way. Great efforts are currently going into studies of this sort, and some successes are described in later chapters. So far, however, the potential of these new approaches in terms of improved drugs for neurological and psychiatric diseases remains largely unrealised. Hope, however (and certainly hype), springs eternal.

- The pathophysiology of neurodegeneration is beginning to be understood (see Ch. 31), which has led to realistic—though as yet theoretical—new strategies for treating some disabling brain diseases. Other areas

of brain research (e.g. the neurobiology of epilepsy, schizophrenia, depressive illnesses) are advancing less rapidly, but there is still progress to report.

DRUG ACTION IN THE CENTRAL NERVOUS SYSTEM

As we have already emphasised, the molecular and cellular mechanisms underlying synaptic processes in the CNS and in the periphery are essentially similar. Understanding how interference with these processes affects brain function is, however, made difficult by several factors. One of these is the complexity of neuronal interconnections in the brain—the wiring diagram. Figure 28.2 illustrates in a very simplified way the kind of interconnections that typically exist for, say, a noradrenergic neuron in the locus ceruleus (see Ch. 30), shown as neuron 1 in the diagram, releasing transmitter a at its terminals. Release of a affects neuron 2 (which releases transmitter b), and also affects neuron 1 by direct feedback and indirectly by affecting presynaptic inputs impinging on neuron 1. The firing pattern of neuron 2 also affects the system, partly through interneuronal connections (neuron 3, releasing transmitter c). It is clear that the effects on the system of blocking or enhancing the release or actions of one or other of the transmitters will be difficult to predict, and will depend greatly on the relative strength of the various excitatory and inhibitory synaptic connections, and on external inputs (x and y in the diagram). A second important complicating factor is that a range of secondary, adaptive responses is generally set in train by any drug-induced perturbation of the system. Typically, an increase in transmitter release, or interference with transmitter reuptake, is countered by inhibition of transmitter synthesis, enhanced transporter expression, or decreased receptor expression. These changes, some of which involve altered gene expression, generally take time (hours, days or weeks) to develop, and are not evident when drug effects are studied in acute experiments.

In the clinical situation, it may be these secondary changes that are responsible for the beneficial and unwanted effects. This is particularly true of antidepressant drugs (Ch. 35) and some antipsychotic drugs (Ch. 34). The development of dependence on drugs such as opiates, benzodiazepines and psychostimulants is similarly gradual (Ch. 39). Thus, one has to take into account not only the primary interaction of the drug with its target, but also the secondary response of the brain to this primary effect; indeed it may be the secondary response, rather than the primary effect, which leads to clinical benefit.

Chemical transmission in the nervous system

- The basic processes of synaptic transmission in the central nervous system are essentially similar to those operating in the periphery (Ch. 6).
- The terms 'neurotransmitter', 'neuromodulator' and 'neurotrophic factor' refer to chemical mediators which operate over different timescales. In general:
  - Neurotransmitters are released by presynaptic terminals and produce rapid excitatory or inhibitory responses in postsynaptic neurons.
  - Neuromodulators are released by neurons, and produce slower pre- or postsynaptic responses, mediated mainly by G-protein-coupled receptors.
  - Neurotrophic factors are released mainly by non-neuronal cells and act on tyrosine-kinase-linked linked receptors which regulate gene expression, and control neuronal growth and phenotypic characteristics.
- Neurotransmitters may be broadly divided into:
  - Fast neurotransmitters, operating through ligand-gated ion channels (e.g. glutamate, GABA)
  - Slow neurotransmitters and neuromodulators, operating mainly through G-protein-coupled receptors (e.g. dopamine, neuropeptides).
- The same agent (e.g. glutamate, 5-HT, acetylcholine) may act through both ligand-gated channels and G-protein-coupled receptors.
- Other neuromodulators, including nitric oxide and arachidonic acid metabolites, may be produced by non-neuronal cells as well as neurons.
- Many other mediators (e.g. cytokines, chemokines, growth factors, steroids) are postulated to control long-term changes in the brain (e.g. synaptic plasticity, remodelling, etc.), mainly by affecting gene transcription.

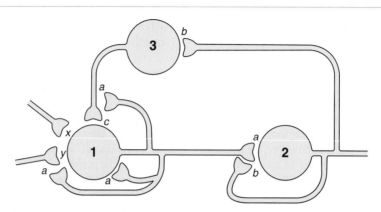

Fig 28.2 Simplified scheme of neuronal interconnections in the CNS. Neurons 1, 2 and 3 are shown releasing transmitters *a*, *b* and *c*, respectively, which may be excitatory or inhibitory. Boutons of neuron 1 terminate on neuron 2, but also on neuron 1 itself, and on presynaptic terminals of other neurons which make synaptic connections with neuron 1. Neuron 2 also feeds back on neuron 1 via interneuron 3. Transmitters (*x* and *y*), released by other neurons are also shown impinging on neuron 1. Even with a such a simple network, the effects of drug-induced interference with specific transmitter systems can be difficult to predict.

Drug action in the central nervous system

- The basic types of drug target (ion channels, receptors, enzymes and transporter proteins) described in Chapter 2 apply in the CNS as elsewhere.
- Most of these targets occur in many different molecular isoforms, the functional significance of which is, in most cases, unclear.
- Many of the currently available neuroactive drugs are relatively non-specific, affecting several different targets, the principal ones being receptors, ion channels and transporters.
- The relationship between the pharmacological profile and the therapeutic effect of neuroactive drugs is often unclear.
- Slowly developing secondary responses to the primary interaction of the drug with its target are often important (e.g. the delayed efficacy of antidepressant drugs, tolerance and dependence with opiates, etc.).

THE CLASSIFICATION OF PSYCHOTROPIC DRUGS

Psychotropic drugs are defined as those that affect mood and behaviour. Because these are extremely complex functions, the classification of drug effects is far from straightforward, and no single basis for classification has been found to be satisfactory. Thus, classification on a chemical basis, which produces categories such as **benzodiazepines**, **butyrophenones**, etc. does not give much guide to pharmacological effects. A pharmaco-logical or biochemical classification, on the other hand, is appealing for drugs whose mechanism of action is reasonably well understood (e.g. **monoamine oxidase inhibitors**, **amine reuptake inhibitors**, **opiates**, etc.), but there are still many instances (e.g. **hallucinogens**) where the mechanism of action is too poorly understood to form the basis of a reliable classification. Another possibility is to adopt an empirical classification based on overall pharmacological effect (e.g. **psychomotor stimulant**) or clinical use (e.g. **antidepressants**, **anti-psychotic agents**, **antiepileptic drugs**, etc.), but this has the weakness that the uses of psychotropic drugs often change according to clinical fashion. **Amphetamine**, for example, a drug with well-characterised effects on mood and behaviour, has had a chequered history and would have been dismissed, revived and reclassified many times if a purely clinical classification had been adopted.

Because no single basis for classifying psychotropic drugs is satisfactory, different authorities tend to offer a variety of hybrid, and often incompatible schemes.

The following classification is based on that suggested in 1967 by the World Health Organization; although not watertight it provides a useful basis for the material presented later (Chs 33–40).

- **Anxiolytics and sedatives**
  Synonyms: hypnotics, sedatives, minor tranquillisers
  Definition: drugs that cause sleep and reduce anxiety
  Examples: barbiturates, benzodiazepines and ethanol
      See Chapters 33 and 39.

- **Antipsychotic drugs**

    Synonyms: neuroleptic* drugs, antischizophrenic drugs, major tranquillisers

    Definition: drugs that are effective in relieving the symptoms of schizophrenic illness

    Examples: clozapine, chlorpromazine, haloperidol
    See Chapter 34.

- **Antidepressant drugs**

    Synonym: thymoleptics*

    Definition: drugs that alleviate the symptoms of depressive illness

    Examples: monoamine oxidase inhibitors and tricyclic antidepressants
    See Chapter 35.

- **Psychomotor stimulants**

    Synonym: psychostimulants

    Definition: drugs that cause wakefulness and euphoria

    Examples: amphetamine, cocaine and caffeine
    See Chapter 38.

- **Psychotomimetic drugs**

    Synonyms: hallucinogens, psychodysleptics*

    Definition: drugs that cause disturbance of perception (particularly visual hallucinations) and of behaviour in ways that cannot be simply characterised as sedative or stimulant effects

    Examples: lysergic acid diethylamide (LSD), mescaline and phencyclidine
    See Chapter 38.

- **Cognition enhancers**

    Synonyms: nootropic drugs

    Definition: drugs that improve memory and cognitive performance

---

*These strange terms are the remnants of a classification proposed by Javet in 1903, who distinguished psycholeptics (depressants of mental function), psychoanaleptics (stimulants of mental function), and psychodysleptics (drugs that produce disturbed mental function). The term neuroleptic (literally 'nerve-seizing') was coined 50 years later to describe chlorpromazine-like drugs (see Ch. 34). It gained favour, presumably by virtue of its brevity rather than its literal meaning.

Examples: tacrine, donepezil, ?piracetam
See Chapter 31.

This is more of a wishful than a real category, intended to encompass drugs that improve learning and memory.

Some drugs defy classification in this scheme; for example, **lithium** (see Ch. 35), which is used in the treatment of manic-depressive psychosis, and **ketamine** (see Ch. 32), which is classed as a dissociative anaesthetic, but produces psychotropic effects rather similar to those produced by phencyclidine.

CLINICAL USE OF PSYCHOTROPIC DRUGS

The term *psychosis* refers to a group of mental disorders (e.g. schizophrenia, manic-depressive psychosis) (see Chs 34 and 35) which are considered to be endogenous in origin (i.e. they represent some inherent malfunction of the brain), as distinct from neurosis, typified by anxiety states, phobias, and so on, which is regarded as an abnormal reaction to external circumstances (see Ch. 33). Though still useful, this distinction is not clear cut. Thus many, if not most, patients complaining of anxiety also show features of depression, and schizophrenic patients frequently appear depressed or anxious in addition to showing the characteristics of schizophrenia. Correspondingly, the use of drugs in psychiatric illness often ignores the conventional demarcations of the specific therapeutic categories that are listed above. The simple-minded pharmacologist, confronted with the realities of clinical practice, may find this confusing. Here we will adhere to the conventional pharmacological categories, but it needs to be emphasised that in clinical use these distinctions are often disregarded.

An added complication with many psychotropic drugs is that, although they produce their pharmacological effects rapidly (e.g. receptor block, inhibition of transporters, etc.), their clinical effect commonly takes days or weeks to develop.

REFERENCES AND FURTHER READING

Bloom F E, Kupfer D J (eds) 1995 Psychopharmacology: a fourth generation of progress. Raven Press, New York *(A 2000-page monster, with excellent and authoritative articles on basic and clinical aspects)*

Carvey P M 1998 Drug action in the central nervous system. Oxford University Press, New York *(Good general textbook)*

Cooper J R, Bloom F E, Roth R H 1996 Biochemical basis of neuropharmacology. Oxford University Press, New York

(Excellent and readable account, focusing on basic, rather than clinical aspects)

Kandel E, Jessel T M, Schwartz J H 1993 Principles of neural science. Elsevier, New York *(Excellent and detailed standard text on neurobiology—little emphasis on pharmacology)*

Levitan I B, Kaczmarek L K 1997 The neuron: cell and molecular biology. Oxford University Press, New York *(Good general account at cellular and molecular level)*

Amino acid transmitters

In this chapter, we discuss the main fast neurotransmitters in the CNS, namely the excitatory transmitter, **glutamate**, and the inhibitory transmitters, **GABA** and **glycine**.

EXCITATORY AMINO ACIDS (EAAs)

EAAs AS CNS TRANSMITTERS

L-glutamate is the principal and ubiquitous excitatory transmitter in the central nervous system (see Cotman et al. 1995 for general review). Aspartate plays a similar role, and possibly also homocysteate, but this is controversial. The realisation of their importance came slowly. By the 1950s (in the words of Krnjevic, one of the glutamate pioneers, 'the era of Prehistory'), work on the peripheral nervous system had highlighted the transmitter roles of acetylcholine and catecholamines, and as the brain also contained these substances, there seemed little reason to look further. The presence of γ-aminobutyric acid (GABA; see below) in the brain, and its powerful inhibitory effect on neurons, were discovered in the 1950s, and its transmitter role was postulated. At the same time, work by Curtis' group in Canberra showed that glutamate and various other acidic amino acids produced a strong excitatory effect, but it seemed inconceivable that such workaday metabolites could actually

be transmitters. Through the 1960s ('the Dark Ages'), neither GABA nor EAAs were thought to be more than pharmacological curiosities, even by their discoverers. In the 1970s ('the Renaissance'), the humblest amino acid, glycine, was established as an inhibitory transmitter in the spinal cord, giving the lie to the idea that the transmitters had to be exotic molecules, too beautiful for any role but to sink into the arms of a receptor. Once glycine had been accepted, the rest quickly followed (the 'Baroque era', an apt phrase to describe the somewhat overwhelming detail which has since been added to the basic discovery). A major advance was the discovery of EAA antagonists, based on the work of Watkins in Bristol, which enabled the physiological role of glutamate to be established unequivocally, and also led to the realisation that EAA receptors are heterogeneous.

To do justice to the wealth of discovery in this field in the last two decades is beyond the range of this book, but interested readers can find their way through many excellent reviews, for example Barnard (1997), Kemp & Leeson (1993), Schoep & Conn (1993), Seeburg (1993), Sucher et al. (1996). Here we will concentrate on pharmacological aspects. Disappointingly, no therapeutic drugs have yet been introduced on the basis of EAA mechanisms, in spite of the many potential applications that exist. The 'Industrial revolution' seems to be running late.

METABOLISM AND RELEASE OF AMINO ACIDS

Glutamate is widely and fairly uniformly distributed in the CNS, and its concentration there is much higher than it is in other tissues. It has an important metabolic role, the metabolic and neurotransmitter pools being linked by transaminase enzymes that catalyse the interconversion of glutamate and α-oxoglutarate (Fig. 29.1). The glutamate in the CNS neurons comes mainly from either glucose, via the Krebs cycle, or glutamine, which is synthesised by glial cells and taken up by the neurons.

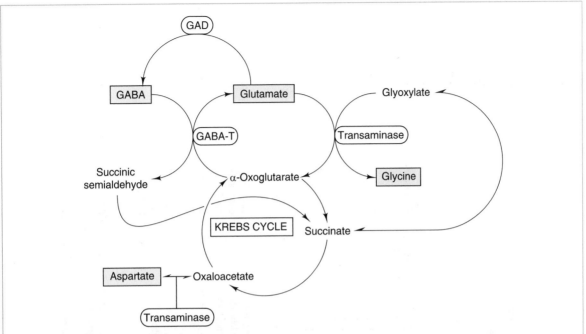

Fig. 29.1 Metabolism of transmitter amino acids in the brain. (GABA = gamma-aminobutyric acid; GAD = glutamic acid decarboxylase; GABA-T = GABA transaminase.) Transmitter substances are marked with light blue boxes.

The synthetic reactions occur in virtually all cells, so they have not been particularly useful in understanding the transmitter function of EAAs. The interconnection between the pathways for the synthesis of EAAs and inhibitory amino acids (GABA and glycine), shown in Figure 29.1, also makes it difficult to use experimental manipulations of transmitter synthesis to study the functional role of individual amino acids.

In common with other transmitters, glutamate is stored in synaptic vesicles and released by calcium-dependent exocytosis, and specific transporter proteins account for its uptake by neurons and other cells, and for its accumulation by synaptic vesicles (see Ch. 6). In contrast to the situation with monoamine synthesis and transport (Chs 7 and 30), few drugs are known (and none are in clinical use) which interfere specifically with glutamate metabolism.

The action of glutamate is terminated mainly by carrier-mediated reuptake into the nerve terminals and neighbouring glial cells. This transport can, under some circumstances (e.g. depolarisation by increased extracellular potassium), operate in reverse and constitute a source of glutamate release (see Takahashi et al. 1997); a process which may occur under pathological conditions such as brain ischaemia (see Ch. 31).

GLUTAMATE RECEPTORS—STRUCTURE AND PHARMACOLOGY

On the basis of studies with selective agonists and antagonists, four main subtypes of EAA receptors can be distinguished, namely *NMDA*, *AMPA*, *kainate* and *metabotropic* receptors (Table 29.1), all of which have been cloned and studied in great detail (see Schoep & Conn 1993, Seeburg 1993). The first three (often called *ionotropic receptors*) are ligand-gated ion channels, named according to their specific agonists (Fig 29.2),* and they have a pentameric structure similar to that described in Chapter 2. NMDA receptors are assembled from two types of subunit, NR1 and NR2, each of which can exist in different isoforms and splice variants, giving rise to many different receptor isoforms in the brain, whose significance is not yet understood—a scenario by now familiar to our readers. The subunits comprising AMPA and kainate receptors, termed $GluR_{1-7}$ and $KA_{1,2}$, are closely related, but distinct from NMDA receptor subunits. AMPA receptors consist of combinations of

---

*NMDA = N-methyl-D-aspartate; AMPA = α-amino-3-hydroxy-5-methyl-isoxazole; kainate is a compound isolated from seaweed.

Table 29.1 Properties of excitatory amino acid receptors

	NMDA			AMPA		Kainate	Metabotropic
	Receptor site	Modulatory site (glycine)	Modulatory site (polyamine)	Receptor site	Modulatory site		
Endogenous agonists	Glutamate Aspartate	Glycine	Spermine Spermidine	Glutamate	??	Glutamate	Glutamate
Other agonists	NMDA	D-serine		AMPA Quisqualate	Cyclothiazide Aniracetam 'Ampakines'**	Kainate Quisqualate	D-AP4 ACPD
Antagonists	AP-5, AP-7 CGS 19755 (selfotel) CPP SDZ EAA 494	Kynurenate Chloro-kynurenate HA-466	Ifenprodil	NBQX CNQX	–	–	MCPG
Channel blockers	Dizocilpine (MK801) Phencyclidine Ketamine Dextromethorphan Mg^{2+}			–		–	Not applicable
Effector mechanisms	Ligand-gated cation channel (slow kinetics, high Ca^{2+} permeability)			Ligand-gated cation channel (fast kinetics, low Ca^{2+} permeability)		Ligand-gated cation channel (fast kinetics, low Ca^{2+} permeability)	G-protein-coupled (IP_3 formation and release of Ca^{2+})
Location	Postsynaptic (also glial) Wide distribution			Postsynaptic		Pre- and postsynaptic	Pre- and postsynaptic
Function	Slow EPSP Synaptic plasticity (LTP, LTD) Excitotoxicity			Fast EPSP Wide distribution		Fast EPSP ?presynaptic inhibition Limited distribution	Synaptic modulation Excitotoxicity

ACPD = 1-aminocyclopentane-1,3-dicarboxylic acid; AP-5 = 2-amino-5-phosphonopentanoic acid; AP-7 = 2-amino-7-phosphonoheptanoic acid; CNQX = 6-cyano-7-nitroquinoxaline-2,3-dione; CPP = 3-(2-carboxypirazin-4-yl)-propyl-1-phosphonic acid; NBQX = 2,3-dihydro-6-nitro-7-sulfamoyl-benzoquinoxaline; MCPG = α-methyl-4-carboxyphenylglycine. Other structures are shown in Table 29.2.

**'Ampakine' is a term invented to describe a number of compounds which appear to enhance the action of AMPA-receptor agonists.

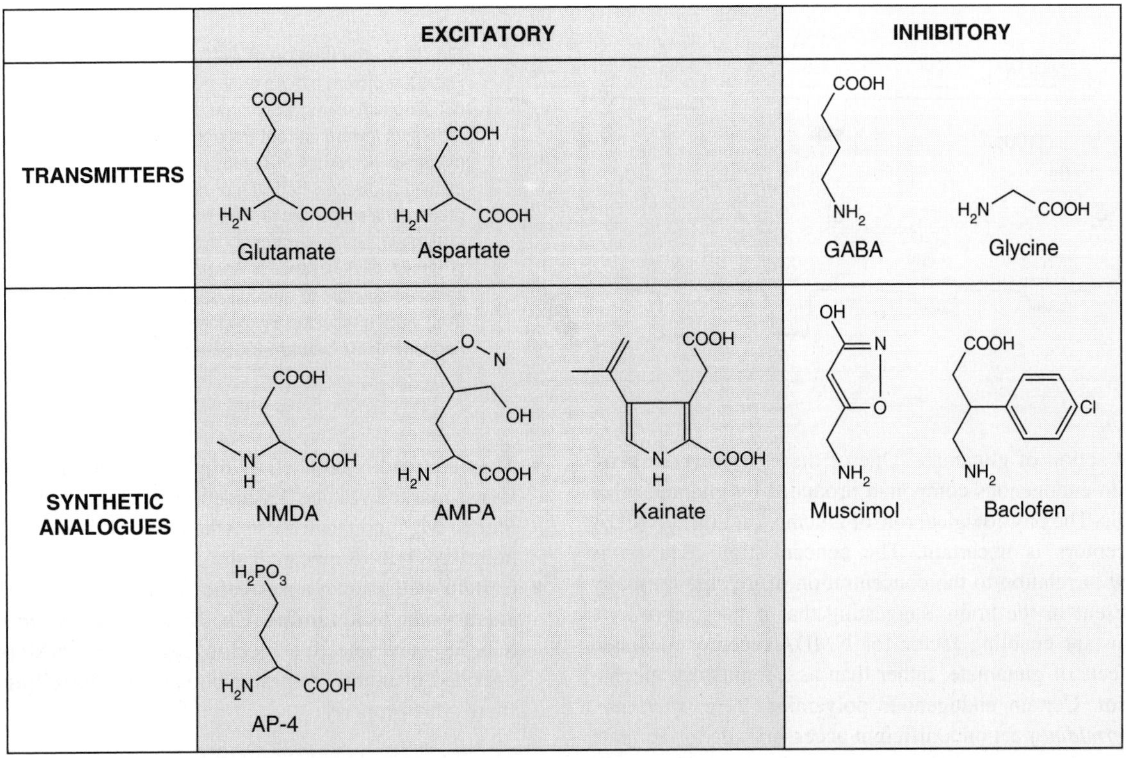

Fig. 29.2 **Structures of agonists acting on glutamate, GABA and glycine receptors.** The receptor specificity of these compounds is shown in Tables 29.1 and 29.2.

$GluR_{1-4}$, each of which can be expressed in two splice variants, described memorably as 'flip' and 'flop', which vary subtly in their physiological and pharmacological properties. The metabotropic receptors are monomeric G-protein-coupled receptors, linked to intracellular second messenger systems (see Ch. 2), and again multiple subtypes (eight, so far) have been detected (see Conn & Pin 1997). They are unusual in showing no sequence homology with other G-protein-coupled receptors, and in having a very large extracellular N-terminal tail, which contains the glutamate binding site, in contrast to most amine receptors in which the agonist binding site is buried amongst the transmembrane helices (Ch. 2).

Binding studies show that glutamate receptors are most abundant in the cortex, basal ganglia and sensory pathways. NMDA and AMPA receptors are generally co-localised, but kainate receptors have a much more restricted distribution. Expression of the many different receptor subtypes in the brain also shows distinct regional differences, but we have hardly begun to understand the significance of this extreme organisational complexity.

Agonists, antagonists and modulators

Specific agonists and antagonists for glutamate receptors are given in Table 29.1. The first antagonists, for NMDA receptors, were the phosphonate analogues, AP-5 and AP-7, which have been used in many studies; later and more potent derivatives such as CPP and CGS 19755 have been used in clinical trials (see below). Selective receptor antagonists for other types of glutamate receptor are shown in Table 29.1.

Both NMDA and AMPA receptors are subject to facilitation by modulators that act at sites distinct from the glutamate binding site. In the case of NMDA receptors, channel opening requires *glycine* as well as glutamate (Fig. 29.3). The binding site for glycine is distinct from the glutamate binding site, and both have to be occupied for the channel to open. This discovery caused a stir, because glycine had hitherto been recognised as an inhibitory transmitter (see below), so to find it facilitating excitation ran counter to the prevailing doctrine. Competitive antagonists are known (see Table 29.1), which block this action of glycine, and thus indirectly inhibit

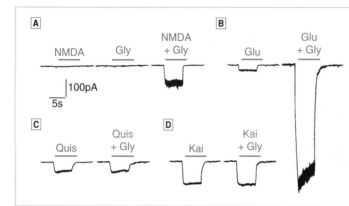

Fig. 29.3   Facilitation of NMDA by glycine.
Recordings from mouse brain neurons in culture (whole patch-clamp technique). Downward deflections represent inward current through EAA-activated ion channels. [A] NMDA (10 µmol/l) or glycine (1 µmol/l) applied separately had little or no effect, but together produced a response. [B] The response to glutamate (10 µmol/l, Glu) was strongly potentiated by glycine (1 µmol/l, Gly). [C] and [D] Responses of AMPA and kainate receptors to quisqualate (Quis) and kainate (Kai) were unaffected by glycine. (From: Johnson J W, Ascher P 1987 Nature 325: 529–531)

the action of glutamate. One of these, **kynurenic acid**, is an endogenous compound produced by glia and other cells. The physiological role of glycine's action at NMDA receptors is uncertain. The concentration required is low in relation to the concentration of glycine normally present in the brain, suggesting that it may serve as a constant enabling factor for NMDA-receptor-mediated effects of glutamate, rather than as a regulatory mechanism. Certain endogenous polyamines (e.g. *spermine*, *spermidine*) act on a different accessory site to facilitate channel opening. The experimental drugs, **ifenprodil** and **eliprodil**, block their action. The physiological role of modulation of NMDA channels by kynurenic acid and polyamines remains uncertain.

Compounds that facilitate agonist action at AMPA receptors include **cyclothiazide** (a compound related to the thiazide diuretics Ch. 20), which inhibits the fast desensitisation produced by glutamate; **aniracetam** and other experimental compounds (rather pretentiously* called '*ampakines*'). Drugs of this type are of interest as possible 'cognition enhancers' (see Ch. 28), since they have this effect in animal models. They are as yet unproven in humans.

Special features of NMDA receptors

NMDA receptors and their associated channels have been studied in more detail than the other types, and show special pharmacological properties, summarised in Figure 29.4, which are postulated to play a role in pathophysiological mechanisms:

- They are highly permeable to Ca^{2+}, as well as to other cations, so activation of NMDA receptors is particularly effective in promoting Ca^{2+} entry.

---

*Confusingly, as well, since they in no way resemble cytokines.

- They are readily blocked by Mg^{2+} ions, and this block shows marked voltage dependence. It occurs at physiological Mg^{2+} concentrations when the cell is normally polarised, but disappears if the cell is depolarised.
- Certain well-known anaesthetic and psychotomimetic agents, such as **ketamine** (Ch. 32) and **phencyclidine** (Ch. 38), are selective blocking agents for NMDA-operated channels. A newer compound, **dizocilpine**, shares this property.

FUNCTIONAL ROLE OF GLUTAMATE RECEPTORS

Studies with selective AMPA receptor antagonists, such as CNQX, show that these receptors are mainly responsible for fast excitatory synaptic transmission in the CNS. In some regions kainate receptors may also serve this role, but the evidence is incomplete. NMDA receptors (which often coexist with AMPA receptors) contribute a slow component to the excitatory synaptic potential (Fig. 29.5), the magnitude of which varies in different pathways. Metabotropic glutamate receptors are linked either to IP_3 production and release of intracellular Ca^{2+} or to inhibition of adenylate cyclase (see Ch. 2). They are located both pre- and postsynaptically, as well as on non-neuronal cells. Their effects on transmission are modulatory, rather than direct, comprising mainly postsynaptic excitatory effects (by inhibition of potassium channels) and presynaptic inhibition (by inhibition of calcium channels).

NMDA and metabotropic glutamate receptors participate in various adaptive and pathophysiological events. Three such roles which are now generally accepted are:

- *synaptic plasticity*
- *excitotoxicity* (discussed in Ch. 31)
- the *pathogenesis of epilepsy* (discussed in Ch. 36).

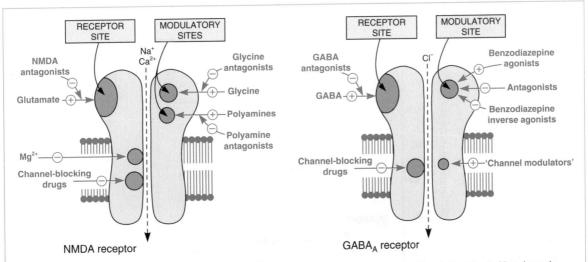

Fig. 29.4 Main sites of drug action on NMDA and GABA$_A$-receptors. Both receptors are multimeric ligand-gated ion channels. Drugs can act as agonists or antagonists at the neurotransmitter receptor site, or at modulatory sites associated with the receptor. They can also act to block the ion channel at one or more distinct sites. In the case of the GABA$_A$-receptor, the mechanism by which 'channel modulators' (e.g. ethanol, anaesthetic agents) facilitate channel opening is uncertain; they may affect both ligand binding and channel sites.

The location of the different binding sites shown in the figure is largely imaginary, though study of mutated receptors is beginning to reveal where they actually reside.

Examples of the different drug classes are given in Tables 29.1 and 29.2.

Synaptic plasticity

Long-term potentiation (*LTP*; see Bliss & Collingridge 1993, Malenka & Nicoll 1993) is the term used to describe a long-lasting (hours in vitro, days or weeks in vivo) enhancement of synaptic transmission that occurs at various CNS synapses following a short (conditioning) burst of presynaptic stimulation, typically at about 100 Hz for 1 second. Its counterpart is *long-term depression* (*LTD*) which is produced by a longer train of stimuli at lower frequency. These phenomena, which are postulated to underlie certain aspects of learning, memory and habituation, have been studied in great detail in the hippocampus (Fig. 29.5), which plays a central role in learning and memory. It has been argued that 'learning', in the synaptic sense, can occur if synaptic strength is enhanced following *simultaneous* activity in both pre- and postsynaptic neurons. LTP shows this characteristic; it does not occur if presynaptic activity fails to excite the postsynaptic neuron, or if the latter is activated independently, for instance by different presynaptic input. Thus LTP initiation involves both the presynaptic and postsynaptic components of EAA synapses. The facilitatory process also appears to involve both pre- and postsynaptic elements (though the small-print argument on this point rumbles on); the release of glutamate is increased, and so is the sensitivity of the postsynaptic membrane to glutamate. The following experimental results have led to the model shown in Figure 29.6.

- NMDA antagonists prevent LTP, without affecting normal, non-potentiated transmission (which depends on AMPA/kainate receptors). Disruption of the NMDA receptor gene has the same effect.
- LTP occurs only if the postsynaptic cell is depolarised at the time when the conditioning burst of stimulation is delivered.
- Antagonists at metabotropic glutamate receptors reduce the duration of LTP; LTP is also impaired in transgenic mice lacking the mGluR1 receptor.
- Calcium entry into the postsynaptic cell is required, and there is evidence that activation of protein kinase C (see Ch. 2) is involved in the mechanism of potentiation.
- LTP is reduced by agents which block the synthesis or effects of nitric oxide or arachidonic acid (see Ch. 30). One or both of these mediators may be the hitherto elusive 'retrograde messenger' through which events in the postsynaptic cell are able to influence the presynaptic nerve terminal.

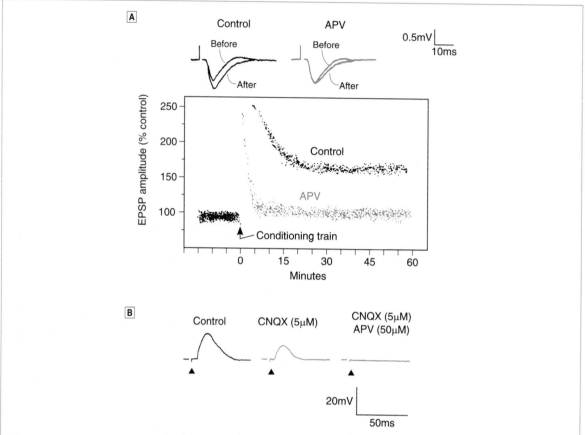

Fig. 29.5   Effects of EAA receptor antagonists on synaptic transmission. ⒜ APV (NMDA antagonist) prevents long-term potentiation (LTP) in the rat hippocampus without affecting the fast epsp. Top records show the extracellularly recorded fast epsp (downward deflection) before, and 50 minutes after, a conditioning train of stimuli (100 Hz for 2 s). The presence of LTP in the control preparation is indicated by the increase in epsp amplitude. In the presence of APV (50 μmol/l), the normal epsp is unchanged, but LTP does not occur. Lower trace shows epsp amplitude as a function of time. The conditioning train produces a short-lasting increase in epsp amplitude which still occurs in the presence of APV, but the long-lasting effect is prevented. ⒝ Block of fast and slow components of epsp by CNQX (AMPA-receptor antagonist) and APV (NMDA-receptor antagonist). epsp (upward deflection) in hippocampal neuron recorded with intracellular electrode is partly blocked by CNQX (5 μmol/l), leaving behind a slow component, which is blocked by APV (50 μmol/l). (From: (A) Malinow R, Madison D, Tsien R W 1988 Nature 335: 821; (B) Andreasen M, Lambert J D, Jensen M S 1989 J Physiol 414: 317–336)

Two special properties of the NMDA receptor and channel underlie its involvement in LTP, namely voltage-dependent channel block by Mg^{2+} and its high Ca^{2+}-permeability. At normal membrane potentials the NMDA channel is blocked by Mg^{2+}; a sustained postsynaptic depolarisation produced by glutamate acting repeatedly on AMPA/kainate receptors, however, removes the Mg^{2+} block, and NMDA receptor activation then allows Ca^{2+} to enter the cell. This rise in $[Ca^{2+}]_i$ in the postsynaptic cell activates protein kinases, phospholipases and nitric oxide synthase, which act jointly (by mechanisms that are

not yet elucidated) to facilitate transmission via AMPA/ kainate receptors. The metabotropic EAA receptor also contributes to the increase in $[Ca^{2+}]_i$.

Though LTP is well established as a synaptic phenomenon, its relationship to learning and memory remains controversial. Some evidence is suggestive: for example, NMDA receptor antagonists applied to the hippocampus impair learning in rats; also, 'saturation' of LTP by electrical stimulation of the hippocampus has been found to impair the ability of rats to learn a maze. On the other hand, LTP-like changes have not been detected after

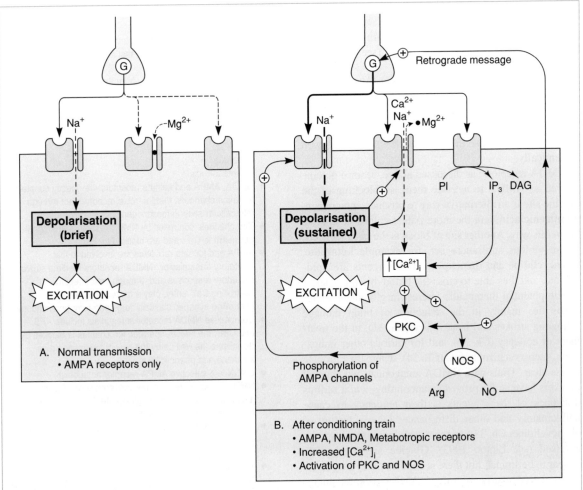

Fig. 29.6 Mechanisms of long-term potentiation LTP. [A] With infrequent synaptic activity, glutamate activates mainly AMPA receptors. There is insufficient glutamate to activate metabotropic receptors, and NMDA-receptor channels are blocked by Mg^{2+}. [B] After a conditioning train of stimuli, enough glutamate is released to activate metabotropic receptors, and NMDA channels are unblocked by the sustained depolarisation. The resulting increase in $[Ca^{2+}]_i$ activates PKC and NOS. PKC phosphorylates various proteins, including AMPA receptors (causing facilitation of transmitter action) and other signal transduction molecules controlling gene transcription (not shown) in the postsynaptic cell. Release of NO facilitates glutamate release (retrograde signalling, otherwise known as *NO turning back*). (G = glutamate; A = AMPA receptor; N = NMDA receptor; M = metabotropic receptor; PI = phosphatidylinositol; IP_3 = (1,4,5) inositol triphosphate; DAG = diacylglycerol; PKC = protein kinase; NOS = nitric oxide synthase)

learning has taken place. Nevertheless, pharmacologists are actively seeking drugs capable of enhancing LTP in the hope that they will improve learning and memory.

LTP is just one manifestation of synaptic plasticity whereby neuronal connections respond to changes in the activity of the nervous system. Other phenomena, including *short-term potentiation* and *long-term depression* also occur, and they too appear to involve glutamate receptors (see Malenka & Nicoll 1993).

GLUTAMATE ANTAGONISTS

Much effort, particularly by Watkins and his colleagues, has gone into the search for selective glutamate antagonists, partly to provide tools for better understanding the physiological roles of the different types of EAA receptor, and partly as potential therapeutic agents with which to treat, for example, epilepsy and neurodegenerative disorders.

477

The main types of EAA antagonists are shown in Table 29.1 and Figure 29.2. They show selectivity with respect to the main receptor types, but drugs which can distinguish the multitude of subtypes (see above) are not yet available.

At the receptor level, selective antagonists exist for NMDA, AMPA and metabotropic gluatamate receptors. Many of these compounds, though very useful as experimental tools in vitro, are unable to penetrate the blood–brain barrier, so they are not effective when given systemically.

NMDA receptors, as discussed above, require glycine as well as NMDA to activate them, so blocking of the glycine site is an alternative way to produce antagonism. **Kynurenic acid**, and the more potent chloro- analogue, act in this way. Another site of block is the channel itself, where various substances act, for example **ketamine**, **phencyclidine** and **dizocilpine**. These agents are lipid-soluble, and thus able to cross the blood–brain barrier.

The potential therapeutic interest in glutamate antagonists lies mainly in the reduction of brain damage following strokes and head injury (Ch. 31), in the treatment of epilepsy (Ch. 36), and for various other indications, such as schizophrenia (Ch. 34), where the rationale is less clear. Trials with NMDA antagonists and channel blockers have so far proved disappointing, and a serious drawback of these agents is their tendency to cause hallucinatory and other disturbances (also a feature of phencyclidine; Ch. 38), so their usefulness remains to be assessed (see Lipton 1993). Glycine site antagonists appear to be similar, but there is hope that they may show an improved margin of safety. AMPA-receptor antagonists seem unpromising as therapeutic agents, since the available agents (as might be expected) produce overall CNS depression, including respiratory depression and motor incoordination, with little margin of safety. Only if subtype selectivity can be achieved is this approach likely to succeed. Against this unpromising background, antagonists at metabotropic receptors may offer the best hope (see Nicoletti et al. 1996), but such compounds are not yet available for clinical use. As in other areas, the profusion of molecular subtypes of glutamate receptors is held to be the shining path leading to the discovery of more selective drugs.

GAMMA-AMINOBUTYRIC ACID (GABA)

GABA is the main inhibitory transmitter in the brain. In the spinal cord and brainstem, glycine is also important.

Excitatory amino acids

- EAAs, namely glutamate, aspartate, and possibly homocysteate, are the main fast excitatory transmitters in the CNS.
- Glutamate is formed mainly from the Krebs cycle intermediate, α-oxoglutarate, by the action of GABA-aminotransferase.
- There are four main EAA receptor subtypes (Table 29.1):
  —NMDA
  —AMPA
  —kainate
  —metabotropic.
- NMDA, AMPA and kainate receptors are directly coupled to cation channels; metabotropic receptors act through intracellular second messengers.
- The channels controlled by NMDA receptors are highly permeant to Ca^{2+} and are blocked by Mg^{2+}.
- AMPA and kainate receptors are involved in fast excitatory transmission; NMDA receptors mediate slower excitatory responses and, through their effect in controlling Ca^{2+} entry, play a more complex role in controlling synaptic plasticity (e.g. long-term potentiation).
- Competitive NMDA receptor antagonists include AP5, and CPP; the NMDA-operated ion channel is blocked by dizocilpine, as well as by the psychotomimetic drugs, ketamine and phencyclidine.
- CNQX is a selective AMPA-receptor antagonist.
- NMDA receptors require low concentrations of glycine as a co-agonist, in addition to glutamate; 7-chlorokynurenate blocks this action of glycine.
- NMDA receptor activation is increased by endogenous polyamines, such as spermine, acting on a modulatory site which is blocked by ifenprodil.
- The entry of excessive amounts of Ca^{2+} produced by NMDA receptor activation can result in cell death—excitotoxicity (see Ch. 31).
- Metabotropic receptors are G-protein-coupled receptors, linked to IP_3 formation and intracellular Ca^{2+} release. They play a part in glutamate-mediated synaptic plasticity and excitotoxicity. Specific agonists and antagonists are known.
- EAA receptor antagonists have yet to be developed for clinical use.

SYNTHESIS, STORAGE AND FUNCTION

GABA occurs in brain tissue, but not in other mammalian tissues, except in trace amounts. In the brain it is particularly abundant (about 10 μmol/g tissue) in the nigrostriatal system, but occurs at lower concentrations (2–5 μmol/g) throughout the grey matter.

GABA is formed from glutamate (Fig. 29.1) by the action of *glutamic acid decarboxylase* (GAD), an enzyme found only in GABA-synthesising neurons in the brain.

Immunohistochemical labelling of GAD is used to map the GABA pathways in the brain. GABA is destroyed by a transamination reaction, in which the amino group is transferred to α-oxoglutaric acid (to yield glutamate), with the production of succinic semialdehyde, and then succinic acid. This reaction is catalysed by *GABA-transaminase* (GABA-T), which is inhibited by **vigabatrine**, a compound used to treat epilepsy (Ch. 36). GABA-ergic neurons have an active GABA uptake system, and it is this, rather than GABA-T, which removes the GABA after it has been released. There are no specific inhibitors of GABA uptake.

GABA functions as an inhibitory transmitter in many different CNS pathways. It is released mainly from short interneurons, the only long GABA-ergic tracts being those running to the cerebellum and striatum. The widespread distribution of GABA, and the fact that virtually all neurons are sensitive to its inhibitory effect, suggest that its function is ubiquitous in the brain. It has been estimated that GABA serves as a transmitter at about 30% of all the synapses in the CNS.

GABA RECEPTORS–STRUCTURE AND PHARMACOLOGY

In common with glutamate, and several other CNS transmitters, GABA acts on two distinct types of receptor, one (the GABA$_A$-receptor) being a ligand-gated channel, the other (GABA$_B$) being a G-protein-coupled receptor. Both receptor types have been cloned, and they show many features in common with glutamate receptors. GABA$_A$-receptors are located postsynaptically, and they mediate fast postsynaptic inhibition. The associated channel is selectively permeable to chloride ions. Because the equilibrium membrane potential for chloride ions is usually somewhat negative to the resting potential of the cell, increasing chloride permeability hyperpolarises the cell, thereby reducing its excitability.

GABA$_A$-receptors are pentamers, composed of three different subunits (α, β, γ) forming an array of α-helices around a central pore (the ion channel) with a large extracellular portion which incorporates the GABA binding site. The receptor subunits each exist in several subtypes, giving the familiar pattern of heterogeneity (as yet unlinked to function) typical of neurotransmitter receptors.

GABA$_B$-receptors are located pre- and postsynaptically, and they closely resemble metabotropic glutamate receptors. They were cloned in 1997, and so far, only two subtypes have been identified, though pharmacological evidence suggests that more may exist. They exert their effects by inhibiting voltage-gated calcium channels (thus reducing transmitter release), and by opening potassium channels (thus reducing postsynaptic excitability) these actions resulting from inhibition of adenylate cyclase.

It is believed that glutamate and GABA, and their receptors, evolved very early, so these receptors probably represent the venerable aristocrats from which upstarts such as the neuropeptide receptors evolved much later.

DRUGS ACTING ON GABA RECEPTORS

GABA$_A$-receptors

GABA$_A$-receptors resemble NMDA receptors in that drugs may act at several different sites (Fig. 29.4; see Johnston 1996, Smith & Olsen 1995). These include:

- the GABA binding site
- one or more modulatory sites
- the ion channel.

GABA$_A$-receptors are the target for several important centrally acting drugs, notably **benzodiazepines**, **barbiturates** and **neurosteroids** (see below). The main agonists, antagonists and modulatory substances that act on GABA receptors are shown in Table 29.2.

Muscimol, derived from a hallucinogenic mushroom, is a powerful GABA$_A$-receptor agonist, which hyperpolarises GABA-sensitive neurons. **Bicuculline**, a naturally occurring convulsant compound, is a specific antagonist, which blocks the fast inhibitory synaptic potential in most CNS synapses. These compounds are useful experimental tools, but have no therapeutic uses.

Benzodiazepines, which have powerful sedative and anxiolytic effects (see Ch. 33) selectively potentiate the effects of GABA on GABA$_A$-receptors. They bind with high affinity to an accessory site (the 'benzodiazepine receptor') on the GABA$_A$-receptor, in such a way that the binding of GABA is facilitated and its agonist effect is enhanced. Studies on recombinant GABA$_A$-receptors have shown that a small region of the γ-subunit confers benzodiazepine sensitivity, and mutations in this region affect the level of constitutive activity (see Ch. 1) at this site, and its sensitivity to benzodiazepines. Sedative benzodiazepines, such as **diazepam**, are agonists (enhancing the action of GABA), whereas convulsant analogues, such as **flumazenil** (Ch. 33) are antagonists.

Modulators which also enhance the action of GABA, but whose site of action is less well defined than that of benzodiazepines (shown as 'channel modulators' in Fig. 29.4) include other CNS depressants such as **barbiturates** (see Ch. 33) and **neurosteroids**. Neurosteroids (see Lambert et al 1995) are compounds which are related

Table 29.2 Properties of inhibitory amino acid receptors

	GABA$_A$			GABA$_B$	Glycine
	Receptor site	Modulatory site (benzodiazepine)	Modulatory site (others)		
Endogenous agonists	GABA	? diazepam binding inhibitor	Progesterone metabolites	GABA	Glycine β-alanine, taurine
Other agonists	Muscimol	Anxiolytic benzodiazpines (e.g. diazepam)	Steroid anaesthetics (e.g. alphaxolone)	Baclofen	–
Antagonists	Bicuculline	Flumazenil	–	Phaclofen CGP 35348 and others	Strychnine
Channel blockers	Picrotoxin			Not applicable	–
Effector mechanisms	Ligand-gated chloride channel			G-protein-coupled receptor; inhibition of adenylate cyclase	Ligand-gated chloride channel
Location	Widespread. Mainly GABA-ergic interneurons			Pre- and postsynaptic Widespread	Postsynaptic Mainly in brainstem and spinal cord
Function	Postsynaptic inhibition (fast ipsp)			Presynaptic inhibition (↓ Ca^{2+} entry) Postsynaptic inhibition (↑ K$^+$ permeability)	Postsynaptic inhibition (fast ipsp)

to steroid hormones, but do not act on conventional intracellular steroid receptors. Interestingly, they include metabolites of progesterone and androgens which are formed in the nervous system, and may have a physiological role. Synthetic neurosteroids include **alphaxolone**, developed as an anaesthetic agent (Ch. 32). Another putative endogenous modulator of GABA-mediated transmission is a peptide, *diazepam binding inhibitor (DBI)*, which occurs in the brain and elsewhere, but whose physiological role is unclear.

Picrotoxin (Ch. 38) is a convulsant which acts by blocking the chloride channel associated with the GABA$_A$-receptor, thus blocking the postsynaptic inhibitory effect of GABA. It has no therapeutic uses.

GABA$_B$-receptors

When the importance of GABA as an inhibitory transmitter was recognised, it was thought that a GABA-like substance might prove to be effective in controlling epilepsy and other convulsive states; since GABA itself fails to penetrate the blood–brain barrier, more lipophilic GABA analogues were sought, one of which, **baclofen**, was introduced in 1972. Unlike GABA, baclofen has little postsynaptic inhibitory effect, and its actions are

not blocked by bicuculline. These findings led to the recognition of the GABA$_B$-receptor, for which baclofen is a selective agonist (see Bowery 1993). Baclofen is used to treat spasticity and related motor disorders (Ch. 36).

Competitive antagonists for the GABA$_B$-receptor include a number of experimental compounds (e.g. saclofen, and more potent compounds with improved brain penetration, such as CGP 35348). Tests in animals have shown that these compounds produce only slight effects on CNS function (in contrast to the powerful convulsant effects of GABA$_A$ antagonists). The main effect observed, paradoxically, was an anticonvulsant action, specifically in an animal model of absence seizures (see Ch. 36) together with enhanced cognitive performance. Whether such compounds will prove to have therapeutic uses remains to be seen.

GLYCINE

Glycine is present in particularly high concentration (5 μmol/g) in the grey matter of the spinal cord. Applied ionophoretically to motoneurons or interneurons it produces an inhibitory hyperpolarisation that is indistinguishable from the inhibitory synaptic response. **Strychnine** (see Ch. 38), a convulsant poison that acts mainly on the spinal cord, blocks both the synaptic inhibitory response and the response to glycine. This, together with direct measurements of glycine release in response to nerve stimulation, provides strong evidence for its physiological transmitter role. β-alanine has pharmacological effects and a pattern of distribution very similar to glycine, but its action is not blocked by strychnine.

The inhibitory effect of glycine is quite distinct from its role in facilitating excitatory responses mediated by NMDA (see p. 473).

The glycine receptor (see Rajendra et al 1997) resembles the GABA$_A$-receptor; it is a multimeric ligand-gated chloride channel, of which a number of subtypes have been identified by cloning, and mutations of the receptor have been identified in some inherited neurological disorders associated with muscle spasm and reflex hyperexcitability. There are no therapeutic drugs which act by modifying glycinergic transmission. Tetanus toxin, a bacterial toxin resembling botulinum toxin (Ch. 7) acts selectively to prevent glycine release from inhibitory interneurons in the spinal cord, causing excessive reflex hyperexcitability and violent muscle spasms ('lockjaw').

Inhibitory amino acids: GABA and glycine

- GABA is the main inhibitory transmitter in the brain.
- It is present fairly uniformly throughout the brain; there is very little in peripheral tissues.
- GABA is formed from glutamate, by the action of GAD (glutamic acid decarboxylase). Its action is terminated mainly by reuptake, but also by deamination, catalysed by GABA-transaminase.
- There are two types of GABA receptor, GABA$_A$ and GABA$_B$.
- GABA$_A$-receptors, which occur mainly postsynaptically, are directly coupled to chloride channels, opening of which reduces membrane excitability. Muscimol is a specific GABA$_A$ agonist, and the convulsant, bicuculline, is an antagonist.
- Other drugs that interact with GABA$_A$-receptors and channels include:
  — benzodiazepine tranquillisers, which act at an accessory binding site to facilitate the action of GABA

- — convulsants such as picrotoxin, which block the anion channel
- — neurosteroids, including endogenous progesterone metabolites, and other CNS depressants, such as barbiturates, which facilitate the action of GABA.
- GABA$_B$ receptors are G-protein-coupled receptors, linked to inhibition of cAMP formation. They cause pre- and postsynaptic inhibition by inhibiting Ca^{2+} channel opening and increasing K$^+$ conductance. Baclofen is a GABA$_B$-receptor agonist, used to treat spasticity. GABA$_B$ antagonists are not yet in clinical use.
- Glycine is an inhibitory transmitter mainly in the spinal cord, acting on its own receptor, which functionally resembles the GABA$_A$ receptor.
- The convulsant drug, strychnine, is a competitive glycine antagonist. Tetanus toxin acts mainly by interfering with glycine release.

REFERENCES AND FURTHER READING

References cited are short authoritative review articles on different aspects of amino acid transmitters and receptors.

Barnard E A 1997 Ionotropic glutamate receptors: new types and new concepts. Trends Pharmacol Sci 18: 141–148

Bliss T V P, Collingridge G L 1993 A synaptic model of memory: long-term potentiation in the hippocampus. Nature 361: 31–38

Bormann J 1988 Electrophysiology of GABA$_A$ and GABA$_B$ receptor subtypes. Trends Neurosci 11: 112–116

Bowery N G 1993 GABA$_B$ receptor pharmacology. Ann Rev Pharmacol Toxicol 33: 109–147

Conn P J, Pin J-P 1997 Pharmacology and functions of metabotropic glutamate receptors. Ann Rev Pharmacol 37: 205–237

Cotman C W, Kahle J S, Miller S E, Ulas J, Bridges R J 1995 Excitatory amino acid transmission. In: Bloom F E, Kupfer D J (eds) Psychopharmacology: a fourth generation of progress. Raven Press, New York, pp 75–85

Johnston G A R 1996 GABA$_A$-receptor pharmacology. Pharmacol

Ther 69: 173–198

Kemp J A, Leeson P D 1993 The glycine site of the NMDA receptor—five years on. Trends Pharmacol Sci 14: 20–25

Lambert J J, Belelli D, Hill-Venning C, Peters J A 1995 Neurosteroids and GABA$_A$-receptor function. Trends Pharmacol Sci 16: 295–303

Lipton S A 1993 Prospects for clinically tolerated NMDA antagonists: open-channel blockers and alternative redox states of nitric oxide. Trends Neurosci 16: 527–532

Lodge D, Collingridge G 1990 Les agents provocateurs: a series on the pharmacology of excitatory amino acids. Trends Pharmacol Sci 11: 22–24 (Series of reviews in this journal published in 1990)

Malenka R C, Nicoll R A 1993 NMDA-receptor-dependent synaptic plasticity: multiple forms and mechanisms. Trends Neurosci 16: 521–527

Nicoletti F, Bruno V, Copani A, Caasabona G, Knopfel T 1996 Metabotropic glutamate receptors: a new target for the therapy of neurodegenerative disorders? Trends Neurosci 19: 267–271

Rajendra S, Lynch J W, Schofield P R 1997 The glycine receptor. Pharmacol Ther 73: 121–146

Schoep D D, Conn P J 1993 Metabotropic glutamate receptors in brain function and pathology. Trends Pharmacol Sci 14: 13–20

Seeburg P H 1993 The molecular biology of mammalian glutamate receptor channels. Trends Neurosci 16: 359–365

Smith G B, Olsen R W 1995 Functional domains of GABA$_A$-receptors. Trends Pharmacol Sci 16: 162–168

Sucher N J, Awobuluyi M, Choi Y-B, Lipton S A 1996 NMDA receptors: from genes to channels. Trends Pharmacol Sci 17: 348–355

Takahashi M, Billups B, Rossi D, Sarantis M, Hamann M, Attwell D 1997 The role of gluatamate transporters in glutamate homeostasis in the brain. J Exp Biol 200(2): 401–409

30

Other transmitters and modulators

In this chapter we discuss the principal monoamine transmitters in the central nervous system, namely, dopamine. 5-hydroxytryptamine (5-HT) and acetylcholine, as well as other mediators about which less is currently known, such as histamine, melatonin and purines. The monoamines were the first CNS transmitters to be identified, and rapid advances came in the mid-1960s, during a remarkable decade of progress—the 'monoamine years'—when a combination of neurochemistry and neuropharmacology led to many important discoveries about the role of CNS transmitters, and about the ability of drugs to influence these systems. Many of the currently used psychotropic drugs that are discussed in later chapters owe their effects to mechanisms that are related to these mediators. They differ from the amino acid transmitters discussed in Chapter 29 in being more localised in particular neurons and tracts, and they are broadly associated with high-level behaviours (for example the stereotypic behaviour associated with enhanced dopamine activity; see below), rather than with overall synaptic excitation or inhibition. More recently, some 'atypical' chemical mediators, such as nitric oxide (Ch. 11) and arachidonic acid metabolites (Ch. 12) have come on the scene, and they are discussed at the end of the chapter. Information on the other major class of CNS mediators, the neuropeptides, is given in Chapter 10, and specific neuropeptides are discussed in Chapters 23, 24, 26, 33 and 37.

The picture currently is of a profusion of different mediators and an even greater motley of receptor subtypes, converging on well-characterised effector mechanisms at the cellular level. Yet, we generally describe their effects on brain function only in relatively crude terms—psychopharmacologists will be at our throats for so underrating the sophistication of their measurements—such as 'motor incoordination', 'arousal', 'cognitive impairment', etc. The gap between these two levels of understanding (the Grand Canyon referred to in Ch. 28) still frustrates the best efforts to link drug action at the molecular level to drug action at the therapeutic level. More detail on the content of this chapter can be found in Cooper et al (1996).

NORADRENALINE

Many aspects of noradrenergic transmission have been discussed in Chapter 8. The basic processes responsible for the synthesis, storage, release and reuptake of noradrenaline are the same in the brain as in the periphery, and the same types of adrenoceptor are also found in pre- and postsynaptic locations in the brain. Here we will consider anatomical and functional aspects of central noradrenergic pathways and their possible involvement in different types of mental disorder.

NORADRENERGIC PATHWAYS IN THE CNS

Though the transmitter role of noradrenaline in the brain was suspected in the 1950s, detailed analysis of its neuronal distribution only became possible when the fluorescence technique, based on the formation of a fluorescent derivative of catecholamines when tissues are exposed to formaldehyde, was devised by Falck & Hillarp. Detailed maps of the pathways of noradrenergic, dopaminergic and serotonergic neurons in laboratory animals were produced, and the same basic features have since been confirmed in human brains. The cell bodies of noradrenergic neurons are restricted to a number of small clusters in the pons and medulla, which send extensively branching axons to many other parts of the brain (Fig. 30.1) including the cerebral cortex, limbic system, hypothalamus, cerebellum and spinal cord. The most prominent cluster of noradrenergic neurons is the *locus ceruleus (LC)*, which is found in the grey matter of the pons. Although it contains only about 10 000 neurons in humans, the axons, running in a discrete *medial forebrain bundle*, give rise to many millions of noradrenergic nerve terminals throughout the cortex, hippocampus and cerebellum. The nerve terminals in this very diffuse system do not form distinct synaptic contacts, but appear to release transmitter at some distance from the target cell. Thus the noradrenergic system resembles a neural aerosol—a touch on the LC push-button and large areas of the brain are sprayed with noradrenaline.

Other noradrenergic neurons lie close to the LC in the pons and medulla. Axons from these cells innervate the hypothalamus, hippocampus and other parts of the forebrain, and also project to the cerebellum and spinal cord. There are also a smaller number of *adrenergic* neurons, whose cell bodies lie more ventrally in the brainstem. Their fibres run mainly to the pons and medulla and hypothalamus, and release adrenaline rather than noradrenaline. Rather little is known about them, but they are believed to be important in cardiovascular control.

FUNCTIONAL ASPECTS

Noradrenaline applied to individual cells in the brain usually causes inhibition, and in most cases this is produced by activation of β-adrenoceptors, linked to cAMP accumulation. In some situations, however, noradrenaline has an excitatory effect, which is mediated by either α- or β-adrenoceptors.

Arousal and mood

Attention has focused mainly on the LC, which is the source of most of the noradrenaline released in the brain, and from which neuronal activity can be measured by implanted electrodes. There is generally a good correlation between LC activity and behavioural arousal. LC neurons are silent during sleep. 'Wake-up' stimuli of an unfamiliar or threatening kind excite these neurons much more effectively than familiar stimuli. Amphetamine-like

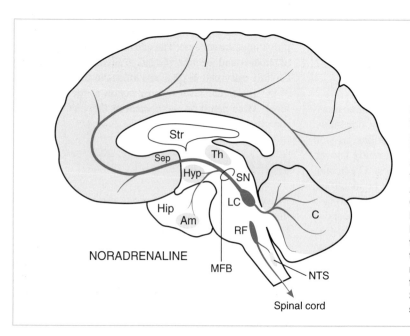

Fig. 30.1 Noradrenaline pathways in the brain. The location of the main groups of cell bodies and fibre tracts is in solid colour. Light shaded areas show the location of noradrenergic terminals. (Ac = Nucleus accumbens; Am = Amygdaloid nucleus; C = cerebellum; LC = locus ceruleus; Hip = hippocampus; Hyp = hypothalamus; MFB = medial forebrain bundle; NTS = nucleus of the tractus solitarius (vagal sensory nucleus); RF = brainstem reticular formation; Sep = septum; SN = substantia nigra; Str = corpus striatum; Th = thalamus)

drugs, which release catecholamines in the brain, increase wakefulness, alertness and exploratory activity (though, in this case, firing of LC neurons is actually reduced, by feedback mechanisms; see Ch. 38).

There is a close relationship between *mood* and state of arousal; depressed individuals are usually lethargic and unresponsive to external stimuli. The catecholamine hypothesis of affective disorders (see Ch. 35) suggested that *depression* results from a functional deficiency of noradrenaline in certain parts of the brain, while mania results from an excess. This remains controversial, and subsequent findings suggest that 5-HT may be more important than noradrenaline in relation to mood.

Blood pressure regulation

The role of central, as well as peripheral, noradrenergic synapses in blood pressure control is shown by the action of hypotensive drugs such as **clonidine** and **methyldopa** (see Chs 8 and 15), which decrease the discharge of sympathetic nerves emerging from the central nervous system. They cause hypotension when injected locally into the medulla or fourth ventricle, in much smaller amounts than are required when the drugs are given systemically. Noradrenaline, and other α_2-adrenoceptor agonists, have the same effect when injected locally. Noradrenergic synapses in the medulla probably form part of the baroreceptor reflex pathway, since stimulation or antagonism

---

Noradrenaline in the CNS

- Mechanisms for synthesis, storage, release and reuptake of noradrenaline in the CNS are essentially the same as in the periphery, as are the receptors (Ch. 8).
- Noradrenergic cell bodies occur in discrete clusters, mainly in the pons and medulla, one important such cell group being the locus ceruleus.
- Noradrenergic pathways, running mainly in the medial forebrain bundle, and descending spinal tracts, terminate diffusely in the cortex, hippocampus, hypothalamus, cerebellum and spinal cord.
- The actions of noradrenaline are mainly inhibitory (β-receptors), but some are excitatory (α- or β-receptors).
- Noradrenergic transmission is believed to be important in the 'arousal' system, controlling wakefulness and alertness; blood pressure regulation: control of mood (functional deficiency contributing to depression), and function of 'reward system'.
- Psychotropic drugs that act partly or mainly on noradrenergic transmission in the CNS include: antidepressants, cocaine, amphetamine. Some antihypertensive drugs (e.g. clonidine, methyldopa) act mainly on noradrenergic transmission in the CNS.

---

of α_2-adrenoceptors in this part of the brain has a powerful effect on the activity of baroreceptor reflexes.

Ascending noradrenergic fibres run to the hypothalamus, and descending fibres run to the lateral horn region of the spinal cord, acting to increase sympathetic discharge in the periphery. It has been suggested that these regulatory neurons may release adrenaline, rather than noradrenaline. Some catecholamine-containing cells in the brainstem contain PNMT (the enzyme that converts noradrenaline to adrenaline; see Ch. 8) and inhibition of this enzyme interferes with the baroreceptor reflex.

DOPAMINE

The distribution of dopamine in the brain is more restricted than that of noradrenaline. A large proportion of the dopamine content of the brain is found in the *corpus striatum*, a part of the extrapyramidal motor system concerned with the coordination of movement (see Ch. 31), and there is also a high concentration in certain parts of the *limbic system* and in the *hypothalamus*.

The synthesis of dopamine follows the same route as that of noradrenaline (see Ch. 8), namely conversion of tyrosine to dopa (the rate-limiting step) followed by decarboxylation to form dopamine (Fig. 30.2). Dopaminergic neurons lack dopamine β-hydroxylase, and thus do not produce noradrenaline.

Dopamine is largely recaptured, following its release from nerve terminals, by a specific dopamine transporter, similar to that for other monoamines (see Giros & Caron 1993). It is metabolised by MAO and COMT (see Ch. 8), the main products being *dihydroxyphenylacetic acid* (DOPAC) and *homovanillic acid* (HVA, the methoxyderivative of DOPAC). The brain content of HVA is often used as an index of dopamine turnover. Drugs that cause the release of dopamine increase HVA, often without changing the concentration of dopamine. DOPAC and HVA, and their sulphate conjugates, are excreted in the urine, which provides an index of dopamine release in human subjects.

DOPAMINERGIC PATHWAYS IN THE CNS

Dopaminergic neurons form three main systems (Fig. 30.3). About 75% of the dopamine in the brain, occurs in the *nigrostriatal pathway*, with cell bodies in the *substantia nigra* (forming the A9 cell group in rats) and the axons terminating in the *corpus striatum*. These fibres run in the medial forebrain bundle along with many noradrenaline- and 5-HT-containing fibres. The abundance of dopamine-

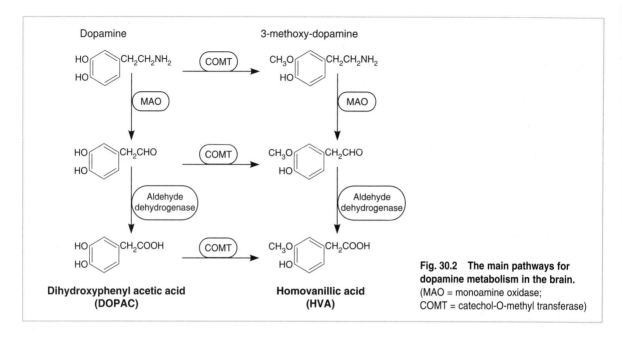

Fig. 30.2 (from image): Dopamine → 3-methoxy-dopamine

Dopamine   3-methoxy-dopamine

HO–[ring]–CH₂CH₂NH₂ → (COMT) → CH₃O–[ring]–CH₂CH₂NH₂ (HO)

(MAO) ↓   ↓ (MAO)

HO–[ring]–CH₂CHO → (COMT) → CH₃O–[ring]–CH₂CHO (HO)

(Aldehyde dehydrogenase) ↓   ↓ (Aldehyde dehydrogenase)

HO–[ring]–CH₂COOH → (COMT) → CH₃O–[ring]–CH₂COOH (HO)

Dihydroxyphenyl acetic acid (DOPAC)   **Homovanillic acid (HVA)**

Fig. 30.2 The main pathways for dopamine metabolism in the brain. (MAO = monoamine oxidase; COMT = catechol-O-methyl transferase)

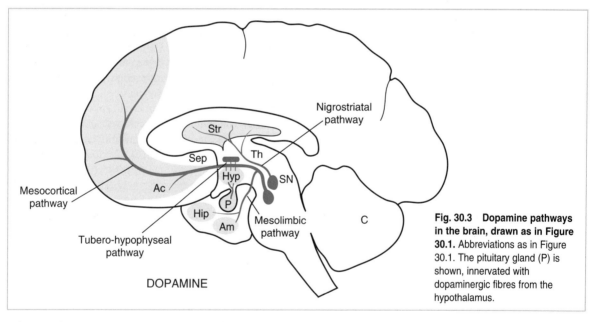

DOPAMINE

Fig. 30.3 Dopamine pathways in the brain, drawn as in Figure 30.1. Abbreviations as in Figure 30.1. The pituitary gland (P) is shown, innervated with dopaminergic fibres from the hypothalamus.

containing neurons in the human striatum can be appreciated from the image shown in Figure 30.4, which was obtained by injecting a dopa derivative containing radioactive fluorine, and scanning for radioactivity 3 hours later by positron emission tomography (PET). The second important system is the *mesolimbic/mesocortical pathway*, whose cell bodies occur in groups in the midbrain (mainly the A10 cell group) with fibres projecting, also via the

medial forebrain bundle, to parts of the limbic system, especially the *nucleus accumbens* and the *amygdaloid nucleus* and to the cortex. Finally, the *tuberohypophyseal system* is a group of short neurons running from the arcuate nucleus of the hypothalamus to the median eminence and pituitary gland, the secretions of which they regulate. There are also many local dopaminergic interneurons in the olfactory cortex and medulla, and in the retina.

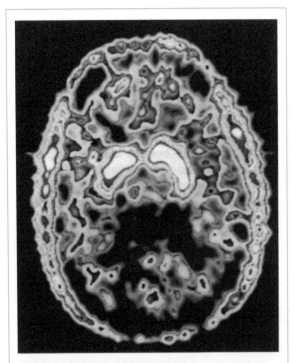

Fig. 30.4 Dopamine in the basal ganglia of a human subject. The subject was injected with 5-fluoro-dopa labelled with the positron-emitting isotope ^{18}F, which was localised 3 hours later by the technique of positron emission tomography. The isotope is accumulated (white areas) by the dopa-uptake system of the neurons of the basal ganglia, and to a smaller extent in the frontal cortex. It is also seen in the scalp and temporalis muscles. (From: Garnett E S et al. Nature 305: 137)

DOPAMINE RECEPTORS

Two types of receptor, D_1 and D_2 (linked, respectively, to activation and inhibition of adenylate cyclase) were originally distinguished on pharmacological and biochemical grounds. Gene cloning has revealed further subgroups, D_1 to D_5 (for review, see Jaber et al. 1996, Seeman & Van Tol 1994). The original D_1 family now includes D_1 and D_5, while the D_2 family, which is pharmacologically more important in the CNS, consists of D_2, D_3 and D_4 (see Table 30.1), of which further splice variants, leading to long and short forms of D_2, and genetic polymorphisms, particularly of D_4 (see below) have subsequently been identified. All belong to the family of G-protein-coupled transmembrane receptors described in Chapter 2, and their signal transduction mechanisms, linked via adenylate cyclase and/or phospholipid hydrolysis to the control of K^+ and Ca^{2+} channels,

arachidonic acid release etc., are similar to those of other such receptors. They are expressed in the brain in distinct but overlapping areas. D_1-receptors are the most abundant and widespread in areas receiving a dopaminergic innervation (namely the striatum, the limbic system, thalamus and hypothalamus: Fig. 30.3), as are D_2-receptors, which also occur in the pituitary gland. D_3-receptors occur in the limbic system, but not in the striatum. Since dopamine antagonists used as antipsychotic drugs (Ch. 34) owe their actions to effects in the mesolimbic system, but often cause motor side-effects by blocking receptors in the striatum, there is interest in targeting the D_3- and D_4-receptors as a means of avoiding these side-effects. The D_4-receptor is much more weakly expressed, mainly in the cortex and limbic systems, but is a focus of interest because of its possible relationship to the mechanism of schizophrenia (Ch. 34) and drug dependence (Ch. 39).

The dopamine receptors relevant to the actions of antipsychotic drugs (Ch. 34) mainly belong to the D_2 family, but the cellular mechanisms remain unclear, because the cells are difficult to study in isolation. In the anterior pituitary, where D_2-receptors cause inhibition of prolactin secretion (see Ch. 24), the cellular mechanism involves inhibition of calcium mobilisation and opening of potassium channels, as well as other ion channel effects.

The D_4-receptor displays an unexpected polymorphism in humans, with a varying number (from 2 to 10) of 16 amino acid repeat sequences being expressed in the third intracellular loop, which participates in G-protein coupling (Ch. 2). However, neither this polymorphism, nor the long/short splice variants in the D_2-receptor are associated with significant changes in receptor function. Expectations that D_4-receptor polymorphism might be related to the occurrence of schizophrenia in man were disappointed after several studies failed to find any correlation. The possible connection with drug dependence is discussed in Chapter 39.

Dopamine, like many other transmitters and modulators, acts presynaptically as well as postsynaptically. Presynaptic D_3-receptors occur mainly on dopaminergic neurons, for example those in the striatum and limbic system, where they act to inhibit dopamine synthesis and release. Dopamine antagonists, by blocking these receptors, increase dopamine synthesis and release, and cause accumulation of dopamine metabolites in these parts of the brain. They also cause an increase in the rate of firing of dopaminergic neurons (see Cooper et al. 1996), probably by blocking a neuronal feedback pathway.

Dopamine receptors also mediate various effects in the periphery, (mediated by D_1-receptors) notably renal

Table 30.1 Dopamine receptors

Distribution	Functional role	D₁ type		D₂ type		
		D_1	D_5	D_2	D_3	D_4
Distribution	**Functional role**					
Cortex	Arousal, mood	++	–	++	–	–
Limbic system	Emotion, stereotypic behaviour	+++	–	+++	+	+
Basal ganglia	Motor control	++	+	+++	+	+
Hypothalamus	Autonomic and endocrine control	++	+	–	–	–
Pituitary gland	Endocrine control	–	–	+++	–	–
Agonists	Dopamine	+ (low potency)		+ (high potency)		
	Apomorphine	PA (low potency)		+ (high potency)		
	Bromocriptine	PA (low potency)		+ (high potency)		
Antagonists	Chlorpromazine	+	+	+++	+++	+
	Haloperidol	++	+	+++	+++	+++
	Spiperone	–	–	+++	+++	+++
	Sulpiride	–	–	+++	++	–
	Clozapine	+	+	+	+	++
Signal transduction		Increase cAMP		Decrease cAMP and/or increase IP₃		
Effect		Mainly postsynaptic inhibition		Pre- and postsynaptic inhibition Stimulation/inhibition of hormone release		

PA = partial agonist

vasodilatation and increased myocardial contractility, and dopamine itself is used clinically in the treatment of circulatory shock (see Ch. 15).

FUNCTIONAL ASPECTS

The functions of dopaminergic pathways divide broadly into:

- motor control (nigrostriatal system)
- behavioural effects (mesolimbic and mesocortical systems)
- endocrine control (tuberohypophyseal system).

Dopamine and motor systems

Ungerstedt showed, in 1968, that bilateral ablation of the *substantia nigra* in rats, which destroys the nigrostriatal neurons, causes profound catalepsy, the animals becoming so inactive that they die of starvation unless artificially fed. Unilateral lesions produced by 6-hydroxydopamine injection caused the animal to turn in circles *towards* the lesioned side, because of an imbalance of dopamine action in the *corpus striatum* between the two sides of the brain. Thus, unilateral injection of **apomor-**

phine (a dopamine-like agonist) into the striatum causes circling away from the injected side. If apomorphine is given systemically to normal rats it causes, as one would expect, no asymmetrical pattern of locomotion, but if given systemically to animals with unilateral lesions of the substantia nigra made days or weeks earlier, apomorphine causes circling *away* from the lesioned side. This is thought to be due to denervation supersensitivity (see Ch. 6), which arises because the destruction of dopaminergic terminals on one side causes a proliferation of dopamine receptors, and hence supersensitivity to apomorphine, of the cells on that side of the striatum. In these animals, administration of drugs that act by releasing dopamine (e.g. **amphetamine**) cause turning *towards* the lesioned side, since the dopaminergic nerve terminals are only present on the normal side. This 'turning model' has been extremely useful in investigating the action of drugs on dopaminergic neurons and dopamine receptors.

Parkinson's disease (Ch. 31) is a disorder of motor control, associated with a deficiency of dopamine in the nigrostriatal pathway.

Many antipsychotic drugs (see Ch. 34) are D₂-receptor antagonists, whose major side-effect is to cause movement disorders, probably associated with block of D_2-receptors in the nigrostriatal pathway.

Transgenic mice lacking D_2-receptors show greatly reduced spontaneous movement, resembling Parkinson's disease.

Behavioural effects

Administration of **amphetamine** to rats, which releases both dopamine and noradrenaline, causes a cessation of normal 'ratty' behaviour (exploration and grooming) and the appearance of repeated 'stereotyped' behaviour (rearing, gnawing and so on) unrelated to external stimuli. These effects are prevented by **dopamine antagonists**, and by destruction of dopamine-containing cell bodies in the midbrain, but not by drugs that inhibit the noradrenergic system. These amphetamine-induced motor disturbances in rats probably reflect hyperactivity in the nigrostriatal dopaminergic system.

Amphetamine also causes a general increase in motor activity, which can be measured, for example, by counting electronically the frequency at which a rat crosses from one part of its enclosure to another. This effect, in contrast to stereotypy, appears to be related to the mesolimbic and mesocortical dopaminergic pathways. There is some evidence (see Ch. 34) that schizophrenia in humans is associated with dopaminergic hyperactivity, but attempts to detect behavioural effects of dopamine in animals that might be related to the symptoms of human schizophrenia have been generally unsuccessful. Chronic administration of amphetamine to a few rats in a large colony produces various types of abnormal social interaction, including withdrawal and aggressive behaviour, but it is difficult to quantify such effects or to establish their relationship to schizophrenia in man.

Surprisingly, deletion of the D_1-receptor gene in mice causes a marked increase in locomotor activity (an effect opposite to that of D_2-receptor deletion), coupled with an insensitivity of the animals to amphetamine and cocaine (which enhances dopamine activity in the brain; see Ch. 38).

Neuroendocrine function

The tuberohypophyseal dopaminergic pathway (see Fig. 30.3) is involved in the control of *prolactin* secretion. The hypothalamus secretes various mediators (mostly small peptides; see Ch. 24), which control the secretion of different hormones from the pituitary gland. One of these, which has an inhibitory effect on prolactin release, is dopamine. This system is of clinical importance. Many antipsychotic drugs (see Ch. 34), by blocking D_2 receptors, increase prolactin secretion, and can cause breast de-

velopment and lactation, even in males. **Bromocriptine**, a dopamine receptor agonist derived from ergot, is used clinically to suppress prolactin secretion by tumours of the pituitary gland.

Growth hormone is increased in normal subjects by dopamine, but bromocriptine paradoxically inhibits the excessive secretion responsible for acromegaly, and has a useful therapeutic effect, provided it is given before excessive growth has taken place (see Ch. 24).

Vomiting

Pharmacological evidence strongly suggests that dopaminergic neurons have a role in the production of nausea and vomiting. Thus, nearly all dopamine receptor agonists (e.g. bromocriptine) and other drugs that increase dopamine release in the brain (e.g. levodopa; Ch. 31) cause nausea and vomiting as side-effects, while many

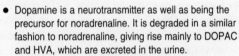

Dopamine in the CNS

- Dopamine is a neurotransmitter as well as being the precursor for noradrenaline. It is degraded in a similar fashion to noradrenaline, giving rise mainly to DOPAC and HVA, which are excreted in the urine.
- There are three main dopaminergic pathways:
  — nigrostriatal pathway, important in motor control
  — mesolimbic/mesocortical pathways, running from groups of cells in the midbrain to parts of the limbic system, especially the nucleus accumbens, and to the cortex; they are involved in emotion and drug-induced reward systems
  — tuberohypophyseal neurons running from the hypothalamus to the pituitary gland, whose secretions they regulate.
- There are two main families of dopamine receptor, D_1 and D_2, linked, respectively, to stimulation and inhibition of adenylate cyclase. The D_1 family comprises D_1 and D_5 subtypes. The D_2 family comprises D_2, D_3 and D_4 subtypes. The known functions of dopamine appear to be mediated mainly by receptors of the D_2 family.
- Receptors of the D_2 family may be implicated in schizophrenia. The D_4-receptor shows marked polymorphism in humans.
- Parkinson's disease is associated with a deficiency of nigrostriatal dopaminergic neurons.
- Behavioural effects of an excess of dopamine activity consist of stereotyped behaviour patterns, and can be produced by dopamine-releasing agents (e.g. amphetamine) and dopamine agonists (e.g. apomorphine).
- Hormone release from the anterior pituitary gland is regulated by dopamine, especially prolactin release (inhibited) and growth hormone release (stimulated).
- Dopamine acts on the chemoreceptor trigger zone to cause nausea and vomiting.

dopamine antagonists (e.g. phenothiazines, metoclopramide; Ch. 21) have anti-emetic activity. D_2-receptors occur in the area of the medulla (*chemoreceptor trigger zone*) associated with the initiation of vomiting (Ch. 21), and are assumed to mediate this effect.

5-HYDROXYTRYPTAMINE

The occurrence and functions of 5-HT in the periphery are described in Chapter 9. Interest in 5-HT as a possible CNS transmitter dates from 1953, when Gaddum found that *lysergic acid diethylamide* (LSD), a drug known to be a powerful hallucinogen, acted as a 5-HT antagonist on peripheral tissues, and suggested that its central effects might also be related to this action. Its presence in the brain was demonstrated a few years later. Even though brain accounts for only about 1% of the total body content, 5-HT is an important CNS transmitter (see Cooper et al. 1996).

In its formation, storage and release 5-HT resembles noradrenaline (see Fig. 9.1). Its precursor is *tryptophan*, an amino acid derived from dietary protein, the plasma content of which varies considerably according to food intake and time of day. Tryptophan is actively taken up into neurons, converted by tryptophan hydroxylase to *5-hydroxytryptophan* and then decarboxylated by a nonspecific amino acid decarboxylase to 5-HT. Tryptophan hydroxylase can be selectively and irreversibly inhibited by *p-chlorophenylalanine* (PCPA). Availability of tryptophan, and the activity of tryptophan hydroxylase are thought to be the main processes that regulate 5-HT synthesis. The decarboxylase is very similar, if not identical, to DOPA decarboxylase, and does not play any role in regulating 5-HT synthesis. Following release, 5-HT is largely recovered by neuronal uptake, this mechanism being inhibited by many of the same drugs (e.g. **tricyclic antidepressants**) that inhibit catecholamine uptake. The carrier is not identical, however, and inhibitors show varying degrees of specificity between the two. Specific serotonin reuptake inhibitors (SSRIs; see Ch. 35) constitute an important group of antidepressant drugs. 5-HT is degraded almost entirely by MAO (Fig. 9.1), which converts it to 5-hydroxyindole acetaldehyde, most of which is dehydrogenated to form 5-hydroxyindole acetic acid (5-HIAA), which is excreted in the urine.

5-HT PATHWAYS IN THE CNS

The distribution of neurons containing 5-HT is very widespread (Fig. 30.5), and is similar to that of noradrenergic neurons. The cells occur in several large clusters in the pons and upper medulla, which lie close to the midline (raphe) and are often referred to as *raphe nuclei*. The rostrally situated nuclei project, via the medial forebrain bundle, to many parts of the cortex, hippocampus, basal ganglia, limbic system and hypothalamus. The caudally situated cells project to the cerebellum, medulla and spinal cord.

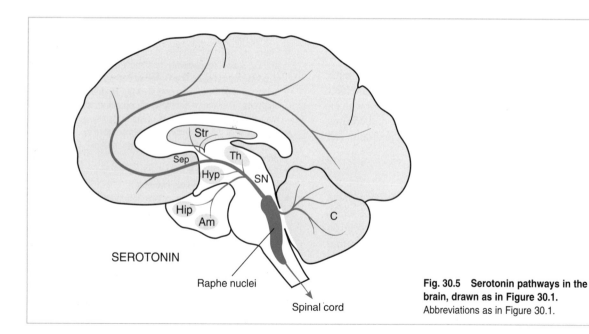

Fig. 30.5 Serotonin pathways in the brain, drawn as in Figure 30.1.
Abbreviations as in Figure 30.1.

5-HT RECEPTORS IN THE CNS

The main 5-HT receptor types are shown in Table 9.1. All are G-protein-coupled receptors except for 5-HT$_3$, which is a ligand-gated cation channel. All are expressed in the CNS, but most of the functional data relate to the three most venerable members of the clan, namely 5-HT$_1$, 5-HT$_2$ and 5-HT$_3$.

5-HT$_1$-receptors are predominantly inhibitory in their effects. 5-HT$_{1A}$-receptors are expressed as autoreceptors by the 5-HT neurons in the raphe nuclei, and their auto-inhibitory effect tends to limit the rate of firing of these cells. They are also widely distributed in the cortex and amygdala, and are believed to be the main target of drugs used to treat anxiety and depression (see Chs 33 and 35). 5-HT$_{1B}$- and 5-HT$_D$-receptors are found mainly as presynaptic inhibitory receptors in the basal ganglia.

5-HT$_2$-receptors (mostly 5-HT$_{2A}$ in the brain) exert an excitatory postsynaptic effect, and are abundant in the cortex and hippocampus. They are believed to be the target of various hallucinogenic drugs (see Ch. 38). The use of 5-HT$_2$-receptor antagonists in treating migraine is discussed in Chapter 9.

5-HT$_3$-receptors are found chiefly in the *area postrema* (a region of the medulla involved in vomiting; see Ch. 21) and other parts of the brainstem, extending to the dorsal horn of the spinal cord. They are also widely, but more sparsely, present in certain parts of the cortex.

Although the remaining members of the 5-HT receptor family are known to be expressed in discrete areas of the brain, little is known so far about their function. Specific agonists and antagonists at these receptors are being investigated, but none are currently in clinical use.

FUNCTIONAL ASPECTS

The precise localisation of 5-HT neurons in the brainstem has allowed their electrical activity to be studied in detail, and correlated with behavioural and other effects produced by drugs thought to affect 5-HT-mediated transmission. 5-HT cells show an unusual, highly regular slow discharge pattern, and are strongly inhibited by 5-HT$_1$-receptor agonists, suggesting a local inhibitory feedback mechanism.

In vertebrates, certain physiological and behavioural functions relate particularly to 5-HT pathways (see Marsden & Heal 1992), namely:

- hallucinations and behavioural changes
- sleep, wakefulness and mood
- control of sensory transmission.

Hallucinatory effects

Many centrally acting 5-HT analogues (e.g. LSD) are hallucinogenic (see Ch. 38), and depress the firing of brainstem 5-HT neurons. These neurons exert an inhibitory influence on cortical neurons, and it is suggested that the loss of cortical inhibition resulting from suppression of activity in these neurons underlies the hallucinogenic effect, as well as certain behavioural effects in experimental animals, such as the 'wet-dog shakes' that occur in rats when the 5-HT precursor, 5-HTP, is administered.

Sleep, wakefulness and mood

Lesions of the raphe nuclei, or depletion of 5-HT by PCPA administration abolish sleep in experimental animals, whereas micro-injection of 5-HT at specific points in the brainstem induces sleep. Attempts to cure insomnia in humans by giving 5-HT precursors (tryptophan or 5-hydroxytryptophan) have, however, proved unsuccessful. There is evidence that 5-HT, as well as noradrenaline, may be involved in the control of mood (see Ch. 35), and the use of tryptophan to enhance 5-HT synthesis has been tried in depression, with equivocal results.

Sensory transmission

After lesions of the raphe nuclei or administration of PCPA, animals show exaggerated responses to many forms of sensory stimulus. They are startled much more easily, and also quickly develop avoidance responses to stimuli that would not normally produce this effect. It appears that the normal ability to disregard irrelevant forms of sensory input requires intact 5-HT pathways. The 'sensory enhancement' produced by hallucinogenic drugs may be partly due to antagonism of 5-HT. 5-HT also exerts an inhibitory effect on transmission in the pain pathway, both in the spinal cord and in the brain, and there is a synergistic effect between 5-HT and analgesics such as morphine (see Ch. 37). Thus depletion of 5-HT by PCPA, or selective lesions to the descending 5-HT-containing neurons that run to the dorsal horn, antagonise the analgesic effect of morphine, while inhibitors of 5-HT uptake have the opposite effect. Other functions in which 5-HT has been implicated include the control of food intake and various autonomic and endocrine functions, such as the regulation of body temperature, blood pressure, and sexual function. Further information can be found in Azmitia & Whitaker-Azmitia (1995) and Cooper et al. (1996).

It will be realised that 5-HT is involved in many very important physiological processes, and there is clearly scope for new drugs that influence 5-HTergic transmission in a selective way. Current examples include SSRIs (Ch. 36); **buspirone**, a 5-HT$_{1A}$-receptor agonist (Ch. 9), is effective in treating anxiety (Ch. 33); 5-HT$_3$-receptor antagonists, such as **ondansetron** (Ch 9), which are used principally as anti-emetic agents (see Ch. 21), are also active in animal models of anxiety, and may prove to be clinically useful in this context. It is possible that some antipsychotic drugs (e.g. clozapine, Ch. 34) owe their efficacy partly to an action on 5-HT receptors.

5-hydroxytryptamine in the CNS

- The processes of synthesis, storage, release, reuptake and degradation of 5-HT in the brain are very similar to events in the periphery (Ch. 9).
- Availability of tryptophan is the main factor regulating synthesis.
- Urinary excretion of 5-HIAA provides a measure of 5-HT turnover.
- 5-HT neurons are concentrated in the midline raphe nuclei in the pons and medulla, projecting diffusely to the cortex, limbic system, hypothalamus and spinal cord, similar to the noradrenergic projections.
- Functions associated with 5-HT pathways include:
  — various behavioural responses (e.g. hallucinatory behaviour, 'wet-dog shakes')
  — feeding behaviour
  — control of mood and emotion
  — control of sleep/wakefulness
  — control of sensory pathways, including nociception
  — control of body temperature
  — vomiting.
- 5-HT can exert inhibitory or excitatory effects on individual neurons, acting either presynaptically or postsynaptically.
- The main receptor subtypes (see Table 9.1) in the CNS are: 5-HT$_{1A}$, 5-HT$_{1B}$, 5-HT$_{1D}$, 5-HT$_2$, 5-HT$_3$. Associations of behavioural and physiological functions with these receptors have been partly worked out. Other receptor types (5-HT$_{4-7}$) also occur in the CNS, but little is known about their function.

ACETYLCHOLINE

There are numerous cholinergic neurons in the central nervous system, and the basic processes by which acetylcholine is synthesised, stored and released are the same as in the periphery (see Ch. 7). Various biochemical markers have been used to locate cholinergic neurons in the brain, the most useful being choline acetyltransferase (CAT), the enzyme responsible for ACh synthesis, which can be labelled by immunofluorescence. Biochemical studies on acetylcholine precursors and metabolites are generally more difficult than corresponding studies on other amine transmitters, because the relevant substances, choline and acetate, are involved in many processes other than acetylcholine metabolism.

CHOLINERGIC PATHWAYS IN THE CNS

Acetylcholine is very widely distributed in the brain, occurring in all parts of the forebrain (including the cortex), midbrain and brainstem, though there is little in the cerebellum. Some of the main cholinergic pathways in the brain are shown in Figure 30.6. The anterior horns and roots of the spinal cord, and the motor nuclei of the cranial nerves contain much more acetylcholine than other parts of the CNS, reflecting the presence of cholinergic motoneurons supplying skeletal muscle. There is a diffuse cholinergic innervation supplying all areas of the forebrain, and the cell bodies of these cholinergic neurons lie in a small area of the basal forebrain, forming the *magnocellular forebrain nuclei* (so-called because the cell bodies are conspicuously large). Other groups of cholinergic neurons occur in the septum, from which the septohippocampal projection arises, and in the pons, from which fibres run to the thalamus and cortex.

Short cholinergic interneurons occur in many areas, particularly in the striatum and in the nucleus accumbens. The role of the striatal cholinergic neurons in connection with parkinsonism and Huntington's chorea is discussed in Chapter 31.

ACETYLCHOLINE RECEPTOR

Acetylcholine has mainly excitatory effects, which are mediated by various subtypes of either nicotinic (ligand-gated channels) or muscarinic (G-protein-coupled) receptors (see Ch. 7). Some muscarinic receptors are inhibitory.

The muscarinic receptors in the brain are predominantly of the M$_1$ type (see Ch. 7), and the central actions of muscarinic antagonists and anticholinesterases depend on block and stimulation of these receptors, respectively. Muscarinic receptors act presynaptically to inhibit acetylcholine release from cholinergic neurons, and muscarinic antagonists, by blocking this inhibition, markedly increase acetylcholine release. Many of the behavioural effects associated with cholinergic pathways seem to be produced by acetylcholine acting on muscarinic receptors.

Nicotinic receptors, are also widespread in the brain, but much sparser than muscarinic receptors. They resemble peripheral nicotinic receptors in their molecular

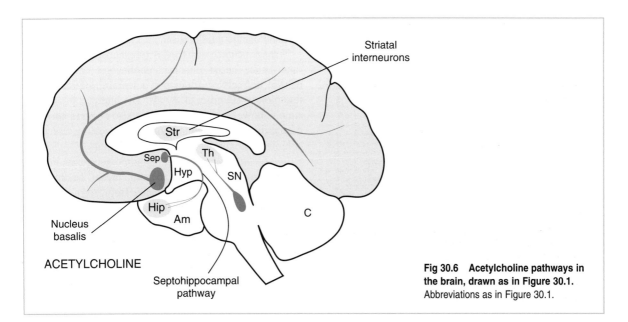

Fig 30.6 Acetylcholine pathways in the brain, drawn as in Figure 30.1. Abbreviations as in Figure 30.1.

structure (Ch. 2; for review see, Galzi & Changeux 1995, Role 1992), comprising pentameric assemblies of α- and β-subunits, each of which come in several patterns (α_{2-9}, and β_{2-5} being expressed in the brain) giving rise to the familiar picture of extensive molecular heterogeneity. Though nicotinic ACh receptors participate in fast excitatory transmission in the periphery, there are only a few situations where this has been observed in the CNS; mostly, these receptors appear to be located presynaptically, and to facilitate the release of other transmitters, such as glutamate and dopamine. Nicotine (see Ch. 39) exerts its central effects by agonist action on nicotinic ACh receptors.

Many of the drugs that block nicotinic receptors (e.g. **tubocurarine**; see Ch. 7) do not cross the blood–brain barrier, and even those that do (e.g. **mecamylamine**) produce no major CNS side-effects.

FUNCTIONAL ASPECTS

The first cholinergic synapse to be investigated in the CNS was that of the Renshaw cell in the ventral horn of the spinal cord. These small interneurons receive an excitatory cholinergic innervation from a branch of the axon of the motoneuron. This synapse works through nicotinic receptors, and its pharmacological properties are very similar to those of the neuromuscular junction (Ch. 7). The Renshaw cell in turn activates inhibitory interneurons that synapse with motoneurons.

Other functional characteristics of cholinergic path-

ways have been deduced mainly from studies of the action of drugs that mimic, accentuate or block the actions of acetylcholine on muscarinic receptors, so the evidence tends to be indirect and circumstantial.

The main functions ascribed to cholinergic pathways are related to arousal and learning, and motor control. Electroencephalographic (EEG) recording can be used to monitor the state of arousal in humans or in experimental animals. A drowsy, inattentive state is associated with a large amplitude, low-frequency EEG record, which switches to a low-amplitude, high-frequency pattern on arousal by any sensory stimulus. Administration of **physostigmine** (an anticholinesterase that crosses the blood–brain barrier) produces EEG arousal, whereas **atropine** has the opposite effect. It is presumed that the cholinergic projection from the ventral forebrain to the cortex mediates this response. The relationship of this response to behaviour is confusing, however, for physostigmine in humans causes a state of lethargy and anxiety, and in rats it depresses exploratory activity, whereas atropine causes excitement and agitation in humans, and increases exploratory activity in rats, effects opposite to what one might expect.

There is evidence that cholinergic pathways, in particular the septohippocampal pathway, are involved in learning and short-term memory (see Hagan & Morris 1988). For example (Fig. 30.7), mice may be trained to execute a maze-running manoeuvre in response to a buzzer, and many will remember the correct response when retested 7 days later. Intracerebral injection of a

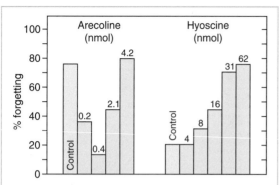

Fig 30.7 Effect of arecoline and hyoscine on learning.
Mice were trained to perform a behavioural feat in order to avoid an electric shock and tested for their ability to remember it 7 days later. The group that performed least well (left) were given the cholinergic agonist **arecoline** by intracerebroventricular injection; at low doses, their performance improved markedly, but at higher doses, their performance declined. The group that performed best in the initial test were given the muscarinic-receptor antagonist **hyoscine**, which caused a deterioration of their performance. (From Flood et al. 1981 Brain Res 215: 177–185)

muscarinic agonist, **arecoline**, immediately after the training session, reduces the percentage of animals which forget the correct response when retested, whereas an injection of the muscarinic antagonist, **hyoscine** (scopolamine), has the opposite effect. In the experiment shown in Figure 30.7 a deliberate bias was introduced, in that the mice selected for the arecoline test were particularly dim (the fast-learners having been excluded), and the training was brief, so that the forgetting rate in the control group was about 70%; an optimal dose of arecoline reduced this to about 15%. The hyoscine test was done on the cleverest mice (the no-hopers being excluded), and the training was more thorough, so the forgetting rate in the control group was only about 20%, and this was increased by hyoscine. More recently, synthetic muscarinic agonists have been shown partially to restore learning and memory deficits induced in experimental animals by lesions of the septohippocampal cholinergic pathway. Hyoscine also impairs memory in human subjects, and causes amnesia when used as preanaesthetic medication. **Nicotine** (see Ch. 39) increases alertness, and can also enhance learning and memory, as can various synthetic agonists at neuronal nicotinic receptors (see Arnevic et al. 1995). Nevertheless, transgenic mice with disruption of brain nicotinic receptors perform normally in a simple spatial learning task. In conclusion, both nicotinic and muscarinic receptors may play a role

in learning and memory, while nicotinic receptors also mediate behavioural arousal.

Transgenic mice which *overexpress* acetylcholinesterase (and hence show impaired cholinergic transmission) behave normally, but develop a learning deficit after a few months (Beeri et al. 1995). The interpretation is not simple, however, since these mice also respond poorly to muscarinic and nicotinic agonists, suggesting that more complex secondary effects were produced.

Involvement of neuronal nicotinic receptors in pain transmission is suggested by the recent finding that **epibatidine**, a compound extracted from frog skin, which is a selective agonist at these receptors, has powerful analgesic properties (Ch. 37).

The significance of cholinergic neurons in neuro-degenerative conditions such as dementia and Parkinson's disease is discussed in Chapter 31.

Secreted acetylcholinesterase

In addition to its well-established role as a membrane enzyme responsible for the rapid hydrolysis of acetylcholine (see Ch. 7), there is evidence that acetylcholinesterase may itself be released by neuronal activity, particularly in the substantia nigra, and can modulate various processes (see Appleyard 1992, Greenfield 1996).

Acetylcholine in the CNS

- Synthesis, storage and release of acetylcholine in the CNS are essentially the same as in the periphery (Ch. 7).
- ACh is widely distributed in the CNS, important pathways being:
  — basal forebrain (magnocellular) nuclei, which send a diffuse projection to most forebrain structures
  — septohippocampal projection
  — short interneurons in the striatum and nucleus accumbens
  — recurrent inhibitory pathway from spinal motoneurons.
- Certain neurodegenerative diseases, especially dementia and parkinsonism (see Ch. 31) are associated with abnormalities in cholinergic pathways.
- Both nicotinic and muscarinic ACh receptors occur in the CNS. The former mediate the central effects of nicotine. Nicotinic receptors are mainly located presynaptically; there are few examples of transmission mediated by postsynaptic nicotinic receptors.
- Muscarinic receptors appear to mediate the main behavioural effects associated with ACh, namely effects on arousal, and on learning and short-term memory.
- Muscarinic antagonists (e.g. hyoscine) cause amnesia.
- Acetylcholinesterase released from neurons may have functional effects distinct from cholinergic transmission.

This view, somewhat heretical, is supported by evidence suggesting that injection of purified AChE into regions of the brain devoid of cholinergic synapses can cause various behavioural effects. One possibility is that AChE possesses some protease activity, and that its effects are secondary to the production of peptide fragments from local protein substrates. Whatever the mechanism, the concept of an enzyme functioning as a released neural mediator is a novel one, whose implications remain to be explored.

HISTAMINE

The role of histamine as a neurotransmitter is reviewed by Schwartz et al. (1995). It is present in the brain in much smaller amounts than in other tissues, such as skin and lung, and part of the brain content is due to mast cells. Histaminergic pathways have, however, been described, with cell bodies mainly in a small region of the hypothalamus, and axons running in the medial forebrain bundle to large areas of the cortex and midbrain. Stimulation of the medial forebrain bundle produces an inhibitory response in cortical and hippocampal neurons, which is partly blocked by metiamide, an H_2-receptor antagonist.

Applied ionophoretically to central neurons, histamine produces either excitatory or inhibitory effects, via H_1-, H_2- or H_3-receptors (see Ch. 12), all of which are typical G-protein-coupled receptors (see Leurs et al. 1995). H_1-receptors are coupled to phospholipase C, and produce mainly excitatory effects, whereas H_2-receptors act through cAMP formation, and are mainly inhibitory. H_3-receptors serve as inhibitory autoreceptors on histaminergic neurons.

Although many selective agonists and antagonists of the various histamine receptor subtypes are known (see Ch. 12), the role of histamine in the CNS is poorly understood. Blocking H_1-receptors causes sedation (the main side-effect of histamine antagonists used to treat allergies; Ch. 12), and also has an anti-emetic effect (Ch. 21). At present, histamine remains a minor player on the neurotransmitter stage, but this may change.

OTHER CNS MEDIATORS

We now move from the rather familiar neuropharmacological territory of the 'classical' monoamines to some of the frontier towns, bordering on the Wild West. Useful drugs are still few and far between in this area, and if applied pharmacology is your main concern, you can safely skip the next part, and wait a few years for law and order to be established.

PURINES

It is likely that both adenosine and ATP act as transmitters and/or modulators in the CNS (for review, see Brundege & Dunwiddie 1997, Williams 1995) as they do in the periphery (Ch. 9). Mapping the pathways is difficult, because purinergic neurons are not easily identifiable histochemically, and most of the information comes from pharmacological studies.

As discussed in Chapter 9, adenosine produces its effects through G-protein-coupled -receptors (A_1, A_2 and A_3), while ATP acts on P_2-receptors, P_{2X} being ligand-gated cation channels, P_{2Y} being G-protein-coupled. G-protein-coupled purine receptors produce, as in the systems that we have discussed above, mainly (but not exclusively) inhibitory effects, while the P_{2X}-receptors are excitatory, producing both pre- and postsynaptic effects in much the same way as nicotinic receptors.

The overall effect of adenosine, or of various A_1-receptor agonists, is inhibitory, leading to effects such as drowsiness, motor incoordination, analgesia and anticonvulsant activity. Xanthines, such as caffeine (Ch. 38), which are antagonists at A_2-receptors, produce arousal and alertness. Many synthetic adenosine agonists have been developed, since such drugs could be useful in treating conditions such as epilepsy, pain and sleep disorders. A further possible use is in neuroprotection, since the inhibitory effect of adenosine on neuronal excitability and glutamate release is able, in experimental models, to protect the brain against ischaemic damage (see Ch. 31).

Even less is known about the function of ATP as a chemical mediator in the brain, mainly because ATP itself is quickly metabolised to ADP and adenosine, which makes its pharmacological actions difficult to unravel, and also because there are few selective agonists or antagonists for ATP receptors. One of its roles may be in nociception, since ATP is released by tissue damage, and causes pain by stimulating unmyelinated afferent nerve terminals, which express P_{2X}-receptors.

MELATONIN

Melatonin is a mediator that breaks the mould of those that we have discussed so far (reviewed by Brzezinski 1997). It is synthesised exclusively in the pineal, an endocrine gland which plays a role in establishing circadian rhythms. The gland contains two enzymes, not found elsewhere, which convert 5-HT by acetylation and O-methylation to melatonin, its hormonal product. Melatonin secretion (in all animals, whether diurnal or nocturnal in their habits) is high at night, and low by day. This rhythm is controlled by input from the retina, via a noradrenergic retinohypothalamic tract which terminates in the *suprachiasmatic nucleus* (SCN) in the hypothalamus, a structure often termed the 'biological clock', which generates the circadian rhythm. The SCN controls the pineal, not directly, but via sympathetic fibres supplying the gland. The effect of this retinal control system is to inhibit melatonin secretion when the light intensity is high. This mechanism does not itself generate the circadian rhythm, but rather 'entrains' it to the light–dark cycle. Circadian rhythms, including the rhythmic secretion of melatonin, continue even in the absence of light–dark cues, but usually with a periodicity rather longer than 24 hours.

Melatonin receptors (as you will have guessed) are widespread, and come in different types. The main ones are typical G-protein-coupled receptors, found mainly in the brain and retina, but also in peripheral tissues. Another type has been identified as one of the previous 'orphan receptors' (see Ch. 2), a member of the retinoic acid intracellular receptor family which regulates gene transcription. We currently know very little about the physiological processes that are controlled by melatonin, though there is intense research activity in this area.

The use of melatonin for medicinal purposes has become rather widespread, and something of an 'alternative medicine' fad, though there are few properly controlled trials of its efficacy. Given orally, melatonin is well absorbed, but quickly metabolised, its plasma half-life being a few minutes. It has been promoted as a means of controlling jet-lag, or of improving the performance of night-shift workers, based on its ability to reset the circadian clock, and controlled studies have confirmed that melatonin given in the evening can alleviate the effects of jet-lag. A single dose appears to have the effect of resynchronising the physiological secretory cycle, though it is not clear how this occurs. It causes sleepiness, and there is some disagreement about whether its actions are distinguishable from those of conventional hypnotic drugs (see Ch. 33). Claims that melatonin produces other effects (e.g. on mood and immune function) have yet to be confirmed.

NITRIC OXIDE

Nitric oxide (NO) as a peripheral mediator is discussed in Chapter 11. Its significance as an important chemical mediator in the nervous system became apparent only about 10 years ago, and demanded a considerable readjustment of our views about neurotransmission and neuromodulation (for review, see Dawson & Snyder 1994). The main defining criteria for transmitter substances—namely that neurons should possess machinery for synthesising and storing the substance, that it should be released from neurons by exocytosis, that it should interact with specific membrane receptors, and that there should be mechanisms for its inactivation—do not apply to NO. Moreover, it is an inorganic toxic gas, not at all like the kind of molecule we are used to. The mediator function of NO, and probably also carbon monoxide, is now well established, however (see Bredt & Snyder 1992, Vincent 1995). NO diffuses rapidly through cell membranes, and its action is not highly localised. Its half-life depends greatly on the chemical environment, ranging from seconds in blood to several minutes in normal tissues. The presence of superoxide, with which NO reacts (see below), shortens its half-life considerably.

NO in the nervous system is produced mainly by the constitutive neuronal form of nitric oxide synthase (nNOS; see Ch 11), which can be detected either histochemically or by immunolabelling. It is present in roughly 2% of neurons, both short interneurons and long-tract neurons, in virtually all brain areas, with particular concentrations in the cerebellum and hippocampus. It occurs in cell bodies and dendrites, as well as in axon terminals, suggesting (since NO is not stored, but released as it is made) that the release of NO is not restricted to conventional neurotransmitter release sites. nNOS is calmodulin-dependent, and is activated by a rise in intracellular calcium concentration, which can occur by many mechanisms, including action potential conduction and neurotransmitter action. Many studies have shown that NO production is increased by activation of synaptic pathways, or by other events, such as brain ischaemia (see Ch. 31).

NO exerts its effects in two main ways:

- By activation of soluble guanylate cyclase, leading to the production of cGMP, leading to various phosphorylation cascades (Ch. 2). This 'physiological' control mechanism operates at low NO concentrations of about 0.1 µM.
- By reacting with the superoxide free radical, to generate peroxynitrite, a highly toxic anion, which acts by oxidising various intracellular proteins. This requires concentrations of 1–10 µM, which are achieved in brain ischaemia.

There is good evidence that NO plays a role in long-term

potentiation and depression (see Ch. 29), since these phenomena are reduced or prevented by NOS inhibitors, and are absent in transgenic mice in which the nNOS gene has been disrupted.

Based on the same kind of evidence, NO is also believed to play an important part in the mechanisms by which ischaemia causes neuronal death (see Ch. 31), and there is speculation that it may be involved in other kinds of neurodegeneration, such as Parkinson's disease, senile dementia and amyotrophic lateral sclerosis. If substantiated, these theories will open up major new therapeutic possibilities in hitherto intractable disease areas.

Carbon monoxide (CO) is best known as a poisonous gas present in vehicle exhaust, which binds strongly to haemoglobin, causing tissue anoxia. However, it is also formed endogenously, and has many features in common with NO (see Verma et al. 1993). Neurons and other cells contain a CO-generating enzyme, haem oxygenase, and CO also activates guanylate cyclase.

The role of carbon monoxide (CO) as a CNS mediator is less well established, but there is some evidence that

it plays a role in the cerebellum, and also in olfactory neurons, where cGMP-sensitive ion channels are involved in the transduction process

Undoubtedly, further functions of NO and CO in the brain will soon be identified, and novel therapeutic approaches may come from targeting the different steps in the synthetic and signal transduction pathways for these surprising mediators. We may have to endure the ponderous whimsy of many 'NO' puns, but it should be worth it in the end.

ARACHIDONIC ACID

The formation of arachidonic acid (AA), and its conversion to eicosanoids (mainly prostaglandins, leukotrienes and HETEs; see Ch. 12), and to the endogenous cannabinoid receptor ligand, anandamide (see Ch. 39) are known to take place in the CNS. They doubtless play an important role, though our knowledge in this area is still fragmentary (for review, see Piomelli 1995), partly because there are few selective inhibitors which can be used to

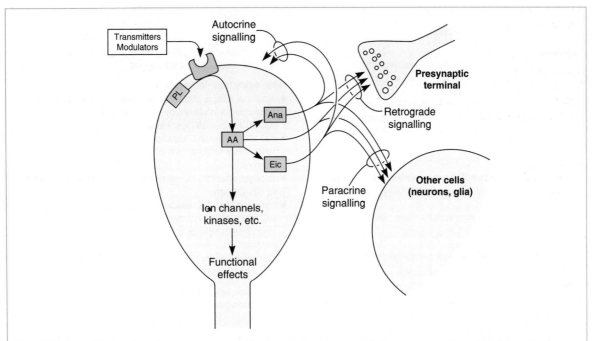

Fig. 30.8   Postulated modes of signalling by arachidonic acid. Arachidonic acid is formed by receptor-mediated cleavage of membrane phospholipid. It can act directly as an intracellular messenger, on ion channels or components of different kinase cascades, producing various long- and short-term effects. It can also be converted to eicosanoids (prostaglandins, leukotrienes or HETEs) or to anandamide. HETEs can also act directly as intracellular messengers. All of these mediators diffuse out of the cell, and exert effects on presynaptic terminals and neighbouring cells, acting either on extracellular receptors, or intracellularly. There are examples of most of these modes of signalling, but only limited information about their functional significance in the nervous system. (AA = arachidonic acid; Ana = anandamide; Eic = eicosanoids; PL = membrane phospholipid)

probe the various steps in the rather lengthy biochemical pathways through which the mediators are formed and exert their effects. Figure 30.8 shows a schematic view of the different possibilities, but it should be realised that evidence as to the functional importance of these pathways is still very limited.

It is known that phospholipid cleavage, leading to AA production, occurs in neurons in response to receptor activation by many different mediators, including neurotransmitters. The AA so formed can act directly as an intracellular messenger, controlling both ion channels and various parts of the protein kinase cascade (see Ch. 2), producing both rapid and delayed effects on neuronal function. AA can also be metabolised to anandamide and to eicosanoids, some of which (principally the HETEs) can also act as intracellular messengers acting in the same cell. Eicosanoids can also exert an autocrine effect via membrane receptors expressed by the cell. Both AA itself, and its products, escape readily from the cell of origin, and can affect neighbouring structures, including presynaptic terminals (retrograde signalling)

and adjacent cells (paracrine signalling) by acting on receptors, or by acting directly as intracellular messengers. Theoretically, the possibilities are endless, but there are so far only a few instances where this system is known to play a significant role. These include our old friend LTP, one component of which is prevented by inhibition of phospholipase A_2, where AA is believed to serve as a retrograde messenger causing facilitation of transmitter release by the presynaptic nerve terminal. A second well-studied system is the *Aplysia* sensory neuron, where the effects of various inhibitory mediators, acting on membrane receptors, are exerted through the intracellular actions of arachidonic acid and its products.

A FINAL MESSAGE

At the end of this long and confusing tour through the brain and its chemistry, our advice is: Hang in there— good things will come out of all this sooner than you might suppose.

Other transmitters and modulators

Histamine
- Histamine fulfils the criteria for a neurotransmitter. Histaminergic neurons originate mainly in the hypothalamus, and have a widespread distribution.
- H_1-, H_2- and H_3-receptors are widespread in the brain.
- The functions of histamine are not well understood, the main clues being that H_1-receptor antagonists are strongly sedative and anti-emetic.

Purines
- Both adenosine and ATP function as transmitters and/or neuromodulators, but the neuronal pathways have not yet been defined.
- Adenosine exerts mainly inhibitory effects, through A_1- and A_2-receptors, resulting in sedative, anticonvulsant and neuroprotective effects.
- Methylxanthines (e.g. caffeine) are antagonists at A_2-receptors, and increase wakefulness.

Melatonin
- Melatonin is synthesised from 5-HT, mainly in the pineal gland, from which it is released as a circulating hormone.
- Secretion is controlled by light intensity, being low by day and high by night. Fibres from the retina run to the suprachiasmatic nucleus ('biological clock'), which controls the pineal gland via its sympathetic innervation.
- Melatonin acts on several types of receptor in the brain and periphery. Given orally, it causes sedation, and also 'resets' the biological clock, being used for this purpose to counter jet-lag.

- Other claimed actions of melatonin (e.g. on mood and immune function) are controversial.

Nitric oxide (see Ch. 11)
- Neuronal NOS is present in many CNS neurons, and NO production is increased by mechanisms (e.g. transmitter action) which raise intracellular Ca^{2+}.
- NO affects neuronal function by increasing cGMP formation, producing both inhibitory and excitatory effects on neurons.
- In larger amounts, NO forms peroxynitrite, which contributes to neurotoxicity.
- Inhibition of nNOS reduces LTP and LTD, probably because NO functions as a retrograde messenger. Inhibition of nNOS also protects against ischaemic brain damage in animal models.
- Carbon monoxide shares many properties with NO, and may also be a neural mediator.

Arachidonic acid metabolites
- Arachidonic acid is produced in neurons by receptor-mediated hydrolysis of phospholipid. It is converted to various eicosanoids and to anandamide.
- AA itself, as well as its active products, can produce rapid and slow effects by regulation of ion channels and protein kinase cascades.
- Such effects can occur in the donor cell, or in adjacent cells and nerve terminals.
- The functional role of the AA pathway in the CNS is still poorly understood.

REFERENCES AND FURTHER READING

Appleyard M E 1992 Secreted acetylcholinesterase: non-classical aspects of a classical enzyme. Trends Neurosci 15: 485–490 (*Review of the controversial function of acetylcholinesterase as a secreted mediator*)

Arnevic S P, Sullivan J P, Williams M 1995 Neuronal nicotinic acetylcholine receptors. In: Bloom F E, Kupfer D J (eds) Psychopharmacology: a fourth generation of progress. Raven Press, New York (*General review article*)

Azmitia E C, Whitaker-Azmitia P M 1995 Anatomy, cell biology and plasticity of the serotonergic system. In: Bloom F E, Kupfer D J (eds) Psychopharmacology: a fourth generation of progress. Raven Press, New York (*General review article*)

Beeri R, Andres C, Lev-Lehman E et al. 1995 Transgenic expression of human acetylcholinesterase induces progressive cognitive deterioration in mice. Curr Biol 5: 1063–1071 (*Describes a transgenic mouse model with impaired cholinergic transmission, leading to cognitive changes*)

Bredt D S, Snyder S H 1992 Nitric oxide, a novel neuronal messenger. Neuron 8: 3–11 (*Widely quoted review article which anticipates many later discoveries*)

Brundege J M, Dunwiddie T V 1997 Role of adenosine as a modulator of synaptic activity in the central nervous system. Adv Pharmacol 39: 353–391 (*General review article*)

Brzezinski A 1997 Melatonin in humans. New Engl J Med 336: 186–195 (*Clear and well-referenced review article. Recommended as an introduction*)

Cooper J R, Bloom F E, Roth R H 1996 Biochemical basis of neuropharmacology. Oxford University Press, New York (*Clear and well-written textbook, giving more detailed information on many topics covered in this chapter*)

Dawson T M, Snyder S H 1994 Gases as biological messengers: nitric oxide and carbon monoxide in the brain. J Neurosci 14: 5147–5159 (*Excellent introductory review, summarising ideas in a new area*)

Galzi J-L, Changeux J-P 1995 Neuronal nicotinic receptors: molecular organization and regulations. Neuropharmacology 34: 563–582 (*General review article, focusing on molecular aspects*)

Giros B, Caron M 1993 Molecular characterization of the dopamine transporter. Trends Pharmacol Sci 14: 43–49 (*Good introductory review*)

Greenfield S A 1996 Non-classical actions of cholinesterases: role in cellular differentiation, tumorigenesis and Alzheimer's disease. Neurochem Int 28: 485–490 (*Review of possible functions of secreted acetylcholinesterase*)

Hagan J J, Morris R G M 1988 The cholinergic hypothesis of memory: a review of animal experiments. In: Iversen L L, Iversen S, Snyder S H (eds) Handbook of psychopharmacology. Plenum, New York, vol 20, pp 237–323 (*Useful summary, now rather dated, of evidence implicating acetylcholine in learning and memory*)

Jaber M, Robinson S W, Missale C, Caron M G 1996 Dopamine receptors and brain function. Neuropharmacology 35: 1503–1519 (*Useful general review*)

Leurs R, Smit M J, Timmerman H 1995 Molecular pharmacological aspects of histamine receptors. Pharmacol Ther 66: 413–463 (*Information on cloning, signal transduction and distribution of histamine receptors*)

Marsden C A, Heal D J (eds) 1992 Central serotonin receptors and psychotropic drugs. Blackwell, Oxford (*Compendium of articles focusing on pharmacology*)

Piomelli D 1995 Arachidonic acid. In: Bloom F E, Kupfer D J (eds) Psychopharmacology: a fourth generation of progress. Raven Press, New York (*Excellent review article*)

Role L W 1992 Diversity in primary structure and function of nicotinic acetylcholine receptor channels. Curr Opin Neurobiol 2: 254–262 (*Review focusing on receptor diversity—relationship with function is not clear*)

Schwartz J-C, Arrang J-M, Garbarg M, Traiffort E 1995 Histamine. In: Bloom F E, Kupfer D J (eds) Psychopharmacology: a fourth generation of progress. Raven Press, New York (*Review on the role of histamine in the CNS by one of the main pioneers in this Cinderella field*)

Seeman P, Van Tol H H M 1994 Dopamine receptor pharmacology. Trends Pharmacol Sci 15: 264–270 (*Introductory review article*)

Verma A, Hirsch D J, Glatt C E, Ronnett G V, Snyder S H 1993 Carbon monoxide: a putative neural messenger. Science 259: 381–384 (*Speculative review, which points out similarities with NO*)

Vincent S R (ed) 1995 Nitric oxide in the nervous system. Academic Press, London (*Useful compendium of review articles on all aspects of NO in the nervous system*)

Williams M 1995 Purinoceptors in central nervous system function. In: Bloom F E, Kupfer D J (eds) Psychopharmacology: a fourth generation of progress. Raven Press, New York (*General review article*)

31

Neurodegenerative disorders

INTRODUCTION

With few exceptions, CNS neurons cannot divide, nor can they regenerate when their axons are interrupted. Thus, any pathological process causing neuronal loss generally has irreversible consequences. At first sight, this appears to be very unpromising territory for pharmacological intervention, and indeed drug therapy currently has rather little to offer, except in the case of Parkinson's disease (see below). Nevertheless, the incidence and social impact of neurodegenerative brain disorders in ageing populations has resulted in a massive research effort in recent years, and the advances made may be translated into therapeutic progress in the not-too-distant future. In this chapter, we discuss:

- mechanisms responsible for neuronal death, focusing on **excitotoxicity**, **oxidative stress** and **apoptosis**
- pharmacological approaches (so far hypothetical) to preventing neuronal loss;
- pharmacological approaches to compensation for neuronal loss.

The discussion focuses mainly on three common neurodegenerative conditions, namely dementia (Alzheimer's disease), ischaemic brain damage (stroke) and Parkinson's disease. The hurried reader may safely skip straight to page 507 without missing anything of current therapeutic importance.

MECHANISMS OF NEURONAL DEATH

Acute injury to cells causes them to undergo *necrosis*, recognised pathologically by cell swelling, vacuolisation and lysis, and associated with calcium overload of the cells and membrane damage (see below). Necrotic cells typically evoke an inflammatory response. Cells can also die by *apoptosis* (programmed cell death), a slower process which occurs normally during development, and is essential for many processes throughout life, for example immune regulation and tissue remodelling (see Ch. 42). Apoptosis, as well as necrosis, occurs in many neurodegenerative disorders (including acute conditions, such as stroke and head injury; for review, see Bredesen 1995). The distinction between necrosis and apoptosis as processes leading to neurodegeneration is not absolute, for there is evidence that challenges such as excitotoxicity and oxidative stress can cause cells to undergo apoptosis, as well as killing them directly. Both processes therefore represent possible targets for putative neuroprotective drug therapy. Pharmacological interference with the apoptotic pathway may become possible in the future, but for the present, most efforts are directed at the processes involved in cell necrosis, and at compensating pharmacologically for the neuronal loss.

EXCITOTOXICITY

In spite of its ubiquitous role as a neurotransmitter (Ch. 29), glutamate is highly toxic to neurons, a phenomenon dubbed *excitotoxicity* (see Choi 1988). A low concentration of glutamate applied to neurons in culture kills the cells, and the finding in the 1970s that glutamate given orally produces neurodegeneration *in vivo* caused considerable alarm, because of the widespread use of glutamate as a 'taste-enhancing' food additive. The 'Chinese restaurant syndrome'—an acute attack of neck stiffness and chest pain—is well known, but so far the possibility of more serious neurotoxicity is only hypothetical.

Local injection of kainic acid, is used experimentally to produce neurotoxic lesions. It acts by excitation of local glutamate-releasing neurons, and the release of glutamate, acting on NMDA, and also metabotropic receptors (Ch. 29) leads to neuronal death.

Calcium overload is the essential factor in excitotoxicity. The mechanisms by which this occurs and leads to cell death are as follows (Fig. 31.1):

- Glutamate activates NMDA, AMPA and metabotropic receptors (Sites 1, 2 and 3). Activation of AMPA receptors depolarises the cell, which unblocks the NMDA-channels (see Ch. 29), permitting calcium entry. Depolarisation also opens voltage-activated Ca^{2+} channels (Site 4), releasing more glutamate. Metabotropic receptors cause the release of intracellular Ca^{2+} from the endoplasmic reticulum. Sodium entry further contributes to Ca^{2+} entry by stimulating Ca^{2+}/Na^+ exchange (Site 5). Depolarisation inhibits or reverses glutamate uptake (Site 6), thus increasing the extracellular glutamate concentration.
- The mechanisms that normally operate to counteract the rise in $[Ca^{2+}]_i$ include the calcium efflux pump (Site 7) and, indirectly, the sodium pump (Site 8).
- The mitochondria and endoplasmic reticulum act as capacious sinks for Ca^{2+}, and normally keep $[Ca^{2+}]_i$ under control. Loading of the mitochondrial stores beyond a certain point, however, disrupts mitochondrial function, reducing ATP synthesis, thus reducing the energy available for the membrane pumps and for Ca^{2+} accumulation by the endoplasmic reticulum. Formation of reactive oxygen species (ROS) is also enhanced. This represents the danger point at which positive feedback exaggerates the process.
- Raised $[Ca^{2+}]_i$ affects many processes, the chief ones relevant to neurotoxicity being:
  —increased glutamate release
  —activation of proteases (calpains) and lipases, causing membrane damage
  —activation of nitric oxide synthase (NOS), which, together with ROS, generates peroxynitrite and hydroxyl free radicals, which react with several cellular molecules, including membrane lipids, proteins and DNA
  —increased arachidonic acid release, which increases free radical production, and also inhibits glutamate uptake (Site 6).

Glutamate and calcium are arguably the two most ubiquitous chemical signals, extracellular and intracellular respectively, underlying brain function, so it is disconcerting that such cytotoxic mayhem can be unleashed when they get out of control. Defence against excitotoxicity is clearly essential if our brains are to have any chance of staying alive. The central role of mitochondrial energy metabolism in providing the main line of defence (see above) suggests that impaired ATP production, rendering neurons vulnerable to excitotoxic damage, may be a common precipitating factor in various neurodegenerative conditions.

The role of excitotoxicity in ischaemic brain damage is well established (see below), and it is also believed to be a factor in other neurodegenerative diseases, such as those discussed below (see Lipton & Rosenberg 1994).

There are several examples of neurodegenerative conditions caused by environmental toxins, acting as agonists on glutamate receptors (see Olney 1990). Domoic acid is a glutamate analogue produced by mussels, which was identified as the cause of an epidemic of severe mental and neurological deterioration in a group of Newfoundlanders in 1987. On the island of Guam, a syndrome combining the features of dementia, paralysis and Parkinson's disease has been tracked down to an excitotoxic amino acid, β-methylamino-alanine, present in the seeds of a local plant. Discouraging the consumption of these seeds has largely eliminated the disease.

APOPTOSIS

Apoptosis can be initiated by various cell surface signals (see review by Steller 1995), and is recognised by nuclear changes (chromatin aggregation and DNA fragmentation) and cell shrinkage. Apoptotic cells can be identified by a staining technique which detects the characteristic DNA breaks. The cell remnants are removed by macrophages without causing inflammation. In general, neural apoptosis is initiated by the absence of particular growth factors, resulting in altered gene transcription, and the activation of specific 'cell death' proteins. Apoptosis is often associated with excitotoxicity, even in acute neurodegenerative conditions in humans, though the link is not well understood. The final process in apoptotic cell death appears to be the activation of a family of proteases

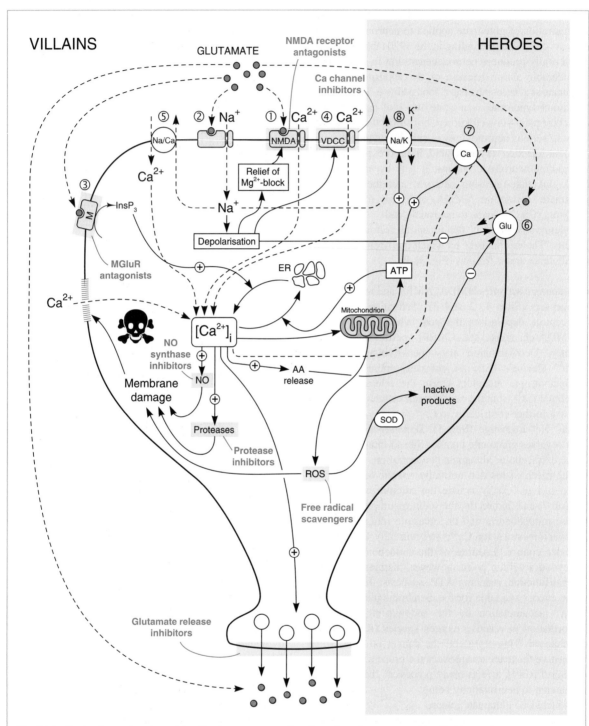

Fig. 31.1 Mechanisms of excitotoxicity. Membrane receptors, ion channels and transporters, identified by numbers 1–8, are discussed in the text. Possible sites of action of neuroprotective drugs (not yet of proven clinical value) are highlighted. Mechanisms on the left (villains) are those which favour cell death, while those on the right (heroes) are protective. See text for details. (ER = endoplasmic reticulum; AA = arachidonic acid; ROS = reactive oxygen species; SOD = superoxide dismutase)

(*caspases*), which inactivate various intracellular proteins. Neural apoptosis is normally prevented by neuronal growth factors, including *nerve growth factor* (NGF) and *brain-derived neurotrophic factor* (BDNF), secreted proteins which are required for the survival of different populations of neurons in the CNS. These growth factors regulate the expression of the two gene products *Bax* and *Bcl-2*, Bax being pro-apoptotic and Bcl-2 being anti-apoptotic (see Davies 1995; also Fig. 42.2). Attention is being focused on the regulation of growth factors, and of the pro- and anti-apoptotic regulatory proteins, in neurodegenerative disorders (see Merry & Korsmeyer 1997), with a view to new therapeutic approaches.

OXIDATIVE STRESS

The brain derives nearly all its energy from mitochondrial oxidative phosphorylation, which generates ATP at the same time as reducing molecular O_2 to H_2O. Under certain conditions, highly reactive species, for example oxygen and hydroxyl free radicals, and H_2O_2 may be generated as side-products of this process (see Coyle & Puttfarken 1993). Oxidative stress is the result of excessive production of these reactive species. They can also be produced as a by-product of other biochemical pathways, including NO synthesis and arachidonic acid metabolism (which are implicated in excitotoxicity; see above), as well as the mixed function oxidase system (see Ch. 4). Unchecked, reactive oxygen radicals attack many key molecules, including enzymes, membrane lipids and DNA. Not surprisingly, defence mechanisms are provided, in the form of enzymes such as superoxide dismutase (SOD) and catalase, as well as antioxidants, such as ascorbic acid, glutathione and α-tocopherol (vitamin E), which normally keep these reactive species in check. Some cytokines, especially TNF-α, which is produced in conditions of brain ischaemia or inflammation (Ch. 12), exert a protective effect, partly by increasing the expression of SOD (see Rothwell et al. 1996). Transgenic animals lacking TNF receptors show enhanced susceptibility to brain ischaemia. Mutations of the gene encoding superoxide dismutase (SOD; Fig. 31.1) are associated with a progressive form of motor neuron disease known as *amyotrophic lateral sclerosis*, a fatal paralytic disease resulting from progressive degeneration of motoneurons, and transgenic mice expressing mutated SOD develop a similar condition (see Louvel et al. 1997). It is possible that accumulated or inherited mutations in enzymes such as those of the mitochondrial respiratory chain lead to a congenital or age-related increase in susceptibility to oxidative stress, which is manifest in different kinds of inherited neurodegenerative disorders (such as Huntington's disease), and in age-related neurodegeneration (see Beal et al. 1993).

Several possible targets for therapeutic intervention with neuroprotective drugs are shown in Figure 31.1. Activity in this area is intense, but with little practical outcome so far. One recent, though modest, success is **riluzole**, a compound which inhibits both the release and the postsynaptic action of glutamate, and retards to some degree the deterioration of patients with amyotrophic lateral sclerosis. For reviews of hopes and achievements in various neurodegenerative diseases, see Green & Cross (1997), Lipton & Rosenberg (1994), Louvel et al. (1997), Olanow et al. (1996a).

Excitotoxicity and oxidative stress

- Excitatory amino acids (e.g. glutamate) can cause neuronal death.
- Excitotoxicity is associated mainly with activation of NMDA receptors, but other types of EAA receptors also contribute.
- Excitotoxicity results from a sustained rise in intracellular calcium concentration (calcium overload).
- Excitotoxicity can occur under pathological conditions (e.g. cerebral ischaemia) in which excessive glutamate release occurs. It can also occur when chemicals such as kainic acid are administered.
- Raised intracellular calcium causes cell death by various mechanisms, including activation of proteases, formation of free radicals, and lipid peroxidation. Formation of NO and arachidonic acid are also involved.
- Various mechanisms act normally to protect neurons against excitotoxicity, the main ones being calcium transport systems, mitochondrial function and the production of free radical scavengers.
- Oxidative stress refers to conditions (e.g. hypoxia) in which the protective mechanisms are compromised, and neurons become more susceptible to excitotoxic damage.
- Excitotoxicity due to environmental chemicals may contribute to some neurodegenerative disorders.
- Measures designed to reduce excitotoxicity include the use of glutamate antagonists, calcium channel blocking drugs and free radical scavengers; none are yet proven for clinical use.

ISCHAEMIC BRAIN DAMAGE

After heart disease and cancer, strokes are the commonest cause of death in Europe and North America, and non-fatal strokes are the commonest cause of disability. Interruption of blood supply to the brain initiates the cascade of neuronal events shown in Figure 31.1, which lead in turn to later consequences, including cerebral oedema and inflammation, which can also contribute to brain damage (see Kogure et al. 1993). Further damage can occur following reperfusion, possibly because of the production of free radicals and other reactive species when the oxygenation is restored. Reperfusion injury may be an important component in stroke patients. These secondary processes often take hours to develop, and controlling them currently offers the best hope for therapeutic intervention.* The lesion produced by occlusion of a major cerebral artery consists of a central core in which the neurons quickly undergo irreversible damage, from which neurodegeneration spreads over hours or even longer, to affect neighbouring areas. The possibility is that neuroprotective therapies, given within a few hours, might inhibit this spread and improve functional recovery.

Glutamate excitotoxicity plays a critical role in brain ischaemia. Thus, it is known that ischaemia causes depolarisation of neurons, and the release of large amounts of glutamate. Ca^{2+} accumulation occurs, partly as a result of glutamate acting on NMDA receptors, for both Ca^{2+} entry and cell death following cerebral ischaemia are inhibited by drugs that block NMDA receptors or channels (see Ch. 29). NO also builds up, to levels much higher than can be produced by electrical stimulation (i.e. to levels that are toxic, rather than modulatory).

In animal models involving cerebral artery occlusion, a long list of drugs targeted at the mechanisms shown in Figure 31.1 can reduce the size of the infarct. These include glutamate antagonists, calcium and sodium channel inhibitors, free radical scavengers, anti-inflammatory drugs, protease inhibitors, and others. It seems that almost anything works.

However, attempts to develop drugs for therapeutic use have so far been disappointing (see Koroshetz & Moskowitz 1996, Wahlgren 1997 for reviews). Controlled clinical trials on stroke patients are problematic and very expensive, partly because of the large variability of outcome in terms of functional recovery, which means that large groups of patients (typically several hundred) need to be followed for several months. The need to start therapy within hours of the attack is an additional problem. **Nimodipine** (a calcium channel antagonist; see Ch. 15), proved ineffective in clinical trials; it actually increased the risk of cerebral haemorrhage, possibly by causing vasodilatation. Trials of NMDA antagonists and channel-blocking drugs (selfotel, eliprodil, dextro-

---

*Some neurologists favour the use of early fibrinolytic therapy (Ch. 17) to limit the degree of ischaemic damage, but this is controversial, and not universally practised.

methorphan) were unsuccessful because of lack of efficacy, or side-effects. Other trials are continuing, including drugs which inhibit glutamate release (adenosine analogues, lobeluzole) or lipid peroxidation (tirilazad) or enhance GABA effects (chlormethiazole).

ALZHEIMER'S DISEASE

Loss of intellectual ability with age is considered to be a normal process, whose rate and extent is very variable. Alzheimer's disease was originally defined as *presenile* dementia, but it now appears that the same pathology underlies the dementia irrespective of the age of onset. Alzheimer's disease (AD) refers to dementia that does not have an antecedent cause, such as stroke, brain trauma or alcohol. Its prevalence rises sharply with age, from about 5% at 65 to 90% or more at 95. Until recently, age-related dementia was considered to result from the steady loss of neurons that normally goes on throughout life, possibly accelerated by a failing blood supply associated with atherosclerosis. Studies over the last decade have, however, revealed specific genetic and molecular mechanisms underlying AD (reviewed by Selkoe 1993, 1997, Yankner 1996), which have opened new therapeutic opportunities (see Aisen & Davis 1997).

PATHOGENESIS OF ALZHEIMER'S DISEASE

AD is associated with a shrinkage of brain tissue, with localised loss of neurons, mainly in the hippocampus and basal forebrain. Two microscopic features are characteristic of the disease, namely extracellular *amyloid plaques*, consisting of amorphous extracellular deposits of β-amyloid protein, and intraneuronal *neurofibrillary tangles*, comprising filaments of a phosphorylated form of a microtuble-associated protein (Tau). These appear also in normal brains, though in smaller numbers. The early appearance of amyloid deposits presages the development of AD, though symptoms may not develop for many years. Altered processing of amyloid protein from its precursor (APP; see below) is now recognised as the key to the pathogenesis of AD. This conclusion is based on several lines of evidence, particularly the genetic analysis of families with familial dementia, a relatively rare form of AD, in which mutations of the APP gene (see below), or of other genes which control amyloid processing, have been discovered. The APP gene resides on chromosome 21, which is duplicated in Down syndrome, which causes early AD-like dementia, associated with overexpression of APP.

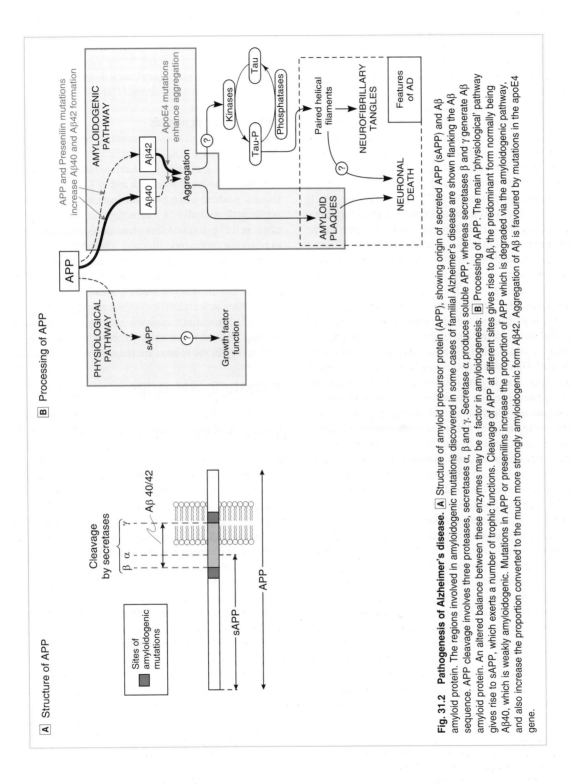

A Structure of APP

B Processing of APP

Fig. 31.2 Pathogenesis of Alzheimer's disease. **A** Structure of amyloid precursor protein (APP), showing origin of secreted APP (sAPP) and Aβ amyloid protein. The regions involved in amyloidogenic mutations discovered in some cases of familial Alzheimer's disease are shown flanking the Aβ sequence. APP cleavage involves three proteases, secretases α, β and γ. Secretase α produces soluble APP, whereas secretases β and γ generate Aβ amyloid protein. An altered balance between these enzymes may be a factor in amyloidogenesis. **B** Processing of APP. The main 'physiological' pathway gives rise to sAPP, which exerts a number of trophic functions. Cleavage of APP at different sites gives rise to Aβ, the predominant form normally being Aβ40, which is weakly amyloidogenic. Mutations in APP or presenilins increase the proportion of APP which is degraded via the amyloidogenic pathway, and also increase the proportion converted to the much more strongly amyloidogenic form Aβ42. Aggregation of Aβ is favoured by mutations in the apoE4 gene.

505

Amyloid deposits consist of aggregates of *amyloid β-protein* (Aβ; Fig. 31.2), containing 40 or 42 residues. Aβ40 is produced normally in small amounts, whereas Aβ42 is overproduced as a result of the genetic mutations mentioned above. Both proteins aggregate to form amyloid plaques, but Aβ42 shows a stronger tendency than Aβ40 to do so, and appears to be the main culprit in amyloid formation. Aβ40 and 42 are produced by proteolytic cleavage of a much larger *amyloid precursor protein* (APP), a membrane protein normally expressed by many cells, including CNS neurons. Mostly, the large extracellular domain is released as soluble APP by the action of secretase α; APP serves various poorly understood trophic functions. Formation of Aβ involves cleavage at two different points, including one in the intramembrane domain of APP, by secretases β and γ (Fig. 31.2). Mutations in the APP gene, or expression of the unrelated *presenilin* genes, facilitates Aβ formation, particularly of Aβ42, resulting in increased plaque formation.* The altered ratio of Aβ42 : Aβ40 can be detected in plasma, which serves as a marker for familial AD. Mutations in the apolipoprotein gene ApoE4, also predispose to AD, probably because expression of abnormal ApoE4 proteins facilitate the aggregation of Aβ. It is uncertain exactly how Aβ accumulation causes neurodegeneration. There is some evidence that the cells die by apoptosis, though an inflammatory response is also evident. Expression of Alzheimer mutations in transgenic animals causes plaque formation and neurodegeneration, and also increases the susceptibility of CNS neurons to other challenges, such as ischaemia, excitotoxicity and oxidative stress, and this increased vulnerability may be the cause of the progressive neurodegeneration in AD. These transgenic models will be of great value in testing potential drug therapies aimed at retarding the neurodegenerative process.

The other main player on the biochemical stage is *tau*, the protein of which the neurofibrillary tangles are composed (Fig. 31.2), though its exact role in the pathogenesis is unclear. Tau is a normal constituent of neurons, being associated with intracellular microtubules. In AD it becomes abnormally phosphorylated, and is deposited intracellularly as *paired helical filaments* with a characteristic microscopic appearance. When the cells die, these filaments aggregate as extracellular neurofibrillary

tangles. It is possible, but not proven, that tau phosphorylation is enhanced by the presence of Aβ plaques. Whether hyperphosphorylation and intracellular deposition of tau harms the cell is not certain, though it is known that tau-phosphorylation impairs fast axonal transport, a process that depends on microtubules.

Loss of cholinergic neurons

Though changes in many transmitter systems have been observed, mainly from measurements on post-mortem brain tissue, a relatively selective loss of cholinergic neurons in the basal forebrain nuclei (a region in which lesions produce cognitive and learning deficits in experimental animals) is characteristic. This discovery, made in 1976, implied that pharmacological approaches to restoring cholinergic function might be feasible.

Choline acetyl transferase (CAT) activity in the cortex and hippocampus is reduced considerably (30–70%) in AD but not in other disorders, such as depression or schizophrenia; acetylcholinesterase activity is also greatly reduced. Muscarinic receptor density, determined by binding studies, is not affected, but nicotinic receptors, particularly in the cortex, are reduced.

THERAPEUTIC APPROACHES

In spite of the recent advances in understanding the mechanism of neurodegeneration in AD, there are still no effective therapies. The main approaches are summarised in Table 31.1 (see also Aisen & Davis 1997). Many are at the experimental stage, and have yet to be tested in humans. The cholinesterase inhibitor, **tacrine**, was recently introduced in the USA, on the basis that enhancement of cholinergic transmission might compensate for the cholinergic deficit that occurs in AD. Trials have shown modest improvements in tests of memory and cognition in about 40% of AD patients, but no improvement in other functional measures which affect quality of life. Tacrine has to be given four times daily, and produces cholinergic side-effects, such as nausea and abdominal cramps, as well as hepatotoxicity in some patients, so it is far from an ideal drug. Other cholinesterase inhibitors include **donepezil**, which was recently introduced in the UK; it is not hepatotoxic, and may have advantages over tacrine.

Much current effort is directed towards measures to retard the neurodegenerative process (reviewed by Aisen & Davis 1997). Epidemiological studies show that lifelong smokers have a reduced probability of developing AD, and nicotine is known to produce both cognitive improvement in man and, surprisingly, neuroprotective effects in vitro. The many adverse effects of

---

*Recently, it was reported (De Strooper et al. 1998) that knocking out the presenilin-1 gene *prevents* Aβ formation by abolishing secretase γ activity, and it is believed that PS-1 amyloidogenic mutants produce excessive secretase γ activity. If so, inhibition of secretase γ could provide a future therapeutic approach.

Table 31.1 Therapeutic approaches in dementia

Approach	Mechanism	Drugs and therapies	Status
Available or in development			
Improved blood flow/ psychostimulation	Vasodilatation Effects on monoamine receptors	Dihydroergotoxine Pentoxyfylline	Many trials of vasodilators, psychostimulants, antidepressants, etc. Efficacy not proven in humans
Nootropic agents*	? Potentiation of glutamate	Piracetam Aniracetam	Improved learning and memory in animal models Efficacy not proven in humans
Cholinergic replacement therapy	Cholinesterase inhibitors	Physostigmine Tacrine Donepezil	Modest efficacy in humans Hepatotoxicity with tacrine Unwanted side-effects
	Muscarinic agonists	Arecoline Pilocarpine M_1-selective compounds in development	Some efficacy in animal models Peripheral side-effects Not yet tested in humans
Hypothetical			
Improved neuronal survival	Neurotrophic factors	Nerve growth factor (NGF) and other growth factors	Improved forebrain cholinergic function in animal models Special delivery systems needed for human use
Halting disease process	Inhibition of amyloid formation	Secretase inhibitors Inhibitors of APP phosphorylation	Not yet developed
	Inhibition of τ-protein deposition	Inhibitors of τ-phosphorylation	Not yet developed
	Inhibition of excitotoxicity	Glutamate antagonists Ca-channel blockers Protease inhibitors, etc.	Being developed mainly in other indications (e.g. stroke)
	Anti-inflammatory drugs	NSAIDs	Clinical efficacy reported
	Antioxidants	α-tocopherol	Efficacy not yet tested

*Drugs which enhance mental performance (see p. 469)

nicotine, as well as its addictiveness, preclude its use for this purpose. There is also evidence that anti-inflammatory drugs, such as indomethacin can improve symptoms and retard the disease progression of AD patients. Though indomethacin is unsuitable for long-term use in the elderly, the principle of using such drugs may prove valuable. Other possibilities include drugs aimed at preventing excitotoxicity (see above), but the prospects seem less good, since the evidence implicating excitotoxicity in the pathogenesis of AD is not very strong.

In the longer term, approaches based on growth factors may be possible, on the basis that shortage of growth factors (particularly nerve growth factor, which is required for survival of the forebrain cholinergic neurons that degenerate in AD) favours neuronal apoptosis. Administering growth factors into the brain is not realistic for routine therapy, but alternative approaches, such as implanting cells engineered to secrete NGF are under investigation.

PARKINSON'S DISEASE

PATHOGENESIS OF PARKINSON'S DISEASE

Parkinson's disease (PD) is a progressive disorder of movement that occurs mainly in the elderly. The chief symptoms are:

- tremor at rest, usually starting in the hands ('pill-rolling' tremor), which tend to diminish during voluntary activity

Dementia and Alzheimer's disease

- Alzheimer's disease (AD) is a common age-related dementia, distinct from vascular dementia associated with brain infarction.
- The main pathological features of AD comprise amyloid plaques, neurofibrillary tangles, and a loss of neurons (particularly cholinergic neurons of the basal forebrain).
- Amyloid plaques consist of the Aβ fragment of amyloid precursor protein (APP), a normal neuronal membrane protein. The causes of excessive Aβ formation are not known, but may include: mutations affecting APP; excessive phosphorylation of APP; abnormal APP proteases. There is some evidence that Aβ is neurotoxic.
- Neurofibrillary tangles comprise aggregates of a highly phosphorylated form of a normal neuronal protein. The relationship of these structures to neurodegeneration is not known.
- Loss of cholinergic neurons is believed to account for much of the learning and memory deficit in AD.
- Currently available therapies for AD are only marginally effective at best; most have shown little or no benefit in controlled trials. Anticholinesterases (tacrine, donepezil) give proven, though limited, benefit.
- Other drugs, including putative vasodilators (dihydroergotoxine), muscarinic agonists (arecoline, pilocarpine) and cognition enhancers (piracetam, aniracetam), give no demonstrable benefit, and are not officially approved.

- muscle rigidity, detectable as an increased resistance in passive limb movement
- suppression of voluntary movements (hypokinesis), due partly to muscle rigidity, and partly to an inherent inertia of the motor system, which means that motor activity is difficult to stop as well as to initiate.

Parkinsonian patients walk with a characteristic fast shuffling gait. They find it hard to start, and once in progress they cannot quickly stop or change direction. PD is commonly associated with dementia, probably because the degenerative process is not confined to the basal ganglia, but also affects other parts of the brain.

PD often occurs with no obvious underlying cause, but it may be the result of cerebral ischaemia, viral encephalitis or other types of pathological damage. The symptoms can also be drug-induced, the main drugs involved being those that reduce the amount of dopamine in the brain (e.g. **reserpine**; see Ch. 8), or block dopamine receptors (e.g. antipsychotic drugs, such as **chlorpromazine**; see Ch. 34). In contrast to schizophrenia and many other neurological and behavioural disorders,

PD shows no hereditary tendency, and an environmental cause seems more likely (see below).

Neurochemical changes

PD affects the basal ganglia, and its neurochemical origin was discovered by Hornykiewicz in 1960 (reviewed by Hornykiewicz & Kish 1986), who showed that the dopamine content of the substantia nigra and corpus striatum (see Ch. 30) in post-mortem brains of PD patients was extremely low (usually less than 10% of normal), and this was later correlated with an almost complete loss of dopaminergic neurons from the substantia nigra and degeneration of nerve terminals in the striatum. Other monoamines, such as noradrenaline and 5-HT contents were much less affected than dopamine. Later studies (e.g. with PET scanning to reveal dopamine transport in the striatum; see Fig. 30.4) have shown a loss of dopamine over several years, with symptoms of PD appearing only when the striatal dopamine content has fallen to 20–40% of normal. Lesions of the nigrostriatal tract or chemically induced depletion of dopamine in experimental animals also produce symptoms of PD. The symptom most clearly related to dopamine deficiency is hypokinesia, which occurs immediately and invariably in lesioned animals. Rigidity and tremor involve more complex neurochemical disturbances of other transmitters (particularly acetylcholine, noradrenaline, 5-HT and GABA) as well as dopamine. In experimental lesions, two secondary consequences follow damage to the nigrostriatal tract, namely a hyperactivity of the remaining dopaminergic neurons, which show an increased rate of transmitter turnover, and an increase in the number of dopamine receptors, which produces a state of denervation hypersensitivity (see Ch. 6). These compensatory mechanisms presumably act to preserve transmission in spite of the neuronal loss, and are important in relation to the therapeutic effectiveness of levodopa (see below). PET scanning of patients suggests that D_1-receptors proliferate in PD, and are down-regulated during treatment with levodopa. The striatum expresses mainly D_1- (excitatory) and D_2- (inhibitory) receptors (see Ch. 30), but few D_3- or D_4-receptors.

Action of MPTP

New light was thrown on the possible aetiology of PD by a chance event. In 1982 a group of young drug addicts in California suddenly developed an exceptionally severe form of PD (known as the 'frozen addict' syndrome), and the cause was traced to the compound 1-methyl 4-phenyl 1,2,3,6-tetrahydropyridine (MPTP), which was a contaminant in a preparation used as a heroin substitute (see

Langston 1985). MPTP causes irreversible destruction of nigrostriatal dopaminergic neurons in various species, and produces a PD-like state in primates. MPTP acts by being converted to a toxic metabolite, MPP$^+$, by the enzyme monoamine oxidase (specifically by the MAO-B subtype; see Ch. 35). MPP$^+$ is taken up by the dopamine transport system, and thus acts selectively on dopaminergic neurons; it inhibits mitochondrial oxidation reactions, producing oxidative stress (see above; Tipton & Singer 1993). MPTP appears to be selective in destroying nigrostriatal neurons, and does not affect dopaminergic neurons elsewhere—the reason for this is unknown. **Selegiline**, a selective MAO-B inhibitor (see below), prevents MPTP-induced neurotoxicity by blocking its conversion to MPP$^+$. It is also used in treating PD (see below); as well as inhibiting dopamine breakdown, it might also work by blocking the metabolic activation of a putative endogenous, or environmental, MPTP-like substance,* which is involved in the causation of PD. Whether or not its action reflects the natural pathogenesis of PD, MPTP is a very useful experimental tool for testing possible therapies.

The intrinsic cholinergic neurons of the corpus striatum (which has the highest content of ACh, CAT and AChE in the brain) are also involved in PD (as well as Huntington's disease; see below). ACh release from the striatum is strongly inhibited by dopamine, and it is suggested that hyperactivity of these cholinergic neurons (associated with the lack of dopamine) leads to the symptoms of PD, whereas hypoactivity (associated with a surfeit of dopamine, secondary to a deficiency of GABA)

---

*It is possible that dopamine itself could be the culprit, since oxidation of dopamine gives rise to potentially toxic metabolites.

> **Parkinson's disease**
>
> - Degenerative disease of the basal ganglia causing tremor at rest, muscle rigidity hypokinesia, often with dementia.
> - Often idiopathic, but may follow stroke, virus infection, can be drug-induced (neuroleptic drugs).
> - Associated with marked loss of dopamine from basal ganglia.
> - Can be induced by MPTP, a neurotoxin affecting dopamine neurons in the corpus striatum.

results in the hyperkinetic movements and hypotonia characteristic of Huntington's disease (Fig. 31.3). In both conditions, therapies aimed at redressing the balance between the dopaminergic and cholinergic neurons are, up to a point, beneficial.

DRUG TREATMENT OF PARKINSON'S DISEASE

For general reviews of current and future approaches, see Hagan et al. (1997), Stern (1997). The drugs that are effective in the treatment of PD fall into the following categories:

- drugs that replace dopamine (e.g. **levodopa**, usually used concomitantly with peripherally acting dopa decarboxylase inhibitors, e.g. **carbidopa**, **benserazide**)
- drugs that mimic the action of dopamine (e.g. **bromocriptine**, **pergolide**, **lisuride** and others in development)
- MAO-B inhibitors (e.g. **selegiline**)
- drugs that release dopamine (e.g. **amantadine**)
- acetylcholine antagonists (e.g. **benztropine**).

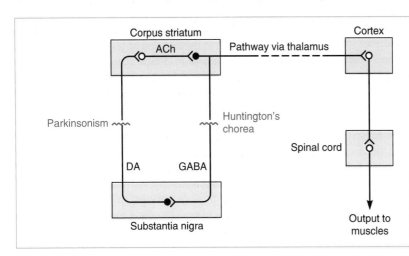

Fig. 31.3 Simplified diagram of the organisation of the extrapyramidal motor system, and the lesions that are believed to occur in Parkinson's disease and Huntington's disease.

Levodopa

Levodopa is the first-line treatment for PD, and is nearly always combined with a peripheral dopa decarboxylase inhibitor, either **carbidopa** or **benserazide**, which reduces the dose needed by about 10-fold, and diminishes the peripheral side-effects. It is well absorbed from the small intestine, a process which relies on active transport, though much of it is inactivated by monoamine oxidase in the wall of the intestine. The plasma half-life is short (about 2 hours). Conversion to dopamine in the periphery, which would otherwise account for about 95% of the levodopa dose, and cause troublesome side-effects, is largely prevented by the decarboxylase inhibitor. Decarboxylation occurs rapidly within the brain, since the decarboxylase inhibitors do not penetrate the blood–brain barrier. It is not certain whether the effect depends on an increased release of dopamine from the few surviving dopaminergic neurons or to a 'flooding' of the synapse with exogenous dopamine. Animal studies suggest that levodopa can act even when no dopaminergic nerve terminals are present. On the other hand, the therapeutic effectiveness of levodopa decreases as the disease advances, so part of its action may rely on the presence of functional dopaminergic neurons. Combination of levodopa with an inhibitor of catechol O-methyl transferase (COMT; see Ch. 8) such as **entacapone**, in order to inhibit its degradation, is under investigation.

Therapeutic effectiveness and unwanted effects of levodopa

At the beginning of treatment with levodopa, with optimisation of the dose, about 80% of patients show improvement, particularly of rigidity and hypokinesia, and about 20% are restored virtually to normal motor function. As time progresses, the effectiveness of levodopa gradually declines (Fig. 31.4). In a typical study of 100 patients treated with levodopa for 5 years, only 34 were better than they had been at the beginning of the trial, 32 patients having died and 21 having withdrawn from the trial. It is likely that the loss of effectiveness of levodopa mainly reflects the natural progression of the disease, but receptor down-regulation and other compensatory mechanisms may also contribute. The possibility that levodopa could actually accelerate the neurodegenerative process through overproduction of dopamine (see above) is currently being assessed in a large-scale trial. Levodopa nevertheless increases the life expectancy of Parkinson patients, probably as a result of improved motor function.

Unwanted effects

There are two main types of unwanted effect:

- Involuntary writhing movements (*dyskinesia*), which

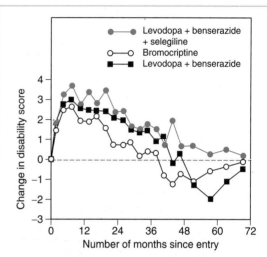

Fig. 31.4 Comparison of levodopa/benserazide, levodopa/ benserazide/selegiline and bromocriptine on progression of Parkinson's disease symptoms. Patients (249–271 in each treatment group) were assessed on a standard disability rating score. Before treatment, the average rate of decline was 0.7 units/year. All three treatments produced improvement over the initial rating for 2–3 years, but the effect declined, either because of refractoriness to the drugs, or to disease progression. Bromocriptine appeared slightly less effective than levodopa regimes, and there was a higher drop-out rate due to side-effects in this group. (Parkinson's Disease Research Group 1993)

develop in the majority of patients within 2 years of starting levodopa therapy. These movements usually affect the face and limbs, and can become very severe. They disappear if the dose of levodopa is reduced, but this causes rigidity to return. Thus, the margin between the beneficial and the unwanted effect becomes progressively narrower, an effect that appears to be related to the duration of levodopa treatment.

- Rapid fluctuations in clinical state, where hypokinesia and rigidity may suddenly worsen for anything from a few minutes to a few hours, and then improve again. This 'on–off effect' is not seen in untreated PD patients or with other anti-PD drugs. The 'off effect' can be so sudden that the patient stops while walking and feels rooted to the spot, or is unable to rise from a chair in which he had sat down normally a few moments earlier. The mechanism of this remarkable effect is not understood. In some patients, the fluctuations reflect the changing plasma levodopa concentration, and it is suggested that as the disease advances, the ability of neurons to store dopamine is lost, so the therapeutic benefit of levodopa depends increasingly on the continuous formation of extraneuronal dopamine, which is dependent on a continuous supply of levodopa. The use of sustained-release preparations, or co-administration of COMT inhibitors such as **entacapone** (see above) may be used to counteract the fluctuations in plasma concentration of levodopa.

In addition to these slowly developing side-effects, levodopa produces several acute effects, which are experienced by most patients at first but tend to disappear after a few weeks. The main ones are:

- *Nausea and anorexia.* **Domperidone**, a peripherally acting dopamine antagonist, may be useful in preventing this effect.
- *Hypotension*, usually of minor importance, but may cause postural hypotension in patients on antihypertensive drugs.
- *Psychological effects.* Levodopa, by increasing dopamine activity in the brain, can produce a schizophrenia-like syndrome (see Ch. 34) with delusions and hallucinations. More commonly, in about 20% of patients, it causes confusion, disorientation, insomnia or nightmares.

Selegiline

Selegiline is a monoamine oxidase (MAO) inhibitor that is selective for MAO-B, which predominates in dopamine-containing regions of the central nervous system. It therefore lacks the unwanted peripheral effects of non-selective MAO inhibitors, and, in contrast to them, does not provoke the 'cheese reaction' or interact so frequently with other drugs (see Ch. 35). Inhibition of MAO-B protects dopamine from intraneuronal degradation, and was initially used as an adjunct to levodopa. Long-term trials showed that the combination of selegiline and levodopa was more effective than levodopa alone in relieving symptoms and prolonging life. Recognition of the role of MAO-B in neurotoxicity (see above) suggested that selegiline might be neuroprotective, rather than merely enhancing the action of levodopa, but clinical studies have given inconclusive results on this point (see Stern 1997). A large-scale trial (Fig. 31.4) showed no difference when selegiline was added to levodopa/benserazide treatment.

Other drugs used in Parkinson's disease

Dopamine receptor agonists.

Bromocriptine, derived from the ergot alkaloids (see Ch. 9), is a potent agonist at dopamine (D_2) receptors

in the central nervous system, and a weak partial agonist at D_1-receptors. Activity at D_2-receptors is thought to underlie its efficacy in PD. It inhibits the anterior pituitary gland, and was first introduced for the treatment of galactorrhoea and gynaecomastia (Ch. 24), but is effective also in PD (Fig. 31.4). Its duration of action is longer (plasma half-life 6–8 hours) than that of levodopa, so that it does not need to be given so frequently. It was hoped that bromocriptine might be effective in patients who had become refractory to levodopa through loss of dopaminergic neurons, but this has not been clearly established. **Apomorphine**, given subcutaneously, sometimes with a continuous pump, is also used. Other dopamine-receptor agonists, such as **lisuride** and **pergolide**, have been developed and are undergoing trial. The side-effects of these drugs are similar to those of levodopa, and limit the doses that can be used. They are not expected to share the (so far theoretical) risk with levodopa of accelerating the neurodegenerative process. Newer drugs, with differing receptor profiles are also being developed (see Hagan et al 1997).

Amantadine

Amantadine was introduced as an antiviral drug, and discovered by accident in 1969 to be beneficial in PD. Many possible mechanisms for its action have been suggested, based on neurochemical evidence of increased dopamine release, inhibition of amine uptake or a direct action on dopamine receptors. Most authors now suggest, although not with much conviction, that increased dopamine release is primarily responsible for the clinical effects.

Amantadine is less effective than levodopa or bromocriptine, and its action declines with time. Its side-effects are considerably less severe, though qualitatively similar to those of levodopa.

Acetylcholine antagonists

For more than a century, until levodopa was discovered, atropine and related drugs were the main form of treatment for PD. Muscarinic acetylcholine receptors exert an excitatory effect, opposite to that of dopamine, on striatal neurons (see Fig. 31.3) and also exert a presynaptic inhibitory effect on dopaminergic nerve terminals. Suppression of these effects thus makes up, in part, for a lack of dopamine. The action of muscarinic antagonists is more limited than that of levodopa, and they diminish tremor more than rigidity or hypokinesia (which are more disabling in their effects). Furthermore, their side-effects—dry mouth, constipation, impaired vision, urinary retention—are often troublesome. They are used mainly to treat PD in patients receiving antipsychotic drugs (which are dopamine antagonists and thus nullify the effect of L-dopa; see Ch. 34). The drugs used for this purpose (e.g. **benztropine**) have less peripheral effect in relation to their central effect than does atropine. Drowsiness and confusion are the main unwanted effects. Patients suffering from PD very often show some degree of dementia, and acetylcholine antagonists would be expected to exacerbate this (see above).

NEW APPROACHES

Because PD results from the loss of a specific group of dopaminergic neurons, it was the first neurodegenerative disease for which neural transplantation was attempted, amid much publicity. Various transplantation approaches have been tried, based on the injection of dissociated foetal cells directly into the substantia nigra. Studies on animals with lesions of the substantia nigra have shown that the transplanted cells are able to survive and re-establish appropriate connections, as well as bringing about a degree of functional recovery. Trials in patients with PD have mainly involved injection of midbrain neurons from aborted human foetuses. The success rate has been very variable, and the benefit generally short-lived, but post-mortem studies have shown that such transplants are able to survive and establish synaptic connections. The use of foetal material is, of course, fraught with difficulties (usually cells from five or more foetuses are needed for one transplant). Hopes for the future rest mainly on the possibility of developing pre-

parations of immortalised neuronal precursor cells, which can be multiplied in culture, and which will differentiate into functional post-mitotic neurons after transplantation. Alternative approaches for treating PD as well as other neurodegenerative conditions include the use of non-neuronal cells (e.g. fibroblasts) genetically modified so that they will secrete missing mediators, such as dopamine or growth factors. Activity in this area is intense (for reviews, see Brustle & McKay 1996, Olanow et al. 1996b).

HUNTINGTON'S DISEASE

Huntington's disease is an inherited (autosomal dominant) disorder resulting in progressive brain degeneration, starting in adulthood and causing rapid deterioration and death. It is one of a group of so-called 'CAG-repeat' neurodegenerative diseases, associated with the expansion of the number of repeats of this trinucleotide sequence in the Huntington's disease gene, and hence the number (50 or more) of consecutive Glu residues in the expressed protein. The protein coded by this gene, *huntingtin*, interacts with various regulatory proteins, including one of the caspases (see above) which participates in excitotoxicity and apoptosis. Some of these interactions are enhanced by the poly-Glu repeat in the mutant protein, and this may account for the neuronal loss, which affects mainly the cortex and the striatum, resulting in progressive dementia and severe involuntary sudden jerky (choreiform) movements. Studies on post-mortem brains showed that the dopamine content of the striatum was normal or slightly increased, while there was a 75% reduction in the activity of glutamic acid decarboxylase, the enzyme responsible for GABA synthesis (Ch. 29). It is believed that the loss of GABA-mediated inhibition in the striatum produces a hyperactivity of dopaminergic synapses, so the syndrome is in some senses a mirror image of PD (Fig. 31.3). The effects of drugs that influence dopaminergic transmission are correspondingly the opposite of those that are observed in PD, dopamine antagonists being effective in reducing the involuntary movements, while drugs such as levodopa and bromocriptine make them worse. Drugs used to alleviate the symptoms include dopamine antagonists, such as **chlorpromazine** (Ch. 34), and the GABA agonist, **baclofen** (Ch. 29). These do not affect the course of the disease, and it is possible that drugs which inhibit excitotoxicity, when these become available (see above), may prove useful.

Drugs used in Parkinson's disease

- Drugs act by counteracting deficiency of dopamine in basal ganglia or by blocking muscarinic receptors.
- The most effective drug is levodopa, a dopamine precursor which passes the blood–brain barrier; it is given with an inhibitor of peripheral dopa decarboxylase (e.g. carbidopa) to minimise side-effects.
- Levodopa is effective in most patients initially, but often loses efficacy after about 2 years.
- Main unwanted effects of levodopa are: involuntary movements, which occur in most patients within 2 years; unpredictable 'on–off effect'. Others are: nausea, postural hypotension and occasionally psychotic symptoms.
- Other useful drugs include: bromocriptine (dopamine agonist), selegiline (MAO-B inhibitor), amantadine (? enhances dopamine release) and benztropine (muscarinic receptor antagonist, used for parkinsonism caused by antipsychotic drugs).

NEURODEGENERATIVE PRION DISEASES

A group of human and animal diseases associated with a characteristic type of neurodegeneration, known as *spongiform encephalopathy* because of the vacuolated appearance of the affected brain, has recently been the focus of intense research activity (reviewed by Haywood, 1997). A key feature of these diseases is that they are transmissible through an infective agent, though not, in general, across species. The recent upsurge of interest has been spurred partly by evidence suggesting that the bovine form of the disease, *bovine spongiform encephalopathy (BSE)*, may actually be transmissible to humans through eating beef. Different human forms of the disease include Creutzfeldt–Jakob disease (CJD, which is unrelated to BSE), and a new variant form (nvCJD) which, as yet very rare, is likely to result from eating, or close contact with, infected beef. Another human form is *kuru*, a neurodegenerative disease affecting cannibalistic tribes in Papua New Guinea. These diseases cause a progressive, and sometimes rapid, dementia and loss of motor coordination, for which no therapies currently exist. *Scrapie*, a common disease of domestic sheep, is another example, and it may have been the practice of feeding sheep offal to domestic cattle that initiated an epidemic of BSE in Britain during the 1980s, leading to the appearance of a few cases of nvCJD in humans in the mid-1990s. Although the BSE epidemic has been controlled, there is concern that many more human cases may develop in its wake, since the incubation period—known to be long—is uncertain. The infectious agent responsible for spongiform encephalopathies could be an unusual virus (see Ch. 44), but most evidence suggests that it is actually a protein without associated nucleic acids, known as a *prion* (see Caughey & Cheseboro, 1997; Prusiner et al, 1998), implying an unusual—indeed heretical—mechanism of infectivity and replication, which remains highly controversial.

The biochemical pathogenesis of prion diseases bears some similarity to that of AD, in that the brain accumulates an abnormal form of a normally-expressed protein. Normal prion proteins (termed PrP^C) are expressed by many cells throughout the body, and their function is unknown. Deletion of the PrP^C gene in mice produces only minor abnormalities. Animals or humans with spongiform encephalopathies accumulate in their brains a truncated and less soluble form, PrP^{SC}, derived by post-translational modification of PrP^C. PrP^{SC} has a strong tendency to aggregate and accumulate as fibrillary structures in the brain, and these appear to produce the neurodegenerative change (probably by mechanisms similar to those responsible for neurotoxicity associated with $A\beta$ formation). There is good evidence that PrP^{SC} itself is the infective prion, since injection of purified PrP^{SC} induces the disease in normal animals. PrP^C knockout animals are not susceptible, however, and it appears that administration of PrP^{SC} somehow catalyses the production of more PrP^{SC} from the normally-expressed PrP^C in the brain. Exactly how this happens remains unclear (see Prusiner et al, 1998), but there is hope that clarification of this unusual molecular process may be the key to preventive therapeutic measures in the future.

REFERENCES AND FURTHER READING

Aisen P S, Davis K L 1997 The search for disease-modifying treatment of Alzheimer's disease. Neurology 48 (suppl 6): S35–41 (*Good review article on current and prospective therapies*)

Beal M F, Hyman B T, Koroshetz W 1993 Do defects in mitochondrial energy metabolism underlie the pathology of neurodegenerative diseases? Trends Neurosci 16: 125–131

Bredesen D E 1995 Neural apoptosis. Ann Neurol 38: 839–851 (*Useful review, with discussion of relevance to clinical disorders*)

Brustle O, McKay R D G 1996 Neuronal progenitors as tools for cell replacement in the nervous system. Curr Opin Neurobiol 6: 688–695 (*Reviews progress in high-tech therapeutic approaches*)

Caughey B, Cheseboro B 1997 Prion protein and the transmissible spongiform encephalopathies. Trends in Cell Biogy 7: 56–62 (*Well-balanced review on the strengths and weaknesses of the prion hypothesis*)

Choi D W 1988 Calcium-mediated neurotoxicity: relationship to specific channel types and role in ischaemic damage. Trends Neurosci 11: 465–469

Coyle J T, Puttfarken P 1993 Oxidative stress, glutamate and neurodegenerative disorders. Science 262: 689–695 (*Good review article*)

Davies A M 1995 The Bcl-2 family of proteins, and the regulation of neuronal survival. Trends Neurosci 18: 355–358 (*Introductory review article on a family of proteins which control apoptosis*)

De Strooper D, Saftig P, Craessmaerts K et al. 1998 Deficiency of presenilin-1 inhibits the normal cleavage of amyloid precursor protein. Nature 391: 387–390

Green R A, Cross A J (eds) 1997 Neuroprotective agents in cerebral ischaemia. Int Rev Neurobiol 40 (*Compendium of articles summarising preclinical and clinical data*)

Hagan J J, Middlemiss D N, Sharpe PC, Poste G H 1997 Parkinson's disease: prospects for improved therapy. Trends Pharmacol Sci 18: 156–163 (*Excellent review of current trends*)

Haywood A M 1997 Transmissible spongiform encephalopathies. New Eng J Med 337: 1821–1828 *(General review article, emphasising some of the epidemiological issues)*

Hornykiewicz O, Kish S J 1986 Biochemical pathology of Parkinson's disease. Adv Neurol 45: 19–34, 183–190 *(Account of the discovery of dopamine deficiency in PD)*

Kogure K, Hossmann K-A, Siesjo B K (eds) 1993 Neurobiology of ischaemic brain damage. Elsevier, Amsterdam *(Comprehensive compendium)*

Koroshetz W J, Moskowitz M A 1996 Emerging treatments for stroke in humans. Trends Pharmacol Sci 17: 227–233 *(Excellent review of the slow progress, and emerging ideas in a difficult area)*

Langston W J 1985 MPTP and Parkinson's disease. Trends Neurosci 8: 79–83 *(Readable account of the MPTP story by its discoverer)*

Lipton S A, Rosenberg P A 1994 Excitatory amino acids as a final common pathway for neurologic disorders. New Engl J Med 330: 613–622 *(Review emphasising central role of glutamate in neurodegeneration)*

Louvel E, Hugon J, Doble A 1997 Therapeutic advances in amyotrophic lateral sclerosis. Trends Pharmacol Sci 18: 196–203 *(Recent summary of research and clinical trials data—mostly negative—on neuroprotective strategies in a progressive neurodegenerative disease)*

Merry D E, Korsmeyer S J 1997 Bcl-2 gene family in the nervous system. Annu Rev Neurosci 20: 245–267 *(Discusses role of proteins controlling apoptosis in neural development and response to injury)*

Olanow C W, Jenner P, Youdim M (eds) 1996a Neurodegeneration and neuroprotection in Parkinson's disease. Academic Press, London *(Compendium of articles on basic and clinical aspects)*

Olanow C W, Kordower J H, Freeman T B 1996b Fetal nigral transplantation as a therapy for Parkinson's disease. Trends Neurosci 19: 102–109 *(Update by one of the pioneers in neural transplantation)*

Olney J W 1990 Excitotoxic amino acids and neuropsychiatric disorders. Annu Rev Pharmacol Toxicol 30: 47–71 *(Dated, but comprehensive review, covering psychiatric as well as neurological diseases)*

Parkinson's Disease Research Group 1993 Comparisons of therapeutic effects of levodopa, levodopa and selegiline, and bromocriptine in patients with early, mild Parkinson's disease: three year interim report. Br Med J 307: 469–472 *(Definitive study, showing little difference in efficacy of different dopamine replacement strategies)*

Prusiner S B, Scott M R, DeArmond S J, Cohen F E 1998 Prion protein biology. Cell 93: 337–348 *(Informative discussion by the Nobel-prizewinning pioneer in this field of the mechanisms underlying the infectivity of prions and the link between CJD and BSE)*

Rothwell N J, Luheshi G, Toulmond S 1996 Cytokines and their receptors in the central nervous system: physiology, pharmacology and pathology. Pharmacol Ther 69: 85–95 *(Useful short review of an emerging area)*

Selkoe D J 1993 Physiological production of the β-amyloid protein and the mechanism of Alzheimer's disease. Trends Neurosci 16: 403–409 *(Introductory review by one of the pioneers of the amyloid theory)*

Selkoe D J 1997 Alzheimer's disease: genotypes, phenotype and treatments. Science 275: 630–631 *(Short but informative summary of recent advances in Alzheimer genetics)*

Steller H 1995 Mechanisms and genes of cellular suicide. Science 267: 1445–1449 *(Review on apoptosis, not only neuronal)*

Stern M B 1997 Contemporary approaches to the pharmacotherapeutic management of Parkinson's disease. Neurology 49 (suppl 1): S2–9 *(Good review of current and future approaches)*

Tipton K F, Singer T P 1993 Advances in our understanding of the mechanisms of neurotoxicity of MPTP and related compounds. J Neurochem 61: 1191–1206 *(Reviews mechanism of action of MPTP in context of neurotoxicity as a basis of neurodegenerative diseases)*

Wahlgren N G 1997 A review of earlier clinical studies on neuroprotective agents and current approaches ischaemia. Int Rev Neurobiol 40: 337–363 *(Review of clinical data)*

Yankner B A 1996 Mechanisms of neuronal degeneration in Alzheimer's disease. Neuron 16: 921–932 *(Review focusing on reasons why neurons are damaged by amyloid deposition)*

32

General anaesthetic agents

General anaesthetics are used as an adjunct to surgical procedures in order to render the patient unaware of, and unresponsive to, painful stimulation. They are given systemically, and exert their main effects on the central nervous system, in contrast to local anaesthetics (see Ch. 40) which work by blocking conduction of impulses in peripheral sensory nerves. Though we now take them for granted, general anaesthetics are the drugs that paved the way for much of modern surgery.

Many drugs, including, for example, **ethanol** and **morphine**, can produce a state of insensibility and obliviousness to pain, but are not used as anaesthetics. For a drug to be useful as an anaesthetic it must be readily controllable, so that induction and recovery are rapid, allowing the level of anaesthesia to be adjusted as required during the course of the operation. For this reason it was only when inhalation anaesthetics were first discovered, in 1846, that surgical operations under controlled anaesthesia became a practical possibility. Until that time surgeons relied on being able to operate at lightning speed, and most operations were amputations. Inhalation is still the commonest route of administration for anaesthetics, though there are now drugs that are sufficiently rapidly metabolised or redistributed in the body to be used as anaesthetics by the intravenous route.

The use of **nitrous oxide** to relieve the pain of surgery was suggested by Humphrey Davy in 1800. He was the first person to make nitrous oxide and he tested its effects on several people, including himself and the Prime Minister, noting that it caused euphoria, analgesia and loss of consciousness. The use of nitrous oxide, billed as 'laughing gas', became a popular fairground entertainment, and came to the notice of an American dentist, Horace Wells, who had a tooth extracted under its influence, while he himself squeezed the inhalation bag. **Ether** also first gained publicity in a disreputable way, through the spread of 'ether frolics' at which it was used to produce euphoria among the guests (explosions, too, one might have thought). William Morton, also a dentist and a student at Harvard Medical School, used it successfully to extract a tooth in 1846 and then suggested to Warren, the chief surgeon at Massachusetts General Hospital, that he should administer it for one of Warren's operations. Warren grudgingly agreed, and on 16 October 1846 a large audience was gathered in the main operating theatre; after some preliminary fumbling, Morton's demonstration was a spectacular success. 'Gentlemen, this is no humbug' was the most gracious comment that Warren could bring himself to make to the assembled audience. A more wordy appreciation came later from Oliver Wendell Holmes (1847), the neurologist–poet–philosopher who first coined the word 'anaesthesia'. 'The knife is searching for disease, the pulleys are dragging back dislocated limbs—Nature herself is working out the primal curse which doomed the tenderest of her creatures to the sharpest of her trials, but the fierce extremity of suffering has been steeped in the waters of forgetfulness, and the deepest furrow in the knotted brow of agony has been smoothed forever'. Morton subsequently sank into an endless and bitter dispute over the patent rights, and contributed nothing more to medical science. In the same year James Simpson, professor of obstetrics in Glasgow, used **chloroform** to relieve the pain of childbirth, bringing on himself fierce denunciation from the clergy, one of whom wrote: 'Chloroform is a decoy of Satan, apparently offering itself to bless women; but in the end it will harden society and rob God of the deep, earnest cries which arise in time of trouble, for help'. Opposition was effectively silenced in 1853 when Queen Victoria gave birth to her seventh child under the influence of chloroform, and the procedure became known as 'anaesthésie à la reine'.

PHYSICOCHEMICAL THEORIES OF ANAESTHESIA

Unlike most drugs, inhalation anaesthetics, which include substances as diverse as **halothane**, **nitrous oxide** and **xenon**, belong to no recognisable chemical class. The shape and electronic configuration of the molecule is evidently unimportant, and the pharmacological action requires only that the molecule has certain physico-chemical properties. The lack of chemical specificity argues against there being any distinctive 'receptor' for anaesthetics (see Ch. 1); instead we need to consider in which 'phase' of the cell the drugs are acting. Anaesthetics appear to act principally on the cell membrane (see below), and theories of anaesthesia focus on interactions with the two main components of the membrane, namely lipids and proteins.

Accounts of the different theories of anaesthesia are given by Halsey (1989), Little (1996), Franks & Lieb (1994).

LIPID THEORY

The lipid theory derives from the extensive work of Overton & Meyer at the turn of the century, who showed a close correlation between *anaesthetic potency* and *lipid solubility* in a diverse group of simple and unreactive organic compounds that were tested for their ability to immobilise tadpoles. This led to the theory, formulated by Meyer in 1937: 'Narcosis commences when any chemically indifferent substance has attained a certain molar concentration in the lipids of the cell.'

The relationship between anaesthetic activity and lipid solubility has been repeatedly confirmed. Figure 32.1

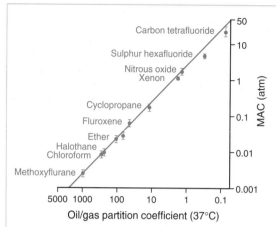

Fig. 32.1 Correlation of anaesthetic potency with oil : gas partition coefficient. Anaesthetic potency in man is expressed as minimum alveolar partial pressure (MAC) required to produce surgical anaesthesia. There is a close correlation with lipid solubility, expressed as the oil : gas partition coefficient. (From: Halsey 1989)

shows results obtained in humans where the *minimal alveolar concentration* (MAC; inversely proportional to potency) required to produce a lack of response to painful stimulation is plotted against lipid solubility, expressed as oil : water partition coefficient, for a wide range of inhalation anaesthetics. The Overton–Meyer studies did not suggest any particular mechanism, but revealed an impressive correlation which any theory of anaesthesia needs to take into account. Oil : water partition should predict partition into membrane lipids, in agreement with abundant evidence that anaesthesia is caused by an alteration of membrane function.

How might the introduction of inert foreign molecules into the cell membrane cause a functional disturbance? Some evidence, notably the phenomenon of *pressure reversal* of anaesthesia, suggests that *volume expansion* is the underlying mechanism. If animals, such as newts, are immobilised by addition of anaesthetic to the water, application of hydrostatic pressure to about 100 atmospheres immediately restores their mobility, and anaesthesia returns as soon as the pressure is lowered. The results are compatible with the theory that anaesthesia occurs when the volume of the lipid phase is expanded by about 0.4% as a result of the intrusion of anaesthetic molecules. Pressure is thought to act simply by opposing this volume expansion. Further work has revealed discrepancies, however, so the interpretation is not clear at present (see Little 1996).

Another theory involves an *increase in membrane*

fluidity due to disordering of the packing array of membrane phospholipids. Physicochemical measurements confirm that this does occur, though relatively high concentrations of anaesthetics are needed, and the effects are small by comparison with those of a modest (< 1°C) rise in temperature, so the relevance of this phenomenon to the pharmacological actions of anaesthetics is not clear.

PROTEIN THEORY

Anaesthetics can bind to proteins, as well as lipids. Work on purified *luciferase* (the enzyme responsible for the luminescent reaction of fireflies) has shown a striking parallel between enzyme inhibition and anaesthetic potency for a wide range of compounds. Evidence for similar interactions of anaesthetics with functional membrane proteins, particularly ligand-gated ion channels, has been obtained more recently (see Franks & Lieb 1994). Many anaesthetic agents are able, at concentrations reached during anaesthesia, to inhibit the function of excitatory receptors, such as the ionotropic glutamate, acetylcholine or 5-HT receptors, as well as enhancing the function of inhibitory receptors, such as $GABA_A$ and glycine (see Harris et al. 1995). Studies with genetically engineered receptors (Mihic et al. 1997) show that these effects depend on the presence of particular domains in the receptor protein, which appear to comprise specific 'modulatory sites' (see Ch. 30) through which the anaesthetic drugs exert their effects on channel function. The test of whether these sites actually mediate anaesthetic action will come when the effect of anaesthetics on transgenic mice expressing such anaesthetic-resistant mutations is determined.

Holding the middle ground (both metaphorically and literally) between the opposing lipid and protein theories of general anaesthetic action are proponents of the view that anaesthetics concentrate at the lipid–protein interface within the membrane, and thereby affect the functioning of membrane proteins. As Little (1996) emphasises, most anaesthetics exert several distinct cellular actions, so it is likely that more than one type of interaction contributes to their effects.

THE EFFECTS OF ANAESTHETICS ON THE NERVOUS SYSTEM

At the cellular level, the effect of anaesthetics is mainly to inhibit synaptic transmission, any effects on axonal conduction probably being unimportant in practice (see Pocock & Richards 1993).

Inhibition of synaptic transmission could be due to reduction of transmitter release, inhibition of the action of the transmitter, or reduction of the excitability of the postsynaptic cell. Though all three effects have been described, most studies suggest that reduced transmitter release and reduced postsynaptic response are the main factors. A reduction of acetylcholine release has been shown in studies on peripheral synapses, and reduced sensitivity to excitatory transmitters (due to inhibition of ligand-gated ion channels; see above) occurs at both peripheral and central synapses.

The action of inhibitory synapses may be enhanced or reduced by anaesthetics. Enhancement of inhibitory synaptic action occurs particularly with barbiturates, though similar effects also occur with volatile anaesthetics (see Little 1996).

Much effort has gone into identifying a particular brain region on which anaesthetics act to produce their effect (see Angel 1993). The most sensitive region appears to be the thalamic sensory relay nuclei and the deep layer of the cortex to which these nuclei project. This constitutes the route taken by sensory impulses reaching the cortex, so inhibition can result in a lack of awareness of sensory input.

Anaesthetics, even in low concentrations, cause short-term *amnesia*, i.e. experiences occurring during the influence of the drug are not recalled later even though the subject was responsive at the time.* It is likely that

---

> **Theories of anaesthesia**
>
> - Many simple, unreactive compounds produce narcotic effects.
> - Anaesthetic potency is closely correlated with lipid solubility (Overton–Meyer correlation), not with chemical structure, suggesting that anaesthesia involves interaction with a hydrophobic domain of the cell.
> - The two main theories of anaesthesia postulate interaction either with the lipid membrane bilayer or with hydrophobic binding sites on protein molecules.
> - The main lipid theory postulates volume expansion as the mechanism by which membrane function is altered. The phenomenon of pressure reversal of anaesthesia is consistent with this, but can be explained in other ways.
> - There is increasing evidence that anaesthetics may act by binding to discrete hydrophobic domains of protein molecules, particularly ion channels.

---

*The benzodiazepine, flunitrazepam, recently achieved a nasty notoriety, since its amnesia-producing and tranquillising effect led to its use as a rapists' aid.

interference with hippocampal function produces this effect, for it is known that the hippocampus is involved in short-term memory and that certain hippocampal synapses are highly susceptible to inhibition by anaesthetics.

As the anaesthetic concentration is increased, all brain functions are affected, including motor control and reflex activity, respiration and autonomic regulation. Thus it is not possible to identify a critical 'target site' in the brain responsible for all the phenomena of anaesthesia.

STAGES OF ANAESTHESIA

When a slowly acting anaesthetic, such as **ether**, is given on its own, certain well-defined stages are passed through as its concentration in the blood increases.

- *Stage I—Analgesia.* The subject is conscious but drowsy. Responses to painful stimuli are reduced. The degree of analgesia actually varies greatly with different agents; it is pronounced with ether and nitrous oxide, but not with halothane.
- *Stage II—Excitement.* The subject loses consciousness, and no longer responds to non-painful stimuli, but responds in a reflex fashion to painful stimuli. Other reflexes, for example the cough reflex, and gagging in response to pharyngeal stimulation, are present and often exaggerated. The subject may move, talk incoherently, hold his breath, choke or vomit. Irregular ventilation may affect the absorption of the anaesthetic agent. It is a dangerous state, and modern anaesthetic procedures are designed to eliminate it.
- *Stage III—Surgical anaesthesia.* Spontaneous movement ceases and respiration becomes regular. If anaesthesia is light, some reflexes (e.g. responses to pharyngeal and peritoneal stimulation) are still present, and muscles show appreciable tone. With deepening anaesthesia, these reflexes disappear, and the muscles relax fully. Respiration becomes progressively shallower, with the intercostal muscles failing before the diaphragm.
- *Stage IV—Medullary paralysis.* Respiration and vasomotor control cease, and death occurs within a few minutes.

Single anaesthetic agents are rarely used on their own, and progression through these stages is seldom observed in practice. The anaesthetic state, for clinical purposes, consists of three main components, namely *loss of consciousness*, *analgesia*, and *muscle relaxation*, and in practice these effects are produced with a combination of drugs rather than with a single anaesthetic agent. Thus, a common procedure would be to produce uncon-

sciousness rapidly with an intravenous induction agent (e.g. **thiopentone**), to maintain unconsciousness and produce analgesia with one or more inhalation agents (e.g. **nitrous oxide** and **halothane**), which might be supplemented with an intravenous analgesic agent (e.g. an opiate; see Ch. 37), and to produce muscle paralysis with a neuromuscular blocking drug (e.g. **atracurium**; see Ch. 7). Such a procedure results in much faster induction and recovery, avoiding long (and hazardous) periods of semiconsciousness, and it enables surgery to be carried out with relatively little impairment of homeostatic reflexes.

EFFECTS ON THE CARDIOVASCULAR AND RESPIRATORY SYSTEMS

Though all anaesthetics decrease the contractility of isolated heart preparations, their effects on cardiac output and blood pressure in humans vary, mainly because of concomitant actions on the sympathetic nervous system. Some agents (e.g. nitrous oxide) cause an increased sympathetic discharge and increased plasma noradrenaline concentration and tend to increase blood pressure, whereas others (e.g. **halothane** and other halogenated anaesthetics) have the opposite effect.

Many anaesthetics, particularly halogenated agents,

Pharmacological effects of anaesthetic agents

- Anaesthesia involves three main neurophysiological changes: unconsciousness, loss of response to painful stimulation and loss of reflexes.
- At supra-anaesthetic doses, all anaesthetic agents can cause death by loss of cardiovascular reflexes and respiratory paralysis.
- At the cellular level, anaesthetic agents affect synaptic transmission rather than axonal conduction. The release of excitatory transmitters and the response of the postsynaptic receptors are both inhibited. GABA-mediated inhibitory transmission is enhanced by some anaesthetics.
- Though all parts of the nervous system are affected by anaesthetic agents, the main targets appear to be the thalamus, cortex and hippocampus.
- Most anaesthetic agents (with exceptions, such as ketamine and benzodiazepines) produce similar neurophysiological effects, and differ mainly in respect of their pharmacokinetic properties and toxicity.
- Most anaesthetic agents cause cardiovascular depression, by effects on the myocardium and blood vessels, as well as on the nervous system. Halogenated anaesthetic agents are likely to cause cardiac dysrhythmias, accentuated by circulating catecholamines.

cause cardiac dysrhythmias, particularly ventricular extra-systoles. The mechanism is not well understood, but involves sensitisation to adrenaline. The usual manifestation is the appearance of ventricular ectopic beats, and careful ECG monitoring shows that these occur very commonly in patients under halothane anaesthesia, without producing any harmful effect. If catecholamine secretion is excessive, however, there is a risk of precipitating ventricular fibrillation, which is a particular hazard if stage II of the induction process is unduly prolonged.

With the exception of nitrous oxide and ketamine, all anaesthetics depress respiration markedly, and increase arterial P_{CO_2}. Nitrous oxide has much less effect, mainly because its low potency prevents very deep anaesthesia from being produced with this drug (see below).

INHALATION ANAESTHETICS

PHARMACOKINETIC ASPECTS

An important characteristic of an inhalation anaesthetic is the speed at which the arterial blood concentration, which governs the pharmacological effect, follows changes in the concentration of the drug in the inspired air. Ideally, the blood concentration should follow as quickly as possible, so that the depth of anaesthesia can be controlled rapidly. In particular, the blood concentration should fall to a sub-anaesthetic level rapidly when administration is stopped, so that the patient recovers consciousness with minimal delay. A prolonged semi-comatose state, in which respiratory reflexes are weak or absent, represents a distinct hazard to life.

The only quantitatively important route by which inhalation anaesthetics enter and leave the body is via the lungs. Metabolic degradation of anaesthetics (see below), though important in relation to their toxicity, is generally insignificant in determining their duration of action. Anaesthetics are all small, lipid-soluble molecules, which cross the alveolar membrane with great ease. It is therefore the rate of delivery of drug to and from the lungs, via the inspired air and the bloodstream, that determines the overall kinetic behaviour of an anaesthetic. The reason that anaesthetics vary in their kinetic behaviour is that their relative solubilities in blood, and in body fat, vary between one drug and another.

The main factors that determine the speed of induction and recovery can be summarised as follows:

● Properties of the anaesthetic
—blood : gas partition coefficient (i.e. solubility in blood)
—oil : gas partition coefficient (i.e. solubility in fat)

● Physiological factors
—alveolar ventilation rate
—cardiac output.

THE SOLUBILITY OF ANAESTHETICS

For practical purposes anaesthetics can be regarded physicochemically as ideal gases: their solubility in different media is expressed as *partition coefficients*, defined as the ratio of the concentration of the agent in two phases at equilibrium.

The blood : gas partition coefficient is the main factor that determines the *rate of induction and recovery* of an inhalation anaesthetic, and the lower the blood : gas partition coefficient the faster the induction and recovery.

The *oil : gas partition coefficient*, a measure of fat solubility, determines the *potency* of an anaesthetic (as already discussed) and also influences the kinetics of its distribution in the body, the main effect being that high lipid solubility tends to delay recovery from the effects of anaesthesia. Values of blood : gas and oil : gas partition coefficients for some anaesthetics are given in Table 32.1.

INDUCTION AND RECOVERY

The brain has a large blood flow, and the blood–brain barrier is freely permeable to anaesthetics, so the concentration of anaesthetic in the brain closely tracks that in the arterial blood. The kinetics of transfer of anaesthetic between the inspired air and the arterial blood therefore determine the kinetics of the pharmacological effect.

If an anaesthetic is added to the inspired air at a concentration which, *at equilibrium*, will produce surgical anaesthesia, the rate at which this equilibrium is approached depends mainly on the blood : gas partition coefficient. Contrary to what one might intuitively suppose, the *lower* the solubility in blood, the *faster* is the process of equilibration. This is because less drug has to be transferred via the lungs to the blood in order to achieve a given partial pressure. Thus a single lungful of air containing a low-solubility agent will bring the partial pressure in the blood closer to that of the inspired air than is the case for a high-solubility agent, and a smaller number of breaths (i.e. a shorter time) will be needed to reach equilibrium. The same principle applies in reverse for washout of the drug, recovery being faster with a low-solubility agent. Figure 32.2 shows the much faster equilibration for nitrous oxide—a low-solubility agent—than for ether—a high solubility agent (now obsolete).

The transfer of anaesthetic between blood and tissues

Table 32.1 Characteristics of inhalation anaesthetics

Drug	Partition coefficients Blood : gas	Oil : gas	MAC (% v/v)	Induction/ recovery	Main adverse effects	Notes
Ether	12.0	65	1.9	Slow	Respiratory irritation Nausea and vomiting Explosion risk	Now obsolete, except where facilities are minimal
Halothane	2.4	220	0.8	Medium	Hypotension Cardiac dysrhythmias Hepatotoxicity (with repeated use) Malignant hyperthermia (rare)	In common use, but declining in favour of newer agents Significant metabolism to trifluoracetate
Nitrous oxide	0.5	1.4	100*	Fast	Few adverse effects Risk of anaemia (with prolonged or repeated use)	Good analgesic effect Low potency precludes use as sole anaesthetic agent—normally combined with other inhalation agents
Enflurane	1.9	98	0.7	Medium	Risk of convulsions (slight) Malignant hyperthermia (rare)	Widely used Similar characteristics to halothane, with less risk of hepatic toxicity
Isoflurane	1.4	91	1.2	Medium	Few adverse effects Possible risk of coronary ischaemia in susceptible patients	Widely used as alternative to halothane
Desflurane	0.4	23	6.1	Fast	Respiratory tract irritation, cough, bronchospasm	Used for day-case surgery, because of fast onset and recovery (comparable to nitrous oxide)
Sevoflurane	0.6	53	2.1	Fast	Few reported Theoretical risk of renal toxicity due to fluoride	Recently introduced Similar to desflurane

*Theoretical value, based on experiments under hyperbaric conditions

also affects the kinetics of equilibration. Figure 32.3 shows a very simple model of the circulation in which two tissue compartments are included. Body fat has a low blood flow and often a high anaesthetic solubility (see Table 32.1), and constitutes about 20% of the volume of a normal male. Thus for a drug such as halothane, which is about 100 times more soluble in fat than in water, the amount present in fat after complete equilibration would be roughly 95% of the total amount in the body. Because of the low blood flow it takes many hours for the drug to enter and leave the fat, which results in a pronounced slow phase of equilibration following the rapid phase associated with the blood–gas exchanges (Fig. 32.2). The more fat-soluble the anaesthetic and the fatter the patient, the more pronounced this slow phase becomes.

Of the physiological factors affecting the rate of equilibration of inhalation anaesthetics, alveolar ventilation is the most important. The greater the ventilation rate, the faster is the process of equilibration, particularly for drugs that have high blood : gas partition coefficients. The use of respiratory depressant drugs, such as **morphine** (see Ch. 37) can thus retard recovery from anaesthesia. Changes in cardiac output produce complex effects. Increasing the cardiac output tends to slow down the early phase of induction, but speed up the later phase of equilibration.

Recovery from anaesthesia involves the same processes as induction but in reverse (Fig. 32.2), the rapid phase of recovery being followed by a slow phase. If anaesthesia with a highly fat-soluble drug has been maintained for a long time, so that the fat has had time

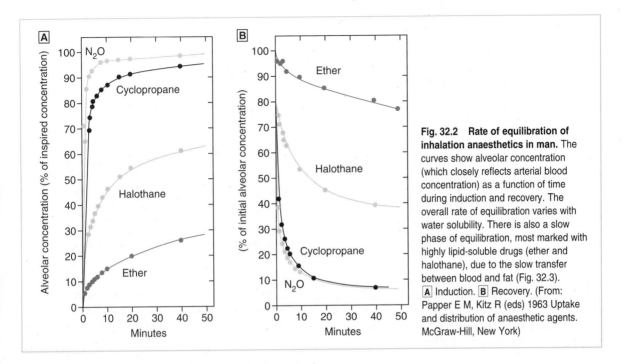

Fig. 32.2 Rate of equilibration of inhalation anaesthetics in man. The curves show alveolar concentration (which closely reflects arterial blood concentration) as a function of time during induction and recovery. The overall rate of equilibration varies with water solubility. There is also a slow phase of equilibration, most marked with highly lipid-soluble drugs (ether and halothane), due to the slow transfer between blood and fat (Fig. 32.3). **A** Induction. **B** Recovery. (From: Papper E M, Kitz R (eds) 1963 Uptake and distribution of anaesthetic agents. McGraw-Hill, New York)

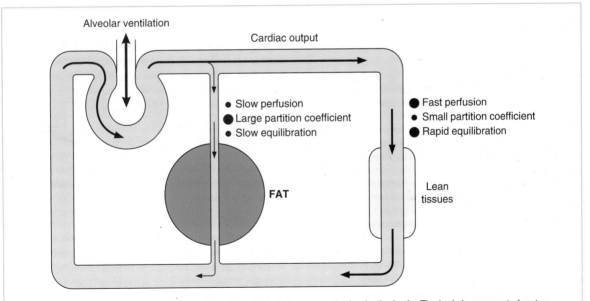

Fig. 32.3 Factors affecting the rate of equilibration of inhalation anaesthetics in the body. The body is represented as two compartments. Lean tissues have a large blood flow and low partition coefficient for anaesthetics, and therefore equilibrate rapidly with the blood. Fat tissues have a small blood flow and large partition coefficient, and therefore equilibrate slowly, acting as a reservoir of drug during the recovery phase.

to accumulate a substantial amount of the anaesthetic, this slow phase of recovery can become very pronounced and the patient may remain drowsy for some hours. Because of these kinetic factors, the search for improved inhalation anaesthetics has focused on agents with low blood and tissue solubility. Newer drugs, which show kinetic properties similar to those of nitrous oxide, but have higher potency, include **sevoflurane** and **desflurane** (Table 32.1).

METABOLISM AND TOXICITY OF INHALATION ANAESTHETICS

It was originally thought that anaesthetics were too unreactive to be metabolised in the body, but in fact the metabolism of halogenated anaesthetics can be considerable, and the resulting metabolites contribute appreciably to certain toxic effects. **Chloroform** (now obsolete) produces hepatotoxicity associated with free radical formation in liver cells. **Methoxyflurane**, a halogenated ether, is now very rarely used, because about 50% is metabolised, generating fluoride and oxalate, which cause renal toxicity. **Enflurane** also generates fluoride, but at much lower (non-toxic) levels (Table 32.1). **Halothane** is the only volatile anaesthetic in current use which undergoes substantial metabolism, about 30% being converted to bromide, trifluoroacetic acid and other metabolites which may be responsible for the rare occurrence of liver toxicity (see below).

Pharmacokinetic properties of inhalation anaesthetics

- Rapid induction and recovery are important properties of an anaesthetic agent, allowing flexible control over the depth of anaesthesia.
- Speed of induction and recovery are determined by two properties of the anaesthetic: solubility in blood (blood : gas partition coefficient) and solubility in fat (lipid solubility).
- Agents with low blood : gas partition coefficients produce rapid induction and recovery (e.g. nitrous oxide, desflurane), agents with high blood : gas partition coefficients show slow induction and recovery (e.g. halothane).
- Agents with high lipid solubility (e.g. halothane) accumulate gradually in body fat, and may produce a prolonged hangover if used for a long operation.
- Some halogenated anaesthetics (especially halothane and methoxyflurane) are metabolised. This is not very important in determining their duration of action, but contributes to toxicity (e.g. renal toxicity associated with fluoride production with methoxyflurane—no longer used).

The problem of toxicity of low concentrations of anaesthetics inhaled over long periods by operating theatre staff causes much concern, following the demonstration that such chronic low-level exposure leads to liver toxicity (associated with metabolite formation) in experimental animals. Epidemiological studies of operating theatre staff have shown increased incidence of liver disease and of certain types of leukaemia, and of spontaneous abortion and congenital malformations, compared with similar groups of subjects not exposed to anaesthetic agents. Though causation has not been clearly established, strict measures are used to minimise the escape of anaesthetics into the air of operating theatres.

INDIVIDUAL INHALATION ANAESTHETICS

The inhalation anaesthetics currently used in developed western countries are **halothane**, **nitrous oxide**, **enflurane** and **isoflurane**. **Ether**, used for many years but now largely obsolete, is still used in some parts of the world. It is explosive, and highly irritant, and commonly causes postoperative nausea and respiratory complications. **Methoxyflurane** (see above) is rarely used because of its renal toxicity. **Desflurane** and **sevoflurane** have been introduced recently.

HALOTHANE

Halothane is a widely used inhalation anaesthetic, but its use is now declining in favour of isoflurane and other drugs (see below). It is non-explosive and non-irritant; induction and recovery are relatively fast; it is highly potent, and can easily produce respiratory and cardiovascular failure, so the concentration administered needs to be controlled accurately. Even in normal anaesthetic concentrations, halothane causes a fall in blood pressure, partly due to myocardial depression and partly to vasodilatation. Halothane is not analgesic, and has a relaxant effect on the uterus, which limits its usefulness for obstetric purposes.

Adverse effects

In common with other halogenated anaesthetics, halothane sensitises the heart to adrenaline, and tends to cause cardiac dysrhythmias, particularly ventricular extrasystoles. Though this does not normally matter, it can be important in special circumstances, e.g. in operations for phaeochromocytoma (see Ch. 8), where there is a risk of precipitating ventricular fibrillation.

Two rare, but serious, adverse reactions are associated with halothane, namely *hepatotoxicity* and *malignant hyperthermia.* In a major study in 1986 of 850 000 cases involving anaesthesia with different agents, nine deaths from liver failure not attributable to any other recognisable cause were reported, seven of which had received halothane. Subsequent reports suggest that the risk is associated with repeated administration of halothane. In the UK a study of 62 cases of unexplained serious liver disease showed that 66% were associated with *repeated* halothane administration. Halothane undergoes metabolism (see above), partly by oxidation to trifluoroacetic acid, which reacts covalently with many proteins. This happens particularly in liver cells, where halothane metabolism takes place, and the mechanism of hepatotoxicity is thought to involve an immune response to certain fluoroacetylated liver enzymes.

Malignant hyperthermia results from excessive metabolic heat production in skeletal muscle, due to excessive release of Ca^{2+} from the sarcoplasmic reticulum. The result is a dramatic rise in body temperature, associated with muscle contractures and acidosis, which can be fatal unless treated promptly. Malignant hyperthermia can be triggered by a number of drugs, including other halogenated anaesthetics, and neuromuscular blocking drugs (see Ch. 7). Susceptibility to it has a genetic basis, being associated with mutations in the gene encoding the Ca^{2+} channel (known as the *ryanodine receptor*, because it is activated by this alkaloid), which controls Ca^{2+} release from the sarcoplasmic reticulum. Why such mutations induce sensitivity of the channel to anaesthetics and other drugs is not clear. Malignant hyperthermia is treated with **dantrolene**, a muscle relaxant drug which blocks these Ca^{2+} channels.

NITROUS OXIDE

Nitrous oxide is an odourless gas with many advantageous features for anaesthesia, and is in widespread use. It is rapid in action, because of its low blood : gas partition coefficient (Table 32.1), and is also an effective analgesic agent in concentrations too low to cause unconsciousness. It is used in this way to reduce pain during childbirth. The potency of nitrous oxide is low; even at a concentration of 80% in the inspired gas mixture (the maximum possible without reducing the oxygen content) nitrous oxide does not produce surgical anaesthesia. It is not therefore used on its own as an anaesthetic, but is very often used (as 70% nitrous oxide in oxygen) as an adjunct to volatile anaesthetics, allowing them to be used at lower concentrations. During recovery from nitrous oxide anaesthesia, the transfer of the gas from the blood into the alveoli can be sufficient to reduce, by dilution,

the alveolar partial pressure of oxygen, producing a transient hypoxia (known as the *second gas effect*), but this is only important in patients with respiratory disease.

Given for brief periods, nitrous oxide is devoid of any serious toxic effects, but prolonged exposure (> 6 h) causes inactivation of methionine synthase, an enzyme required for DNA and protein synthesis, resulting in bone marrow depression which leads to anaemia and leukopenia. This does not normally occur with brief exposure to nitrous oxide, but prolonged or repeated use needs to be avoided. It should also be avoided in patients with anaemia related to vitamin B_{12} deficiency. Prolonged exposure to very low concentrations of nitrous oxide, far below the level causing anaesthesia, may affect protein and DNA synthesis very markedly, and nitrous oxide has been suspected to be a cause of the increased frequency of abortion and foetal abnormality among operating theatre staff.

ENFLURANE

Enflurane is a halogenated ether, similar to halothane in its potency and moderate speed of induction. It was introduced as an alternative to methoxyflurane, its advantages being that it causes little production of fluoride (and therefore lacks renal toxicity) and is less fat-soluble than methoxyflurane so that recovery is faster. The main drawback to enflurane, which otherwise has many favourable characteristics, is that it can cause seizures, either during induction or following recovery from anaesthesia. In this connection it is interesting that a related substance, the fluorine-substituted diethyl-ether, hexafluoroether, is a powerful convulsant agent, though the mechanism is not understood. Enflurane, in common with other halogenated anaesthetics, can induce malignant hyperthermia.

ISOFLURANE

Isoflurane, which is now the most widely used volatile anaesthetic, is similar to enflurane in many respects. It is not appreciably metabolised, and shows little sign of toxicity; it also lacks the proconvulsive property of enflurane. It is an expensive drug, because of the difficulty in separating isomers formed during synthesis. It tends to cause hypotension, and is a powerful coronary vasodilator. Paradoxically, this can exacerbate cardiac ischaemia in patients with coronary disease, because of the 'steal' phenomenon (see Ch. 14).

Desflurane, introduced recently, is chemically similar to isoflurane, but its lower solubility in blood and fat means that induction and recovery are faster, so it is gaining in use as an anaesthetic for day-case surgery. It is not appreciably metabolised. Its potency is lower than that of the drugs described above, the MAC being about 6%. At the concentrations used for induction (about 10%) desflurane causes some respiratory tract irritation, which can lead to coughing and bronchospasm.

Sevoflurane, another recent introduction, resembles desflurane, but is more potent and therefore less likely to cause respiratory irritation. It is partially (about 3%) metabolised, and detectable levels of fluoride are produced, though this does not appear to be sufficient to cause toxicity.

Individual inhalation anaesthetics

- The main agents in current use in developed western countries are halothane, nitrous oxide, isoflurane and enflurane. Ether is still used in some countries.
- **Halothane:**
  — widely used agent
  — potent, non-explosive and non-irritant hypotensive; may cause dysrhythmias; about 30% metabolised
  — hangover likely, due to high lipid solubility
  — risk of liver damage if used repeatedly.
- **Nitrous oxide:**
  — low potency, therefore must be combined with other agents
  — rapid induction and recovery
  — good analgesic properties
  — risk of bone marrow depression due to inhibition of methionine synthase with prolonged administration.
- **Enflurane:**
  — halogenated anaesthetic similar to halothane
  — less metabolism than halothane, therefore less risk of toxicity
  — faster induction and recovery than halothane (less accumulation in fat)
  — some risk of epilepsy-like seizures.
- **Isoflurane:**
  — similar to enflurane, but lacks epileptogenic property
  — may precipitate myocardial ischaemia in patients with coronary disease.
  Desflurane and sevoflurane are similar, with faster onset and recovery, advantageous for day-case surgery.
- **Ether:**
  — obsolete except where modern facilities are not available
  — easy to administer and control
  — slow onset and recovery, with postoperative nausea and vomiting
  — analgesic and muscle relaxant properties
  — highly explosive
  — irritant to respiratory tract
  — long and hazardous stage II if used on its own.

Many inhalation anaesthetics have been introduced and gradually superseded, mainly because of their inflammable nature or because of toxicity. They include **chloroform** (hepatotoxicity and cardiac dysrhythmias), **diethyl ether** (explosive and highly irritant to the respiratory tract, leading to postoperative complications), **vinyl ether** (explosive), **cyclopropane** (explosive, strongly depressant to respiration, and hypotensive), **trichloroethylene** (chemically unstable, no special advantages), **methoxyflurane** (slow recovery and renal toxicity).

Further information is available in many excellent textbooks of anaesthesia (e.g. Bowdle et al. 1994, Miller 1994).

INTRAVENOUS ANAESTHETIC AGENTS

Even the fastest-acting inhalation anaesthetics, such as nitrous oxide, take a few minutes to act, and cause a period of excitement before anaesthesia is produced. Intravenous anaesthetics act much more rapidly, producing unconsciousness in about 20 seconds, as soon as the drug reaches the brain from its site of injection. These drugs (e.g. **thiopentone**, **etomidate**, **propofol**; see below) are normally used for *induction of anaesthesia*. They are preferred by patients, since injection generally lacks the menacing quality associated with a face-mask in an apprehensive individual.

Other drugs used as intravenous induction agents include certain benzodiazepines (see Ch. 33), such as **diazepam** and **midazolam** which act rather less rapidly than the drugs listed above. Though intravenous anaesthetics on their own are generally unsatisfactory for producing maintained anaesthesia because their elimination from the body is relatively slow compared to that of inhalation agents, **propofol** can be used in this way, and the duration of action of **ketamine** is sufficient that it can be used for short operations without the need for an inhalation agent.

The combined use of **droperidol**, a dopamine antagonist related to antipsychotic drugs (Ch. 34) and an opiate analgesic, such as **fentanyl** (Ch. 37) can be used to produce a state of deep sedation and analgesia (known as *neuroleptanalgesia*) in which the patient remains responsive to simple commands and questions, but does not respond to painful stimuli or retain any memory of the procedure. This is used for minor surgical procedures, such as endoscopy.

The properties of the main intravenous anaesthetics are summarised in Table 32.2. Agents now withdrawn because of a high incidence of acute allergic reactions,

Table 32.2 Properties of intravenous anaesthetic agents

Drug	Speed of induction and recovery	Main unwanted effects	Notes
Thiopentone	Fast (cumulation occurs, giving slow recovery)	Cardiovascular and respiratory depression. Hangover	Widely used as induction agent for routine purposes
Etomidate	Fast onset. Fairly fast recovery	Excitatory effects during induction and recovery Adrenocortical suppression	Less cardiovascular and respiratory depression than with thiopentone Causes pain at injection site
Propofol	Fast onset. Very fast recovery	Cardiovascular and respiratory depression	Rapidly metabolised. Possible to use as continuous infusion. Causes pain at injection site
Ketamine	Slow onset. After-effects common during recovery	Psychotomimetic effects following recovery Postoperative nausea, vomiting and salivation	Produces good analgesia and amnesia
Midazolam	Slower than other agents		Little respiratory or cardiovascular depression

producing hypotension and bronchoconstriction, include **propanidid** and **althesin**.

THIOPENTONE

Thiopentone belongs to the barbiturate class of central nervous system depressants (Ch. 33), and is the only one of major importance in anaesthesia. It has very high lipid solubility, and this accounts for the speed and transience of its effect when it is injected intravenously (see below). The free acid is insoluble in water, so thiopentone is given as the sodium salt. This solution is strongly alkaline, and is unstable, so the drug must be dissolved immediately before it is used.

Pharmacokinetic aspects

On intravenous injection, thiopentone causes unconsciousness within about 20 seconds, and lasting for 5–10 minutes. The anaesthetic effect closely parallels the concentration of thiopentone in the blood reaching the brain, because its high lipid solubility allows it to cross the blood–brain barrier without noticeable delay.

The blood concentration of thiopentone declines rapidly, by about 80% within 1–2 minutes, following the initial peak after intravenous injection, because the drug is redistributed, first to tissues with a large blood flow (liver, kidneys, brain, etc.) and more slowly to muscle. Uptake into body fat, though favoured by the high lipid solubility of thiopentone, occurs only slowly, because of the low blood flow to this tissue. After several hours, however, most of the thiopentone present in the body will have accumulated in body fat, the rest having been

metabolised. Recovery from the anaesthetic effect occurs within about 5 minutes, governed entirely by redistribution of the drug to well-perfused tissues; very little is metabolised in this time. After the initial rapid decline the blood concentration drops more slowly, over several hours, as the drug is taken up by body fat and metabolised. Consequently, thiopentone produces a long-lasting 'hangover'; furthermore, repeated intravenous doses cause progressively longer periods of anaesthesia, since the plateau in blood concentration becomes progressively more elevated as more drug accumulates in the body. For this reason, thiopentone cannot be used to maintain surgical anaesthesia, but only as an induction agent.

Thiopentone binds to plasma albumin (roughly 70% of the blood content normally being bound). The fraction bound is less in states of malnutrition, liver disease or renal disease, which affect the concentration and drug-binding properties of plasma albumin, and this can appreciably reduce the dose needed for induction of anaesthesia.

Actions and side-effects

The actions of thiopentone on the nervous system are very similar to those of inhalation anaesthetics, though it has no analgesic effect, and can cause profound respiratory depression even in amounts that fail to abolish reflex responses to painful stimuli.

Its long after-effect, associated with a slowly declining plasma concentration, means that drowsiness and some degree of respiratory depression persist for some hours.

Accidental injection of thiopentone around, rather than into, the vein, or into an artery, can cause local tissue necrosis and ulceration or severe arterial spasm which can result in gangrene. Immediate injection of procaine, through the same needle, is the recommended procedure if this accident occurs. The risk is small, now that lower concentrations of thiopentone are used for intravenous injection. Thiopentone, like other barbiturates, can precipitate an attack of porphyria in susceptible individuals (see Ch. 49).

ETOMIDATE

Etomidate has gained favour over thiopentone on account of the larger margin between the anaesthetic dose and the dose needed to produce respiratory and cardiovascular depression. It is also more rapidly metabolised than thiopentone, and thus less likely to cause a prolonged hangover. In other respects, etomidate is very similar to thiopentone, though it appears more likely to cause involuntary movements during induction, and to cause postoperative nausea and vomiting. With prolonged use, etomidate appears to suppress the adrenal cortex, which has been associated with an increase in mortality in severely ill patients. It is therefore only used as an induction agent, and is preferable to thiopentone in patients at risk of circulatory failure.

PROPOFOL

Propofol, introduced in 1983, is also similar in its properties to thiopentone, but has the advantage of being very rapidly metabolised, and therefore giving rapid recovery without any hangover effect. This enables it to be used as a continuous infusion to maintain surgical anaesthesia without the need for any inhalation agent. Propofol lacks the tendency to cause involuntary movement and adrenocortical suppression seen with etomidate. It is particularly useful for the growing practice of day-case surgery.

OTHER INDUCTION AGENTS

Ketamine

Ketamine closely resembles, both chemically and pharmacologically, **phencyclidine**, which is a 'street-drug' with a pronounced effect on sensory perception (see Ch. 38). Both drugs produce a similar anaesthesia-like state, but ketamine produces considerably less euphoria and sensory distortion than phencyclidine and is thus more useful in anaesthesia. Both drugs are believed to act by blocking activation of one type of excitatory amino acid receptor (the NMDA-receptor; see Ch. 30).

Given intravenously, ketamine takes effect more slowly (2–5 minutes) than thiopentone, and produces a different effect, known as 'dissociative anaesthesia' in which there is a marked sensory loss and analgesia, as well as amnesia and paralysis of movement, without actual loss of consciousness. During induction and recovery, involuntary movements and peculiar sensory experiences often occur. Ketamine does not act simply as a depressant, and it produces cardiovascular and respiratory effects quite different from those of most anaesthetics. Blood pressure and heart rate are usually increased, and respiration is unaffected by effective anaesthetic doses. The main drawback of ketamine, in spite of the safety associated with a lack of overall depressant activity, is that hallucinations, and sometimes

---

Intravenous anaesthetic agents

- Most commonly used for induction of anaesthesia, followed by inhalation agent.
- Thiopentone is most commonly used; etomidate and propofol are alternatives, all act within 20–30 s if given intravenously.
- **Thiopentone:**
  — barbiturate with very high lipid solubility
  — rapid action due to rapid transfer across blood–brain barrier; short duration (about 5 min) due to redistribution, mainly to muscle
  — slowly metabolised, and liable to accumulate in body fat; therefore may cause prolonged effect if given repeatedly
  — no analgesic effect
  — narrow margin between anaesthetic dose and dose causing cardiovascular depression
  — risk of severe vasospasm if accidentally injected into artery.
- **Etomidate:**
  — similar to thiopentone, but more quickly metabolised
  — less risk of cardiovascular depression
  — may cause involuntary movements during induction
  — possible risk of adrenocortical suppression.
- **Propofol:**
  — rapidly metabolised
  — very rapid recovery; no cumulative effect
  — useful for day-case surgery
- **Ketamine:**
  — analogue of phencyclidine, with similar properties
  — action differs from other agents; probably related to effect on NMDA-type glutamate receptors
  — onset of effect is relatively slow (2–5 min)
  — produces 'dissociative' anaesthesia, in which patient may remain conscious, though amnesic and insensitive to pain
  — high incidence of dysphoria, hallucinations, etc. during recovery; used mainly for minor procedures in children.

delirium and irrational behaviour, are common during recovery. These after-effects limit the usefulness of ketamine, but are said to be less marked in children;* thus,

ketamine, often in conjunction with a benzodiazepine, is often used for minor procedures in paediatrics.

---

*A cautionary note: Many adverse effects are claimed to be less marked in children, perhaps because they cannot verbalise their experiences. Until recently muscle relaxants alone were used without anaesthesia during cardiac surgery in neonates. The babies did not complain of pain, but their circulating catecholamine levels were astronomical.

Midazolam

Midazolam is appreciably slower in the onset and offset of its action than the drugs discussed above, but lacks the tendency to cause respiratory and cardiovascular depression, which can be an advantage in some patients.

REFERENCES AND FURTHER READING

Angel A 1993 Central neuronal pathways and the process of anaesthesia. Br J Anaesth 71: 148–163 (*Review of effects of anaesthetics at the neurophysiological level*)

Bowdle T A, Horita A, Kharasch E D 1994 The pharmacologic basis of anesthesiology. Churchill Livingstone, New York (*Comprehensive textbook*)

Franks N P, Lieb W R 1994 Molecular and cellular mechanisms of general anaesthesia. Nature 367: 607–614 (*Good discussion of the opposing 'lipid' and 'protein' theories by pioneers from the protein camp*)

Halsey M J 1989 Physicochemical properties of inhalation anaesthetics. In: Nunn J F, Utting J E, Brown B R (eds) General anaesthesia. Butterworth, London (*Good summary of evidence supporting lipid theories of anaesthesia*)

Harris R A, Mihic S J, Dildy-Mayfield J E, Machu T K 1995 Actions of anesthetics on ligand-gated ion channels: role of receptor subunit composition. FASEB J 9: 1454–1462 (*Review of evidence in favour of ligand-gated ion channels as site of action of anaesthetics*)

Little H J 1996 How has molecular pharmacology contributed to our understanding of the molecular mechanism(s) of general anaesthesia? Pharmacol Ther 69: 37–58 (*Balanced account of the strengths and shortcomings of current theories*)

Mihic S J, Ye Q, Wick M J et al. 1997 Sites of volatile anaesthetic action on $GABA_A$ and glycine receptors. Nature 389: 385–389 (*Use of site-directed mutagenesis to identify channel domains involved in binding of anaesthetic to enhance channel opening*)

Miller R D (ed) 1994 Anaesthesia. Churchill Livingstone, New York (*Comprehensive textbook*)

Pocock G, Richards C D 1993 Excitatory and inhibitory synaptic mechanisms in anaesthesia. Br J Anaesth 71: 134–147 (*Summary of evidence showing that anaesthetics can enhance as well as inhibit synaptic function*)

33

Anxiolytic and hypnotic drugs

In this chapter we discuss **anxiolytic drugs** (used to treat the symptoms of anxiety) and **hypnotic drugs** (used to treat insomnia). Though the clinical objectives are different, the same drugs are often used for both purposes. This is a reflection of the fact that drugs that relieve anxiety generally cause a degree of sedation and drowsiness, which is one of the main drawbacks in the clinical use of anxiolytic drugs. In high doses, all of these drugs cause unconsciousness, and eventually death from respiratory and cardiovascular depression. Benzodiazepines form the most important group, though anxiolytic and hypnotic drugs from an earlier era are still in use. In recent years, a number of drugs acting on 5-HT receptors in the brain, which do not have strong sedative activity, have been introduced as anxiolytic agents. Possible new approaches, based on neuropeptide mediators, are also discussed briefly.

THE NATURE OF ANXIETY AND MEASUREMENT OF ANXIOLYTIC ACTIVITY

The distinction between a 'pathological' and a 'normal' state of anxiety is hard to draw, but in spite of (or perhaps because of) this uncertainty, anxiolytic drugs are among the most frequently prescribed substances, used regularly by upwards of 10% of the population in most developed countries.

The chief manifestations of anxiety are:

- *expressed complaint*—presentation with anxiety as a symptom
- *somatic and autonomic effects*—restlessness and agitation, tachycardia, sweating, weeping, gastrointestinal disorders, sleep disturbance, etc.
- *interference with normal productive activities.*

Clinical conditions related to anxiety include *phobic anxiety* and *panic disorder*. In phobic states, anxiety is triggered by specific circumstances, such as open spaces, social interactions or spiders. In panic disorder, attacks of overwhelming fear occur in association with marked somatic symptoms, such as sweating, tachycardia, chest pains, trembling, choking, etc. Such attacks can be induced even in normal individuals by infusion of sodium lactate, and the condition appears to have a genetic component, so an underlying biochemical abnormality is suspected. The distinction between these conditions and generalised anxiety disorders is not a sharp one, and anxiolytic drugs are used to treat all of them.

Anxiety is a subjective human phenomenon and, except for some of the associated somatic and autonomic changes, it has no obvious counterpart in experimental animals. In biological terms, anxiety may be regarded as a particular form of behavioural inhibition that occurs in response to environmental events that are *novel, non-rewarding* (under conditions where reward is expected) or *punishing*. In animals this behavioural inhibition may take the form of immobility, or suppression of a behavioural response such as bar-pressing to obtain food (see below). To develop new anxiolytic drugs it is essential to have animal tests that give a good guide to activity in man, and considerable effort has gone into developing and validating such tests.

ANIMAL MODELS OF ANXIETY

Various types of behavioural test may be used to measure anxiolytic activity. For example, a rat placed in an unfamiliar environment normally responds by remaining immobile, though alert ('behavioural suppression') for a time, which may represent 'anxiety' produced by the strange environment. This immobility is reduced if anxiolytic drugs are administered. The 'elevated cross' is a widely used test model. Two arms of the cross are closed in, and the others are open. Normally rats spend most of their time in the closed arms and avoid the open arms (afraid, possibly, of falling off). Administration of anxiolytic drugs increases the time spent in the open arms, and also increases the mobility of the rats as judged by the frequency of crossing the transection.

Conflict tests can also be used. For example, a rat trained to press a bar repeatedly to obtain a food pellet normally achieves a high and consistent response rate. A conflict element is then introduced: at intervals, indicated by an auditory signal, bar pressing results in an occasional 'punishment' in the form of an electric shock in addition to the reward of a food pellet. Normally, the rat ceases pressing the bar (behavioural inhibition), and thus avoids the shock, during the period when the signal is sounding. The effect of an anxiolytic drug is to relieve this suppressive effect, so that the rats continue bar-pressing for reward in spite of the 'punishment'. Other types of psychotropic drug are not effective, nor are analgesic drugs. Other evidence confirms that anxiolytic drugs affect the level of behavioural inhibition produced by the 'conflict situation', rather than simply raising the pain threshold.

In other tests, aggressive behaviour is produced experimentally by lesions of the midbrain septum, or by housing mice in individual cages and then introducing a stranger. Anxiolytic drugs reduce the amount of aggressive behaviour displayed, in a quantifiable way. They also increase the amount of 'social' interaction occurring between pairs of rats placed in an unfamiliar environment, this being a situation in which social interaction is greatly decreased in control animals. In many of these tests, the response is an increase in behavioural activity, so it is clear that the anxiolytic drugs are producing something more than a non-specific sedation.

TESTS ON HUMANS

Various 'anxiety scale' tests have been devised, based on standard patient questionnaires. These have confirmed the efficacy of many anxiolytic drugs, but placebo treatment often also produces highly significant responses.

Other tests rely on measurement of the somatic and autonomic effects associated with anxiety. An example is the *galvanic skin response* (GSR) in which the electrical conductivity of the skin is used as a measure of sweat production. Any novel stimulus, whether pleasant or unpleasant, causes a response. This forms the basis of the lie-detector test. If an innocuous stimulus is repeated at intervals, the magnitude of the response decreases (habituation). The rate of habituation is less in anxious patients than in normal subjects, and is increased by anxiolytic drugs.

A human version of the conflict test described above involves the substitution of money for food pellets, and the use of graded electric shocks as punishment. As with rats, administration of diazepam increases the rate of button-pressing for money during the periods when the punishment was in operation, though the subjects reported no change in the painfulness of the electric shock. Subtler forms of torment and reward are not hard to imagine.

Measurement of anxiolytic activity

- Behavioural tests in animals are based on measurements of the behavioural inhibition (considered to reflect 'anxiety') in response to conflict or novelty.
- Human tests for anxiolytic drugs employ psychiatric rating scales or measures of autonomic responses, such as the galvanic skin response.
- Tests such as these can distinguish between anxiolytic drugs (benzodiazepines, 5-HT agonists, etc.) and other types of psychotropic drug.

CLASSIFICATION OF ANXIOLYTIC AND HYPNOTIC DRUGS

The main groups of drugs are:

- *Benzodiazepines.* This is the most important group, used as anxiolytic and hypnotic agents.
- *5-HT$_{1A}$-receptor agonists* (e.g. **buspirone**). These agents, recently introduced, are anxiolytic but not appreciably sedative.
- *Barbiturates.* These are now largely obsolete, superseded by benzodiazepines. Their use is now confined to anaesthesia (Ch. 32) and the treatment of epilepsy (Ch. 36).
- *β-adrenoceptor antagonists* (e.g. **propranolol**; Ch. 8). These are used to treat some forms of anxiety, particularly where physical symptoms, such as sweating,

tremor and tachycardia, are troublesome. Their effectiveness depends on block of peripheral sympathetic responses rather than on any central effects. They are sometimes used by actors and musicians to reduce the symptoms of stage fright, but their use by snooker players to minimise tremor is banned as unsportsmanlike.

- *Miscellaneous other drugs* (e.g. **chloral hydrate**, **meprobamate** and **paraldehyde**). They are no longer recommended, but therapeutic habits die hard, and chloral hydrate and paraldehyde are still used, mainly in hospitals. Sedative antihistamines (see Ch. 13), such as **diphenhydramine**, are sometimes used as sleeping pills, particularly for wakeful children.

Classes of anxiolytic and hypnotic drugs

- Benzodiazepines: the most important class, used for treating both anxiety states and insomnia.
- 5-HT$_{1A}$-receptor agonists: recently introduced, showing anxiolytic activity with little sedation.
- Barbiturates: now largely obsolete as anxiolytic/sedative agents, though still occasionally prescribed.
- β-adrenoceptor antagonists: used mainly to reduce physical symptoms of anxiety (tremor, palpitations, etc.); no effect on affective component.
- Miscellaneous other agents are still used occasionally to treat insomnia (benzodiazepines are preferable in most cases).

BENZODIAZEPINES

The first benzodiazepine, **chlordiazepoxide**, was synthesised by accident in 1961, the unusual 7-membered ring having been produced as a result of an unplanned reaction in the laboratories of Hoffman la Roche. Its unexpected pharmacological activity was recognised in a routine screening procedure, and benzodiazepines quite soon became the most widely prescribed drugs in the pharmacopoeia.

CHEMISTRY AND STRUCTURE–ACTIVITY RELATIONSHIPS

The basic chemical structure of benzodiazepines consists of an unusual 7-membered ring fused to an aromatic ring, with four main substitutent groups which can be modified without loss of activity. Thousands of compounds have been made and tested, and about 20 are available for clinical use, the most important ones being listed in Table 33.1. They are basically similar in their pharmacological

actions, though some degree of selectivity has been reported. For example, some, such as **clonazepam** show anticonvulsant activity with less marked sedative effects. It is possible that selectivity with respect to two types of benzodiazepine receptor (see below) may account for these differences, but this remains conjectural. From a clinical point of view, differences in pharmacokinetic behaviour among different benzodiazepines (see below) are more important than differences in profile of activity. Drugs with a similar structure have been discovered which specifically antagonise the effects of the benzodiazepines, e.g. **flumazenil** (see below).

PHARMACOLOGICAL EFFECTS

The most important effects of the benzodiazepines are on the central nervous system and consist of:

- reduction of anxiety and aggression
- sedation and induction of sleep
- reduction of muscle tone and coordination
- anticonvulsant effect.

Reduction of anxiety and aggression

The measurement of anxiolytic effects in animals and man has been discussed above. Benzodiazepines show activity in this type of assay, and also exert a marked 'taming' effect, allowing animals to be handled more easily.* If given to the dominant member of a pair of animals (e.g. mice or monkeys) housed in the same cage, benzodiazepines reduce the number of attacks by the dominant individual and increase the number of attacks made upon him. With the possible exception of **alprazolam** (Table 33.1), benzodiazepines do not have antidepressant effects. Benzodiazepines may paradoxically produce an increase in irritability and aggression in some individuals. This appears to be particularly pronounced with the ultra-short-acting drug **triazolam** (and led to its withdrawal in the UK and some other countries), and is generally more common with short-acting compounds. It is probably a manifestation of the benzodiazepine withdrawal syndrome, which occurs with all of these drugs (see below), but is more acute with drugs whose action wears off rapidly.

The use of benzodiazepines as anxiolytic agents is reviewed by Shader & Greenblatt (1993).

---

*This depends on the species. Cats actually become more excitable, as a colleague of one of the authors discovered to his cost when attempting to sedate a tiger in the Baltimore zoo.

Sedation and induction of sleep

Benzodiazepines decrease the time taken to get to sleep, and increase the total duration of sleep, though the latter effect occurs only in subjects who normally sleep for less than about 6 hours each night. Both effects tend to decline when benzodiazepines are taken regularly for 1–2 weeks.

On the basis of EEG measurements, several levels of sleep can be recognised. Of particular psychological importance are 'rapid eye movement' (REM) sleep, which is associated with dreaming, and 'slow wave' (SW) sleep, which corresponds to the deepest level of sleep when the metabolic rate and adrenal steroid secretion are at their lowest and the secretion of growth hormone is at its highest (see Ch. 24). All hypnotic drugs reduce the proportion of REM sleep, though benzodiazepines affect it less than other hypnotics. Artificial interruption of REM sleep causes irritability and anxiety, even if the total amount of sleep is not reduced, and the lost REM sleep is made up for at the end of such an experiment by a rebound increase. The same rebound in REM sleep is seen at the end of a period of administration of benzodiazepines or other hypnotics. It is therefore assumed that REM sleep has a function, and that the relatively slight reduction of REM sleep by benzodiazepines is a point in their favour.

The proportion of SW sleep is significantly reduced by benzodiazepines, though growth hormone secretion is unaffected.

Figure 33.1 shows the improvement of subjective ratings of sleep quality produced by a benzodiazepine, and the rebound decrease at the end of a 32-week period of drug treatment. It is notable that, though tolerance to objective effects such as reduced sleep latency occurs within a few days, this is not obvious in the subjective ratings.

In general, the sedative effects of benzodiazepines appear to go hand in hand with their anxiolytic effects, so it has not yet been possible to develop a non-sedative anxiolytic agent.

Reduction of muscle tone and coordination

Benzodiazepines reduce muscle tone by a central action that is independent of their sedative effect. Cats are particularly sensitive to this action, and some benzodiazepines (e.g. **clonazepam**, **flunitrazepam**) reduce decerebrate rigidity in doses that are much smaller than those needed to produce behavioural effects. In other species, the effect is less clear. Coordination can be tested by measuring the length of time for which mice can stay on a slowly rotating horizontal plastic rod, or the time taken for them

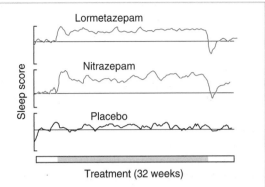

Fig. 33.1 Effects of long-term benzodiazepine treatment on sleep quality. 100 poor sleepers were given, under double-blind conditions, lormetazepam 5 mg, nitrazepam 2 mg, or placebo nightly for 24 weeks, the test period being preceded and followed by 4 weeks of placebo treatment. They were asked to assess, on a subjective rating scale, the quality of sleep during each night, and the results are expressed as a 5-day rolling average of these scores. The improvement in sleep quality was maintained during the 24-week test period, and was followed by a 'rebound' worsening of sleep when the test period ended. (From: Oswald I et al. 1982 Br Med J 284: 860–864)

to escape from confinement by climbing up the inside of a tubular chimney. Performance in these acrobatic tricks is impaired by benzodiazepines and other sedatives, but it is not clear that particular drugs show selectivity in this respect in species other than the cat. Studies in humans have failed to show differences between benzodiazepines.

Increased muscle tone is a common feature of anxiety states in humans, and may contribute to the aches and pains, including headache, which often trouble anxious patients. The relaxant effect of benzodiazepines may therefore be clinically useful. A reduction of muscle tone appears to be possible without appreciable loss of coordination.

Anticonvulsant effects

All of the benzodiazepines have anticonvulsant activity in experimental animal tests. They are highly effective against chemically induced convulsions caused by leptazol, bicuculline and similar drugs (see Chs 36 and 38) but less so against electrically induced convulsions. Benzodiazepines do not affect strychnine-induced convulsions in experimental animals. Both bicuculline and strychnine are believed to act by blocking the action of inhibitory transmitters in the central nervous system; strychnine exerts its effect on glycine receptors (see Ch. 38), whereas bicuculline and several other chemical convulsant agents act on $GABA_A$-receptors (Ch. 29). Since benzodiazepines enhance the action of GABA but not glycine, the selectivity of their anticonvulsant action is explicable. **Clonazepam** (see above), because of its selective anticonvulsant action, is used to treat epilepsy (Ch. 36), as is **diazepam**, which is given intravenously to control life-threatening seizures in *status epilepticus*.

MECHANISM OF ACTION

Benzodiazepines (once thought, in the absence of evidence to the contrary, to be acting as 'non-specific depressants') act very selectively on GABA$_A$-receptors (Ch. 29), which mediate the fast inhibitory synaptic response produced by activity in GABA-ergic neurons. The effect of benzodiazepines is to enhance the response to GABA, by facilitating the opening of GABA-activated chloride channels (Fig. 33.2). As described in Chapter 29, benzodiazepines bind specifically to a regulatory site on the receptor, distinct from the GABA binding site, and act allosterically to increase the affinity of GABA for the receptor, which can be measured in binding studies. Single channel recordings show an increase in the frequency of channel opening by a given concentration of GABA, but no change in the conductance or mean open time, consistent with an effect on GABA binding rather than the channel-gating mechanism. Benzodiazepines do not affect receptors for other amino acids, such as glycine or glutamate (Fig. 33.2). For unknown reasons, the enhancement of neuronal response to applied GABA, shown in Figure 33.2, appears to be more pronounced than the enhancement of actual synaptic responses; furthermore, the GABA-enhancing effect of benzodiazepines reaches a maximum at low concentrations, and is reduced when the concentration is increased, so it is possible that other mechanisms may contribute to their overall effects.

The GABA$_A$-receptor is a ligand-gated ion channel (see Ch. 2) consisting of a pentameric assembly of subunits. Studies on expressed receptors show that GABA binding requires the presence of α and β subunits, whereas benzodiazepine binding requires α and γ subunits. Each of the subunits exists in different isoforms which are expressed in different brain regions. Of the three isoforms of the γ-subunit, only two confer benzodiazepine sensitivity on the receptor complex. It is known that GABA$_A$-mediated synaptic transmission is potentiated by benzodiazepines in some parts of the brain, but not in others (or in peripheral neurons that express GABA$_A$-receptors), and these differences may reflect the different patterns of γ-subunit expression.*

The distribution of diazepam binding sites in the brain is highest in the cerebral cortex, less in the limbic system and midbrain, and still less in the brainstem and spinal cord. It roughly, but not exactly, agrees with counts of GABA$_A$ receptors, though the number of benzodiazepine sites is consistently less.**

The emergence of multiple molecular subtypes of the GABA and benzodiazepine receptors is an example of a (by now) familiar pharmacological scenario. The

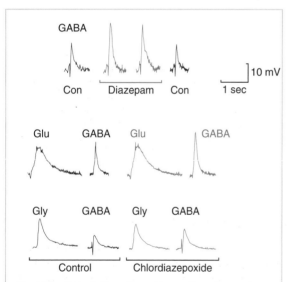

Fig. 33.2 Potentiating effect of benzodiazepines and pentobarbitone on the action of GABA in mouse spinal cord neurons grown in tissue culture. Drugs were applied by ionophoresis to mouse spinal cord neurons grown in tissue culture, from micropipettes placed close to the cells. The membrane was hyperpolarised to –90 mv, and the cells were loaded with chloride ions from the recording microelectrode, so inhibitory amino acids (GABA and glycine), as well as excitatory ones (glutamate), caused depolarising responses. The potentiating effect of diazepam is restricted to GABA responses, glutamate and glycine responses being unaffected.

---

*There is some pharmacological evidence for two different classes of benzodiazepine receptor in the brain, BZD$_1$ and BZD$_2$. This is based mainly on the activity of a different class of compounds typified by **zolpidem** (see below) which is tentatively classified as BZD$_1$-selective, and exerts sedative and anxiolytic effects but lacks anticonvulsant and muscle-relaxant properties. Recent studies suggest that the BZD$_1$/BZD$_2$ receptors represent assemblies of different α and γ subunits.

**Peripheral benzodiazepine binding sites, not associated with GABA receptors, are known to exist in many tissues, but their function and pharmacological significance are unknown.

pharmacological complexities are beginning to be explained in terms of this molecular diversity, but much still remains unclear. Being lost in a labyrinth is surely an advance on being lost in a featureless fog.

Is there an endogenous benzodiazepine-like mediator?

Whether there is an endogenous ligand for the benzodiazepine receptors, whose function is to regulate the action of GABA, is still uncertain. The main candidate is a 10 kDa peptide, diazepam-binding inhibitor (DBI) isolated from rat brain. This peptide binds strongly to the benzodiazepine binding site of the $GABA_A$ receptor, and has the opposite effect to benzodiazepines; i.e. it inhibits chloride channel opening by GABA, and when injected into the brain, has an anxiogenic and pro-convulsant effect. Other possible endogenous modulators of $GABA_A$-receptors include steroid metabolites (see Ch. 29). There is also evidence that benzodiazepines themselves may occur naturally in the brain. At present there is no general agreement on the identity and function of an endogenous ligand.

Benzodiazepine inverse agonists and antagonists

The term 'inverse agonist' (Ch. 1) is applied to drugs which bind to benzodiazepine receptors and exert the opposite effect to that of conventional benzodiazepines, producing signs of increased anxiety and convulsions. DBI is an example, and some benzodiazepine analogues act similarly. It is possible (see Fig. 33.3) to explain these complexities in terms of the two-state model discussed in Chapter 1, by postulating that the benzodiazepine receptor exists in two distinct conformations, only one of which (A) can bind a GABA molecule and open the chloride channel. The other conformation (B) cannot bind GABA. Normally, with no benzodiazepine receptor ligand present, there is an equilibrium between these two conformations; sensitivity to GABA is present, but submaximal. Benzodiazepine agonists (e.g. diazepam) are postulated to bind preferentially to conformation A, thus shifting the equilibrium in favour of A and enhancing GABA sensitivity. Inverse agonists bind selectively to B, and have the opposite effect. Competitive antagonists, such as **flumazenil** (see below), bind equally to A and B, and consequently do not disturb the conformational equilibrium but antagonise the effect of both agonists and inverse agonists. Some of the molecular variants of the $GABA_A$-receptor (see above) seem to show different relative affinities for agonists, antagonists and inverse agonists, and it is possible that this reflects differences in the equilibrium between the A and B states as a function of the subunit composition of the receptor.

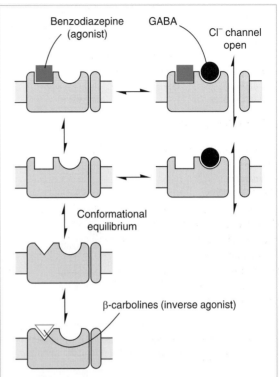

Fig. 33.3 Model of benzodiazepine/GABA receptor interaction. Benzodiazepine agonists (e.g. diazepam) and antagonists (e.g. flumazenil) are believed to bind to a site on the GABA receptor distinct from the GABA binding site. A conformational equilibrium exists between states in which the benzodiazepine receptor exists in its agonist-binding conformation (above) and in its antagonist-binding conformation (below). In the latter state, the GABA receptor has a much reduced affinity for GABA, so that the chloride channel remains closed.

PHARMACOKINETIC ASPECTS

Benzodiazepines are well absorbed when given orally, usually giving a peak plasma concentration in about 1 hour. Some (e.g. oxazepam, lorazepam) are absorbed more slowly. They bind strongly to plasma protein, and their high lipid solubility causes many of them to accumulate gradually in body fat. These two factors result in distribution volumes not far from 1 l/kg body weight for most benzodiazepines. They are normally given by mouth, but can be given intravenously (e.g. diazepam in status epilepticus, midazolam in anaesthesia). Intramuscular injection often results in slow absorption.

Benzodiazepines are all metabolised, and eventually excreted as glucuronide conjugates in the urine. They vary greatly in duration of action, and can be roughly

Table 33.1 Characteristics of benzodiazepines in man

Drug	Half-life of parent compound (h)	Active metabolite	Half-life of metabolite (h)	Overall duration of action	Main uses
Triazolam* Midazolam	2–4	Hydroxylated derivative	2	Ultra-short (< 6 h)	Hypnotic* Midazolam used as intravenous anaesthetic
Zolpidem†	2	No		Ultra-short (~ 4 h)	Hypnotic
Lorazepam, oxazepam, temazepam, lormetazepam	8–12	No		Short (12–18 h)	Anxiolytic, hypnotic
Alprazolam	6–12	Hydroxylated derivative	6	Medium (24 h)	Anxiolytic, antidepressant
Nitrazepam	16–40	No		Medium	Hypnotic, anxiolytic
Diazepam, chlordiazepoxide	20–40	Nordazepam	60	Long (24–48 h)	Anxiolytic, muscle relaxant Diazepam used i.v. as anticonvulsant
Flurazepam	1	Desmethyl-flurazepam	60	Long	Anxiolytic
Chlonazepam	50	No		Long	Anticonvulsant, anxiolytic (especially mania)

*Triazolam has been withdrawn from use in UK on account of side-effects.
†Zolpidem is not a benzodiazepine, but acts at the same site.

divided into short-, medium- and long-acting compounds (Table 33. 1). Several are converted to active metabolites, such as N-desmethyldiazepam (**nordazepam**) which has a half-life of about 60 hours, and which accounts for the tendency of many benzodiazepines to produce cumulative effects and long hangovers when they are given at regular intervals. The short-acting compounds are those that are metabolised directly by conjugation with glucuronide. The main pathways are shown in Figure 33.4. Figure 33.5 shows the gradual build-up and slow disappearance of nordazepam from the plasma of a human subject given diazepam daily for 15 days.

Advancing age affects the rate of oxidative reactions more than that of conjugation reactions. Thus the effect of the long-acting benzodiazepines, which may be used regularly as hypnotics or anxiolytic agents for many years, tends to increase with age, and it is common for drowsiness and confusion to develop insidiously for this reason.*

*At the age of 91, the grandmother of one of the authors was growing increasingly forgetful and mildly dotty, having been taking nitrazepam for insomnia regularly for years. To the author's lasting shame, it took a canny general practitioner to diagnose the problem. Cancellation of the nitrazepam prescription produced a dramatic improvement.

UNWANTED EFFECTS

These may be divided into:

- toxic effects resulting from acute overdosage
- unwanted effects occurring during normal therapeutic use
- tolerance and dependence.

Acute toxicity

Benzodiazepines in acute overdose are considerably less dangerous than other anxiolytic/hypnotic drugs. Since such agents are often used in attempted suicide, this is an important advantage. In overdose, benzodiazepines cause prolonged sleep, without serious depression of respiration or cardiovascular function. However, in the presence of other CNS depressants, particularly alcohol, benzodiazepines can cause severe, even life-threatening, respiratory depression. The availability of an effective antagonist, **flumazenil**, means that the effects of an acute overdose can be counteracted,** which is not possible for most CNS depressants.

**In practice, patients are usually left to sleep it off, since there is a risk of seizures with flumazenil; however, flumazenil may be useful diagnostically to rule out coma of other causes.

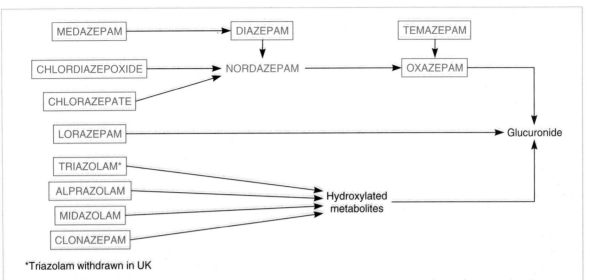

*Triazolam withdrawn in UK

Fig. 33.4 The metabolism of benzodiazepines. The N-demethylated metabolite, nordazepam, is formed from a number of benzodiazepines, and is important because it is biologically active and has a very long half-life. Compounds with pharmacological activity are shown in blue. Drugs available for clinical use are shown in boxes.

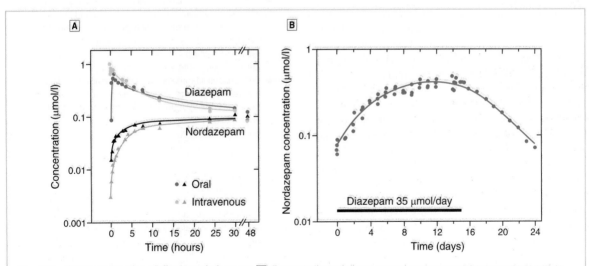

Fig. 33.5 Pharmacokinetics of diazepam in humans. Ⓐ Concentrations of diazepam and nordazepam following a single oral or intravenous dose. Note the very slow disappearance of both substances after the first 20 hours. Ⓑ Accumulation of nordazepam during 2 weeks' daily administration of diazepam, and slow decline (half-life about 3 days) after cessation of diazepam administration. (Data from; Kaplan S A et al. 1973 J Pharmacol Sci 62: 1789)

Side-effects during therapeutic use

The main side-effects of benzodiazepines are drowsiness, confusion, amnesia and impaired coordination, which considerably affects manual skills such as driving performance. An interaction with alcohol is often claimed, whereby a low plasma concentration of a benzodiazepine can enhance the depressant effect of alcohol in a more than additive way. The long and unpredictable duration of action of many benzodiazepines is important in relation to side-effects. Long-acting drugs such as nitrazepam are no longer used as hypnotics, and even shorter-acting compounds such as lorazepam can produce a substantial day-after impairment of job performance and driving skill.

Tolerance and dependence

Tolerance (i.e. a gradual escalation of dose needed to produce the required effect) occurs with all benzodiazepines, as does dependence, which is their main drawback. They share these properties with other hypnotics and sedatives. Tolerance is less marked than it is with barbiturates, which produce pharmacokinetic tolerance because of induction of hepatic drug-metabolising enzymes—this does not occur with benzodiazepines. Such tolerance as does occur appears to represent a change at the receptor level, but the mechanism is not well understood.

The sleep-inducing effect shows relatively little tolerance (Fig. 33.1). In a study with intravenous diazepam in normal subjects, its euphoric effect was not present in those taking oral diazepam daily. It is not clear whether tolerance to the anxiolytic effect is significant.

In spite of early claims that benzodiazepines cannot produce dependence, this is a major problem. In human subjects and patients, stopping benzodiazepine treatment after weeks or months causes an increase in symptoms of anxiety, together with tremor and dizziness. Though animals show only a weak tendency to self-administration of benzodiazepines, withdrawal after chronic administration causes physical symptoms similar to those that follow opiate withdrawal (see Ch. 39), namely nervousness, tremor, loss of appetite and sometimes convulsions, The withdrawal syndrome, in both animals and humans, is slower in onset and less intense than with barbiturates, probably because of the long plasma half-life of most benzodiazepines. Short-acting benzodiazepines cause more abrupt withdrawal effects. With triazolam, a very short-acting drug and no longer in use, the withdrawal effect occurred within a few hours, even after a single dose, producing early-morning insomnia and daytime anxiety when the drug was used as a hypnotic.

The physical withdrawal symptoms make it difficult for patients to give up taking benzodiazepines, but severe psychological dependence, such as readily occurs with many drugs of abuse (Ch. 39) is not a major problem.

BENZODIAZEPINE ANTAGONISTS

Competitive antagonists of benzodiazepines were first discovered in 1981. The best-known compound is **flumazenil**. This compound was originally reported to lack effects on behaviour or on drug-induced convulsions when given on its own, though it was later found to possess some 'anxiogenic' and pro-convulsant activity. Flumazenil is used (see Broaden & Goa 1988), mainly to reverse the sedative action of benzodiazepines used during anaesthesia, and also in the treatment of acute benzodiazepine overdose. Flumazenil acts quickly and effectively when given by injection, but its action lasts for only about 2 hours, so drowsiness tends to return. It is often used in treating comatose patients suspected of having overdosed with benzodiazepines even before the diagnosis is confirmed on the basis of a blood sample. Convulsions may rarely occur in patients treated with flumazenil, and this is more common in patients receiving tricyclic antidepressants (Ch. 35). Reports that

---

Benzodiazepines

- Act by binding to a specific regulatory site on the $GABA_A$-receptor, thus enhancing the inhibitory effect of GABA. Subtypes of the $GABA_A$-receptor exist in different regions of the brain, and differ in their sensitivity to benzodiazepines.
- Anxiolytic benzodiazepines are *agonists* at this regulatory site. Other benzodiazepines (e.g. flumazenil) are *antagonists*, and prevent the actions of the anxiolytic benzodiazepines. A further class of *inverse agonists* is recognised, which reduce the effectiveness of GABA and are anxiogenic; they are not used clinically.
- Endogenous ligands for the benzodiazepine binding site are believed to exist. They include peptide and steroid molecules, but their physiological function is not yet understood.
- Benzodiazepines cause:
  —reduction of anxiety and aggression
  —sedation, leading to improvement of insomnia
  —muscle relaxation and loss of motor coordination
  —suppression of convulsions (antiepileptic effect).
- Differences in the pharmacological profile of different benzodiazepines are minor; clonazepam appears to have more anticonvulsant action in relation to its other effects.
- Benzodiazepines are active orally, and differ mainly in respect of their duration of action. Short-acting agents (e.g. lorazepam and temazepam $t_{1/2}$ 8–12 h) are metabolised to inactive compounds, and are used mainly as sleeping pills. Some long-acting agents (e.g. diazepam and chlordiazepoxide) are converted to a long-lasting active metabolite (nordazepam).
- Some are used intravenously, e.g. diazepam in status epilepticus; midazolam in anaesthesia.
- Zolpidem is a short-acting drug which is not a benzodiazepine, but acts similarly.
- Benzodiazepines are relatively safe in overdose. Their main disadvantages are interaction with alcohol, long-lasting hangover effects and the development of dependence

flumazenil improves the mental state of patients with severe liver disease (hepatic encephalopathy) and alcohol intoxication have not been confirmed in controlled trials.

BUSPIRONE

Besides the GABA pathways discussed so far, many other transmitters and modulators have been implicated in anxiety and panic disorders, particularly 5-HT (see Blackburn 1992), noradrenaline (Charney et al. 1995) and neuropeptides, such as CCK (see below).

The importance of 5-HT is reflected in the clinical use of **buspirone**, a potent agonist at 5-HT_{1A}-receptors (Ch. 9) to treat anxiety. Buspirone also binds to dopamine receptors, but it is likely that its 5-HT-related actions are important in relation to anxiety suppression, since related anxiolytic compounds (e.g. **ipsapirone** and **gepirone**; see Traber & Glaser 1987) show high specificity for 5-HT_{1A}-receptors. Exactly how these 5-HT anxiolytic drugs work is still unclear (see Lucki 1992). It is possible that they act on inhibitory presynaptic receptors, thus reducing the release of 5-HT and other mediators. They also inhibit the activity of noradrenergic locus ceruleus neurons (Ch. 30), and thus interfere with arousal reactions. However, buspirone takes days or weeks to produce its effect in man, suggesting a more complex indirect mechanism of action. Buspirone is ineffective in controlling panic attacks.

Buspirone, ipsapirone and gepirone have side-effects quite different from those of benzodiazepines. They do not cause sedation or motor incoordination, nor have withdrawal effects been reported. Their main side-effects are nausea, dizziness, headache and restlessness, which generally seem to be less troublesome than the side-effects of benzodiazepines.

5-HT_{1A} agonists as anxiolytic drugs

- **Buspirone** is a potent (though non-selective) agonist at 5-HT_{1A}-receptors. **Ipsapirone** and **gepirone** are similar.
- Anxiolytic effects take days or weeks to develop.
- Side-effects appear less troublesome than with benzodiazepines; they include dizziness, nausea, headache, but not sedation or loss of coordination.

BARBITURATES

The sleep-inducing properties of barbiturates were discovered early in this century, and hundreds of compounds

were made and tested. Until the 1960s, they formed the largest group of hypnotics and sedatives in clinical use. Barbiturates all have depressant activity on the central nervous system, producing effects similar to those of inhalation anaesthetics. They cause death from respiratory and cardiovascular depression if given in large doses, which is one of the main reasons that they are now little used as anxiolytic and hypnotic agents. **Pentobarbitone**, and similar typical barbiturates with a duration of action of 6–12 hours are still very occasionally used as sleeping pills and anxiolytic drugs, but they are less safe than benzodiazepines.

Barbiturates which remain in widespread use are those which have specific properties, such as **phenobarbitone**, used for its anticonvulsant activity (see Ch. 36), and **thiopentone**, which is widely used as an intravenous anaesthetic agent (see Ch. 32).

Barbiturates share with benzodiazepines the ability to enhance the action of GABA, but they bind to a different site on the GABA-receptor/chloride channel, and their action seems to be much less specific.

Apart from the risk of dangerous overdose, the main disadvantages of barbiturates are that they induce a high degree of tolerance and dependence, and that they strongly induce the synthesis of hepatic cytochrome P450 and conjugating enzymes and thus increase the rate of metabolic degradation of many other drugs, giving rise to a number of potentially troublesome drug interactions (Ch. 48).

Barbiturates

- Non-selective CNS depressants which produce effects ranging from sedation and reduction of anxiety, to unconsciousness and death from respiratory and cardiovascular failure. Therefore dangerous in overdose.
- Act partly by enhancing action of GABA, but less specific than benzodiazepines.
- Mainly used in anaesthesia and treatment of epilepsy; use as sedative/hypnotic agents is no longer recommended.
- Potent inducers of hepatic drug-metabolising enzymes, especially cytochrome P450 system, so liable to cause drug interactions. Also precipitate attacks of acute porphyria in susceptible individuals.
- Tolerance and dependence occur.

OTHER POTENTIAL ANXIOLYTIC DRUGS

In addition to the 5-HT_{1A} agonists described above, drugs acting on other 5-HT receptors may also be useful as anxiolytic agents (see Blackburn 1992). 5-HT$_3$-receptor antagonists, such as **ondansetron** (Ch. 9) show anxiolytic activity in animal models, but have not proved efficacious in controlled human trials. Both 5-HT uptake inhibitors, such as **fluoxetine**, and mixed 5-HT/noradrenaline uptake inhibitors, which are used mainly as antidepressant drugs (Ch. 35), also show efficacy in anxiety disorders as well as in panic attacks.

Antagonists to the neuropeptide, cholecystokinin (CCK; see Ch. 10) have been tested as anxiolytic drugs. CCK, which is expressed in many areas of the brainstem and midbrain that are involved in arousal, mood and emotion, has been considered as a possible mediator of panic attacks (see Harro et al. 1993). Intravenous injection of a CCK-related tetrapeptide (which is able to cross the blood–brain barrier) induces panic attacks in patients with this condition. Non-peptide CCK antagonists were developed, but proved ineffective in clinical trials.

REFERENCES AND FURTHER READING

*All are review articles on different aspects of anxiety and
anxiolytic drugs.*

Blackburn T P 1992 5-HT receptors and anxiolytic drugs. In:
Marsden C A, Heal D J (eds) Central serotonin receptors and
psychotropic drugs. Blackwell Scientific Publications, Oxford,
pp 175–197
Broaden R N, Goa K L 1988 Flumazenil. A preliminary review of
its benzodiazepine antagonist properties, intrinsic activity and
clinical use. Drugs 35: 448–467
Charney D S, Bremner J D, Redmond D E 1995 Noradrenergic
neural substrates for anxiety and fear. In: Bloom F E, Kupfer
D J (eds) Psychopharmacology: a fourth generation of progress.
Raven Press, New York
Harro J, Vasar E, Bradwejn J 1993 CCK in animal and human
research on anxiety. Trends Pharmacol Sci 14: 244–249
Lucki I 1992 5-HT$_1$ receptors and behaviour. Neurosci Behav Rev
16: 83–93
Shader R I, Greenblatt D J 1993 Use of benzodiazepines in
anxiety disorders. New Engl J Med 328: 1398–1405
Traber J, Glaser T 1987 5-HT$_{1A}$ receptor-related anxiolytics.
Trends Pharmacol Sci 8: 432–437

34

Antipsychotic drugs

Antipsychotic drugs are also known as *neuroleptic drugs*, *anti-schizophrenic drugs*, or *major tranquillisers*. Pharmacologically, they are characterised as dopamine receptor antagonists, though many of them also act on other targets, particularly 5-HT receptors, which may contribute to their clinical efficacy.

The most important types of psychosis are:

- schizophrenia
- affective disorders (e.g. depression, mania)
- organic psychoses (mental disturbances caused by head injury, alcoholism, or other kinds of organic disease).

Antipsychotic drugs are used mainly in the treatment of schizophrenia and other behavioural emergencies, but they are also used for other psychotic illnesses. The principal drugs used to treat affective disorders are discussed in Chapter 35.

THE NATURE OF SCHIZOPHRENIA

Schizophrenia (see Crow 1982) affects about 1% of the population. It is one of the most important forms of psychiatric illness because it often affects people from an early age, is often chronic and usually highly disabling.

There is a strong hereditary factor in its aetiology, and evidence suggestive of a fundamental biological disorder (see below). The main clinical features of the disease are as follows:

Positive symptoms:

- *Delusions* (often paranoid in nature)
- *Hallucinations*, usually in the form of voices, and often exhortatory in their message
- *Thought disorder*, comprising wild trains of thought and irrational conclusions, often associated with the feeling that thoughts are inserted or withdrawn by an outside agency.

Negative symptoms:

- *Withdrawal* from social contacts
- *Flattening of emotional responses.*

Schizophrenia often begins in adolescence or young adult life; it can follow a relapsing and remitting course, or be chronic and progressive, particularly in cases with a later onset. Chronic schizophrenia used to account for most of the patients in long-stay psychiatric hospitals; following the closure of many of these in the UK, it now accounts for many of society's outcasts.

THEORIES OF SCHIZOPHRENIA

The cause of schizophrenia remains unclear, but involves a combination of genetic and environmental factors (see Egan & Weinberger 1997). The disease shows a strong, but incomplete, hereditary tendency. In first degree relatives, the risk is about 10%; even in monozygotic twins, one of whom has schizophrenia, the probability of the other being affected is only about 50%. There is substantial evidence suggesting that schizophrenia is associated with a neurodevelopmental disorder, affecting mainly the cerebral cortex, and occurring in the first few months of prenatal development (see Harrison 1997). Brain imaging in chronic schizophrenia shows cortical atrophy, with enlargement of the cerebral ventricles. This was originally ascribed to progressive neuro-degeneration, but it was later shown to be present in pre-schizophrenic subjects, and not to be progressive. Studies of post-mortem schizophrenic brains show evidence of misplaced cortical neurons with abnormal morphology, suggestive of defective cell migration during early development. Additional evidence suggests that environmental factors, such as maternal virus infections during pregnancy, may contribute. Schizophrenia is therefore now viewed as a *neurodevelopmental*, rather than a neurodegenerative, disorder. Psychological factors, such as stress, may precipitate acute episodes, but are not the underlying cause.

The search for neurochemical abnormalities in schizophrenia has been unsuccessful for many years (for a catalogue of the failures, see Lieberman & Koreen 1993). Though it was hoped that a neurochemical theory would provide the basis for rational drug treatment, the opposite has occurred: drugs found by chance to be effective have provided the main clues about the nature of the disorder. The main neurochemical theories are discussed below.

Few animal models of schizophrenia are available for testing prospective therapies. A characteristic feature of schizophrenia is a defect in 'selective attention'. Whereas a normal individual quickly accommodates to stimuli of a familiar or inconsequential nature, and responds only to stimuli that are unexpected or significant, the ability of schizophrenic patients to discriminate between significant and insignificant stimuli seems to be impaired. Thus, the ticking of a clock may command as much attention as the words of a companion; a chance thought, which a normal person would dismiss as inconsequential, may become an irresistible imperative. 'Latent inhibition' is a form of behavioural testing in animals which can be used as a model for this type of sensory habituation. Latent inhibition is impaired by **amphetamine**, and by psychotomimetic drugs such as LSD, this effect being inhibited by many antipsychotic drugs (see Ellenbroek & Cools 1990).

Dopamine theory

The dopamine theory was proposed in 1965 (see Meltzer & Stahl 1976), and is supported by a good deal of indirect evidence. The best evidence comes from pharmacological observations in man and experimental animals. **Amphetamine** releases dopamine in the brain, and can produce in man a behavioural syndrome indistinguishable from an acute schizophrenic episode—very familiar to doctors who treat drug-users. In animals dopamine release causes a specific pattern of stereotyped behaviour, which resembles the repetitive behaviours often seen

in schizophrenic patients. Potent D_2-receptor agonists (e.g. **apomorphine** and **bromocriptine**; Ch. 30) produce similar effects in animals, and these drugs, like amphetamine, exacerbate the symptoms of schizophrenic patients. Furthermore, dopamine antagonists and drugs that block neuronal dopamine storage (e.g. **reserpine**) are effective in controlling the positive symptoms of schizophrenia, and in preventing amphetamine-induced behavioural changes. There is a strong correlation between clinical antipsychotic potency and activity in blocking D_2-receptors (Fig. 34.1), and receptor imaging studies have shown that clinical efficacy of antipsychotic drugs is consistently achieved when D_2-receptor occupancy reaches about 80%.

There is little direct biochemical evidence that hyperactivity of dopamine, specifically at D_2-receptors, occurs in schizophrenia; many studies have given negative or inconsistent results. The amount of homovanillic acid (HVA, the main dopamine metabolite; see Ch. 30) in the CSF of schizophrenic patients is normal or low, rather than high. In post-mortem brains, dopamine or its metabolites are not present in abnormally high concentrations, nor is the activity of dopamine-metabolising enzymes abnormal. Furthermore, the production of prolactin, which might be expected to be abnormally low if dopaminergic transmission was facilitated, is normal in schizophrenic patients. One difficulty in interpreting such studies is that nearly all schizophrenic patients are treated with drugs that are known to affect dopamine metabolism, whereas the non-schizophrenic control group are not. Even where it has been possible to allow for this factor, however, the results are still generally negative. A well-controlled study by Reynolds (1983), however, showed a raised dopamine content post-mortem in the amygdala of schizophrenic subjects, the nor-adrenaline content being normal. Most surprisingly the increased dopamine content was confined to the left side of the brain, which makes it most unlikely that it could have been the result of antipsychotic drug treatment. Recent studies have shown that dopamine release may be increased in schizophrenic, compared with control subjects (Laruelle et al. 1996). A radioligand imaging technique was used to measure binding of a specific antagonist (**raclopride**) to D_2-receptors in the striatum. Injection of amphetamine caused dopamine release, and thus displacement of raclopride, measured as a reduction of the signal intensity. This reduction was significantly greater in schizophrenic than control subjects, implying a greater amphetamine-induced release of dopamine.

An increase in dopamine receptor density in schizophrenia has been reported in some studies, but not

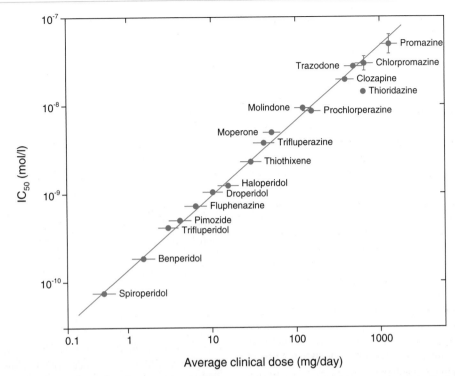

Fig. 34.1 Correlation between the clinical potency and affinity for dopamine D$_2$-receptors among neuroleptic drugs. Clinical potency is expressed as the daily dose used in treating schizophrenia, and binding activity is expressed as the concentration needed to produce 50% inhibition of haloperidol binding. (From: Seeman P et al. 1976 Nature 261: 717)

consistently, and the interpretation is complicated by the fact that antipsychotic drug treatment is known to increase dopamine receptor expression. A large increase in D$_4$-receptors was found in one study (Seeman et al. 1993), but the conclusion relied on an indirect estimate of D$_4$-receptor labelling, and in later experiments no difference in D$_4$-receptor mRNA was detected, so the finding remains equivocal.

The D$_4$-receptor has also attracted attention on account of the high degree of genetic polymorphism that it shows in human subjects, and because some of the newer antipsychotic drugs (e.g. clozapine; see below) turn out to have a high affinity for this receptor subtype. Genetic studies have, however, failed to show any relationship between schizophrenia and D$_4$-receptor polymorphism. Moreover, a specific D$_4$-receptor antagonist (L745870) proved ineffective in clinical trials.

Other theories

Several other transmitters, particularly 5-HT, noradrenaline and glutamate, interact strongly with dop-

amine pathways, and may be important in relation to the actions of antipsychotic drugs, and possibly also in the aetiology of schizophrenia. The complexity of neurotransmitter interactions and the ingenuity of theorists are such that the possibilities tend to outnumber the facts in a somewhat dispiriting way.

The idea that 5-HT dysfunction could be involved in schizophrenia was based on the fact that **lysergic acid diethylamide (LSD**; see Ch. 38) produces schizophrenia-like symptoms, and has drifted in and out of favour many times (see Busatto & Kerwin 1997).

Though there is no clear biochemical evidence suggesting any alteration in 5-HT metabolism or 5-HT receptor function in schizophrenia, many effective antipsychotic drugs, in addition to blocking dopamine receptors (see below) also act as 5-HT$_2$-receptor antagonists. 5-HT has a modulatory effect on dopamine pathways, so the two theories are not incompatible. Affinity for 5-HT$_2$-receptors is a feature of many of the recently-developed 'atypical' antipsychotic drugs (see below), which produce fewer extrapyramidal side-effects than the earlier dopamine-selective compounds, so it is postulated that a degree of $5\text{-}HT_2$-receptor block can counteract the undesirable side-effects associated with D_2-receptor antagonists. It is also possible that 5-HT receptor antagonism contributes directly to the antipsychotic profile of these drugs, but opinions on this differ sharply.

Another transmitter to be implicated in the pathophysiology of schizophrenia is—you will not be surprised to learn—glutamate. In favour of this view is the fact that various compounds that block NMDA receptor effects (for example **phencyclidine**, **ketamine**, **dizocilpine**; see Ch. 29) all produce subjective effects in humans (e.g. hallucinations, thought disorder) that closely resemble the mental state changes in schizophrenia, suggesting that diminished glutamate transmission might be a factor in the disease. According to this view (see Lidsky & Bannerjee 1996), glutamate and dopamine exert excitatory and inhibitory effects respectively on GABA-ergic striatal neurons which project to the thalamus and constitute a sensory 'gate' (see above). Too little glutamate, or too much dopamine, disables the gate, allowing uninhibited sensory input to reach the cortex. Though such pathways exist, there is so far little evidence for loss of glutamate function in schizophrenia.

In conclusion, the dopamine hyperactivity theory of schizophrenia is supported by considerable—mostly indirect—evidence. Though it is undoubtedly an oversimplification, it provides the best framework for understanding the action of antipsychotic drugs, though effects on 5-HT receptors contribute significantly to the clinical profile of some of the newer drugs.

The nature of schizophrenia

- Psychotic illness characterised by delusions, hallucinations and thought disorder (positive symptoms), together with social withdrawal and flattening of emotional responses (negative symptoms).
- Acute episodes (mainly positive symptoms) frequently recur and develop into chronic schizophrenia, with predominantly negative symptoms.
- Incidence is about 1% of population, with a strong, but not invariable, hereditary component.
- Pharmacological evidence is generally consistent with dopamine overactivity hypothesis, but most neurochemical evidence is negative or equivocal. Increase in dopamine receptors in limbic system (especially in left hemisphere) is consistently found.
- There is some evidence for involvement of 5-HT, and possibly other mediators, such as glutamate.

ANTIPSYCHOTIC DRUGS

CLASSIFICATION OF ANTIPSYCHOTIC DRUGS

More than 20 different antipsychotic drugs are available for clinical use, but with certain exceptions the differences between them are minor.

An important distinction is drawn between the main group, often referred to as *classical* or *typical antipsychotic drugs*, and the more recently developed agents (e.g. dibenzodiazepines, diphenylbutylpiperazines and benzamides) which are termed *atypical antipsychotic drugs*. These terms are widely used, but not clearly defined. 'Atypical' commonly refers to the diminished tendency of some newer compounds to cause unwanted motor side-effects (see below), but it is also used to describe compounds with a pharmacological profile somewhat different from that of 'classical' compounds, or compounds which improve the negative as well as the positive symptoms. In practice, it suffices to distinguish the large group of ('classical') pre-1980 drugs (phenothiazines, thioxanthines and butyrophenones) which are very similar in their properties, from a more diverse group of newer compounds described below.

Table 34.1 summarises the main drugs that are in clinical use.

Classification of antipsychotic drugs

- Main categories are:
  - *typical antipsychotics* (e.g. **chlorpromazine, haloperidol, fluphenazine, thioridazine, flupenthixol, clopenthixol**)
  - *atypical antipsychotics* (e.g. **clozapine, risperidone, sulpiride, olanzapine**)
- Distinction between 'typical' and 'atypical' groups is not clearly defined, but rests on:
  - incidence of exrapyramidal side-effects (less in 'atypical' group)
  - efficacy in treatment-resistant group of patients
  - efficacy against negative symptoms.

GENERAL PROPERTIES OF ANTIPSYCHOTIC DRUGS

The therapeutic activity of the prototype drug, chlorpromazine, in schizophrenic patients was discovered through the acute observations of a French surgeon, Laborit, in 1947. He tested various substances, including **promethazine**, for their ability to alleviate signs of stress in patients undergoing surgery, and concluded that

Table 34.1 Characteristics of antipsychotic drugs

Drug	Receptor affinity						EPS	Sed.	Hypo.	Main side-effects Other	Notes
	D_1	D_2	α-adr	H_1	mACh	$5\text{-}HT_2$					
Classical											
Chlorpromazine	++	+++	+++	++	++	+	++	++	++	Increased prolactin (gynaecomastia) Hypothermia Anticholinergic effects Hypersensitivity reactions Obstructive jaundice	Phenothiazine class **Fluphenazine, trifluperazine** are similar, but: • do not cause jaundice • less hypotension • more EPS Fluphenazine available as depot preparation
Thioridazine	+	++	+++	–	++	++	+	++	++	As chlorpromazine, but does not cause jaundice	Phenothiazine class First drug with lower EPS tendency
Haloperidol	+	+++	±	+	±	+	+++	–	++	As chlorpromazine, but does not cause jaundice Fewer anticholinergic side-effects	Butyrophenone class Widely used antipsychotic drug Strong EPS tendency
Flupenthixol	++	+++	++	–	–	+++	++	+	+	Increased prolactin (gynaecomastia) Restlessness	**Clopenthixol** is similar Available as depot preparations
Atypical											
Sulpiride	–	+++	–	–	–	–	+	+	–	Increased prolactin (gynaecomastia)	Benzamide class Selective D_2/D_3 antagonist Less EPS than haloperidol Poorly absorbed. **Remoxipride and pimozide** (long-acting) are similar
Clozapine	++	++	++	++	++	+++	–	++	+	Risk of agranulocytosis (~1%)—regular blood counts required Seizures Salivation Anticholinergic side-effects Weight gain	Dibenzodiazepine class Antagonist at D_4-receptors No EPS Shows efficacy in 'treatment-resistant' patients Effective against negative and positive symptoms **Olanzapine** is similar, without risk of agranulocytosis
Risperidone	–	+++	++	–	–	+++	+	+	+	Weight gain EPS at high doses Hypotension	Benzixazole class ? Effective against negative symptoms
Sertindole	–	+++	++	–	–	+++	+	+	++	Ventricular dysrhythmias (ECG checks advisable) Weight gain Nasal congestion	Long plasma half-life (~3 days) ? Effective against negative symptoms
Seroquel	–	+++	+++	–	++	+	+	++	++	Tachycardia Agitation Dry mouth	Novel type, acting mainly on α-adrenoceptors Not yet fully evaluated

EPS = extrapyramidal side-effects; Sed. = sedation; Hypo. = hypotension

promethazine had a calming effect that was different from mere sedation. Elaboration of the phenothiazine structure produced **chlorpromazine**, the antipsychotic effect of which was demonstrated, at Laborit's instigation, by Delay & Deniker in 1953. This drug was unique in controlling the symptoms of psychotic patients without excessively sedating them. The clinical efficacy of phenothiazines was discovered long before their mechanism of action was understood.

Pharmacological investigation showed that phenothiazines blocked the actions of many different mediators, including histamine, catecholamines, acetylcholine and 5-HT, and this multiplicity of actions led to the trade name Largactil for chlorpromazine. It is now clear (see Fig. 34.1) that antagonism at dopamine receptors is the main determinant of antipsychotic action.

MECHANISM OF ACTION

DOPAMINE RECEPTORS AND DOPAMINERGIC NEURONS

The classification of dopamine receptors in the CNS is discussed in Chapter 30 (see Table 30.1). There are two main receptor types: D_1, which increases adenylate cyclase activity, and D_2, which mediates the main presynaptic and postsynaptic inhibitory actions of dopamine. D_3- and D_4-receptors belong to the same group as D_2. The antipsychotic drugs probably owe their therapeutic effects mainly to blockade of D_2-receptors. As stated above, antipsychotic effects require about 80% block of D_2-receptors. Antagonism at D_2-receptors can be measured in experimental animals by various tests, such as inhibition of amphetamine-induced stereotypic behaviour, or of apomorphine-induced turning behaviour in animals with unilateral striatal lesions (see Ch. 30), and in vitro by ability to inhibit the binding of a radioactive D_2 antagonist (e.g. **spiroperidol**) to brain membrane fragments. The main groups, phenothiazines, thioxanthines and butyrophenones, show some preference for D_2- over D_1-receptors; some of the newer agents (e.g. **sulpiride**, **remoxipride**) are highly selective for D_2-receptors, whereas **clozapine** is relatively non-selective between D_1 and D_2, but has high affinity for D_4.

All antipsychotic drugs have been found initially to increase the rate of production of dopamine in regions containing dopaminergic nerve terminals (see O'Donnell & Grace 1996). This is detectable by an increase in tyrosine hydroxylase activity, and an increase in the concentration of the dopamine metabolites, homovanillic acid and DOPAC. At the same time electrical recording has shown that the activity of midbrain dopaminergic

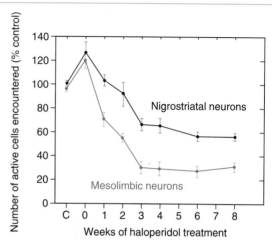

Fig. 34.2 Effect of chronic haloperidol treatment on the activity of dopaminergic neurons in the rat brain. In both regions the activity of dopaminergic neurons, recorded with microelectrodes from anaesthetised animals, initially increases and then declines, reaching a steady level after 3 weeks. (From: White F J, Wang R Y 1983 Life Sci 32: 983)

neurons in the substantia nigra and ventral tegmentum is initially increased by these drugs. Effects on the latter are believed to correlate with antipsychotic effects, whereas effects on the former are responsible for the unwanted motor effects produced by antipsychotic drugs (see below). Thus **haloperidol**, a classical drug with marked unwanted motor effects, acts on both sets of dopamine neurons, whereas **clozapine**, an atypical drug which lacks motor effects, affects only the ventral tegmental neurons.

Antipsychotic drugs, like many neuroactive compounds, take several weeks to take effect, even though their receptor-blocking action is immediate.* When antipsychotic drugs are administered chronically, the increase in activity of dopaminergic neurons is transient, and gives way after about 3 weeks to inhibition (Fig. 34.2), at which time both the biochemical and electrophysiological markers of activity decline.

Another delayed effect seen with chronic administration of antipsychotic drugs is proliferation of dopamine receptors, detectable as an increase in haloperidol binding (see Seeman 1987), and also a pharmacological supersensitivity to dopamine, somewhat akin to the phenomenon of denervation supersensitivity. At present neither

---

*Their sedating effect is also immediate, allowing them to be used in acute behavioural emergencies.

the mechanism of the delayed effects nor their relationship to the clinical response is at all well understood.

Antipsychotic drugs show varying patterns of selectivity in their receptor-blocking effects (Table 34.1), some having high affinity for 5-HT and/or D_4-receptors. The connection between their receptor specificity and their functional and therapeutic effects, despite a wealth of fine argument, remains hidden. Were it understood, we should not have to fall back in desperation on words like 'atypical' to hide our uncertainty.

Mechanism of action of antipsychotic drugs

- All antipsychotic drugs are antagonists at dopamine D_2-receptors, but most also block other monoamine receptors, especially 5-HT$_2$. Clozapine also blocks D_4-receptors.
- Antipsychotic potency generally runs parallel to activity on D_2-receptors, but other activities may determine side-effect profile.
- Antipsychotics take days or weeks to work, suggesting that secondary effects (e.g. increase in number of D_2-receptors in limbic structure) may be more important than direct effect of D_2-receptor block.

PHARMACOLOGICAL EFFECTS OF ANTIPSYCHOTIC DRUGS

BEHAVIOURAL EFFECTS

Antipsychotic drugs produce many behavioural effects in experimental animals (see Ögren 1996), but no single test is known that distinguishes them clearly from other types of psychotropic drug. Antipsychotic drugs reduce spontaneous motor activity and in larger doses cause *catalepsy*, a state in which the animal remains immobile even when placed in an unnatural position. Inhibition of the hyperactivity induced by amphetamine is used as an indicator of the required antipsychotic action of these drugs, whereas ability to cause catalepsy is used as an indicator of their tendency to cause unwanted extrapyramidal symptoms in clinical use (see below). These effects probably reflect dopamine antagonism in the mesocortical/mesolimbic and the striatonigral pathways respectively. Other tests reveal effects that are not associated with motor inhibition. For example, in a conditioned avoidance model, a rat may be trained to respond to a conditioned stimulus, such as a buzzer, by remaining immobile and thereby avoiding a painful shock; chlorpromazine impairs performance in this test, as well as

in tests that demand active motor responses. In doses too small to reduce spontaneous motor activity, chlorpromazine reduces social interactions (grooming, mating, fighting, etc.), and also impairs performance in discriminant tests (e.g. requiring the animal to respond differently to red and green lights).

Inhibition of amphetamine-induced behavioural changes occurs with all of the 'classical' antipsychotic drugs, reflecting their action on D_2-receptors. Some of the atypical drugs, which have less activity on D_2-receptors are less active in such models, and also in the catalepsy model, but are equally efficacious in conditioned avoidance tests. Both classical and atypical drugs, moreover, reduce the hyperactivity caused by phencyclidine (a glutamate antagonist; Ch. 29) which causes a schizophrenia-like syndrome in humans. Conditioned avoidance, and phencyclidine tests in animals are therefore used as guides to antipsychotic activity in man.

In man, the effect of antipsychotic drugs is to produce a state of apathy and reduced initiative. The subject displays few emotions, is slow to respond to external stimuli and tends to drowse off. He is, however, easily aroused and can respond to questions accurately, with no marked loss of intellectual function. Aggressive tendencies are strongly inhibited. The effects in humans differ from those of hypnotic and anxiolytic drugs, which cause drowsiness and confusion, with euphoria rather than apathy.

Many antipsychotic drugs show anti-emetic activity (see Ch. 21), reflecting antagonism at dopamine receptors. The antihistamine activity of many phenothiazines is also important.

UNWANTED EFFECTS

Extrapyramidal motor disturbances and tardive dyskinesia

Antipsychotic drugs produce two main kinds of motor disturbance in humans, collectively termed extrapyramidal side-effects (EPS), which result directly or indirectly from D_2-receptor blockade. EPS constitute one of the main disadvantages of all of the 'classical' antipsychotic drugs. The term 'atypical' was originally applied to some of the newer compounds that show much less tendency to produce EPS.

The effects comprise *acute dystonias* and *tardive dyskinesia*.

Acute dystonias are involuntary movements (muscle spasms, protruding tongue, torticollis, etc.), and often a Parkinson-type syndrome (Ch. 31). They occur commonly in the first few weeks, often declining with time, and they are reversible on stopping drug treatment. The occurrence of acute dystonias is consistent with block of the dopaminergic nigrostriatal pathway, and there is evidence that the relative selectivity of atypical antipsychotic drugs for the mesolimbic/mesocortical pathway accounts for the diminished risk of acute dystonias.

Tardive dyskinesia (see Klawans et al. 1988) develops after months or years (hence 'tardive') in 20–40% of patients treated with classical antipsychotic drugs, and is one of the main problems of antipsychotic therapy. Its seriousness lies in the fact that it is a disabling and often irreversible condition, which often gets worse when antipsychotic therapy is stopped, and is resistant to treatment. The syndrome consists of involuntary movements, often of the face and tongue, but also of the trunk and limbs, which can be severely disabling. It resembles that seen after prolonged treatment of parkinsonian patients with levodopa. The incidence depends greatly on the drug dosage, the age of the patient (commonest in patients over 50) and on the drug used. The reason why atypical antipsychotic drugs (e.g. **clozapine**, **olanzapine**, **sertindole**) are better in this regard is not clear. Sparing of the nigrostriatal pathway (see above) is important, but not well explained in pharmacological terms. Clozapine has relatively high affinity for D_1 and D_4, compared with D_2, receptors, and also has marked antimuscarinic activity, as do some other antipsychotic drugs, such as **thioridazine**, which may counteract its effects on the motor system.

There are several theories about the mechanism of tardive dyskinesia (see Casey 1995). One is that it is associated with a gradual increase in the number of D_2-receptor sites in the striatum, which is less marked with the atypical antipsychotic drugs. Another possibility is that chronic block of inhibitory dopamine receptors enhances catecholamine and/or glutamate release in the striatum, leading to excitotoxic neurodegeneration (Ch. 31).

Endocrine effects

Dopamine, released in the median eminence by neurons of the tuberohypophyseal pathway (see Chs 24, 30) acts physiologically via D_2-receptors as an inhibitor of prolactin secretion, being transported from its site of release in the median eminence to the anterior pituitary gland via the hypophyseal portal vascular system. The result of blocking D_2-receptors by antipsychotic drugs is thus to increase the plasma prolactin concentration (Fig. 34.3), resulting in *breast swelling*, *pain* and *lactation*, which can occur in men as well as women. As can be seen from Figure 34.3, the effect is maintained during chronic antipsychotic administration, without any habituation.

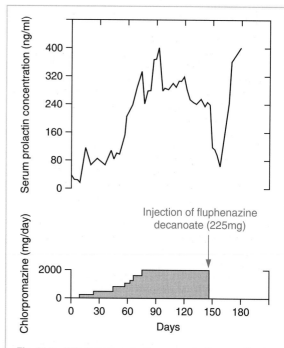

Fig. 34.3   Effect of neuroleptics on prolactin secretion in a schizophrenic patient. When daily dosage with chlorpromazine was replaced with a depot injection of fluphenazine the plasma prolactin initially dropped, because of the delay in absorption, and then returned to a high level. (From: Meltzer H Y et al. 1978 In: Lipton et al. (eds) Psychopharmacology. A generation of progress. Raven Press, New York)

Unwanted effects of antipsychotic drugs

- Important side-effects common to most drugs are extrapyramidal motor disturbances (see separate box), endocrine disturbances (increased prolactin release); these are secondary to dopamine receptor block. Sedation, hypotension and weight gain are also common.
- Obstructive jaundice sometimes occurs with phenothiazines.
- Other side-effects (dry mouth, blurred vision, hypotension, etc.) are due to block of other receptors, particularly α-adrenoceptors and muscarinic ACh receptors.
- Some antipsychotics cause agranulocytosis as a rare and serious idiosyncratic reaction. With clozapine, leukopenia is common, and requires routine monitoring.
- Antipsychotic malignant syndrome is a rare but potentially dangerous idiosyncratic reaction.

Other less pronounced endocrine changes have also been reported, including a decrease of growth hormone secretion, but these, unlike the prolactin response, are unimportant clinically.

Other unwanted effects

Sedation, which tends to decrease with continued use, occurs with many antipsychotic drugs. Antihistamine (H_1) activity is a property of phenothiazines, and contributes to their sedative and anti-emetic properties (Ch. 21), but not to their antipsychotic action.

Phenothiazines and, to a variable extent, other antipsychotic drugs, block a variety of receptors, particularly acetylcholine (muscarinic), histamine (H_1), noradrenaline (α) and 5-HT (Table 34.1).

Blocking muscarinic receptors produces a variety of peripheral effects, including *blurring of vision and increased intraocular pressure*, *dry mouth and eyes*, *constipation* and *urinary retention* (see Ch. 7). It may, however, also be beneficial in relation to extrapyramidal side-effects. Acetylcholine acts in opposition to dopamine in the basal ganglia (see Ch. 31) and it is possible that the relative lack of extrapyramidal side-effects with **clozapine** and **thioridazine** is due to their high antimuscarinic potency (see above).

Blocking α-adrenoceptors results in the important side-effect in humans of *orthostatic hypotension* (see Ch. 15), but does not seem to be important for their antipsychotic action.

Weight gain is a common and troublesome side-effect, probably related to 5-HT antagonism.

Various idiosyncratic and hypersensitivity reactions can occur, the most important being:

- *Jaundice*, which occurs with older phenothiazines, such as chlorpromazine. The jaundice is usually mild, and of obstructive origin, and disappears quickly when the drug is stopped or substituted by a antipsychotic of a different class.
- *Leukopenia* and *agranulocytosis* are rare, but potentially fatal, and occur in the first few weeks of treatment. The incidence of leukopenia (usually reversible) is less than 1 in 10 000 for most antipsychotics, but much higher (1–2%) with **clozapine**, whose use therefore requires regular monitoring of blood cell counts. Provided the drug is stopped at the first sign of leukopenia or anaemia, the effect is reversible. **Olanzapine** appears to be free of this disadvantage.
- *Urticarial skin reactions* are common but usually mild. Excessive sensitivity to ultraviolet light may also occur.
- *Neuroleptic malignant syndrome* is a rare but serious complication, similar to the malignant hyperthermia syndrome seen with certain anaesthetics (see Ch. 32). Muscle rigidity is accompanied by a rapid rise in body temperature and mental confusion. It is usually reversible, but death from renal or cardiovascular failure occurs in 10–20% of cases.

PHARMACOKINETIC ASPECTS

Chlorpromazine, which is typical of many phenothiazines, is erratically absorbed into the bloodstream after oral administration. Figure 34.4 shows the wide range of variation of the peak plasma concentration as a function of dosage in 14 patients. Among four patients treated at the high dosage level of 6–8 mg/kg, the variation in peak plasma concentration was nearly 90-fold; two showed marked side-effects, one was correctly controlled and one showed no clinical response.

The relationship between the plasma concentration and the clinical effect of antipsychotic drugs is also highly variable, and the dosage has to be adjusted on a trial-and-error basis. This is made even more difficult by the fact that at least 40% of schizophrenic patients fail to take drugs as prescribed. It is remarkably fortunate that the acute toxicity of antipsychotic drugs is slight, given the unpredictability of the clinical response.

The plasma half-life of most antipsychotic drugs is 15–30 hours, clearance depending entirely on hepatic

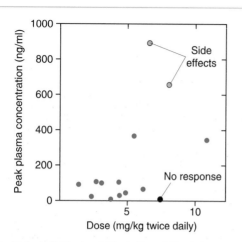

Fig. 34.4 Individual variation in the relation between dose and plasma concentration of chlorpromazine in a group of schizophrenic patients. (Data from: Curry S H et al. 1970 Arch Gen Psychiat 22: 289)

transformation by a combination of oxidative and conjugative reactions. The metabolism of phenothiazines is complex, but metabolites do not appear to contribute much to the pharmacological response.

Most antipsychotic drugs can be given orally or by intramuscular injection, once or twice a day. Slow-release (depot) preparations of many are available, in which the active drug is esterified with heptanoic or decanoic acid and dissolved in oil. Given as an intra-muscular injection, the drug acts for 2–4 weeks, but initially may produce acute side-effects. These preparations are widely used as a means of overcoming compliance problems.

CLINICAL USE AND CLINICAL EFFICACY

The major use of antipsychotic drugs is in the treatment of schizophrenia and acute behavioural emergencies, but they are also widely used as adjunct therapy in the treatment of other illnesses, such as psychotic depression and mania. Some of the newer antipsychotics (e.g. **sulpiride**) have been claimed to have specific antidepressant actions. Phenothiazines are also useful as anti-emetics (see Ch. 21). Minor uses include the treatment of Huntington's chorea (mainly **haloperidol**; see Ch. 31).

The clinical efficacy of antipsychotic drugs in enabling schizophrenic patients to lead more normal lives has been demonstrated in many controlled trials. The inpatient population (mainly chronic schizophrenics) of mental hospitals declined sharply in the 1950s and 1960s. The efficacy of the newly introduced antipsychotic drugs was a significant enabling factor, as well as the changing public and professional attitudes towards hospitalisation of the mentally ill.

Classical antipsychotic drugs, apart from their side-effects, have two main shortcomings:

- They are effective in only about 70% of schizophrenic patients. The remaining 30% are classed as 'treatment-resistant', and present a major therapeutic problem. The reason for the difference between responsive and unresponsive patients is unknown at present.
- While they control the positive symptoms (thought disorder, hallucinations, delusions, etc.) effectively, they are ineffective in relieving the negative symptoms (emotional flattening, social isolation).

Some of the atypical antipsychotic drugs, particularly **clozapine**, overcome both of these shortcomings to some degree, showing efficacy in treatment-resistant patients, and improving negative, as well as positive symptoms (see Meltzer & Ranjan 1996). More recent compounds, such as **risperidone** and **sertindole**, plus others in the pipeline, have yet to be fully evaluated.

Clinical efficacy of antipsychotic drugs

- Antipsychotic drugs are effective in controlling symptoms of acute schizophrenia, when large doses may be needed.
- Long-term antipsychotic treatment is often effective in preventing recurrence of schizophrenic attacks, and is a major factor in allowing schizophrenic patients to lead normal lives.
- Depot preparations are often used for maintenance therapy.
- Antipsychotic drugs are not generally effective in improving negative schizophrenic symptoms.
- Approximately 40% of chronic schizophrenic patients are poorly controlled by antipsychotic drugs; clozapine may be effective in some of these 'antipsychotic-resistant' cases.

REFERENCES AND FURTHER READING

Busatto G F, Kerwin R W 1997 Perspectives on the role of serotonergic mechanisms in the pharmacology of schizophrenia. J Psychopharmacol 11: 3–12 (*Assesses the evidence implicating 5-HT as well as dopamine in the action of antipsychotic drugs*)

Casey D E 1995 Tardive dyskinesia: pathophysiology. In: Bloom F E, Kupfer D J (eds) Psychopharmacology: a fourth generation of progress. Raven Press, New York

Crow T J 1982 Schizophrenia. In: Crow T J (ed) Disorders of neurohumoral transmission. Academic Press, London (*Useful introduction to schizophrenia*)

Csernansky J G (ed) 1996 Antipsychotics. Handbook of experimental pharmacology. Springer, Berlin, vol 120 (*Comprehensive collection of recent review articles. Contains much information, but not exciting to read*)

Egan M F, Weinberger D R 1997 Neurobiology of schizophrenia. Curr Opin Neurobiol 7: 701–707 (*Excellent short review on biological basis of schizophrenia, including recent neuroimaging and genetic studies*)

Ellenbroek B A, Cools A R 1990 Animal models with construct validity for schizophrenia. Behav Pharmacol 1: 469–490

Harrison P J 1997 Schizophrenia: a disorder of development. Curr Opin Neurobiol 7: 285–289 (*Reviews persuasively the evidence favouring abnormal early brain development as the basis of schizophrenia*)

Klawans H L, Tanner C M, Goetz C G 1988 Epidemiology and pathophysiology of tardive dyskinesias. Adv Neurol 49: 185–197

Laruelle M, Abi-Dargham A, van Dyck C H et al. 1996 Single photon emission computerised tomography imaging of amphetamine-induced dopamine release in drug-free schizophrenic subjects. Proc Natnl Acad Sci USA 93: 9235–9240 (*One of the few convincing pieces of evidence to show an abnormality in dopamine function in schizophrenia*)

Lidsky T I, Bannerjee S P 1996 Contribution of glutamatergic dysfunction to schizophrenia. Drug News Perspect 9: 453–459 (*Pulls together the so-far slender evidence implicating glutamate in schizophrenia*)

Lieberman J A, Koreen A R 1993 Neurochemistry and neuroendocrinology of schizophrenia: a selective review. Schizophr Bull 19: 371–429 (*Compilation of a large amount of mostly negative results of studies which have attempted to define the neurochemical phenotype of schizophrenia*)

Meltzer H Y, Ranjan R 1996 Efficacy of novel antipsychotic drugs in treatment-refractory schizophrenia. In: Csernansky J G (ed) Antipsychotics. Handbook of experimental pharmacology. Springer, Berlin, vol 120 (*Useful summary of trials data with atypical antipsychotic drugs*)

Meltzer H, Stahl S M 1976 The dopamine hypothesis of schizophrenia: a review. Schizophr Bull 2: 19–76 (*Review by one of the pioneers in this field*)

O'Donnell P, Grace A A 1996 Basic neurophysiology of antipsychotic drug action. In: Chernansky J G (ed) Antipsychotics. Handbook of experimental pharmacology. Springer, Berlin, vol 120 (*Review of effects of antipsychotic drugs at the neurophysiological level, emphasising distinction between acute and chronic effects*)

Ögren S O 1996 The behavioural pharmacology of typical and atypical antipsychotic drugs. In: Csernansky J G (ed) Antipsychotics. Handbook of experimental pharmacology. Springer, Berlin, vol 120

Reynolds G P 1983 Increased concentrations and lateral asymmetry of amygdala dopamine in schizophrenia. Nature 305: 527–529. (*Demonstrates unilateral increase of brain dopamine in post-mortem schizophrenic brains—one of the few positive neurochemical findings*)

Reynolds G P 1992 Developments in the drug treatment of schizophrenia. Trends Pharmacol Sci 13: 116–121 (*Optimistic review of new approaches*)

Seeman P 1987 Dopamine receptors and the dopamine hypothesis of schizophrenia. Synapse 1: 133–152 (*Convincing, and widely quoted, review of role of dopamine receptors in schizophrenia*)

Seeman P, Guan H-C, Van Tol H H M 1993 Dopamine D_4 receptors elevated in schizophrenia. Nature 365: 441–445 (*Controversial study claiming large increase in specific receptor subtype*)

Drugs used in affective disorders

THE NATURE OF AFFECTIVE DISORDERS

Affective disorders are characterised primarily by changes of mood (depression or mania) rather than by thought disturbances. Depression is the most common manifestation, and it may range from a very mild condition, bordering on normality, to severe depression—sometimes called psychotic depression—accompanied by hallucinations and delusions.

The symptoms of depression include emotional and biological components:

- Emotional symptoms:
  —misery, apathy and pessimism
  —low self-esteem: feelings of guilt, inadequacy and ugliness
  —indecisiveness, loss of motivation.
- Biological symptoms:
  —retardation of thought and action
  —loss of libido
  —sleep disturbance and loss of appetite.

Mania is in most respects exactly the opposite, with excessive exuberance, enthusiasm and self-confidence, accompanied by impulsive actions, these signs often being combined with irritability impatience and aggression, and sometimes with grandiose delusions of the Napoleonic kind. As with depression, the mood and actions are inappropriate to the circumstances.

There are two distinct types of depressive syndrome, namely *unipolar depression*, in which the mood swings are always in the same direction, and *bipolar affective disorder*, in which depression alternates with mania. Unipolar depression is commonly (about 75% of cases) non-familial, clearly associated with stressful life-events, and accompanied by symptoms of anxiety and agitation; this type is sometimes termed *reactive* depression. Other cases (about 25%, sometimes termed *endogenous* depression) show a familial pattern, unrelated to external stresses, and with a somewhat different symptomatology. This distinction is made clinically, but there is little evidence that antidepressant drugs show significant selectivity between these conditions. Bipolar depression, which usually appears in early adult life, and is much less common, results in oscillating depression and mania over a period of a few weeks. There is a strong hereditary tendency, but attempts to pinpoint the gene or genes responsible, by genetic linkage studies of affected families, have so far failed.

THE MONOAMINE THEORY OF DEPRESSION

The main biochemical theory of depression is the monoamine hypothesis, proposed by Schildkraut in 1965, which states that depression is caused by a functional deficit of monoamine transmitters at certain sites in the brain, while mania results from a functional excess. For reviews of the evolving status of the theory, see Baker & Dewhurst (1985), Maes & Meltzer (1995), Schatzberg & Schildkraut (1995).

The monoamine hypothesis grew originally out of associations between the clinical effects of various drugs which cause or alleviate symptoms of depression and their known neurochemical effects on monoaminergic transmission in the brain. Initially the monoamine hypothesis was formulated in terms of noradrenaline, but subsequent work showed that most of the observations were equally consistent with 5-HT being the key substance. This pharmacological evidence, which is summarised below, gives general support to the monoamine hypothesis, though there are several anomalies. Attempts to obtain more direct evidence, by studying monoamine metabolism in depressed patients, or by measuring changes in the number of monoamine receptors in post-mortem brain tissue, have given mainly inconsistent and equivocal results, and the interpretation of these studies is often problematic. Similarly, investigation by functional tests of the activity of known monoaminergic pathways (e.g. those controlling pituitary hormone release) in depressed patients have also given equivocal results.

Pharmacological evidence

Table 35.1 summarises the main drugs that are known to affect monoamine metabolism, and compares their predicted effect on mood with the observed effect. In general, there is reasonable support for the theory, though there are several examples of drugs that might have been predicted to improve or worsen depressive symptoms, but fail to do so convincingly. It has to be recognised that

the basis for predicting the effects of drugs on mood is, at best, very simple-minded. Thus, supplying a transmitter precursor will not necessarily increase the release of transmitter unless availability of the precursor is rate-limiting. Similarly, a drug that releases monoamines from normal nerve terminals may fail to do so if the nerve terminals are functionally defective. The absence of a useful antidepressant action of amphetamine is therefore not strong evidence against the monoamine theory. The pharmacological evidence does not enable a clear distinction to be drawn between the noradrenaline and 5-HT theories of depression. Clinically, it seems that inhibitors of noradrenaline reuptake and of 5-HT reuptake are equally effective as antidepressants (see below) though individual patients may respond better to one or the other.

More difficult to reconcile with the monoamine theory in any simple way is the fact that the biochemical actions of antidepressant drugs appear very rapidly, whereas their antidepressant effects take days or weeks to develop. A similar situation exists in relation to antipsychotic drugs (Ch. 34) and some anxiolytic drugs (Ch. 33), suggesting that the secondary, adaptive changes in the brain, rather than the primary drug effect, are responsible for the clinical improvement. Evidence for such adaptive changes in monoamine receptor function is discussed below (p. 555). This change in the interpretation of the mechanism of action of antidepressant drugs clearly undermines one of the original key arguments on which the monoamine theory was based. The general conclusion that

Table 35.1 Pharmacological evidence relating to the monoamine hypothesis of depression

Drug	Principal action	Effect in depressed patients
Effects consistent with the hypothesis		
Tricyclic antidepressants	Block NA and 5-HT reuptake	Mood ↑
MAO inhibitors	Increase stores of NA and 5-HT	Mood ↑
α-methyltyrosine	Inhibits NA synthesis	Mood ↓ Calming of manic patients
Methyldopa	Inhibits NA synthesis	Mood ↓
Reserpine	Inhibits NA and 5-HT storage	Mood ↓
Electroconvulsive therapy	?Increases CNS responses to NA and 5-HT	Mood ↑
Effects that do not support hypothesis		
Amphetamine	Releases NA and blocks reuptake	None. Euphoria in normal subjects
Cocaine	Inhibits NA reuptake	None. Euphoria in normal subjects
Tryptophan (5-hydroxytryptophan)	Increase 5-HT synthesis	Mood? ↑ in some studies
α- and β-adrenoceptor antagonists	Block actions of NA	Mood slightly ↓ with β-antagonists No effect on manic patients
Methysergide	5-HT antagonist	None
L-dopa	Increases NA synthesis	None
Iprindole	No effect on amine metabolism	Mood ↑

monoamines are in some way important remains reasonably firm, but recent studies have done more to confuse than to clarify the original theory.

Biochemical studies

Many studies have sought to test the amine hypothesis by looking for biochemical abnormalities in CSF, blood or urine, or in post-mortem brain tissue, from depressed or manic patients. They have included studies of monoamine metabolites, receptors, enzymes and transporters, largely with negative results. The major metabolites of noradrenaline and 5-HT, respectively, are 3-methoxy-4-hydroxyphenylglycol (MHPG) and 5-hydroxyindoleacetic acid (5-HIAA). These appear in the CSF, blood and urine (see Chs 8, 9 and 30). There are two fundamental problems in relating changes in the concentration of these metabolites in body fluids to changes in transmitter function in the brain. One is that many secondary factors can affect their concentration, such as diet, transport between CSF, blood and urine, or release of monoamines from non-cerebral sites. The second is that many patients receive drug treatment, which affects the metabolite concentrations markedly.

Studies of urinary MHPG excretion in normal and depressed subjects have shown convincingly that the level is reduced in bipolar depressive patients, and is lower during the depressive than during the manic phase. In unipolar depression, however, MHPG excretion, though highly variable between patients, is not significantly lower than in controls, so support for the monoamine theory is at best equivocal. Plasma noradrenaline actually tends to be higher in depressed than in normal subjects, possibly because it reflects peripheral sympathetic activity, which increases with the anxiety that often accompanies depression. It too shows a cyclic variation in bipolar depressive patients.

Results pertaining to altered 5-HT metabolism are also highly variable (see Maes & Meltzer 1995). Studies of 5-HIAA in CSF and urine have generally failed to find any clear correlation with depression. Low levels of 5-HIAA occur in the brain and CSF of suicide victims, but the association is believed to be with violent behaviour rather than with depression. More consistent changes have been reported in the plasma concentration of L-tryptophan (TRP, the precursor of 5-HT). Though the resting levels are not significantly different in depressed patients, the rise in plasma TRP following an intravenous or oral dose is reduced, implying lower 'TRP-availability'.

Other evidence in support of the monoamine theory is that agents known to block NA or 5-HT synthesis respectively consistently reverse the therapeutic effects of antidepressant drugs that act selectively on these two transmitter systems (see below).

Functional studies

Various attempts have been made to test for a functional deficit of monoamine pathways in depression. Hypothalamic neurons controlling pituitary function receive noradrenergic and 5-HT inputs, which control the discharge of these cells and thus regulate the secretion of pituitary hormones such as ACTH and growth hormone. The plasma cortisol concentration is usually high in depressed patients and it fails to respond with the normal fall when a synthetic steroid, such as dexamethasone, is given. This formed the basis of a clinical test, the *dexamethasone suppression test* (also used in the diagnosis of Cushing's syndrome; see p. 424). Other hormones in plasma are also affected; e.g. growth hormone concentration is reduced and prolactin is increased. In general, these changes are consistent with deficient monoamine transmission, but they are not specific to depressive syndromes.

In summary, there is a good deal of circumstantial evidence to suggest that Schildkraut's monoamine theory is basically correct, though it requires a good deal of special pleading to accommodate many of the clinical observations. There are, however, some glaring inconsistencies, of which the most obvious are the following:

- Neither amphetamine nor cocaine have antidepressant actions, despite their ability to enhance monoamine transmission.
- Antidepressant drugs have a delayed therapeutic effect, which coincides in time with an apparent inhibition rather than facilitation of monoaminergic transmission.
- Some clinically effective antidepressants seem to lack any actions that could enhance monoamine transmission.
- The biochemical changes associated with depression have, in several studies, been identical with changes observed in manic patients.

Recognising these inconsistencies, many authors (see reviews by Ashton 1992, Maj et al. 1984) have suggested more complicated mechanisms than a simple transmitter deficit, and have invoked dopamine, acetylcholine and peptides in delicately balanced arrays in attempts to account for all the facts. Receptor down-regulation and its counterpart, denervation supersensitivity, as long-term effects of agents that enhance or inhibit transmitter function are also often invoked. The complexities of these models generally go beyond the experimental data, and, despite its shortcomings, Schildkraut's basic hypothesis remains the best basis for understanding the actions of antidepressant drugs. It clearly needs to be modified and elaborated, but clinical and experimental studies in the last few years have generated much more prose than progress in this direction, possibly because the methodology for studying transmitter function in humans lacks sufficient precision.

Monoamine theory of depression

- The monoamine theory, proposed in 1965, suggests that depression results from functionally deficient monoaminergic (noradrenaline and/or 5-HT) transmission in the CNS.
- The theory was based on the ability of known antidepressant drugs (TCA and MAOI) to facilitate monoaminergic transmission, and of drugs such as reserpine to cause depression.
- Other pharmacological evidence fails to support the monoamine hypothesis.
- Biochemical studies on depressed patients do not, in general, support the monoamine hypothesis in its simple form.
- An abnormally weak response of plasma cortisol to exogenous steroid (dexamethasone suppression test) is common in depression, and may reflect defective monoamine transmission in the hypothalamus.
- Though the monoamine hypothesis in its simple form is no longer tenable as an explanation of depression, pharmacological manipulation of monoamine transmission remains the most successful therapeutic approach.

ANIMAL MODELS OF DEPRESSION

Progress in unravelling the neurochemical mechanisms is, as in so many areas of psychopharmacology, considerably limited by the lack of good animal models of the clinical condition. There is no known animal condition corresponding to the inherited condition of depression in man, but various procedures have been described which produce in animals behavioural states (withdrawal from social interaction, loss of appetite, reduced motor activity, etc.) typical of human depression (see review by Porsolt 1985). For example, the delivery of repeated inescapable painful stimuli leads to a state of 'learned helplessness', in which even when the animal is free to escape it fails to do so. Mother–infant separation in monkeys, and administration of amine-depleting drugs, such as reserpine, also produce states that superficially resemble human depression. As well as being inherently distasteful, these experiments often require elaborate and

expensive experimental protocols, and there is only a limited amount of information about the similarity of these states to human depression. However, it has been reported that the learned helplessness state and the effect of mother–infant separation can be reversed by tricyclic antidepressants, and increased by small doses of α-methyl p-tyrosine (which inhibits noradrenaline synthesis), suggesting a basic similarity to the human state.

ANTIDEPRESSANT DRUGS

TYPES OF ANTIDEPRESSANT DRUG

Antidepressant drugs fall into the following categories:

- *Tricyclic antidepressants* (TCA), e.g. **imipramine**, **amitriptyline**. These are non-selective (or in some cases noradrenaline-selective) inhibitors of monoamine uptake
- *Selective 5-HT uptake inhibitors*, e.g. **fluoxetine**, **fluvoxamine**, **paroxetine**, **sertraline**.
- *Monoamine oxidase inhibitors* (MAOI), e.g. **phenelzine**, **tranylcypromine**, which are non-selective with respect to the MAO-A and B subtypes (see below), **clorgyline**, **moclobemide**, which are MAO-A-selective.
- *'Atypical' antidepressants*. This group includes (a) compounds that act similarly to TCA but have a different chemical structure (e.g. **nomifensine** and **maprotiline**), and (b) compounds with different pharmacological actions (e.g. **mianserin**, **bupropion**, **trazodone**).

Table 35.2 summarises the main features of these types of drug. A recent update is provided by Frazer (1997).

Mention should also be made of electroconvulsive therapy (ECT) which is effective, and usually acts more rapidly than antidepressant drugs (see later section).

MEASUREMENT OF ANTIDEPRESSANT ACTIVITY

The clinical effectiveness of the first MAOI and TCA drugs was discovered by chance when these drugs were given to patients for other reasons. **Iproniazid**, the first MAOI, was originally used to treat tuberculosis, being chemically related to isoniazid (see Ch. 43); **imipramine**, the first TCA, resembles chlorpromazine (see Ch. 34) and was first tried as an antipsychotic drug. Later, the monoamine hypothesis of depression produced a kind of biochemical rationale for their antidepressant actions and, hence, ways of testing new compounds as a preliminary to clinical trials. The results of such

Table 35.2 Characteristics of the main classes of antidepressant drugs

	TCA	MAOI	5-HT uptake inhibitors	Atypical (see Table 35.5)
Examples	Imipramine Desipramine Amitriptyline Protriptyline Clomipramine	Phenelzine Tranylcypromine Isocarboxazid Moclobemide	Fluoxetine Fluvoxamine Paroxetine Sertraline Citalopram	Maprotiline Bupropion Mianserin Trazodone Venlafaxine
Duration of action	1–3 days	2–4 weeks (except moclobemide ~12 hours)	1–3 days	12–24 hours
Delay in therapeutic effect	2–4 weeks	2–4 weeks	2–4 weeks	2–4 weeks (some claimed faster)
Immediate effect on mood	Sedation, dysphoria	Euphoria	None	Variable, usually slight
Main unwanted effects	Sedation Anticholinergic effects (dry mouth, constipation, blurred vision) Postural hypotension Seizures Mania Impotence	Sedation Postural hypotension Insomnia Weight gain Liver damage (rare)	Nausea Diarrhoea Anxiety and restlessness Insomnia	Variable Generally no anticholinergic effects Hypotension (trazodone) Sedation (trazodone) Seizures (maprotiline, bupropion)
Risk with acute overdose	High (cardiac dysrhythmias, seizures, mania)	Moderate (seizures, mania)	Low	Variable. Some cause seizures or dysrhythmias
Risk of drug interactions	Many	Many, especially sympathomimetic drugs and tyramine-containing foods	Must not be used with MAOI	Few

biochemical tests are successful in predicting clinical efficacy for conventional TCA and MAOI, but fail to predict efficacy with the newer group of atypical antidepressant drugs. Various behavioural tests have also been used (see above), though there is no animal model that satisfactorily resembles depressive illness in man. Some of the most useful tests are the following:

- *Potentiation of noradrenaline effects in the periphery.* Stimulation of sympathetic nerves or administration of noradrenaline causes contraction of smooth muscle, which is enhanced if the noradrenaline reuptake mechanism of the nerve terminal is blocked (see Ch. 8). This test gives positive results with monoamine uptake inhibitors, but does not reveal MAOI or atypical antidepressant activity.
- *Potentiation of the central effects of amphetamine.* Amphetamine works partly by releasing noradrenaline in the brain, and its actions are enhanced both by MAOI and by uptake inhibitors. Some atypical anti-

depressants also give a positive response, making it a useful test for predicting activity in man.

- *Antagonism of reserpine-induced depression.* Reserpine depletes the brain of both noradrenaline and 5-HT, causing various measurable effects (hypothermia, bradycardia, reduced motor activity, etc.) which are reduced by antidepressant drugs. This test also reveals activity among the atypical antidepressants.
- *Block of amine uptake in vitro.* Among TCA there is a fairly good correlation between antidepressant activity and potency in inhibiting noradrenaline or 5-HT uptake, but MAOI and many atypical antidepressants have no effect.

A general point that has to be borne in mind when using in vitro tests to assess potential antidepressants is that many drugs (particularly TCA) are metabolised to pharmacologically active substances in vivo, and it is often unclear whether the parent drug or the metabolite is actually responsible for the clinical effect.

MECHANISM OF ACTION OF ANTIDEPRESSANT DRUGS

In the absence of a simple mechanistic theory to account for antidepressant action (see above), it is useful to look for pharmacological effects that the various drugs have in common, concentrating more on the slow adaptive changes that follow a similar time-course to the therapeutic effect. This approach (see Stahl & Palazidou 1986) has led to the discovery that certain monoamine receptors, in particular β_1- and α_2-adrenoceptors, are

consistently down-regulated following chronic antidepressant treatment. This can be demonstrated in experimental animals as a reduction in the number of binding sites, as well as by a reduction in the functional response to agonists (e.g. stimulation of cAMP formation by β-adrenoceptor agonists). Receptor down-regulation probably also occurs in man, since endocrine responses to **clonidine**, an α_2-adrenoceptor agonist, are reduced by long-term antidepressant treatment. Other receptors have also been studied; α_1-adrenoceptors are not consistently affected, but 5-HT$_2$-receptors are also down-regulated.

How these findings relate to the monoamine theory is far from clear at present. Loss of β-adrenoceptors as a factor in alleviating depression does not fit comfortably with theory, since β-adrenoceptor antagonists are not antidepressant, though it is the most consistent change reported. Impaired presynaptic inhibition, secondary to down-regulation of α_2-adrenoceptors might, it is argued, facilitate monoamine release and thus facilitate transmission.

TRICYCLIC ANTIDEPRESSANT DRUGS

Tricyclic antidepressants are an important group of antidepressants in clinical use. They are, however, far from ideal in practice, and it was the need for drugs which act more quickly and reliably and produce fewer side-effects that led to the introduction of newer 5-HT reuptake inhibitors and 'atypical' antidepressants (see below).

Chemical aspects

TCA are closely related in structure to the phenothiazines (Ch. 34) and were initially produced (in 1949) as potential antipsychotic drugs. **Imipramine** was found to be of no use in schizophrenia, but effective in relieving depression, so other compounds, such as **clomipramine**, were synthesised. They differ from phenothiazines principally in the incorporation of an extra atom into the central ring (Fig. 35.1), which twists the structure so that the molecule is no longer planar as in phenothiazines.

Similar changes to the structure of thioxanthine-type antipsychotic drugs resulted in drugs such as **amitriptyline**. All of these compounds are tertiary amines, with two methyl groups attached to the basic nitrogen atom. They are quite rapidly demethylated in vivo (Fig. 35.2) to the corresponding secondary amines (**desipramine**, **nortriptyline**, etc.), which are themselves active and may be administered as drugs in their own right. Other tricyclic derivatives with slightly modified bridge structures include **protriptyline** and **doxepin**. The pharmacological differences between these drugs are not very

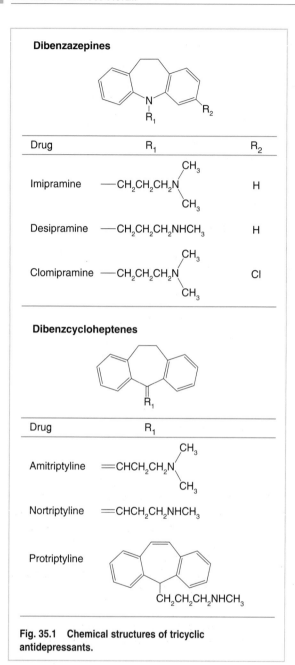

Fig. 35.1 Chemical structures of tricyclic antidepressants.

Table (from figure):

Dibenzazepines

Drug	R_1	R_2
Imipramine	—$CH_2CH_2CH_2N(CH_3)_2$	H
Desipramine	—$CH_2CH_2CH_2NHCH_3$	H
Clomipramine	—$CH_2CH_2CH_2N(CH_3)_2$	Cl

Dibenzcycloheptenes

Drug	R_1
Amitriptyline	=$CHCH_2CH_2N(CH_3)_2$
Nortriptyline	=$CHCH_2CH_2NHCH_3$
Protriptyline	$CH_2CH_2CH_2NHCH_3$

great, and relate mainly to their side-effects, which are discussed below.

Mechanism of action

As discussed above, the main effect of TCA is to block the uptake of amines by nerve terminals, by competition for the binding site of the carrier protein (Ch. 8). Syn-

thesis of amines, storage in synaptic vesicles, and release are not directly affected, though some TCA appear to increase transmitter release indirectly by blocking presynaptic α_2-adrenoceptors. Most TCA inhibit noradrenaline and 5-HT uptake by brain synaptosomes to a similar degree (Fig. 35.3), but have much less effect on dopamine uptake. It has been suggested that improvement of emotional symptoms reflects mainly an enhancement of 5-HT-mediated transmission, whereas relief of biological symptoms results from facilitation of noradrenergic transmission. Interpretation is made difficult by the fact that the major metabolites of TCA have considerable pharmacological activity (in some cases greater than that of the parent drug) and often differ from the parent drug in respect of their noradrenaline/5-HT selectivity (Table 35.3).

In addition to their effects on amine uptake, most TCA affect one or more types of neurotransmitter receptor, including muscarinic ACh receptors, histamine receptors and 5-HT receptors (see Frazer 1997). The antimuscarinic effects of TCA do not contribute to their antidepressant effects, but are responsible for various troublesome side-effects (see below).

The down-regulation of β-adrenoceptors and 5-HT$_2$-receptors that is consistently produced by TCA (Sulser 1983) may be essential for their clinical effects, but the mechanism has not been elucidated (see p. 555).

Actions and unwanted effects

In non-depressed human subjects, TCA cause sedation, confusion and motor incoordination. These effects occur also in depressed patients in the first few days of treatment, but tend to wear off in 1–2 weeks as the antidepressant effect develops. In experimental animals, TCA produce sedation, but they are able to reverse the depressant effect of reserpine treatment.

Unwanted effects with normal clinical dosage

TCA produce a number of troublesome side-effects, mainly due to interference with autonomic control.

Atropine-like effects include dry mouth, blurred vision, constipation and urinary retention. These effects are strong with **amitriptyline**, and much weaker with **desipramine**. *Postural hypotension* occurs with TCA. This may seem anomalous for drugs which enhance noradrenergic transmission, and possibly results from an effect on adrenergic transmission in the medullary vasomotor centre. The other common side-effect is sedation (see above), and the long duration of action means that daytime performance is often affected by drowsiness and difficulty in concentrating.

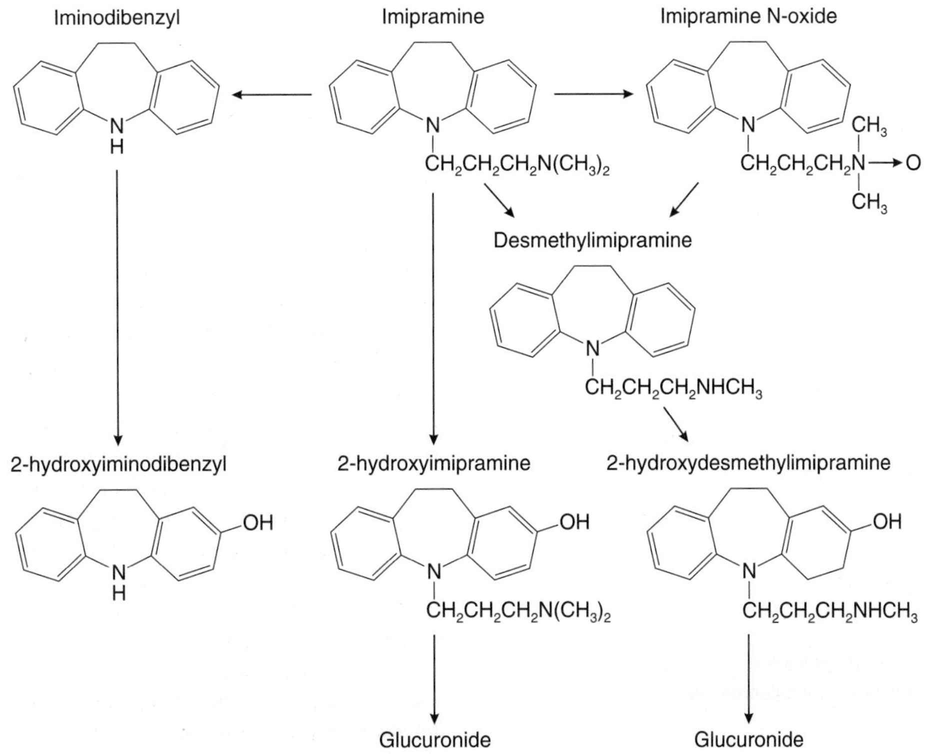

Fig. 35.2 Metabolism of imipramine, which is typical of that of other tricyclic antidepressants.

Interactions with other drugs

TCA are particularly likely to cause adverse effects when given in conjunction with other drugs (see Ch. 48). They are strongly bound to plasma protein, so their effects tend to be enhanced by competing drugs (e.g. **aspirin** and **phenylbutazone**). They rely on hepatic microsomal metabolism for elimination from the body, and this may be inhibited by competing drugs (e.g. antipsychotics and some steroids).

TCA cause a strong potentiation of the effects of alcohol, for reasons that are not well understood, and deaths have occurred as a result of this, when severe respiratory depression has followed a bout of drinking. TCA also interact with various antihypertensive drugs (see Ch. 15) with potentially dangerous consequences, so their use in hypertensive patients requires close monitoring.

Acute toxicity

Antidepressant drugs (most commonly TCA) are often used for attempted suicide, so their acute toxic effects are a matter of some practical importance. In the UK, TCA overdose is estimated to cause about 400 deaths annually. The main effects are on the central nervous system and the heart. The initial effect of TCA overdosage is to cause excitement and delirium, which may be accompanied by convulsions. This is followed by coma and respiratory depression lasting for some days before a gradual recovery. Pronounced atropine-like effects are produced, with flushing, dry mouth and skin, and inhibition of gut and bladder.

Table 35.3 Inhibition of neuronal noradrenaline and 5-HT uptake by tricyclic antidepressants and their metabolites

Drug/metabolite	NA uptake	5-HT uptake
Imipramine	+++	++
Desmethylimipramine (DMI)	++++	+
Hydroxy-DMI	+++	–
Clomipramine (CMI)	++	+++
Desmethyl-CMI	+++	+
Amitriptyline (AMI)	++	++
Nortriptyline (desmethyl-AMI)	+++	++
Hydroxy-nortriptyline	++	++

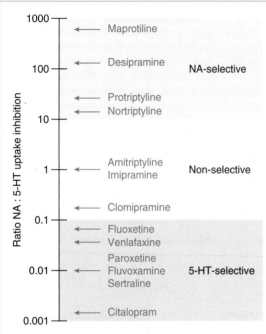

Fig. 35.3 Selectivity of inhibition of noradrenaline and 5-HT uptake by various antidepressants.

Tricyclic antidepressants (TCA)

- TCA are chemically related to phenothiazines, and some have similar receptor-blocking actions.
- Important examples are: imipramine, amitriptyline and clomipramine.
- Widely used as antidepressants.
- Most are long-acting, and they are often converted to active metabolites.
- Important side-effects: sedation (H_1-block); postural hypotension (α-adrenoceptor block); dry mouth, blurred vision, constipation (muscarinic block); occasionally mania and convulsions.
- Dangerous in acute overdose: confusion and mania; cardiac dysrhythmias.
- Liable to interact with other drugs: e.g. alcohol, anaesthetics, hypotensive drugs and NSAIDs, should not be given with MAOI.

Cardiac dysrhythmias are common, usually atrial or ventricular extrasystoles, and sudden death may occur from ventricular fibrillation. The mechanism is not understood, but the dysrhythmias often fail to respond to β-adrenoceptor-blocking drugs, so it is not very likely that enhanced noradrenaline effects on the heart are responsible.

One form of treatment that has been reported to control the main CNS effects is the use of the anticholinesterase, **physostigmine** (see Ch. 7), though this is not recommended routinely. This suggests that the antimuscarinic effects of TCA may be partly responsible, and indeed the symptoms produced closely resemble those of atropine poisoning.

Pharmacokinetic aspects

TCA are all rapidly absorbed when given orally and bind strongly to plasma albumin, most being 90–95% bound at therapeutic plasma concentrations. They bind to extra-vascular tissues, which accounts for their generally large distribution volumes (usually 10–50 l/kg; see Ch. 4) and low rates of elimination. This extravascular sequestration means that extracorporeal dialysis is ineffective in acute overdosage.

TCA are metabolised in the liver by two main routes (Fig. 35.2), namely *N-demethylation*, whereby tertiary amines are converted to secondary amines (e.g. **imipramine** to **desmethylimipramine**, **amitriptyline** to **nortriptyline**) and *ring hydroxylation*. Both the desmethyl and the hydroxylated metabolites commonly retain biological activity (see Table 35.3). During prolonged treatment with TCA, the plasma concentration of these metabolites is usually comparable to that of the parent drug, though there is wide variation between individuals. Inactivation of the drugs occurs by glucuronide conjugation of the hydroxylated metabolites, the glucuronides being excreted in the urine.

The overall half-times for elimination of TCA are generally long, ranging from 10 to 20 hours for **imipramine** and **desipramine** to about 80 hours for **protriptyline**. They are even longer in elderly patients. Thus, gradual accumulation is possible, leading to slowly developing side-effects. The relationship between plasma concentrations and the therapeutic effect may not be simple, according to a study on nortriptyline (Fig. 35.4) which shows that too high a plasma concentration actually reduces the antidepressant effect, and there is quite a narrow 'therapeutic window'. Whether this is true for other antidepressant drugs is not known.

SELECTIVE 5-HT UPTAKE INHIBITORS

Drugs of this type (often termed SSRIs—selective serotonin reuptake inhibitors) include **fluoxetine, fluvoxamine, paroxetine** and **sertraline** (see Table 35.2). Fluoxetine is currently the most prescribed antidepressant. As well as showing selectivity with respect to 5-HT over noradrenaline uptake, they are less likely

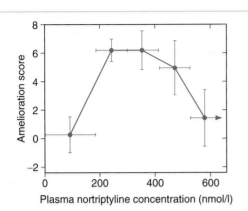

Fig. 35.4 'Therapeutic window' for nortriptyline. The antidepressant effect, determined from subjective rating scales, is optimal at plasma concentrations between 200 nmol/l and 400 nmol/l, and declines at higher levels.

5-HT uptake inhibitors are used in a variety of psychiatric disorders, as well as in depression, including anxiety disorders, panic attacks, and obsessive–compulsive disorder.

5-HT uptake inhibitors (SSRI)

- Examples include fluoxetine, fluvoxamine, paroxetine, sertraline, citalopram.
- Antidepressant actions are similar in efficacy and timecourse to those of TCA.
- Acute toxicity is less than that of MAOI or TCA, so overdose risk is reduced.
- Side-effects include nausea, insomnia. and sexual dysfunction.
- No food reactions, but dangerous 'serotonin reaction' (hyperthermia, muscle rigidity, cardiovascular collapse) can occur if given with MAOI.
- Currently the most commonly prescribed antidepressants; also used for some other psychiatric indications.

---

than TCA to cause anticholinergic side-effects, and are less dangerous in overdose. In contrast to MAOI (see below) they do not cause 'cheese reactions'. They are as effective as TCA and MAOI in treating depression of moderate degree, but probably less effective than TCA in treating severe depression. There is some evidence (see Maes & Meltzer 1995) that patients with low plasma TRP availability respond preferentially to SSRIs.

Pharmacokinetic aspects

SSRIs are well absorbed orally, and have plasma half-lives of 15–24 hours, fluoxetine being longer-acting (24–96 hours). The delay of 2–4 weeks before the therapeutic effect develops is similar to that seen with other antidepressants. Paroxetine and fluoxetine are not used in combination with TCA, whose hepatic metabolism they inhibit, for fear of increasing TCA toxicity.

Unwanted effects

Common side-effects are nausea, anorexia, insomnia, loss of libido and failure of orgasm.

In combination with MAOI, SSRIs can result in 'serotonin syndrome' associated with tremor, hyperthermia and cardiovascular collapse, from which deaths have occurred.

There have been reports of increased aggression, and occasionally violence, in patients treated with fluoxetine, but these have not been confirmed by controlled studies.

In spite of the apparent advantages of 5-HT uptake inhibitors over TCA in terms of side-effects, the combined results of many trials show no overall difference in terms of patient acceptability (Song et al. 1993).

MONOAMINE OXIDASE INHIBITORS (MAOI)

Drugs of the MAOI type were among the first to be introduced clinically as antidepressants, but were largely superseded by tricyclic and other types of antidepressants whose clinical efficacies were considered better and whose side-effects are generally less than those of MAOI. The main examples are **phenelzine**, **tranylcypromine** and **iproniazid**. These drugs cause irreversible inhibition of the enzyme, and do not distinguish between the two main isozymes (see below). Recently, the discovery of reversible inhibitors that show isozyme selectivity has rekindled interest in this class of drug. Though several studies have shown a reduction in platelet MAO activity in certain groups of depressed patients, there is no clear evidence that abnormal MAO activity is involved in the pathogenesis of depression.

MAO (see Ch. 8) is found in nearly all tissues, and exists in two similar molecular forms, coded by separate genes (see Table 35.4). MAO-A has a substrate preference for 5-HT, and is the main target for the antidepressant MAOI. MAO-B has a substrate preference for phenylethylamine, and both enzymes act on noradrenaline and dopamine. Type B is selectively inhibited by **selegiline**, which is used in the treatment of parkinsonism (see Ch. 31). Disruption of the MAO-A gene in mice causes increased brain accumulation of 5-HT and, to a lesser extent, noradrenaline, along with aggressive behaviour (Cases et al. 1995). A family has been reported with an inherited mutation leading to loss of MAO-A

Table 35.4 Substrates and inhibitors for type A and type B monoamine oxidase

	Type A	Type B
Preferred substrates	Noradrenaline 5-HT	Phenylethylamine Benzylamine
Non-specific substrates		Dopamine Tyramine
Specific inhibitors	Clorgyline Moclobemide	Selegiline
Non-specific inhibitors		Pargyline Tranylcypromine Iproniazid

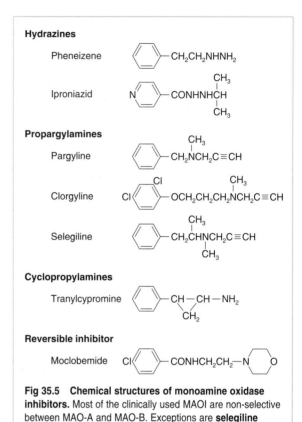

Fig 35.5   Chemical structures of monoamine oxidase inhibitors. Most of the clinically used MAOI are non-selective between MAO-A and MAO-B. Exceptions are **selegiline** (MAO-B-specific, and not used as in antidepressant) and **clorgyline** (MAO-A-specific and effective in depression).

activity, whose members showed mental retardation and violent behaviour patterns. Most antidepressant MAOI act on both forms of MAO, but clinical studies with subtype-specific inhibitors have shown clearly that antidepressant activity, as well as the main side-effects of MAOI, is associated with MAO-A inhibition. MAO is located intracellularly, mostly associated with mitochondria, and has two main functions:

- Within nerve terminals, MAO regulates the free intraneuronal concentration of noradrenaline or 5-HT and hence the releasable stores of these transmitters. It is not involved in the inactivation of released transmitter. The biochemical role of MAO in noradrenergic nerves, and the effect of MAOI on transmitter metabolism are discussed in Chapter 8.
- MAO is important in the inactivation of endogenous and ingested amines which would otherwise produce unwanted effects. An example is tyramine, an ingested amine which is a substrate for both MAO-A and MAO-B, and is important in producing some of the side-effects of MAOI (see below).

Chemical aspects

MAOI possess a phenylethylamine-like structure, similar to MAO substrates (Fig. 35.5); most contain a reactive group (e.g. hydrazine, propargylamine, cyclopropylamine) which enables the inhibitor to bind covalently to the enzyme, resulting in a non-competitive and long-lasting inhibition. Recovery of MAO activity after inhibition takes several weeks with most drugs, but is quicker after tranylcypromine which forms a less stable bond with the enzyme. **Moclobemide** acts as a reversible competitive inhibitor.

MAOI are not particularly specific in their actions and inhibit a variety of other enzymes as well as MAO, including many enzymes involved in the metabolism of other drugs. This is responsible for some of the many clinically important drug interactions associated with MAOI.

Pharmacological effects

MAOI cause a rapid and sustained increase in the 5-HT, noradrenaline and dopamine content of the brain, 5-HT being affected most and dopamine least. Similar changes occur in peripheral tissues such as heart, liver and intestine, and increases in the plasma concentrations of these amines are also detectable. Although these increases in tissue amine content are largely due to accumulation within neurons, transmitter release in response to nerve activity is not increased. In contrast to the effect of TCA, MAOI do not increase the response of peripheral organs, such as the heart and blood vessels, to sympathetic nerve stimulation. The main effect of MAOI is to increase the cytoplasmic concentration of monoamines in nerve terminals, without greatly affecting the vesicular stores which form the pool that is releasable by nerve stimulation. The increased cytoplasmic pool results in an increased rate of spontaneous leakage of monoamines, and also an increased release by indirectly acting sympathomimetic amines such as amphetamine and tyramine (see Ch. 8). This occurs because these amines work by displacing noradrenaline from the vesicles into the nerve terminal cytoplasm, from which it may either leak out and produce a response, or be degraded by MAO (see Fig. 8.9). Inhibition of MAO increases the proportion that escapes, and thus enhances the response. Tyramine thus causes a much greater rise in blood pressure in MAOI-treated animals than in controls. This mechanism is important in relation to the 'cheese reaction' produced by MAOI in humans (see later section).

In normal human subjects, MAOI cause an immediate increase in motor activity, and euphoria and excitement develop over the course of a few days. This is in contrast to TCA which cause only sedation and confusion when given to non-depressed subjects. MAOI (like TCA) are also effective in reversing the behavioural effects of reserpine treatment. The effects of MAOI on amine metabolism develop rapidly, and the effect of a single dose lasts for several days. There is a clear discrepancy, as with TCA, between the rapid biochemical response and the delayed antidepressant effect.

The mechanisms underlying the antidepressant effects of MAOI are not well understood; as discussed above, the superficially similar actions of MAOI and TCA in protecting monoamines from removal or destruction may be misleading, since their effects on neurotransmission appear to be very different. Some evidence for a common, if poorly understood, mechanism of action comes from studies demonstrating that MAOI and TCA produce a similar delayed down-regulation of β-adrenoceptors and 5-HT$_2$-receptors.

Unwanted effects and toxicity

Many of the unwanted effects of MAOI result directly from MAO inhibition, but some are produced by other mechanisms.

Hypotension is a common side-effect; indeed **pargyline** was at one time used as an antihypertensive drug. One possible explanation for this effect—the opposite of what might have been expected—is that amines such as dopamine or octopamine are able to accumulate within peripheral sympathetic nerve terminals and displace noradrenaline from the storage vesicles, thus reducing noradrenaline release associated with sympathetic activity.

Excessive central stimulation may cause tremors, excitement, insomnia, and, in overdose, convulsions.

Weight gain, associated with increased appetite, occurs in a proportion of patients, and can be so extreme as to require the drug to be discontinued.

Atropine-like side-effects (dry mouth, blurred vision, urinary retention, etc.) are common with MAOI, though they are less of a problem than with TCA.

MAOI of the hydrazine type (e.g. **phenelzine** and **iproniazid**) produce, very rarely (less than 1 in 10 000), *severe hepatotoxicity* which seems to be due to the hydrazine moiety of the molecule. Their use in patients with liver disease is therefore unwise.

Interaction with other drugs and foods

Interaction with other drugs and foods is the most serious problem with MAOI, and is the main factor that caused their clinical use to decline. The special advantage claimed for the new reversible MAOI, such as moclobemide, is that these interactions are reduced.

The '*cheese reaction*' is a direct consequence of MAO inhibition, and occurs when normally innocuous amines produced during fermentation (mainly **tyramine**) are ingested. Tyramine is normally metabolised by MAO in the gut wall and liver and so little dietary tyramine reaches the systemic circulation. MAO inhibition allows tyramine to be absorbed, and also enhances its sympathomimetic effect, as discussed above. The result is acute hypertension, giving rise to a severe throbbing headache, and occasionally even to intracranial haemorrhage. Though many foods contain some tyramine, it appears that at least 10 mg of tyramine needs to be ingested to produce such a response and the main danger is from ripe cheeses and from concentrated yeast products such as Marmite. Administration of indirectly acting sympathomimetic amines (e.g. **ephedrine**, **amphetamine**) is also likely to cause severe hypertension in patients receiving MAOI; directly acting agents, such as **noradrenaline** used in conjunction with local anaesthetic injection (see Ch. 40), are not hazardous.

Hypertensive episodes have also been reported in patients given TCA and MAOI simultaneously. The probable explanation is that inhibition of noradrenaline reuptake further enhances the cardiovascular response to dietary tyramine, thus accentuating the cheese reaction. This combination of drugs can also produce excitement and hyperactivity.

MAOIs interact with some drugs to cause not merely an enhancement of their action, but an abnormal syndrome. An important example is the opioid analgesic **pethidine** (see Ch. 37) which may cause severe hyperpyrexia, with restlessness, coma and hypotension when given in combination with MAOI. The mechanism is not known for certain, but it is likely that an abnormal pethidine metabolite is produced because of inhibition of the normal demethylation pathway.

A comparison of the main characteristics of MAOI and other antidepressant drugs is given in Table 35.2.

Monoamine oxidase inhibitors (MAOI)

- Main examples are phenelzine, tranylcypromine, iproniazid and moclobemide.
- Have tended to be superseded by TCA, mainly because of interactions and doubts about efficacy; currently undergoing a revival.
- Action is long-lasting (weeks) because of irreversible inhibition of MAO. Moclobemide has a short duration of action.
- Main side-effects: postural hypotension (sympathetic block); atropine-like effects (as with TCA); weight gain; CNS stimulation, causing restlessness, insomnia, liver damage (rare).
- Acute overdose causes CNS stimulation, sometimes convulsions.
- May cause severe hypertensive response to tyramine-containing foods ('cheese reaction'); should not be given simultaneously with TCA or SSRI. This does not occur with moclobemide.
- Interact with pethidine, causing hyperpyrexia and hypotension.

'ATYPICAL' ANTIDEPRESSANT DRUGS

Uncertainty about the exact biochemical mode of action of antidepressants has meant that the development of new drugs has often been empirical. This has resulted in the introduction of a heterogeneous group of compounds, only distantly related to conventional TCA though sharing some of their biochemical actions. The main claims made for these newer agents are:

- fewer side-effects (e.g. sedation and anticholinergic effects)
- lower acute toxicity in overdose
- action with less delay
- efficacy in patients non-responsive to TCA or MAOI.

In practice, the newer drugs may definitely be better than TCA in respect of side-effects and acute toxicity, but have not proved to be more rapid in action, nor more efficacious.

The properties of some of the more important drugs in this class are summarised in Table 35.5.

They can be divided into two broad categories:

- Non-tricyclic structures with similar noradrenaline-

uptake blocking effects to TCA (e.g. **nomifensine** and **maprotiline**). These drugs are all relatively inactive against 5-HT uptake (see Fig. 35.3), but nomifensine is unusual in being highly active as a dopamine uptake inhibitor.

- Drugs that do not affect amine reuptake (e.g. **mianserin**, **trazodone** and **bupropion**). The mechanism of action of these drugs is uncertain. One possibility is that mianserin increases noradrenaline release by blocking α_2-adrenoceptors on noradrenergic nerve terminals, thus reducing the inhibitory feedback control of noradrenaline release. Bupropion does not, however, work in this way, and indeed seems to lack every expected property of an antidepressant drug except for clinical efficacy.

Atypical antidepressant drugs

- Heterogeneous group, including maprotiline, venlafaxine, trazodone, mianserin and bupropion.
- No common mechanism of action. Some are weak monoamine uptake blockers, but others (e.g. bupropion) act by unknown mechanisms.
- Delay in therapeutic response is similar to TCA and MAOI. Venlafaxine may act more rapidly.
- Most are fairly short-acting.
- Unwanted effects and acute toxicity vary, but are generally less than with TCA.

ELECTROCONVULSIVE THERAPY (ECT)

A tortuous line of reasoning, namely that schizophrenia and epilepsy were considered to be mutually exclusive, led to the use of induced convulsions as therapy for psychological disorders in the 1930s, and its efficacy in treating severe depression has been repeatedly confirmed. ECT in humans involves stimulation through electrodes placed on either side of the head, with the patient lightly anaesthetised, paralysed with a neuromuscular-blocking drug so as to avoid physical injury, and artificially ventilated. Controlled trials have shown ECT to be at least as effective as antidepressant drugs, with response rates ranging between 60% and 80%; it appears to be the most effective treatment for severe suicidal depression. The main disadvantage of ECT is that it often causes confusion and memory loss lasting for days or weeks.

The effect of ECT on experimental animals has been carefully analysed to see if it provides clues as to the mode of action of antidepressant drugs (see Grahame-

Table 35.5   Properties of 'atypical' antidepressant drugs

Drug	Mechanism	Unwanted effects	Advantages	Pharmacokinetics	Notes
Maprotiline	Selective NA* uptake blocker	Atropine-like effects Sedation Seizures Allergic rashes Acute toxicity similar to TCA[†]	No major advantages	Long-acting $t_{1/2}$ ~40 h	Similar to imipramine, with long duration of action
Trazodone	Weak 5-HT uptake blocker Also blocks 5-HT$_2$- and α_2-receptors	Sedation Confusion Hypotension Cardiac dysrhythmias	No atropine-like effects Safe in overdose	Fairly short-acting $t_{1/2}$ 6–12 h	Anxiolytic activity Nefazodone is similar
Mianserin	Blocks α_2-, 5-HT$_2$-, and H$_1$-receptors No effect on monoamine uptake	Sedation Seizures Hypersensitivity reactions including agranulocytosis	No atropine-like effects No cardiovascular effects Safe in overdose	Medium duration of action $t_{1/2}$ ~12 h	
Bupropion	No effect on amine uptake Increase NA release	Dizziness, anxiety, seizures	Safe in overdose	$t_{1/2}$ ~12 h	Relatively safe. Main disadvantage is seizure risk
Venlafaxine	Weak 5-HT uptake inhibitor	As SSRIs, i.e. nausea, anxiety, sexual dysfunction	Claimed to produce rapid effect (~1 week)	$t_{1/2}$ 6–12 h	

*NA = noradrenaline
[†]TCA = tricyclic antidepressant drugs

Smith 1984), but the clues it gives are distinctly enigmatic. 5-HT synthesis and uptake are unaltered, and noradrenaline uptake is somewhat increased (in contrast to the effect of TCA). Decreased β-adrenoceptor responsiveness, both biochemical and behavioural, occurs with both ECT and long-term administration of antidepressant drugs, but changes in 5-HT-mediated responses tend to go in opposite directions (see Maes & Meltzer 1995).

CLINICAL EFFECTIVENESS OF ANTIDEPRESSANT TREATMENTS

The overall clinical efficacy of antidepressants has been established in many well-controlled clinical trials. However, it is clear that a substantial proportion of patients recover spontaneously, and that 30–40% of patients fail to improve with drug treatments. The effects of the drugs are significant, but not miraculous.

The results of a Medical Research Council trial in 1965 showed ECT to be the most effective treatment. **Imipramine** also produced significant improvement, but the MAOI **phenelzine** appeared to be no better than the placebo. The reported ineffectiveness of phenelzine in this trial (together with the incidence of severe hypertensive episodes), caused MAOI to lose favour clinically. Subsequent trials showed that with larger dosage, MAOI may be significantly better than TCA for patients with mild depression, particularly those with symptoms of anxiety. The overall conclusion of many individual trials is that there is little to choose in terms of overall efficacy between any of the drugs currently in use. Nonetheless, individual patients may respond better to one drug than to another.*

Even the most favourable trials show that about 30% of depressed patients fail to show improvement. Attempts to identify which patients will respond on the basis of behavioural or biochemical measurements (e.g. platelet MAO activity, MHPG excretion) have not been successful.

---

*Placebo responses are particularly evident in antidepressant trials, patients being influenced by the attitude of the prescriber, who is in turn influenced by claims for the latest in a long line of drugs. A nightmare for hospital formulary committees!

MOOD STABILISERS

LITHIUM

Lithium is different in its effects from the antidepressant drugs discussed so far, in that it controls the manic phase of manic-depressive (bipolar) illness and is also effective in unipolar depression. Used prophylactically in bipolar depression, lithium is able to prevent the swings of mood and thus to reduce both the depressive and the manic phases of the illness. Given in an acute attack, lithium is effective only in reducing mania and has no effect during the depressive phase. Other drugs (e.g. antipsychotics) are equally effective in treating acute mania; they act more quickly and are considerably safer, so the clinical use of lithium is mainly confined to prophylactic control of manic-depressive illness.

The psychotropic effect of lithium was discovered in 1949 by Cade, who had predicted that urate salts should prevent the induction by uraemia of a hyper-excitability state in guinea pigs. He found lithium urate to produce an effect, quickly discovered that it was due to lithium rather than urate, and went on to show that lithium produced a rapid improvement in a group of manic patients.

Pharmacological effects and mechanism of action

Lithium is clinically effective at a plasma concentration of 0.5–1 mmol/l, and above 1.5 mmol/l it produces a variety of toxic effects, so the therapeutic window is narrow. In normal subjects, 1 mmol/l lithium in plasma has no appreciable psychotropic effects. It does, however, produce many detectable biochemical changes, and it is still extremely unclear how these may be related to its therapeutic effect.

Lithium is a monovalent cation, which can mimic the role of sodium in excitable tissues, being able to permeate the fast voltage-sensitive channels that are responsible for action potential generation (see Ch. 40). It is, however, not pumped out by the Na^+/K^+-ATPase and therefore tends to accumulate inside excitable cells, leading to a partial loss of intracellular potassium, and depolarisation of the cell. Its effects on monoamine metabolism are complex. Given acutely, lithium increases noradrenaline and 5-HT turnover in the brain, but seems to inhibit depolarisation-evoked release. These changes apparently subside during long-term administration, though, clinically, the drug remains effective, so their significance is unclear.

The biochemical effects of lithium are complex, but its therapeutic actions are generally ascribed to two mechanisms (see Atack et al. 1995, Nahorski et al. 1991):

- The phosphatidyl inositol (PI) pathway (see Ch. 2) is blocked at the point where inositol phosphate is hydrolysed to free inositol. This step is required for the regeneration of PI in the membrane after it has been hydrolysed by agonist action, as described in Chapter 2. Lithium thus causes a depletion of membrane PI and accumulation of intracellular inositol phosphate. The result is inhibition of agonist-stimulated IP_3 formation through various PI-linked receptors, and therefore block of many receptor-mediated effects.
- Hormone-induced cAMP production is usually reduced (e.g. the response of renal tubular cells to ADH, and of the thyroid to TSH; see Chs 20 and 25). This is not, however, a pronounced effect in the brain.

It is believed that the effects of lithium on these two important second messenger systems account for its therapeutic effect, and that its cellular selectivity depends on the uptake of lithium in varying amounts reflecting the activity of sodium channels in different cells. This could explain its relatively selective action in the brain and kidney, even though many other tissues use the same second messengers.

Pharmacokinetic aspects and toxicity

Lithium is given by mouth as the carbonate salt, and is excreted by the kidney. About half of an oral dose is excreted within about 12 hours—the remainder, which presumably represents lithium taken up by cells, is excreted over the next 1–2 weeks. This very slow phase means that, with regular dosage, lithium accumulates slowly over approximately 2 weeks before a steady state is reached. The narrow therapeutic limit for the plasma concentration (approximately 0.5–1.5 mmol/l) means that monitoring is essential. Sodium depletion reduces the rate of excretion by increasing the reabsorption of lithium by the proximal tubule, and thus increases the likelihood of toxicity. Diuretics which act distal to the proximal tubule (Ch. 20) also have this effect, and renal disease also predisposes to lithium toxicity.

The main toxic effects that may occur during treatment are:

- Nausea, vomiting and diarrhoea.
- Tremor.
- Renal effects: polyuria (with resulting thirst) resulting from inhibition of the action of antidiuretic hormone. At the same time there is some sodium retention, associated with increased aldosterone

secretion. With prolonged treatment, serious renal tubular damage may occur, making it essential to monitor renal function regularly in lithium-treated patients.

- Thyroid enlargement, sometimes associated with hypothyroidism.
- Weight gain.

Acute lithium toxicity results in various neurological effects, progressing from confusion and motor impairment, to coma, convulsions and death if the plasma concentration reaches 3–5 mmol/l.

OTHER MOOD-STABILISING DRUGS

The toxicity of lithium and need for regular monitoring have led to alternatives being sought for the treatment of bipolar disorder. Drugs currently under investigation include certain antiepileptic drugs–notably **carbamazepine** and **valproate** (see Ch. 36).

Lithium

- Inorganic ion taken orally as lithium carbonate.
- Mechanism of action is not understood. The main biochemical possibilities are:
  —interference with IP_3 formation.
  —interference with cAMP formation.
- Effects on neurotransmitter systems are numerous and complex.
- Acts to control mania as well as depression; Mainly used prophylactically in bipolar depression.
- Long plasma half-life and narrow therapeutic window. Hence, side-effects are common, and monitoring of plasma concentration essential.
- Main unwanted effects: nausea, thirst and polyuria, hypothyroidism, tremor, weakness, mental confusion, teratogenesis. Acute overdose causes confusion, convulsions and cardiac dysrhythmias.
- Action enhanced by diuretic drugs.
- Alternative mood-stabilising drugs include carbamazepine, valproate.

REFERENCES AND FURTHER READING

Atack J R, Broughton H B, Pollack S J 1995 Inositol monophosphatase—a putative target for Li+ in the treatment of bipolar disorder. Trends Neurosci 18: 343–349 (*Review of evidence suggesting that lithium action depends on interference with inositol recycling, and hence role of inositol phosphate in intracellular signalling*)

Ashton H 1992 Brain systems, disorders and psychotropic drugs. Blackwell Scientific Publications, Oxford (*Comprehensive monograph*)

Baker G B, Dewhurst W G 1985 Biochemical theories of affective disorders. In: Dewhurst W G, Baker G B (eds) Pharmacotherapy of affective disorders. Croom Helm, Beckenham (*Useful review of earlier hypotheses relating monoamine disturbances to mood disorders*)

Cases O, Seif I, Grimsby J et al. 1995 Aggressive behaviour and altered amounts of brain serotonin and norepinephrine in mice lacking MAOA. Science 268: 1763–1766 (*Studies on transgenic mice lacking MAO-A, confirming association of monoamine disturbances with behavioural changes*)

Frazer A 1997 Pharmacology of antidepressants. J Clin Psychopharmacol 17: 2S–18S (*Good general review*)

Grahame-Smith D G 1984 The neuropharmacological effects of electroconvulsive shock and their relationship to the therapeutic effect of electroconvulsive therapy in depression. In: Usdin E et al. (eds) Frontiers in biochemical and pharmacological research in depression. Raven Press, New York (*Attempts to correlate biochemical effects of ECT with therapeutic benefit*)

Maes M, Meltzer H Y 1995 The serotonin hypothesis of major depression. In: Bloom F E, Kupfer D J (eds) Psychopharmacology: the fourth generation of progress. Raven Press, New York (*Review showing how emphasis has shifted*

towards the involvement of 5-HT, rather than noradrenaline, in the aetiology of depression*)

Maj J, Przegalinski E, Mogilnicka E 1984 Hypotheses concerning the mechanism of action of antidepressant drugs. Rev Physiol Biochem Pharmacol 100: 1–74 (*General review article, now rather outdated*)

Nahorski S R, Ragan C I, Challiss R A J 1991 Lithium and the phosphoinositide cycle: an example of uncompetitive inhibition and its pharmacological consequences. Trends Pharmacol Sci 12: 297–303 (*Short review article; see also Atack et al. 1995*)

Porsolt R D 1985 Animal models of affective disorders. In: Dewhurst W G, Baker G B (eds) Pharmacotherapy of affective disorders. Croom Helm, Beckenham (*Useful review of animal models, still mainly valid despite date*)

Schatzberg A F, Schildkraut J J 1995 Recent studies on norepinephrine systems in mood disorders. In: Bloom F E, Kupfer D J (eds) Psychopharmacology: the fourth generation of progress. Raven Press, New York (*Review by the father of the monoamine hypothesis; see also Maes & Meltzer 1995*)

Song F, Freemantle N, Sheldon T A et al. 1993 Selective serotonin reuptake inhibitors: meta-analysis of efficacy and acceptability. Br Med J 306: 683–687 (*Summary of clinical trials data, showing limitations as well as advantages of SSRIs*)

Stahl S M, Palazidou L 1986 The pharmacology of depression: studies of neurotransmitter receptors lead the search for biochemical lesions and new drug therapies. Trends Pharmacol Sci 7: 349–354 (*Review emphasising role of secondary receptor changes in the delayed efficacy of antidepressants*)

Sulser F 1983 Mode of action of antidepressant drugs. J Clin Psychiat 44: 14–20 (*General review article*)

36

Antiepileptic drugs and centrally acting muscle relaxants

EPILEPSY

Epilepsy is a very common disorder, affecting 0.5–1% of the population. Usually there is no recognisable cause, although it often develops after brain damage, such as trauma, infection or tumour growth, or other kinds of neurological disease Detailed coverage is given in the textbook by Hopkins et al. (1995).

The characteristic event in epilepsy is the *seizure*, which is associated with the episodic high-frequency discharge of impulses by a group of neurons in the brain. What starts as a local abnormal discharge may then spread to other areas of the brain. The site of the primary discharge and the extent of its spread determines the symptoms that are produced, which range from a brief lapse of attention to a full-blown convulsive fit lasting for several minutes. The particular symptoms produced depend on the function of the region of the brain that is affected. Thus involvement of the motor cortex causes convulsions; involvement of the hypothalamus causes peripheral autonomic discharge, and involvement of the reticular formation in the upper brainstem leads to loss of consciousness.

Abnormal electrical activity during a seizure can be detected by electroencephalograph (EEG) recording from electrodes distributed over the surface of the scalp. Various types of seizure can be recognised on the basis of the nature and distribution of the abnormal discharge (Fig. 36.1).

TYPES OF EPILEPSY

The agreed clinical classification of epilepsy recognises two major categories, namely *partial* and *generalised* seizures, though there is some overlap and many varieties of each.

Partial seizures

Partial seizures are those in which the discharge begins locally, and often remains localised. These may produce relatively simple symptoms without loss of consciousness, such as involuntary muscle contractions, abnormal sensory experiences or autonomic discharge, or they may cause more complex effects on consciousness, mood and behaviour, often termed psychomotor epilepsy. The localised EEG discharge in this type of epilepsy is shown in Figure 36.1D. Partial seizures can often be attributed to local cerebral lesions, and their incidence increases with age.

An epileptic focus in the motor cortex results in attacks, sometimes called *Jacksonian epilepsy*, consisting of repetitive jerking of a particular muscle group, which spreads and may involve much of the body within about 2 minutes before dying out. Though the patient loses voluntary control of the affected parts of the body, he does not lose consciousness. In *psychomotor epilepsy*, which is often associated with a focus in the temporal lobe, the attack may consist of stereotyped purposive movements such as rubbing or patting movements, or much more complex behaviour such as dressing or walking or hair-combing. The seizure usually lasts for a few minutes, after which the patient recovers with no recollection of the event. The behaviour during the

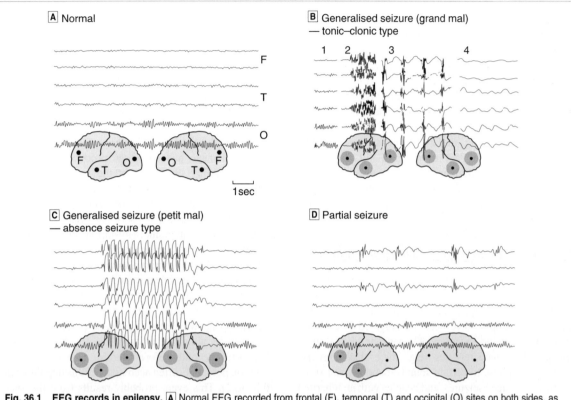

Fig. 36.1 EEG records in epilepsy. **A** Normal EEG recorded from frontal (F), temporal (T) and occipital (O) sites on both sides, as shown in the inset diagram. The α-rhythm (10/s) can be seen in the occipital region. **B** Sections of EEG recorded during a generalised tonic–clonic (grand mal) seizure. 1. Normal record. 2. Onset of tonic phase. 3. Clonic phase. 4. Post-convulsive coma. **C** Generalised absence seizure (petit mal) showing sudden brief episode of 3/s 'spike and wave' discharge. **D** Partial seizure with synchronous abnormal discharges in left frontal and temporal regions. (From: Eliasson S G et al. 1978 Neurological pathophysiology, 2nd edn. Oxford University Press, New York)

seizure can be bizarre and accompanied by a strong emotional response.

Generalised seizures

Generalised seizures involve the whole brain, including the reticular system, thus producing abnormal electrical activity throughout both hemispheres. Immediate loss of consciousness is characteristic of generalised seizures. The main categories are *tonic–clonic seizures* (*grand mal*) and *absences* (*petit mal*). A tonic–clonic seizure consists of an initial strong contraction of the whole musculature, causing a rigid extensor spasm. Respiration stops and defaecation, micturition and salivation often occur. This tonic phase lasts for about 1 minute and is followed by a series of violent, synchronous jerks which gradually dies out in 2–4 minutes. The patient stays unconscious for a few more minutes and then gradually recovers, feeling ill and confused. Injury may occur during the convulsive

episode. The EEG shows generalised continuous high-frequency activity in the tonic phase, and an intermittent discharge in the clonic phase (Fig. 36.1B).

Absence seizures occur in children; they are much less dramatic, but may occur more frequently (many seizures each day), than tonic–clonic seizures. The patient abruptly ceases whatever he or she was doing, sometimes stopping speaking in mid-sentence, and stares vacantly for a few seconds, with little or no motor disturbance. The patient is unaware of his or her surroundings, and recovers abruptly with no after-effects. The EEG pattern shows a characteristic synchronous discharge during the period of the seizure (Fig. 36.1C). A particularly severe kind of epilepsy (Lennox–Gastaut syndrome) that occurs in children is associated with progressive mental retardation, possibly a reflection of excitotoxic neurodegeneration (see Ch. 31). About one-third of cases of epilepsy are familial, but in only one rare type has a gene defect been identified. The mutation turned out to be in a ubiquitous endogenous protease inhibitor, cystatin B, previously unsuspected of any connection with neuronal function.*

Pharmacologically there is a clear distinction between drugs that are effective in absence seizures and those that are effective in other types of epilepsy, though most drugs show little selectivity with respect to the other clinical subdivisions.

With optimal drug therapy, epilepsy is controlled completely in about 75% of patients, but about 10% (50 000 in Britain) continue to have seizures at intervals of 1 month or less, which severely disrupts their life and work. There is therefore a need to improve the efficacy of therapy.

CELLULAR MECHANISMS UNDERLYING EPILEPSY

The underlying neuronal abnormality in epilepsy is poorly understood. Because detailed studies are difficult to carry out on epileptic patients, many different animal models of epilepsy have been investigated (see Upton 1994). These include a variety of genetic strains that show epilepsy-like characteristics (e.g. mice that convulse briefly in response to certain sounds, baboons that show photically induced seizures, and beagles with an inherited abnormality that closely resembles human epilepsy). Local cortical damage (e.g. by applying aluminium oxide paste or crystals of a cobalt salt) results in focal epilepsy. Local application of penicillin crystals has a similar effect, probably by interfering with inhibitory synaptic transmission. Convulsant drugs, such as **leptazol** (see Ch. 38) are often used, particularly in the testing of anti-epileptic agents, and seizures caused by electrical stimulation of the whole brain are used for the same purpose. It has been found empirically that drugs which inhibit leptazol-induced convulsions and raise the *threshold* for production of electrically induced seizures are generally effective against absence seizures, whereas those that reduce the *duration and spread* of electrically induced convulsions are effective in controlling other types of epilepsy, such as tonic–clonic seizures.

An interesting form of experimental epilepsy is the so-called *kindling response* (see review by Mosh & Ludvig 1988). Low-intensity electrical stimulation of certain regions of the limbic system such as the amygdala with implanted electrodes normally produces no seizure response. If a brief period of stimulation is repeated

daily for several days, however, the response gradually increases until very low levels of stimulation will evoke a full seizure. This change is prevented by NMDA-receptor antagonists, and may involve processes similar to those that cause long-term potentiation of synaptic transmission in the hippocampus (see Ch. 29). Kindling may be relevant to human epilepsy (see Mosh & Ludvig 1988). Thus it is often found that surgical removal of a damaged region of cortex fails to cure the epilepsy, as though the abnormal discharge from the region of primary damage had somehow produced a secondary hyperexcitability elsewhere in the brain. Prophylactic treatment with antiepileptic drugs for 2 years following severe head injury reduces the subsequent incidence of post-traumatic epilepsy (Servit & Musil 1981), which suggests that a phenomenon similar to kindling may underlie this form of epilepsy.

By intracellular recording techniques it was shown in 1963 that the group of neurons from which the epileptic discharge originates display an unusual type of electrical behaviour, termed the '*paroxysmal depolarising shift*' (PDS), during which the membrane potential suddenly decreases by about 30 mV and remains depolarised for up to a few seconds before returning to normal. A burst of action potentials often accompanies this depolarisation (Fig. 36.2). This event probably results from the abnor-

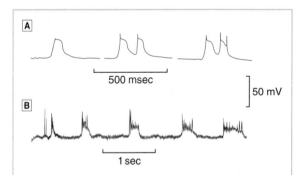

Fig. 36.2 '**Paroxysmal depolarising shift**' compared to experimental activation of glutamate receptors of the N-methyl D-aspartate type. [A] PDS recorded with an intracellular microelectrode from cortical neurons of anaesthetised cats. Seizure activity was induced by topical application of penicillin. [B] Intracellular recording from caudate nucleus of anaesthetised cat. The glutamate analogue, N-methyl D-aspartate was applied by ionophoresis from a nearby micropipette. Note the periodic waves of depolarisation, associated with a burst of action potentials, which closely resemble the paroxysmal depolarising shift. (From: (A) Matsumoto H, Marsan C A 1964 Exp Neurol 9: 286, (B) Herrling P L et al. 1983 J Physiol 339: 207)

---

*Comment of an expert in epilepsy genetics, quoted in *Science*: 'Boy, what a surprising thing!'

mally exaggerated and prolonged action of an excitatory transmitter, and it is interesting that activation of gluta-mate receptors of the NMDA type (see Ch. 29) produces 'plateau-shaped' depolarising responses very similar to the PDS (Fig. 36.2), as well as initiating seizure activity. This membrane response probably occurs because of the voltage-dependent blocking action of Mg^{2+} on channels operated by NMDA receptors (see Ch. 29). Glutamate must undoubtedly participate in the epileptic discharge, and efforts—so far unsuccessful—have been made to develop glutamate antagonists as antiepileptic drugs. It is known that repeated seizure activity can lead to neuronal degeneration, possibly due to 'excitotoxicity' (Ch. 31). Attention is currently focused mainly on an abnormal balance of excitatory and inhibitory synaptic influences as the mechanism underlying epilepsy, though a primary defect leading to membrane instability, such as altered potassium or sodium channel function, cannot be ruled out.

Attempts to find a common neurochemical basis for human or experimental epilepsy have been disappointing, though there are some clues. The quest has focused mainly on a possible deficit in GABA-mediated inhibi-tory transmission, or on an excess of excitatory amino acids (see reviews by Chapman 1988, Porter et al. 1992). The epileptic focus has been reported to contain more glutamate than normal, though the GABA content is not affected. Potassium-stimulated glutamate release from slices of cortex removed surgically from epileptic patients is increased in the epileptic focus compared with normal tissue. There are, however, no major abnor-malities in the activity of enzymes involved in amino acid synthesis or degradation, or in the number of glutamate or GABA receptors, either in the brains of epileptic patients or in the various animal models of epilepsy. Direct evidence favouring an abnormality of amino acid transmission as the underlying cause of seizures is therefore limited.

MECHANISM OF ACTION OF ANTIEPILEPTIC DRUGS

Two main mechanisms appear to be important in the action of anticonvulsant drugs:

- enhancement of GABA action
- inhibition of sodium channel function.

Other mechanisms that may operate with some drugs (see Meldrum 1996) are inhibition of calcium channels and glutamate receptors. Many of the current antiepileptic drugs were developed empirically on the basis of activity in animal models, such as the electroshock seizure test, and their mechanism of action at the cellular level was only clarified later. Some recent drugs (see below) were designed to enhance GABA function in different ways.

Enhancement of GABA action

Several antiepileptic drugs (e.g. **phenobarbitone** and **benzodiazepines**) enhance the activation of $GABA_A$-receptors, thus facilitating the GABA-mediated opening of chloride channels (see Chs 29 and 33). A recently introduced drug **vigabatrin** (see below) acts by inhibiting the enzyme GABA-transaminase which is responsible for inactivating GABA, and **tiagabine** inhibits GABA uptake; both thereby enhance the action of GABA as an inhibitory transmitter. **Gabapentin** (see below) was designed as an agonist at $GABA_A$-receptors, but ironi-cally was found to be an effective antiepileptic drug in spite of having little or no effect on GABA receptors or on the transporter; its mechanism of action remains uncertain (see Macdonald & Kelly 1995).

Nature of epilepsy

- Epilepsy affects about 0.5% of the population.
- The characteristic event is the seizure, which is often associated with convulsions, but may occur in many other forms.
- The seizure is caused by an abnormal high-frequency discharge of a group of neurons, starting locally and spreading to a varying extent to affect other parts of the brain.
- Seizures may be partial or generalised depending on the location and spread of the abnormal neuronal discharge. The attack may involve mainly motor, sensory or behavioural phenomena. Unconsciousness occurs when the reticular formation is involved.
- Two common forms of generalised epilepsy are the tonic–clonic fit (grand mal) and the absence seizure (petit mal). Status epilepticus is a life-threatening condition in which seizure activity is uninterrupted.
- Many animal models have been devised, including electrically and chemically induced generalised seizures, production of local chemical damage, and kindling. These provide good prediction of antiepileptic drug effects in humans.
- The neurochemical basis of the abnormal discharge is not well understood. It may be associated with enhanced excitatory amino acid transmission, impaired inhibitory transmission, or abnormal electrical properties of the affected cells. The glutamate content in areas surrounding an epileptic focus is often raised.
- Repeated epileptic discharge can cause neuronal death (excitotoxicity).
- Current drug therapy is effective in 70–80% of patients.

Inhibition of sodium channel function

Several of the most important antiepileptic drugs (e.g. **phenytoin, carbamazepine, valproate, lamotrigine**) affect membrane excitability by an action on voltage-dependent sodium channels (see Ch. 40) which carry the inward membrane current necessary for the generation of an action potential. Their blocking action shows the property of *use-dependence* (see Ch 40); in other words they block preferentially the excitation of cells that are firing repetitively, and the higher the frequency of firing, the greater the block produced. This characteristic, which is relevant to the ability of drugs to block the high-frequency discharge that occurs in an epileptic fit without unduly interfering with the low-frequency firing of neurons in the normal state, arises from the ability of blocking drugs to discriminate between sodium channels in their *resting*, *open* and *inactivated* states. Depolari-sation of a neuron (such as occurs in the PDS described above) increases the proportion of the sodium channels in the inactivated state. Antiepileptic drugs bind pre-ferentially to channels in this state, preventing them from returning to the resting state, and thus reducing the number of functional channels available to generate action potentials. The same mechanism accounts for the actions of some antidysrhythmic drugs (see Ch. 14), and indeed, phenytoin was previously used for its cardiac, as well as for its antiepileptic effect.

Other mechanisms

In many cases the mechanism of action of antiepileptic drugs remains poorly understood (see Levy et al. 1995, Macdonald & Kelly 1995, Meldrum 1996 for further information). **Phenobarbitone** is a barbiturate (see Ch. 33) which has a considerably greater antiepileptic effect in relation to its sedative action than most other barbiturates, though it is no more effective than other barbiturates in potentiating the action of GABA. Further-more, phenobarbitone is as effective against electrically induced convulsions as it is against leptazol-induced con-vulsions in rats or mice, whereas benzodiazepines, which are known to work by increasing the action of GABA, are without effect on electrically induced convulsions. Phenobarbitone reduces the electrical activity of neurons within a chemically induced epileptic focus within the cortex, whereas diazepam (a benzodiazepine) does not suppress the focal activity but appears to prevent it from spreading. The action of phenobarbitone cannot therefore be due solely to its interaction with GABA, and it is likely that it also acts by inhibiting excitatory synaptic responses, though little is known about the mechanism.

Phenytoin has been studied in great detail. It not only causes use-dependent block of sodium channels (see above), but also affects other aspects of membrane func-tion, including calcium channels, and post-tetanic poten-tiation, as well as intracellular protein phosphorylation by calmodulin-activated kinases, which could also interfere with membrane excitability and synaptic function.*

Obvious targets for potential antiepileptic drugs are the receptors for excitatory amino acids (see Ch. 29), and antagonists acting on NMDA, AMPA or metabotropic glutamate receptors all show anticonvulsant activity in various animal models. Few of these drugs have yet been tested in humans, but in general they show a narrow margin between the desired anticonvulsant effect and un-acceptable side-effects, such as loss of motor coordination.

Mechanism of action of antiepileptic drugs

- Current antiepileptic drugs are thought to act mainly by two main mechanisms:
  — reducing electrical excitability of cell membranes, possibly through use-dependent block of sodium channels
  — enhancing GABA-mediated synaptic inhibition. This may be achieved by an enhanced postsynaptic action of GABA, by inhibiting GABA-transaminase, or by drugs with direct GABA-agonist properties.
- A few drugs appear to act by a third mechanism, namely inhibition of T-type calcium channels.
- Newer drugs act by other mechanisms, yet to be elucidated.
- Drugs that block excitatory amino acid receptors are effective in animal models, but not yet developed for clinical use.

ANTIEPILEPTIC DRUGS

The term 'antiepileptic' is used synonymously with 'anti-convulsant' to describe drugs that are used to treat epilepsy (which does not necessarily cause convulsions) as well as non-epileptic convulsive disorders.

Antiepileptic drugs are fully effective in controlling seizures in 50–80% of patients, though unwanted effects are common (see below). Patients with epilepsy usually need to take drugs continuously for many years, so avoi-dance of side-effects is particularly important. There is clearly a need for more specific and effective drugs, and

---

*The highly complex actions of established antiepileptic drugs are apt to make discouraging reading for those engaged in trying to develop new drugs on simple rational principles. Serendipity, not science, appears to be the path to therapeutic success.

several new drugs have been recently introduced for clinical use. The main well-established antiepileptic drugs (see Table 36.1) are **phenytoin**, **carbamazepine**, **valproate**, **ethosuximide** and **phenobarbitone**, together with various benzodiazepines, such as **diazepam**, **clonazepam** and **clobazam**. The newer drugs, whose place in therapy is still being evaluated, include **vigabatrin**, **gabapentin**, **lamotrigine**, **felbamate**, **tiagabine** and **topiramate**.

PHENYTOIN

Phenytoin is the most important member of the hydantoin group of compounds, which are structurally related to the barbiturates. It is highly effective in reducing the intensity and duration of electrically induced convulsions in mice, though ineffective against leptazol-induced convulsions. Clinically, in spite of its many side-effects and unpredictable pharmacokinetic behaviour, phenytoin is one of the most useful antiepileptic drugs, being effective against various forms of partial and generalised seizures, but not against absence seizures, which may even get worse.

Pharmacokinetic aspects

Phenytoin has certain pharmacokinetic peculiarities that need to be taken into account when it is used clinically. It is well absorbed when given orally, and about 80–90% of the plasma content is bound to albumin. Other drugs, such as **salicylates**, **phenylbutazone** and **valproate**, inhibit this binding competitively (see Ch. 48). This increases the free phenytoin concentration, but also increases hepatic clearance of phenytoin, so may enhance or reduce the effect of the phenytoin in an unpredictable way. Phenytoin is metabolised by the hepatic mixed function oxidase system and excreted mainly as glucuronide. It causes induction, and thus increases the rate of metabolism of other drugs (e.g. oral anticoagulants). The metabolism of phenytoin itself can be either enhanced or competitively inhibited by various other drugs that share the same hepatic enzymes. **Phenobarbitone** produces both effects, and since competitive inhibition is immediate whereas induction takes time, it initially enhances and later reduces the pharmacological activity of phenytoin. **Ethanol** has a similar dual effect.

The metabolism of phenytoin shows the characteristic of *saturation* (see Ch. 4), which means that over the therapeutic plasma concentration range the rate of inactivation does not increase in proportion to the plasma concentration. The consequences of this are:

- The plasma half-life (approximately 20 hours) increases as the dose is increased.

- The steady-state mean plasma concentration, achieved when a patient is given a constant daily dose, varies disproportionately with the dose.

This can be a striking phenomenon. Figure 36.3 shows that in one patient increasing the dose by 50% caused the steady-state plasma concentration to increase more than four-fold.

The range of plasma concentration over which phenytoin is effective without causing excessive unwanted effects is quite narrow (approx. 40–100 µmol/l). The very steep relationship between dose and plasma concentration, and the many interacting factors, mean that there is considerable individual variation in the plasma concentration achieved with a given dose. A radioimmunoassay for phenytoin in plasma is available, and its use has helped considerably in achieving an optimal therapeutic effect. The past tendency was to add further drugs in cases where a single drug failed to give adequate control. It is now recognised that much of the unpredictability can be ascribed to pharmacokinetic variability, and regular plasma monitoring has reduced the use of polypharmacy.

Unwanted effects

Side-effects of phenytoin begin to appear at plasma concentrations exceeding 100 µmol/l and may be severe above about 150 µmol/l. The milder side-effects include vertigo, ataxia, headache and nystagmus, but not sedation. At higher plasma concentrations, marked confusion with intellectual deterioration occurs; these effects occur acutely and are quickly reversible. Hyperplasia of the gums, which is disfiguring rather than harmful, often develops gradually, as does hirsutism, which probably results from increased androgen secretion. Megaloblastic anaemia, associated with a disorder of folate metabolism, sometimes occurs, and can be corrected by giving folic acid (Ch. 18). Hypersensitivity reactions, mainly rashes, are quite common. Phenytoin has also been implicated as a cause of the increased incidence of foetal malformations in children born to epileptic mothers, particularly the occurrence of cleft palate; this appears to be due to the formation of an epoxide metabolite (see Yerby 1988). Severe idiosyncratic reactions, including hepatitis and skin reactions, occur in a small proportion of patients

CARBAMAZEPINE

Carbamazepine is chemically derived from the tricyclic antidepressant drugs (see Ch. 35), and was found in a routine screening test to inhibit electrically evoked seizures in mice. Pharmacologically and clinically its

Table 36.1 Properties of the main antiepileptic drugs

Drug	Cellular mechanisms	Effect on discharge	Main uses	Main unwanted effects	Pharmacokinetics
Phenytoin	Use-dependent block of Na$^+$ channels	Inhibits spread	All types **except** absence seizures	Ataxia, vertigo Gum hypertrophy Hirsutism Megaloblastic anaemia Foetal malformation Hypersensitivity reactions	Half-life approx. 24 h Saturation kinetics; therefore unpredictable plasma levels Plasma monitoring often required
Carbamazepine	Use-dependent block of Na$^+$ channels	Inhibits spread	All types **except** absence seizures Especially temporal lobe epilepsy (Also used in trigeminal neuralgia) Most widely used antiepileptic drug	Sedation, ataxia Blurred vision Water retention Hypersensitivity reactions Leukopenia, liver failure (rare)	Half-life 12–18 h (longer initially) Strong induction of microsomal enzymes; therefore risk of drug interactions
Valproate	Uncertain. Weak effect on GABA-transaminase and on Na$^+$ channels	Unknown	Most types, especially absence seizures	Generally less than with other drugs Nausea Hair loss Weight gain Foetal malformations	Half-life 12–15 h
Ethosuximide*	Inhibition of T-type Ca^{2+} channels	Inhibits 3/s thalamic 'spike and wave' discharge	Absence seizures May exacerbate tonic–clonic seizures	Nausea, anorexia Mood changes Headache	Long plasma half-life (approx. 60 h)
Phenobarbitone†	Enhanced GABA action ? Inhibition of glutamate-mediated excitation	Inhibits initiation of discharge	All types **except** absence seizures	Sedation, depression	Long plasma half-life (> 60 h) Strong induction of microsomal enzymes; therefore risk of drug interactions (e.g. with phenytoin)
Benzodiazepines: e.g. clonazepam, clobazam, diazepam	Enhanced GABA action	Inhibits spread	All types Diazepam used i.v. to control status epilepticus	Sedation Withdrawal syndrome (see Ch. 33)	See Ch. 33
Vigabatrin	Inhibits GABA-transaminase Increases brain GABA content	Inhibits spread	All types Appears to be effective in patients resistant to other drugs	Sedation Behavioural and mood changes (occasionally psychosis)	Short plasma half-life, but enzyme inhibition is long-lasting

*Trimethadione is similar to ethosuximide in that it acts selectively against absence seizures. Its greater toxicity (especially the risk of severe hypersensitivity reactions) means that ethosuximide has largely replaced it in clinical use.
†Primidone is pharmacologically similar to phenobarbitone, and is converted to phenobarbitone in the body. It has no clear advantages, and is more liable to produce hypersensitivity reactions, so is now rarely used.
See text for details of newer antiepileptic drugs (**lamotrigine, felbamate, gabapentin, tiagabine, topiramate**), not yet fully evaluated.

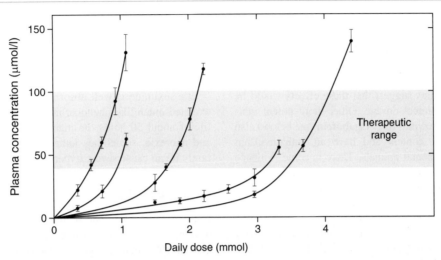

Fig. 36.3 Non-linear relationship between daily dose of phenytoin and steady-state plasma concentration in five individual human subjects. Although the therapeutic range is quite broad (40–100 µmol/l) the daily dose required varies greatly between individuals, and for any one individual the dose has to be adjusted rather precisely to keep within the acceptable plasma concentration range. (Redrawn from: Richens A, Dunlop A 1975 Lancet 2: 247)

actions resemble those of phenytoin, though it appears to be particularly effective in treating complex partial seizures (e.g. psychomotor epilepsy). It is also used to treat various types of neuropathic pain (see Ch. 37), including trigeminal neuralgia, an exceedingly painful condition which is probably associated with a paroxysmal discharge of neurons associated with the trigeminal sensory pathway. Though not obviously associated with epilepsy, this condition probably involves similar neuronal mechanisms. Carbamazepine is now one of the most widely used antiepileptic drugs, and is occasionally used in treating manic-depressive illness (see Ch. 35).

Pharmacokinetic aspects

Carbamazepine is well absorbed. Its plasma half-life is about 30 hours when it is given as a single dose, but it is a strong inducing agent, and the plasma half-life shortens to about 15 hours when it is given repeatedly. A slow-release preparation is used for patients who experience dose-related side-effects (see below).

Unwanted effects

Carbamazepine produces a variety of unwanted effects, ranging from drowsiness, dizziness and ataxia to more severe mental and motor disturbances. It can also cause water retention and a variety of gastrointestinal and cardiovascular side-effects. The incidence and severity of these effects is relatively low, however, compared with

other drugs. Treatment is usually started with a low dose, which is built up gradually to avoid dose-related toxicity. Severe bone marrow depression, causing neutropenia, and other severe forms of hypersensitivity reaction have occurred, but are very rare.

Carbamazepine is a powerful inducer of hepatic microsomal enzymes, and thus accelerates the metabolism of many other drugs, such as phenytoin, oral contraceptives, warfarin, corticosteroids, etc. In general it is inadvisable to combine it with other antiepileptic drugs.

VALPROATE

Valproate is a simple monocarboxylic acid, chemically unrelated to any other class of antiepileptic drug, and in 1963 it was discovered quite accidentally to have anticonvulsant properties in mice. It inhibits most kinds of experimentally induced convulsions, and is effective in many kinds of epilepsy, being particularly useful in certain types of infantile epilepsy, where its low toxicity and lack of sedative action are important, and in adolescents in whom grand mal and petit mal coexist, since valproate (unlike most antiepileptic drugs) is effective against both.

Mechanism of action

Valproate has many effects, and probably works by several mechanisms—a familiar refrain in many areas of neuropharmacology—of which the details remain uncertain (see Macdonald & Kelly 1995)

Valproate causes a significant increase in the GABA content of the brain, and is a weak inhibitor of two enzyme systems that inactivate GABA, namely GABA-transaminase and succinic semialdehyde dehydrogenase, but in vitro studies suggest that these effects would be very slight at clinical dosage. Other more potent inhibitors of these enzymes (e.g. **vigabatrin**; see below) also increase GABA content and have an anticonvulsant effect in experimental animals, There is some evidence that it enhances the action of GABA by a postsynaptic action, but no clear evidence that it affects inhibitory synaptic responses. It also has effects on sodium channels, weaker than those of phenytoin.

Valproate is well absorbed orally and excreted, mainly as the glucuronide, in the urine, the plasma half-life being about 15 hours.

Unwanted effects

Compared with most antiepileptic drugs, valproate is relatively free of unwanted effects. It causes thinning and curling of the hair in about 10% of patients. The most serious side-effect is hepatotoxicity. An increase in serum glutamic oxaloacetic transaminase (SGOT), which signals liver damage of some degree, commonly occurs, but proven cases of valproate-induced hepatitis are rare. The few cases of fatal hepatitis in valproate-treated patients may well have been caused by other factors. Valproate is teratogenic, causing spina bifida and other neural tube defects.

ETHOSUXIMIDE

Ethosuximide, which belongs to the succinimide class, is another drug developed empirically by modifying the barbituric acid ring structure. Pharmacologically and clinically, however, it is different from the drugs so far discussed, in that it is active against leptazol-induced convulsions in animals and against absence seizures in man, with little or no effect on other types of epilepsy. **Trimethadione**, the first drug found to be effective in absence seizures, has now been supplanted by ethosuximide, which has fewer unwanted effects, especially sedation and hypersensitivity reactions, which were a major problem with trimethadione. Ethosuximide is used clinically for its selective effect on absence seizures, but is said to precipitate tonic–clonic seizures in susceptible patients.

The mechanism of action of ethosuximide and trimethadione appears to differ from that of other antiepileptic drugs. The main effect described is inhibition of a particular calcium channel subtype (the T-channel), which may play a role in generating the 3/second firing rhythm in thalamic relay neurons which is a feature of absence seizures (see Macdonald & Kelly 1995, Meldrum 1996).

Ethosuximide is well absorbed, and metabolised and excreted much like phenobarbitone, with a plasma half-life of about 50 hours. Its main side-effects are nausea and anorexia, sometimes lethargy and dizziness. Very rarely it can cause severe hypersensitivity reactions.

PHENOBARBITONE

Phenobarbitone was one of the first barbiturates to be developed and its antiepileptic properties were recognised in 1912. In its action against experimentally induced convulsions and clinical forms of epilepsy it closely resembles phenytoin; it affects the duration and intensity of artificially induced seizures, rather than the seizure threshold, and is correspondingly (like phenytoin) ineffective in treating absence seizures. **Primidone**, now rarely used, acts by being metabolised to phenobarbitone. It often causes hypersensitivity reactions. The clinical uses of phenobarbitone are virtually the same as those of phenytoin, though phenytoin is preferred because of the absence of sedation.

Pharmacokinetic aspects

The pharmacokinetic behaviour of phenobarbitone is straightforward. It is well absorbed and about 50% of the drug in the blood is bound to plasma albumin. It is eliminated slowly from the plasma (half-life, 50–140 hours). About 25% is excreted unchanged in the urine. Since phenobarbitone is a weak acid, its ionisation and hence renal elimination are increased if the urine is made alkaline (see Ch. 5). The remaining 75% is metabolised, mainly by oxidation and conjugation, by the hepatic microsomal enzymes. Phenobarbitone is a particularly effective inducer, and by this mechanism it lowers the plasma concentration of several other drugs (e.g. steroids, oral contraceptive, warfarin, tricyclic antidepressants) to an extent that is clinically important.

Unwanted effects

The main unwanted effect of phenobarbitone is sedation, which often occurs at plasma concentrations within the therapeutic range for seizure control. This is a serious drawback, since the drug may have to be used for years on end. Some degree of tolerance to the sedative effect seems to occur, but objective tests of cognition and motor performance show impairment even after long-term treatment. Other unwanted effects that may occur with clinical dosage include megaloblastic anaemia (similar to that caused by phenytoin), mild hypersensitivity reactions and osteomalacia. Like other barbiturates (see Ch. 48) it must not be given to patients with porphyria. In overdose, phenobarbitone produces coma and respiratory and circulatory failure, as do all barbiturates.

BENZODIAZEPINES

Diazepam, given intravenously, is used to treat *status epilepticus*, a life-threatening condition in which epileptic seizures occur almost without a break. Its advantage in this situation is that it acts very rapidly compared with other antiepileptic drugs. With most benzodiazepines (see Ch. 33), the sedative effect is too pronounced for them to be used as maintenance antiepileptic therapy. **Clonazepam**, and the related compound, **clobazam**, are claimed to be relatively selective as antiepileptic drugs. Sedation is the main side-effect of these compounds, and an added problem may be the withdrawal syndrome, which results in an exacerbation of seizures if the drug is stopped.

NEWER ANTIEPILEPTIC DRUGS

For about 25 years, from the mid-1960s, the inventiveness of the pharmaceutical industry in producing improved antiepileptic drugs dried up. New drugs began to appear from 1990 onwards, the motivation being that existing antiepileptic drug therapy failed to achieve control of seizures in about 25% of cases, and was limited by unwanted effects. Several of these newer drugs are now in use, and more are under evaluation (see reviews by Dichter & Brodie 1996, Perucca 1996, Upton 1994).

Vigabatrin

Vigabatrin, the first 'designer drug' in the epilepsy field, is a γ-vinyl-substituted analogue of GABA that was designed as an inhibitor of the GABA metabolising enzyme, GABA-transaminase. Vigabatrin is extremely specific for this enzyme, and works by forming an irreversible covalent bond. In animal studies, vigabatrin increases the GABA content of the brain, and also increases the stimulation-evoked release of GABA, implying that GABA-transaminase inhibition can increase the releasable pool of GABA and effectively enhance inhibitory transmission. In humans, vigabatrin increases the content of GABA in the CSF. Although its plasma half-life is short, it produces a long-lasting effect, because the enzyme is

> **The major antiepileptic drugs**
>
> - The main drugs in current use are: phenytoin, carbamazepine, valproate and ethosuximide.
> - **Phenytoin**
>   - Acts mainly by use-dependent block of sodium channels
>   - Effective in many forms of epilepsy, but not absence seizures
>   - Metabolism shows saturation kinetics, therefore plasma concentration can vary widely; monitoring is therefore needed
>   - Drug interactions are common
>   - Main unwanted effects are sedation, confusion, gum hyperplasia, skin rashes, anaemia, teratogenesis
>   - Widely used in treatment of epilepsy; also used as antidysrhythmic agent
> - **Carbamazepine**
>   - Derivative of tricyclic antidepressants
>   - Similar profile to that of phenytoin, but with fewer unwanted effects
>   - Effective in most forms of epilepsy (except absence seizures); particularly effective in psychomotor epilepsy; also useful in trigeminal neuralgia
>   - Strong inducing agent; therefore many drug interactions
>   - Low incidence of unwanted effects; principally sedation, ataxia, mental disturbances, water retention
> - **Valproate**
>   - Chemically unrelated to other antiepileptic drugs
>   - Mechanism of action not clear; weak inhibition of GABA-transaminase; some effect on sodium channels
>   - Relatively few unwanted effects; baldness, teratogenicity, liver damage (rare, but serious)
> - **Ethosuximide**
>   - The main drug used to treat absence seizures, may exacerbate other forms
>   - Acts by blocking T-type Ca^{2+}-channels
>   - Relatively few unwanted effects, mainly nausea and anorexia
> - Secondary drugs include:
>   - Phenobarbitone: highly sedative
>   - Various benzodiazepines (e.g. clonazepam); diazepam used in treating status epilepticus.

blocked irreversibly, and so can be given by mouth once daily. Evidence of neurotoxicity was found in animals, but has not been found in humans, removing one of the main question marks hanging over this drug.

The main drawback of vigabatrin is the occurrence of depression, and occasionally psychotic disturbances, in a minority of patients; otherwise it is relatively free from side-effects.

Vigabatrin has been reported to be effective in a substantial proportion of patients resistant to the established drugs, and may represent an important therapeutic advance.

Lamotrigine

Lamotrigine, though chemically unrelated, resembles phenytoin and carbamazepine in its pharmacological effects, acting on sodium channels, and inhibiting the release of excitatory amino acids. It appears that, despite its similar mechanism of action, lamotrigine has a broader therapeutic profile than the earlier drugs, with significant efficacy against absence seizures. Its main side-effects are nausea, dizziness and ataxia, and hypersensitivity reactions (mainly mild rashes, but occasionally more severe). Its plasma half-life is about 24 hours, with no particular pharmacokinetic anomalies, and it is taken orally.

Felbamate

Felbamate is an analogue of an obsolete anxiolytic drug, meprobamate. It is active in many animal seizure models, and has a broader clinical spectrum than earlier antiepileptic drugs, but its mechanism of action at the cellular level is uncertain. It has only a weak effect on sodium channels, and little effect on GABA, combined with some inhibition at the facilitatory glycine site of the NMDA receptor (Ch. 29). Its acute side-effects are mild, mainly nausea, irritability and insomnia, but it occasionally causes severe reactions, resulting in aplastic anaemia or hepatitis. For this reason, its recommended use is limited to a form of intractable epilepsy in children (Lennox–Gastaut syndrome) that is unresponsive to other drugs. Its plasma half-life is about 24 hours, and it can enhance the plasma concentration of other antiepileptic drugs given concomitantly.

Gabapentin

Gabapentin was designed as a simple analogue of GABA that would be sufficiently lipid-soluble to penetrate the blood–brain barrier. It turned out to be an effective anticonvulsant in several animal models, but, surprisingly, not a GABA-mimetic. It has no effect on any of the major neurotransmitter mechanisms, or on sodium or calcium channels, but binds with high affinity to a specific site in the brain, which appears to be the amino acid transporter system that occurs in many neurons and other cells. The mechanistic implications of this are unknown, and its mode of action remains an intriguing mystery. The side-effects of gabapentin (mainly sedation and ataxia) are less severe than with many antiepileptic drugs. The absorption of gabapentin from the intestine depends on the amino acid carrier system (see Ch. 4), and shows the property of saturability, which means that increasing the dose does not proportionately increase the amount absorbed. This makes gabapentin relatively safe, and free

of side-effects associated with overdosing. Its plasma half-life is about 6 hours, requiring dosing two to three times daily. It is free of interactions with other drugs. Efficacy in patients resistant to conventional drugs has been claimed, but the clinical role of gabapentin remains to be established.

Tiagabine

Tiagabine, an analogue of GABA which is able to penetrate the blood–brain barrier, acts by inhibiting GABA uptake, and was the product of rational drug design. It binds selectively to one of the four known molecular subtypes of the GABA transporter, which is expressed in both neurons and glial cells. It enhances the extracellular GABA concentration, as measured in microdialysis experiments, and also potentiates and prolongs GABA-mediated synaptic responses in the brain. It has a short plasma half-life, and its main side-effects are drowsiness and confusion. The clinical usefulness of tiagabine has not yet been fully assessed.

Topiramate

Topiramate is a recently introduced drug which, mechanistically, appears to do a little of everything, blocking sodium channels, enhancing the action of GABA, blocking AMPA receptors and, for good measure, weakly inhibiting carbonic anhydrase. Its spectrum of action resembles that of phenytoin, and it is claimed to produce less severe side-effects, as well as being devoid of the pharmacokinetic properties that cause trouble with phenytoin. Its main drawback is that (like many antiepileptic drugs) it is teratogenic in animals, so it should not be used in women of child-bearing age. Currently, it

---

Clinical uses of antiepileptic drugs

- *Tonic–clonic (grand mal) seizures*: **carbamazepine** preferred because of low incidence of side-effects), **phenytoin, valproate**. Use of single drug is preferred when possible, because of risk of pharmacokinetic interactions. Newer agents (not yet fully assessed) include **vigabatrin, lamotrigine, felbamate, gabapentin**.
- *Partial (focal) seizures*: **carbamazepine, valproate**; **clonazepam** or **phenytoin** are alternatives.
- *Absence seizures (petit mal)*: **ethosuximide** or **valproate**. Valproate is used when absence seizures coexist with tonic–clonic seizures, since most drugs used for tonic–clonic seizures may worsen absence seizures.
- *Myoclonic seizures*: **valproate** or **clonazepam**.
- *Status epilepticus*: must be treated as an emergency, with diazepam intravenously or (in infants with no accessible veins) rectally.

is recommended for use as add-on therapy in refractory cases of epilepsy.

MUSCLE SPASM AND CENTRALLY ACTING MUSCLE RELAXANTS

Many diseases of the brain and spinal cord produce an increase in muscle tone which can be painful and disabling. Spasticity, resulting from birth injury or cerebral vascular disease, and the paralysis produced by spinal cord lesions are examples. Local injury or inflammation, as in arthritis, can have the same effect, and chronic back pain is also often associated with local muscle spasm.

Certain centrally acting drugs are available which have the effect of reducing the background tone of the muscle without seriously affecting its ability to contract transiently under voluntary control. The distinction between voluntary movements and 'background tone' is not clear cut, and the selectivity of those drugs is not complete. Postural control, for example, is usually jeopardised by centrally acting muscle relaxants. Furthermore, drugs that affect motor control generally produce rather widespread effects on the central nervous system, and drowsiness and confusion turn out to be very common side-effects of these agents. The main group of drugs that have been used to control muscle tone are:

- **mephenesin** and related drugs
- **baclofen**
- **benzodiazepines** (see Ch. 33)
- **botulinum toxin** (see Ch. 7). Injected into a muscle, this neurotoxin causes long-lasting paralysis confined to the site of injection. Its use to treat local muscle spasm is increasing.

Mephenesin

Mephenesin is an aromatic ether, which acts mainly on the spinal cord, causing a selective inhibition of poly-synaptic excitation of motor neurons. Thus it strongly inhibits the flexor reflex without affecting the tendon jerk reflex, which is monosynaptic, and it abolishes de-cerebrate rigidity. Its mechanism of action at the cellular level is unknown. Mephenesin is little used clinically, though it is sometimes given as an intravenous injection to reduce acute muscle spasm resulting from injury.

Baclofen

Baclofen (see Ch. 29) is a chlorophenyl derivative of GABA, originally prepared as a lipophilic GABA-like agent in order to assist penetration of the blood–brain barrier, which GABA itself does not do. Baclofen is a selective agonist at presynaptic $GABA_B$-receptors (see Ch. 29). The antispastic action of baclofen is exerted mainly on the spinal cord, where it inhibits both mono-synaptic and polysynaptic activation of motor neurons. It is effective when given by mouth, and is used in the treatment of spasticity associated with multiple sclerosis or spinal injury. However, it is ineffective in cerebral spasticity caused by birth injury.

Baclofen produces various unwanted effects, particularly drowsiness, motor incoordination and nausea, and it may also have behavioural effects. It is not useful in epilepsy.

REFERENCES AND FURTHER READING

Chapman A G 1988 Amino acid abnormalities in plasma, CSF and brain in epilepsy. In: Pedley T A, Meldrum B S (eds) Recent advances in epilepsy. Churchill Livingstone, Edinburgh, vol 4 *(Evidence for enhanced glutamate-mediated transmission in epileptic brains)*

Dichter M A, Brodie M J 1996 New antiepileptic drugs. N Engl J Med 334: 1583–1590 *(Review of clinical pharmacology of new drugs)*

Hopkins A, Shorvon S, Cascino G 1995 Epilepsy, 2nd edn. Chapman & Hall, London *(Comprehensive general textbook)*

Levy R H, Mattson R H, Meldrum B S, Dreifuss F E, Penry J K (eds) 1995 Antiepileptic drugs, 4th edn. Raven Press, New York *(Comprehensive general textbook)*

Macdonald R L, Kelly K M 1995 Antiepileptic drug mechanisms of action. Epilepsia 36 (suppl 2): S2–S12 *(Excellent review article summarising current knowledge on mechanisms)*

Meldrum B S 1996 Update on the mechanism of action of antiepileptic drugs. Epilepsia 37 (suppl 6): S4–S11 *(Excellent review article summarising current knowledge on mechanisms)*

Mosh S L, Ludvig N 1988 Kindling. In: Pedley T A, Meldrum B S (eds) Recent advances in epilepsy. Churchill Livingstone, Edinburgh, vol 4 *(Describes kindling model in relation to epileptic syndromes)*

Perucca E 1996 The new generation of antiepileptic drugs: advantages and disadvantages. Br J Clin Pharmacol 42: 531–543 *(Review of clinical pharmacology of recently introduced drugs)*

Porter R J, Schmidt D, Treiman D M, Nadi N S 1992 Pharmacologic approaches to the treatment of focal seizures. Adv Neurol 57: 607–634 *(Focuses mainly on glutamate antagonists—disappointing so far)*

Servit Z, Musil F 1981 Prophylactic treatment of post-traumatic epilepsy: results of a long-term follow-up in Czechoslovakia. Epilepsia 22: 15–20 *(Important study showing that early use of antiepileptic drugs improves prognosis after head injury)*

Upton N 1994 Mechanisms of action of new antiepileptic drugs: rational design and serendipitous findings. Trends Pharmacol Sci 15: 456–463 *(Useful review article)*

Yerby M S 1988 Teratogenicity of antiepileptic drugs. In: Pedley T A, Meldrum B S (eds) Recent advances in epilepsy. Churchill Livingstone, Edinburgh, vol 4 *(Reviews data relating to teratogenic risk of antiepileptic drugs—an important problem)*

37

Analgesic drugs

The control of pain is one of the most important uses to which drugs are put. Analgesic drugs fall into four main categories:

- Morphine-like drugs (**opioids**)
- Non-steroidal anti-inflammatory drugs (**aspirin** and related substances; see Ch. 13)
- **Local anaesthetics** (see Ch. 40)
- Various centrally acting non-opioid drugs, for example:
  —Antidepressants (e.g. **amitriptyline**), which appear to have an analgesic action in patients who are not suffering from depression. This may be related to

their effect of enhancing monoaminergic transmission (see Ch. 35), since inhibitory monoaminergic pathways are known to be important in modulating pain transmission (see below).
  —Drugs used for specific painful conditions, for example, **carbamazepine** (used in trigeminal neuralgia; Ch. 36), **ergotamine** (used in migraine; Ch. 9).

Morphine-like drugs, as well as most of the drugs in the last group, produce analgesia by acting mainly on the central nervous system; local anaesthetics act peripherally, while aspirin-like drugs appear to act by both central and peripheral effects. In this chapter we consider first some physiological aspects of pain perception, and then present the pharmacology of the opioid drugs in detail. Finally, new pharmacological approaches are briefly discussed.

NEURAL MECHANISMS OF PAIN SENSATION

Excellent detailed accounts of the neural basis of pain can be found in Besson & Chaouch (1987), Fields (1987), and Wall & Melzack (1994).

NOCICEPTIVE AFFERENT NEURONS

Under normal conditions, pain is associated with electrical activity in small diameter primary afferent fibres of peripheral nerves. These nerves have sensory endings in peripheral tissues, and are activated by stimuli of various kinds (mechanical, thermal, chemical; Cesare & McNaughton 1997, Kress & Reeh 1996). They are distinguished from other sorts of mechanical and thermal receptors by their higher threshold, since they are normally activated only by stimuli of noxious intensity— sufficient to cause some degree of tissue damage. Recordings of activity in single afferent fibres in human subjects have shown that stimuli sufficient to excite these small afferent fibres also evoke a painful sensation. Many of these fibres are non-myelinated C-fibres with low conduction velocities (<1 m/s); this group is known as *C-polymodal nociceptors* (PMN). Others are fine myelinated (Aδ) fibres, which conduct more rapidly but respond to similar peripheral stimuli. Though there are some species differences, the majority of the C-fibres are associated with polymodal nociceptive endings. Afferents from muscle and viscera also convey nociceptive information. In the nerves from these tissues, the small myelinated fibres are connected to high-threshold mechanoreceptors, while the unmyelinated fibres are connected to polymodal nociceptors, as in the skin.

Experiments on human subjects, in which recording or stimulating electrodes are applied to cutaneous sensory nerves, have shown that activity in the Aδ-fibres causes a sensation of sharp, well-localised pain, whereas C-fibre activity causes a dull burning pain.

The mechanism by which a variety of different stimuli can evoke activity in nociceptive nerve terminals is only partly understood. With many pathological conditions, tissue injury is the immediate cause of the pain, and this results in the local release of a variety of chemical agents which are assumed to act on the nerve terminals, either activating them directly or enhancing their sensitivity to other forms of stimulation. The pharmacological properties of nociceptive nerve terminals are discussed in more detail below.

The cell bodies of spinal nociceptive afferent fibres lie in dorsal root ganglia; fibres enter the spinal cord via the dorsal roots, ending in the grey matter of the dorsal horn (Fig. 37.1). Most of the nociceptive afferents terminate in the superficial region of the dorsal horn, the C-fibres and some Aδ-fibres innervating cell bodies in laminae I and II, while other A-fibres penetrate deeper into the dorsal horn (lamina V). Cells in laminae I and V give rise to the main projection pathways from the dorsal horn to the thalamus.

The non-myelinated afferent neurons contain several neuropeptides (see Ch. 10), particularly substance P and calcitonin gene-related peptide (CGRP) These are released as mediators at both the central and peripheral terminals, and play an important role in the pathology of pain.

MODULATION IN THE NOCICEPTIVE PATHWAY

Acute pain is generally well accounted for in terms of *nociception*—an excessive noxious stimulus giving rise to an intense and unpleasant sensation. In contrast, most chronic pain states* are associated with aberrations of

---

*Defined as pain which outlasts the precipitating tissue injury. Many clinical pain states fall into this category. The dissociation of pain from noxious input is most evident in 'phantom limb' pain which occurs after amputations and may be very severe. The pain is usually not relieved by local anaesthetic injections, implying that electrical activity in afferent fibres is not an essential component. At the other extreme, noxious input with no pain, there are many well-documented reports of mystics and showmen who subject themselves to horrifying ordeals with knives, burning embers, nails and hooks (undoubtedly causing massive afferent input) without apparently suffering pain.

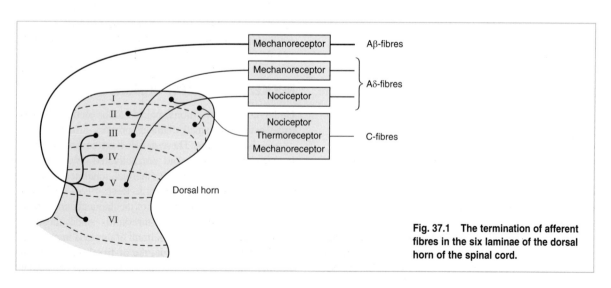

Fig. 37.1 The termination of afferent fibres in the six laminae of the dorsal horn of the spinal cord.

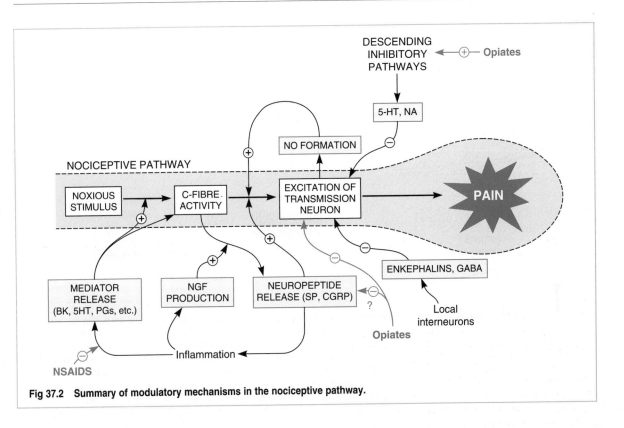

Fig 37.2   Summary of modulatory mechanisms in the nociceptive pathway.

the normal physiological pathway, giving rise to *hyperalgesia* (an increased amount of pain associated with a mild noxious stimulus), *allodynia* (pain evoked by a non-noxious stimulus), or spontaneous spasms of pain with no precipitating stimulus. An analogy is with an old radio set that plays uncontrollably loudly (hyperalgesia), receives two stations at once (allodynia), or produces random shrieks and whistles (spontaneous pain spasms). These distortions in the transmission line are beginning to be understood in terms of various types of positive and negative modulation in the nociceptive pathway, discussed in more detail below. Some of the main mechanisms are summarised in Figure 37.2.

HYPERALGESIA AND ALLODYNIA

Anyone with a burn or a sprained ankle has experienced hyperalgesia and allodynia. Hyperalgesia involves both sensitisation of peripheral nociceptive nerve terminals and central facilitation of transmission at the level of the dorsal horn and thalamus—changes defined by the term *neuroplasticity* (Ch. 29). The peripheral component is due to the action of mediators such as *bradykinin*, *prostaglandins*, etc. acting on the nerve terminals (see

below). The central component reflects facilitation of synaptic transmission. This has been well studied in the dorsal horn (see McMahon et al. 1993). The synaptic responses of dorsal horn neurons to nociceptive inputs display the phenomenon of 'wind-up'—i.e. the synaptic potentials steadily increase in amplitude with each stimulus—when repeated stimuli are delivered at physiological frequencies (see Fig. 37.3). This activity-dependent facilitation of transmission has many features in common with the phenomenon of long-term potentiation (LTP) in the hippocampus, described in Chapter 29, and the chemical mechanisms underlying it also appear to be similar (see McMahon et al. 1993; Fig. 37.3). In the dorsal horn, the facilitation is blocked by NMDA-receptor antagonists, also by antagonists of *substance P*, a slow excitatory transmitter released by nociceptive afferent neurons (see above), and by inhibitors of NO synthesis. Substance P produces a slow depolarising response in the postsynaptic cell, which builds up during repetitive stimulation, and (as with LTP; see Fig 29.6) is believed to enhance NMDA-receptor-mediated transmission. This results in calcium influx and activation of NO synthase (see Ch. 11), the released NO acting to facilitate transmission by mechanisms that have yet to be

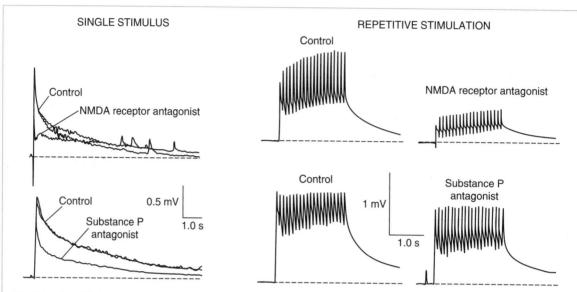

SINGLE STIMULUS

Control

NMDA receptor antagonist

Control

Substance P
antagonist

0.5 mV

1.0 s

REPETITIVE STIMULATION

Control

NMDA receptor antagonist

Control

Substance P
antagonist

1 mV

1.0 s

Fig 37.3   Effect of glutamate and substance P antagonist on nociceptive transmission in the rat spinal cord. The rat paw was inflamed by ultraviolet irradiation 2 days before the experiment, a procedure which induces hyperalgesia and spinal cord facilitation. The synaptic response was recorded from the ventral root, in response to stimulation of C-fibres in the dorsal root with single stimuli (left) or repetitive stimuli (right). The effect of the NMDA-receptor antagonist D-AP5 (see Ch. 29) and the substance P antagonist RP 67580 (NK_2-receptor-selective) are shown. The slow component of the synaptic response is reduced by both antagonists (left-hand traces), as is the 'wind-up' in response to repetitive stimulation (right-hand traces). These effects are much less pronounced in the normal animal. Thus both glutamate, acting on NMDA receptors, and substance P, acting on NK_2-receptors, are involved in nociceptive transmission, and their contribution increases as a result of inflammatory hyperalgesia. (Records kindly provided by L Urban and S W Thompson)

elucidated. Substance P and CGRP released from primary afferent neurons also act in the periphery, promoting inflammation by their effects on blood vessels and cells of the immune system (Ch. 12). This mechanism, known as *neurogenic inflammation*, acts to amplify and sustain the inflammatory reaction, and the accompanying activation of nociceptive afferent fibres. There is evidence that these processes (summarised in Fig. 37.2) are also involved in pathological hyperalgesia (e.g. that associated with inflammatory responses), in which central facilitation is known to occur (see Coderre et al. 1993). The importance of repetitive C-fibre activity in setting up a long-lasting state of hyperexcitability in the spinal cord has led to the concept of *pre-emptive analgesia*, whereby, in the anaesthetised patient, the field of a surgical operation is treated with local anaesthetic in order to block the intense C-fibre discharge associated with the incision and operation, thus preventing, it is argued, the spinal cord hyperexcitability from being established, and thereby reducing postoperative pain. Clinical reports on the efficacy of this procedure give conflicting views (see Dahl & Kehlet 1993). Other mechanisms can also

contribute to central facilitation. Nerve growth factor (NGF) a cytokine-like mediator produced by peripheral tissues, particularly in inflammation, acts specifically on nociceptive afferent neurons, increasing their electrical excitability, chemosensitivity and peptide content, and also promoting the formation of synaptic contacts. Increased NGF production may be an important mechanism by which nociceptive transmission becomes facilitated by tissue damage, leading to hyperalgesia (see McMahon 1996). Increased gene expression in dorsal horn neurons (particularly of the opioid peptide dynorphin) accompanies peripheral inflammation and activity in the nociceptive pathway; this peptide, which has both excitatory and inhibitory effects in the spinal cord, also plays a part in long-term modulation, though its exact role is unclear (see Dubner & Ruda 1992).

THE SUBSTANTIA GELATINOSA AND THE GATE CONTROL THEORY

Cells of lamina II of the dorsal horn (the substantia gelatinosa, SG) are mainly short inhibitory interneurons projecting to lamina I and lamina V, and they regulate transmission at the first synapse of the nociceptive pathway, between the primary afferent fibres and the spinothalamic tract transmission neurons. This gatekeeper function gave rise to the term 'gate control theory', proposed by Wall & Melzack in 1965. According to this view (summarised in Fig. 37.4) the SG cells respond both to the activity of afferent fibres entering the cord (thus allowing the arrival of impulses via one group of afferent fibres to regulate the transmission of impulses via another pathway) and to the activity of descending pathways (see below). The SG is rich in both opioid peptides and opioid receptors and may be an important site of action for morphine-like drugs (see later section).

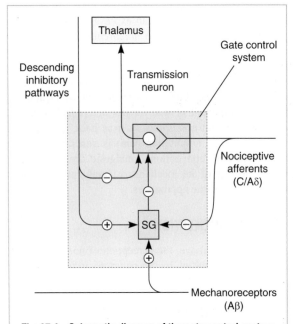

Fig. 37.4 Schematic diagram of the gate control system. This system regulates the passage of impulses from the peripheral afferent fibres to the thalamus via transmission neurons originating in the dorsal horn. Neurons in the *substantia gelatinosa* (SG) of the dorsal horn act to inhibit the transmission pathway. Inhibitory interneurons are activated by descending inhibitory neurons or by non-nociceptive afferent input. They are inhibited by nociceptive C-fibre input, so the persistent C-fibre activity facilitates excitation of the transmission cells by either nociceptive or non-nociceptive inputs. This autofacilitation causes successive bursts of activity in the nociceptive afferents to become increasingly effective in activating transmission neurons. Details of the interneuronal pathways are not shown. (From: Melzack R, Wall P D 1982 The challenge of pain. Penguin, Harmondsworth)

Further studies have added extra detail to the dorsal horn circuitry shown schematically in Figure 37.4 (see Fields & Basbaum 1994), and it is evident that similar 'gate' mechanisms also operate in the thalamus.

From the spinothalamic tracts, the projection fibres form synapses mainly in the ventral and medial parts of the thalamus with cells whose axons run to the somatosensory cortex. In the medial thalamus in particular, many cells respond specifically to noxious stimuli in the periphery and lesions in this area cause analgesia. Functional imaging studies in conscious subjects (see Rainville et al. 1997) suggest that the affective component of pain sensation involves a specific region of the cingulate cortex, distinct from the somatosensory cortex (lesions of which do not prevent the sensation of pain, though they can alter its quality).

DESCENDING INHIBITORY CONTROLS

As mentioned above, descending pathways constitute one of the gating mechanisms that control impulse transmission in the dorsal horn (see Fields & Basbaum 1994). A key part of this descending system is the *periaqueductal grey* (PAG) area of the midbrain, a small area of grey matter surrounding the central canal. In 1969 Reynolds found that electrical stimulation of this brain area in the rat caused analgesia sufficiently intense that abdominal surgery could be performed without anaesthesia and without eliciting any marked response. Non-painful sensations were unaffected. The PAG receives inputs from many other brain regions, including the hypothalamus, cortex and thalamus, and is thought to represent the mechanism whereby cortical and other inputs act to control the nociceptive 'gate' in the dorsal horn.

The main neuronal pathway activated by PAG stimulation runs first to an area of the medulla close to the midline, known as the *nucleus raphe magnus* (NRM), and thence via fibres running in the dorsolateral funiculus of the spinal cord, which form synaptic connections on dorsal horn interneurons. The major transmitter at these synapses is 5-HT, and the interneurons in turn act to inhibit the discharge of spinothalamic neurons (Fig. 37.5). The NRM itself receives an input from spinothalamic neurons, via the adjacent *nucleus reticularis paragigantocellularis* (NRPG), so this descending inhibitory system may form part of a regulatory feedback loop whereby transmission through the dorsal horn is controlled according to the amount of activity reaching the thalamus.

The descending inhibitory pathway is probably an important site of action for opioid analgesics (see below).

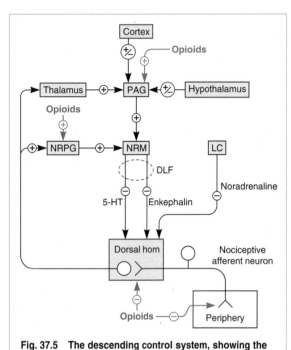

Fig. 37.5 **The descending control system, showing the main sites of action of opioids on pain transmission.** Opioids excite neurons in the periaqueductal grey matter (PAG) and in the *nucleus reticularis paragigantocellularis* (NRPG), which in turn project to the rostroventral medulla, which includes the *nucleus raphe magnus* (NRM). From the NRM, 5-HT- and enkephalin-containing neurons run to the *substantia gelatinosa* of the dorsal horn, and exert an inhibitory influence on transmission. Opioids also act directly on the dorsal horn, as well as on the peripheral terminals of nociceptive afferent neurons. The *locus ceruleus* (LC) sends noradrenergic neurons to the dorsal horn, which also inhibit transmission. The pathways shown in this diagram represent a considerable oversimplification, but depict the general organisation of the supraspinal control mechanisms. Blue shaded boxes represent areas rich in opioid peptides. (DLF = dorsolateral funiculus) (For more detailed information, see Fields & Basbaum 1994.)

Both PAG and SG are particularly rich in enkephalin-containing neurons, and opioid antagonists, such as naloxone (see later section) can prevent electrically induced analgesia, which would suggest that opioid peptides may function as transmitters in this system. The physiological role of opioid peptides in regulating pain transmission has been controversial, mainly because under normal conditions naloxone has relatively little effect on pain threshold. Under pathological conditions, however, when stress is present, naloxone causes hyperalgesia, implying that the opioid system is active.

There is also a noradrenergic pathway from the *locus*

ceruleus (see Ch. 30), which has a similar inhibitory effect on transmission in the dorsal horn (Fig. 37.5).

NEUROPATHIC PAIN

Neurological disease affecting the sensory pathway can produce severe chronic pain—termed *neuropathic pain*—unrelated to any peripheral tissue injury. This occurs with CNS disorders, such as stroke and multiple sclerosis, or with conditions associated with peripheral nerve damage, such as mechanical injury, diabetic neuropathy or herpes zoster infection (shingles). The pathophysiological mechanisms underlying this kind of pain are poorly understood, though spontaneous activity in damaged sensory neurons is thought to be a factor. The sympathetic nervous system also plays a part, since damaged sensory neurons can express α-adrenoceptors, and develop a sensitivity to noradrenaline that they do not possess under normal conditions. Thus physiological stimuli that evoke sympathetic responses can produce severe pain, a phenomenon described clinically as *sympathetically mediated pain*. Neuropathic pain, which appears to be a component of many types of clinical pain (including common conditions such as back pain, cancer pain, as well as amputation pain) is generally difficult to control with conventional analgesic drugs. A better understanding of its mechanism should provide more rational therapeutic approaches.

PAIN AND NOCICEPTION

As emphasised above, the perception of noxious stimuli (termed 'nociception' by Sherrington) is not the same

---

Modulation of pain transmission

- Transmission in the dorsal horn is subject to various modulatory influences, constituting the 'gate control' mechanism.
- Descending pathways from the midbrain and brainstem exert a strong inhibitory effect on dorsal horn transmission. Electrical stimulation of the midbrain PAG causes analgesia through this mechanism.
- The descending inhibition is mediated mainly by enkephalins, 5-HT, noradrenaline and adenosine. Opioids cause analgesia partly by activating these descending pathways, partly by inhibiting transmission in the dorsal horn, and partly by inhibiting excitation of sensory nerve terminals in the periphery.
- Repetitive C-fibre activity facilitates transmission through the dorsal horn ('wind-up') by mechanisms involving activation of NMDA and substance P receptors.

thing as pain, which is a subjective experience, and includes a strong emotional (affective) component. The amount of pain that a particular stimulus produces depends on many factors other than the stimulus itself. A stabbing sensation in the chest will cause much more pain if it occurs spontaneously in a middle-aged man than if it is due to a 2-year-old poking him in the ribs with a sharp stick. The nociceptive component may be much the same, but the affective component is quite different. Animal tests of analgesic drugs commonly measure nociception, and involve testing the reaction of an animal to a mildly painful stimulus, often mechanical or thermal. Such measures include the tail-flick test (measuring the time taken for a rat to withdraw its tail when a standard radiant heat stimulus is applied) or the paw pressure test (measuring the withdrawal threshold when a normal or inflamed paw is pinched with increasing force). Similar tests can be used on human subjects, who simply indicate when a stimulus begins to feel painful, but the pain in these circumstances lacks the affective component. Clinically, spontaneous pain of neuropathic origin is coming to be recognised as particularly important, but this is difficult to model in animal studies for both technical and ethical reasons. It is recognised clinically that many analgesics, particularly those of the morphine-type can greatly reduce the distress associated with pain even though the patient reports no great change in the intensity of the actual sensation. It is much more difficult to devise tests that measure this affective component, and important to realise that it may be at least as significant as the antinociceptive component in the action of these drugs. There is often a poor correlation between the activity of analgesic drugs in animal tests (which mainly assess antinociceptive activity) and their clinical effectiveness.

CHEMICAL MEDIATORS IN THE NOCICEPTIVE PATHWAY

CHEMOSENSITIVITY OF NOCICEPTIVE NERVE ENDINGS

In most cases stimulation of nociceptive endings in the periphery is chemical in origin. Excessive mechanical or thermal stimuli can obviously cause acute pain, but the persistence of such pain after the stimulus has been removed, or the pain resulting from inflammatory or ischaemic changes in tissues, generally reflects an altered chemical environment of the pain afferents. Much of our current knowledge comes from the early work of Keele & Armstrong, who developed a simple method for measuring the pain-producing effect of various substances that act on cutaneous nerve endings. They pro-

duced small blisters on the forearm of human subjects, and applied chemicals to the blister base. Pain was recorded subjectively, and with practice the subjects could achieve reproducible responses.

The main groups of substances that stimulate pain endings in the skin (see Rang et al. 1994) are discussed below.

Various neurotransmitters including 5-HT, histamine and acetylcholine

5-HT is the most active; histamine is much less active and tends to cause itching rather than actual pain. Both of these substances are known to be released locally in inflammation (see Ch. 12).

Kinins

The most active substances are *bradykinin* and *kallidin* (see Ch. 12), two closely related peptides produced under conditions of tissue injury by the proteolytic cleavage of the active kinins from a precursor protein contained in the plasma (reviewed by Dray & Perkins 1993). Bradykinin is a potent pain-producing substance, acting partly by release of prostaglandins, which strongly enhance the direct action of bradykinin on the nerve terminals (Fig. 37.6). Bradykinin acts by combining with specific receptors of the G-protein-coupled type (Ch. 2), and produces its cellular effects through production of various intracellular messengers (see Cesare & McNaughton 1997). Specific competitive antagonists, based on the peptide structure of bradykinin, such as **icatibant** (Ch. 12) have recently been developed, and these show analgesic and anti-inflammatory properties. Such peptides are not suitable for clinical use as analgesics, but may provide a new principle on which to base future analgesic drugs.

Various metabolites and substances released from active cells, such as lactic acid, ATP and ADP, K+

Low pH excites nociceptive afferent neurons specifically by opening proton-activated cation channels similar or identical to those activated by capsaicin (see below). ATP acts similarly. A type of ATP receptor restricted to sensory neurons, termed P_{2X3} (see Ch. 9), which mediates this response, was recently identified (see Burnstock & Wood 1996). These agents are mainly of interest as potential mediators of ischaemic pain.

Prostaglandins

Prostaglandins do not themselves cause pain, but they strongly enhance the pain-producing effect of other agents such as 5-HT or bradykinin (Fig. 37.6). Prostaglandins of the E and F series are released in inflammation (Ch. 12) and also during tissue ischaemia. They sensitise nerve terminals to other agents partly by inhibiting potassium

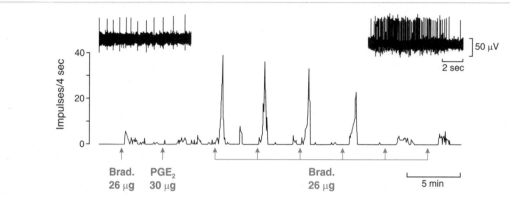

Fig 37.6 Response of a nociceptive afferent neuron to bradykinin and prostaglandin. Recordings were made from a nociceptive afferent fibre supplying a muscle, and drugs were injected into the arterial supply. *Upper records:* single fibre recordings showing discharge caused by bradykinin alone (left), and by bradykinin following injection of prostaglandin (right). *Lower trace:* ratemeter recording of single fibre discharge showing long-lasting enhancement of response to bradykinin after an injection of prostaglandin E_2. Prostaglandin itself did not evoke a discharge. (From: Mense S 1981 Brain Res 225: 95)

channels, and partly by facilitating—through second-messenger-mediated phosphorylation reactions (see Ch. 2)—the cation channels opened by noxious agents. It is of interest that bradykinin itself causes prostaglandin release, and thus has a powerful 'self-sensitising' effect on nociceptive afferents. Other eicosanoids, including prostacyclins, leukotrienes and the unstable HETE derivatives (Ch. 12), may also be important, but information is sparse (see Rang et al. 1998).

Capsaicin and related irritant substances

Capsaicin is the active substance in chilli peppers and is responsible for their burning taste. Other spicy plants (ginger, black pepper, etc.) also contain similar agents, but capsaicin is the most potent and most thoroughly studied. It is a highly potent pain-producing substance, which selectively stimulates nociceptive and temperature-sensitive nerve endings in tissues.

There are several very interesting features of the action of capsaicin (for reviews, see Wood 1993).

- Capsaicin acts on membrane receptors that were recently cloned (Caterina et al. 1997) and are specifically expressed by nociceptive sensory neurons. The receptors are directly coupled to cation channels (see Ch. 2), which have a high permeability to calcium. Calcium entry may account for many of the cellular effects produced by capsaicin. Interestingly, the capsaicin receptor also responds to temperatures above about 45°C, and its physiological function may be related to thermal pain.
- After a few applications the pain-producing effect

disappears and nociceptive responses to other stimuli disappear as well; capsaicin applied topically to the skin is sometimes used to treat certain kinds of neuropathic pain.

Mechanisms of pain and nociception

- Nociception is the mechanism whereby noxious peripheral stimuli are transmitted to the central nervous system. Pain is a subjective experience, not always associated with nociception.
- Polymodal nociceptors (PMN) are the main type of peripheral sensory neuron that responds to noxious stimuli. The majority are non-myelinated C-fibres whose endings respond to thermal, mechanical and chemical stimuli.
- Chemical stimuli acting on PMN to cause pain include bradykinin, 5-HT, and capsaicin. PMN are sensitised by prostaglandins, which explains the analgesic effect of aspirin-like drugs, particularly in the presence of inflammation.
- Nociceptive fibres terminate in the superficial layers of the dorsal horn, forming synaptic connections with transmission neurons running to the thalamus.
- PMN neurons release glutamate (fast transmitter) and various peptides (especially substance P) which act as slow transmitters. Peptides are also released peripherally and contribute to neurogenic inflammation.
- Neuropathic pain, associated with damage to neurons of the nociceptive pathway rather than an excessive peripheral stimulus, is frequently a component of chronic pain states, and may respond poorly to opioid analgesics.

- It causes release of substance P from afferent neurons (see above), both peripherally and within the spinal cord. In adult animals the afferent neurons are depleted of substance P and take days or weeks to recover.
- In newborn animals, capsaicin selectively destroys C-fibre neurons in the periphery, and the animals grow up with a greatly reduced response to painful and thermal stimuli. It has therefore been widely used as an experimental tool for investigating the function of C-fibre afferents.

TRANSMITTERS AND MODULATORS IN THE NOCICEPTIVE PATHWAY

TACHYKININS

Substance P (SP), discovered in 1931 by von Euler & Gaddum, was the first neuropeptide to be discovered, and it still enjoys *prima donna* status. In 1931 there was no simple way to purify or determine the structure of a peptide, and SP remained a pharmacological curiosity. Nearly 20 years later, Erspamer found another peptide, *eledoisin*, in a Mediterranean octopus, which had very similar actions to SP. He purified this from nearly 2 tons of octopus, and elucidated its sequence (Fig. 37.7). Encouraged, he did the same for some amphibian peptides, which turned out to have very similar sequences. He called them tachykinins (fast-acting) to distinguish them from bradykinin (see Ch. 12), which has a much

slower action on smooth muscle. In 1970, SP was purified from hypothalamus, and shown to belong to the tachykinin family, which are characterised by the terminal sequence –Phe X Gly Leu Met NH_2 (unblushingly referred to as the 'canonical sequence' by peptide pundits). More recently, two less-abundant mammalian tachykinins, neurokinin A (NKA) and neurokinin B, were identified. As often happens in the peptide field, several groups converged on these substances, and called them by different names, causing a merry confusion. The tachykinins, like other neuropeptides (Ch. 10), are formed by cleavage of larger protein precursors, preprotachykinins. SP and NKA are represented in the same preprotachykinin gene, and tissue-specific splicing patterns allow either SP alone, or both peptides, to be formed in different situations. Detailed information on the tachykinins can be found in various reviews (e.g. Maggi et al. 1993, Maggio 1988).

Distribution

Substance P and NKA, which are derived from the same gene, are distributed widely in the nervous system, but especially in nociceptive primary afferent neurons. Nociceptive sensory neurons express several neuropeptides, which are released at both the central and the peripheral terminals when the neurons are activated. Release of peptides at the peripheral terminals of these neurons is thought to play a part in 'neurogenic inflammation' (see Holzer 1988). SP-containing terminals are abundant in the walls of many blood vessels, including

Opioid peptides

Leu-enkephalin	Tyr	Gly	Gly	Phe	Leu										
Dynorphin A	Tyr	Gly	Gly	Phe	Leu	Arg	Arg	Ile	Arg	Pro	Lys	Leu	Lys	Trp	Asp	Asn	Gln
Met-enkephalin	Tyr	Gly	Gly	Phe	Met										
β-endorphin	Tyr	Gly	Gly	Phe	Met	Thr	Ser	Glu	Lys	Ser	Gln	Thr	Pro	Leu	Val	Thr	Leu	+9 residues
Nociceptin	Phe	Gly	Gly	Phe	Thr	Gly	Ala	Arg	Lys	Ser	Ala	Arg	Lys	Leu	Ala	Asn	Gln

Tachykinins

Substance P	Arg	Pro	Lys	Pro	Gln	Gln	Phe	Phe	Gly	Leu	Met	NH₂
Neurokinin A		His	Lys	Thr	Asp	Ser	Phe	Val	Gly	Leu	Met	NH₂
Neurokinin B		Asp	Met	His	Asp	Phe	Phe	Val	Gly	Leu	Met	NH₂

Mammalian

Eledoisin	pGlu	Pro	Ser	Lys	Asp	Ala	Phe	Ile	Gly	Leu	Met	NH₂
Physalaemin	pGlu	Ala	Asp	Pro	Asn	Lys	Phe	Phe	Gly	Leu	Met	NH₂

Amphibian

Fig. 37.7 Structure of opioid and tachykinin peptides, with common amino acids highlighted.

cerebral vessels, and it has been postulated that peptide release is involved in migraine and other types of headache (see Ch. 9).

Tachykinin receptors

Three tachykinin receptor subtypes exist, NK_1, NK_2 and NK_3, the preferred agonists being SP, NKA and NKB, respectively. Most of the known effects of tachykinins are mediated by NK_1- or NK_2-receptors, with much inter-species variation. Less is known about NK_3-receptors, and their role seems to be more limited. Substance P, acting on NK_1-receptors, and NKA, acting on NK_2-receptors, elicit very slow excitatory synaptic potentials in dorsal horn neurons, which are insufficient on their own to excite the postsynaptic neuron, but may build up during repetitive activity to produce a burst of action potentials lasting for a few seconds in response to each stimulus. Inflammation, through the action of NGF, increases the substance P content of nociceptive neurons, and enhances these slow excitatory responses in the spinal cord, an adaptive change which may be an important factor in hyperalgesia (Fig. 37.6). The presence of abundant NK_1-receptors in the superficial layers of the dorsal horn can be revealed by immunofluorescent labelling. Using this technique, Mantyh et al. (1995) showed that a noxious stimulus to the rat's paw, which releases SP from primary afferent terminals, causes internalisation of these surface receptors, due to agonist-induced endocytosis (see Ch. 2). The physiological significance of this remains uncertain, but the result confirms the postulated modulatory role of SP in the nociceptive pathway.

Tachykinins elicit a wide range of responses from cells of many types, including neurons, smooth muscle, vascular endothelium, exocrine gland cells, mast cells and cells of the immune system (see review by Maggi et al. 1993), the overall pattern of effects being similar to that seen with agents such as bradykinin (Ch. 12) or 5-HT (Ch. 9). Most types of smooth muscle, including that of the gastrointestinal tract and airways, contract in response to tachykinins. Blood vessels show a mixture of constrictor and dilator responses (endothelium-dependent; see Ch. 10), together with increased permeability, leading to oedema formation. Many neurons, including central and autonomic neurons, show a slow excitatory response, as described above. Intrathecal application of SP causes a scratching response in conscious animals, and may produce hyperalgesia, consistent with the postulated transmitter role of SP in the nociceptive pathway. Mast cells are activated, and release histamine, and various exocrine glands, including salivary glands,

are also stimulated. Receptor cloning has shown that, as expected, tachykinin receptors belong to the family of G-protein-coupled receptors described in Chapter 2, and act through various second messengers.

There is evidence to suggest that substance P is involved not only in the nociceptive pathway, but also in inflammatory conditions, such as arthritis, asthma, hay fever, inflammatory bowel disease and migraine (see Maggi et al. 1993).

Tachykinin antagonists

Modifications of the amino acid sequence of SP, the significant change being the incorporation of D-amino acids, led to the first generation of competitive antagonists, in particular **spantide** (D-Arg[1] D-Trp[7,9] Leu[11]-SP), which acts selectively on the NK_1-receptor. In 1991, the first non-peptide tachykinin antagonist (CP 96345) made its appearance. This potent compound, which bears no resemblance to substance P, was developed by Pfizer from a lead which emerged from random screening. Others quickly followed, and there are now several peptide and non-peptide tachykinin antagonists which distinguish between the receptor subtypes (see Maggi et al. 1993), and which are active in animal models of inflammatory pain, though none are yet in clinical use. Besides analgesia, other potential indications for tachykinin antagonists include emesis and migraine, and (more speculatively) anxiety states (see Longmore et al. 1997).

Tachykinins

- There are three endogenous tachykinins—substance P (SP), neurokinin A (NKA) and neurokinin B (NKB), which are widely distributed in the central and peripheral nervous systems.
- Nociceptive sensory neurons express SP and NKA, and release them in the periphery and in the dorsal horn. Inflammation increases SP expression.
- SP release in the periphery when nociceptors are activated contributes to neurogenic inflammation. SP release in the dorsal horn contributes to the wind-up phenomenon.
- There are three tachykinin receptors—NK_1, NK_2 and NK_3—whose preferred agonists are SP, NKA and NKB, respectively.
- Nociceptive transmission and neurogenic inflammation are mediated mainly through NK_1-receptors.
- Selective NK_1-receptor antagonists may be developed as future analgesic compounds.

OPIOID PEPTIDES

In 1975, Hughes & Kosterlitz succeeded in isolating from the brain two pentapeptides, which compete strongly with morphine-like drugs for binding to receptors in the brain, and which have pharmacological actions closely resembling those of morphine itself. This outstanding work showed that the hitherto mysterious actions of morphine (see below) stemmed from its ability to mimic the actions of a family of endogenous mediators, the opioid peptides. This very satisfying result fuelled the expectation that the discovery of other neuropeptides might similarly illuminate the actions of other types of drug that affect the central nervous system; to date, however, morphine-like drugs remain the only class known to act by mimicking peptides. For general reviews of opioid peptides, see Cooper et al. (1996), Wagner & Chavkin (1995).

Opioid peptides, defined as peptides with opiate-like pharmacological effects, are coded by three distinct genes, whose products are respectively *preproopiomelano-cortin* (*POMC*), *preproenkephalin* and *preprodynorphin* (see Ch. 10).* The mediators about which most is known are β-endorphin, met-enkephalin, leu-enkephalin and dynorphin. In the brain, these peptides are widely distributed. In the spinal cord, dynorphin occurs mainly in interneurons, while the enkephalins are found mainly in long descending pathways from the midbrain to the dorsal horn. Opioid peptides are also produced by many non-neuronal cells, including endocrine and exocrine glands and cells of the immune system, as well as in brain areas distinct from those involved in nociception, and correspondingly, they play a regulatory role in many different physiological systems, as reflected in the rather complex pharmacological properties of opiate drugs (see below).

The receptors through which opioid peptides exert their effects are described below.

---

*Recently, a fourth class of opioid peptide, **nociceptin**, was discovered (see Henderson & McKnight 1997), whose structure (Fig. 37.7) derives from a distinct precursor, whose gene has not yet been cloned. Nociceptin was identified as the endogenous ligand for a novel opioid receptor-like protein (ORL) which had been detected by screening for homologues of the known opioid receptors. Because none of the then-known opioid peptides recognised ORL, it was classed as an 'orphan receptor' (Ch. 2). The discovery of nociceptin means that it is no longer an orphan, but little is yet known about the function of this system. The name 'nociceptin' was coined because earlier studies showed that it caused hyperalgesia when injected into the brain—the opposite of other opioid peptides. Later studies showed, however, that its effects on nociception are more complex, and can go in either direction (see Henderson & McKnight 1997).

OTHER MEDIATORS

- Glutamate (see Ch. 29) is released from primary afferent neurons and, acting on AMPA receptors, is responsible for fast synaptic transmission at the first synapse in the dorsal horn. There is also a slower NMDA-receptor-mediated response, which is important in relation to the wind-up phenomenon (see Fig. 37.6).
- GABA (see Ch. 29) is released by spinal cord interneurons, and inhibits transmitter release by primary afferent terminals in the dorsal horn (see Malcangio & Bowery 1996)
- 5-HT is the transmitter of inhibitory neurons running from NRM to the dorsal horn.
- Noradrenaline is the transmitter of the inhibitory pathway from the locus ceruleus to the dorsal horn, and possibly also in other antinociceptive pathways.
- Adenosine plays a dual role in regulating nociceptive transmission, activation of A_1-receptors causing analgesia, while activation of A_2-receptors does the reverse. There is evidence for descending inhibitory purinergic pathways acting on pain transmission through A_1-receptors (see Sawynok & Sweeney 1996).

ANALGESIC DRUGS

MORPHINE-LIKE DRUGS

The term **opioid** applies to any substance, whether endogenous or synthetic, that produces morphine-like effects that are blocked by antagonists such as naloxone. The older term, **opiate**, is restricted to synthetic morphine-like drugs with non-peptidic structures. The field is reviewed thoroughly by Herz (1993).

Opium is an extract of the juice of the poppy *Papaver somniferum*, which has been used for social and medicinal purposes for thousands of years, as an agent to produce euphoria, analgesia and sleep, and to prevent diarrhoea. It was introduced in Britain at the end of the 17th century, usually taken orally as 'tincture of laudanum', addiction to which acquired a certain social cachet during the next 200 years. The situation changed when the hypodermic syringe and needle were invented in the mid-19th century and opiate dependence began to take on a more sinister significance.

CHEMICAL ASPECTS

Opium contains many alkaloids related to morphine. The structure of morphine (Fig. 37.8) was determined in 1902 and since then many semisynthetic compounds

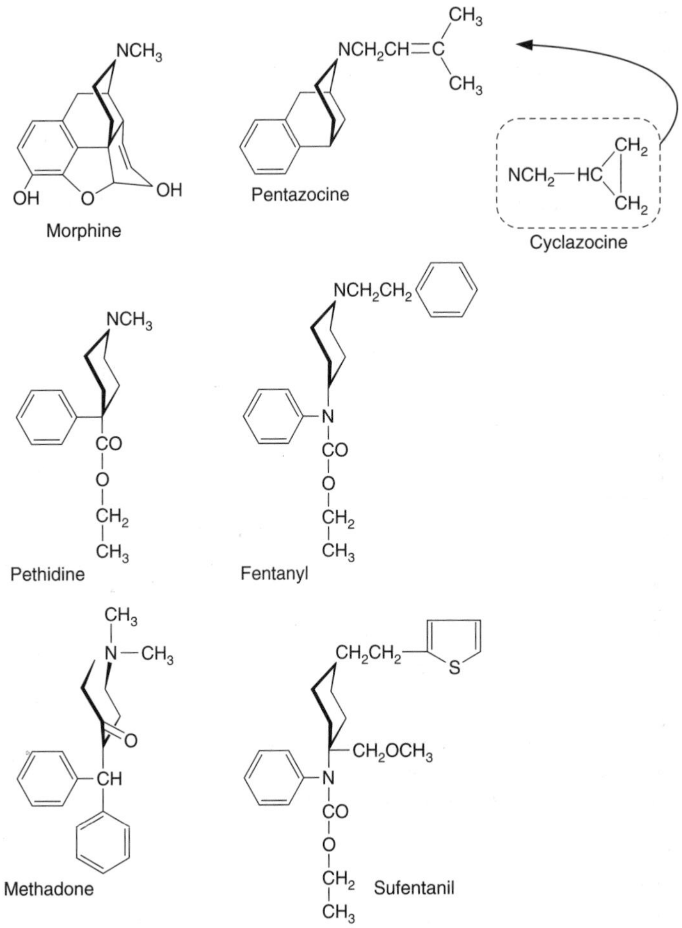

Fig 37.8   Structures of some opiate analgesics.

(produced by chemical modification of morphine) and fully synthetic opiates have been studied. In addition to morphine-like compounds, opium also contains papaverine, a smooth muscle relaxant (see Ch. 15).

The main groups of drugs that are discussed in this section are:

- *Morphine analogues.* These are compounds closely related in structure to morphine, and often synthesised from it. They may be agonists (e.g. **morphine**, **diamorphin**e (heroin) and **codeine**), partial agonists (e.g. **nalorphine** and **levallorphan**), or antagonists (e.g. **naloxone**).
- *Synthetic derivatives with structures unrelated to morphine:*
  —phenylpiperidine series, e.g. **pethidine** and **fentanyl**
  —methadone series, e.g. **methadone** and **dextropropoxyphene**

—benzomorphan series, e.g. **pentazocine** and **cyclazocine**
—semisynthetic thebaine derivatives, e.g. **etorphine** and **buprenorphine**.

Mention should also be made of **loperamide**, an opiate that does not enter the brain, and therefore lacks analgesic activity. Like other opiates (see below) it inhibits peristalsis, and is used to control diarrhoea (see Ch. 21).

Morphine analogues

Morphine is a **phenanthrene** derivative (see Table 37.1), with two planar rings (A and B) and two aliphatic ring structures (C and D), which occupy a plane roughly at right angles to A and B. Variants of the morphine molecule have been produced by substitution at one or both of the hydroxyl groups (the phenolic OH at position 3 and the alcoholic OH at position 6), and by substitution at

Table 37.1 Morphine analogues

Drug	Substituents			
	3	6	N	14
Morphine	—OH	—OH	—CH$_3$	—H
Diamorphine (heroin)	—OCO · CH$_3$	—OCO · CH$_3$	—CH$_3$	—H
Codeine	—OCH$_3$	—OH	—CH$_3$	—H
Levorphanol	—OH	—H	—CH$_3$	—H (lacks —O— at C$_4$–C$_5$)
Dihydrocodeine	—OCH$_3$	—OH	—CH$_3$	—H (lacks double bond C$_7$–C$_8$)
Nalorphine	—OH	—OH	—CH$_2$CH=CH$_2$	—H
Nalbuphine	—OH	—OH	—CH$_2$—cyclobutyl	—OH (lacks double bond C$_7$–C$_8$)
Butorphanol	—OH	—H	—CH$_2$—cyclobutyl	—H (lacks —O— at C$_4$–C$_5$ and double bond C$_7$–C$_8$)
Naloxone	—OH	=O	—CH$_2$CH=CH$_2$	—HO (lacks double bond C$_7$–C$_8$)

Buprenorphine

the nitrogen atom at position 17. Some of the most important analogues are shown in Table 37.1.

Synthetic derivatives

Phenylpiperidine series. **Pethidine** (known as meperidine in USA), the first fully synthetic morphine-like drug, was discovered accidentally when new atropine-like drugs were being sought. It is chemically simpler than morphine, though its pharmacological actions are very similar.

Fentanyl and **sufentanil** are more potent and shorter-acting derivatives which are used intravenously to treat severe pain or as an adjunct to anaesthesia.

Methadone series. Methadone, though its structural formula bears no obvious chemical relationship to that of morphine, assumes a similar conformation in solution, and was designed by reference to the common three-dimensional structural features of morphine and pethidine (Fig. 37.8). It is longer-acting than morphine, but otherwise very similar to it. **Dextropropoxyphene** is very similar and used clinically for treating mild or moderate pain.

Benzomorphan series. The most important members of this class are **pentazocine** and **cyclazocine** (Fig. 37.8). These drugs differ from morphine in their receptor-binding profile (see below), and so have somewhat different actions and side-effects.

Thebaine derivatives. **Etorphine** is a highly potent morphine-like drug, used mainly in veterinary practice. **Buprenorphine** resembles morphine, but is a partial agonist (see below); thus, although very potent, its maximal effect is less than that of morphine, and it antagonises the effect of other opioids.

OPIOID RECEPTORS

Direct evidence that opioids are recognised by specific receptors came from binding studies by Snyder and his colleagues in 1973, though the existence of specific antagonists had earlier suggested that such receptors must exist. Various pharmacological observations implied that more than one type of receptor was involved, the original suggestion of multiple receptor types arising from in vivo

Opioid analgesics

- There are three main families of endogenous opioid peptides; these have analgesic activity and have many physiological functions, but they are not used as drugs.
- Opioid drugs include:
  — phenanthrene derivatives, structurally related to morphine
  — synthetic compounds with dissimilar structures but similar pharmacological effects.
- Important morphine-like agonists include diamorphine, codeine; other structurally related compounds are partial agonists (e.g. nalorphine and levallorphan) or antagonists (e.g. naloxone).
- The main groups of synthetic analogues are the piperidines (e.g. pethidine and fentanyl), the methadone-like drugs, the benzomorphans (e.g. pentazocine) and the thebaine derivatives (e.g. buprenorphine).
- Opioid analgesics may be given orally, by injection, or intrathecally to produce analgesia with limited side-effects.

Table 37.2 Functional effects associated with the main types of opioid receptor

	μ	δ	κ
Analgesia			
Supraspinal	+++	–	–
Spinal	++	++	+
Peripheral	++	–	++
Respiratory depression	+++	++	–
Pupil constriction	++	–	+
Reduced GI motility	++	++	+
Euphoria	+++	–	–
Dysphoria	–	–	+++
Sedation	++	–	++
Physical dependence	+++	–	+

studies of the spectrum of actions (analgesia, sedation, pupillary constriction, bradycardia, etc.) produced by different drugs. It was also found that some opioids, but not all, were able to relieve withdrawal symptoms in morphine-dependent animals, and this was interpreted in terms of distinct receptor subtypes. The conclusion (see Dhawan et al. 1996) from these and many subsequent pharmacological studies, now confirmed by receptor cloning, is that three types of opioid receptor, termed μ, δ and κ, mediate the main pharmacological effects of opiates, as summarised in Table 37.2.* There is pharmacological evidence, not yet confirmed by cloning, for further subdivisions of each of these subtypes, and their significance remains uncertain. Recent studies on the characteristics of transgenic mouse strains lacking functional μ-receptors (see Childers 1997) confirm that the major pharmacological effects of morphine, including analgesia, are mediated by this receptor.

The interaction of various opioid drugs and peptides with the various receptor types is summarised in Table

37.3. In addition to endogenous peptides and drugs in clinical use, some agents that are used as experimental tools for distinguishing the different receptor subtypes are also shown.

AGONISTS AND ANTAGONISTS

Opioids vary not only in their receptor specificity, but also in their efficacy at the different types of receptor. Thus some agents act as agonists on one type of receptor and antagonists or partial agonists at another, producing a very complicated pharmacological picture.

Three main categories may be distinguished (Table 37.3):

- *Pure agonists.* This group includes most of the typical morphine-like drugs. They all have high affinity for μ-receptors and generally lower affinity for δ- and κ-sites. Some drugs of this type, notably **codeine**, **methadone** and **dextropropoxyphene**, are sometimes referred to as *weak agonists*, since their maximal effects, both analgesic and unwanted, are less than those of morphine, and they do not cause dependence. Whether they are truly partial agonists is not established.
- *Partial agonists and mixed agonist–antagonists.* These drugs typified by **nalorphine** and **pentazocine** combine a degree of agonist and antagonist activity on different receptors. **Nalorphine**, for example, is an agonist when tested on guinea-pig ileum, but it also inhibits competitively the effect of morphine on this tissue (consistent with a partial agonist profile; see Ch. 1). In vivo it shows a similar mixture of agonist and antagonist actions. **Pentazocine** and **cyclazocine**,

*A fourth subtype, σ, was also postulated in order to account for the 'dysphoric' effects (anxiety, hallucinations, bad dreams, etc.) produced by some opiates. These are, however, not true opioid receptors, since many other types of psychotropic drug also interact with them, and their biological role remains unclear (see Walker et al. 1990). Of the opiate drugs, only benzomorphans, such as **pentazocine** and **cyclazocine**, bind appreciably to σ-receptors, which is consistent with their known psychotomimetic properties.

Table 37.3 Selectivity of opioid drugs and peptides for receptor subtypes

	μ	δ	κ
Endogenous peptides			
β-endorphin	+++	+++	+++
Leu-enkephalin	+	+++	–
Met-enkephalin	++	+++	–
Dynorphin	++	+	+++
Opiate drugs			
Pure agonists			
Morphine, codeine, oxymorphone, dextropropoxyphene	+++	+	+
Methadone	+++	–	–
Pethidine	++	+	+
Etorphine, bremazocine	+++	+++	+++
Fentanyl, sufentanil	+++	+	–
Partial/mixed agonists			
Pentazocine, ketocyclazocine	+	+	++
Nalbuphine	+	+	(++)
Nalorphine	++	–	(++)
Buprenorphine	(+++)	–	++
Antagonists			
Naloxone	+++	+	++
Naltrexone, diprenorphine	+++	+	+++
Research tools (receptor-selective)			
DAMGO*	+++	–	–
DPDPE*	–	++	–
U50488	–	–	+++
CTOP*	+++	–	–
Naltrindole	–	+++	–
Nor-binaltorphimine	+	+	+++

Note: Blue + symbols represent **agonist** activity; partial agonists in brackets
Black + symbols denote **antagonist** activity.
– symbols represent weak or no activity.
*DAMGO, DPDPE and CTOP are synthetic opioid-like peptides, more receptor-selective than endogenous opioids. U50488 is a synthetic opiate.

MECHANISM OF ACTION OF OPIOIDS

The opioids have probably been studied more intensively than any other group of drugs in the effort to understand their powerful effects in molecular, biochemical and physiological terms, and to use this understanding to develop opioid drugs as analgesics with significant advantages over morphine. While the receptor biology is well worked out, the physiological pathways that are regulated by opioids, which underlie their analgesic and other actions, are only partly understood. Even so, morphine*—the grandfather of the opioid family—remains the standard against which any new analgesic is assessed. It is rather as though mercurials were still the standard diuretic drugs, or Ehrlich's salvarsan the standard drug for treating syphilis. Useful reviews on the neuropharmacology of opiates include Duggan & North (1984), Pasternak (1993), Yaksh (1997).

Cellular actions

Opioid receptors belong to the family of G-protein-coupled receptors, and inhibit adenylate cyclase, so reducing the intracellular cAMP content (see Dhawan et al. 1996). All three receptor subtypes exert this effect, and they also exert effects on ion channels through a direct G-protein coupling to the channel. By these means, opioids promote the opening of potassium channels and inhibit the opening of voltage-gated calcium channels (see review by North 1993), which are the main effects seen at the membrane level. These membrane effects reduce both neuronal excitability (since the increased potassium conductance causes hyperpolarisation of the membrane) and transmitter release (due to inhibition of calcium entry). The overall effect is therefore inhibitory at the cellular level. Nonetheless, opioids increase activity in some neuronal pathways (see below), presumably by suppressing the firing of inhibitory interneurons. At the cellular level, all three receptor subtypes mediate very similar effects, though the heterogeneous distribution of the receptors means that particular neurons and pathways are affected selectively by different agonists.

Effects on the nociceptive pathway

Opioid receptors are widely distributed in the brain, and their relationship to the nociceptive pathway is summarised in Figure 37.5. Opioids are effective as analgesics when given intrathecally in minute doses, implying that a central action can account for their analgesic effect. Injection of morphine into the PAG region

on the other hand, are antagonists at μ-receptors, but partial agonists on δ- and κ-receptors. Most of the drugs in this group tend to cause dysphoria, rather than euphoria, an effect which may be due to an interaction with the non-opioid σ-receptor.

- *Antagonists.* These drugs produce very little effect when given on their own, but block the effects of opioids. The most important examples are **naloxone** and **naltrexone**.

*Described by Osler as 'God's own medicine'.

causes marked analgesia, which can be prevented by surgical interruption of the descending pathway to NRM or by blocking 5-HT synthesis pharmacologically with p-chlorophenylalanine. This latter procedure interrupts the 5-HT pathway running from NRM to the dorsal horn. Moreover, systemic morphine is rendered less effective in suppressing nociceptive spinal reflexes by transection of the spinal cord in the neck, and the firing of neurons associated with the descending inhibitory pathways is increased by morphine, implying that there is a significant supraspinal component of the overall effect.

At the spinal level, morphine inhibits transmission of nociceptive impulses through the dorsal horn, and suppresses nociceptive spinal reflexes, even in patients with spinal cord transection. It inhibits release of substance P from dorsal horn neurons in vitro and in vivo (Fig. 37.9), by a presynaptic inhibitory effect on the central terminals of nociceptive afferent neurons. Microinjection of morphine into the dorsal horn also produces this effect. However, direct measurement of substance P release (by an antibody-covered microprobe inserted directly into the dorsal horn) failed to show any inhibition of release when morphine was given systemically in

analgesic doses, implying that an action on primary afferent terminals may not be important in producing its therapeutic effect.

There is also evidence (see Stein & Yassouridis 1997) that opiates inhibit the discharge of nociceptive afferent terminals in the periphery, particularly under conditions of inflammation, in which the expression of opioid receptors by sensory neurons is increased. Injection of morphine into the knee joint following surgery to the joint provides effective analgesia, undermining the age-old principle that opioid analgesia is exclusively a central phenomenon.

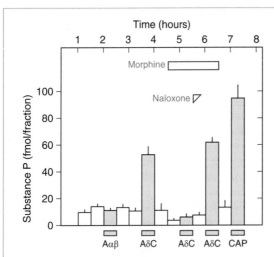

Fig. 37.9 Morphine inhibits the release of substance P from cat spinal cord. Substance P was measured by radioimmunoassay in the fluid superfusing the spinal cord. Stimulation of the sciatic nerve at low intensity stimulates large myelinated fibres (Aα and Aβ) only and evokes no release. Increasing the stimulus strength to recruit Aδ and C fibres causes substance P release. The release is blocked by morphine, this effect being antagonised by naloxone. Capsaicin (CAP) added to the fluid superfusing the spinal cord also releases substance P. (From: Yaksh T L et al. 1980 Nature 286: 155)

> **Opioid receptors**
>
> - μ-receptors are thought to be responsible for most of the analgesic effects of opioids, and for some major unwanted effects (e.g. respiratory depression, euphoria, sedation and dependence). Most of the analgesic opioids are μ-receptor agonists.
> - δ-receptors are probably more important in the periphery, but may also contribute to analgesia.
> - κ-receptors contribute to analgesia at the spinal level, and may elicit sedation and dysphoria, but produce relatively few unwanted effects, and do not contribute to dependence. Some analgesics are relatively κ-selective.
> - σ-receptors are not true opioid receptors, but are the site of action of certain psychotomimetic drugs, with which some opioids interact.
> - All opioid receptors are linked through G-proteins to inhibition of adenylate cyclase. They also facilitate opening of K^+ channels (causing hyperpolarisation), and inhibit opening of Ca^{2+} channels (inhibiting transmitter release). These membrane effects are not linked to the decrease in cAMP formation.

PHARMACOLOGICAL ACTIONS

Morphine is typical of many opioid analgesics, and will be taken as the reference compound.

The most important effects of morphine are on the central nervous system and the gastrointestinal tract, though numerous effects of lesser significance on many other systems have been described.

Effects on the central nervous system

Analgesia

Morphine is effective in most kinds of acute and chronic pain, though opioids in general are less useful in neuropathic pain syndromes (such as phantom limb and other types of deafferentation pain, trigeminal neuralgia, etc.)

than in pain associated with tissue injury, inflammation or tumour growth.

As well as being antinociceptive, morphine also reduces the affective component of pain. This reflects its supraspinal action, possibly at the level of the limbic system, which is probably involved in the euphoria-producing effect. Drugs such as nalorphine and pentazocine share the antinociceptive actions of morphine but have much less effect on the psychological response to pain.

Euphoria

Morphine causes a powerful sense of contentment and well-being. This is an important component of its analgesic effect, since the agitation and anxiety associated with a painful illness or injury are thereby reduced. If morphine or **diamorphine** ('heroin') is given intravenously, the result is a sudden 'rush' likened to an 'abdominal orgasm'. The euphoria produced by morphine depends considerably on the circumstances. In patients who are distressed, it is pronounced, but in patients who become accustomed to chronic pain, morphine causes analgesia with little or no euphoria. Some patients report restlessness rather then euphoria under these circumstances.

Euphoria appears to be mediated through μ-receptors, and to be balanced by the dysphoria associated with κ-receptor activation (see Table 37.2). Thus, different opioid drugs vary greatly in the amount of euphoria that they produce. It does not occur with codeine or with pentazocine to any marked extent, and nalorphine, in doses sufficient to cause analgesia, produces dysphoria.

Respiratory depression

Respiratory depression, resulting in increased arterial Pco_2, occurs with a normal analgesic dose of morphine or related compounds. Analgesia and respiratory depression are both mediated by μ-receptors, and the balance between them is thus the same for most opioids. The depressant effect is associated with a decrease in the sensitivity of the respiratory centre to Pco_2. Neurons in the medullary respiratory centre itself do not appear to be directly depressed, but opioids applied to the ventral surface of the medulla in the region where CO_2 chemosensitivity is maximal, have a powerful depressant effect on respiration.

Respiratory depression by opioids is *not* accompanied by depression of the medullary centres controlling cardiovascular function (in contrast to the action of anaesthetics and other general depressants). This means that respiratory depression produced by opioids is much better tolerated than a similar degree of depression caused

by, say, a barbiturate. Nonetheless, respiratory depression is the most troublesome unwanted effect of these drugs, and, unlike that due to general CNS depressant drugs, it occurs at therapeutic doses. It is the commonest cause of death in acute opioid poisoning.

Depression of cough reflex

Cough suppression, surprisingly, does not correlate closely with the analgesic and respiratory depressant actions of opioids, and its mechanism at the receptor level is unclear. In general, increasing substitution on the phenolic –OH group of morphine (position 3; see Table 37.1) increases antitussive relative to analgesic activity. Thus **codeine** suppresses cough in subanalgesic doses, and is often used in cough medicines (see Ch. 19). **Pholcodine**, with a much larger substituent group at position 3, is even more selective, though these agents cause constipation as an unwanted effect.

Nausea and vomiting

Nausea and vomiting occur in up to 40% of patients to whom morphine is given, and do not seem to be separable from the analgesic effect among a range of opioid analgesics. The site of action is the *area postrema* (*chemoreceptor trigger zone*) a region of the medulla where chemical stimuli of many kinds may initiate vomiting (see Ch. 21).* Nausea and vomiting following morphine injection are usually transient, and disappear with repeated administration.

Pupillary constriction

Pupillary constriction is a centrally mediated effect, caused by μ- and κ-receptor-mediated stimulation of the oculomotor nucleus. Pinpoint pupils are an important diagnostic feature in overdosage with morphine and related drugs, because most other causes of coma and respiratory depression produce pupillary dilatation.

Effects on the gastrointestinal tract

Morphine increases tone and reduces motility in many parts of the gastrointestinal system, resulting in constipation which may be severe, and very troublesome to the patient. The resulting delay in gastric emptying can considerably retard the absorption of other drugs. Pressure in the biliary tract increases because of contraction of the gall bladder and constriction of the biliary sphincter. This effect is harmful in patients suffering

---

*The chemically related compound, apomorphine, is more strongly emetic than morphine, through its action as a dopamine agonist; despite its name, it is inactive on opioid receptors. It was at one time used as a conditioned 'aversion therapy' for treating various kinds of unwanted behaviour.

from biliary colic due to gallstones, in whom pain may be increased rather than relieved. The rise in intrabiliary pressure can cause a transient increase in the concentration of amylase and lipase in the plasma.

The action of morphine on visceral smooth muscle is probably mediated mainly through the intramural nerve plexuses, since the increase in tone is reduced or abolished by atropine. It is partly mediated by a central action of morphine, since intraventricular injection of morphine inhibits propulsive gastrointestinal movements. The local effect of morphine and other opioids on neurons of the myenteric plexus is inhibitory, associated with hyperpolarisation resulting from an increased potassium conductance. The receptors involved in these effects are of the μ, κ and δ type, with much variation between different preparations and different species.

Other actions of opioids

Morphine releases histamine from mast cells, by an action unrelated to opioid receptors. This release of histamine can cause local effects, such as *urticaria* and *itching* at the site of the injection, or systemic effects, namely *bronchoconstriction* and *hypotension*. The bronchoconstrictor effect can have serious consequences for asthmatic patients, to whom morphine should not be given. Pethidine does not produce this effect.

Hypotension and bradycardia occur with large doses of most opioids, due to an action on the medulla. With morphine and similar drugs, histamine release may contribute to the hypotension.

Effects on smooth muscle other than that of the gastro-intestinal tract and bronchi are slight, though spasm of the ureters, bladder and uterus sometimes occur. The Straub tail reaction, one of the more improbable phenomena in pharmacology, consists of a raising and stiffening of the tail of rats or mice given opioid drugs, and is due to spasm of a muscle at the base of the tail. It was through this effect that the analgesic action of pethidine was discovered.

Opioids also exert complex *immunosuppressant* effects, which may be important as a link between the nervous system and immune function (see Sibinga & Goldstein 1988). The pharmacological significance of this is not yet clear, but there is evidence in humans that the immune system is depressed by long-term opioid abuse, leading to increased susceptibility to infections.

TOLERANCE AND DEPENDENCE

Tolerance to opioids (i.e. an increase in the dose needed to produce a given pharmacological effect) develops rapidly, and is readily demonstrated. *Dependence* is a different phenomenon, much more difficult to define and measure, which involves two separate components, namely *physical* and *psychological dependence* (see Ch. 39). Physical dependence is associated with a physiological *withdrawal syndrome* (or *abstinence syndrome*), which can be reproduced in experimental animals, and appears to be closely related to tolerance. Morphine also produces *strong psychological dependence*, expressed as craving for the drug, which is probably more important than the physical withdrawal syndrome as a factor causing dependence in humans, but is far harder to study.

Tolerance

Tolerance can be detected within 12–24 hours of morphine administration. Figure 37.10 shows the increase in the equianalgesic dose of morphine (measured by the hot-plate test) that occurred when a slow-release pellet of morphine was implanted subcutaneously in mice. The pellet was removed 8 hours before the test, to allow its effect to disappear before the test was carried out. Within 3 days the equianalgesic dose increased about five-fold. Sensitivity returned to normal within about 3 days of removing the pellet. Tolerance extends to most of the pharmacological effects of morphine, including analgesia, emesis, euphoria, and respiratory depression, but affects the constipating and pupil-constricting actions much less. Thus, addicts may take 50 times the normal analgesic dose of morphine with relatively little respiratory depression, but marked constipation and pupillary constriction.

Actions of morphine

- The main pharmacological effects are:
  — analgesia
  — euphoria and sedation
  — respiratory depression and suppression of cough
  — nausea and vomiting
  — pupillary constriction
  — reduced gastrointestinal motility, causing constipation
  — histamine release, causing bronchoconstriction and hypotension.
- The most troublesome unwanted effects are constipation and respiratory depression.
- Morphine may be given by injection (intravenous or intramuscular), or by mouth, often as slow-release tablets.
- Acute overdosage with morphine produces coma and respiratory depression.
- Morphine is metabolised to morphine-6-glucuronide, which is more potent as an analgesic.

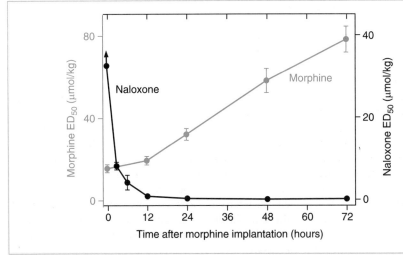

Fig 37.10 Development of morphine tolerance in mice. The ED_{50} for analgesia (hot-plate test) produced by subcutaneous injection of a test dose of morphine (dark blue circles) was measured at intervals after implantation of a slow-release pellet of morphine, the pellet being removed 8 hours before the assay in order to allow the circulating morphine concentration to fall to zero before the test dose was given. The ED_{50} increases about five-fold after 72 hours. Simultaneously, the dose of naloxone needed to precipitate withdrawal symptoms (black circles) decreases very markedly. (From: Way E L et al. 1969 J Pharmacol Exp Ther 167: 1)

The cellular mechanisms responsible for tolerance are discussed in Chapter 39. Certain possibilities can be excluded, such as increased metabolic degradation, reduced affinity of opioids for their receptors, down-regulation of opioid receptors and inhibition of the release of endogenous opioids. Tolerance is a general phenomenon of opioid receptor ligands, irrespective of which type of receptor they act upon. Cross-tolerance occurs between drugs acting at the same receptor, but not between opioids that act on different receptors. In clinical settings, the opiate dose required for effective pain relief may increase as a result of developing tolerance, but it does not constitute a major problem.

Physical dependence

Physical dependence is characterised by a clear-cut *abstinence syndrome*. In experimental animals (for example, rats) abrupt withdrawal of morphine after chronic administration for a few days causes an increased irritability, loss of weight and a variety of abnormal behaviour patterns, such as body shakes, writhing, jumping and signs of aggression. These reactions decrease after a few days, but abnormal irritability and aggression persist for many weeks. Human addicts show a similar abstinence syndrome, somewhat resembling severe influenza, with yawning, pupillary dilatation, fever, sweating, piloerection,* nausea, diarrhoea and insomnia.

Patients are extremely restless and distressed and have a strong craving for the drug. The symptoms are maximal in about 2 days and largely disappear in 8–10 days, though some residual symptoms and physiological abnormalities persist for several weeks. Re-administration of morphine rapidly abolishes the abstinence syndrome.

Many physiological changes have been described in relation to the abstinence syndrome. For example, reflex hyperexcitability is demonstrable in the spinal cord of morphine-dependent animals, and can be produced by

---

Tolerance and dependence

- Tolerance develops rapidly, accompanied by physical withdrawal syndrome.
- The mechanism of tolerance may involve adaptive up-regulation of adenylate cyclase. It is not pharmacokinetic in origin and receptor down-regulation is not a major factor.
- Dependence is satisfied by μ-receptor agonists, and the withdrawal syndrome is precipitated by μ-receptor antagonists.
- Dependence comprises two components: (a) physical dependence, associated with the withdrawal syndrome, lasting for a few days; (b) psychological dependence, associated with craving, lasting for months or years. Psychological dependence rarely occurs in patients being given opioids as analgesics.
- Weak, long-acting μ-receptor agonists, such as methadone, may be used to relieve withdrawal symptoms.
- Certain opioid analgesics, such as codeine, pentazocine and buprenorphine, are much less likely to cause physical or psychological dependence.

---

*Causing goose pimples. This is the origin of the phrase 'cold turkey' used to describe the effect of morphine withdrawal.

chronic intrathecal as well as systemic administration of morphine. The noradrenergic pathways emanating from the *locus ceruleus* (see above) may also play an important role in causing the abstinence syndrome, and the α_2-adrenoceptor agonist, clonidine, is sometimes used to alleviate it. The rate of firing of *locus ceruleus* neurons is reduced by opioids, and increased during the abstinence syndrome. Similar changes affect dopaminergic neurons in the *ventral tegmental area* which project to the *nucleus accumbens*. These cells receive input from opioid-containing neurons, and constitute the 'reward pathway' responsible for the strong reinforcing effect of opioids (see Ch. 39).

PHARMACOKINETIC ASPECTS

Table 37.4 summarises the pharmacokinetic properties of the main opioid analgesics. The absorption of morphine congeners by mouth is variable. **Morphine** itself is slowly and erratically absorbed, and is commonly given by intravenous or intramuscular injection to treat acute severe pain; oral morphine is, however, often used in treating chronic pain, and slow-release preparations are available to increase its duration of action. **Codeine** is well absorbed, and normally given by mouth. Most morphine-like drugs undergo considerable first-pass metabolism, and are therefore markedly less potent when taken orally than when injected.

The plasma half-life of most morphine analogues is 3–6 hours. Hepatic metabolism is the main mode of inactivation, usually by conjugation with glucuronide. This occurs at the 3- and 6-OH groups, and these glucuronides constitute a considerable fraction of the drug in the bloodstream. Morphine-6-glucuronide is, surprisingly, more active as an analgesic than morphine itself, and contributes substantially to the pharmacological effect. Morphine-3-glucuronide has been claimed to antagonise the analgesic effect of morphine, but the significance of this experimental finding is uncertain. Morphine glucuronides are excreted in the urine, so the dose needs to be reduced in cases of renal failure. Glucuronides also reach the gut via biliary excretion, where they are hydrolysed, most of the morphine being reabsorbed (enterohepatic circulation). Because of low conjugating capacity in neonates, morphine-like drugs have a much longer duration of action; because even a small degree of respiratory depression can be hazardous, morphine congeners should not be used in the neonatal period, nor used as analgesics during childbirth. **Pethidine** (see below) is a safer alternative for this purpose.

Analogues that have no free –OH in the 3-position (i.e.

diamorphine, **codeine**) are metabolised to morphine, which accounts for at least part of their pharmacological activity.

Morphine produces very effective analgesia when administered intrathecally, and is often used in this way by anaesthetists, the advantage being that the sedative and respiratory depressant effects are reduced, though not completely avoided.

For the treatment of chronic or postoperative pain, opioids are being increasingly used 'on demand' (patient-controlled analgesia). The patients are provided with an infusion pump which they control, the maximum possible rate of administration being limited to avoid acute toxicity. Contrary to fears, patients show little tendency to use excessively large doses and become dependent; instead the dose is adjusted to achieve analgesia without excessive sedation, and is reduced as the pain subsides. Being in control of their own analgesia, the patients' anxiety and distress is reduced, and analgesic consumption actually tends to decrease.

UNWANTED EFFECTS

The main unwanted effects of morphine and related drugs are listed in Table 37.4.

Acute overdosage with morphine results in coma and respiratory depression, with characteristically constricted pupils. It is treated by giving **naloxone** intravenously. This also serves as a diagnostic test, for failure to respond to naloxone indicates a cause other than opioid poisoning for the comatose state. There is a danger of precipitating a severe withdrawal syndrome with naloxone, since opioid poisoning occurs mainly in addicts.

OTHER OPIOID ANALGESICS

Diamorphine is the diacetyl derivative of morphine. A strong smell of vinegar commonly provides the lead to illicit heroin producers, at least in fiction. It is pharmacologically very similar to morphine, and somewhat more active, and is converted to morphine in the body. Because of its greater lipid solubility it crosses the blood–brain barrier more rapidly than morphine, and gives a greater 'rush' when injected intravenously. It is said to be less emetic than morphine, but the evidence for this is slight. It is still available in Britain for clinical use as an analgesic though it is banned in many countries. Its only advantage over morphine is its greater solubility, which allows smaller volumes to be given orally. It exerts the same respiratory depressant effect as morphine, and if given intravenously is more likely to cause de-

Table 37.4 Characteristics of the main opioid analgesic drugs

Drug	Uses	Route of administration	Pharmacokinetic aspects	Main adverse effects	Notes
Morphine	Widely used for acute and chronic pain	Oral, including sustained-release form Injection* Intrathecal	Half-life 3–4 h Converted to active metabolite (morphine-6-glucuronide)	Sedation, respiratory depression Constipation Nausea and vomiting Itching (histamine release) Tolerance and dependence Euphoria	Tolerance and withdrawal effects not common when used for analgesia
Heroin	Acute and chronic pain	Oral Injection	Acts more rapidly and more briefly than morphine Metabolised partly to morphine	As morphine	Not available in all countries Considered (irrationally) to be analgesic of last resort
Hydromorphone	Acute and chronic pain	Oral Injection	Half-life 2–4 h No active metabolites	As morphine, but allegedly less sedative	**Levorphanol** is similar, with longer duration of action
Methadone	Chronic pain Maintenance of addicts	Oral Injection	Long half-life (> 24 h) Slow onset	As morphine, but little euphoric effect Cumulation may occur due to long half-life	Slow recovery results in attenuated withdrawal syndrome
Pethidine	Acute pain	Oral Intramuscular injection	Half-life 2–4 h Active metabolite (norpethidine) may account for stimulatory effects	As morphine Anticholinergic effects Risk of excitement and convulsions	Known as **meperidine** in US Severe interaction with monoamine oxidase inhibitors
Buprenorphine	Acute and chronic pain	Sublingual Injection Intrathecal	Half-life about 12 h Slow onset Inactive orally owing to first-pass metabolism	As morphine but less pronounced Respiratory depression not reversed by naloxone (therefore not suitable for obstetric use)	Useful in chronic pain with patient-controlled injection systems
Pentazocine	Mainly acute pain	Oral Injection	Half-life 2–4 h	Psychotomimetic effects (dysphoria) Irritation at injection site May precipitate morphine withdrawal syndrome (μ-antagonist effect)	**Butorphanol** (not available in UK) and **nalbuphine** are similar Butorphanol is not active orally Nalbuphine less likely than pentazocine to cause euphoria
Fentanyl	Acute pain Anaesthesia	Intravenous Epidural Transdermal patch	Half-life 1–2 h	As morphine	High potency allows transdermal administration **Sufentanil** is similar
Codeine	Mild pain	Oral	Acts as pro-drug. Metabolised to morphine and other active opioids	Mainly constipation No dependence liability	Effective only in mild pain Also used to suppress cough **Dihydrocodeine** is similar
Dextropropoxyphene	Mild pain	Mainly oral	Half-life ~4 h. Active metabolite (norpropoxyphene) with half-life ~24 h	Respiratory depression May cause convulsions (possibly due to norpropoxyphene)	Similar to codeine **Tramadol** is similar, but may also act by non-opioid mechanisms (e.g. inhibition of amine uptake)

*Injections may be given intravenously, intramuscularly or subcutaneously for most drugs.

pendence. Its duration of action (about 2 hours) is shorter than that of morphine.

Codeine (3-methylmorphine) is more reliably absorbed by mouth than morphine, but has only 20% or less of the analgesic potency. Furthermore, its analgesic effect does not increase appreciably at higher dose levels. It is therefore used mainly as an oral analgesic for mild types of pain (headache, backache, etc.). Unlike morphine, it causes little or no euphoria, and is rarely addictive, so is available freely without prescription. It is often combined with paracetamol in proprietary analgesic preparations. In relation to its analgesic effect, codeine produces the same degree of respiratory depression as morphine, but the limited response even at high doses means that it is seldom a problem in practice. It does, however, cause constipation. Codeine has marked antitussive activity and is often used in cough mixtures (see Ch. 19). **Dihydro-codeine** is pharmacologically very similar, having no substantial advantages or disadvantages over codeine.

Dextropropoxyphene is similar to codeine, but has a longer duration of action. It was thought to be safe in overdose and free from dependence liability, but experience has shown that neither is the case.

Pethidine is very similar to morphine in its pharmacological effects, except that it tends to cause restlessness rather than sedation, and it has an additional anti-muscarinic action which may cause dry mouth and blurring of vision as side-effects. It produces a very similar euphoric effect, and is equally liable to cause dependence. Its duration of action is appreciably shorter than that of morphine, and the route of metabolic degradation is different. Pethidine is partly N-demethylated in the liver to norpethidine, which has a hallucinogenic and convulsant effect. This becomes significant with large oral doses of pethidine, producing an overdose syndrome rather different from that of morphine. Pethidine is preferred to morphine for analgesia during labour, because it is shorter-acting. The difference in the duration of action of morphine and pethidine is particularly marked in the neonate. This is because the conjugation reactions, on which the excretion of morphine, but not of pethidine, depends, are deficient in the newborn. Severe reactions, consisting of excitement, hyperthermia and convulsions, have been reported when pethidine is given to patients receiving monoamine oxidase inhibitors. This seems to be due to inhibition of an alternative metabolic pathway, leading to increased norpethidine formation, but the details are not known.

Fentanyl and **sufentanil** are highly potent phenyl-piperidine derivatives, with actions similar to morphine, but short-lasting, particularly sufentanil. Their main use is in anaesthesia, and they may be given intrathecally. They are also used in patient-controlled infusion systems, where a short duration of action is advantageous.

Etorphine is a morphine analogue of remarkable potency, more than 1000 times that of morphine, but otherwise very similar in its actions. Its high potency confers no particular clinical advantage, but it is used successfully to immobilise wild animals for trapping and research purposes, since the required dose, even for an elephant, is small enough to be incorporated into a dart or pellet.

Methadone is also pharmacologically similar to morphine, the main difference being that its duration of action is considerably longer (plasma half-life > 24 hours) and it is claimed to have less sedative action. The increased duration seems to occur because the drug is bound in the extravascular compartment, and slowly released. One consequence is that the physical abstinence syndrome is less acute than with morphine or other short-acting drugs, though the psychological dependence is no less pronounced. For this reason, methadone is widely used as a means of treating morphine and diamorphine addiction. In the presence of methadone, an injection of morphine does not cause the normal euphoria, nor is there a physical abstinence syndrome, so it is often possible to wean addicts from morphine or diamorphine by giving regular oral doses of methadone—an improvement if not a cure.*

Pentazocine is a mixed agonist–antagonist (see earlier section). In low doses its potency and effects are very similar to those of morphine, but increasing the dose does not cause a corresponding increase in the effects produced. Thus, at high doses, pentazocine causes only slight respiratory depression, and it causes marked dysphoria, with nightmares and hallucinations, rather than euphoria. It also tends to raise, rather than lower, arterial blood pressure. These differences mean that pentazocine has less tendency to cause dependence, and its acute toxicity is much less than that of morphine. Its antagonist activity is apparent in the fact that, given concurrently with morphine, pentazocine actually reduces the analgesic and other actions of morphine, and can even precipitate an abstinence syndrome in morphine addicts. Binding studies show that it has a higher affinity for κ- than for μ-receptors, and also acts on non-opioid σ-receptors, this spectrum being somewhat different from that of conventional opioid drugs. Though clearly much less addictive than the conventional opioids, pentazocine

---

*The benefits come mainly from removing the risks of self-injection and the need to finance the drug habit through crime.

still has an appreciable tendency to cause dependence, and is far from the ideal morphine substitute that it was originally thought to be.

Buprenorphine is a partial agonist on μ-receptors. It is less liable to cause dysphoria than pentazocine, but more liable to cause respiratory depression. It has a long duration of action. Its abuse liability is probably less than that of morphine.

Meptazinol and **dezocine** are recently introduced opiates of unusual chemical structure. Meptazinol can be given orally or by injection, and has a short plasma half-life. It seems to be relatively free of morphine-like side-effects, causing neither euphoria nor dysphoria, nor causing severe respiratory depression. It does, however produce nausea, sedation and dizziness, and has atropine-like side-effects. Because of its short duration of action and lack of respiratory depression, it may have advantages for obstetric analgesia. Dezocine is a partial agonist at μ-receptors, with analgesic activity similar to that of morphine, but with respiratory depressant activity that reaches a 'ceiling' at high doses. It has not yet been fully evaluated.

OPIOID ANTAGONISTS

Nalorphine (Table 37.1) is closely related in structure to morphine, and was the first specific antagonist to be discovered, and the first clear evidence in favour of a specific receptor for morphine, recognition of which led to the successful search for endogenous mediators. Nalorphine has, in fact, a more complicated action than that of a simple competitive antagonist (Table 37.3). In low doses it is a competitive antagonist, and blocks most actions of morphine in whole animals or isolated tissues. Higher doses, however, are analgesic, and mimic the effects of morphine. These effects probably reflect an antagonist action on μ-receptors, coupled with a partial agonist action on δ- and κ-receptors, the latter causing dysphoria, which makes it unsuitable for use as an analgesic. Nalorphine can itself produce physical dependence, but can also precipitate a withdrawal syndrome in morphine or diamorphine addicts. Nalorphine now has few clinical uses. At one time it was the most effective antidote available in cases of acute morphine or diamorphine overdosage, but had the disadvantage that, if large doses were needed, nalorphine itself caused respiratory depression. It has therefore been superseded by naloxone, which has no such effect.

Naloxone was the first pure opioid antagonist, with affinity for all three opioid receptors. It blocks the actions of endogenous opioid peptides as well as those of morphine-like drugs, and has been extensively used as an experimental tool to determine the physiological role of these peptides, particularly in pain transmission.

Given on its own, naloxone produces very little effect in normal subjects, but produces a rapid reversal of the effects of morphine and other opioids, including partial agonists such as pentazocine and nalorphine. It has little effect on pain threshold under normal conditions, but causes hyperalgesia under conditions of stress or inflammation, when endogenous opioids are produced. This occurs, for example in patients undergoing dental surgery, or in animals subjected to physical stress. Naloxone also inhibits acupuncture analgesia, which is known to be associated with the release of opioid peptides. Analgesia produced by PAG stimulation is also prevented.

The main clinical use of naloxone is to treat respiratory depression caused by opioid overdosage, and occasionally to reverse the effect of opioid analgesics, used during labour, on the respiration of the newborn baby. It is usually given intravenously and its effects are produced immediately. It is rapidly metabolised by the liver, and its effect lasts only 2–4 hours, which is considerably shorter than that of most morphine-like drugs. Thus it may have to be given repeatedly.

Naloxone has no important unwanted effects of its own, but precipitates withdrawal symptoms in addicts. It can be used to detect opioid addiction.

Naltrexone is very similar to naloxone but with the advantage of a much longer duration of action (half-life about 10 hours). It may be of value in addicts who have been 'detoxified', since it nullifies the effect of a dose of opiate should the patient's resolve fail. Its use in other conditions, such as alcoholism and septic shock, is being

---

Opioid antagonists

- Pure antagonists include naloxone (short-acting) and naltrexone (long-acting). They block μ-, δ- and κ-receptors more-or-less equally.
- Other drugs, such as nalorphine and pentazocine, produce a mixture of agonist and antagonist effects.
- Naloxone does not affect pain threshold normally, but blocks stress-induced analgesia, and can exacerbate clinical pain.
- Naloxone rapidly reverses opioid-induced analgesia and respiratory depression, and is used mainly to treat opioid overdose or to improve breathing in newborn babies affected by opioids given to the mother.
- Naloxone precipitates withdrawal symptoms in morphine-dependent patients or animals. Pentazocine may also do this.

Clinical use of analgesic drugs

- The choice and route of administration of analgesic drugs depends on the nature and duration of the pain.
- A progressive approach is often used, starting with non-steroidal anti-inflammatory drugs, supplemented first by weak opioid analgesics, and then by strong opioids.
- In general, severe acute pain (e.g. trauma, burns, post-operative pain) is treated with strong opioid drugs (e.g. morphine, fentanyl) given by injection. Mild inflammatory pain (e.g. arthritis) is treated with non-steroidal anti-inflammatory drugs (e.g. aspirin) supplemented by weak opioid drugs (codeine, dextropropoxyphene, pentazocine) given orally if required. Severe pain (e.g. cancer pain, severe arthritis or back pain) is treated with strong opioids given orally, intrathecally, epidurally or by subcutaneous injection. Patient-controlled infusion systems are commonly used.
- Chronic neuropathic pain is often unresponsive to opioids, and treated with tricyclic antidepressants (e.g. amitriptyline), or other drugs, such as carbamazepine.

investigated, though the role of opioid peptides in these conditions is controversial.

Specific antagonists at μ-, δ- and κ-receptors are available for experimental use (Table 37.3), but not yet for clinical purposes.

NEW APPROACHES

It can be seen from the earlier discussion of the neural mechanisms involved in pain and nociception that there are many potential sites at which drugs might act to inhibit transmission of information from the periphery to the thalamus and cortex. Attempts to develop new types of drug have tended to be dominated by opioid agonists on the one hand and NSAIDs on the other, but other possibilities are now being considered (see Rang & Urban 1995), and may find their way into clinical use. They include:

- *Enkephalinase inhibitors*, such as **thiorphan** and the experimental drug RB120 act by inhibiting the metabolic degradation of endogenous opioid peptides, and have been shown to produce analgesia, together with other morphine-like effects, without causing dependence.
- Various neuropeptides, such as *somatostatin* (see Ch. 24) and *calcitonin* (see Ch. 25), produce powerful analgesia when applied intrathecally, and there are clinical reports suggesting that they may have similar effects when used systemically to treat endocrine disorders.
- Non-peptide *antagonists of substance P*, which modulates transmission through the dorsal horn (see above), have recently been developed and may prove to be useful analgesic drugs.
- *Adenosine analogues*, and *adenosine kinase inhibitors*, which mimic or enhance the inhibitory effect of adenosine on nociceptive pathways.
- Agonists at nicotinic ACh receptors, based on *epibatidine* (an alkaloid from frog skin, which is a potent nicotinic agonist, and—unexpectedly—a potent analgesic as well). Derivatives with fewer side-effects are under investigation.
- Transplantation of *enkephalin-secreting adrenal medullary cells* into the spinal canal.

REFERENCES AND FURTHER READING

Besson J-M, Chaouch A 1987 Peripheral and spinal mechanisms of nociception. Physiol Rev 67: 67–186

Burnstock G, Wood J N 1996 Purinergic receptors: their role in nociception and primary afferent neurotransmission. Curr Opin Neurobiol 6: 526–532 *(Review of a novel cloned ATP receptor which is expressed selectively by nociceptive sensory neurons)*

Caterina M J, Schumacher M A, Tominaga M, Rosen T A, Levine J D, Julius D 1997 The capsaicin receptor: a heat-activated ion channel in the pain pathway. Nature 389: 816–824 *(The cloning of the long-sought capsaicin receptor, which turned out to be an unusual type of ligand-gated channel, also showing heat-sensitivity)*

Cesare P, McNaughton P 1997 Peripheral pain mechanisms. Curr Opin Neurobiol 7: 493–499 *(Review article discussing recent work on sensitisation of heat responses by other agents)*

Childers S R 1997 Opioid receptors: pinning down the opiate targets. Curr Biol 7: R695–R697 *(News on results obtained with opiate receptor knock-outs)*

Coderre T J, Katz J, Vaccarino A L, Melzack R 1993 Contribution of central neuroplasticity to pathological pain: review of clinical and experimental evidence. Pain 52: 259–285

Cooper J R, Bloom F E, Roth R H 1996 The biochemical basis of neuropharmacology. Oxford University Press, New York *(Excellent textbook, with good account of opioid peptides)*

Dahl J B, Kehlet H 1993 The value of pre-emptive analgesia in the treatment of post-operative pain. Br J Anaesth 70: 434–439 *(Assesses evidence supporting the efficacy or otherwise of pre-emptive local anaesthesia)*

Dhawan B N, Cesselin F, Raghubir R et al. 1996 Classification of opioid receptors. Pharmacol Rev 48: 567–592 *(The last word on opioid receptor classification, from the International Union of Pharmacology subcommittee entrusted with the task)*

Dray A, Perkins M 1993 Bradykinin and inflammatory pain. Trends Neurosci 16: 99–104

Dubner R, Ruda M A 1992 Activity-dependent neuronal plasticity following tissue injury and inflammation. Trends Neurosci 15: 96–102

Duggan A W, North R A 1984 Electrophysiology of opioids. Pharmacol Rev 35: 219–281 *(Good review article on effects of opiates at the membrane level)*

Fields H L 1987 Pain. McGraw-Hill, New York *(Excellent introductory textbook)*

Fields H L, Basbaum A I 1994 Central nervous system mechanisms of pain modulation. In: Wall P D, Melzack R (eds) Textbook of pain. Churchill Livingstone, Edinburgh

Henderson G, McKnight A T 1997 The orphan opioid receptor and its endogenous ligand—nociceptin/orphanin FQ. Trends Pharmacol Sci 18: 293–300 *(Review article summarising what we know about the newly discovered opioid peptide and its receptor)*

Herz A (ed) 1993 Opioids. (2 vols) Handbook of experimental pharmacology. Springer-Verlag, Berlin, vol 104 *(Definitive compendium of reviews on all aspects of opioid pharmacology)*

Holzer P 1988 Local effector functions of capsaicin-sensitive sensory nerve endings: involvement of tachykinins, calcitonin gene-related peptide and other neuropeptides. Neuroscience 24: 739–768 *(Review of neurogenic inflammation and other peripheral effector roles of peptidergic afferent neurons)*

Kress M, Reeh P W 1996 Chemical excitation and sensitization in nociceptors. In: Belmonte C, Cervero F (eds) Neurobiology of nociceptors. Oxford University Press, Oxford, pp 258–297 *(Review of peripheral modulation of nociceptors)*

Longmore J, Hill R G, Hargreaves R J 1997 Neurokinin-receptor antagonists: pharmacological tool and therapeutic drugs. Can J Physiol Pharmacol 75: 612–621 *(Review article on new tachykinin antagonists)*

McMahon S B 1996 NGF as a mediator of inflammatory pain. Philos Trans R Soc Lond 351: 431–440 *(Review of evidence implicating NGF as a mediator of inflammatory pain and hyperalgesia, including studies of a novel type of NGF inhibitor)*

McMahon S B, Lewin G R, Wall P D 1993 Central hyper-excitability triggered by noxious inputs. Curr Opin Neurobiol 3: 602–610 *(Review of mechanisms of dorsal horn plasticity)*

Maggi C A, Pattachini R, Rovero P, Giachetti A 1993 Tachykinin receptors and tachykinin receptor antagonists. J Autonom Pharmacol 13: 23–93 *(Comprehensive review)*

Maggio J E 1988 Tachykinins. Ann Rev Neurosci 11: 13–28 *(General review)*

Malcangio M, Bowery N 1996 GABA and its receptors in the spinal cord. Trends Pharmacol Sci 17: 457–462 *(Review article on role of GABA in the nociceptive pathway)*

Mantyh P et al. 1995 Receptor endocytosis and dendrite reshaping in spinal neurons after somatosensory stimulation. Science 268: 1629–1632 *(Elegant study with immunofluorescent receptor labelling, revealing SP-mediated receptor plasticity in dorsal horn neurons)*

North R A 1993 Opioid actions on membrane ion channels. In: Herz A (ed) Opioids. Handbook of experimental pharmacology. Springer-Verlag, Berlin, vol 104

Pasternak G W 1993 Pharmacological mechanisms of opioid analgesics. Clin Neuropharmacol 16: 1–18 *(Review of physiological mechanisms of opiate analgesia)*

Rainville P, Duncan G H, Price D D, Carrier B, Bushnell M C 1997 Pain affect encoded in human anterior cingulate but not somatosensory cortex. Science 277: 968–971 *(Imaging study showing cortical area involved in affective component of pain)*

Rang H P, Urban L 1995 New molecules in analgesia. Br J Anaesth 75: 145–156 *(Review of novel pharmacological approaches to analgesia)*

Rang H P, Bevan S, Dray A 1994 Nociceptive peripheral neurons: cellular properties. In: Wall P D, Melzack R (eds) Textbook of pain. Churchill Livingstone, Edinburgh *(Review of chemosensitivity of primary afferent neurons)*

Rang H P, Bevan S J, Perkins M N 1998 Peripherally acting analgesic agents. In: Sawynok J, Cowan A (eds) Novel aspects of pain management: opioids and beyond. John Wiley, New York

Sawynok J, Sweeney M I 1996 The role of purines in nociception. Neuroscience 32: 557–569 *(Review article drawing attention to role of adenosine as a modulator in nociceptive transmission)*

Sibinga N E S, Goldstein A 1988 Opioid peptides and opioid receptors in cells of the immune system. Annu Rev Immunol 16: 219–249 *(Summarises evidence implicating opioid peptides in control of immune system)*

Snyder S H, Pasternak G W, Pert C 1973 In: Iversen L L, Iverson S D, Synder S H (eds) Handbook of psychopharmacology. Plenum, New York, vol 5: 329–360

Stein C, Yassouridis A 1997 Peripheral morphine analgesia. Pain 71: 119–121 *(Short polemic emphasising that opioid analgesia has a significant peripheral component)*

Wagner J J, Chavkin C 1995 Neuropharmacology of endogenous opioid peptides. In: Bloom F E, Kupfer D J Psychopharmacology: the fourth generation of progress. Raven Press, New York *(General review article)*

Walker J M, Bowen W D, Walker F O, Matsumoto R R, De Costa B, Rice K C 1990 Sigma receptors: biology and function. Pharmacol Rev 42: 355–402

Wall P D, Melzack R (eds) 1994 Textbook of pain. Churchill Livingstone, Edinburgh *(Large multi-author reference book)*

Wood J N (ed) 1993 Capsaicin in the study of pain. Academic Press, London *(Collection of articles on capsaicin and sensory neurons)*

Yaksh T L 1997 Pharmacology and mechanisms of opioid analgesic activity. Acta Anaesthesiol Scand 41: 94–111 *(Review of evidence relating to sites of action and receptor specificity of analgesic effect of opioids)*

38

Central nervous system stimulants and psychotomimetic drugs

Drugs that have a predominantly stimulant effect on the central nervous system fall into three broad categories:

- convulsants and respiratory stimulants
- psychomotor stimulants
- psychotomimetic drugs.

Drugs in the first category (e.g. **doxapram**, **nikethamide**, **leptazol** and **strychnine**) have relatively little effect on mental function, and appear to act mainly on the brainstem and spinal cord, producing exaggerated reflex excitability, an increase in activity of the respiratory and vasomotor centres, and with higher dosage, convulsions.

Drugs in the second category (e.g. **amphetamine**, **caffeine** and **cocaine**) have a marked effect on mental function and behaviour, producing excitement and euphoria, reduced sensation of fatigue and an increase in motor activity.

Drugs in the third category (e.g. **lysergic acid diethylamide** (LSD), **phencyclidine** and **cannabinoids**) mainly affect thought patterns and perception, distorting cognition in a complex way and producing effects that superficially resemble psychotic illness.

The distinctions between these three categories are not completely clear cut. Amphetamine, for example, can produce psychotomimetic effects as well as excitement and euphoria. Table 38.1 summarises the classification of the drugs that are discussed in this chapter.

Cannabinoids (see Ch. 39) has predominantly depressant rather than stimulant actions; in addition, certain of its effects resemble those of psychotomimetic drugs.

CONVULSANTS AND RESPIRATORY STIMULANTS

Convulsants and respiratory stimulants (sometimes called *analeptics*), are a chemically diverse group of substances whose mechanisms of action are, with some exceptions, not well understood. Such drugs were once used to treat patients in terminal coma or with severe respiratory failure. Although temporary restoration of function could sometimes be achieved, mortality was not reduced, and the treatment carried a considerable risk of causing convulsions which left the patient more deeply comatose than before. They were used mainly to give the impression that something was being done for a patient *in extremis*. There remains a very limited clinical use for respiratory stimulants in treating acute ventilatory failure (see Ch. 19), **amiphenazole** and **doxapram** (Table 38.1) being most commonly used since these drugs carry less risk of causing convulsions than earlier compounds.

Also included in this group are various compounds, such as **strychnine**, **picrotoxin** and **leptazol**, which are of interest as experimental tools, but have no clinical uses.

Strychnine is an alkaloid found in the seeds of an Indian tree, which has been used for centuries as a poison (mainly vermin, but also human; it is much favoured in detective stories of a certain genre). It is a powerful convulsant, and acts throughout the central nervous system but particularly on the spinal cord, causing violent extensor spasms that are triggered by minor sensory stimuli, the head being thrown back and the face fixed, we are told, in a hideous grin. These effects result from blocking receptors for glycine, which is the main inhibitory transmitter acting on motoneurons. The action of strychnine superficially resembles that of tetanus toxin, a protein neurotoxin produced by the anaerobic bacterium *Clostridium tetani*, which blocks the release of glycine from inhibitory interneurons. This is very similar to the action

Table 38.1 Central nervous system stimulants and psychotomimetic drugs

Category	Examples	Mode of action	Clinical significance
Convulsants and respiratory stimulants (analeptics)			
Respiratory stumulants	Amiphenazole	Not known	Occasionally used as respiratory stimulant Risk of convulsions less than with nikethamide
	Doxapram	Not known	Short-acting respiratory stimulant sometimes given by intravenous infusion to treat acute respiratory failure
Miscellaneous convulsants	Strychnine	Antagonist of glycine Main action is to increase reflex excitability of spinal cord	No clinical uses
	Bicuculline	Competitive antagonist of GABA	No clinical uses
	Picrotoxin	Non-competitive antagonist of GABA	Clinical use as respiratory stimulant; now obsolete
	Nikethamide	Not known	Risk of convulsions
	Leptazol	Not known	No clinical use. Convulsant activity in experimental animals provides a useful model for testing anticonvulsant drugs (see Ch. 36)
Psychomotor stimulants			
	Amphetamine and related compounds, e.g. dexamphetamine, methylamphetamine, methylphenidate, fenfluramine, MDMA	Release of catecholamines Inhibition of catecholamine uptake	Very limited clinical use owing to dependence liability, peripheral sympathomimetic effects, and risk of pulmonary hypertension Some agents used as appetite suppressants Mainly important as drugs of abuse
	Cocaine	Inhibition of catecholamine uptake Local anaesthetic	Important as drug of abuse Risk of foetal damage Occasionally used for nasopharyngeal and ophthalmic anaesthesia (see Ch. 40)
	Methylxanthines, e.g. caffeine, theophylline	Inhibition of phosphodiesterase Antagonism of adenosine (relevance of these actions to central effects is not clear)	Clinical uses unrelated to stimulant activity, though caffeine is included in various 'tonics'. Theophylline used for action on cardiac and bronchial muscle. Constituents of beverages
Psychotomimetic drugs (hallucinogens)			
	Lysergic acid diethylamide (LSD)	Mixed agonist/antagonist at 5-HT receptors (see Ch. 9)	No clinical use Important as drug of abuse
	Mescaline	Not known. Chemically similar to amphetamine	
	Psilocybin	Chemically related to 5-HT. Probably acts on 5-HT receptors	
	Tetrahydrocannabinol (THC)	Acts as CNS depressant with mild psychotomimetic effects	No established clinical use* See Chapter 39
	Phencyclidine	Chemically similar to ketamine (see Ch. 32) Acts on σ-receptors. Also blocks NMDA-receptor-operated ion channels (see Ch. 29)	Originally proposed as an anaesthetic, now important as drug of abuse and as a model for schizophrenia

*Nabilone**, a synthetic cannabinoid, is sometimes used as an anti-emetic to reduce nausea during cancer chemotherapy.
MDMA = methylenedioxymethamphetamine

of a closely related toxin, **botulinum toxin** (see Ch. 7), which is produced by another bacterium of the *Clostridium* genus, and causes paralysis by blocking acetylcholine release. In small doses, strychnine causes a measurable improvement in visual and auditory acuity; it was until quite recently included in various 'tonics', on the basis that CNS stimulation should restore both the weary brain and the debilitated body.

Bicuculline is another plant alkaloid which somewhat resembles strychnine in its effects, but acts by blocking receptors for GABA rather than glycine. Its action is confined to GABA$_A$-receptors, which control chloride permeability, and it does not affect GABA$_B$-receptors (see Ch. 29). Its main effects are on the brain rather than the spinal cord, and it is a useful experimental tool for studying GABA-mediated transmission; it has no clinical uses.

Picrotoxin (obtained from the fishberry) also blocks the action of GABA on chloride channels, though not competitively. The plant's name reflects the native practice in the East Indies of incapacitating fish by throwing berries into the water. Picrotoxin, like bicuculline, causes convulsions and has no clinical uses.

Leptazol (**pentylenetetrazole**) acts similarly, though its mode of action is unknown. Inhibition of leptazol-induced convulsions by antiepileptic drugs (see Ch. 36) correlates quite well with their effectiveness against absence seizures, and leptazol has occasionally been used diagnostically in man, since it can precipitate the typical EEG pattern of absence seizures in susceptible patients.

Amiphenazole and **doxapram** are similar to the above drugs, but have a bigger margin of safety between respiratory stimulation and convulsions. Doxapram also causes nausea, coughing and restlessness, which limit its usefulness. It is rapidly eliminated, and it is occasionally used as an intravenous infusion in patients with acute respiratory failure.

PSYCHOMOTOR STIMULANTS

AMPHETAMINES AND RELATED DRUGS

Amphetamine, and its active dextro-isomer **dextro-amphetamine**, together with **methamphetamine** and **methylphenidate** comprise a group of drugs with very similar pharmacological properties (see Fig. 38.1), which includes 'street drugs' such as methylenedioxymethamphetamine (MDMA or 'ecstasy'; see below). **Fenfluramine**, though chemically similar, has slightly different pharmacological effects. All of these drugs act by releasing monoamines from nerve terminals in the brain. Noradrenaline and dopamine are the most important mediators in this connection, but 5-HT release also occurs, particularly with fenfluramine.

Pharmacological effects
The main central effects of amphetamine-like drugs are:

- locomotor stimulation
- euphoria and excitement
- stereotyped behaviour
- anorexia.

In addition, amphetamines have peripheral sympathomimetic actions, producing a rise in blood pressure and inhibition of gastrointestinal motility.

In experimental animals, amphetamines cause increased alertness and locomotor activity, and increased grooming; they also increase aggressive activity. On the other hand, systematic exploration of novel objects by unrestrained rats is reduced by amphetamine. The animals run around more but appear less attentive to their surroundings. Studies of conditioned responses suggest that amphetamines increase the overall rate of responding without affecting the training process markedly. Thus, in a fixed interval schedule where a reward for lever-pressing is forthcoming only after a fixed interval (say 10 minutes) following the last reward, trained animals normally press the lever very infrequently in the first few minutes after the reward, and increase the rate towards the end of the 10-minute interval when another reward is due. The effect of amphetamine is to increase the rate of unrewarded responses at the beginning of the 10-minute interval without affecting (or even reducing) the rate towards the

---

Convulsants and respiratory stimulants

- This is a diverse group of drugs which have little clinical use.
- Certain short-acting respiratory stimulants (e.g. doxapram, amiphenazole) can be used in respiratory failure.
- Strychnine is a convulsant poison that acts mainly on the spinal cord, by blocking receptors for the inhibitory transmitter, glycine.
- Picrotoxin and bicuculline act as GABA$_A$-antagonists; bicuculline blocks the GABA$_A$-receptor site, whereas picrotoxin appears to block the ion channel.
- Leptazol works by an unknown mechanism. Leptazol-induced convulsions provide an animal model for testing anticonvulsant drugs, giving good correlation with effectiveness in preventing absence seizures.

end of the period. The effects of amphetamine on more sophisticated types of conditioned response, for example those involving discriminative tasks, are not clear cut, and there is no clear evidence that either the rate of learning of such tasks or the final level of performance that can be achieved is affected by the drug. Put crudely, amphetamine makes the animals busier rather than brighter.

With large doses of amphetamines, stereotyped behaviour occurs. This consists of repeated actions, such as licking, gnawing, rearing or repeated movements of the head and limbs. These activities are generally inappropriate to the environment, and with increasing doses of amphetamine they take over more and more of the behaviour of the animal. These behavioural effects are evidently produced by the release of catecholamines in the brain, since pretreatment with **6-hydroxydopamine**, which depletes the brain of both noradrenaline and dopamine, abolishes the effect of amphetamine, as does pretreatment with α-**methyltyrosine**, an inhibitor of catecholamine biosynthesis (see Ch. 8). Similarly, **tricyclic antidepressants** and **MAO inhibitors** (see Ch. 35) potentiate the effects of amphetamine, presumably by blocking noradrenaline reuptake or metabolism. Interestingly, **reserpine**, which inhibits vesicular storage of catecholamines (see Ch. 8), does not block the behavioural effects of amphetamine. This is probably because amphetamine releases cytosolic rather than vesicular catecholamines

Table 38.2	Behavioural effects of amphetamines			
Drug	Euphoria	Locomotor stimulation	Stereotyped behaviour	Anorexia
Amphetamine	++	+++	+++	++
MDMA	+++	+++	+++	+
Methylphenidate	+	+++	+++	+
Fenfluramine	–	–	–	+++

(see Ch. 8). The behavioural effects of amphetamine are probably due mainly to release of dopamine rather than noradrenaline. The evidence for this is that destruction of the central noradrenergic bundle does not affect locomotor stimulation produced by amphetamine, whereas destruction of the dopamine-containing *nucleus accumbens* (see Ch. 30) or administration of antipsychotic drugs which antagonise dopamine (see Ch. 34) inhibits this response.

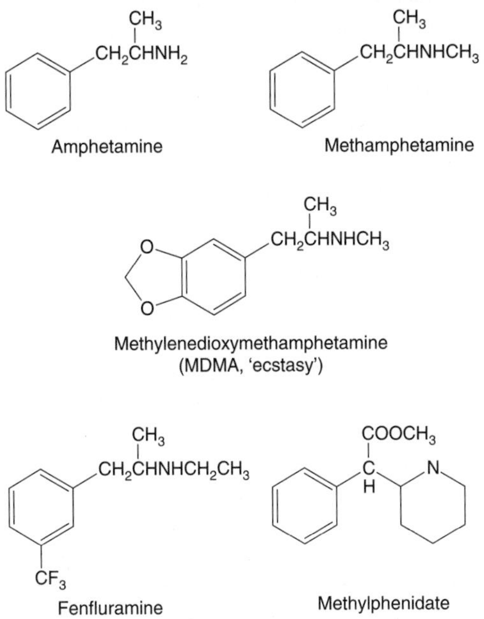

Amphetamine-like drugs cause marked anorexia, but with continued administration this effect wears off in a few days and food intake returns to normal. Amphetamine-like drugs differ in their relative activity in causing locomotor stimulation and anorexia (see Table 38.2). **Fenfluramine** and its D-isomer **dexfenfluramine**, cause anorexia without stimulation (actually being somewhat sedative), and pharmacological studies suggest that this action may depend more on 5-HT release than on release of noradrenaline or dopamine. The same effect can be produced by local injection of amphetamine into the lateral hypothalamus.

In man, amphetamine causes euphoria; with intravenous injection, this can be so intense as to be described as 'orgasmic'. Subjects become confident, hyperactive and talkative, and sex drive is said to be enhanced. Fatigue, both physical and mental, is reduced by amphetamine, and many studies have shown improvement of both mental and physical performance in fatigued, though not in well-rested subjects. Mental performance is improved for simple tedious tasks much more than for difficult tasks, and amphetamines have been used to improve the performance of soldiers, military pilots and others who need to remain alert under extremely fatiguing conditions. It has also been in vogue as a means of helping students to concentrate before and during examinations, but the improvement caused by reduction of fatigue can be offset by the mistakes of overconfidence.*

Fig. 38.1 Structures of amphetamine-like drugs.

*Pay heed to the awful warning of the medical student who, it is said, having taken copious amounts of dextroamphetamine, left the examination hall in confident mood, having spent 3 hours writing his name over and over again.

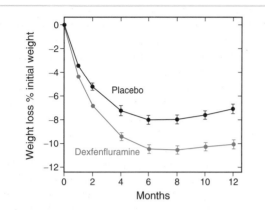

Fig. 38.2 Effect of an amphetamine analogue (dexfenfluramine) on weight loss by patients undergoing treatment for obesity. Dexfenfluramine (1–5 mg twice daily) or placebo were given under double-blind conditions. (From: Guy-Grand B et al. 1989 Lancet 1: 142–145)

Amphetamine-like drugs bring about a small but significant improvement of athletic performance, particularly in endurance events. They are banned in sporting events, and easily detected in urine.

As appetite suppressants in humans, for use in treating obesity, amphetamine derivatives have not generally been successful, mainly because their effectiveness is too short-lived and the risk of producing dependence is too great. However, a placebo-controlled trial on 822 obese Europeans (*imagine!*) showed that dexfenfluramine treatment significantly improved weight loss under a dietary and educational regime, measured over a 12-month period (Fig. 38.2), without serious immediate side-effects.*

Tolerance and dependence

If amphetamine is taken repeatedly over the course of a few days, which occurs when users seek to maintain the euphoric 'high' that a single dose produces, a state of 'amphetamine psychosis' can develop, which closely resembles an acute schizophrenic attack (see Ch. 34), with hallucinations, accompanied by paranoid symptoms and aggressive behaviour. At the same time, repetitive stereotyped behaviour may develop (e.g. polishing shoes or stringing beads). The close similarity of this condition to schizophrenia, and the effectiveness of antipsychotic drugs in controlling it, is consistent with the dopamine theory of schizophrenia discussed in Chapter 34. When

---

*There is, however, serious concern about the association between the use of these drugs and pulmonary hypertension, which can be so severe as to necessitate heart–lung transplantation.

the drug is stopped after a few days, there is usually a period of deep sleep, and on awakening, the subject feels extremely lethargic, depressed and anxious (sometimes even suicidal), and is often very hungry. Even a single dose of amphetamine, which produces euphoria rather than acute psychotic symptoms, usually leaves the subject later feeling tired and depressed. These after-effects may be the result of depletion of the normal stores of noradrenaline and dopamine, but the evidence for this is not clear cut. A state of amphetamine dependence can be produced in experimental animals—thus, rats quickly learn to press a lever in order to obtain a dose of amphetamine, and also become inactive and irritable in the withdrawal phase. These effects do not occur with fenfluramine.

Tolerance develops rapidly to the peripheral sympathomimetic and anorexic effects of amphetamine, but more slowly to the other effects (locomotor stimulation and stereotyped behaviour). Dependence on amphetamine appears to be a consequence of the unpleasant after-effect that it produces, and the insistent memory of euphoria, which leads to a desire for a repeat dose. There is no clear-cut physical withdrawal syndrome such as occurs with opiates. It is estimated that only about 5% of users progress to full-blown dependence, the usual pattern being that the dose is increased as tolerance develops, and then uncontrolled 'binges' occur in which the user takes the drug repeatedly over a period of a day or more, remaining continuously intoxicated. Large doses may be consumed in such binges, with a high risk of acute toxicity, and the demand for the drug displaces all other considerations.

Experimental animals, given unlimited access to amphetamine, take it in such large amounts that they die from the cardiovascular effects within a few days. Given limited amounts, they too develop a 'binge' pattern of dependence.

Pharmacokinetic aspects

Amphetamine is readily absorbed from the gastrointestinal tract, and freely penetrates the blood–brain barrier. It does this more readily than other indirectly acting sympathomimetic amines, such as **ephedrine** or **tyramine** (Ch. 8), which probably explains why it produces more marked central effects than those drugs. It is also readily absorbed from the nasal mucosa, and is often taken by 'snorting'. Amphetamine is mainly excreted unchanged in the urine, and the rate of excretion is increased when the urine is made more acidic (see Ch. 5). The plasma half-life of amphetamine varies from about 5 hours to 20–30 hours, depending on urine flow and urinary pH.

Clinical use and unwanted effects

The uses of amphetamines are very few. Their use in treating obesity is very suspect, because of the risk of pulmonary hypertension (see above).

Paradoxically, amphetamines (particularly methylphenidate, the preferred drug in this indication) are effective in controlling *attention deficit* and *hyperactivity disorder* in children, whose incessant overactivity and very limited attention span disrupt their education and social development. The mechanism of this effect is unknown.

Narcolepsy is a disabling condition, probably a form of epilepsy, in which the patient suddenly and unpredictably falls asleep at frequent intervals during the day. Amphetamine is helpful but not completely effective.

The limited clinical usefulness of amphetamine is offset by its many unwanted effects, including hypertension, insomnia, tremors, risk of exacerbating schizophrenia and risk of dependence.

Sudden deaths have occurred in 'ecstasy' users, even after a single, moderate dose. The drug can induce a condition resembling 'heat-stroke' associated with muscle damage and renal failure, and also causes inappropriate secretion of antidiuretic hormone, leading to dehydration and hyponatraemia.

COCAINE

Cocaine (see reviews by Gawin & Ellinwood 1988, Johanson & Fischman 1989) is found in the leaves of a South American shrub, coca. These leaves are used for their stimulant properties by natives of South America, particularly those living at high altitude, who use it to reduce fatigue during work at high altitude. Considerable mystical significance was attached to the powers of cocaine to boost the flagging human spirit, and Freud experimented with it on his patients. As a result of Freud's experiments with cocaine, his ophthalmologist colleague, Köller, obtained supplies of the drug and discovered its local anaesthetic action (Ch. 40), but the psychostimulant effects of cocaine have not proved to be clinically useful. On the other hand, they led to it becoming at one time the most frequently abused substance in western countries, though its use has decreased somewhat since 1990. The mechanisms and treatment of cocaine abuse are discussed in Chapter 39.

Pharmacological effects

Cocaine is a potent inhibitor of catecholamine uptake by noradrenergic nerve terminals (uptake 1; see Ch. 8), and strongly enhances the peripheral effects of sympathetic nerve activity. It has a marked psychomotor stimulant effect, causing euphoria, garrulousness, increased motor activity and a magnification of pleasure, similar to the effects of amphetamine. These effects are due mainly to inhibition of neuronal dopamine reuptake (Ch. 30), though cocaine also inhibits noradrenaline and 5-HT reuptake. Cocaine has less tendency than amphetamines to produce stereotyped behaviour, delusions, hallucinations and paranoia. With excessive dosage, tremors and convulsions, followed by respiratory and vasomotor depression, may occur. The peripheral sympathomimetic actions lead to tachycardia, vasoconstriction and an increase in blood pressure. Body temperature may increase, owing to the increased motor activity coupled with reduced heat loss. Like amphetamine, cocaine produces no clear-cut physical dependence syndrome, but tends to cause depression and dysphoria, coupled with craving for the drug (see Ch. 39), following the initial stimulant effect. Withdrawal of cocaine after administration for a few days causes a marked deterioration of motor performance and learned behaviour, which are restored by resuming dosage with the drug. There is thus a considerable degree of psychological dependence. The pattern of dependence, evolving from occasional use through escalating dosage to compulsive binges, is identical to that seen with amphetamines.

The duration of action of cocaine (about 30 minutes when given intravenously) is much shorter than that of amphetamine.

Pharmacokinetic aspects

Cocaine is readily absorbed by many routes. For many years, illicit supplies consisted of the hydrochloride salt, which could be given by nasal inhalation or intravenously. The latter route produces an intense and immediate euphoria, whereas nasal inhalation produces a less dramatic sensation, and also tends to cause atrophy and necrosis of the nasal mucosa and septum. Cocaine use increased dramatically when the free base form ('crack') became available as a street drug. Unlike the salt, this can be smoked, giving a very rapid, intense effect with less risk and inconvenience than intravenous or nasal administration. The social, economic, and even political consequences of this small change in formulation have been far-reaching.

A cocaine metabolite is deposited in hair, and analysis of its content along the hair shaft allows the pattern of cocaine consumption to be monitored, a technique which has revealed a much higher incidence of cocaine use than was voluntarily reported. Cocaine exposure in utero can be estimated from analysis of the hair of neonates.

Cocaine is still occasionally used topically as a local

anaesthetic, mainly in ophthalmology and minor nose and throat surgery, but has no other clinical uses. It is a valuable pharmacological tool for the study of catecholamine release and reuptake, because of its relatively specific action in blocking uptake 1.

Adverse effects

Toxic effects occur commonly in cocaine abusers. The main acute dangers are cardiac dysrhythmias and coronary or cerebral thrombosis. Slowly developing damage to the myocardium can also occur, leading to heart failure, even in the absence of acute cardiac effects.

Cocaine can severely impair brain development in utero (see Volpe 1992). The brain size is significantly reduced in babies exposed to cocaine in pregnancy, and the incidence of neurological and limb malformations is also increased. The incidence of ischaemic and haemorrhagic brain lesions, and of sudden infant death, is also higher in cocaine-exposed babies. Interpretation of the data is difficult because many cocaine-abusers also take other illicit drugs which may affect foetal development, but the probability is that cocaine is highly detrimental.

Effects of amphetamines and cocaine

Amphetamines
- The main effects are:
  — increased motor activity
  — euphoria and excitement
  — anorexia
  — with prolonged administration, stereotyped and psychotic behaviour.
- Effects are due mainly to release of catecholamines, especially noradrenaline and dopamine.
- Stimulant effect lasts for a few hours, and is followed by depression and anxiety.
- Tolerance to the stimulant effects develops rapidly, though peripheral sympathomimetic effects may persist.
- Amphetamines may be useful in treating narcolepsy, and also (paradoxically) to control hyperkinetic children. **Dexfenfluramine** is used as an appetite-suppressant.
- Their main importance is in drug abuse.

Cocaine
- Cocaine acts by inhibiting catecholamine uptake (especially dopamine) by nerve terminals.
- Behavioural effects of cocaine are very similar to those of amphetamines, though psychotomimetic effects are rarer. Duration of action is shorter.
- Cocaine used in pregnancy impairs foetal development, and may produce foetal malformations.
- As drugs of abuse, amphetamines and cocaine produce strong psychological dependence, and carry a high risk of severe adverse reactions.

METHYLXANTHINES

Various beverages, particularly tea, coffee and cocoa, contain methylxanthines to which they owe their mild central stimulant effects. The main compounds responsible are **caffeine** and **theophylline**. The nuts of the cola plant also contain caffeine, which is present in cola-flavoured soft drinks. However, the most important sources, by far, are coffee and tea, which account for more than 90% of caffeine consumption. A cup of instant coffee or strong tea contains 5–70 mg caffeine, while filter coffee contains about twice as much. Among adults in tea and coffee drinking countries, the average daily caffeine consumption is about 200 mg. Further information on the pharmacology and toxicology of caffeine is presented by Arnaud (1987) and Nehlig et al (1992).

Pharmacological effects

Methylxanthines have the following major pharmacological actions:

- CNS stimulation
- diuresis (see Ch. 20)
- stimulation of cardiac muscle (see Ch. 14)
- relaxation of smooth muscle, especially bronchial muscle (see Ch. 19).

The latter two effects resemble those of β-adrenoceptor stimulation (see Ch. 8). This is thought to be because methylxanthines (especially theophylline) inhibit phosphodiesterase, which is responsible for the intracellular metabolism of cAMP (Ch. 2). They thus increase intracellular cAMP and produce effects that mimic those of mediators that stimulate adenylate cyclase. Methylxanthines also antagonise many of the effects of adenosine, acting on both A_1- and A_2-receptors (see Ch. 9). Transgenic mice lacking functional A_2-receptors are abnormally active and aggressive, and fail to show increased motor activity in response to caffeine (Ledent et al. 1997), suggesting that antagonism at A_2-receptors accounts for part, at least of its CNS stimulant action. The concentration of caffeine reached in plasma and brain after 2–3 cups of strong coffee—about 100 μM—is sufficient to produce appreciable adenosine receptor block, and a small degree of phosphodiesterase inhibition. The diuretic effect probably results from vasodilatation of the afferent glomerular arteriole, causing an increased glomerular filtration rate.

Caffeine and theophylline have very similar stimulant effects on the central nervous system. Human subjects experience a reduction of fatigue, leading to insomnia, with improved concentration and a clearer flow of thought. This is confirmed by objective studies which have shown that caffeine reduces reaction time, and produces an increase in the speed at which simple calculations can be performed (though without much improvement in accuracy). Performance at motor tasks, such as typing and simulated driving, is also improved, particularly in fatigued subjects. Mental tasks, such as syllable-learning, association tests and so on, are also facilitated by moderate doses (up to about 200 mg caffeine, or about 3 cups of coffee) but inhibited by larger doses. By comparison with amphetamines, methylxanthines produce less locomotor stimulation and do not induce euphoria, stereotyped behaviour patterns or a psychotic state, but their effects on fatigue and mental function are similar.

Tolerance and habituation develop to a small extent, but much less than with amphetamines, and withdrawal effects are slight. Caffeine does not lead to self-administration in animals, and it cannot be classified as a dependence-producing drug.

Clinical use and unwanted effects

There are few clinical uses for caffeine. It is included with aspirin in some preparations for treating headaches and other aches and pains, and with ergotamine in some antimigraine preparations, the object being to produce a mildly agreeable sense of alertness. Theophylline is used mainly as a bronchodilator in treating severe asthmatic attacks (see Ch. 19). Caffeine has few unwanted side-effects, and is safe even in very large doses. In vitro tests show that it has a quite strong mutagenic effect, and there is evidence that large doses are teratogenic in animals. However, epidemiological studies have so far not revealed any carcinogenic or teratogenic effect of tea or coffee drinking in humans.

Methylxanthines

- Caffeine and theophylline produce psychomotor stimulant effects.
- Average caffeine consumption from beverages is about 200 mg/day.
- Main psychological effect is reduced fatigue and improved mental performance, without euphoria. Even large doses do not cause stereotyped behaviour or psychotomimetic effects.
- Methylxanthines act mainly by antagonism at A_2 purine receptors, and partly by inhibiting phosphodiesterase, thus producing effects similar to those of β-adrenoceptor agonists.
- Peripheral actions are exerted mainly on heart, smooth muscle and kidney.
- Theophylline is used clinically as a bronchodilator; caffeine is not used clinically.

PSYCHOTOMIMETIC DRUGS

Psychotomimetic drugs (also referred to as *psychedelic* or *hallucinogenic* drugs) are characterised by the fact that they affect thought, perception and mood, without causing marked psychomotor stimulation or depression. Thoughts and perceptions tend to become distorted and dream-like, rather than being merely sharpened or dulled, and the change in mood is likewise more complex than a simple shift in the direction of euphoria or depression. Not surprisingly, the categorisation of these drugs is very imprecise, and there is no sharp dividing line between the effects of, say, cocaine and those of LSD or cannabis. Psychotomimetic drugs fall broadly into two groups:

- Those with a chemical resemblance to known neurotransmitters (catecholamines or 5-HT). These include **LSD** and **psilocybin**, which are related to 5-HT; **mescaline** and **MDMA** ('ecstasy'; see above), which are related to amphetamine.
- Drugs unrelated to monoamine neurotransmitters, e.g. **cannabis** (see Ch. 39) and **phencyclidine**.

LSD, PSILOCYBIN AND MESCALINE

LSD is an exceptionally potent psychotomimetic drug, capable of producing very marked effects in humans in doses less than 1 µg/kg. It is a chemical derivative of lysergic acid, which occurs in the cereal fungus, ergot (see Ch. 9), and was first synthesised by Hoffman in 1943. Hoffman deliberately swallowed about 250 µg of LSD, and wrote 30 years later of the experience: 'the faces of those around me appeared as grotesque coloured masks ... marked motoric unrest, alternating with paralysis ... heavy feeling in the head, limbs and entire body, as if they were filled with lead ... clear recognition of my condition, in which state I sometimes observed, in the manner of an independent observer, that I shouted half insanely.' These effects lasted for a few hours, after which Hoffman fell asleep, 'and awoke next morning feeling perfectly well'. Apart from these dramatic psychological effects, LSD has few physiological effects. **Mescaline**, which is derived from a Mexican cactus and has been known as a hallucinogenic agent for many centuries, was made famous by Aldous Huxley in *The Doors of Perception*. **Psilocybin** is obtained from a fungus, and has very similar properties. Both have basically similar effects to LSD but are much less potent.

Pharmacological effects

The main effects of these drugs are on mental function, most notably an alteration of perception in such a way that sights and sounds appear distorted and fantastic. Hallucinations visual, auditory, tactile or olfactory also occur, and sensory modalities may become confused, so that sounds are perceived as visions. Thought processes tend to become illogical and disconnected, but subjects generally retain insight into the fact that their disturbance is drug-induced. Occasionally, LSD produces a syndrome that is extremely disturbing to the subject (the 'bad trip') in which the hallucinatory experience takes on a menacing quality, and may be accompanied by paranoid delusions. This sometimes goes so far as to produce homicide or suicide attempts, and in many respects, the state has features in common with acute schizophrenic illness. Furthermore, 'flashbacks' of the hallucinatory experience have been reported weeks or months later.

LSD acts on various 5-HT receptor subtypes (see Ch. 9), and in the central nervous system it is believed to work mainly as a 5-HT$_2$-receptor agonist (see Cooper et al. 1996). It inhibits the firing of 5-HT-containing neurons in the raphe nuclei (see Ch. 30), apparently by acting as an agonist on the inhibitory autoreceptors of these cells. The action of mescaline is apparently different, however, and exerted mainly on noradrenergic neurons. It is still quite unclear how changes in cell firing rates might be related to the psychotomimetic action of these drugs.

The main effects of psychotomimetic drugs are subjective, so it is not surprising that animal tests which reliably predict psychotomimetic activity in man have not been devised. Attempts to measure changes in perception by behavioural conditioning studies have given variable results, but some authors have claimed that effects consistent with increased sensory 'generalisation' (i.e. a tendency to respond similarly to any sensory stimulus) can be detected in this way. One of the more bizarre tests involves disorganisation of web-spinning patterns in spiders, whose normal elegantly symmetrical webs become jumbled and erratic if the animals are treated with LSD.

Dependence and adverse effects

Neither LSD nor other psychotomimetic agents (except for **phencyclidine**; see below) are self-administered by experimental animals. Indeed, they can be shown to have aversive rather than reinforcing properties in behavioural tests, which stands in marked contrast to most of the drugs that are widely abused by humans. Tolerance to the effects of LSD develops quite quickly, and there is cross-tolerance between it and most other psychotomimetics.

There is no physical withdrawal syndrome in animals or man.

There has been much concern over reports that LSD and other psychotomimetic drugs, as well as causing potentially dangerous 'bad trips', can lead to more persistent mental disorder (see Abraham & Aldridge 1993). There are recorded instances in which altered perception and hallucinations have lasted for up to 3 weeks following a single dose of LSD, and of precipitation of attacks in schizophrenic patients. Furthermore, it is believed that LSD can occasionally initiate long-lasting schizophrenia. This, coupled with the fact that the occasional 'bad trip' can result in severe injury through violent behaviour, means that LSD and other psychotomimetics must be regarded as highly dangerous drugs, far removed from the image of peaceful 'experience enhancers' that the hippy subculture* of the 1960s so enthusiastically espoused.

PHENCYCLIDINE

Phencyclidine was originally synthesised as a possible intravenous anaesthetic agent, but was found to produce in many patients a period of disorientation and hallucinations following recovery of consciousness. **Ketamine** (see Ch. 32), a close analogue of phencyclidine, is better as an anaesthetic, though it too can cause symptoms of disorientation. Phencyclidine is now of interest mainly as a drug of abuse (now declining in popularity).

Pharmacological effects

The effects of phencyclidine resemble those of other psychotomimetic drugs (see Johnson & Jones 1990), but also include analgesia, which was one of the reasons for its introduction as an anaesthetic agent. It can also cause stereotyped motor behaviour, like amphetamine. It has the same reported tendency as LSD to cause occasional 'bad trips', and to lead to recurrent psychotic episodes. Its mode of action at a cellular level is not well understood. Specific high-affinity binding sites occur on neuronal membranes, particularly in the frontal cortex and hippocampus, and it appears to have two distinct sites of action. One site is the σ-receptor recognised by various opioids of the benzomorphan type (Ch. 37), while the other is the glutamate-operated ion channel (the NMDA-receptor channel; see Ch. 29) which is blocked by phencyclidine, as well as by ketamine. The σ-receptor is generally believed to mediate the effects of dysphoria and hallucinations produced by certain opiates, and may account for the psychotomimetic effects of phencyclidine. At

---

*You may recall the Beatles' lyric 'Lucy in the Sky with Diamonds', also the phrase 'Drop out; tune in; turn on' coined by Timothy Leary, whose ashes were sent into orbit in 1997.

present it is unclear whether the NMDA-channel action is important. However, studies with **dizocilpine**, an NMDA channel-blocker (see Ch. 29) that lacks affinity for the σ-receptor, suggest that it has much less psychotomimetic activity than phencyclidine, though other behavioural effects are similar. Which, if either, of the two phencyclidine-binding sites is the key to its behavioural effects remains undecided. One prominent question, however, is whether there may be an endogenous ligand for either of the phencyclidine-binding sites, and, if so, whether such substances might be involved in the causation of schizophrenia (see Debonnel 1993).

Psychotomimetic drugs

- The main types are:
  - LSD, psilocybin and mescaline (actions related to 5-HT and catecholamines)
  - phencyclidine.
- Their main effect is to cause sensory changes, hallucinations and delusions, resembling symptoms of acute schizophrenia.
- They are not used clinically, but are important as drugs of abuse.
- LSD is exceptionally potent, producing a long-lasting sense of dissociation and disordered thought, sometimes with frightening hallucinations and delusions which can lead to violence. Hallucinatory episodes can recur after a long interval.

- LSD and phencyclidine precipitate schizophrenic attacks in susceptible patients, and LSD may cause long-lasting psychopathological changes.
- LSD appears to act as an agonist at 5-HT receptors, and suppresses electrical activity in 5-HT raphe neurons, an action which appears to correlate with psychotomimetic activity.
- They do not cause physical dependence, and tend to be aversive, rather than reinforcing, in animal models.
- The mechanism of action of phencyclidine is complex; it binds to the σ-receptor, and also blocks the glutamate-activated NMDA-receptor channel, as well as interacting with other neurotransmitter systems.

REFERENCES AND FURTHER READING

Except where otherwise indicated, all are general review articles.

Abraham H D, Aldridge A M 1993 Adverse consequences of lysergic acid diethylamide. Addiction 88: 1327–1334

Arnaud M J 1987 The pharmacology of caffeine. Prog Drug Res 31: 273–313

Cooper J R, Bloom F E, Roth R H 1996 The biochemical basis of neuropharmacology. Oxford University Press, New York *(Good coverage on mode of action of LSD and amphetamines)*

Debonnel G 1993 Current hypotheses on sigma receptors and their physiological role: possible implications in psychiatry. J Psychiatr Neurosci 18: 157–172

Gawin F H, Ellinwood E H 1988 Cocaine and other stimulants. N Engl J Med 318: 1173–1182

Henderson G 1982 Phenylcyclidine, a widely used but little understood psychotomimetic agent. Trends Pharmacol Sci 3: 248–250

Johanson C-E, Fischman M W 1989 The pharmacology of cocaine related to its abuse. Pharmacol Rev 41: 3–47

Johnson K M, Jones S M 1990 Neuropharmacology of phencyclidine: basic mechanisms and therapeutic potential. Annu Rev Pharmacol Toxicol 30: 707–750

Ledent C et al. 1997 Aggressiveness, hypoalgesia and high blood pressure in mice lacking the adenosine A₂ₐ receptor. Nature 388: 674–678 *(Study of transgenic mice, showing loss of stimulant effects of caffeine in mice lacking A₂-receptors)*

Nehlig A, Daval J-L, Debry G 1992 Caffeine and the central nervous system: mechanisms of action, biochemical, metabolic and psychostimulant effects. Brain Res Rev 17: 139–170

Sonders M S, Keana J F W, Weber E 1988 Phencyclidine and psychotomimetic sigma opiates: recent insights into their biochemical and physiological sites of action. Trends Neurosci 11: 37–40

Volpe J J 1992 Effect of cocaine on the fetus. N Engl J Med 327: 399–407

39

Drug dependence and drug abuse

There are many drugs that human beings consume because they choose to, and not because they are advised to by doctors. Society in general disapproves, because in most cases there is a social cost; for certain drugs, this is judged to outweigh the individual benefit, and their use is banned in many countries. In western societies, the three most commonly-used non-therapeutic drugs are **caffeine**, **nicotine** and **ethanol**, all of which are legally and freely available. A much larger number of drugs are widely used, though their manufacture, sale and consumption has been declared illegal in most western countries, except when it is under the direction of the medical profession. A list of the more important ones is given in Table 39.1. This list does not include the increasing number of drugs that are used illicitly by body-builders and sportsmen to enhance their performance, an account of which is presented by Mottram (1988).

The reasons why particular drugs should come to be used in a way that constitutes a problem to society are complex and largely outside the scope of this book. The drug and its pharmacological activity are only the starting point, though drug-taking is clearly seen by society in a quite different light from other forms of addictive self-gratification, such as opera-going, football or sex. At first sight, the 'drugs of abuse' form an extremely heterogeneous pharmacological group; we can find little in common at the molecular and cellular level between say, morphine, cocaine and barbiturates. What links them is that people find their effect pleasurable (hedonic) and tend to want to repeat it, an action which reflects the effect—common to all dependence-producing drugs—of activating mesolimbic dopaminergic neurons (see below). This hedonic effect becomes a problem when:

- the want becomes so insistent that it dominates the lifestyle of the individual and becomes burdensome
- the habit itself causes actual harm to the individual or the community.

Examples of the latter are the mental incapacity and liver damage caused by ethanol, the many diseases associated with smoking, the high risk of infection (especially with HIV), the serious risk of overdosage with most narcotics, and the criminal behaviour resorted to when an addict needs to finance his habit.

In this chapter we discuss some general aspects of drug dependence and drug abuse, and describe the pharmacology of three important drugs which have no place in therapy but are consumed in large amounts, namely **nicotine**, **ethanol** and **cannabis**. Other drugs with abuse potential are described elsewhere in this book (see Table 39.1). For further information on various aspects of drug abuse, see Shuckit (1995), Winger et al. (1992).

THE NATURE OF DRUG DEPENDENCE

Drug dependence describes the state when drug-taking becomes compulsive, taking precedence over other needs.

Table 39.1 The main drugs of abuse

Type	Examples	Dependence liability	Discussed in
Narcotic analgesics	Morphine	V. strong	Ch. 37
	Diamorphine	V. strong	Ch. 37
General CNS depressants	Ethanol	Strong	This chapter
	Barbiturates	Strong	Ch. 33
	Methaqualone	Moderate	Ch. 33
	Glutethimide	Moderate	Ch. 33
	Anaesthetics	Moderate	Ch. 32
	Solvents	Strong	–
Anxiolytic drugs	Benzodiazepines	Moderate	Ch. 33
Psychomotor stimulants	Amphetamines	Strong	Ch. 38
	Cocaine	V. strong	Ch. 38
	Caffeine	Weak	Ch. 38
	Nicotine	V. strong	This chapter
Psychotomimetic agents	LSD	Weak or absent	Ch. 38
	Mescaline	Weak or absent	Ch. 38
	Phencyclidine	Moderate	Ch. 38
	Cannabis	Weak or absent	This chapter

The older term *drug addiction* is not clearly defined, but generally implies a state of physical dependence (see below). *Drug abuse* and *substance abuse* are more general terms, meaning any use of illicit substances. *Tolerance*—the decrease in pharmacological effect on repeated administration of the drug—often accompanies the state of dependence, and it is possible that related mechanisms account for both phenomena (see below).

The common feature of the various types of psychoactive drugs that can engender dependence is that all produce a *rewarding* effect. In animal studies, where this cannot be inferred directly, it is manifest as *positive reinforcement* (i.e. an increase in the probability of occurrence of any behaviour that results in the drug being administered). Thus, with all dependence-producing drugs, the phenomenon of spontaneous self-administration can be demonstrated in animal studies. Coupled with the direct rewarding effect of the drug, there is usually also a process of *habituation*, or adaptation, when the drug is given repeatedly or continuously, such that cessation of the drug has an aversive effect, *negative reinforcement*, from which the subject will attempt to escape by self-administration of the drug. The physical withdrawal syndrome, associated with the state of physical dependence, is one manifestation of this type of habituation; the intensity and nature of physical withdrawal symptoms varies from one class of drug to another, being particularly marked with opioids. It is less important in sustaining drug-seeking behaviour than psychological habituation, which is associated with a craving that is not related to physical symptoms. A degree of physical dependence is often produced when patients receive opioid analgesics in hospital for several days, but this almost never leads to addiction. On the other hand, addicts who are nursed through and recover fully from the physical abstinence syndrome are still extremely likely to revert to drug-taking later. Thus, physical dependence does not seem to be the major factor in long-term drug dependence. In addition to the positive and negative reinforcement associated with drug administration and withdrawal, *conditioning* plays a significant part in sustaining drug dependence. When a particular environment or location, or the sight of a syringe or cigarette, becomes associated with the pleasurable experience of drug-taking, the antecedent stimulus itself evokes the response, as with Pavlov's dogs. The same happens in reverse, so that the antecedents of *not* taking the drug become aversive. This kind of conditioning is generally more persistent and less easily extinguished than unconditioned reinforcement, and probably accounts for the high relapse rate of 'weaned' addicts. The psychological factors in drug dependence are discussed by Koob (1996), and summarised in Figure 39.1.

Animal models provide some insight into the neurobiological basis of reward and habituation, but in man the drug habit is evidently sustained by processes that are more complex and long-lasting than the neurobiological changes observed in experimental animals.

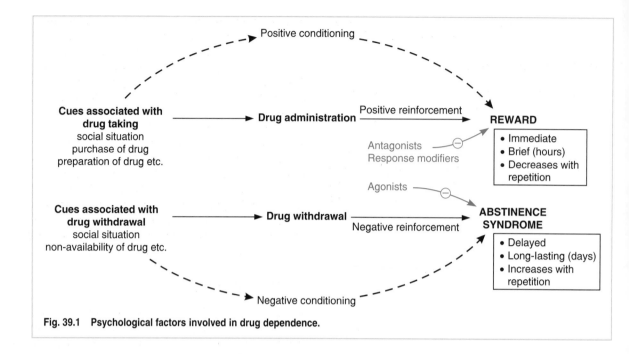

Fig. 39.1 **Psychological factors involved in drug dependence.**

Drug dependence

- Dependence is defined as an excessive craving which develops as a result of repeated administration of the drug.
- Dependence occurs with a wide range of psychotropic drugs, acting by many different mechanisms.
- The common feature of dependence-producing drugs is that they have a positive reinforcing action ('reward') associated with activation of the mesolimbic dopaminergic pathway.
- Dependence is often associated with (a) tolerance to the drug, which can arise by various biochemical mechanisms; (b) a physical abstinence syndrome, which varies in type and intensity for different classes of drug; (c) psychological dependence (craving), which may be associated with the tolerance-producing biochemical changes.
- Psychological dependence, which usually outlasts the physical withdrawal syndrome, is the major factor leading to relapse among treated addicts.

REWARD PATHWAYS

An important reward pathway involved in drug dependence is the mesolimbic dopaminergic pathway (see Ch. 30) running, via the medial forebrain bundle, from the ventral midbrain (A10 cell group) to the *nucleus accumbens* and limbic region. All dependence-producing

drugs so far tested, including opioids, nicotine, amphetamines, ethanol and cocaine, increase the release of dopamine in the nucleus accumbens, as shown by microdialysis and other techniques. Some of these stimulate firing of A10 cells, whereas others, such as amphetamine and cocaine, act to cause dopamine release or prevent its reuptake (see Ch. 8). Chemical or surgical interruption of this dopaminergic pathway consistently impairs drug-seeking behaviours in many experimental situations (see Koob 1992). Deletion of D_2-receptors in a transgenic mouse strain eliminated the reward properties of morphine administration, without eliminating other opiate effects, and it did not prevent the occurrence of physical withdrawal symptoms in morphine-dependent animals (Maldonado et al. 1997) suggesting that the dopaminergic pathway is responsible for the positive reward, but not for the negative withdrawal effects. There is evidence that other mediators, particularly 5-HT, glutamate and GABA, influence the mesolimbic dopamine pathway, and possibly other reward pathways. In general, manipulations that increase 5-HT activity (e.g. 5-HT agonists or uptake blockers; see Chs 9 and 35), reduce drug-seeking behaviour. 5-HT uptake inhibitors (e.g. **zimeldine**) or 5-HT agonists (e.g. **buspirone**) reduce slightly the alcohol consumption in alcoholic patients, as does **camprosate**, an inhibitor of glutamate-mediated transmission, recently introduced for treating alcoholism (see below). These approaches, based on the neurochemical manipulation of the reward pathway, are yet to be fully evaluated.

HABITUATION MECHANISMS

The cellular mechanisms involved in habituation to the effects of drugs such as opioids and cocaine have been studied in some detail (see Nestler & Aghajanian 1997). Both classes of drug produce, on chronic administration, an increase in the activity of adenylate cyclase in brain regions such as the *nucleus accumbens*, which compensates for their acute inhibitory effect on cAMP formation, and produces a rebound increase in cAMP when the

drug is terminated (Fig. 39.2). Chronic opioid treatment increases the amount, not only of adenylate cyclase itself, but also of other components of the signalling pathway, including the G-proteins and various protein kinases. This increase in cAMP affects many cellular functions through the increased activity of various cAMP-dependent protein kinases, which control the activity of ion channels (making the cells more excitable), as well as various enzymes and transcription factors. Similar effects also occur with cocaine, but much less is known about other dependence-producing drugs. These changes (see Fig. 39.3) probably account for the relatively short-term (days to weeks) phenomena of tolerance and dependence, but the long-term processes responsible for craving and relapse—the major issues in human addiction—are very poorly understood at the neurochemical level.

GENETIC FACTORS

Epidemiological studies, particularly in alcoholism, show clear evidence of a genetic component in the pathogenesis of drug abuse. Twin studies suggest that genetic factors contribute up to 60% of an individual's susceptibility to alcohol abuse. There are also well-characterised genetic strains of rats and mice which differ in their tendency to self-administer alcohol, or in the intensity of withdrawal symptoms following chronic opioid administration. Genetic analysis of alcoholics and multiple drug abusers have suggested a higher frequency of a particular mutation of the dopamine D_2-receptor gene in these patients compared with controls (see Crabbe et al. 1994). This is of interest in relation to the proposed role of dopaminergic pathways in drug-induced reward (see above), but the finding has not been consistently replicated, and its significance is not known at present.

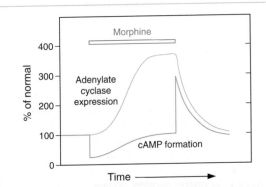

Fig. 39.2 Biochemical mechanism postulated to explain morphine tolerance and dependence. Morphine inhibits adenylate cyclase thus reducing cAMP formation (grey line). A secondary rise in adenylate cyclase expression occurs (blue line), so that cAMP production recovers in the presence of morphine (i.e. tolerance develops). On cessation of morphine treatment excessive cAMP production occurs, causing withdrawal symptoms, until the high level of adenylate cyclase expression returns to normal. (From: Sharma S K et al. 1975 Proc Natl Acad Sci USA 72: 3092)

	Drug-taking		Drug withdrawal	
State produced:	Acute drugged state	Chronic drugged state	Acute abstinence	Chronic abstinence
Effect:	Reward	Tolerance, dependence	Withdrawal syndrome	Craving
Mechanism:	Activation of mesolimbic DA pathway. ? Other reward pathways.	Adaptive changes in receptors, transporters, 2nd messengers, etc. (e.g. ↑adenylate cyclase, ↑DA transporter)	Uncompensated adaptive changes (e.g.↓DA, ↑glutamate)	Not known

Drug-taking: *Days–weeks* (arrow). Drug withdrawal: *Months–years* (arrow).

Fig. 39.3 Cellular and physiological mechanisms involved in drug dependence.

PHARMACOLOGICAL APPROACHES TO TREATING DRUG DEPENDENCE

From the discussion above, it will be clear that drug dependence involves many psychosocial, and some genetic factors, as well as neuropharmacological mechanisms, so drug treatment is only one component of the therapeutic approaches that are used.

The main pharmacological approaches (see O'Brien 1997) are summarised in Table 39.2.

NICOTINE AND TOBACCO

Tobacco growing, chewing and smoking was indigenous throughout the American subcontinent and Australia at the time that European explorers first visited these places. Smoking spread through Europe during the 16th century, coming to England mainly as a result of its enthusiastic espousal by Raleigh at the court of Elizabeth I. James I strongly disapproved of both Raleigh and tobacco, and initiated the first antismoking campaign in the early 17th century with the support of the Royal College of Physicians. Parliament responded by imposing a substantial duty on tobacco, thereby setting up the dilemma (from which we show no sign of being able to escape) of giving the State an economic interest in the continuation of smoking at the same time that its official expert advisers were issuing emphatic warnings about its dangers.

Until the latter half of the 19th century, tobacco was smoked in pipes, and by men. Cigarette manufacture began at the end of the 19th century, and now cigarettes account for more than 90% of tobacco consumption. The trend in cigarette consumption this century is shown in Figure 39.4. From a peak level in the early 1970s, cigarette consumption in the UK dropped by about 50%, the main factors being increased price, adverse publicity, restrictions on advertising, and the compulsory publication of health warnings. Filter cigarettes (which give a somewhat lower delivery of tar and nicotine than standard cigarettes) and low-tar cigarettes (which are also low in nicotine) constitute an increasing proportion of the total. The proportion of cigarette smokers in the UK is currently just under 30% with little difference between men and women. About 10% of children aged 10–15 are regular smokers. Currently, there are about 1 billion smokers in the world.

For reviews on nicotine and smoking, see Balfour & Fagerstrom (1996), Benowitz (1996).

PHARMACOLOGICAL EFFECTS OF SMOKING

Nicotine is the only pharmacologically active substance in tobacco smoke, apart from carcinogenic tars and carbon monoxide (see below). The acute effects of smoking can be mimicked by injection of nicotine, and are blocked by **mecamylamine**, an antagonist at neuronal nicotinic acetylcholine receptors (see Ch. 7).

Effects on the central nervous system

The central effects of nicotine are complex and cannot be summed up overall simply in terms of stimulation or inhibition. At the cellular level, nicotine acts on nicotinic acetylcholine receptors (brain nAChRs, which are molecular variants of peripheral nAChRs; see Ch. 2), opening cation channels and causing neuronal excitation, exactly as it does in autonomic ganglia and the neuromuscular synapse (Ch. 7). As well as activating the receptors,

Table 39.2 Pharmacological approaches to treating drug dependence	
Effect sought	Examples
To alleviate acute withdrawal symptoms	Short-term use of methadone to blunt acute opiate withdrawal symptoms Use of benzodiazepines to assist in the acute phase of alcohol withdrawal
As a long-term substitute for the abused drug	Methadone substitution for opiate addiction Nicotine patches or gum
To block the acute rewarding effect of the drug (used after the acute withdrawal phase has been overcome)	Naltrexone, to block the effect of opiates (also claimed to reduce effect of alcohol) Disulfiram to produce an unpleasant reaction to alcohol Immunisation against cocaine (circulating antibodies inactivate cocaine and abolish its effects—not yet approved for clinical use)
To diminish craving—a poorly understood mechanism	Antidepressants (especially SSRIs, bupropion; see Ch. 35) Acamprosate, to reduce alcohol craving (poorly characterised mechanism related to NMDA receptors)

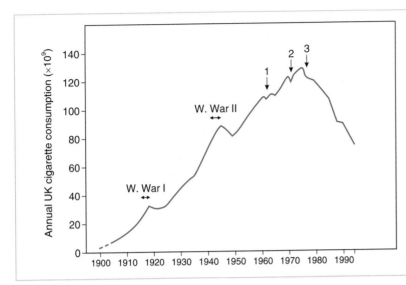

Fig. 39.4 Cigarette consumption in UK 1900–1994. Numbers 1, 2 and 3 refer to publication of Royal College of Physicians reports on smoking and health. Since 1980, drop in consumption has closely followed price increases. (Data from: Ashton H, Stepney R 1982 Smoking psychology and pharmacology. Tavistock Publications, London; Townsend 1996 Price and consumption of tobacco. Br Med Bull 52: 132–142)

nicotine also causes desensitisation, which may be an important component of its effects, since the effects of a dose of nicotine are diminished in animals after sustained exposure to the drug. Chronic nicotine administration leads to a substantial *increase* in the number of nAChRs (an effect opposite to that produced by sustained administration of most receptor agonists), which may represent an adaptive response to prolonged receptor desensitisation. It is likely that the overall effect of nicotine reflects a balance between activation of nicotinic acetylcholine receptors, causing neuronal excitation, and desensitisation, causing synaptic block.

At the spinal level, nicotine inhibits spinal reflexes, causing skeletal muscle relaxation which can be measured by electromyography. It is probably due to stimulation of the inhibitory Renshaw cells in the ventral horn of the spinal cord (see Ch. 28). The higher level functioning of the brain, as reflected in the subjective sense of alertness or by the EEG pattern, can be affected in either direction by nicotine, according to dose and circumstances. Smokers report that smoking wakes them up when they are drowsy and calms them down when they are tense, and EEG recordings broadly bear this out. It also seems that small doses of nicotine tend to cause arousal, whereas large doses do the reverse. Tests of motor and sensory performance (e.g. reaction time measurements or vigilance tests) in humans generally show improvement after smoking, and nicotine enhances learning in rats. Some extremely elaborate tests have been conducted to see, for example, whether the effect of nicotine on performance and aggression varies according

to the amount of stress. In one the subject first has to name the colours of a series of squares (low stress), and then has to name the colours in which the names of other colours are written (high stress). The difference between the scores, reflecting the extent by which performance is affected by stress, was diminished by smoking. Some tests border on nasty-mindedness, such as one in which subjects played a complicated logical game with a computer which initially played fair and then began to cheat randomly, causing stress and aggression in the subjects and a decline in their performance. Smoking, it was reported, did not reduce the anger, but did reduce the decline in performance.

Peripheral effects

The peripheral effects of small doses of nicotine result from stimulation of autonomic ganglia (see Ch. 7) and of peripheral sensory receptors, mainly in the heart and lungs. Stimulation of these receptors elicits various autonomic reflex responses, causing tachycardia, increased cardiac output and increased arterial pressure, reduction of gastrointestinal motility and sweating. When people smoke for the first time, they usually experience nausea and sometimes vomit, probably because of stimulation of sensory receptors in the stomach. All of these effects decline with repeated dosage, though the central effects remain. Secretion of adrenaline and noradrenaline from the adrenal medulla contribute to the cardiovascular effects, and release of antidiuretic hormone from the posterior pituitary causes a decrease in urine flow. The plasma concentration of free fatty acids is increased, probably owing to sympathetic stimulation and adrenaline secretion.

Smokers weigh, on average, about 4 kg less than non-smokers, mainly because of reduced food intake; giving up smoking usually causes weight gain associated with increased food intake.

PHARMACOKINETIC ASPECTS

An average cigarette contains about 0.8 g of tobacco and 9–17 mg of nicotine, of which about 10% is normally absorbed by the smoker. This fraction varies greatly with the habits of the smoker and the type of cigarette.

Nicotine in cigarette smoke is rapidly absorbed from the lungs, but poorly from the mouth and nasopharynx. Thus, inhalation is required to give appreciable absorption of nicotine, each puff delivering a distinct bolus of drug to the central nervous system. Pipe or cigar smoke is less acidic than cigarette smoke, and the nicotine tends to be absorbed from the mouth and nasopharynx, rather than the lungs. Absorption is considerably slower than from inhaled cigarette smoke, and a later and longer-lasting peak in the plasma nicotine concentration occurs with pipe or cigar smoking than with cigarette smoking (Fig. 39.5). An average cigarette, smoked over 10 minutes, causes the plasma nicotine concentration to rise to 20–30 ng/ml (130–200 nmol/l), falling to about half within 10 minutes and then more slowly over the next 1–2 hours. The rapid decline results mainly from redistribution between the blood and other tissues; the slower decline is due to hepatic metabolism, mainly by oxidation to an inactive ketone metabolite, **cotinine**. This has a long

plasma half-life, and measurement of plasma cotinine concentration provides a useful measure of smoking behaviour. A nicotine patch applied for 24 hours causes the plasma concentration to rise to 75–150 nmol/l over 6 hours and to remain fairly constant for about 20 hours.

Tobacco smoking

- Cigarette consumption in the UK is now declining, after reaching a peak in the mid-1970s.
- The prevalence of smoking is now less than 30% of the adult population, and equal in both sexes.
- Nicotine is the only pharmacologically active agent in tobacco, apart from carcinogenic tars and carbon monoxide.
- The amount of nicotine absorbed from an average cigarette is about 1.5 mg, which causes the plasma nicotine concentration to reach 130–200 nmol/l. These values depend greatly on the type of cigarette, and on the extent of inhalation of the smoke.

TOLERANCE AND DEPENDENCE

As with all drugs of abuse, three separate but related processes—tolerance, physical dependence and psychological dependence—contribute to the overall state of dependence, in which taking the drug becomes compulsive.

The effects of nicotine associated with peripheral ganglionic stimulation show rapid tolerance, perhaps as a result of desensitisation of nicotinic acetylcholine receptors by nicotine. With large doses of nicotine this

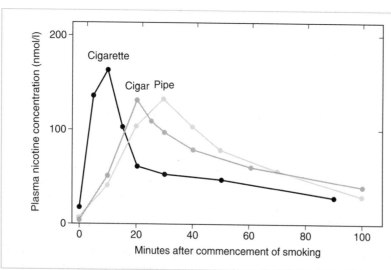

Fig. 39.5 Nicotine concentration in plasma during smoking. The subjects were habitual smokers who smoked a cigarette, cigar or pipe according to their usual habit. (From: Bowman W C, Rand M 1980 Textbook of pharmacology. Blackwell, Oxford, Ch. 4)

desensitisation produces a block of ganglionic, transmission rather than stimulation (see Ch. 7). Tolerance to the central effects of nicotine (e.g. in the arousal response), is much less than in the periphery. The increase in the number of nicotinic receptors in the brain produced by chronic nicotine administration in animals (see above) also occurs in heavy smokers. Since the cellular effects of nicotine are diminished, it is possible that the additional binding sites represent desensitised, rather than functional receptors.

The addictiveness of smoking is due to nicotine, whose addictive properties have been clearly demonstrated in animal experiments. Thus, rats choose to drink dilute nicotine solution in preference to water if given a choice, and will perform various tasks to obtain nicotine as a reward. In a situation in which lever-pressing causes an injection of nicotine to be delivered, rats quickly learn to self-administer it. Similarly, monkeys who have been trained to smoke, by providing a reward in response to smoking behaviour, will continue to do so spontaneously (i.e. unrewarded) if the smoking medium contains nicotine, but not if nicotine-free tobacco is offered instead. Like other dependence-producing drugs (see above) nicotine causes excitation of the mesolimbic pathway, and increased dopamine release in the *nucleus accumbens*. Brain nAChRs comprise pentamers of α-and β-subunits (see Ch. 2), each of which exists in several isoforms (α_{2-7}, β_{1-4}), and many combinations are expressed in different brain regions. Knocking out the β_2-subunit in transgenic mice eliminates both the reward properties, and the increase in dopamine release caused by nicotine (Picciotto et al. 1998), confirming the role of nAChRs and mesolimbic dopamine release in the response to nicotine. In contrast to normal mice, the mutant mice could not be induced to self-administer nicotine, even though they did so with cocaine. Further evidence implicating brain nAChRs in the addictive property of nicotine comes from experiments with mecamylamine, an antagonist at nAChRs. If monkeys are habituated to tobacco-smoking so that they choose to puff smoke in preference to air, administration of mecamylamine causes them to switch to puffing air instead of smoke.

A physical withdrawal syndrome occurs in both humans and experimental animals accustomed to regular nicotine administration. Its main features are increased irritability, impaired performance of psychomotor tasks, aggressiveness and sleep disturbance. The withdrawal syndrome is much less severe than that produced by opiates, and it can be alleviated not only by nicotine but also by amphetamine, a finding consistent with the postulated role of dopamine in the reward pathway.

The nicotine withdrawal syndrome lasts for 2–3 weeks, though the craving for cigarettes persists for much longer than this; relapses during attempts to give up cigarette smoking occur most commonly at a time when the physical withdrawal syndrome has long since subsided.

Pharmacology of nicotine

- At a cellular level, nicotine acts on nicotinic acetylcholine receptors (nAChRs) to cause neuronal excitation. Its central effects are blocked by receptor antagonists such as mecamylamine.
- Brain nAChRs differ from peripheral nAChRs, and a variety of subtypes occur in different brain regions.
- At the behavioural level, nicotine produces a mixture of inhibitory and excitatory effects.
- Nicotine shows reinforcing properties, associated with increased activity in the mesolimbic dopaminergic pathway, and self-administration can be elicited in animal studies.
- EEG changes show an arousal response, and subjects report increased alertness, accompanied by a reduction of anxiety and tension.
- Learning, particularly under stress, is facilitated by nicotine.
- Peripheral effects of nicotine are due mainly to ganglionic stimulation: tachycardia, increased blood pressure and reduced gastrointestinal motility. Tolerance develops rapidly to these effects.
- Nicotine is metabolised, mainly in the liver, within 1–2 hours. The inactive metabolite, cotinine, has a long plasma half-life, and can be used as a measure of smoking habits.
- Nicotine gives rise to tolerance, physical dependence and psychological dependence (craving), and is highly addictive. Attempts at long-term cessation succeed in only about 20% of cases.
- Nicotine replacement therapy (chewing gum or skin patch preparations) improves the chances of giving up smoking, but only when combined with active counselling.

HARMFUL EFFECTS OF SMOKING

The life expectancy of smokers is shorter than that of non-smokers. For example, in a 1971 study of British doctors, the proportion of heavy smokers dying between the ages of 35 and 65 was estimated to be 40% compared with 15% for non-smokers. For a recent analysis, see Peto et al (1996).

The main health risks are:

- *Cancer*, particularly of the lung and upper respiratory tract, but also of the oesophagus, pancreas and bladder.

Smoking 20 cigarettes per day is estimated to increase the risk of lung cancer about 10-fold. Lung cancer accounts for about half of the total cancer deaths in men, and about 90% is estimated to be caused by smoking. Pipe and cigar smoking carry much less risk than cigarette smoking, though the risk is still appreciable. Tar, rather than nicotine, is responsible for the cancer risk.

- *Coronary heart disease*, and other forms of peripheral vascular disease. The mortality among men aged 55–64 from coronary thrombosis is about 60% greater in men who smoke 20 cigarettes per day than in non-smokers. Though the increase in risk is less than it is for lung cancer, the actual number of excess deaths associated with smoking is larger, because coronary heart disease is so common. Other kinds of peripheral vascular disease (e.g. stroke, intermittent claudication and diabetic gangrene) are also strongly smoking-related. Many studies have suggested that nicotine is mainly responsible for the adverse effect of smoking on the incidence of cardiovascular disease. Another factor may be carbon monoxide (see below). Surprisingly, there is no clear increase in ischaemi heart disease in pipe and cigar smokers, even though similar blood nicotine and carboxyhaemoglobin concentrations are reached, suggesting that nicotine and carbon monoxide may not be the only causative factors.
- *Chronic bronchitis.* There is a much higher incidence of chronic bronchitis in smokers than non-smokers. Nonetheless, in contrast to lung cancer, chronic bronchitis has declined in prevalence over the past 50 years. This is generally attributed to cleaner air and other social changes, and smoking now appears to be the most important remaining cause. Its effect is probably due to tar and other irritants, rather than nicotine.
- *Deleterious effects in pregnancy.* Smoking, particularly during the latter half of pregnancy, significantly reduces birth weight (by about 8% in women who smoke 25 or more cigarettes per day during pregnancy) and increases perinatal mortality (by an estimated 28% in babies born to mothers who smoke in the last half of pregnancy). There is evidence that children born to smoking mothers remain behind, in both physical and mental development, for at least 7 years. By 11 years of age, the difference is no longer significant. These effects of smoking, though measurable, are much smaller than the effects of other factors, such as social class and birth order. Various other complications of pregnancy are also more common in women who smoke, including spontaneous abortion (increased

30–70% by smoking), premature delivery (increased about 40%) and placenta praevia (increased 25–90%). Nicotine is excreted in breast milk in sufficient amounts to cause tachycardia in the infant.

Beneficial effects of smoking include a significant (approximately twofold) reduction in the incidence of Parkinson's disease, and a smaller (doubtfully significant) reduction in the incidence of Alzheimer's disease. These effects are postulated to result from activation of nicotinic receptors, which benefits Parkinson's disease by causing dopamine release, and counters the cholinergic deficit in Alzheimer's disease (see Ch. 31). A reduction of symptoms in inflammatory bowel disease has also been reported.

The agents probably responsible for the harmful effects are:

- *Tar and irritants*, such as NO_2, formaldehyde, etc. Cigarette smoke tar contains many known carcinogenic hydrocarbons, as well as tumour promoters, which account for the high cancer risk. It is likely that the various irritant substances are also responsible for the increase in bronchitis and emphysema.
- *Nicotine* probably accounts for retarded foetal development, because of its vasoconstrictor properties, but it is not known whether it also causes the increase in cardiovascular risk.
- *Carbon monoxide.* The average carbon monoxide content of cigarette smoke is about 3%. Carbon monoxide has a high affinity for haemoglobin and the average carboxyhaemoglobin content in the blood of cigarette smokers has been estimated at about 2.5% (compared with 0.4% for non-smoking urban dwellers). In very heavy smokers, up to 15% of haemoglobin may be complexed with carbon monoxide, a level which has been shown to cause retardation of foetal development in rats. It is possible that this factor also contributes to the increased incidence of heart and vascular disease. Foetal haemoglobin has a higher affinity for carbon monoxide than adult haemoglobin, and the proportion of carboxyhaemoglobin is higher in foetal than maternal blood.

'Low tar' cigarettes give a lower yield of both tar and nicotine than standard cigarettes. However, it has been shown that smokers puff harder, inhale more, and smoke more cigarettes when low tar brands are substituted for standard brands. The end result may be a slightly reduced intake of tar and nicotine, but an increase in carbon monoxide intake, with no net gain in terms of safety.

Pharmacological approaches to treatment of nicotine dependence

Most smokers would like to quit, but few succeed. The most successful smoking-cure clinics, using a combination of psychological and pharmacological treatments, achieve a success rate of about 25%, measured as the percentage of patients still abstinent after 1 year. The main pharmacological approach used is **nicotine replacement therapy** (see Benowitz 1993), though **clonidine** and the nicotinic receptor antagonist **mecamylamine**, have also been used.

Nicotine replacement therapy is used mainly to assist smokers to quit by relieving the psychological and physical withdrawal syndrome. Because nicotine is relatively short-acting, and not well absorbed from the gastrointestinal tract, it is given either in the form of chewing gum, used several times daily, or as a transdermal patch which is replaced daily. These preparations cause various side-effects, particularly nausea and gastrointestinal cramps, cough, insomnia and muscle pains. Because of the risk of coronary spasm, nicotine should not be used in patients with heart disease. Transdermal patches often cause local irritation and itching. The conclusion of many double-blind trials of nicotine against placebo is that these preparations, combined with professional counselling and supportive therapy, roughly double the chances of successfully breaking the smoking habit, but the success rate measured as abstinence 1 year after ceasing treatment is still only about 25%. Nicotine on its own, without counselling and support, is no more effective than placebo, so its use as an over-the-counter smoking remedy has little justification. Though of limited value as an aid to abstinence, the long-term use of nicotine can significantly reduce cigarette consumption by smokers. In Sweden, the use of 'smokeless tobacco' (i.e. nicotine by inhalation) is widespread, and the tobacco consumption and smoking-related death rate is much lower than elsewhere in Europe or North America.

The elucidation of the role of nAChR subtypes in the brain may allow novel agonists with selectivity for particular subtypes to be developed as nicotine substitutes with fewer side-effects, but this remains theoretical at present.

Clonidine, an α_2-adrenoceptor agonist (see Ch. 8) reduces the withdrawal effects of several dependence-producing drugs, including opioids and cocaine, as well as nicotine.* Clonidine may be given orally or as a transdermal patch, and is about as effective as nicotine

---

*It also reduces postmenopausal flushing, which may represent a physiological oestrogen withdrawal response.

substitution in assisting abstinence. The side-effects of clonidine (hypotension, dry mouth, drowsiness) are troublesome, however, and it is not widely used.

The use of **mecamylamine** which antagonises the effects of nicotine, is not promising. Small doses actually increase smoking, presumably because the antagonism can be overcome by increasing the amount of nicotine. Larger doses of mecamylamine, which abolish the effects of nicotine more effectively, have so many autonomic side-effects (see Ch. 7) that compliance is poor.

Harmful effects of smoking

- Smoking reduces life expectancy, mainly through increased risk of:
  — cancer, especially lung cancer, of which about 90% of cases are smoking-related; carcinogenic tars are responsible
  — ischaemic heart disease; both nicotine and CO may be responsible
  — chronic bronchitis; tars are mainly responsible.
- Smoking in pregnancy reduces birth weight and retards childhood development. It also increases abortion rate and perinatal mortality. Nicotine, and possibly carbon monoxide, are responsible.

ETHANOL

Judged on a molar basis, the consumption of ethanol far exceeds that of any other drug. The ethanol content of various drinks ranges from about 2.5% (weak beer) to about 55% (strong spirits), and the size of the normal measure is such that a single drink usually contains about 8–12 g (0.17–0.26 moles) of ethanol. It is by no means unusual to consume 1–2 moles at a sitting, equivalent to about 0.5 kg of most other drugs. Its low pharmacological potency is reflected in the range of plasma concentrations needed to produce pharmacological effects: minimal effects occur at about 10 mmol/l (46 mg/100 ml), and 10 times this concentration may be lethal. The average *per capita* ethanol consumption in the UK is about 8 litres/year (expressed as pure ethanol) a figure that has changed little over the last 20 years, the main change having been a growing consumption of wine in preference to beer.

For calculation of ethanol consumption in the community, ethanol intake is often expressed in terms of units. One unit is equal to 8 g of ethanol, and is the amount contained in ½ pint of normal strength beer, 1 measure of spirits or 1 standard glass of wine. Based on the health

risks described below, the current official recommen-
dation is a maximum of 21 units/week for men and 14
units/week for women. It is estimated that in the UK,
about 25% of men and 7% of women exceed these levels.
The annual government revenue from drink (mainly tax)
amounts to about £7 billion, whereas the social cost is
estimated at £2 billion. Views differ as to whether this
represents a good bargain or a moral outrage.

PHARMACOLOGICAL EFFECTS OF ETHANOL

Effects on the central nervous system

The main effects of ethanol are on the central nervous
system (see review by Charness et al. 1989), where its
depressant actions resemble those of volatile anaesthetics
(Ch. 32). Though ethanol, at pharmacologically effective
concentrations, produces a measurable increase in the
structural disorder (i.e. increased fluidity) of lipid membranes, as do volatile anaesthetics (see Ch. 33), it is
likely that its actions depend mainly on its effects on
specific membrane ion channels and receptors. At a
cellular level, the effect of ethanol is purely depressant,
though it increases impulse activity—presumably by
disinhibition—in some parts of the CNS, notably in the
mesolimbic dopaminergic neurons that are involved in
the reward pathway described above. The main theories
of ethanol action (see reviews by Little 1991, Lovinger
1997, Tabakoff & Hoffman 1996) are:

- enhancement of GABA-mediated inhibition, similar
  to the action of benzodiazepines (see Ch. 33)
- inhibition of calcium entry through voltage-gated
  calcium channels
- inhibition of NMDA receptor function.

Ethanol enhances the action of GABA acting on $GABA_A$-
receptors in a similar way to benzodiazepines (see
Ch. 33). Its effect is, however, smaller and less consistent than that of benzodiazepines, and no clear effect
on inhibitory synaptic transmission in the CNS has been
demonstrated for ethanol. The benzodiazepine antagonist,
flumazenil, reverses the central depressant actions of
ethanol (see Lister & Nutt 1987), but this appears to result
from physiological antagonism, rather than from a direct
pharmacological interaction. The use of flumazenil to
reverse ethanol intoxication and treat dependence has not
found favour for several reasons. It carries a risk of causing
seizures, and could cause an increase in ethanol consumption and thus increase long-term toxic manifestations.

Ethanol inhibits transmitter release in response to nerve
terminal depolarisation, by inhibiting the opening of
voltage-sensitive Ca^{2+} channels in neurons.

The excitatory effects of glutamate are inhibited by
ethanol at concentrations that produce CNS depressant
effects in vivo. NMDA-receptor activation is inhibited at
lower ethanol concentrations than are required to affect
AMPA receptors (see Ch. 30). Other effects produced by
ethanol include an enhancement of the excitatory effects
produced by activation of nicotinic acetylcholine receptors
and 5-HT$_3$-receptors. The relative importance of these
various effects in the overall effects of ethanol on CNS
function is not clear at present.

The effects of acute ethanol intoxication in man are
well known, and include slurred speech, motor incoordination, increased self-confidence and euphoria. The
effect on mood varies among individuals, most becoming
louder and more outgoing, but some becoming morose
and withdrawn. At higher levels of intoxication, the
mood tends to become highly labile, with euphoria and
melancholy, aggression and submission, often occurring
successively. The association between alcohol and violence
is well documented.

Intellectual and motor performance and sensory
discrimination show uniform impairment by ethanol, but
subjects are generally unable to judge this for themselves.
In tests on bus drivers, for example, in which subjects
were asked to drive through a gap which they considered
to be the minimum for their bus to pass through, ethanol
caused them not only to hit the barriers more often at
any given gap setting, but also to set the gap to a narrower
dimension, often narrower than the bus.

Much effort has gone into measuring the effect of
ethanol on driving performance in real life, as opposed
to artificial tests under experimental conditions. In one
American study, large numbers of city drivers were
tested for plasma ethanol concentration, including drivers
who had been involved in an accident and those that
had not. This allowed the relative probability of being
involved in an accident to be calculated as a function
of ethanol concentration. It was found that no significant
change occurred up to 50 mg/100 ml (10.9 mmol/l); by
80 mg/100 ml (17.4 mmol/l) the probability was increased
about fourfold and by 150 mg/100 ml (32.6 mmol/l)
about 25-fold. In the UK, driving with a blood ethanol
concentration greater than 80 mg/100 ml constitutes a
legal offence.

The relationship between plasma ethanol concentration and effect is highly variable. A given concentration
produces a larger effect when the concentration is rising
than when it is steady or falling. A substantial degree
of tissue tolerance develops in habitual drinkers with
the result that a higher plasma ethanol concentration is
needed to produce a given effect (see below). In one

study, 'gross intoxication' (assessed by a battery of tests that measured speech, gait and so on) occurred in 30% of subjects between 50 and 100 mg/100 ml and in 90% of subjects with more than 150 mg/100 ml. Coma generally occurs at about 300 mg/100 ml and death from respiratory failure is likely at 400–500 mg/100 ml.

In addition to the acute effects of ethanol on the nervous system, chronic administration also causes several irreversible neurological syndromes (see Charness et al. 1989). These may be due to ethanol itself, or to metabolites such as acetaldehyde or fatty acid esters. The majority of chronic alcoholics show a degree of dementia associated with ventricular enlargement detectable by brain-imaging techniques. Degeneration in the cerebellum and other specific brain regions can also occur, as well as peripheral neuropathy. Some of these changes are not due to ethanol itself, but to accompanying thiamine deficiency which is common in alcoholics.

Effects on other systems

The main cardiovascular effect of ethanol is to produce cutaneous vasodilatation, central in origin, which causes a warm feeling but actually increases heat loss.

Ethanol increases salivary and gastric secretion. This is partly a reflex effect produced by the taste and irritant action of ethanol. However, heavy consumption of spirits causes damage directly to the gastric mucosa, causing chronic gastritis. Both this and the increased acid secretion are factors in the high incidence of gastric bleeding in alcoholics.

Ethanol produces a variety of endocrine effects. In particular, it increases the output of adrenal steroid hormones, by stimulating the anterior pituitary gland to secrete ACTH. However, the increase in plasma hydrocortisone usually seen in alcoholics (producing a 'pseudo-Cushing's syndrome') is due partly to inhibition by ethanol of hydrocortisone metabolism in the liver.

Diuresis is a familiar effect of ethanol. It is caused by inhibition of ADH secretion, and tolerance develops rapidly, so that the diuresis is not sustained. There is a similar inhibition of oxytocin secretion, which can cause delayed parturition at term. Attempts have been made to use this effect in premature labour, but the dose needed is large enough to cause obvious drunkenness in the mother. If the baby is born prematurely in spite of the ethanol, it too may be intoxicated at birth, sufficiently for respiration to be depressed. The procedure evidently has serious disadvantages.

Chronic male alcoholics are often impotent, and show signs of feminisation. This is associated with impaired testicular steroid synthesis, but induction of hepatic micro-somal enzymes by ethanol, and hence an increased rate of testosterone inactivation, also contributes.

Effects of ethanol on the liver

Together with brain damage, liver damage is the most serious long-term consequence of excessive ethanol consumption (see Lieber 1995). In the sequence of effects, increased fat accumulation (fatty liver) progresses to hepatitis (i.e. inflammation of the liver) and eventually to irreversible hepatic necrosis and fibrosis. Diversion of portal blood flow around the fibrotic liver often causes oesophageal varices to develop, which can bleed suddenly and catastrophically. Increased fat accumulation in the liver occurs, in rats or in man, after a single large dose of ethanol. The mechanism is complex, the main factors being:

- increased release of fatty acids from adipose tissue, which is the result of increased stress, causing sympathetic discharge
- impaired fatty acid oxidation, because of the metabolic load imposed by the ethanol itself.

With chronic ethanol consumption, many other factors contribute to the liver damage. One is malnutrition, for an alcoholic may satisfy much of his calorie requirement from ethanol itself. 300 grams of ethanol (equivalent to one bottle of whisky), provides about 2000 kcal, but, unlike a normal diet, it provides no vitamins, amino acids or fatty acids. Thiamine deficiency is an important factor in causing chronic neurological damage (see above). The hepatic changes occurring in alcoholics are partly due to chronic malnutrition, but mainly to the cellular toxicity of ethanol, which promotes inflammatory changes in the liver.

The overall incidence of chronic liver disease is a function of cumulative ethanol consumption over many years. Thus, overall consumption, expressed as g/kg body weight per day multiplied by years of drinking, provides an accurate predictor of the incidence of cirrhosis. An increase in the plasma concentration of the liver enzyme γ-glutamyl transpeptidase (GGT) provides an index of liver damage, though not specific to ethanol.

Effects on lipid metabolism, platelet function and atherosclerosis

Moderate drinking reduces mortality associated with coronary heart disease, the maximum effect—about 30% reduction of mortality*—being achieved at a level of

---

*The effect is much more pronounced (>50% reduction) in men with high plasma concentrations of LDL cholesterol (see Ch. 16).

2–3 units/day (see Groenbaek et al. 1994). Most evidence suggests that ethanol, rather than any specific beverage, such as red wine, is the essential factor. Two mechanisms have been proposed. The first involves the effect of ethanol on the plasma lipoproteins which are the carrier molecules for cholesterol and other lipids in the bloodstream (see Ch. 16). Epidemiological studies, as well as studies on volunteers, have shown that ethanol, in daily doses too small to produce obvious CNS effects, can over the course of a few weeks increase plasma HDL concentration, thus exerting a protective effect against atheroma formation.

Ethanol may also protect against ischaemic heart disease by inhibiting platelet aggregation. This effect occurs at ethanol concentrations in the range achieved by normal drinking in man (10–20 mmol/l) and probably results from inhibition of arachidonic acid formation from phospholipid. In man, the magnitude of the effect depends critically on dietary fat intake, and it is not yet clear how important it is clinically.

The effect of ethanol on foetal development

The adverse effect of ethanol consumption during pregnancy on foetal development was demonstrated in the early 1970s, when the term foetal alcohol syndrome (FAS) was coined.

The characteristic features of FAS are:

- abnormal facial development, with wide-set eyes, short palpebral fissures and small cheek bones
- reduced cranial circumference
- retarded growth
- mental retardation and behavioural abnormalities, often taking the form of hyperactivity and difficulty with social integration
- other anatomical abnormalities, which may be major or minor (e.g. congenital cardiac abnormalities, malformation of the eyes and ears).

The overall incidence of FAS is 0.5–3 per 1000 live births, but it affects about 30% of children born to alcoholic mothers. Full-blown FAS is rare with mothers who drink less than about 5 units/day; though there is no clearly defined threshold for producing lesser degrees of foetal impairment, there is no evidence that amounts less than about 2 units/day are harmful. It is uncertain whether there is a critical period during pregnancy when ethanol consumption is likely to lead to FAS. One study (Hanson et al. 1978) suggests that FAS incidence correlates most strongly with ethanol consumption very early in pregnancy, even before pregnancy is recognised, implying that not only pregnant women, but also women who are likely to become pregnant, must be advised not to drink heavily. Experiments on rats and mice suggest that the effect on facial development may be produced very early in pregnancy (up to 4 weeks in humans), while the effect on brain development is produced rather later (up to 10 weeks).

Other adverse effects of chronic ethanol consumption include *gastritis*, associated with increased acid secretion and the direct irritant effect of ethanol, *immunosuppression*, leading to increased incidence of infections, such as pneumonia, and *increased cancer risk*, particularly of the mouth, larynx and oesophagus.

Effects of ethanol

- Ethanol consumption is generally expressed in units of 10 ml (8 g) pure ethanol. Per capita consumption in Britain is about 8 l/year.
- Ethanol acts as a general CNS depressant, similar to volatile anaesthetic agents, producing the familiar effects of acute intoxication.
- Several cellular mechanisms are postulated: inhibition of calcium channel opening, enhancement of GABA action and inhibitory action at NMDA-type glutamate receptors.
- Effective plasma concentrations:
  — threshold effects: about 40 mg/100 ml (5 mmol/l)
  — severe intoxication: about 150 mg/100 ml
  — death from respiratory failure: about 500 mg/100 ml.
- Main peripheral effects are: self-limiting diuresis (reduced ADH secretion), cutaneous vasodilatation and delayed labour (reduced oxytocin secretion).
- Neurological degeneration occurs in heavy drinkers, causing dementia and peripheral neuropathies.
- Long-term ethanol consumption causes liver disease, progressing to cirrhosis and liver failure.
- Moderate ethanol consumption has a protective effect against ischaemic heart disease.
- Excessive consumption in pregnancy causes impaired foetal development, associated with small size, abnormal facial development and other physical abnormalities, and mental retardation.
- Tolerance, physical dependence and psychological dependence all occur with ethanol.
- Drugs used to treat alcohol dependence include disulfiram (aldehyde dehydrogenase inhibitor), naltrexone (opiate antagonist), and acamprosate (response modifier).

PHARMACOKINETIC ASPECTS

Metabolism of ethanol

Ethanol, being uncharged and highly lipid-soluble, is rapidly absorbed, an appreciable amount being absorbed from the stomach. A substantial fraction is removed from the portal vein blood by first-pass hepatic metabolism. Hepatic metabolism of ethanol shows saturation kinetics (see Ch. 5) at quite low ethanol concentrations, so the fraction of ethanol removed decreases as the concentration reaching the liver increases. Thus, if ethanol absorption is rapid and portal vein concentration is high, most of the ethanol escapes into the systemic circulation, whereas with slow absorption, more is removed by first-pass metabolism. This is one reason why drinking ethanol on an empty stomach produces a much greater pharmacological effect. Ethanol is quickly distributed throughout the body water, the rate of its redistribution depending mainly on the blood flow to individual tissues, as with volatile anaesthetics (see Ch. 32).

Ethanol is about 90% metabolised, 5–10% being excreted unchanged in expired air and in urine. This fraction is not pharmacokinetically significant, but provides the basis for estimating blood ethanol concentration from measurements on breath or urine. The ratio of ethanol concentrations in blood and alveolar air, measured at the end of deep expiration, is relatively constant, 80 mg/100 ml of ethanol in blood producing 35 µg/100 ml in expired air, this being the basis of the breathalyser test. The concentration in urine is more variable, and provides a less accurate measure of blood concentration.

Ethanol metabolism occurs almost entirely in the liver, and mainly by a pathway involving successive oxidations, first to acetaldehyde and then to acetic acid (Fig. 39.6). Since ethanol is often consumed in large quantities (compared with most drugs), 1–2 moles daily being by no means unusual, it constitutes a substantial load on the hepatic oxidative systems. The oxidation of 2 moles of ethanol consumes about 1.5 kg of the cofactor NAD^+. Availability of NAD^+ limits the rate of ethanol oxidation to about 10 ml/hour in a normal adult, independently of ethanol concentration (Fig. 39.7), causing the process to show saturating kinetics (Ch. 5). It also leads to competition between the ethanol and other metabolic substrates for the available NAD^+ supplies, which may be a factor in ethanol-induced liver damage (see Ch. 49). The intermediate metabolite, acetaldehyde, is a reactive and toxic compound and this may also contribute to the hepatotoxicity. A small degree of esterification of ethanol with various fatty acids also occurs in the tissues, and these esters may also contribute to long-term toxicity.

Alcohol dehydrogenase is a soluble cytoplasmic enzyme, confined mainly to liver cells, which oxidises ethanol at the same time as reducing NAD^+ to NADH (Fig. 39.6). Ethanol metabolism causes the ratio of NAD^+ to NADH to fall, and this has other metabolic consequences (e.g. increased lactate, and slowing down

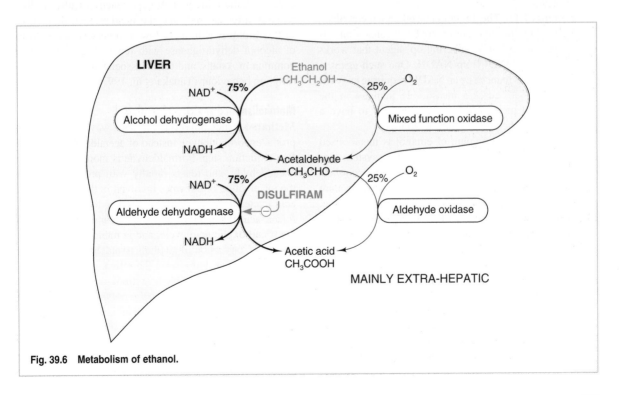

Fig. 39.6 Metabolism of ethanol.

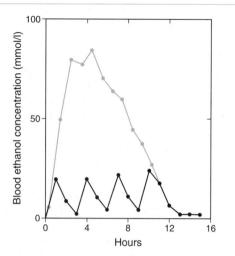

Fig. 39.7 Zero-order kinetics of ethanol elimination in rats. Rats were given ethanol orally (104 mmol/kg) either as a single dose, or as four divided doses. The single dose results in a much higher and more sustained blood ethanol concentration than the same quantity given as divided doses. Note that, after the single dose, ethanol concentration declines linearly, the rate of decline being similar after a small or large dose, because of the saturation phenomenon. (From: Kalant H et al. 1975 Biochem Pharmacol 24: 431)

of the Krebs cycle). The limitation on ethanol metabolism imposed by the limited rate of NAD$^+$ regeneration has led to attempts to find a 'sobering-up' agent that works by regenerating NAD$^+$ from NADH. One such agent is fructose, which is reduced by an NADH-requiring enzyme. In large doses it causes a measurable increase in the rate of ethanol metabolism, but not enough to have a useful effect on the rate of return to sobriety.

Normally, a trivial amount of ethanol is metabolised by the microsomal mixed function oxidase system (see Ch. 5), but induction of this system occurs in alcoholics. Ethanol can affect the metabolism of other drugs that are metabolised by the mixed function oxidase system (e.g. **phenobarbitone**, **warfarin** and **steroids**), with an initial inhibitory effect produced by competition, followed by enhancement due to enzyme induction.

Nearly all of the acetaldehyde produced is converted to acetate in the liver, by *aldehyde dehydrogenase* (Fig. 39.6). Normally, only a little acetaldehyde escapes from the liver, giving a blood acetaldehyde concentration of 20–50 μmol/l after an intoxicating dose of ethanol in humans. The circulating acetaldehyde usually has little or no effect, but the concentration may become much larger under certain circumstances, and produce toxic effects.

This occurs if aldehyde dehydrogenase is inhibited by drugs such as **disulfiram**. In the presence of disulfiram, which produces no marked effect when given alone, ethanol consumption is followed by a severe reaction, comprising flushing, tachycardia, hyperventilation and considerable panic and distress, which is due to excessive acetaldehyde accumulation in the bloodstream. This reaction is extremely unpleasant, but not harmful, and disulfiram can be used as aversion therapy to discourage people from taking ethanol. Some other drugs, notably oral hypoglycaemic agents of the sulphonylurea class (e.g. **chlorpropamide**; see Ch. 22) and certain antibacterial drugs (e.g. **nitrofurantoin**; see Ch. 43) also occasionally produce similar reactions to ethanol. Interestingly, a Chinese herbal medicine, used traditionally to cure alcoholics, contains **daidzin**, recently shown to be a specific inhibitor of aldehyde dehydrogenase. In hamsters (which spontaneously consume alcohol in amounts that would defeat even the hardest two-legged drinker, while remaining, as far as one can tell, completely sober), daidzin markedly inhibits alcohol consumption (see Keung & Vallee 1993).

Genetic factors

In 50% of Asians, an inactive genetic variant of one of the aldehyde dehydrogenase isoforms (ALDH-1) is expressed; these individuals experience a disulfiram-like reaction after alcohol, and the incidence of alcoholism in this group is extremely low. Conversely, an isoform of alcohol dehydrogenase with reduced activity is also common in Asians, and this is associated with excessive drinking behaviour (Tanaka et al. 1997).

Metabolism and toxicity of methanol

Methanol is metabolised in the same way as ethanol, but produces formaldehyde instead of acetaldehyde from the first oxidation step. Formaldehyde is more reactive than acetaldehyde, and reacts rapidly with proteins, causing the inactivation of enzymes involved in the tricarboxylic acid cycle. It is converted to another toxic metabolite, formic acid. This, unlike acetic acid, cannot be utilised in the tricarboxylic acid cycle, and is liable to cause tissue damage. Conversion of alcohols to aldehydes occurs not only in the liver, but also in the retina, catalysed by the dehydrogenase responsible for retinol–retinal conversion. Formation of formaldehyde in the retina accounts for one of the main toxic effects of methanol, namely blindness, which can occur after ingestion of as little as 10 g. Formic acid production, and derangement of the tricarboxylic acid cycle, also produce severe acidosis. Methanol is used as an industrial solvent, and also to adulterate industrial ethanol in order to make it unfit to drink. Methanol poisoning is quite common, and it is treated by administration of large doses of ethanol, which acts to retard methanol metabolism by competition for alcohol dehydrogenase. This is often done in conjunction with haemodialysis to remove unchanged methanol, which has a small volume of distribution.

Metabolism of ethanol

- Ethanol is metabolised mainly by the liver, first by alcohol dehydrogenase to acetaldehyde, then by aldehyde dehydrogenase to acetate. About 25% of the acetaldehyde is metabolised extrahepatically.
- Small amounts of ethanol are excreted in urine and expired air. Hepatic metabolism shows saturation kinetics, mainly because of limited availability of NAD^+. Maximal rate of ethanol metabolism is about 10 ml/hour. Thus, plasma concentration falls linearly rather than exponentially.
- Acetaldehyde may produce toxic effects. Inhibition of aldehyde dehydrogenase by disulfiram accentuates nausea etc., caused by acetaldehyde, and can be used in aversion therapy.
- Methanol is similarly metabolised to formic acid, which is toxic, especially to retina.
- Asian races show a high rate of genetic polymorphism of alcohol and aldehyde dehydrogenase, associated with alcoholism and alcohol intolerance, respectively.

TOLERANCE AND DEPENDENCE

Tolerance to the effects of ethanol can be demonstrated in both humans and experimental animals, to the extent of a two- to threefold reduction in potency occurring over 1–3 weeks of continuing ethanol administration. A small component of this is due to the more rapid elimination of ethanol. The major component is tissue tolerance, which accounts for a roughly twofold decrease in potency and which can be observed in vitro (e.g. by measuring the inhibitory effect of ethanol on transmitter release from synaptosomes) as well as in vivo. The mechanism of this tolerance is not known for certain (see Little 1991), but it is known that ethanol tolerance is associated with tolerance to many anaesthetic agents, and alcoholics are often difficult to anaesthetise with drugs such as halothane.

Chronic ethanol administration produces various changes in CNS neurons, which tend to oppose the acute cellular effects that it produces (see above). There is a small reduction in the density of $GABA_A$-receptors, and a proliferation of voltage-gated Ca^{2+} channels and NMDA

receptors. The effect on Ca^{2+} channels has received particular attention (see Charness et al. 1989), Studies on brain synaptosomes and isolated neurons from ethanol-tolerant rats have revealed various changes. The acute effect of ethanol (see above) is to reduce Ca^{2+} entry through voltage-gated Ca^{2+} channels, and thus to reduce transmitter release. During chronic exposure to ethanol, Ca^{2+} entry recovers owing to a proliferation of Ca^{2+} channels, and when ethanol is withdrawn, depolarisation-evoked Ca^{2+} entry and transmitter release are increased above normal, which is possibly associated with the physical withdrawal symptoms. Consistent with this explanation, Ca^{2+}-channel-blocking drugs of the dihydropyridine type (see Ch. 14) reduce the effects of ethanol withdrawal in experimental animals (see Little 1991).

A well-defined physical abstinence syndrome develops in response to ethanol withdrawal. As with most other dependence-producing drugs, this is probably important as a short-term factor in sustaining the drug habit, but other (mainly psychological) factors are more important in the longer term. The physical abstinence syndrome usually subsides in a few days, but the craving for ethanol and the tendency to relapse last for very much longer.

The physical abstinence syndrome in man, in severe form, develops after about 8 hours. In the first stage, the main symptoms are tremor, nausea, sweating, fever and, sometimes, hallucinations. These last for about 24 hours. This phase may be followed by tonic–clonic convulsions, indistinguishable from grand mal epilepsy. Over the next few days, the condition of '*delirium tremens*' develops, in which the patient becomes confused, agitated and often aggressive, and may suffer much more severe hallucinations. A similar syndrome of central and autonomic hyperactivity can be produced in experimental animals by ethanol withdrawal.

Alcohol dependence ('alcoholism') is common (4–5% of the population) and, as with smoking, difficult to treat effectively. The main pharmacological approaches (see Zernig et al. 1997; Table 39.2) are the following:

- To alleviate the acute abstinence syndrome during 'drying out', **benzodiazepines** (see Ch. 33) are effective; **clonidine** and **propranolol**, are also useful. Clonidine (α_2-adrenoceptor agonist) is believed to act by inhibiting the exaggerated transmitter release that occurs during withdrawal, while propranolol (β-adrenoceptor antagonist) blocks the effects of excessive sympathetic activity.
- To render alcohol consumption unpleasant, **disulfiram** (see above).

- To reduce alcohol-induced reward, **naltrexone** (opiate antagonist) is effective, for reasons that are poorly understood.
- To reduce craving, **acamprosate** is used. This recently introduced compound, a taurine analogue, has complex effects on amino-acid transmission, and the mechanism of its interaction with ethanol is uncertain. Several clinical trials have shown it to improve the success rate in achieving alcohol abstinence, with few unwanted effects.

CANNABIS

Extracts of the hemp plant, *Cannabis sativa*, which grows freely in temperate and tropical regions, contain the active substance Δ^9-tetrahydrocannabinol (**THC**; Fig. 39.8). **Marijuana** is the name given to the dried leaves and flower heads, prepared as a smoking mixture; **hashish** is the extracted resin. For centuries, these substances have been used for various medicinal purposes and as intoxicant preparations. Marijuana was brought to North America by immigrants, mainly in the 19th century, and began to be regarded as a social problem in the early years of this century; it was banned during the 1930s. Its use increased dramatically in the 1960s, and recent figures suggest that about 15% of the adult population in America and Western Europe have taken cannabis at some time, with a much higher proportion (close to 50%) among teenagers and young adults.

CHEMICAL ASPECTS

Cannabis extracts contain numerous related compounds, called cannabinoids, most of which are insoluble in water. The most abundant cannabinoids are Δ^9-**tetrahydrocannabinol** (THC), its precursor **cannabidiol**, and **cannabinol**, which is formed spontaneously from THC. THC is the most active pharmacologically, and also the most abundant, constituting about roughly 1–10% by weight of marijuana and hashish preparations. A metabolite, 11-hydroxy-THC is more active than THC itself, and probably contributes to the pharmacological effect. Radioimmunoassays have been developed for cannabinoids, but they lack sufficient chemical specificity to be able to distinguish THC from numerous other cannabinoids found in crude extracts, and from the various metabolites that are formed in vivo. Thus, the assay of pharmacologically active THC in biological fluids still presents a problem.

PHARMACOLOGICAL EFFECTS

THC acts mainly on the central nervous system, producing a mixture of psychotomimetic and depressant effects, together with various centrally mediated peripheral autonomic effects (see review by Dewey 1986).

The main subjective effects in humans consist of:

- a feeling of relaxation and well-being, similar to the effect of ethanol, but without the accompanying aggression

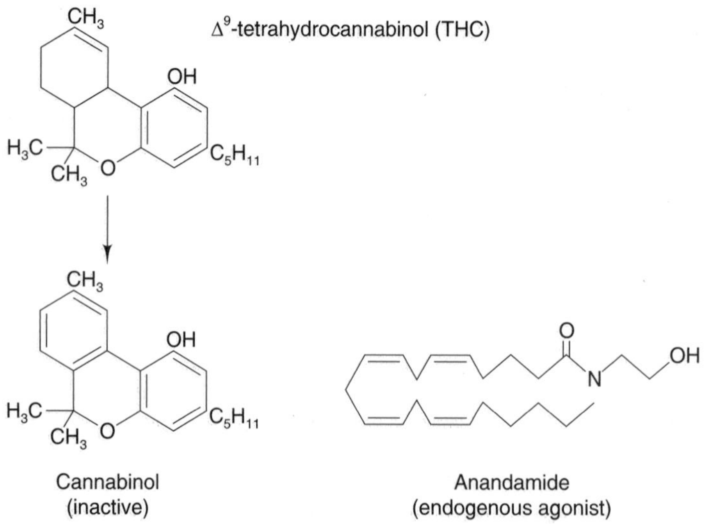

Fig. 39.8   Structure of cannabinoids. Anandamide is an arachidonic acid derivative which is present in the brain and believed to be an endogenous agonist for cannabinoid receptors.

Δ^9-tetrahydrocannabinol (THC)

Cannabinol (inactive)

Anandamide (endogenous agonist)

- a feeling of sharpened sensory awareness, with sounds and sights seeming more intense and fantastic.

These effects are similar to, but usually less pronounced than, those produced by psychotomimetic drugs such as LSD (see Ch. 38). Subjects report that time passes extremely slowly. The alarming sensations and paranoid delusions that often occur with LSD are seldom experienced after cannabis.

Central effects that can be directly measured in human and animal studies include:

- impairment of short-term memory, and simple learning tasks—subjective feelings of confidence and heightened creativity are not reflected in actual performance
- impairment of motor coordination (e.g. driving performance)
- catalepsy—the retention of fixed unnatural postures
- analgesia
- anti-emetic action
- increased appetite.

The main peripheral effects of cannabis are:

- tachycardia, which can be prevented by drugs that block sympathetic transmission
- vasodilatation, which is particularly marked on the scleral and conjunctival vessels, producing a bloodshot appearance characteristic of cannabis smokers
- reduction of intraocular pressure
- bronchodilatation.

RECEPTORS AND ENDOGENOUS LIGANDS

Cannabinoids, being highly lipid-soluble, were originally thought to act in a similar way to general anaesthetic agents, but the identification of specific cannabinoid receptors in the brain and in the periphery dismissed this idea. Subsequent work, including cloning (see Abood & Martin 1996, Pertwee 1997), has shown that cannabinoid receptors are typical members of the family of G-protein-coupled receptors (see Ch. 2), linked to inhibition of adenylate cyclase. The receptors are also coupled to potassium channel activation and calcium channel inhibition, and thereby exert an inhibitory effect on transmitter release. These cellular effects closely resemble those of opioids. The distribution of brain cannabinoid receptors (CB_1 subtype) corresponds to the main pharmacological effects. They occur particularly in the hippocampus (memory impairment), cerebellum and *substantia nigra*

(motor disturbance) and mesolimbic dopamine pathways (reward), as well as in the cortex. The peripheral cannabinoid receptor (CB_2 subtype) shows only about 45% amino acid homology with CB_1, and is located mainly in the lymphoid system. This was an unexpected finding, but may account for the inhibitory effects on immune function that have been reported with cannabis. The discovery of specific cannabinoid receptors in the brain naturally led to a search for an endogenous chemical mediator, and the discovery of **anandamide**, an amide derivative of arachidonic acid (see Fig. 39.8), which produces short-lasting cannabinoid-like effects when injected into the brain. The physiological role of this system, and the mechanism of synthesis and release of anandamide are currently attracting much interest. The peripheral CB_2-receptor shows a different pharmacological specificity from the CB_1-receptor, but so far very little is known about its function. Agonists and antagonists specific for each type have been developed (see Pertwee 1997). A potent CB_1-receptor antagonist, SR141716A, produces effects opposite to those of cannabinoid agonists, namely increased locomotor activity, improved short-term memory, as well as enhanced transmitter release in peripheral tissues. This implies a degree of tonic activation of CB_1-receptors under physiological conditions, which could result either from the presence of endogenous cannabinoids, or from constitutive activation of the receptor in the absence of any ligand, assuming that SR141716A could act as an inverse agonist (see Ch. 1). Much remains to be discovered about the endogenous cannabinoid system, an area of intense current interest.

The effects of cannabis on intraocular pressure, bronchial smooth muscle, pain perception and the vomiting reflex are of potential therapeutic value, and certain cannabinoid derivatives, e.g. **nabilone**, have been developed as therapeutic agents. The pronounced central effects produced by these compounds, including their possible addictive properties (see below), limit their usefulness. As there is little evidence for subtypes of the CB_1-receptor—which might offer the possibility of developing ligands with more selective central effects—therapeutic developments on this front are currently stalled.

TOLERANCE AND DEPENDENCE

Tolerance to cannabis, and physical dependence, occur only to a minor degree, and mainly in heavy users. The abstinence symptoms are similar to those of ethanol or opiate withdrawal, namely nausea, agitation, irritability, confusion, tachycardia, sweating, etc., but are relatively mild and do not result in a compulsive urge to take the drug. Psychological dependence does not seem to occur with cannabis, and overall it cannot be classified as addictive (see review by Abood & Martin 1992).

PHARMACOKINETIC ASPECTS

The effect of cannabis, taken by smoking or by intravenous injection, takes about 1 hour to develop fully, and lasts for 2–3 hours. A small fraction is converted to 11-hydroxy-THC, which is more active than THC itself, but most is converted mainly to inactive metabolites. It is partly conjugated, and undergoes enterohepatic recirculation. Being highly lipophilic, THC and its metabolites are sequestered in body fat, and excretion continues for several days after a single dose.

ADVERSE EFFECTS

THC is relatively safe in overdose, producing drowsiness and confusion, but not respiratory or cardiovascular effects that threaten life. In this respect it is safer than most abused substances, particularly opiates and ethanol. Even in low doses, THC and synthetic derivatives such as nabilone, produce euphoria and drowsiness, sometimes accompanied by sensory distortion and hallucinations. These effects, together with the legal restrictions on the use of THC, preclude the widespread therapeutic use of cannabinoids.

THC produces teratogenic and mutagenic effects in rodents, and an increased incidence of chromosome breaks in circulating white cells has been reported in humans. Such breaks are, however, by no means unique to cannabis, and epidemiological studies have not shown any increased risk of foetal malformation or cancer among cannabis users.

Certain endocrine effects occur in humans, notably a decrease in plasma testosterone and a reduction of sperm count. One study showed a reduction of more than 50% in both plasma testosterone and sperm count in subjects smoking 10 or more marijuana cigarettes per week.

It is very difficult to assess the evidence that cannabis causes long-term psychological changes. It has been sug-

gested that it can cause schizophrenia, and that it leads to a gradually developing state of apathy and underachievement, but it is very difficult to prove causation even where a positive association has been found.

The long-running argument over the legalisation of cannabis centres mainly on the seriousness of these adverse effects. Opponents of legalisation argue that it would be folly to change the law in favour of the use by the public at large of a substance which could turn out to have serious toxic effects. Proponents of a change argue that the present law is clearly ineffective and encourages crime, and that cannabis is undoubtedly safer than either ethanol or tobacco.

Cannabis

- Main active constituent is Δ^9-tetrahydrocannabinol (THC), though pharmacologically active metabolites may be important.
- Actions on CNS include both depressant and psychotomimetic effects.
- Subjectively, subjects experience euphoria and a feeling of relaxation, with sharpened sensory awareness.
- Objective tests show impairment of learning, memory and motor performance.
- THC also shows analgesic and anti-emetic activity, as well as causing catalepsy and hypothermia in animal tests.
- Peripheral actions include vasodilatation, reduction of intraocular pressure and bronchodilatation.
- Cannabinoid receptors belong to the G-protein-coupled receptor family, linked to inhibition of adenylate cyclase and effects on Ca^{2+} and K^+ channel function, causing inhibition of synaptic transmission. The brain receptor (CB_1) differs from the peripheral receptor (CB_2), which is expressed mainly in cells of the immune system. Selective agonists and antagonists have been developed.
- Anandamide, an arachidonic acid derivative, is an endogenous ligand for the CNS cannabinoid receptor; its function has not yet been ascertained.
- Cannabinoids are less liable than opiates, nicotine or alcohol to cause dependence, but may have long-term psychological effects.
- Nabilone, a THC analogue, has been developed for its anti-emetic property; otherwise, cannabinoids are not generally available for clinical use.

REFERENCES AND FURTHER READING

Abood M E, Martin B R 1992 Neurobiology of marijuana abuse. Trends Pharmacol Sci 13: 201–206

Abood M E, Martin B R 1996 Molecular neurobiology of the cannabinoid receptor. Int Rev Neurobiol 39: 197–221

Balfour D J K, Fagerstrom K O 1996 Pharmacology of nicotine and its therapeutic use in smoking cessation and neurodegenerative disorders. Pharmacol Ther 72: 51–81 *(Review of the pharmacology of nicotine and its usefulness as replacement therapy)*

Benowitz N L 1993 Nicotine replacement therapy. Drugs 45: 157–170

Benowitz N L 1996 Pharmacology of nicotine: addiction and therapeutics. Ann Rev Pharmacol 36: 597–613 *(General review article, including information on potential therapeutic uses of nicotine other than reduction of smoking)*

Charness M E, Simon R P, Greenberg D A 1989 Ethanol and the nervous system. N Engl J Med 321: 442–454

Crabbe J C, Belknap J K, Buck K J 1994 Genetic animal models of alcohol and drug abuse. Science 264: 1715–1723 *(Summary of confusing data on genetics of drug abuse. Human studies have implicated a mutation in the D_2-receptor, but not all studies agree on this)*

Dewey W L 1986 Cannabinoid pharmacology. Pharmacol Rev 38: 151–178

Groenbaek M et al. 1994 Influence of sex, age, body mass index and smoking on alcohol intake and mortality. Br Med J 308: 302–306 *(Large-scale Danish study showing reduced coronary mortality at moderate levels of drinking, with increase at high levels)*

Hanson J W, Streissguth A P, Smith D W 1978 The effects of moderate alcohol consumption during pregnancy on fetal growth and morphogenesis. J Pediatr 92: 457–460

Keung W-M, Vallee B L 1993 Daidzin and daidzein suppress free-choice ethanol intake by Syrian golden hamsters. Proc Natl Acad Sci USA 90: 10008–10012

Koob G F 1992 Drugs of abuse: anatomy, pharmacology and function of reward pathways. Trends Pharmacol Sci 13: 177–184

Koob G F 1996 Drug addiction: the yin and yang of hedonic homeostasis. Neuron 16: 893–896

Lieber C S 1995 Medical disorders of alcoholism. N Engl J Med 333: 1058–1065 *(Review focusing on ethanol-induced liver damage in relation to ethanol metabolism)*

Lister R G, Nutt D J 1987 Is Ro 15-4513 a specific alcohol antagonist? Trends Neurosci 6: 223–225

Little H J 1991 Mechanisms that may underlie the behavioural effects of ethanol. Prog Neurobiol 36: 171–194

Lovinger D M 1997 Alcohols and neurotransmitters-gated ion channels: past present and future. Naunyn-Schmiedebergs Arch Pharmacol 356: 267–282 *(Review article arguing that alcohol effects depend on interaction with synaptic ion channels)*

Maldonado R, Saiardi A, Valverde O, Samad T A, Roques B P, Borelli E 1997 Absence of opiate rewarding effects in mice lacking dopamine D2 receptors. Nature 388: 586–589 *(Use of transgenic animals to demonstrate role of dopamine receptors in reward properties of opiates)*

Mottram D 1988 Drugs in sport. E & F N Spon, London

Nestler E J, Aghajanian G K 1997 Molecular and cellular basis of addiction. Science 278: 58–63 *(Short review focusing on adaptive responses of cAMP system in brain)*

O'Brien C P 1997 A range of research-based pharmacotherapies for addiction. Science 278: 66–70 *(Useful overview of pharmacological approaches to treatment)*

Pertwee R G 1997 Pharmacology of cannabinoid CB_1 and CB_2 receptors. Pharmacol Ther 74: 129–180 *(Comprehensive review of properties of cannabinoid receptors and their ligands)*

Peto R, Lopez A D, Boreham J, Thun M, Heath C, Doll R 1996 Mortality from smoking worldwide. Br Med Bull 52: 12–21

Picciotto M R, Zoli M, Rimondini R et al. 1998 Acetylcholine receptors containing the β_2 subunit are involved in the reinforcing properties of nicotine. Nature 391: 173–177 *(Shows that knocking out the β_2 subunit of nAChR, which is expressed by mesolimbic neurons, abolishes the normal reward and self-administration properties of nicotine)*

Royal College of Physicians Reports 1971, 1977 Smoking or health. Pitman Medical Publishing, Tunbridge Wells

Shuckit M A 1995 Drug and alcohol abuse. Plenum Medical Book Company, New York

Tabakoff B, Hoffman P L 1996 Alcohol addiction: an enigma among us. Neuron 16: 909–912 *(Review of alcohol actions at the cellular and molecular level—ignore the silly title)*

Tanaka F, Shiratori Y, Yokusuka O, Imazeki F, Tsukada Y, Omata M 1997 Polymorphism of alcohol-metabolizing genes affects drinking behaviour and alcoholic liver disease in Japanese men. Alcohol Clin Exp Res 21: 596–601 *(Describes polymorphism of aldehyde and alcohol dehydrogenases, and their effect on drinking behaviour)*

Winger G, Hofmann F G, Woods J H 1992 A handbook on drugs and alcohol abuse. Oxford University press, New York

Zernig G, Fabisch K, Fabisch H 1997 Pharmacotherapy of alcohol dependence. Trends Pharmacol Sci 18: 229–231 *(Short review of drug therapies used in alcoholism)*

40

Local anaesthetics and other drugs that affect ion channels

INTRODUCTION

The property of electrical excitability is what enables the membranes of nerve and muscle cells to generate propagated action potentials, which are essential for communication in the nervous system and for the initiation of mechanical activity in cardiac and striated muscle. Electrical excitability depends on the existence of voltage-gated ion channels in the cell membrane, most importantly on Na^+ channels that are gated in such a way that they open, and the membrane becomes selectively permeable to Na^+, when the membrane is depolarised. Also important are the voltage-dependent K^+ channels and Ca^{2+} channels, which function in basically the same way. These channels are membrane proteins, and they all possess a basically similar molecular structure (see below). Their distinct ion selectivity, however, means that they have quite different physiological functions; Na^+, K^+ and Ca^{2+} channels are also selectively affected by quite different classes of drugs. The pharmacology of Ca^{2+} channels, which are particularly important in relation to the heart and vascular smooth muscle, is discussed in Chapters 14 and 15. This chapter focuses on the function and pharmacology of Na^+ and K^+ channels. **Local anaesthetics**, which act mainly by blocking Na^+ channels, are discussed in detail, and other agents that affect Na^+ and K^+ channels (many of which appear in other parts of this book) are also considered. Inherited diseases associated with ion channel malfunction are becoming increasingly recognised (see Ackerman & Clapham 1997).

There are, broadly speaking, two ways in which channel function may be modified, namely *block of the channels* and *modification of gating behaviour*. Either mechanism can cause an increase or a decrease of electrical excitability. Thus, blocking Na^+ channels reduces excitability, whereas block of K^+ channels tends to increase it. Similarly, an agent that affects Na^+ channel gating so as to increase channel opening will tend to increase excitability and vice versa.

SODIUM AND POTASSIUM CHANNELS OF EXCITABLE MEMBRANES

Our present understanding of electrical excitability—the ability of a cell to generate a short-lasting, all-or-nothing depolarisation or reversal of the membrane (known as an *action potential*) in response to electrical stimulation—rests firmly on the work of Hodgkin, Huxley & Katz, published in 1949–1952. Before then it was known that the resting cell membrane was selectively permeable to K^+, that the potential of the interior of the cell was negative to the outside by 60–90 mV, and that the action potential was associated with a large increase in membrane conductance. Hodgkin and his colleagues, in a remarkable tour de force (at a time when valve-operated amplifiers, and even oscilloscopes, had to be painstakingly designed and built by the scientists themselves) devised the *voltage-clamp technique* and applied it successfully to study the mechanism of action potential generation in the squid giant axon. For accounts of these experiments, see Katz (1966), Nicholls et al. (1992). Their analysis showed that the action potential is generated by the interplay of two separate ionic permeability changes:

- a rapid, transient increase in Na^+ permeability which

occurs when the membrane is depolarised beyond about −50 mV

- a slower, sustained increase in K⁺ permeability.

Because of the inequality of Na⁺ and K⁺ concentrations on the two sides of the membrane, an increase in Na⁺ permeability causes an inward current of Na⁺ ions, whereas an increase in K⁺ permeability causes an outward current. The separate nature of these two currents can be most clearly demonstrated by the use of Na⁺- and K⁺-channel-blocking drugs, as shown in Figure 40.1, depicting the currents that flow through the membrane of a single node of Ranvier of a frog axon when the membrane potential is suddenly stepped from −120 mV to a more depolarised level. Stepping to −45 mV produces a transient inward current which decays in about 10 ms. With larger depolarisations, this inward current gets smaller, and a later, sustained outward current is seen. If the membrane is depolarised even further, the transient current reverses in direction. This happens when the internal potential is made positive to the sodium equilibrium potential (E_{Na}) which is a function of the intracellular and extracellular Na⁺ concentrations, and is about +40 mV under normal conditions. The explanation for this complex behaviour is that the sodium current at any moment depends on two factors:

- the *state of activation* of the channels (i.e. the fraction of channels that is open), which is a function of both membrane potential and time
- the *driving force* for Na⁺ ions ($E_m − E_{Na}$).

At potentials negative to about −60 mV, no channels are activated, so no current flows. Between about −50 mV and −30 mV (the activation range for Na⁺ channels) the channels progressively open. With further depolarisation, the peak current decreases because, though activation is complete, $E_m − E_{Na}$ decreases. When the membrane is made more positive than E_{Na} (normally about +40 mV), the driving force changes in direction and the current flows outward.

The Na⁺ current can be seen uncomplicated by K⁺ current (Fig. 40.1) if the K⁺ channels are blocked with **tetraethylammonium** (**TEA**; see below). The Na⁺ current is transient, even if the membrane depolarisation is sustained, and decays to zero in 5–10 ms. This spontaneous closure of the channels, known as *inactivation*, is an important property of the Na⁺ channel. During the physiological initiation or propagation of a nerve impulse, the first event is a small depolarisation of the membrane, produced either by transmitter action or by the approach of an action potential passing along the axon. This opens Na⁺ channels, allowing an inward current of Na⁺ ions to flow, which depolarises the membrane still further. The process is thus a regenerative one, and the increase in Na⁺ permeability is enough to bring the membrane potential close to E_{Na}.

In many types of cell, including most nerve cells, the process of repolarisation is assisted by the opening of voltage-dependent K⁺ channels. These function in much the same way as Na⁺ channels (i.e. they open when the cell is depolarised), but differ in two important ways.

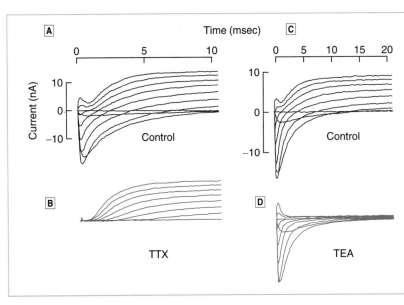

Fig. 40.1 Separation of Na⁺ and K⁺ currents in nerve membrane. Voltage clamp records from the node of Ranvier of a single frog nerve fibre. At time 0 the membrane potential was stepped to a depolarised level, ranging from −60 mV (lower trace in each series) to +60 mV (upper trace in each series) in 15-mV steps. A, C Control records from two fibres. B Effect of tetrodotoxin (TTX) which abolishes Na⁺ currents. D Effect of tetraethylammonium (TEA) which abolishes K⁺ currents. (From: Hille B 1970 Prog Biophys 21: 1)

Firstly, their activation kinetics are about 10 times slower; secondly, they do not inactivate appreciably. This means that the K$^+$ channels open later than the Na$^+$ channels (Fig. 40.2). Because of the high intracellular and low extracellular K$^+$ concentrations, E_K is about -100 mV, so opening K$^+$ channels causes an outward (repolarising) current, which occurs later than the Na$^+$ current, and contributes to the rapid termination of the action potential. The behaviour of the Na$^+$ and K$^+$ channels during an action potential is shown in Figure 40.2, and an overall scheme showing the various regulatory processes and sites of drug action is shown in Figure 40.3.

The function of these voltage-gated ion channels has been intensively studied with the help of molecular bio-

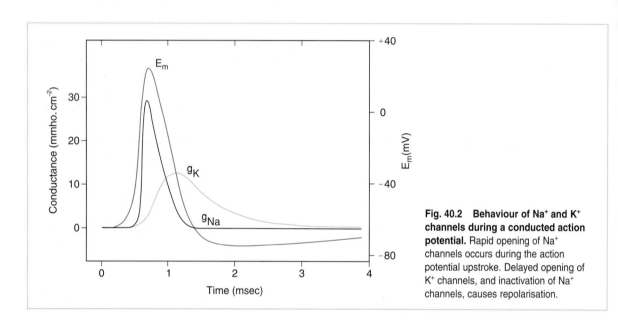

Fig. 40.2 Behaviour of Na$^+$ and K$^+$ channels during a conducted action potential. Rapid opening of Na$^+$ channels occurs during the action potential upstroke. Delayed opening of K$^+$ channels, and inactivation of Na$^+$ channels, causes repolarisation.

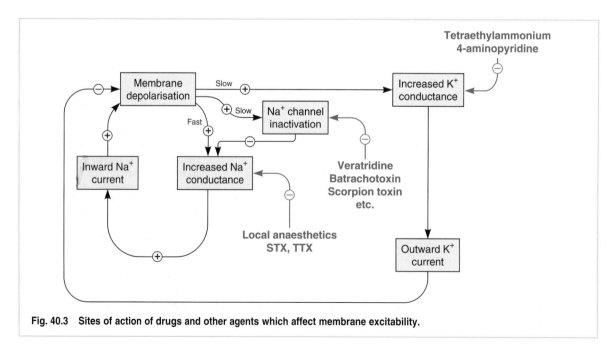

Fig. 40.3   Sites of action of drugs and other agents which affect membrane excitability.

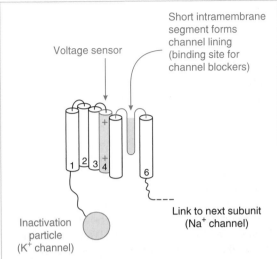

Voltage sensor

Short intramembrane segment forms channel lining (binding site for channel blockers)

1 2 3 4 6

Inactivation particle (K⁺ channel)

Link to next subunit (Na⁺ channel)

Fig. 40.4 Structure of voltage-gated ion channels. The diagram shows one of the four domains of the channel. In Na⁺ channels, the four domains are linked as a single chain; in K⁺ channels, they are separate subunits, and may comprise fewer than 6 membrane-spanning helices. Movement of helix 4 (voltage-sensor) is responsible for channel activation. Inactivation occurs when the intracellular inactivation particle blocks the channel. (In the Na⁺ channel, the inactivating particle is formed from one of the intracellular loops; see text.) The channel pore is formed from the short intramembrane segment, plus adjacent helices; channel-blocking drugs bind in this region.

largely by making selective mutations, and observing their effects on the function and pharmacology of the channels. Part of the lining of the channel is formed by the loops linking S5 and S6 in each of the four domains, and this forms the binding site for some channel-blocking drugs, as well as conferring the ion-selectivity of the channel. The S4 helix contains positively charged residues, and is believed to be the voltage-sensor, which moves outwards as the cell is depolarised, and controls the gating of the channel. Inactivation of the channel depends on the intracellular domain, which functions as a tethered stopper, and physically blocks the channel from the inside. In the case of the K⁺ channel (Fig. 40.4), the stopper is made from the intracellular C-terminal region of each of the four subunits; in the Na⁺ channel; it is formed by one of the intracellular loops linking two adjacent domains. Many molecular variants of the α-subunits have been identified, and these give rise to the physiological differences between the properties of the channels in different tissues, such as the heart, brain, peripheral nervous system, endocrine cells, smooth and skeletal muscle cells, etc., all of whose physiological functions depend on the processes involving ion channels. The details are beyond the scope of this book, but information on the subtypes of K⁺, Na⁺ and Ca²⁺ channels can be found in recent reviews (see Catterall 1993, Mathie et al. 1998, Pongs 1992, Tsien et al. 1995) and is summarised in the TIPS Receptor & Ion Channel Nomenclature Supplement (1996).

logy techniques (see reviews by Catterall 1993, Pongs 1992). The three main types of channel show considerable sequence homology, and have the same basic structure* (Fig. 40.4). The main component is the α-subunit, which consists of an aggregate of four very similar protein domains; these exist either as regions of a single very long peptide chain (as in the Na⁺ channel) or as independent subunits (as in the K⁺ channel). Each of the four domains contains six membrane-spanning α-helices (S1–S6) stacked like sticks of gelignite, and the four domains are arranged symmetrically around a central aqueous pore—the ion channel. The functional organisation of these complex proteins has been elucidated

---

*An exception is a family of K⁺ channels, known as *inward rectifier channels* which includes various K⁺ channels that are regulated by G-protein-coupled receptors, such as the cardiac muscarinic ACh receptor (Ch. 14), and neuronal opiate receptors (Ch. 37), as well as the ATP-gated K⁺ channels of pancreatic islet cells (Ch. 22). These channels are truncated versions of the full structure, lacking S1–S4 (the voltage sensor) but incorporating the channel lining and intracellular domains.

Ionic basis of electrical excitability

- An electrically excitable cell is one that generates an all-or-nothing action potential in response to depolarisation of the membrane.
- In nerve and striated muscle cells, electrical excitability is due to the existence of voltage-activated Na⁺ channels, which open transiently when the membrane is depolarised. Opening of Na⁺ channels causes an inward current of Na⁺ ions across the membrane, which further depolarises it.
- Recovery of the membrane potential is due to:
  — inactivation of Na⁺ channels
  — delayed opening of voltage-activated K⁺ channels, through which outward K⁺ current flows, causing repolarisation.
- Drugs may reduce membrane excitability by:
  — blocking Na⁺ channels (mainly neurons)
  — activating K⁺ channels (more important in smooth muscle and myocardium than in neurons).
- Drugs may enhance membrane excitability by:
  — blocking inactivation of Na⁺ channels
  — blocking K⁺ channels.

DRUGS THAT AFFECT SODIUM CHANNELS

Though many drugs block voltage-sensitive Na^+ channels, and inhibit the generation of the action potential, the only drugs in this category that are clinically useful are the local anaesthetics, various anticonvulsant drugs (see Ch. 36) and class I antidysrhythmic drugs (see Ch. 14). Compounds that are widely used as experimental tools for studying Na^+ channels include **tetrodotoxin** (TTX) and **saxitoxin** (STX), which are highly potent and selective blocking agents, and compounds that affect the gating properties of Na^+ channels such as **veratridine**, **batrachotoxin**, and **pyrethroid** insecticides.

LOCAL ANAESTHETICS

History

Coca leaves have been chewed for their psychotropic effects for thousands of years (see Ch. 38) by South American Indians, who knew about the numbing effect they produced on the mouth and tongue. Cocaine was isolated in 1860 and proposed as a local anaesthetic for surgical procedures. Sigmund Freud sought to make use of its 'psychic energising' power for psychiatric purposes. This was not a success, but his ophthalmologist friend in Vienna, Carl Köller, obtained some cocaine from Freud and showed in 1884 that reversible corneal anaesthesia could be produced by dropping cocaine into the eye. The idea was rapidly taken up, and within a few years cocaine anaesthesia was introduced into dentistry and general surgery. A synthetic substitute, procaine was discovered in 1905, and many other useful compounds were later developed.

Chemical aspects

Local anaesthetic molecules consist of an aromatic part linked by an ester or amide bond to a basic side-chain (Fig. 40.5). They are weak bases, with pK_a values mainly in the range 8–9, so that they are mainly, but not completely, ionised at physiological pH. This is important in relation to their ability to penetrate the nerve sheath and axon membrane; quaternary derivatives, which are fully ionised irrespective of pH, are ineffective as local anaesthetics. **Benzocaine**, an atypical local anaesthetic, has no basic group.

The presence of the ester or amide bond in local anaesthetic molecules is important because of its susceptibility to metabolic hydrolysis. The ester-containing compounds are usually inactivated in the plasma and tissues (mainly liver) by non-specific esterases. Amides are more stable,

and these anaesthetics generally have longer plasma half-lives.

Mechanism of action

Local anaesthetics block the initiation and propagation of action potentials by preventing the voltage-dependent increase in Na^+ conductance (Fig. 40.3). Though they exert a variety of non-specific effects on membrane function, their main action is to block Na^+ channels, which they do by physically plugging the transmembrane pore, interacting with residues of the S6 transmembrane helical domain (see Hille 1992, Ragsdale et al. 1994, Strichartz & Ritchie 1987).

Local anaesthetic activity is strongly pH-dependent, being increased at alkaline pH (i.e. when the proportion of ionised molecules is low) and vice versa. This is because the compound needs to penetrate the nerve sheath and the axon membrane to reach the inner end of the Na^+ channel (where the local anaesthetic binding site resides). Because the ionised form is not membrane-permeant, penetration is very poor at acid pH. Once inside the axon, it is the ionised form of the local anaesthetic molecule which binds to the channel (Fig. 40.6). This pH-dependence can be clinically important, since inflamed tissues are often acidic, and thus somewhat resistant to local anaesthetic agents.

Further analysis of local anaesthesic action (see Strichartz & Ritchie 1987) has shown that many drugs exhibit the property of 'use-dependent' block of Na^+ channels, as well as affecting, to some extent, the gating of the channels. Use-dependence means that the more the channels are opened, the greater the block becomes. It is a prominent feature of the action of many class I antidysrhythmic drugs (Ch. 14) and antiepileptic drugs (Ch. 36), and occurs because the blocking molecule enters the channel much more readily when the channel is open than when it is closed. With quaternary local anaesthetics working from the inside of the membrane, the channels must be cycled through their open state a few times before the blocking effect appears. With tertiary local anaesthetics, on the other hand, block can develop even if the channels are not open, and it is likely that the blocking molecule (uncharged) can enter the channel either directly from the membrane phase or via the open gate (Fig. 40.6). The relative importance of these two blocking pathways—the hydrophobic pathway via the membrane, and the hydrophilic pathway via the inner mouth of the channel—varies according to the lipid solubility of the drug, and the degree of use-dependence varies correspondingly.

As discussed earlier, the channel can exist in three

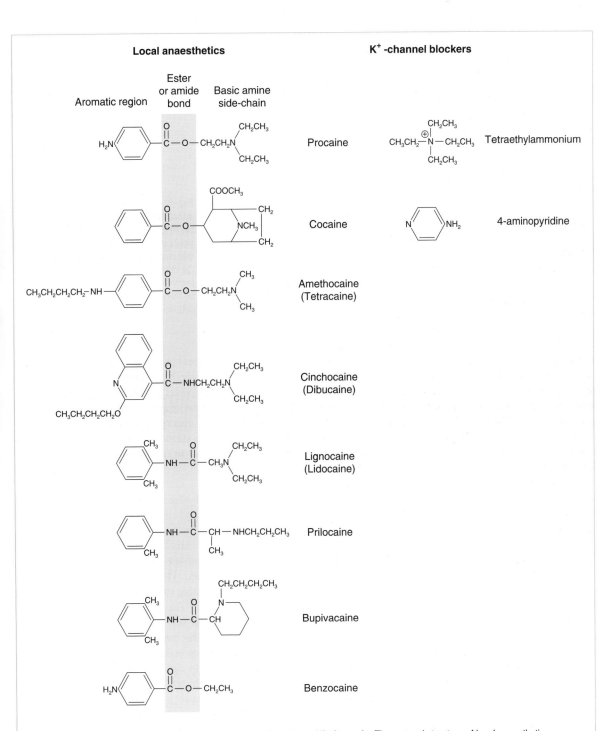

Fig. 40.5   Structures of local anaesthetics and drugs that block K$^+$ channels. The general structure of local anaesthetic molecules consists of aromatic group (left), ester or amide group (shaded) and amine group (right).

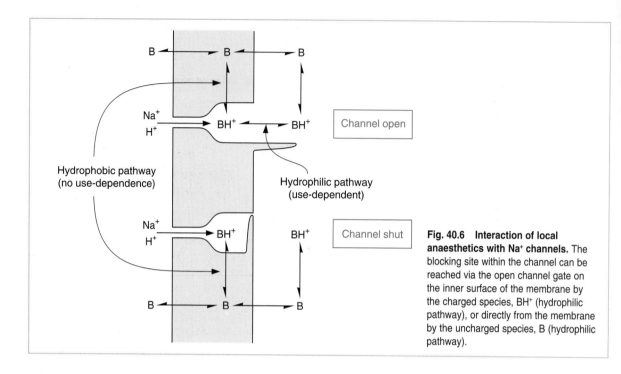

Fig. 40.6 Interaction of local anaesthetics with Na⁺ channels. The blocking site within the channel can be reached via the open channel gate on the inner surface of the membrane by the charged species, BH⁺ (hydrophilic pathway), or directly from the membrane by the uncharged species, B (hydrophilic pathway).

functional states—resting, open and inactivated. Many local anaesthetics have been shown to bind most strongly to the inactivated state of the channel. Thus, at any given membrane potential the equilibrium between resting and inactivated channels will, in the presence of a local anaesthetic, be shifted in favour of the inactivated state, and this factor contributes to the overall blocking effect. The passage of a train of action potentials causes the channels to cycle through the open and inactivated states, both of which are more likely to bind local anaesthetic molecules than the resting state; thus, both mechanisms contribute to 'use-dependence'.

In general, local anaesthetics block conduction in small-diameter nerve fibres more readily than in large fibres. However, the smallest fibres in peripheral nerve are unmyelinated C-fibres, and these are rather less susceptible than the smallest myelinated (Aδ) fibres. Since nociceptive impulses are carried by Aδ- and C-fibres, pain sensation is blocked more readily than other sensory modalities (touch, proprioception, etc.). Motor axons, being large in diameter, are also relatively resistant. The differences in sensitivity among different nerve fibres, though easily measured experimentally, are not of much practical importance, and it is rarely possible to produce a block of pain sensation without affecting other modalities and causing local paralysis.

Local anaesthetics, as their name implies, are mainly used to produce local nerve block. In concentrations too low to cause nerve block, however, they are able to suppress the spontaneous discharge in sensory neurons that is believed to be responsible for *neuropathic pain* (see Ch. 37). Drugs undergoing trial for oral use as analgesics in such pain states include two antidysrhythmic drugs, **tocainide** and **mexiletine** (see Ch. 14).

Unwanted effects

The main unwanted effects of local anaesthetics involve the central nervous and cardiovascular systems, and they constitute the main source of hazard when local anaesthetics are used clinically. The main effect of local anaesthetics on the central nervous system is, paradoxically, to cause stimulation. This produces restlessness and tremor, with subjective effects ranging from confusion to extreme agitation. The tremor can progress to actual convulsions, and further increasing the dose produces CNS depression. The main threat to life comes from respiratory depression in this phase. The only local anaesthetic with markedly different CNS effects is **cocaine** (see Ch. 38), which produces euphoria at doses well below those that cause convulsions. This relates to its specific effect on monoamine uptake; an effect not shared by other local anaesthetics. **Procaine** is particularly liable to produce unwanted central effects, which is one reason for its replacement in clinical use by agents

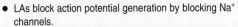

Action of local anaesthetics (LAs)

- LAs block action potential generation by blocking Na^+ channels.
- LAs are amphiphilic molecules, with a hydrophobic aromatic group, and a basic amine group.
- LAs probably act in their cationic form, but must reach their site of action by penetrating the nerve sheath and axonal membrane as unionised species; they therefore have to be weak bases.
- Many LAs show use-dependence (depth of block increases with action potential frequency). This arises:
  — because anaesthetic molecules gain access to the channel more readily when the channel is open
  — because anaesthetic molecules have higher affinity for inactivated than for resting channels.
- Use-dependence is mainly of importance in relation to antidysrhythmic and antiepileptic effects of Na^+ channel blockers.
- LAs block conduction in the following order: small myelinated axons, non-myelinated axons, large myelinated axons. Nociceptive and sympathetic transmission is thus blocked first.
- Drugs selective for specific Na^+ channel subtypes may prove useful in other indications, such as neuro-degenerative disorders, stroke, neuropathic pain, etc.

such as **lignocaine** and **prilocaine**, whose central effects are much less pronounced.

The cardiovascular effects of local anaesthetics are due mainly to myocardial depression and vasodilatation. Reduction of myocardial contractility probably results indirectly from an inhibition of the Na^+ current in cardiac muscle (see Ch. 14). The resulting decrease of $[Na^+]_i$, in turn reduces intracellular Ca^{2+} stores (see Ch. 14), and this reduces the force of contraction. The antidysrhythmic effect of some local anaesthetics (especially **lignocaine**) is clinically useful.

Vasodilatation, mainly affecting arterioles, is due partly to a direct effect on vascular smooth muscle, and partly to inhibition of the sympathetic nervous system. The combined myocardial depression and vasodilatation leads to a fall in blood pressure, which may be sudden and life-threatening. **Cocaine** is an exception in respect of its cardiovascular effects, because of its ability to inhibit noradrenaline reuptake (see Ch. 8). This produces an enhancement of sympathetic activity, leading to tachycardia, increased cardiac output, vasoconstriction and increased arterial pressure.

Though local anaesthetics are usually administered in such a way as to minimise their spread to other parts of the body, they are ultimately absorbed into the

systemic circulation. They may also be injected into veins or arteries by accident. The most dangerous unwanted effects result from actions on the central nervous and cardiovascular systems discussed above, namely restlessness and convulsions followed by respiratory depression, and hypotension, or even cardiac arrest. Hypersensitivity reactions sometimes occur with local anaesthetics, usually in the form of allergic dermatitis, but rarely as an acute anaphylactic reaction. Other unwanted effects that are specific to particular drugs include mucosal irritation (**cocaine**) and methaemoglobinaemia (which occurs after large doses of **prilocaine**, because of the production of a toxic metabolite).

Pharmacokinetic aspects

Local anaesthetics vary a good deal in the rapidity with which they penetrate tissues, and this affects the rate at which they cause nerve block when injected into tissues and the rate of onset of, and recovery from, anaesthesia (Table 40.1). It also affects their usefulness as surface anaesthetics for application to mucous membranes.

Most of the ester-linked local anaesthetics (e.g. **amethocaine**) are rapidly hydrolysed by plasma cholinesterase, so their plasma half-life is short. Procaine—now rarely used—is hydrolysed to *p*-aminobenzoic acid, a folate precursor which interferes with the antibacterial effect of sulphonamides (see Ch. 43). The amide-linked drugs (e.g. **lignocaine** and **prilocaine**) are metabolised mainly in the liver, usually by N-dealkylation rather than cleavage of the amide bond, and the metabolites are often pharmacologically active.

Benzocaine is an unusual local anaesthetic of very low solubility, which is used as a dry powder to dress painful skin ulcers. The drug is slowly released and produces long-lasting surface anaesthesia.

The *routes of administration*, *uses* and *main adverse effects* of local anaesthetics are summarised in Table 40.2.

Future directions

Currently available local anaesthetic agents do not distinguish between the many Na^+-channel subtypes that are known to be expressed in different tissues (see above). It is expected that, with the molecular characterisation of these channels, and a better understanding of their role in pathophysiological situations, selective blocking agents can be developed for use in a wide variety of clinical situations, including epilepsy, neurodegenerative diseases, stroke, neuropathic pain, myopathies, etc., which are discussed elsewhere in this book. There is much activity in this area, so stay tuned.

Table 40.1 Properties of local anaesthetics

Drug	Onset	Duration	Tissue penetration	Plasma half-life	Main unwanted effects	Notes
Cocaine	Medium	Medium	Good	~1 h	Cardiovascular and CNS effects due to block of amine uptake	Rarely used, only as spray for upper respiratory tract
Procaine	Medium	Short	Poor	<1 h	CNS: restlessness, shivering, anxiety, occasionally convulsions followed by respiratory depression CVS: bradycardia and decreased cardiac output, vasodilatation, which can cause cardiovascular collapse	No longer used
Lignocaine (lidocaine)	Rapid	Medium	Good	~2 h	As procaine, but less tendency to cause CNS effects	Widely used for local anaesthesia. Also used i.v. for treating ventricular arrhythmias (Ch. 14). **Mepivacaine** is similar
Amethocaine (tetracaine)	Very slow	Long	Moderate	~1 h	As lignocaine	Used mainly for spinal and corneal anaesthesia
Bupivacaine	Slow	Long	Moderate	~2 h	As lignocaine, but greater cardiotoxicity	Widely used because of long duration of action. **Ropivacaine** is similar, with less cardiotoxicity
Prilocaine	Medium	Medium	Moderate	~2 h	No vasodilator activity Can cause methaemoglobinaemia	Widely used, not for obstetric analgesia because of risk of neonatal methaemoglobinaemia

---

Unwanted effects and pharmacokinetics of LAs

- LAs are either esters or amides. Esters are rapidly hydrolysed by plasma cholinesterase, and amides are metabolised in the liver. Plasma half-lives are generally short, about 1–2 hours.
- Unwanted effects are due mainly to escape of LAs into systemic circulation.
- Main unwanted effects are:
  - CNS effects, agitation, confusion, tremors progressing to convulsions and respiratory depression
  - cardiovascular effects, namely myocardial depression and vasodilatation, leading to fall in blood pressure
  - occasional hypersensitivity reactions.
- LAs vary in the rapidity with which they penetrate tissues, and in their duration of action. Lignocaine penetrates tissues readily, and is suitable for surface application; bupivacaine has a particularly long duration of action.

TETRODOTOXIN AND SAXITOXIN

We should not be surprised that nature, rather than medicinal chemistry, has provided the most potent and selective agents that block Na^+ channels of excitable tissues. **Tetrodotoxin** (TTX) is produced by a marine bacterium, and accumulates in the tissues of a poisonous Pacific fish, the puffer fish, so called because when alarmed it inflates itself to an almost spherical spiny ball. It is evidently a species highly preoccupied with defence, but the Japanese are not easily put off and the puffer fish is regarded by them as a special delicacy. To serve it in public restaurants, however, the chef must be registered as sufficiently skilled in removing the toxic organs (especially liver and ovaries) so as to make the flesh safe to eat. Accidental tetrodotoxin poisoning is quite common, nonetheless. Historical records of long sea-voyages often contained reference to attacks of severe weakness, progressing to complete paralysis and death, caused by eating puffer fish.

Saxitoxin (STX) is produced by a marine microorganism, which sometimes proliferates in very large numbers and even colours the sea, giving the 'red tide' phenomenon. At such times, marine shellfish can accumulate the toxin and become poisonous to humans.

These toxins, unlike conventional local anaesthetics,

Table 40.2   Methods of administration, uses and adverse effects of local anaesthetics (LAs)

Method	Uses	Drugs	Notes and adverse effects
Surface anaesthesia	Nose, mouth, bronchial tree (usually in spray form), cornea, urinary tract Not effective for skin*	Lignocaine, tetracaine, dibucaine, benzocaine	Risk of systemic toxicity when high concentrations and large areas are involved
Infiltration anaesthesia	Direct injection into tissues to reach nerve branches and terminals Used in minor surgery	Most	**Adrenaline** or **felypressin** often added as vasoconstrictors (not with fingers or toes, for fear of causing ischaemic tissue damage) Only suitable for small areas; otherwise, serious risk of systemic toxicity
Intravenous regional anaesthesia	LA injected intravenously distal to a pressure cuff to arrest blood flow; remains effective until the circulation is restored Used for limb surgery	Mainly lidocaine, prilocaine	Risk of systemic toxicity when cuff is released prematurely. Risk is small if cuff remains inflated for at least 20 minutes
Nerve-block anaesthesia	LA is injected close to nerve trunks (e.g. brachial plexus, intercostal or dental nerves), to produce a loss of sensation peripherally Used for surgery, dentistry, analgesia	Most	Less LA needed than for infiltration anaesthesia. Accurate placement of the needle is important Onset of anaesthesia may be slow Duration of anaesthesia may be increased by addition of vasoconstrictor
Spinal anaesthesia	LA injected into the subarachnoid space (containing CSF), to act on spinal roots and spinal cord Glucose sometimes added so that spread of LA can be limited by tilting patient Used for surgery to abdomen, pelvis or leg, mainly when general anaesthesia cannot be used	Mainly lignocaine, tetracaine	Main risks are bradycardia and hypotension (due to sympathetic block), respiratory depression (due to effects on phrenic nerve or respiratory centre). Avoided by minimising cranial spread Postoperative urinary retention (block of pelvic autonomic outflow) is common
Epidural anaesthesia[†]	LA injected into epidural space, blocking spinal roots Uses as for spinal anaesthesia; also for painless childbirth	Mainly lignocaine, bupivacaine	Unwanted effects similar to those of spinal anaesthesia, but less probable, because longitudinal spread of LA is reduced Postoperative urinary retention common

*Surface anaesthesia does not work well on the skin, though recently a non-crystalline mixture of lignocaine and prilocaine (**eutectic mixture of local anaesthetics** or **EMLA**) has been developed for application to the skin, producing complete anaesthesia in about 1 hour.

[†]Intrathecal or epidural administration of LA in combination with an opiate (see Ch. 37) produces more effective analgesia than can be achieved with the opiate alone. Only a small concentration of LA is needed, insufficient to produce appreciable loss of sensation or other side-effects. The mechanism of this synergism is unknown, but the procedure is proving useful in pain treatment.

act exclusively from the outside of the membrane. Both are complex molecules, bearing a positively charged *guanidinium* moiety. The guanidinium ion is able to permeate voltage-sensitive Na^+ channels, and this part of the TTX or STX molecule lodges in the channel, while the rest of the molecule blocks its outer mouth. In contrast to the local anaesthetics, there is no interaction between the gating and blocking reactions with TTX or STX—their association and dissociation are independent of whether the channel is open or closed. Some voltage-sensitive Na^+ channels are insensitive to TTX, notably those of cardiac muscle and nociceptive peripheral sensory neurons, the latter being of interest as a possible target for novel analgesic agents (see Ch. 37).

TTX and STX are unsuitable for clinical use as local anaesthetics, being expensive to obtain from their exotic sources and poor at penetrating tissues because of their very low lipid solubility. They have, however, been important as experimental tools for the isolation and cloning of Na^+ channels (see Catterall 1993).

AGENTS THAT AFFECT SODIUM CHANNEL GATING

Various substances, mostly complex and ornate molecules, are known which modify Na^+ channel gating in such a way as to increase the probability of opening of the channels (see Hille 1992). They include various toxins, mainly from frog skin (e.g. **batrachotoxin**), scorpion or sea anemone venoms; plant alkaloids such as **veratridine**; and insecticides such as **DDT** and the **pyrethrins**. They facilitate Na^+ channel activation, so that Na^+ channels open at the normal resting potential; they also inhibit inactivation, so that the channels fail to close if the membrane remains depolarised. The membrane thus becomes hyperexcitable, and the action potential is prolonged. Spontaneous discharges occur at first, but the cells eventually become permanently depolarised and inexcitable. All of these substances affect the heart, producing extrasystoles and other dysrhythmias, culminating in fibrillation; they also cause spontaneous discharges in nerve and muscle, leading to twitching and convulsions. The very high lipid solubility of substances like DDT makes them effective as insecticides, for they are readily absorbed through the integument. Drugs in this class are useful as experimental tools for studying Na^+ channels, but have no clinical uses.

AGENTS THAT AFFECT POTASSIUM CHANNELS

Many aspects of K^+ channel pharmacology are discussed elsewhere in this book (e.g. Chs 2, 15, 22). The main types of K^+ channel are:

- *Voltage-activated K^+ channels.* Several variants exist, with different kinetic properties. They play an important part in controlling the duration of the action potential, and the repetitive firing patterns of neurons and cardiac muscle fibres. Various venoms and toxins from scorpions, snakes, sea anemones and the like interact specifically with different members of this family.

Tetraethylammonium (TEA) and **4-aminopyridine** (4-AP) block most voltage-gated K^+ channels. Their effects have been helpful in clarifying the role of K^+ channels in nerve conduction, but the compounds are not of clinical use. 4-AP was tested in multiple sclerosis, a demyelinating disease of the central nervous system in which conduction fails because of the loss of myelin. Blocking K^+ channels can enable action potentials to propagate successfully through the demyelinated segments of affected axons. However, the severe side-effects of 4-AP (nausea and convulsions), preclude its use, and more selective drugs are being sought.

- *Ca^{2+}-activated K^+ channels.* These open in response to an increase of intracellular $[Ca^{2+}]$. They probably have a protective function, suppressing membrane excitability when $[Ca^{2+}]_i$ rises. Though various blocking agents are known, including **apamin** (a constituent of bee venom) they are not of clinical importance so far.
- *Receptor-controlled K^+ channels* (see Ch. 2). Examples include the cardiac K^+ channel controlled by muscarinic ACh receptors, and neuronal channels sensitive to opiates and various neurotransmitters (see Ch. 30).
- *ATP-sensitive K^+ channels.* These close when intracellular ATP increases. They occur in many situations, including pancreatic islets (see Ch. 22), where they are involved in the control of insulin secretion, and in vascular smooth muscle cells. They are inhibited by hypoglycaemic drugs of the **sulphonylurea** type, and opened by vasodilators such as **cromokalim**, **pinacidil** and **diazoxide** (Ch. 15).

In general, though K^+ channels clearly play an important role in controlling membrane excitability and the firing pattern of neurons, the details of which channels do what are still very unclear, and the casual observer may wonder weakly why so many are necessary. At present, the pharmacological manipulation of neuronal K^+ channels is of little clinical importance.

REFERENCES AND FURTHER READING

Ackerman M J, Clapham D E 1997 Ion channels—basic science and clinical disease. N Engl J Med 336: 1575–1586 (*Interesting review covering aspects of channel structure and function, and discussing inherited diseases associated with channel malfunction*)

Catterall W A 1993 Structure and function of voltage-gated ion channels. Trends Neurosci 16: 500–506 (*Short review of molecular biology of channels*)

Hille B 1992 Ionic channels of excitable membranes. Sinauer, Sunderland, MA (*Excellent clearly written textbook for those wanting more than the basic minimum*)

Katz B 1966 Nerve, muscle and synapse. McGraw-Hill, New York (*A classic by one of the major pioneers of membrane and synaptic physiology*)

Mathie A, Woolterton J R, Watkins C S 1998 Voltage-activated potassium channels in mammalian neurons and their block by novel pharmacological agents. Gen Pharmacol 30: 13–24 (*Useful review of the complex pharmacology of potassium channels*)

Nicholls J G, Martin A R, Wallace B G 1992 From neuron to brain. Sinauer, Sunderland, MA (*Excellent textbook, which successfully integrates information from the molecular to the functional level*)

Pongs O 1992 Structural basis of voltage-gated K^+-channel pharmacology. Trends Pharmacol Sci 13: 359–365 (*Useful short review of an increasingly complex field*)

Ragsdale D R, McPhee J C, Scheuer T, Catterall W A 1994 Molecular determinants of state-dependent block of Na^+ channels by local anesthetics. Science 265: 1724–1728 (*Use of site-directed mutations of the Na^+ channel to show that local anaesthetics bind to residues in the S6 transmembrane domain*)

Strichartz G R, Ritchie J M 1987 The action of local anaesthetics on ion channels of excitable tissues. In: Strichartz G R (ed) Local anaesthetics. Handbook of experimental pharmacology. Springer-Verlag, Berlin, vol 81. pp 21–52 (*Excellent review of actions of local anaesthetics—other articles in the same volume cover more clinical aspects*)

TIPS Receptor & Ion Channel Nomenclature Supplement 1996 Trends Pharmacol Sci (*Useful tables summarising the pharmacological properties of Na^+, K^+ and Ca^{2+} channel subtypes*)

Tsien R W, Lipscombe D, Madison D, Bley K, Fox A 1995 Reflections on Ca^{2+}-channel diversity, 1988–1994. Trends Neurosci 18: 52–54 (*Short review on calcium channel subtypes*)

CHEMOTHERAPY OF INFECTIOUS AND MALIGNANT DISEASE

Basic principles of chemotherapy

The development of chemotherapy during the past 60 years constitutes one of the most important therapeutic advances in the history of medicine.

The term '**chemotherapy**' was coined by Ehrlich at the beginning of the century to describe the use of synthetic chemicals to destroy infective agents. In recent years the definition of the term has been broadened to include '**antibiotics**'—substances produced by some microorganisms that kill or inhibit the growth of other microorganisms. The term chemotherapy is now also applied to the use of chemicals (either natural or synthetic) used to inhibit the growth of malignant or cancerous cells within the body. Ehrlich had assumed that the development of completely selective agents was an unattainable goal and that the most that could be hoped for was the production of substances that were maximally 'parasitotropic' and minimally 'organotropic'. This view has turned out to be rather more pessimistic than was warranted because some totally selective antibacterial agents have been produced.

THE MOLECULAR BASIS OF CHEMOTHERAPY

Chemotherapeutic agents are chemicals which are intended to be toxic for the infectious organism but innocuous for the host. The feasibility of such selective toxicity depends on the existence of exploitable biochemical differences between the organism and the host.

Living organisms are classified as either prokaryotes—consisting of cells *without* nuclei (the *bacteria*), or eukaryotes—consisting of cells *with* nuclei (e.g. protozoa, fungi, helminths). In a separate category are the *viruses*, which are not, properly speaking, cells at all because they do not have their own biochemical machinery for generating energy or for any sort of synthesis. Viruses need to utilise the metabolic machinery of the host cell and they thus present a particular kind of problem for chemotherapeutic attack.

Before discussing the molecular basis of chemotherapy, we need to define some terms. The word 'microbe' is generally used to describe bacteria, viruses and fungi and the word 'parasite' to describe protozoa and helminths. These categories overlap; for example, *Pneumocystis carinii* is classified by some authorities under protozoa and by others under fungi. In this book we are only concerned with these organisms if they cause disease. The immune response of the human host makes no distinction between the above categories when they cause disease, and the dictionary definition of 'parasite' covers all of them. Accordingly, to simplify discussion, we shall be using the term 'parasite' for any organism that can cause disease.* That leaves the mysterious prions (see Ch. 31) which cause disease but are at present unclassifiable—the despair of taxonomists.

In yet another category are *cancer* cells—host cells that have become malignant, i.e. they have escaped from the regulating devices which control normal cells. Cancer cells can be considered to be, in a special sense, 'foreign' or 'parasitic', but are clearly more similar to normal host cells than are any of the categories considered above, and are an especially difficult problem for selective toxicity.

---

*It is a problem to distinguish between 'commensals'—organisms that are parasitic without causing disease—and disease-causing organisms, since it is now clear that many so-called commensals can cause disease if the immune system of the host is compromised.

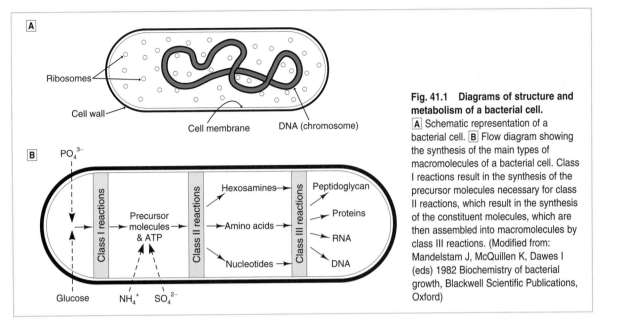

Fig. 41.1 Diagrams of structure and metabolism of a bacterial cell. [A] Schematic representation of a bacterial cell. [B] Flow diagram showing the synthesis of the main types of macromolecules of a bacterial cell. Class I reactions result in the synthesis of the precursor molecules necessary for class II reactions, which result in the synthesis of the constituent molecules, which are then assembled into macromolecules by class III reactions. (Modified from: Mandelstam J, McQuillen K, Dawes I (eds) 1982 Biochemistry of bacterial growth, Blackwell Scientific Publications, Oxford)

All living creatures, host and parasite alike, have the same basic blueprint: DNA; and some biochemical processes are common to many, even all, organisms. Finding agents that affect parasite but not human host necessitates finding either qualitative or quantitative biochemical differences between them. In this introductory chapter to the subject of chemotherapy, we consider, very broadly, the molecular aspects of drug action against 'parasites', giving examples of biochemical differences that have been exploited to develop drugs to treat infectious disease and cancer.

Bacteria cause more infectious disease than any other parasites, so let us start with a bacterial cell and ask what such a cell has to do in order to grow and divide. Figure 41.1 shows in simplified diagrammatic form the main structures and functions of a 'generalised' bacterial cell. Surrounding the cell is the *cell wall*, which characteristically contains *peptidoglycan* in all forms of bacteria except mycoplasma. Peptidoglycan is *unique* to prokaryotic cells and has no counterpart in eukaryotes. Within the cell wall is the *plasma membrane*, which is similar to that of the eukaryotic cell, consisting of a phospholipid bilayer and proteins. However, in bacteria the plasma membrane does not contain any sterols and this may result in differential penetration of chemicals. It functions as a selectively permeable membrane with specific transport mechanisms for various types of nutrients. The function of the cell wall is to support this underlying plasma membrane, which is subject to

an internal osmotic pressure of about 5 atmospheres in Gram-negative organisms, and about 20 atmospheres in Gram-positive organisms.* The plasma membrane and cell wall together comprise the envelope.

Within the plasma membrane is the *cytoplasm*. As in eukaryotic cells, this contains all the soluble proteins (most having enzymic functions), the ribosomes involved in protein synthesis, all the small molecule intermediates involved in metabolism and all the inorganic ions. However, the bacterial cell, unlike the eukaryotic cell, has no nucleus; instead, the genetic material, in the form of a single chromosome that holds all the genetic information of the cell, lies loose in the cytoplasm. In further contrast to eukaryotic cells, the chromosome of the bacterial cell contains no histones, and there are no mitochondria—all the energy generation goes on in the plasma membrane.

These, then, are the essential structures of the generalised bacterial cell. Some bacteria have additional components such as a capsule and/or one or more flagella, but the only additional structure with relevance for chemotherapy is the *outer membrane*, outside the cell wall, which is found in Gram-negative bacteria and which may prevent penetration of antibacterial agents (see Ch. 43, p. 688). It also prevents easy access of

---

*The terms Gram-positive and Gram-negative refer to whether or not the cell stains with a particular combination of dyes. More detail of the differences between Gram-positive and Gram-negative organisms is given in Chapter 43 (p. 685).

lysozyme (an enzyme that can break down cell wall structures and is found in white blood cells and tissue fluids such as tears) to the peptidoglycan of the cell wall.

Having outlined the essential structures of the bacterial cell, we need now to consider the biochemical reactions involved in their formation (Fig. 41.1). There are three general classes of reactions:

- *Class I*. The utilisation of glucose or some alternative carbon source for the generation of energy (ATP) and of simple carbon compounds (such as the intermediates of the citric acid cycle) which are used as precursors in the next class of reactions.
- *Class II*. The utilisation of the energy and precursors to make all the necessary small molecules: amino acids, nucleotides, phospholipids, amino sugars, carbohydrates and growth factors.
- *Class III*. Assembly of the small molecules into macromolecules: proteins, RNA, DNA, polysaccharides and peptidoglycan.

These reactions are potential targets for attack by chemotherapeutic agents. Other potential targets are the formed structures, for example the cell membrane, or, in higher organisms, the microtubules (targets in fungi and cancer cells). Specific types of cells may be targets in some higher organisms (e.g. muscle tissue in helminths).

In considering these targets, emphasis will be placed on bacteria, but reference will also be made to protozoa, helminths, fungi, cancer cells and, where possible, viruses. The classification that follows is clearly not a rigid one; a drug may affect reactions in more than one class or more than one subgroup of reactions within a class.

The molecular basis of chemotherapy

- To be effective, chemotherapeutic drugs should be toxic for invading organisms and innocuous for the host; such selective toxicity depends on there being exploitable biochemical differences between the parasite (e.g. a bacterium) and the host.
- The three general classes of biochemical reactions are potential targets for chemotherapy. The characteristics of each class are as follows:
  — *Class I*, glucose and other carbon sources are used to produce simple carbon compounds.
  — *Class II*, energy and class I compounds are used to make small molecules, e.g. amino acids, nucleotides, etc.
  — *Class III*, small molecules are built into larger molecules, e.g. proteins, nucleic acids, peptidoglycan (in bacteria), etc.

BIOCHEMICAL REACTIONS AS POTENTIAL TARGETS

Class I reactions

Class I reactions are not promising targets, for two reasons. First, there is no very marked difference between bacteria and human cells in the mechanism for obtaining energy from glucose, since both use the Embden–Meyerhof pathway and the citric acid cycle. Second, even if the glucose pathways were to be blocked, a large variety of other compounds (amino acids, lactate, etc.) could be used by bacteria as alternatives.

Class II reactions

Class II reactions are better targets since some pathways involved in class II reactions exist in parasitic but not in human cells. For instance, human cells have in the course of evolution lost the ability, possessed by bacteria, to synthesise some amino acids—the so-called 'essential' amino acids—and also the growth factors or vitamins. Any such difference represents a potential target. Another type of target occurs when a pathway is identical in both bacteria and humans but has differential sensitivity to drugs.

Folate

The *synthesis* of folate is an example of a metabolic pathway found in bacteria but not in man. Folate is required for DNA synthesis in both bacteria and in humans (see Chs 18 and 42). Humans obtain it from the diet and have evolved a transport mechanism for taking it up into the cells. Humans do not need to synthesise it, and indeed cannot do so. By contrast, most species of bacteria, as well as the asexual forms of malarial protozoa, have not evolved the necessary transport mechanisms and they cannot make use of preformed folate. They must, of necessity, synthesise their own folate. This is a prime example of a difference that has proved to be useful for chemotherapy. **Sulphonamides** contain the sulphanilamide moiety—a structural analogue of *p*-aminobenzoic acid (PABA), which is essential in the synthesis of folate (see Figs 18.2 and 43.1). Sulphonamides compete with PABA for the enzyme involved in folate synthesis and thus inhibit the metabolism of the bacteria. They are consequently *bacteriostatic* not *bactericidal* and are therefore only really effective in the presence of adequate host defences (which are discussed in Ch. 12).

The *utilisation* of folate, in the form of tetrahydrofolate (FH$_4$), as a cofactor in thymidylate synthesis (see Figs 18.4 and 42.11) is an example of a pathway in which there is differential sensitivity of human and bacterial enzymes to chemicals (Table 41.1). This pathway is virtually identical in microorganisms and humans, but one of the

Table 41.1 Specificity of inhibitors of dihydrofolate reductase

Inhibitor	C_{50} (µmol/l) for FH_2 reductase		
	Human	Protozoal	Bacterial
Trimethoprim	260	0.07	0.005
Pyrimethamine	0.7	0.0005	2.5
Methotrexate	0.001	Approx. 0.1*	Inactive

*Tested on *P. berghei*, a rodent malaria

key enzymes, dihydrofolate reductase, which reduces dihydrofolate to tetrahydrofolate (Fig. 18.3), is many times more sensitive to the folate antagonist **trimethoprim** in bacteria than in man. In some malarial protozoa this enzyme is somewhat less sensitive to trimethoprim than is the bacterial enzyme. The relative IC_{50} values (the concentration causing 50% inhibition) for bacterial, malarial, protozoal and mammalian enzymes are given in Table 41.1, as are those for **pyrimethamine**, primarily an antimalarial agent (Ch. 46). Another antimalarial drug which inhibits the protozoal enzyme specifically is **proguanil**. The human enzyme on the other hand is very sensitive to the effect of the folate analogue **methotrexate** (Table 41.1), and this compound is used in the chemotherapy of certain cancers (see Ch. 42). Methotrexate is inactive in bacteria because, being very similar in structure to folate, it requires active uptake by cells. Trimethoprim and pyrimethamine enter the cells by diffusion.

The use of sequential blockade with a combination of two drugs which, in the parasite, affect the same pathway at different points, for example **sulphonamides** and the **folate antagonists** (Fig. 43.1, p. 688), may be more successful than the use of either alone (e.g. in the treatment of *Pneumocystis* pneumonia. Furthermore, lower concentrations of each drug are effective when the two are used together. Thus, **pyrimethamine** and a **sulphonamide** (sulphadoxine) are used to treat falciparum malaria (p. 732). An antibacterial formulation that contains both a sulphonamide and trimethoprim is **co-trimoxazole** (p. 689); though this is less effective than when originally introduced because of the development of resistance to the sulphonamide.

Pyrimidine and purine analogues

The pyrimidine analogue, **fluorouracil**, which is used in cancer chemotherapy (Ch. 42) is converted to a fraudulent nucleotide that interferes with thymidylate synthesis. Other cancer chemotherapy agents that give

rise to fraudulent nucleotides are the purine analogues **mercaptopurine** and **thioguanine**. **Flucytosine**, an antifungal drug (Ch. 45), is deaminated to fluorouracil within the cell; selectivity for fungal cells is due to the fact that this deamination occurs to a much lesser extent in humans.

Class III reactions

Class III reactions are particularly good targets for selective toxicity because every cell *has* to make its own macromolecules—these cannot just be picked up from the environment and there are very distinct differences between mammalian cells and parasitic cells in the pathways involved in class III reactions.

The synthesis of peptidoglycan

Peptidoglycan constitutes the cell wall of bacteria and does not occur in eukaryotes. It is the equivalent of a non-stretchable string bag enclosing the whole bacterium. For some bacteria (the Gram-negative organisms), the bag consists of a single thickness, but for others (Gram-positive organisms), it is up to 40 layers thick. Each layer consists of multiple backbones of amino sugars—alternating N-acetyl-glucosamine and N-acetylmuramic acid residues (Fig. 41.2)—the latter having short peptide side-chains which are cross-linked to form a latticework. The cross-links differ in different species. In staphylococci they consist of five glycine residues (Fig. 41.2). This cross-linking is responsible for the strength that allows the cell wall to resist the high internal osmotic pressure. The peptidoglycan is in fact one gigantic molecule with a molecular weight of many millions, constituting up to 10–15% of the dry weight of the cell.

In synthesising the peptidoglycan layer, the cell has the problem of using cytoplasmic components to build up this very large insoluble structure on the outside of the cell membrane. To do this it is necessary to transport the components, which are synthesised within the cell, and which are individually hydrophilic, piecemeal through the hydrophobic cell membrane. This is accomplished by linking them to a very large lipid carrier, containing 55 carbon atoms, which 'tows' them across the membrane. The process of peptidoglycan synthesis is outlined in Figure 41.3. First, N-acetylmuramic acid, which has attached to it both UDP and a pentapeptide, is transferred to the C_{55} lipid carrier in the membrane, with the release of UMP. This is followed by a reaction with UDP-N-acetylglucosamine, resulting in the formation of a disaccharide carrying the pentapeptide and attached to the carrier. This disaccharide with peptide attached is the basic building block of the peptidoglycan. In *Staphylo-*

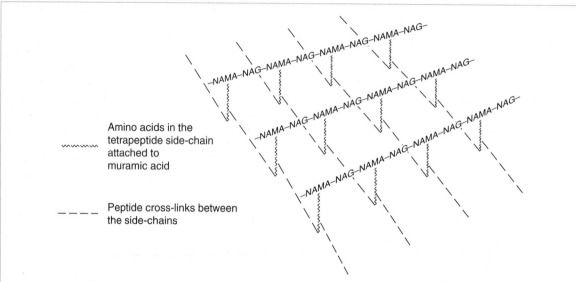

Fig. 41.2   Schematic diagram of a single layer of peptidoglycan from a bacterial cell (e.g. *Staph. aureus*). (NAMA = N-acetylmuramic acid; NAG = N-acetylglucosamine.) In *Staph. aureus* the peptide cross-links consist of five glycine residues. Gram-positive bacteria have several layers of peptidoglycan.

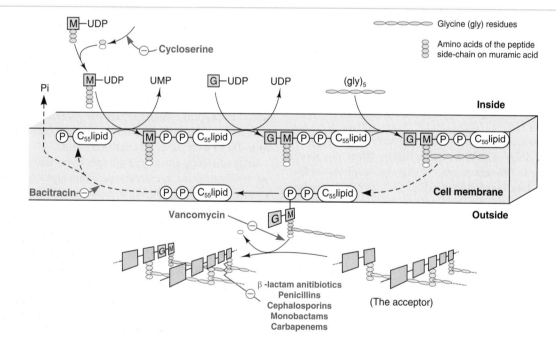

Fig. 41.3   Schematic diagram of the biosynthesis of peptidoglycan in a bacterial cell (e.g. *Staph. aureus*) with the sites of action of various antibiotics. The hydrophilic disaccharide–pentapeptide is transferred across the lipid cell membrane attached to a large lipid (C_{55} lipid) by a pyrophosphate bridge (–P–P–). On the outside, it is enzymically attached to the 'acceptor' (the growing peptidoglycan layer). The final reaction is a transpeptidation, in which the loose end of the $(gly)_5$ chain is attached to a peptide side-chain of an M in the acceptor and during which the terminal amino acid (alanine) is lost. The lipid is regenerated by loss of a phosphate group (Pi) before functioning again as a carrier. (M = N-acetylmuramic acid; G = N-acetylglucosamine)

coccus aureus, the five glycine residues are attached to the peptide chain at this stage, as is shown in Figure 41.3. The 'building block' is now transported to the outside of the cell and added to the growing end of the peptido-glycan, the 'acceptor', with the release of the C_{55} lipid, which still has two phosphates attached. The lipid then loses one phosphate group and thus becomes available for another cycle. Cross-linking between the peptide side-chains of the sugar residues in the peptidoglycan layer then occurs, the hydrolytic removal of the terminal alanine supplying the requisite energy.

This synthesis of peptidoglycan can be blocked at several points by antibiotics (Fig. 41.3 and Ch. 43). **Cycloserine**, which is a structural analogue of D-alanine, prevents the addition of the two terminal alanines to the initial tripeptide side-chain on N-acetylmuramic acid, by competitive inhibition. **Vancomycin** inhibits the release of the building block unit from the carrier, thus preventing its addition to the growing end of the peptido-glycan. **Bacitracin** interferes with the regeneration of the lipid carrier by blocking its dephosphorylation. **Penicillins**, **cephalosporins** and other β-lactams inhibit the final transpeptidation that establishes the cross-links by forming covalent bonds with penicillin-binding proteins that have transpeptidase and carboxypetidase activities.

Protein synthesis

The ribosomes are cytoplasmic nucleoprotein structures that are the basic units of machinery for the synthesis of proteins on messenger RNA templates. They are different in eukaryotes and prokaryotes and this pro-vides the basis for the selective antimicrobial action of some antibiotics. The bacterial ribosome consists of a 50S subunit and a 30S subunit (Fig. 41.4) whereas in the mammalian ribosome, the subunits are 60S and 40S.

A simplified version of protein synthesis in bacteria is as follows:

* Messenger RNA (mRNA), which is transcribed from DNA (see below), becomes attached to the 30S subunit of the ribosome, which moves along the mRNA so that successive codons of the messenger pass along the ribosome from the A position (shown on the right in Fig. 41.4), to the P position. (A codon is a triplet consisting of three nucleotides that codes for a specific amino acid.)
* The 'P site' contains the growing peptide chain attached to a molecule of transfer RNA (tRNA). The next amino acid residue to be added—linked to its specific tRNA, with its distinctive anticodon—moves into the A site, being bound to the site by a codon : anti-codon recognition, which occurs by complementary base-pairing (Fig. 41.4A and B).
* A transpeptidation reaction occurs which links the peptide chain on the tRNA at the P site to the amino acid on the incoming tRNA at the A site (Fig. 41.4C).
* The tRNA from which the peptide chain has been removed is now ejected from the P site (Fig. 41.4D).
* The tRNA at the A site is translocated to the P site, and the ribosome moves on one codon, relative to the messenger (Fig. 41.4D).
* A new tRNA, with amino acid attached and with the relevant anticodon, now moves into the A site, and the whole process is repeated.

Antibiotics may affect protein synthesis at any one of these stages (Fig. 41.4 and Ch. 43).

Nucleic acid synthesis

The nucleic acids of the cell are DNA and RNA. There are three types of RNA: messenger RNA (mRNA), transfer RNA (tRNA) and ribosomal RNA (rRNA). (The ribosomal RNA is an integral part of the ribosome, being necessary for its assembly and having a role in the binding of mRNA.) All are involved in protein synthesis (see above).

DNA is the template for the synthesis of both DNA and RNA. It exists in the cell as a double helix. Each chain or strand is a linear polymer of nucleotides. Each nucleotide consists of a base linked to a sugar (deoxy-ribose) and a phosphate. The bases are adenine (A), cytosine (C), guanine (G) or thymine (T). The chain is made up of alternating sugar and phosphate groups with the bases attached rather like beads on a necklace. Specific hydrogen bonding between G and C and be-tween A and T on each strand (i.e. complementary base-pairing) is the basis of the double-strand structure of DNA (Fig. 41.5). The DNA helix is itself twisted, resulting in 'supercoiling' (Figs 41.6 and 43.5).

Initiation of DNA synthesis requires first the activity of an enzyme that produces local unwinding of the positive 'supercoil' and introduction of a negative supercoil. This enzyme is DNA gyrase (also called topoisomerase II).

During the synthesis of DNA, nucleotide units—each consisting of a base linked to a sugar and three phosphate groups—are added by base-pairing with the comple-mentary residues in the template. Condensation occurs with the elimination of two of the phosphate groups, catalysed by DNA polymerase (Fig. 41.7).

RNA, like DNA, is a polymer of purine and pyrimidine nucleotides, but it exists as a single, not a double strand. The sugar moiety here is ribose, and the ribonucleotides contain the bases adenine, guanine, cytosine and uracil (U).

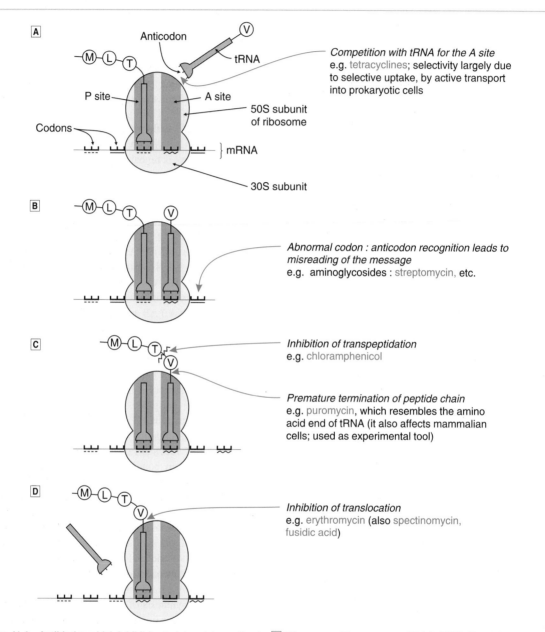

Fig. 41.4 Antibiotics which inhibit bacterial protein synthesis. [A] **Ribosome with messenger RNA (mRNA).** The different mRNA codons (triplets of three nucleotides which code for specific amino acids) are represented by dots, dashes and straight or wavy lines. A transfer RNA with peptide chain Met–Leu–Trp (MLT) attached is in the P site, bound by codon : anticodon recognition (i.e. by complementary base-pairing). The incoming transfer RNA (tRNA) carries valine (V), covalently linked. [B] The incoming tRNA binds to the A site by complementary base-pairing. [C] Transpeptidation occurs. The peptide chain attached to the tRNA in the new A site now consists of Met–Leu–Trp–Val (MLTV). The tRNA in the P site has been 'discharged', i.e. has lost its peptide. [D] The discharged tRNA is ejected from the P site. The tRNA with the peptide chain attached is translocated from the A to the P site leaving the A site free for the next tRNA. The ribosome moves to the next codon on the mRNA, shown as moving to the right along the codons.

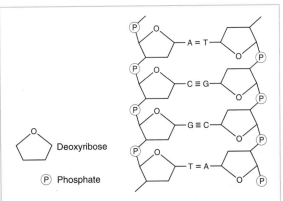

Fig. 41.5   Structure of DNA. Each strand of DNA consists of a sugar–phosphate backbone with purine or pyrimidine bases attached. The purines are adenine (A) or guanine (G) and the pyrimidines are cytosine (C) or thymine (T). The sugar is deoxyribose. Complementarity between the two strands of DNA is maintained by hydrogen bonds (either 2 or 3) between bases.

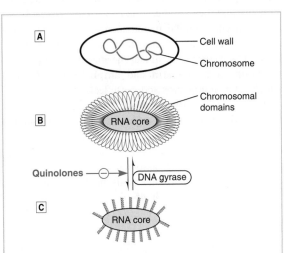

Fig. 41.6   Site of action for quinolone antibacterials.
Ⓐ Conventional diagram used to depict a bacterial cell and chromosome (e.g. *Escherichia coli*). Note that the *E. coli* chromosome is 1300 mm long and is contained in a cell envelope of 2 μ × 1 μ; this is approximately equivalent to a 50-metre length of cotton folded into a matchbox.
Ⓑ Chromosome folded around RNA core, and then
Ⓒ supercoiled by DNA gyrase (topoisomerase II). Quinolone antibacterials interfere with the action of this enzyme.
(Modified from: Smith J T 1985 In: Greenwood D, O'Grady F (eds) Scientific basis of antimicrobial therapy. Cambridge University Press, p. 69)

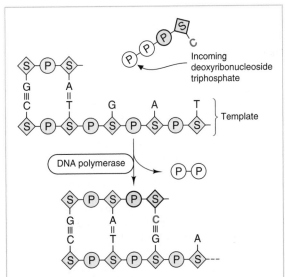

Fig. 41.7   DNA replication. Nucleotides are added, one at a time, by base-pairing to an exposed template strand and are then covalently joined together in a reaction catalysed by DNA polymerase. The units which pair with the complementary residues in the template consist of a base linked to a sugar and three phosphate groups. Condensation occurs with the elimination of two phosphates.
(P = phosphate; S = sugar; A = adenine; T = thymine; G = guanine; C = cytosine)

It is possible to interfere with nucleic acid synthesis in five different ways:

- *By inhibiting the synthesis of the nucleotides.* This can be accomplished by an effect on reactions earlier in the metabolic pathway. Examples of agents that have such an effect have been described under class II reactions.
- *By altering the base-pairing properties of the template.* Agents that intercalate in the DNA have this effect. Examples are the acridines (**proflavine, acriflavine**), which are used topically as antiseptics. The acridines double the distance between adjacent base-pairs and cause a *frame-shift* mutation (Fig. 41.8), whereas some purine and pyrimidine analogues cause mispairing. One example is the antiviral drug **vidarabine** (Ch. 44).
- *By inhibiting either DNA or RNA polymerase.* **Actinomycin D** binds to the guanine residues in DNA and blocks the movement of RNA polymerase, thus preventing transcription and consequently inhibiting protein synthesis. It is used in cancer chemotherapy in man (Ch. 42) and also as an experimental tool, but it is not useful as an antibacterial agent. Specific inhibitors of bacterial RNA polymerase that act by

mRNA (normal)	UCU Ser	UUU Phe	CUU Leu	AUU Ile	GUU Val	UCU... Ser
mRNA (mutant)	UCU Ser	UUG Leu	UCU Ser	UAU Tyr	UGU Cys	UUC... Phe

Fig. 41.8   An example of the effect on RNA and protein synthesis of a frame-shift mutation in the DNA. A frame-shift mutation is one that involves a *deletion* of a base or an *insertion* of an extra base. In the above example an extra cytosine has been inserted in the DNA template with the result that when messenger RNA is formed, it has an additional guanine (G), as indicated in the light blue box. The effect is to alter that codon and all the succeeding ones (shown in blue), so that a completely different protein is synthesised, as indicated by the different amino acids (Leu instead of Phe, Ser instead of Leu, etc.). (G = guanine; C = cytosine; A = adenine; U = uracil)

binding to this enzyme in prokaryotic but not in eukaryotic cells include **rifamycin** and **rifampicin**, which are active, in particular, against *Mycobacterium tuberculosis*, the tubercle bacillus (Ch. 43). **Aciclovir** (an analogue of guanine; see Fig. 44.5) is phosphorylated, in cells infected with herpes virus, the initial phosphorylation being by a virus-specific kinase, the aciclovir triphosphate, which has an inhibitory action on the DNA polymerase of the herpes virus (Ch. 44).

RNA retroviruses have a reverse transcriptase (viral RNA-dependent DNA polymerase) that makes a DNA copy of the viral RNA, the viral DNA copy being integrated into the host cell DNA as a 'provirus'. Various agents (**zidovudine**, **didanosine**) are phosphorylated by cellular enzymes to the triphosphate form which competes with the equivalent host cell triphosphates essential for the formation of proviral DNA by the viral reverse transcriptase.

Cytarabine (cytosine arabinoside) is used in cancer chemotherapy (Ch. 42). Its triphosphate derivative is a potent inhibitor of DNA polymerase in mammalian cells. **Foscarnet** inhibits viral RNA polymerase by attaching to the pyrophosphate binding site.

- *By inhibiting DNA gyrase* (also called topoisomerase II; see Fig. 41.6). This is the mechanism of action of the fluoroquinolones: **cinoxacin**, **ciprofloxacin**, **nalidixic acid** and **norfloxacin**—chemotherapeutic agents used particularly in infections with Gram-negative organisms (Ch. 43, p. 700). These drugs are selective for the bacterial enzyme because it is structurally different from the mammalian enzyme. Some anticancer agents, for example **doxorubicin** (p. 677), act on the mammalian topoisomerase II.

- *By direct effects on DNA itself. Alkylating agents* form covalent bonds with bases in the DNA and prevent replication. Compounds with this action are used only in cancer chemotherapy and include **nitrogen mustard derivatives** and **nitrosoureas** (Ch. 42). **Mitomycin** also binds covalently to DNA. No antibacterial agents work by these mechanisms.

THE FORMED STRUCTURES OF THE CELL AS POTENTIAL TARGETS

The membrane

The plasma membrane of bacterial cells is fairly similar to that in mammalian cells in that it consists of a *phospholipid* bilayer in which proteins are embedded. Nevertheless, this structure can be more easily disrupted in certain bacteria and some fungi than in mammalian cells.

Polymixins are cationic detergent antibiotics that have a selective effect on bacterial cell membranes. They are peptides that contain both hydrophilic and lipophilic groups separated within the molecule. They interact with the phospholipids of the cell membrane and disrupt its structure and they are therefore bactericidal (Ch. 43).

Fungal cells, unlike mammalian and bacterial cells, have large amounts of ergosterol in the plasma membrane. The ergosterol facilitates the attachment of polyene antibiotics (e.g. **nystatin** and **amphotericin**; Ch. 45) which act as ionophores and cause leakage of cations.

Azoles, such as **itraconazole**, have antifungal action by inhibiting synthesis of ergosterol, altering membrane fluidity and thus the function of membrane-associated enzymes. The azoles also affect Gram-positive bacteria, their selectivity being associated with the presence of high levels of free fatty acids in the membrane of susceptible organisms (Ch. 45).

DNA

Bleomycin, an anticancer antibiotic, causes fragmentation of the DNA strands following free radical formation (Ch. 42).

Intracellular organelles

Microtubules and/or microfilaments

The benzimidazoles (e.g. **albendazole**) have anthelminthic action by binding selectively to parasite tubulin and preventing microtubule formation (Ch. 47).

The vinca alkaloids, **vinblastine** and **vincristine**, are anticancer agents which disrupt the functioning of microtubules during cell division (Ch. 42).

Food vacuoles

The erythrocytic form of the malaria plasmodium feeds on host haemoglobin, which is digested by proteases in the parasite food vacuole, the final product, haem, being detoxified by polymerisation. **Chloroquine** has antimalarial action by inhibiting plasmodial haem polymerase (Ch. 46).

Muscle fibres

Some anthelminthic drugs have a selective action on muscle cells in helminths (Ch. 47).

Piperazine acts as an agonist on parasite-specific GABA-gated chloride channels in nematode muscle, hyperpolarising the muscle fibre membrane and paralysing

---

Potential targets for chemotherapy

Biochemical reactions
- *Class I reactions* are poor targets.
- *Class II reactions* are better targets:
  - Folate synthesis in bacteria is inhibited by sulphonamides. Folate utilisation is inhibited by folate antagonists, e.g. trimethoprim in bacteria, pyrimethamine in the malarial parasite, methotrexate (an anticancer drug) in humans.
  - Pyrimidine analogues, e.g. fluorouracil, and purine analogues, e.g. mercaptopurine, give rise to fraudulent nucleotides; they are used to treat cancer.
- *Class III reactions* are important targets:
  - Peptidoglycan synthesis in bacteria can be selectively inhibited by β-lactam antibiotics, e.g. penicillin.
  - Protein synthesis can be selectively inhibited in bacteria by antibiotics that prevent binding of tRNA (e.g. tetracyclines), cause misreading of mRNA (e.g. aminoglycosides), inhibit transpeptidation (e.g. chloramphenicol), inhibit translocation of tRNA from A site to P site (e.g. erythromycin).
  - Nucleic acid synthesis can be inhibited by: (a) altering base-pairing of DNA template (e.g. vidarabine: antiviral agent), (b) inhibiting DNA polymerase (e.g. aciclovir, foscarnet: antiviral agents), (c) inhibiting DNA gyrase (e.g. ciprofloxacin: antibacterial).

Formed structures of the cell
- The plasma membrane:
  - amphotericin acts as an ionophore in fungal cells
  - azoles inhibit fungal membrane ergosterol synthesis.
- Microtubule function is disrupted by:
  - vinca alkaloids (anticancer drugs)
  - benzimidazoles (anthelminthics).
- Muscle fibres:
  - avermectins (anthelminthics) increase chloride permeability
  - pyrantel (anthelminthic) stimulates nematode nicotinic receptors, eventually causing muscle paralysis.

---

the worm; **avermectins** increase chloride permeability in helminth muscle—possibly by a similar mechanism.

Pyrantel and **levamisole** act as agonists at nematode acetylcholine nicotinic receptors on muscle, causing contraction followed by paralysis (Ch. 47).

RESISTANCE TO ANTIBIOTICS

During the last 60 years the development of effective and safe drugs to deal with bacterial infections has revolutionised medical treatment, and the morbidity and mortality from microbial disease have been dramatically reduced. Unfortunately, along with the development of man's chemotherapeutic defences against bacteria has gone the development of bacterial defences against chemotherapeutic agents, resulting in the emergence of *resistance*. This is not unexpected, it being an evolutionary principle that organisms adapt genetically to changes in their environment. Since the doubling time of bacteria can be as short as 20 minutes, there may be many generations in even a few hours and thus plenty of opportunity for evolutionary adaptation. The phenomenon of resistance imposes serious constraints on the options available for the medical treatment of many bacterial infections. Resistance to chemotherapeutic agents can also develop in protozoa, in multicellular parasites and in populations of malignant cells. However, in this chapter, discussion will be confined mainly to the mechanisms of resistance in bacteria.*

Antibiotic resistance in bacteria spreads at three levels:

- by transfer of bacteria between people
- by transfer of resistance genes between bacteria (usually on plasmids)
- by transfer of resistance genes between genetic elements within bacteria, on transposons. (Transposons are defined and explained below.)

Understanding the mechanisms involved in antibiotic resistance is of importance both for the sensible use of these drugs in clinical practice and for the development of new antibacterial drugs to circumvent resistance. One result of the studies of resistance has been the development of new techniques using R plasmids and resistance genes for the cloning of foreign DNA. This cloning has been used rewardingly in many branches of biology and also in the production, by bacteria, of biologically active peptides such as mammalian hormones.

---

*Resistance to anticancer agents is considered in Chapter 42, page 680; resistance to antimalarial drugs is considered in Chapter 46.

GENETIC DETERMINANTS OF ANTIBIOTIC RESISTANCE

Chromosomal determinants—mutations

The spontaneous mutation rate in bacterial populations for any particular gene is very low—about 1 per 10^6–10^8 cells per cell division, i.e. the probability is that 1 cell in, say, 10 million will, on division, give rise to a daughter cell containing a mutation in a particular gene. However, since in an infection there are likely to be very many more cells than this, the probability of a mutation causing a change from drug sensitivity to drug resistance can be quite high with some species of bacteria and with some drugs. Fortunately, with most infective species and with most antibiotics, a few mutants are not sufficient to produce resistance. If an infecting bacterial population containing some mutants resistant to a particular antibiotic is exposed to that antibiotic, the mutants will have an enormous selective advantage. Luckily, in most cases the drastic reduction of the population by the antibiotic enables the host's natural defences (see Ch. 12) to deal effectively with the invading pathogens. However, this will not occur if the infection is caused by a population of microorganisms that are all resistant to the drug.

For most organisms, resistance due to chromosomal mutation is not of great clinical relevance, possibly because the mutants often have reduced pathogenicity; but it is important in methicillin-resistant staphylococcal infections (see below) and in infections due to mycobacteria, particularly tuberculosis.

Extrachromosomal determinants—plasmids

Many species of bacteria contain, in addition to the chromosome, extrachromosomal genetic elements called *plasmids* that exist free in the cytoplasm. These are genetic elements *other* than the chromosome, which can replicate on their own. They consist of closed loops of DNA about 1–3% of the size of the chromosome. There may be 1–40 copies of a particular plasmid present, depending on the type, and there may be more than one type of plasmid in each bacterial cell. Plasmids that carry genes for resistance to antibiotics ('r genes') are referred to as R plasmids. Much of the drug resistance encountered in clinical medicine is plasmid determined. It is not known how these genes arose.

THE TRANSFER OF RESISTANCE GENES BETWEEN GENETIC ELEMENTS WITHIN THE BACTERIUM

Transposons

Some stretches of DNA can be fairly readily transferred (transposed) from one plasmid to another and also from plasmid to chromosome or vice versa. This is because integration of these segments of DNA, which are called *transposons*, into the acceptor DNA can occur independently of the normal mechanism of genetic recombination (i.e. cross-over), which usually requires extensive homology. During the process of integration, the transposon can replicate (Fig. 41.9) and this results in a copy in both the donor and the acceptor DNA molecules. (Note that transposons, unlike plasmids, are not able to replicate on their own and that some transposons do not replicate during transfer.) Transposons may carry one or more resistance genes (see below) and can 'hitch-hike' on a plasmid to a new species of bacterium; and even if the plasmid is unable to replicate in the new host, the transposon may transfer to the new host's chromosome or to its indigenous plasmids. This probably accounts for the widespread distribution of certain of the resistance

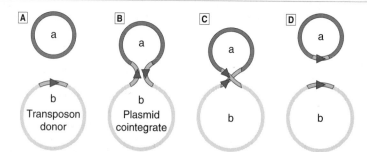

Fig. 41.9 An example of the transfer and replication of a transposon (which may carry genes coding for resistance to antibiotics). [A] Two plasmids, a and b, with plasmid b containing a transposon (shown in blue). [B] An enzyme encoded by the transposon cuts DNA of both donor plasmid and target plasmid a, to form a 'cointegrate'. During this process the transposon replicates. [C] An enzyme encoded by the transposon 'resolves' the cointegrate. [D] Both plasmids now contain the transposon DNA.

genes on different R plasmids and among unrelated bacteria.

Gene cassettes and integrons

Plasmids and transposons do not complete the tally of mechanisms that natural selection has provided to confound the hopes of the microbiologist/chemotherapist. Resistance—in fact, multidrug resistance—can also be spread by another mobile element: the gene cassette, which consists of a resistance gene attached to a small recognition site. Several cassettes may be packaged together in a multicassette array, which can in turn be integrated into a larger mobile DNA unit, termed an 'integron' (an addition to the already arcane terminology of bacterial geneticists). The integron (which can be located on a transposon), contains a gene for the enzyme, an integrase (recombinase), which inserts the cassette(s) at unique sites on the integron. This system—transposon/integron/multiresistance cassette array—allows particularly rapid and efficient transfer of multidrug resistance between genetic elements within the bacterium (and between bacteria on plasmids, see below).

THE TRANSFER OF RESISTANCE GENES BETWEEN BACTERIA

The transfer of resistance genes between bacteria of the same species and of different species is of fundamental importance in the spread of resistance to antibiotics. There are three mechanisms for gene transfer: conjugation, transduction and transformation.

Conjugation

Conjugation involves cell-to-cell contact during which chromosomal or extrachromosomal DNA is transferred from one bacterium to another. It is the main mechanism for the spread of resistance. The ability to conjugate is encoded in *conjugative plasmids*; these are plasmids that contain *transfer genes* which, in coliform bacteria, code for the production, by the host bacterium, of surface tubules of protein that connect the two cells—'sex pili'. The conjugative plasmid then passes across from one bacterium to the other, which is usually of the same species. Many Gram-negative and some Gram-positive bacteria can conjugate. Some plasmids cross the species barrier and, accepting one host as readily as another, are suggestively described as *promiscuous plasmids*. Many R plasmids are conjugative.* Non-conjugative plasmids, if

they coexist in a 'donor' cell with conjugative plasmids, can make use of the sex pili. The transfer of resistance by conjugation is significant in populations of bacteria that are normally found at high densities, as in the gut.

Transduction

Transduction is a process by which plasmid DNA is enclosed in a bacterial virus (or phage) and transferred to another bacterium of the same species. It is a relatively ineffective means of transfer of genetic material, but there is evidence that it is clinically important in the transmission of resistance genes between strains of staphylococci and between strains of streptococci.

Transformation

In a few species, a bacterium can, under natural conditions, undergo transformation by taking up naked DNA from its environment and incorporating it into its genome through the normal cross-over mechanism. This is possible only when the incoming DNA comes from a cell belonging to the same strain as the host bacterium or one that is very closely related. Transformation is probably not of importance in the clinical problem of drug resistance.

Resistance to antibiotics

- Resistance in bacterial populations can be spread from person to person by bacteria, from bacterium to bacterium by plasmids, from plasmid to plasmid (or chromosome) by transposons.
- Plasmids are extrachromosomal genetic elements that can replicate independently and can carry genes coding for resistance to antibiotics (r genes).
- The main method of transfer of r genes from one bacterium to another is by conjugative plasmids, which can cause the bacterium to make a connecting tube between bacteria, through which the plasmid itself (and other plasmids) can pass.
- A less common method of transfer is by transduction, i.e. the transmission of an r-gene-carrying plasmid into a bacterium by a bacterial virus (phage).
- Transposons are stretches of DNA that can be transposed from one plasmid to another, and also from plasmid to chromosome and vice versa. For example an r-gene-carrying transposon in one plasmid codes for enzymes that cause integration of that plasmid into another plasmid, followed by their separation; during this the transposon replicates so that both plasmids will then contain the r-gene-carrying transposon.

---

*The combination of resistance genes with the stretch of DNA which encodes for the sex pilus, which is often referred to as the 'resistance transfer factor' or 'RTF', is sometimes called the 'R factor'.

BIOCHEMICAL MECHANISMS OF RESISTANCE TO ANTIBIOTICS

The production of an enzyme that inactivates the drug

Inactivation of β-lactam antibiotics

The most important example of resistance due to inactivation is that of β-lactams. The enzymes concerned are *β-lactamases*, which cleave the β-lactam ring of **penicillins** and **cephalosporins** (see Ch. 43). Cross-resistance between the two classes of antibiotic is not complete because some lactamases have a preference for penicillins and some for cephalosporins.

Staphylococci are the principal bacteria producing β-lactamase, and the genes coding for the enzymes are on plasmids which are transferred by transduction. In staphylococci the enzyme is inducible, i.e. its synthesis is not expressed in the absence of the drug, but minute, sub-inhibitory, concentrations derepress the gene and result in a 50- to 80-fold increase in production. The enzyme is able to diffuse through the envelope and inactivate antibiotic molecules in the surrounding medium. The serious clinical problem posed by the staphylococci with resistance due to β-lactamase production was tackled by developing semisynthetic penicillins (such as **methicillin**) and new β-lactam antibiotics (**monobactams** and **carbapenems**), which were not susceptible, and cephalosporins (such as **cephamandole**), which were less susceptible to inactivation by these enzymes. (But see below for 'methicillin-resistant' staphylococci.)

Gram-negative organisms can also produce β-lactamases, which are a significant factor in their resistance to the semisynthetic **broad-spectrum β-lactam antibiotics**. In these organisms, the enzymes may be determined by either chromosomal genes or by plasmid genes. In the former case, the enzymes may be inducible. In the latter they are produced constitutively (i.e. they are synthesised even when the substrate is absent) and remain attached to sites in the cell wall, preventing access of the drug to the membrane-associated target site; they do not inactivate the drug in the surrounding medium. Many of these β-lactamases are encoded by transposons, some of which may also carry resistance determinants to several other antibiotics.

Inactivation of chloramphenicol

Chloramphenicol inactivation is brought about by *chloramphenicol acetyltransferase* produced by resistant strains of both Gram-positive and Gram-negative organisms, the resistance gene being plasmid-borne. In Gram-negative bacteria the enzyme is produced constitutively, which results in levels of resistance fivefold higher than in Gram-positive bacteria, in which the enzyme is inducible.

Inactivation of aminoglycosides

Inactivation of aminoglycosides may be brought about by phosphorylation, adenylation or acetylation and the requisite enzymes have been found in both Gram-negative and Gram-positive organisms. The resistance genes are carried on plasmids and several are found on transposons.

Alteration of drug-sensitive site or drug-binding site

The protein on the 30S subunit of the ribosome, which is the binding site for **aminoglycosides**, may be altered as the result of a chromosomal mutation. A plasmid-mediated alteration of the binding-site protein on the 50S subunit underlies resistance to **erythromycin**, and decreased binding of **fluoroquinolones** because of a point mutation in the DNA gyrase A protein has recently been described. An altered DNA-dependent RNA polymerase determined by a chromosomal mutation is the basis for resistance to **rifampicin**.

In addition to resistance to **β-lactams** due to production of β-lactamase (as described above), some strains of *Staph. aureus* have become resistant even to some β-lactams that are not significantly inactivated by β-lactamase (e.g. **methicillin**), owing to expression of an additional β-lactam-binding site coded for by a mutated chromosomal gene.

Decreased drug accumulation in the bacterium

An important example of decreased drug accumulation is the plasmid-mediated resistance to **tetracyclines** in both Gram-positive and Gram-negative bacteria. The resistance genes in the plasmid code for inducible proteins in the bacterial membrane, which promote energy-dependent efflux of the tetracyclines and hence resistance. This type of resistance is common and has reduced the value of the tetracyclines in human and veterinary medicine. A recently described gene in *Staph. aureus* has also been shown to code for a membrane-associated protein that causes active efflux of **fluoroquinolones** from the cell. There is also recent evidence of plasmid-determined inhibition of 'porin' synthesis, which could affect those hydrophilic antibiotics that enter the bacterium by these water-filled channels in the outer membrane.

Altered permeability due to chromosomal mutations involving the polysaccharide components of the outer membrane of Gram-negative organisms may confer enhanced resistance to **ampicillin**.

Mutations affecting envelope components have been reported to affect the accumulation of **aminoglycosides**, **β-lactams**, **chloramphenicol**, **peptide antibiotics** and **tetracycline**.

The development of a pathway that bypasses the reaction inhibited by the antibiotic

Recently, resistance to **trimethoprim** has developed, the mechanism being plasmid-directed synthesis of a dihydrofolate reductase with low or zero affinity for trimethoprim. It is transferred by transduction and may be spread by transposons.

Sulphonamide resistance in many bacteria is plasmid-mediated and is due to the production of a form of dihydropteroate synthetase with a low affinity for sulphonamides but no change in affinity for PABA. Bacteria causing serious infections have been found to carry plasmids with resistance genes to both sulphonamides and trimethoprim.

CURRENT STATUS OF ANTIBIOTIC RESISTANCE IN BACTERIA

The most disturbing development of resistance has been in staphylococci, many strains of which are now resistant to almost all currently available antibiotics. In addition to resistance to some β-**lactams** due to production of β-lactamase and the production of an additional β-lactam-binding site which renders them resistant to **methicillin** (see above), *Staph. aureus* may also manifest resistance to other antibiotics as follows:

- to **streptomycin** (due to chromosomally determined alteration of target site)
- to **aminoglycosides** in general (due to altered target site and plasmid-determined inactivating enzymes)
- to **chloramphenicol** and the **macrolides** (due to plasmid-determined enzymes)
- to **trimethoprim** (due to transposon-encoded drug-resistant dihydrofolate reductase)
- to **sulphonamides** (due to chromosomally determined increased production of PABA)
- to **rifampicin** (thought to be due to chromosomally determined and plasmid-determined increases in efflux of the drug)
- to **fusidic acid** (due to chromosomally determined decreased affinity of the target site or a plasmid-encoded decreased permeability to the drug)
- to **quinolones**, for example ciprofloxacin, norfloxacin (due to chromosomally determined reduced uptake).

Infections with these organisms, referred to as '**m**ethicillin-**r**esistant *Staphylococcus aureus*' (MRSA), have become a serious problem, particularly in hospitals, where they can spread rapidly among elderly and/or seriously ill patients, and patients with burns or wounds. In a number of hospitals, surgical wards have had to be closed because of the high rates of infection among patients. Until recently, the glycopeptide, **vancomycin**, was the antibiotic of last resort against MRSA, but, ominously, in 1997, strains of MRSA resistant to this drug were isolated from hospitalised patients in the USA and Japan. The vancomycin resistance seems to have developed spontaneously. This could have major clinical consequences—and not only for nosocomial* infections with MRSA. It had been thought that antibiotic-resistant bacteria were dangerous only to seriously ill, hospitalised patients in that the genetic load of multiple resistance genes would lead to reduced virulence; but there is now evidence that the spectrum and frequency of disease produced by methicillin-susceptible and methicillin-resistant staphylococci are similar.**

In the last few years, enterococci have been rapidly developing resistance to many chemotherapeutic agents and have emerged as the second most common nosocomial pathogen. Non-pathogenic enterococci are ubiquitously present in the intestine, have intrinsic resistance to many antibacterial drugs and can readily become resistant to other agents by taking up plasmids and transposons carrying the relevant resistance genes; this resistance is easily transferred to invading pathogenic enterococci.

Enterococci, already multiresistant, have recently developed resistance to **vancomycin**, thought to be due to replacement of the last two amino acids, D-Ala–D-Ala, with D-Ala–D-lactate in the *five* amino acid chain attached to N-acetylglucosamine-N-acetylmuramic acid (G-M) in the first steps of peptidoglycan synthesis (see Figs 41.3 and Ch. 43). This is becoming a major problem in hospitalised patients. A particular concern is the possibility of transfer of vancomycin resistance from enterococci to staphylococci, since they can coexist in the same patient.

Furthermore, many other pathogens are developing, or have developed, resistance to commonly used drugs.*** The list includes, among others, *P. aeruginosa*, *Strep. pyogenes*, *Strep. pneumoniae*, *N. meningitidis*, *N. gonorrhoeae*, *H. influenzae*, *H. ducreyi* as well as

---

*Nosocomial infections are those acquired in hospital.

**Reports from Iceland indicate that multidrug-resistant and non-resistant *pneumococci* can be equally virulent; and in South Africa, mortality from meningitis due to penicillin-resistant pneumococci was reported to be higher than that due to penicillin-susceptible pneumococci.

***It should be emphasised that one reason for our current inability to win the war against these microbe foes is that antibiotics are often used indiscriminately and to excess.

Mycobacterium, *Campylobacter*, and *Bacteroides* species (see Jacobi & Archer 1991). Some strains of *Mycobacterium tuberculosis* are now able to evade every antibiotic in the clinician's armamentarium, and tuberculosis, once considered easily treatable, is now reported to be causing more deaths world-wide than malaria and AIDS together.

Extensive efforts are currently under way in many countries to find new antibiotics effective against the rapidly growing ranks of multiresistant bacteria; but nature has endowed microorganisms with fiendishly effective adaptive mechanisms for dealing with our pharmaceutical attack and so far several have been effortlessly keeping pace with our attempts to deal with them.

Biochemical mechanisms of resistance to antibiotics

- Production of enzymes that inactivate the drug: e.g. β-lactamases, which inactivate penicillin; acetyltransferases, which inactivate chloramphenicol; kinases and other enzymes, which inactivate aminoglycosides.
- Alteration of the drug-binding sites: this occurs with aminoglycosides, erythromycin, penicillin.
- Reduction of drug uptake by the bacterium: e.g. tetracyclines.
- Alteration of enzymes: e.g. dihydrofolate reductase becomes insensitive to trimethoprim.

- Many pathogenic bacteria have developed resistance to the commonly used antibiotics; some examples are:
  — Some strains of staphylococci and enterococci are resistant to virtually all current antibiotics—resistance being transferred by transposons and/or plasmids. These organisms can cause serious and virtually untreatable nosocomial infections.
  — Some strains of *Mycobacterium tuberculosis* have become resistant to most antituberculosis agents.

REFERENCES AND FURTHER READING

Amyes S G B, Gemmell C G (eds) 1997 Antibiotic resistance. J Med Microbiol 46: 436–470 *(Review of a symposium)*

Arthur M, Reynolds P, Courvalin P 1996 Glycopeptide resistance in enterococci. Trends Microbiol 4: 401–407

Chopra I, Hodgson J et al. 1997 The search for antimicrobial agents effective against bacteria resistant to multiple antibiotics. Antimicrob Agents Chemother 41: 497–503

Croft S L 1997 The current status of antiparasite chemotherapy. Parasitology 114: S3–S15 *(Comprehensive coverage of current drugs and outline of approaches to possible future agents)*

Courvalin P 1996 Evasion of antibiotic action by bacteria. J Antimicrobial Chemother 37: 855–869

Foley M, Tilley L 1997 Quinoline antimalarials: mechanisms of action and resistance. Int J Parasitol 27: 231–240 *(Good, short review; useful diagrams)*

Franklin T J, Snow G A, Barrett-Bee K J, Nolan R D 1989 Resistance to antimicrobial drugs. In: Franklin T J, Snow G A (eds) Biochemistry of antimicrobial action, 4th edn. Chapman & Hall, London, ch 8

Greenwood D (ed) 1995 Antimicrobial chemotherapy, 3rd edn. Oxford University Press, Oxford, p 428

Harai K, Mitsuhashi S 1992 Mechanisms of resistance to quinolones. Prog Drug Res 38: 107–120

Hawkey P M 1998 The origins and molecular basis of antibiotic resistance. Brit Med J 7159: 657–659 *(Succinct overview of resistance: useful simple diagrams. This is one of 12 papers/articles on resistance in this issue of the journal)*

Jacobi G A, Archer G L 1991 Mechanisms of disease: new mechanisms of bacterial resistance to antimicrobial agents. N Engl J Med 324: 601–612

Jones M E, Peters E et al. 1997 Widespread occurrence of integrons causing multiple antibiotic resistance in bacteria. Lancet 349: 1742–1743

Levy S B 1992 Active efflux mechanisms for antimicrobial resistance. Antimicrob Agents Chemother 36: 695–703

Levy S B 1998 The challenge of antibiotic resistance. Scientific American (March): 32–39 *(Simple, clear up-to-date review by an expert in the field; excellent diagrams)*

Levy S B 1998 Antibacterial resistance: bacteria on the defence. Brit Med J 7159: 612–613 *(Resistance seen from the point of view of the bacterium. This is one of seven editorials on the subject of resistance in this issue of the journal)*

Martin R J, Robertson A P, Bjorn H 1997 Target sites of anthelminthics. Parasitology 114 (suppl): S111–S124

Michel M, Gutman L 1997 Methicillin-resistant *Staphylococcus aureus* and vancomycin-resistant enterococci: therapeutic realities and possibilities. Lancet 349: 1901–1906 *(Excellent review article; good diagrams)*

Noskin G A 1997 Vancomycin-resistant enterococci: clinical, microbiologic, and epidemiologic features. J Lab Clin Med 130: 14–20

Recchia G D, Hall R M 1995 Gene cassettes: a new class of mobile element. Microbiology 141: 3015–3027

Sato K, Hoshino K, Mitsuhashi S 1992 Mode of action of the new quinolones: the inhibitory action on DNA gyrase. Prog Drug Res 38: 121–132

Silver L S, Bostian K A 1993 Discovery and development of new antibiotics: the problem of antibiotic resistance. Antimicrob Agents Chemother 37: 377–383

Smith J T 1985 The 4-quinolone antibacterials. In: Greenwood D, O'Grady F (eds) The scientific basis of antimicrobial therapy. Cambridge University Press, Cambridge, pp 69–94

Tabaqchali S 1997 Vancomycin-resistant *Staphylococcus aureus*: apocalypse now? Lancet 350: 1644

Tomasz A 1994 Multiple-antibiotic-resistant pathogenic bacteria. N Engl J Med 330: 1247–1251 *(A special report based on a Rockefeller workshop)*

42

Cancer chemotherapy

Cancer is a disease in which there is uncontrolled multiplication and spread within the body of abnormal forms of the body's own cells. It is one of the major causes of death in the developed nations—at least one in five of the population of Europe and North America can expect to die of cancer. Figures for the last 100 years or so give the impression that the disease is increasing in these countries, but allowance has to be made for the fact that cancer is largely a disease of the later age groups, and with the advances in public health and medical science many more people live to the age where they are liable to get cancer.

The terms 'cancer', 'malignant neoplasm',* and 'malignant tumour' are synonymous, and are distinguished from benign** tumours by the properties of *dedifferentiation*, *invasiveness* and the *ability to metastasise* (spread to other parts of the body). In this chapter we shall be concerned only with the therapy of malignant neoplasia or cancer. The appearance of these abnormal characteristics reflects altered patterns of gene expression in the cancer cells, resulting from genetic mutations.

There are three main approaches to treating established cancer—*surgical excision*, *irradiation*, and *chemotherapy*—and the role of each of these depends on the type of tumour and the stage of its development. Chemotherapy is the main method of treatment for only a few cancers but it is increasingly used as an adjunct to surgery or irradiation for many types of tumour. A list of cancers in which drug treatment has an important place is given in Table 42.1.

Table 42.1   Some examples of malignant disease in which drug therapy has an important place

Hodgkin's disease
Non-Hodgkin's lymphoma
Chronic granulocytic leukaemia
Acute lymphocytic leukaemia
Hairy cell leukaemia
Germ cell cancer (testis, ovary)
Choriocarcinoma
Prostate cancer

*Neoplasm means 'new growth'.

**Both benign and malignant tumours manifest uncontrolled proliferation.

Other approaches to cancer treatment—immunotherapy, angiogenesis inhibitors, gene therapy, and use of biological response modifiers (e.g. interferons, haemopoietic growth factors, etc.)—are being investigated (see below).

Chemotherapy of cancer, as compared with that of bacterial disease, presents a difficult problem. In biochemical terms, microorganisms are both quantitatively and qualitatively different from human cells (see Ch. 41); but cancer cells and normal cells are so similar in many respects that it has proved difficult to find *general*, *exploitable*, *biochemical* differences between them.

THE BIOLOGY OF CANCER

In the past few years, a prodigious advance in the understanding of cell proliferation has led to better understanding of the biology of the cancer cell; this in turn is beginning to lead to new approaches to the development of anticancer agents. To understand how current anticancer drugs act (and how drugs now in the pipeline and future agents will act), it is important to consider in more detail the special characteristics of the cancer cell.

THE SPECIAL CHARACTERISTICS OF CANCER CELLS

As specified above, cancer cells manifest, to varying degrees, four characteristics that distinguish them from normal cells:

- uncontrolled proliferation
- dedifferentiation and loss of function
- invasiveness
- metastasis.

UNCONTROLLED PROLIFERATION

The proliferation of cancer cells is not controlled by the processes that normally regulate cell division and tissue growth. It is this, rather than their *rate* of proliferation, that distinguishes them from normal cells. Some normal cells (such as neurons) have little or no capacity to divide and proliferate, but others, for example in the bone marrow and the epithelium of the gastrointestinal tract, have the property of continuous rapid division. Some cancer cells multiply slowly (e.g. those in plasma cell tumours) and some fast (e.g. the cells of Burkitt's lymphoma). It is therefore not generally true that cancer cells proliferate faster than normal cells. Consider, for example, the cells of the liver. Under normal conditions only a very small proportion of these are undergoing division at any one time. However, if two-thirds of the liver is removed, the remaining cells will divide fast and continuously until—in 2 weeks in the rat—the liver regains its original size. Growth then stops, because it is controlled by regulatory processes which are as yet ill understood. The significant point about cancer cells is that their proliferation is not subject to these regulatory processes.

The cell cycle

In discussing the difference between the proliferation of normal cells and that of cancer cells, one needs to consider the cell cycle of dividing cells. This starts with the cell 'gearing up' for division by synthesising the components necessary for DNA replication. Figure 42.1 shows the various phases of the cycle—G_1, S (DNA synthesis), G_2, and M (mitosis). There are two check points, one between G_1 and S and one between G_2, and M.

Most anticancer drugs act in S phase (Fig. 42.1), but some act in M phase and some have complex actions in the cycle (see p. 680).

Progress through the cell cycle depends on the balance between various positive and negative regulatory forces (see Karp & Broder 1995).

The positive forces involve growth factors (Chs 2 and 12) that stimulate the cell to start on the cycle, and a series of cyclins and cyclin-dependent kinases (cdks). The cyclins bind to and regulate the cdks which in turn control the enzymes of the cell cycle (Fig. 42.1). The D family of cyclin/cdks stimulate the processes that take the cell through G_1 phase. The D cyclin/cdk complexes plus E/cdk promote progression into and through S phase. Cyclin A/cdk promotes progression through S phase and cyclin B/cdk through G_2 phase.

The action of the cyclin/cdks is modulated by various negative regulatory forces—proteins that bind to the cdks and inhibit their action. These proteins are induced by various genes, e.g. the *p53* gene and the retinoblastoma (*Rb*) gene—which constitute the two 'superbrakes' on the cell cycle. If there is DNA damage, these inhibitors normally halt the cycle at checkpoint 1, allowing for repair (see Fig. 42.1). If repair fails, apoptosis (see Fig. 42.2) is initiated.

In cancer cells, the cell cycle control is disrupted by (1) abnormal growth factor function and/or (2) abnormal cyclin/cdk function and/or (3) abnormal DNA synthesis as a result of oncogene activity and/or (4) abnormal decrease in negative regulatory forces owing to mutation of tumour suppressor genes.

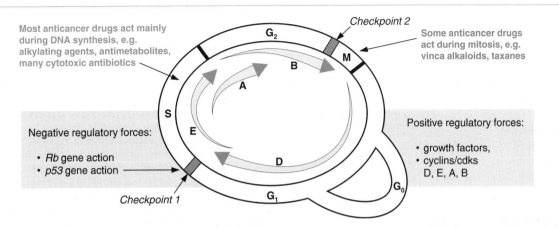

Fig. 42.1 **Diagram of the cell cycle specifying the four phases—G$_1$, S (DNA synthesis), G$_2$ and M (mitosis)—and indicating the main sites of action of most anticancer drugs.** A cell stimulated to divide by growth factors, starts in G$_1$, preparing for DNA synthesis. Progress through the cycle is determined by a cell cycle control system, the two families of proteins—the cyclins and their respective cyclin-dependent kinases (cdks)—coded for by the delayed response nuclear proto-oncogenes (see Fig. 42.3). The cyclins bind to the cdks and regulate their action. Thickness of arrow represents intensity of action of cdks. Proteins induced by various genes, e.g. the *p53* gene and the retinoblastoma (*Rb*) gene, bind to the cdks and inhibit their action. If there is DNA damage, the actions of the tumour suppressor gene, *p53*, stops the cycle at checkpoint 1, allowing for repair. If repair fails, apoptosis (see Fig. 42.2) is initiated. G$_0$ represents a phase in which the cells are not dividing but can re-enter the cycle. As a cell differentiates, it leaves the cycle. (Adapted from Dale et al. 1999)

Apoptosis

Unlike *necrosis*, which is disorganised disintegration of damaged cells, *apoptosis* is the built-in self-destruct mechanism of the cell, consisting of a genetically pro-grammed sequence of biochemical events leading to cell death. Apoptosis protects the organism from fostering superannuated cells and abnormal cells and is important in many aspects of body function. It eliminates cells that become redundant during development and differen-tiation. It is the mechanism involved in the shedding of the intestinal lining, the regression of mammary gland cells after lactation or the death of time-expired neutro-phils. It is the basis for the development of self-tolerance in the immune system (Ch. 12) and is implicated in the pathophysiology of cancer, autoimmune diseases, neuro-degenerative conditions (Ch. 31) and AIDS. It is espe-cially important in the context of malignancy because it acts as a first-line defence against mutations—removing cells with abnormal DNA that could become malignant (see Rudin & Thompson 1997).

There is evidence that apoptosis is a default response, i.e. that continuous active signalling by tissue-specific trophic factors, cytokines, hormones, cell-to-cell contact factors (adhesion molecules, integrins, etc.) may be re-quired for cell survival and viability and that the self-destruct mechanism is automatically triggered unless there is active and continuous inhibition by these anti-apoptotic factors (see Meredith & Schwartz 1997). This has relevance for the propensity of tumours to invade and metastasise (discussed below).

The intracellular pathway of apoptosis involves activation of interleukin-1b enzyme, ceramide, proteases, endonucleases, etc. The action of various gene products, e.g. the *p53* protein, modulates and controls apoptosis (see Fig. 42.1); the *Bcl-2* gene protein represses apoptosis.

Many cytotoxic anticancer agents work in S phase of the cell cycle, causing damage to DNA (Fig. 42.1). There is now evidence that for many, if not most of these agents, the damage initiates apoptosis—resulting in programmed cell death (Fig. 42.2); a list is given in McConkey et al. (1996, p. 62). There is also now increasing evidence that apoptosis-controlling factors are implicated in the development of some types of tumour resistance to anti-cancer agents.

Mechanisms involved in uncontrolled proliferation

In discussing uncontrolled proliferation of the cancer cell, we need to consider the signal transduction mecha-nisms for cell division. Cells in multicellular organisms divide in response to the following:

- *extracellular signals* (growth factors), which act on
- *cell surface receptors* (see Ch. 2), which in turn trigger

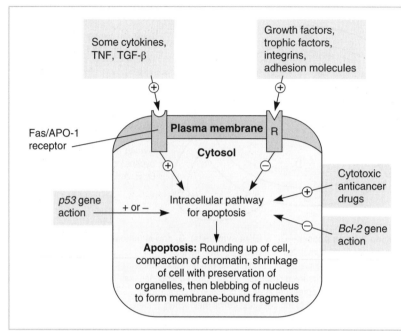

Fig. 42.2 Simplified diagram of the signalling pathway and the sequence of events in apoptosis (cell suicide). The Fas/Apo-1 receptor is the prototype receptor mediating apoptosis and can be stimulated by the factors specified. The receptor labelled 'R' represents the respective receptors for trophic factors, growth factors, cell-to-cell contact factors (adhesion molecules, integrins), etc. Continuous stimulation of these receptors is necessary for cell survival/proliferation; withdrawal of stimulation results in apoptosis. *Bcl-2* gene action inhibits apoptosis. When the DNA is undamaged, *p53* inhibits apoptosis; when it is damaged *p53* halts the cell cycle allowing for repair. If repair fails, *p53* initiates apoptosis. Many anticancer drugs kill cells by triggering apoptosis.

- *intracellular transduction events*—involving both cytosolic and nuclear transducers—which result in
- *the production of the cell cycle transducers*, which lead to *DNA synthesis* and finally to cell division.

Disruption of any of the above—by activation of oncogenes or inactivation of tumour suppressor genes (see below)—could result in uncontrolled proliferation. An outline of these is given in the left-hand section of Figure 42.3.

One reason for the continuous proliferation of cancer cells—their 'immortalisation'—is thought to be that, in contrast to normal cells, their telomeres (specialised structures on the ends of each chromosome) do not shorten with each round of cell division. The shortening and possibly disappearance of telomeres is believed to be the basis for cessation of cell division—leading to senescence. In growing tissue, an enzyme, telomerase, maintains and stabilises the telomeres (see Greider & Blackburn 1996). Most fully differentiated cells do not express telomerase, but about 95% of late-stage malignant tumours do express it and it is suggested that it is this enzyme that confers 'immortality' on a cancer cell; though this is controversial.

Angiogenesis and tumour growth

The actual growth of the tumour depends on the development of its own blood supply. Tumours 1–2 mm in diameter can receive nutrients by diffusion, but any further expansion requires the development of new blood vessels—*angiogenesis*, which occurs in response to vascular growth factors produced by the growing tumour. During angiogenesis, enzymes (e.g. metalloproteinases) break down surrounding tissue—making space for new blood vessels (see Harris 1997).

DEDIFFERENTIATION AND LOSS OF FUNCTION

The multiplication of normal cells involves division of the stem cells in a particular tissue to give rise to daughter cells. These daughter cells eventually differentiate to become the mature cells of the relevant tissue and carry out their programmed functions. Thus, fibroblasts become capable of secreting and organising collagenous extracellular matrix, muscle cells become capable of contraction, and so on. One of the main characteristics of cancer cells is the loss—to a varying degree in different tumours—of the capacity to differentiate. In general, poorly differentiated cancers multiply faster, and have a poorer prognosis than well-differentiated cancers.

INVASIVENESS

Normal cells are not found outside their 'designated' tissue of origin; e.g. liver cells are not found in the

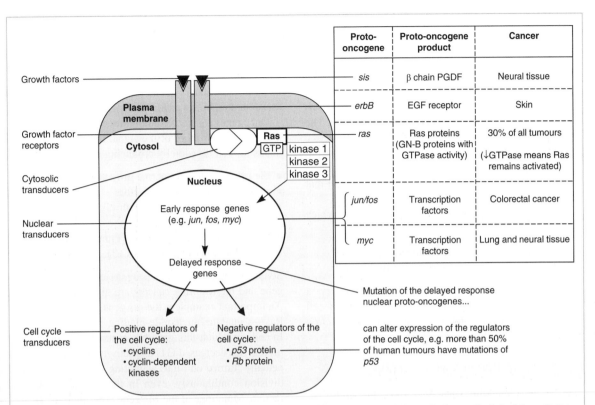

Proto-oncogene	Proto-oncogene product	Cancer
sis	β chain PGDF	Neural tissue
erbB	EGF receptor	Skin
ras	Ras proteins (GN-B proteins with GTPase activity)	30% of all tumours (↓GTPase means Ras remains activated)
jun/fos	Transcription factors	Colorectal cancer
myc	Transcription factors	Lung and neural tissue

Growth factors

Plasma membrane

Growth factor receptors

Cytosol

Ras GTP kinase 1 kinase 2 kinase 3

Cytosolic transducers

Nucleus

Early response genes (e.g. *jun, fos, myc*)

Nuclear transducers

Delayed response genes

Cell cycle transducers

Positive regulators of the cell cycle:
• cyclins
• cyclin-dependent kinases

Negative regulators of the cell cycle:
• *p53* protein
• *Rb* protein

Mutation of the delayed response nuclear proto-oncogenes...

...can alter expression of the regulators of the cell cycle, e.g. more than 50% of human tumours have mutations of *p53*

Fig. 42.3   Simplified diagram of the signal transduction pathway initiated by growth factors, listing on the left of the cell, the classes of substances coded for by proto-oncogenes, and on the right, examples of specific proto-oncogenes and the products they code for. The last column gives examples of the cancers produced when these proto-oncogenes are converted to oncogenes. Many growth factors have integral tyrosine kinase (see Fig. 2.17). These receptors dimerise (form pairs), then phosphorylate each other's tyrosine residues. The cytosolic transducers include proteins that bind to these phosphorylated tyrosine residues. The kinase cascade (1 = Raf, 2 = MEK and 3 = Map kinase) can also be initiated by the phospholipase Cγ/diacylglycerol/protein kinase C pathway. (GN-B protein = guanine nucleotide-binding protein; PDGF = platelet-derived growth factor; EGF = epidermal growth factor) (Adapted from Dale et al. 1998)

bladder, pancreatic cells are not found in the testis. This is because during differentiation and during the growth of tissues and organs, normal cells develop certain spatial relationships with respect to each other, and these are continuously maintained even when the cells are involved in repair processes. These relationships are maintained by various tissue-specific survival factors—the anti-apoptotic factors specified above. Any cells that escape accidentally, lose these survival signals and undergo apoptosis.

Thus, although the cells of the normal mucosal epithelium of the rectum proliferate continuously as the lining is shed, they remain as a lining epithelium. A cancer of the rectal mucosa, on the other hand, invades the tissues in the other layers of the rectum and may invade the tissues of other pelvic organs. Cancer cells have not only

lost, through mutation, the restraints that act on normal cells, they also secrete enzymes, e.g. metalloproteinases (see above), that break down the extracellular matrix enabling the cancer cells to slip through.

METASTASES

These are secondary tumours formed by cells that have been released from the initial or primary tumour and have reached other sites through blood vessels or lymphatics, or as a result of being shed into body cavities. As discussed above, it is now thought that aberrant migration of cells would lead to programmed cell death as a result of withdrawal of the necessary anti-apoptotic factors. Cancer cells which have the ability to metastasise, have undergone a series of genetic changes which alter their responses to the regulatory factors that control the tissue siting of normal cells thus enabling them to establish themselves 'extraterritorially'.

THE GENESIS OF A CANCER CELL

A normal cell turns into a cancer cell because of a mutation in its DNA, which can be inherited* or acquired. The development of cancer is a complex multistage process, involving not only more than one genetic change but usually also other factors that are not in themselves cancer-producing but which increase the likelihood that the genetic mutation(s) will result in cancer.

There are two main categories of genetic change which lead to cancer:

- the inactivation of tumour suppressor genes
- the activation of proto-oncogenes to oncogenes.

Oncogenes are genes which confer malignancy on a cell. Proto-oncogenes are genes that normally control cell division and differentiation but which can be converted to oncogenes. See Weinberg (1996).

INACTIVATION OF TUMOUR SUPPRESSOR GENES

Normal cells contain genes that have the ability to suppress malignant change—termed tumour suppressor genes (anti-oncogenes)—and there is now good evidence that mutations of these genes are involved in many different cancers.

Gene *p53* can be taken as an example. It acts as a molecular policeman in the nucleus, triggering a feedback control mechanism. If the DNA is damaged, the protein products of *p53* gene accumulate and arrest DNA replication at checkpoint 1, allowing time for repair (see Fig. 42.1). If the repair fails, *p53* activity triggers cell suicide by apoptosis. Cells in which *p53* is altered by mutation, or by binding to viral or altered host proteins, cannot stop the abnormal DNA replicating. Such cells will accumulate mutations and chromosomal translocations undisturbed, leading eventually, if other genetic changes occur, to cancer.

Mutations in *p53* are the most commonly found mutations in human cancer cells (see Lane 1994).

The loss of function of tumour suppressor genes can be the critical event in carcinogenesis.

---

*It is not the cancer itself that is inherited but a gene which has mutated and now *predisposes* to cancer. Examples are the tumour suppressor genes *BRCA1* and *BRCA2*; women who inherit a single defective copy of either of these genes have a significantly increased risk of developing breast cancer.

ACTIVATION OF PROTO-ONCOGENES

The host's genes that control normal growth and differentiation—the 'proto-oncogenes'—can promote malignancy when converted into active oncogenes as a result of point mutations, gene amplification or chromosomal translocation, or the action of certain viruses.

Oncogenes can confer autonomy of growth on cells by affecting one or more of the signal transduction mechanisms for cell division by producing abnormalities in:

- the production of autocrine growth factors
- the receptors for growth factors
- receptor-linked signalling pathways—the cytosolic and nuclear transducers
- cell cycle transducers—e.g. cyclins and cyclin-dependent kinases (see Fig. 42.3).

Some examples of proto-oncogene conversion to oncogene and the resulting cancers are given in Figure 42.3. An important example is the *ras* gene; this gene codes for Ras—a guanine nucleotide-binding protein (see Ch. 2). In cells in which this gene has mutated, the altered Ras protein has decreased GTPase activity so that Ras is perpetually 'turned on', thus activating the pathway for cell division continuously, even in the absence of growth factors. Mutations of the *ras* gene contribute to 20–30% of all human cancers.

Oncogenes interfere not only with proliferation but also with differentiation—inducing defects in the execution of differentiation programmes. And it may well be that one of the fundamental effects of oncogene products is to interfere with the action of tumour suppressor genes.

An outline of the factors involved in the genesis of cancer is given in Figure 42.4. For a simple summary of the biology of cancer, see Dale et al. (1998).

GENERAL PRINCIPLES OF ACTION OF CYTOTOXIC ANTICANCER DRUGS

In experiments with rapidly growing transplantable leukaemias in mice, it has been found that a given therapeutic dose of a cytotoxic drug destroys a constant fraction of the malignant cells. Thus a dose which kills 99.99% of cells, if used to treat a tumour with 10^{11} cells, will still leave 10 million (10^7) viable malignant cells. As the same principle holds for similar fast-growing tumours in humans, schedules for chemotherapy of these tumours are necessarily aimed at producing as near a total cell kill as possible, because in contrast to the situation with microorganisms, very little reliance can

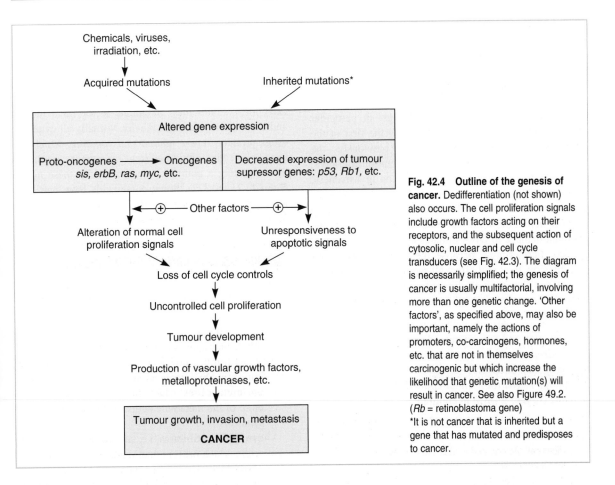

Fig. 42.4 Outline of the genesis of cancer. Dedifferentiation (not shown) also occurs. The cell proliferation signals include growth factors acting on their receptors, and the subsequent action of cytosolic, nuclear and cell cycle transducers (see Fig. 42.3). The diagram is necessarily simplified; the genesis of cancer is usually multifactorial, involving more than one genetic change. 'Other factors', as specified above, may also be important, namely the actions of promoters, co-carcinogens, hormones, etc. that are not in themselves carcinogenic but which increase the likelihood that genetic mutation(s) will result in cancer. See also Figure 49.2. (Rb = retinoblastoma gene) *It is not cancer that is inherited but a gene that has mutated and predisposes to cancer.

be placed on the host's immunological defence mechanisms against the remaining cancer cells.

One of the major difficulties in the use of cancer chemotherapy is that a tumour is usually far advanced before it is diagnosed. Let us suppose that a tumour arises from a single cell and that the growth is exponential—as it may well be in the initial stages. Doubling times vary with different tumours, for example being, very roughly, 24 hours with Burkitt's lymphoma, 2 weeks with some leukaemias, and 3 months with mammary cancers. Approximately 30 doublings would be required to produce a cell mass with a diameter of 2 cm, containing 10^9 cells. A tumour that size is within the limits of diagnostic procedures, though it might be unnoticed in many organs, such as the liver. Another 10 doublings would produce 10^{12} cells—a tumour mass which is likely to be lethal, and which would measure about 20 cm in diameter if it were all in one clump. The neoplasm would therefore be silent for the first three-quarters or more of its existence, and the problem of stopping its development after diagnosis, when there are very large numbers of malignant cells, would be considerable.

However, continuous exponential growth of this sort does not usually occur. With most solid tumours (for example of lung, stomach, uterus and so on, as opposed to leukaemias—the tumours of white blood cells) the growth rate falls as the neoplasm gets larger. This is partly because the tumour tends to outgrow its blood supply with resultant necrosis of some of its bulk, and partly because not all the cells proliferate continuously. The cells of a solid tumour can be considered as belonging to three compartments: compartment A consists of dividing cells, possibly being continuously in cell cycle (Fig. 42.1); compartment B consists of resting cells (in G_0 phase)—cells which, though not dividing, are potentially able to do so; and compartment C consists of cells that are no longer able to divide but which contribute to the tumour volume. Essentially only cells in compartment A, which may form as little as 5% of some solid tumours, are susceptible to the main currently available drugs, as is explained below. The cells in compartment C do not constitute a problem—it is the existence of cells in compartment B that makes cancer chemotherapy difficult, because these cells are not very sensitive to cytotoxic drugs, but are liable to re-enter compartment A following a course of chemotherapy.

Most currently used anticancer drugs, in particular those which are 'cytotoxic', affect only the first of the characteristics of cancer cells outlined previously—the process of cell division, i.e. they are antiproliferative; they have no specific inhibitory effect on invasiveness, the loss of differentiation or the tendency to metastasise. For many, their antiproliferative action results mainly from an action during S phase of the cell cycle, and the resultant damage to DNA initiates apoptosis (see above, p. 665). Furthermore, because their main effect is on cell division, they will affect all rapidly dividing normal tissues and thus they are likely to produce, to a greater or lesser extent, the following general toxic effects:

- *bone marrow toxicity* with decreased leukocyte production and thus decreased resistance to infection
- *impaired wound healing*
- *loss of hair* (alopecia)
- *damage to gastrointestinal epithelium*
- *depression of growth* in children

Cancer cell biology and cancer chemotherapy: general principles

- The term 'cancer' refers to a malignant neoplasm (new growth).
- The cell cycle (G_1, S, G_2, M) is regulated by:
  — positive forces: growth factors, cyclin/cdks
  — negative forces (brakes), e.g. gene *p53* which halts the cycle at checkpoint 1 and triggers apoptosis if the DNA is damaged.
- Cancer cells can manifest:
  — uncontrolled proliferation
  — loss of function due to lack of the capacity to differentiate
  — invasiveness
  — the ability to metastasise.
- Cancer arises as a result of a series of genetic changes in the cell, the main genetic lesions being:
  — inactivation of tumour suppressor genes, e.g. *p53*
  — the activation of oncogenes (mutation of the normal genes controlling cell division).
- Most anticancer drugs are antiproliferative—most damage DNA and thereby initiate apoptosis. They also affect rapidly dividing normal cells and are thus likely to depress bone marrow, impair healing, depress growth, cause sterility and hair loss, and be teratogenic. Most cause nausea and vomiting.

- *sterility*
- *teratogenicity.*

They can also, in certain circumstances, be *carcinogenic* (i.e. they may themselves cause cancer). In addition, if there is rapid cell destruction with extensive purine catabolism, urates may precipitate in the renal tubules and cause *kidney damage*. Finally, virtually all cytotoxic drugs produce *severe nausea and vomiting*, which has been called 'the inbuilt deterrent' to patient compliance in completing a course of treatment with these agents (see Ch. 21, p. 377). Some compounds have particular toxic effects which are specific for them. These will be dealt with under the individual drugs.

DRUGS USED IN CANCER CHEMOTHERAPY

The main anticancer drugs can be divided into the following general categories:

- Cytotoxic drugs:*
  —**alkylating agents and related compounds** which act by forming covalent bonds with DNA and thus impeding DNA replication
  —**antimetabolites**, which block or subvert one or more of the metabolic pathways involved in DNA synthesis
  —**cytotoxic antibiotics**, i.e. substances of microbial origin which prevent mammalian cell division
  —**plant derivatives** (**vinca alkaloids**, **taxanes**, **campothecins**)—most of these specifically affect microtubule function and hence the formation of the mitotic spindle.
  The mechanism of action of these drugs is discussed more fully below and summarised in Figure 42.5.
- Hormones—of which the most important are steroids, namely **glucocorticoids**, **oestrogens** and **androgens**—and drugs that suppress hormone secretion or antagonise hormone action.
- Miscellaneous agents. Agents that do not fit into the above categories are described briefly under this heading.

For detailed coverage of the pharmacology of anticancer drugs see Chabner & Longo (1996) or Foye (1995).

The clinical use of anticancer drugs is the province of the specialist oncologist and is not covered in detail here. An outline of the drugs used in particular tumours and

---

*The term 'cytotoxic drug' applies to any drug that can damage or kill cells. In practice, it is used more restrictively to mean drugs that inhibit cell division and are potentially useful in cancer chemotherapy.

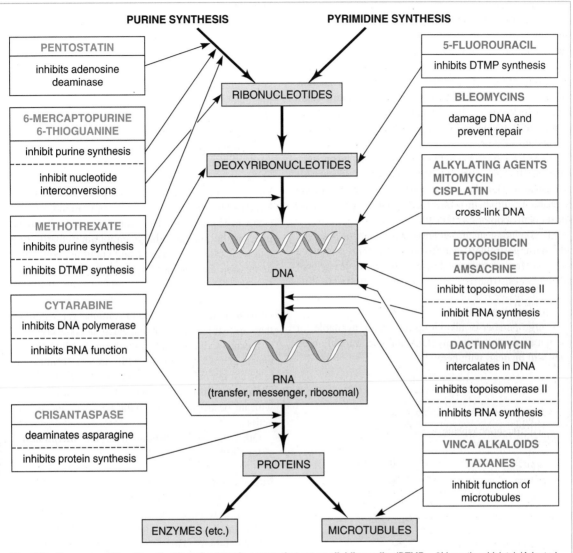

Fig. 42.5 Summary of the sites of action of cytotoxic agents that act on dividing cells. (DTMP = 2′deoxythymidylate) (Adapted from: Calabresi P, Parks R E 1980. In: Gilman A G, Goodman L S, Gilman A (eds) The pharmacological basis of therapeutics, 6th edn. Macmillan, New York)

a detailed list of their toxic effects is given in Laurence et al. (1997). In the following sections we concentrate on mechanisms of action and outline the main unwanted effects of commonly used anticancer agents.

ALKYLATING AGENTS AND RELATED COMPOUNDS

Alkylating agents and related compounds contain chemical groups which have the property of forming covalent bonds with suitable nucleophilic substances in the cell.

With alkylating agents themselves, the main step is the formation of a carbonium ion—a carbon atom with only six electrons in its outer shell (see Fig. 42.7). Such ions are highly reactive and react instantaneously with an electron donor such as amine, –OH, or –SH groups. Most of the cytotoxic anticancer alkylating agents are bifunctional, i.e. they have two alkylating groups.

The 7 nitrogen (N7) of guanine, being strongly nucleophilic, is probably the main molecular target for alkylation in DNA, although N1 and N3 of adenine and N3 of cytosine may also be affected. A bifunctional agent, being able to react with two groups, can cause intra- or interchain cross-linking (Figs 42.6 and 42.7). This can interfere not only with transcription but with replication, which is probably the critical effect of anticancer alkylating agents. Other effects of alkylation at guanine N7 are excision of the guanine base with main chain scission, or pairing of the alkylated guanine with thymine instead of cytosine and eventual substitution of the GC pair by an AT pair.

The main action occurs during replication, when some parts of the DNA are unpaired and more susceptible to alkylation; i.e. the effects are made manifest during S phase, resulting in a block at G_2 (see Fig. 42.1) and subsequent apoptotic cell death.

All alkylating agents depress bone marrow function and cause gastrointestinal disturbances. With prolonged use, two further unwanted effects occur: depression of gametogenesis (particularly in men) leading to sterility, and an increased risk of acute non-lymphocytic leukaemia and other malignancies.

A large number of alkylating agents are available for use in cancer chemotherapy. Only a few commonly used ones will be dealt with here.

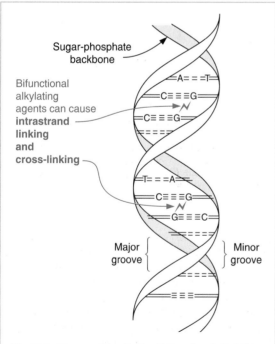

Fig. 42.6 The possible effects of bifunctional alkylating agents on DNA. (G = guanine; C = cytosine; A = adenine; T = thymine)

Sugar-phosphate backbone

Bifunctional alkylating agents can cause **intrastrand linking and cross-linking**

Major groove

Minor groove

Nitrogen mustards

Nitrogen mustards are related to sulphur mustard, the 'mustard gas' used during the First World War, and their basic formula is R-N-bis-(2-chloroethyl). Examples are given in Figure 42.8. In the body, each 2-chloroethyl side-chain undergoes an intramolecular cyclisation with the release of a chloride ion. The highly reactive ethylene immonium derivative so formed can interact with DNA (see Fig. 42.7) and other molecules.

Cyclophosphamide is probably the most commonly used alkylating agent. It is inactive until metabolised in the liver by the P450 mixed function oxidases (see Fig. 42.9 and Ch. 5). It has a pronounced effect on lymphocytes and can be used as an immunosuppressant (see Ch. 12). It is usually given orally or by intravenous injection but may also be given intramuscularly. Important toxic effects are nausea and vomiting, bone marrow depression and haemorrhagic cystitis. This latter effect (which also occurs with the related drug, **ifosfamide**) is due to the metabolite acrolein and can be ameliorated by increasing fluid intake and administering compounds that are sulphydryl donors, such as N-acetylcysteine or **mesna** (sodium-2-mercapto-ethane sulphonate). These agents interact specifically with acrolein, forming a non-toxic compound. See also Chapters 5 and 49.

Estramustine is a combination of mustine (see above) with an oestrogen. It has both cytotoxic and hormonal action.

Other nitrogen mustards used are **melphalan** and **chlorambucil**.

Nitrosoureas

Examples of the nitrosoureas are the chloroethylnitrosoureas, **lomustine** and **carmustine** (see Fig. 42.8), which, because they are lipid-soluble and can thus cross the blood–brain barrier, may be used against tumours of the brain and meninges. However, most nitrosoureas have a severe cumulative depressive effect on the bone marrow that starts 3–6 weeks after initiation of treatment.

Busulphan

Busulphan has a selective effect on the bone marrow, depressing the formation of granulocytes and platelets in low dosage and red cells in higher dosage. It has little or no effect on lymphoid tissue or the gastrointestinal tract. It is used in chronic granulocytic leukaemia.

Other alkylating agents are **thiotepa** and **treosulphan**.

Cisplatin

Cisplatin is a water-soluble planar coordination complex containing a central platinum atom surrounded by two

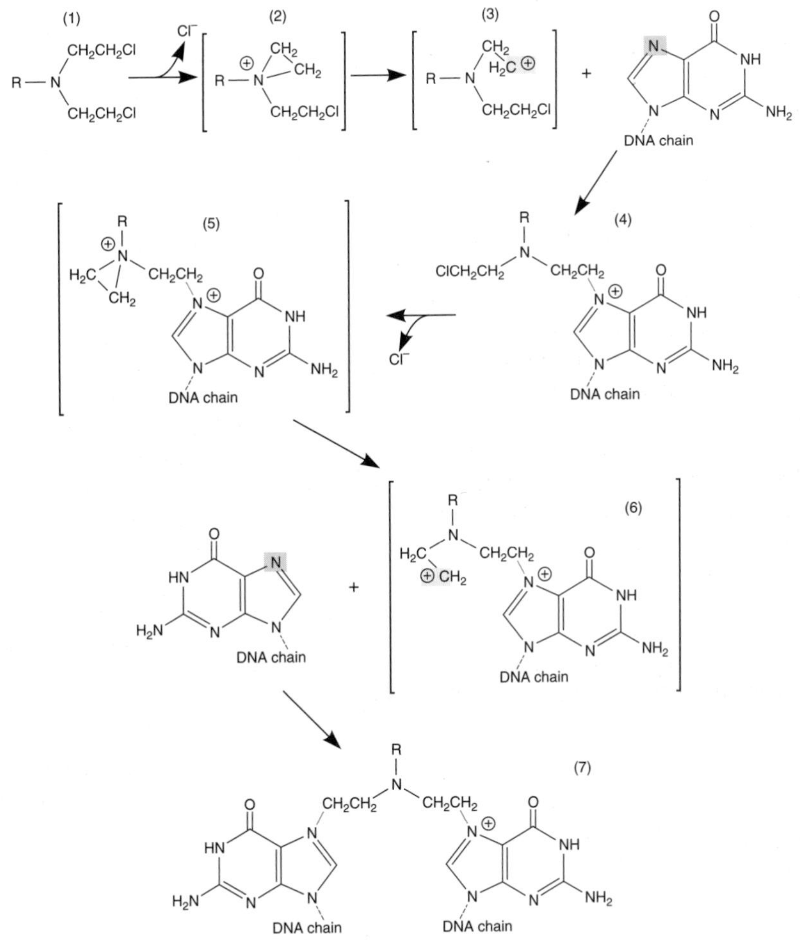

Fig. 42.7   An example of alkylation and cross-linking of DNA by a nitrogen mustard. A bis(chloroethyl)amine (1) undergoes intramolecular cyclisation forming an unstable ethylene immonium cation and releasing a chloride ion (2), the tertiary amine being transformed to a quaternary ammonium compound. The strained ring of the ethylene immonium intermediate opens to form a reactive carbonium ion (in light blue box) (3), which reacts immediately with N7 of guanine (in grey box) to give 7-alkylguanine (bond shown in blue), the N7 being converted to a quaternary ammonium nitrogen (4). A bifunctional alkylating agent may undergo a second cyclisation (5), with carbonium ion formation—in light blue box (6), and interact with another guanine residue—in grey box—thus linking two bases as shown in Figure 42.6 (7).

chlorine atoms and two ammonia groups (Fig. 42.8). Its action is analogous to that of the alkylating agents. When it enters the cell, chloride ions dissociate leaving a reactive diamine–platinum complex which reacts with water and then interacts with DNA. It causes intrastrand cross-linking—probably between N7 and O6 of adjacent guanine molecules—which results in the breaking of the hydrogen bonds between the guanine and cytosine bases and thus local denaturation of the DNA chain.

Cisplatin is given by slow intravenous injection or infusion. It is seriously nephrotoxic unless regimes of hydration and diuresis are instituted. It has low myelotoxicity but causes very severe nausea and vomiting. 5-HT$_3$-receptor antagonists, e.g. **ondansetron** (see Chs 9 and 21), are extremely effective in preventing this and have transformed cancer chemotherapy with this compound. Tinnitus and hearing loss in the high frequency range may occur, as may peripheral neuropathies, hyperuricaemia and anaphylactic reactions.

It has revolutionised the treatment of solid tumours of the testes and ovary.

Carboplatin is a derivative of cisplatin. It causes less

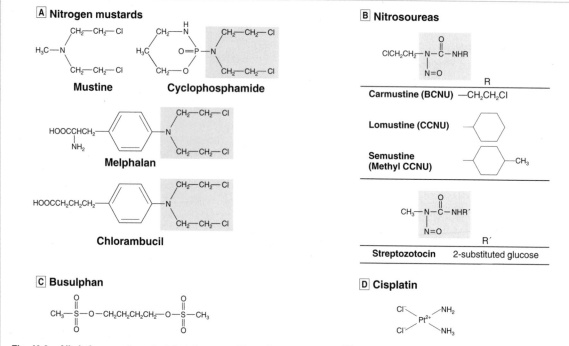

Fig. 42.8 **Alkylating agents and related drugs used in anticancer therapy.** [A] Nitrogen mustards; the portion of the molecule within the light blue box is the nitrogen mustard group. [B] Nitrosoureas; the portion within the grey box is the nitrosourea group. [C] Busulphan (an alkylsulphonate). [D] Cisplatin.

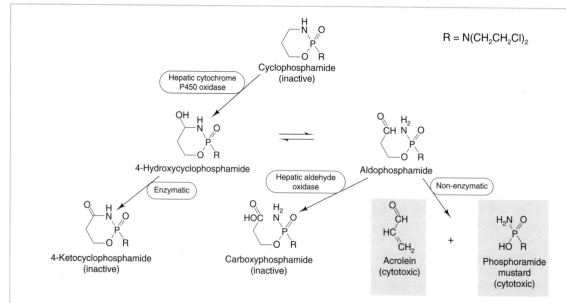

Fig. 42.9 **The metabolism of cyclophosphamide.** Cyclophosphamide is inactive until metabolised in the liver by P450 mixed function oxidases to 4-hydroxycyclophosphamide, which forms aldophosphamide reversibly. Aldophosphamide is conveyed to other tissues where it is converted to phosphoramide mustard (the actual cytotoxic molecule) and acrolein, which is responsible for unwanted effects. The active metabolites are shown in blue boxes.

nephrotoxicity, neurotoxicity and ototoxicity, and less severe nausea and vomiting than cisplatin, but is more myelotoxic.

Dacarbazine, a pro-drug, is activated in the liver, and the resulting compound is subsequently cleaved in the target cell to release an alkylating derivative. *Unwanted*

Anticancer drugs: alkylating agents and related compounds

- Alkylating agents have alkyl groups which can form covalent bonds with cell substituents; a carbonium ion is the reactive intermediate. Most have two alkylating groups and can cross-link two nucleophilic sites such as the N7 of guanine in DNA. Cross-linking can cause defective replication due to pairing of alkylguanine with thymine leading to substitution of AT for GC, or excision of guanine and chain breakage.
- Their principal effect occurs during DNA synthesis; the resulting DNA damage triggers apoptosis.
- Unwanted effects include myelosuppression, sterility and risk of non-lymphocytic leukaemia.
- The main alkylating agents are:
  — Nitrogen mustards: e.g. cyclophosphamide, which is activated to give aldophosphamide, which is then converted to phosphoramide mustard (the cytotoxic molecule) and acrolein (which causes bladder damage that can be ameliorated by mesna). Cyclophosphamide myelosuppression affects particularly the lymphocytes.
  — Nitrosoureas: e.g. lomustine may act on non-dividing cells; can cross the blood–brain barrier; causes delayed, cumulative myelotoxicity.
- Cisplatin causes intrastrand linking in DNA; it has low myelotoxicity but causes severe nausea and vomiting and can be nephrotoxic. It has revolutionised the treatment of germ cell tumours.

effects include myelotoxicity and severe nausea and vomiting.

ANTIMETABOLITES

Folate antagonists

The main folate antagonist is **methotrexate**: it is one of the most widely used antimetabolites in cancer chemotherapy.

Folates are essential for the synthesis of purine nucleotides and thymidylate, which in turn are essential for DNA synthesis and cell division. (This topic is also dealt with in Chs 18, 41 and 46.) In structure, folates consist of three elements: a heterobicyclic pteridine, *p*-aminobenzoic acid (PABA) and glutamic acid (Fig. 42.10). Folates in the blood have a single glutamate residue, but most intracellular folates are converted to polyglutamates. These polyglutamates are preferentially retained within the cells. In order to act as coenzymes, folates must be reduced to tetrahydrofolate (FH_4). This reaction is catalysed by *dihydrofolate reductase* and occurs in two steps, first to dihydrofolate (FH_2), then to FH_4 (Fig. 42.11). Folate polyglutamates have a much higher affinity for dihydrofolate reductase than does folate monoglutamate. FH_4 functions as a cofactor in the transfer of one-carbon units, a process which is essential both for the methylation of uracil in 2-deoxyuridylate (DUMP) to form thymidylate (DTMP) and thus for the synthesis of DNA, and also for the de novo synthesis of purines (see also Fig. 18.4).

During the formation of DTMP from DUMP, FH_4 is converted back to FH_2 (Fig. 42.11). Dihydrofolate reductase has a crucial role in maintaining the level of intracellular FH_4 by reduction of the FH_2 produced from folate reduction and that generated during thymidylate

---

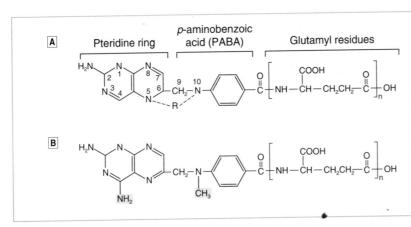

Fig. 42.10 Structure of (A) folic acid and (B) methotrexate. Both compounds are shown as polyglutamates. In tetrahydrofolate, one-carbon groups (R) are transported on N5 or N10 or both (shown dotted). See Figures 18.2, 18.3 and 18.4. The points at which methotrexate differs from endogenous folic acid are shown in the blue boxes.

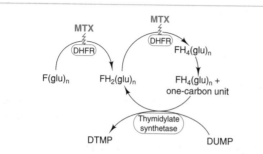

Fig. 42.11 Simplified diagram of action of methotrexate on thymidylate synthesis. Tetrahydrofolate polyglutamate [FH$_4$ (glu)$_n$] functions as a carrier of a one-carbon unit, providing the methyl group necessary for the conversion of 2′deoxyuridylate (DUMP) to 2′deoxythymidylate (DTMP) by thymidylate synthetase. This one-carbon transfer results in the oxidation of FH$_4$(glu)$_n$ to FH$_2$(glu)$_n$. (DHFR = dihydrofolate reductase; MTX = methotrexate)

synthesis. **Methotrexate** has a higher affinity for dihydrofolate reductase than has FH$_2$; it thus inhibits the enzyme (Fig. 42.11) and depletes intracellular FH$_4$. The binding of methotrexate to dihydrofolate reductase involves an additional hydrogen bond or ionic bond not present when FH$_2$ binds. The reaction most sensitive to FH$_4$ depletion is thymidylate synthesis, which is inhibited at a methotrexate concentration of 1 nmol/l, whereas inhibition of purine synthesis requires 10 times this concentration.

Methotrexate is usually given orally but can also be given intramuscularly, intravenously or intrathecally.

The drug has low lipid solubility and thus does not readily cross the blood–brain barrier. It is actively taken up into cells by the transport system used by folate, the rate of uptake of methotrexate being higher than that of the endogenous substance. As with folic acid, intracellular methotrexate is metabolised to polyglutamate derivatives. These polyglutamates are retained in the cell for some time (weeks or months in some tissues) in the absence of extracellular drug.

Resistance to methotrexate may develop in tumour cells, a variety of mechanisms being involved: decreased membrane transport, altered dihydrofolate reductase with reduced affinity for the drug, increased amounts of the enzyme, and, possibly, decreased polyglutamation of the drug.

Unwanted effects are depression of the bone marrow and damage to the epithelium of the gastrointestinal tract; pneumonitis can occur. In addition, when high-dose regimes are used, there may be nephrotoxicity, due to precipitation of the drug or a metabolite in the renal tubules. High-dose regimes (doses 10 times greater than the standard doses), sometimes used in cases of methotrexate resistance, must be followed by 'rescue' with **folinic acid** (a form of tetrahydrofolate).

Pyrimidine analogues

Fluorouracil interferes with thymidylate synthesis and therefore with synthesis of DNA. Its structure is given in Figure 42.12. It is converted into a 'fraudulent' nucleotide fluorodeoxyuridine monophosphate (FDUMP). This interacts with thymidylate synthetase and the folate cofactors, but cannot be converted into thymidylate because, in FDUMP, fluorine has replaced hydrogen at C5 where methylation would take place, and this carbon–fluorine bond is less susceptible to enzymic cleavage than the carbon–hydrogen bond. The result is inhibition of DNA synthesis but not RNA or protein synthesis.

Fluorouracil is usually given parenterally. The main *unwanted effects* are gastrointestinal epithelial damage and myelotoxicity. Cerebellar disturbances can occur.

A newer thymidylate synthesis inhibitor is **tomudex**.

Cytarabine (cytosine arabinoside; Fig. 42.12) is an analogue of the naturally occurring nucleoside, 2′deoxycytidine. Cytarabine enters the target cell and undergoes the same phosphorylation reactions as the physiological nucleoside, to give the triphosphate. The drug is incorporated into both RNA and DNA to a limited extent, but its main cytotoxic action is the inhibition of DNA

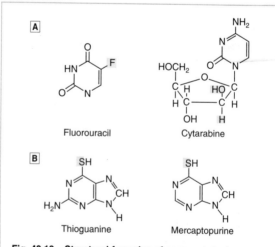

Fig. 42.12 Structural formulae of some cytotoxic antimetabolites. [A] Pyrimidine analogues. [B] Purine analogues. The points at which the drugs differ from endogenous compounds are shown in the blue boxes.

polymerase by its triphosphate. (The DNA polymerases require the triphosphates of the four deoxyribonucleosides for DNA synthesis—illustrated in Fig. 41.7.) Both replication and repair synthesis are inhibited by cytosine arabinoside triphosphate, the former more than the latter.

The main *unwanted effects* are on the bone marrow and the gastrointestinal tract. It causes nausea and vomiting.

Gemcitabine, a promising new analogue of cytarabine, has fewer unwanted actions—an influenza-like syndrome and mild myelotoxicity.

Purine analogues

The main anticancer purine analogues include **fludarabine, pentostatin, cladribine, mercaptopurine** and **thioguanine** (Fig. 42.12).

Fludarabine is metabolised to the triphosphate and inhibits DNA synthesis by actions similar to cytarabine. It is myelosuppressive.

Pentostatin has a different mechanism of action. It inhibits adenosine deaminase, the enzyme that catalyses deamination of adenosine to inosine. This action can interfere with critical pathways in purine metabolism and have significant effects on cell proliferation.

Other purine analogues—the immunosuppressant **azathioprine**, which gives rise to mercaptopurine in vivo (see Fig. 13.3) and the xanthine oxidase inhibitor, **allopurinol** (see Fig. 13.2)—are used for non-malignant conditions. Allopurinol inhibits the breakdown of mercaptopurine and increases both its effect and its toxicity.

Anticancer drugs: antimetabolites

These drugs block or subvert pathways in DNA synthesis.

- Folate antagonists. Methotrexate inhibits dihydrofolate reductase, preventing generation of tetrahydrofolate; the main result is interference with thymidylate synthesis. Methotrexate is taken up into cells by the folate carrier, and, like folate, converted to the polyglutamate form. Normal cells affected by high doses can be 'rescued' by folinic acid. Unwanted effects: myelosuppression, possible nephrotoxicity.
- Pyrimidine analogues. Fluorouracil is converted to a fraudulent nucleotide and inhibits thymidylate synthesis. Cytarabine its triphosphate form inhibits DNA polymerase; potent myelosuppressive.
- Purine analogues. Mercaptopurine is converted into a fraudulent nucleotide. Fludarabine its triphosphate form inhibits DNA polymerase; it is myelosuppressive. Pentostatin inhibits adenosine deaminase—a critical pathway in purine metabolism.

CYTOTOXIC ANTIBIOTICS

Antitumour antibiotics produce their effects mainly by direct action on DNA.

The anthracyclines

The main anticancer anthracycline antibiotic is **doxorubicin**. Others are **idarubicin, epirubicin, aclarubicin,** and **mitozantrone**.

Doxorubicin has several cytotoxic actions. It binds to DNA and inhibits both DNA and RNA synthesis, but its main cytotoxic action appears to be mediated through an effect on *topoisomerase II* (a DNA gyrase; see Ch. 41, p. 656), the activity of which is markedly increased in proliferating cells. The significance of the enzyme lies in the fact that during replication of the DNA helix, reversible swivelling needs to take place around the replication fork in order to prevent the daughter DNA molecule becoming inextricably entangled during mitotic segregation. The swivel is produced by topoisomerase II, which nicks both DNA strands and subsequently reseals the breaks. Doxorubicin intercalates in the DNA and its effect is, in essence, to stabilise the DNA–topoisomerase II complex after the strands have been nicked, thus causing the process to seize up at this point.

It is given by intravenous infusion. Extravasation at the injection site can cause local necrosis.

In addition to the general *unwanted effects* (p. 655), doxorubicin can cause cumulative, dose-related cardiac damage, leading to dysrhythmias and heart failure. This action may be due to generation of free radicals. Marked hair loss frequently occurs.

This drug is widely used but may eventually be replaced by **idarubicin**.

Epirubicin and **mitozantrone** are structurally related to doxorubicin. Mitozantrone has dose-related cardiotoxicity and causes bone marrow suppression. Epirubicin is less cardiotoxic than doxorubicin.

Dactinomycin intercalates, in the minor groove of DNA, between adjacent guanosine–cytosine pairs, interfering with the movement of RNA polymerase along the gene and thus preventing transcription. There is also evidence that it has a similar action to the anthracyclines on topoisomerase II. It can have all the toxic effects outlined previously at the beginning of this chapter.

The **bleomycins** are a group of metal-chelating glycopeptide antibiotics that degrade preformed DNA, causing chain fragmentation and release of free bases. Their action on DNA is thought to involve chelation of ferrous iron and interaction with oxygen, resulting in the oxidation of the iron and generation of superoxide and/or hydroxyl radicals. Bleomycin is most effective in the G_2 phase of the cell cycle and mitosis, but is also active against non-dividing cells, i.e. cells in the G_0 phase (Fig. 42.1). In contrast to most anticancer drugs, bleomycin causes little myelosuppression. Its most serious toxic effect is pulmonary fibrosis, which occurs in 10% of patients treated and is reported to be fatal in 1%. Allergic reactions can occur. About half the patients manifest mucocutaneous reactions (the palms are frequently affected) and many develop hyperpyrexia.

Mitomycin, after enzymatic activation in the cells, functions as a bifunctional alkylating agent, alkylating preferentially at O6 of guanine. It cross-links DNA and may also degrade DNA through the generation of free radicals. It causes marked myelosuppression and can also cause kidney damage and fibrosis of lung tissue.

> **Anticancer drugs: cytotoxic antibiotics**
>
> - Doxorubicin inhibits DNA and RNA synthesis; the DNA effect is mainly due to interference with topoisomerase II action. Unwanted effects: nausea and vomiting, myelosuppression, hair loss; it is cardiotoxic in high doses.
> - Bleomycin causes fragmentation of DNA chains. It can act on non-dividing cells. Unwanted effects: fever, allergies, mucocutaneous reactions, pulmonary fibrosis. Virtually no myelosuppression.
> - Dactinomycin intercalates in DNA, interfering with RNA polymerase and inhibiting transcription. It also interferes with the action of topoisomerase II. Unwanted effects: nausea and vomiting, myelosuppression.
> - Mitomycin is activated to give an alkylating metabolite.

PLANT DERIVATIVES

Vinca alkaloids

Vinca alkaloids are derived from the periwinkle plant, the main alkaloids being **vincristine**, **vinblastine** and **vindesine**. They act by binding to tubulin and inhibit its polymerisation into microtubules, preventing spindle formation in mitosing cells and causing arrest at metaphase. Their effects only become manifest during mitosis. They also inhibit other cellular activities that involve the microtubules, such as leukocyte phagocytosis and chemotaxis as well as axonal transport in neurons.

The vinca alkaloids are relatively non-toxic. Vincristine has very mild myelosuppressive activity, but causes paraesthesias (sensory changes) and neuromuscular abnormalities fairly frequently. Vinblastine is less neurotoxic but causes leukopenia, while vindesine has both moderate myelotoxicity and neurotoxicity.

A new vinca alkaloid is **vinorelbine**.

Etoposide is derived from mandrake root. Its mode of action is not clearly known but may be due to inhibition of mitochondrial function and of nucleoside transport, as well as to an effect on topoisomerase II similar to that seen with doxorubicin (see above).

Unwanted effects include nausea and vomiting, myelosuppression and hair loss.

Taxanes

The taxanes, **paclitaxel** and **docelatel** are derivatives of yew tree bark. They act on microtubules, stabilising them (in effect 'freezing' them) in the polymerised state. This has repercussions similar to those described above for the vinca alkaloids. Unwanted effects, which can be serious, include bone marrow suppression and cumulative neurotoxicity. Hypersensitivity to paclitaxel is liable to occur and requires pretreatment with corticosteroids and antihistamines.

Campothecins

The campothecins, **irinotecan** and **topotecan**, bind to and inhibit topoisomerase I, high levels of which occur throughout the cell cycle. Diarrhoea and reversible bone marrow depression occur, but in general, these drugs have fewer unwanted effects than most other anticancer agents.

> **Anticancer drugs: plant derivatives**
>
> - Vincristine inhibits mitosis at metaphase by binding to tubulin. Relatively non-toxic, but can cause unwanted neuromuscular effects.
> - Etoposide inhibits DNA synthesis by an action on topoisomerase II, and also inhibits mitochondrial function. Common unwanted effects include vomiting, myelosuppression and alopecia.
> - Paclitaxel stabilises microtubules, inhibiting mitosis; relatively toxic, hypersensitivity reactions occur.
> - Irinotecan binds to and inhibits topoisomerase 1; relatively few toxic effects.

HORMONES

Tumours derived from hormone-sensitive tissues may be hormone-dependent. Their growth can be inhibited by hormones with opposing actions, by hormone antagonists or by agents that inhibit the synthesis of the relevant hormones. Hormones or hormone analogues which themselves have inhibitory actions on particular tissues can be used in treatment of tumours of those tissues.

Glucocorticoids have inhibitory effects on lymphocyte proliferation (see Ch. 12) and are used in leukaemias and lymphomas. They are also used in a supportive role in other cancers on the basis of their effect on raised intracranial pressure.

Oestrogens, such as **fosfestrol** (a pro-drug, activated by acid phosphatase in prostatic tissue to yield stilboestrol), block the effect of androgens in androgen-dependent prostatic tumours, though this is a minor use; these tumours are best treated with gonadotrophin-releasing hormone analogues (see below).

One use of oestrogens in anticancer therapy is to employ these steroids to *recruit* resting mammary cancer cells (i.e. cells in compartment B; see above) into the proliferating pool of cells (i.e. into compartment A), thus allowing a greater killing efficacy of the cytotoxic drugs which are then given.

Progestogens have been useful in endometrial neoplasms and have also been used in renal tumours. The main agents used are **megestrol** and **medroxyprogesterone**.

The hormone-dependency of tumours treated with steroids is, in general, related to the presence of steroid receptors in the malignant cells.

Gonadotrophin-releasing hormone analogues

As explained in Chapter 26 (p. 446) analogues of the gonadotrophin-releasing hormones, such as **goserelin**, can, under certain circumstances, inhibit gonadotrophin release. It can be used to treat advanced breast cancer in premenopausal women and prostate cancer. The surge of testosterone secretion which can occur in prostate cancer patients so treated can be prevented by an anti-androgen such as **cyproterone** (p. 445).

An analogue of somatostatin, **octreotide** (see p. 411), is used to treat various hormone-secreting tumours of the gastrointestinal tract such as VIPomas, glucagonomas, carcinoid syndrome and gastrinomas. These tumours express somatostatin receptors, activation of which inhibits cell proliferation, as well as hormone secretion.

Hormone antagonists

Hormone antagonists can be effective in several hormone-sensitive tumours.

Anti-oestrogens

An anti-oestrogen, **tamoxifen** (p. 441), is remarkably effective in some cases of hormone-dependent breast cancer, and may have a role in preventing these cancers. In breast tissue, tamoxifen competes with endogenous oestrogens for the oestrogen receptors and inhibits the transcription of oestrogen-responsive genes. Tamoxifen is also reported to have cardioprotective effects, partly by virtue of its ability to protect low density lipoproteins against oxidative damage.

Anti-androgens

Androgen antagonists, **flutamide** and **cyproterone**, are used in prostate tumours.

Adrenal hormone synthesis inhibitors

Several agents which inhibit synthesis of adrenal hormones have effects in postmenopausal breast cancer. The drugs used are **formestane**, which acts at a late stage of sex hormone synthesis, inhibiting the enzyme, aromatase, which metabolises androgens to oestrogens (see Fig. 26.3), and **trilostane** and **aminoglutethimide** (see Fig. 24.6) which inhibit sex hormone synthesis at an early stage. Replacement of corticosteroids is necessary with these latter two agents.

RADIOACTIVE ISOTOPES

Radioactive isotopes have a place in the therapy of certain tumours; e.g. **radioactive iodine** (^{131}I) is used in treating thyroid tumours (discussed in Ch. 25).

Anticancer agents: hormones and radioactive isotopes

- Hormones or their antagonists are used in hormone-sensitive tumours:
  — Glucocorticoids for leukaemias and lymphomas
  — Tamoxifen for breast tumours
  — GnRH analogues for prostate and breast tumours
  — Antiandrogens for prostate cancers
  — Inhibitors of sex hormone synthesis for postmenopausal breast cancer.
- Radioactive isotopes can be targeted at specific tissues, e.g. ^{131}I for thyroid tumours.

MISCELLANEOUS AGENTS

Procarbazine inhibits DNA and RNA synthesis and interferes with mitosis at interphase. Its effects may be due to the production of active metabolites. It is given orally.

It interacts with some agents: it causes disulfiram-like actions with alcohol (see Ch. 48), exacerbates the effects of CNS depressants and, because it is a weak monoamine oxidase inhibitor, can produce hypertension if given with certain sympathomimetic agents (Ch. 48). It causes the usual unwanted effects (p. 655), thus it can be leukaemogenic, carcinogenic and teratogenic. Allergic skin reactions may necessitate cessation of treatment.

Hydroxyurea is a urea analogue that inhibits ribonucleotide reductase, thus interfering with the conversion of ribonucleotides to deoxyribonucleotides. It has the usual unwanted effects (p. 655), bone marrow depression being significant. Some experts use hydroxyurea in selected patients with sickle cell anaemia because of its ability to promote formation of fetal haemoglobin, which prevents sickling of red blood cells.

Crisantaspase is a preparation of the enzyme asparaginase, given intramuscularly or intravenously. It breaks down asparagine to aspartic acid and ammonia. It is active against tumour cells which, having lost the capacity to synthesise asparagine, now require an exogenous source of it, e.g. acute lymphoblastic leukaemia cells. Most normal body cells are able to synthesise asparagine, and the drug thus has a fairly selective action on certain tumours. It has very little suppressive effect on the bone marrow, or the mucosa of the gastrointestinal tract or hair follicles. It causes nausea and vomiting and it can cause CNS depression, anaphylactic reactions and liver damage.

Mitotane interferes with the synthesis of adrenocortical steroids (Ch. 24) having eventually a cytotoxic action on cells in the adrenal cortex. It is used solely for tumours of these cells.

Amsacrine has a mechanism of action similar to that of doxorubicin (p. 677). Bone marrow depression and cardiac toxicity have been reported.

Biological response modifiers

Agents which enhance the host's response are referred to as **biological response modifiers**. Some, e.g. γ-**interferon**, **aldesleukin** (a preparation of interleukin 2), and **tretinoin** are in use for selected tumours. Tretinoin is a powerful inducer of differentiation in leukaemic cells and is used as an adjunct to chemotherapy.

Anticancer drugs: miscellaneous agents

- Procarbazine inhibits DNA and RNA synthesis and interferes with mitosis.
- Crisantaspase is active against acute lymphoblastic leukaemia cells which cannot synthesise asparagine.
- Hydroxyurea inhibits ribonucleotide reductase.
- Amsacrine acts on topoisomerase II.
- Mitozantrone causes DNA chain breakage.
- Mitotane stops synthesis of adrenocortical steroids.

RESISTANCE TO ANTICANCER DRUGS

The resistance which neoplastic cells manifest to cytotoxic drugs can be primary (present when the drug is first given) or acquired (developing during treatment with the drug). Acquired resistance may be due either to adaptation of the tumour cells or to mutation, with the emergence of cells which are less affected or unaffected by the drug and which consequently have a selective advantage over the sensitive cells. Examples of various mechanisms of resistance are:

- Decreased accumulation of drugs in cells due to the increased expression of a cell surface, energy-dependent drug transport protein, termed P-glycoprotein (see Bellamy 1996). The transporter is coded for by the *mdr* gene and is responsible for *multidrug resistance* to many structurally dissimilar anticancer drugs (doxorubicin, vinblastine, dactinomycin, etc.). The physiological role of P-glycoprotein is thought to be the protection of cells against environmental toxins. The transporter consists of 12 transmembrane domains round a central core or barrel. It functions as a hydrophobic 'vacuum cleaner', picking up drugs as they enter the cell membrane and expelling them through the barrel to the outside. Several non-cytotoxic agents can reverse multidrug resistance (see p. 683).
- A decrease in amount of drug taken up by the cell (methotrexate).
- Insufficient activation of the drug (mercaptopurine, fluorouracil, cytarabine). By this is meant that there may be decreased metabolism of these agents so that they do not enter the pathways where they would normally exert their effects. Thus, fluorouracil may not be converted to FDUMP, cytarabine may not undergo phosphorylation, mercaptopurine may not be converted into a 'fraudulent' nucleotide.
- Increase in inactivation (cytarabine, mercaptopurine).
- Increased concentration of target enzyme (methotrexate).
- Decreased requirement for substrate (crisantaspase).
- Increased utilisation of alternative metabolic pathways (antimetabolites).
- Rapid repair of drug-induced lesions (alkylating agents).
- Altered activity of target, for example modified topoisomerase II (doxorubicin).
- Mutations in the *p53* gene and overexpression of the *Bcl-2* gene family (several cytotoxic drugs).

DRUG EFFECTS ON THE CELL CYCLE AND THE POSSIBLE CLINICAL APPLICATIONS

The mitotic cycle of dividing cells can be considered to consist of four phases (see Fig. 42.1). Cells that are constantly in cell cycle constitute the 'growth fraction' of the tumour.

Anticancer drugs can be classified in terms of their actions on the cycle as:

- *Phase-specific agents*, i.e. acting at a specific phase of the cell cycle. The vinca alkaloids act in mitosis. Cytarabine, hydroxyurea, fluorouracil, methotrexate and mercaptopurine act in S phase. Some of these compounds have some action during G_1 phase and thus may slow the entry of a cell into S phase, where it would be more susceptible to the drug.
- *Cycle-specific agents*, i.e. acting at all stages of the cell cycle and not having much effect on cells out of cycle: alkylating agents, dactinomycin, doxorubicin and cisplatin.
- *Cycle non-specific agents*, i.e. acting on cells whether in cycle or not: bleomycins and nitrosoureas.

It has been proposed that this information could be of value in selecting agents for clinical use. Tumours with a high growth fraction should respond to phase-specific and cycle-specific agents. For tumours with a small growth fraction the use of cycle non-specific agents (together with surgery or X-ray) could be considered. It has been suggested that combinations of cytotoxic drugs should be based on the above classification, but not all authorities agree that treatment schedules based on these principles are better than purely empirical schedules.

TREATMENT SCHEDULES

Treatment with combinations of several anticancer agents increases the cytotoxicity against cancer cells without necessarily increasing the general toxicity. Thus, for example, **methotrexate**, with mainly myelosuppressive toxicity, may be used in a regime with **vincristine**, which has mainly neurotoxicity. The few drugs with low myelotoxicity, such as **cisplatin** and **bleomycin**, are good candidates for combination regimes. Treatment with combinations of drugs also decreases the possibility of the development of resistance to individual agents. Detailed consideration of the combination schedules used in the clinic can be found in clinical pharmacology manuals; the subject is beyond the scope of this book. Drugs are often given in large doses intermittently, in several courses with intervals of 2–3 weeks between courses, rather than in small doses continuously. This is because such a regime permits the bone marrow to regenerate during the intervals. Furthermore, it has been shown that the same total dose of an agent is more effective when given in one or two large doses than in multiple small doses.

TECHNIQUES FOR DEALING WITH EMESIS AND MYELOSUPPRESSION

Emesis

The nausea and vomiting induced by many cancer chemotherapy agents constitutes an 'inbuilt deterrent' to patient compliance (see also Ch. 21, p. 377). It is a particular problem with cisplatin, but also complicates therapy with many other compounds, such as the alkylating agents. 5-HT$_3$-receptor antagonists such as **ondansetron** or **granisetron** (see Chs 9 and 21) are effective against cytotoxic-drug-induced vomiting. Of the other anti-emetic agents available (see p. 377), **metoclopramide** in high dose, given intravenously, has proved useful, and it is often combined with therapy with **dexamethasone** (Ch. 24) or **lorazepam** (Ch. 33). As metoclopramide commonly causes extrapyramidal side-effects in children and young adults, **diphenhydramine** (Ch. 13) can be used instead.

Myelosuppression

Myelosuppression limits the use of many anticancer agents. Regimes to overcome the problem have included removing some of the patient's bone marrow prior to giving the chemotherapy agent, and replacing it afterwards. This has been combined with purging of the bone marrow in vitro (see below). Administering **molgramostim**, then harvesting stem cells from the blood and multiplying them up in vitro with the relevant haemopoietic growth factors (Ch. 23) is now frequently used. The use of haemopoietic growth factors after replacement of the marrow has been successful in some cases. A further possibility is the introduction, into the extracted bone marrow, of the mutated gene which confers multidrug resistance, so that when replaced, the *marrow cells* (but not the cancer cells) will be resistant to the cytotoxic action of the anticancer drugs.

POSSIBLE FUTURE STRATEGIES FOR CANCER CHEMOTHERAPY

Some of the main drawbacks of the current chemotherapy of cancer are:

- the fact that current anticancer drugs are aimed at the destruction of the cancer cell rather than at the basic changes which make a cell malignant (see above, pp. 664–668)
- the lack of selectivity of anticancer drugs against tumour cells as compared with normal cells

- the development of resistance (particularly multidrug resistance) to anticancer drugs (see above)
- the fact that, with many tumours, total elimination of malignant cells is not possible with therapeutic doses, and the host's immune response is often not adequate to deal with the remaining cells.

Attempts are being made to overcome these problems—the first by developing new approaches based on the advances in knowledge of the biology of the cancer cell, the second by using selective targeting of anticancer compounds, the third by developing agents which reverse multidrug resistance and the fourth by boosting or augmenting the host's immune responses to the tumour.

APPROACHES BASED ON THE BIOLOGY OF THE CANCER CELL

As outlined above on page 664, there have been significant advances in our knowledge of the basis of malignancy, particularly as regards the role of oncogenes and tumour suppressor genes. In addition, there is now understanding of the factors underlying infiltration of cancer cells into adjacent tissues, metastasis and the signal transduction pathways for cell division and apoptosis. Compounds that target these aspects are being developed and tested and could well transform the treatment of cancer in the coming decade.

Progress is being made with antisense oligonucleotides (ONs). This topic is covered in Chapter 50 and discussed by Wagner & Flanagan (1997). ONs are small synthetic segments of single-stranded DNA that are complementary to a portion of the mRNA and which can bind to their corresponding sequence on the mRNA. This now double-stranded section—a hybrid of mRNA and ON DNA—prevents translation of the mRNA and thus blocks expression of the particular oncogene. Normal ONs are rapidly hydrolysed by nucleases; however, sulphur analogues (phosphorothioate ONs) are resistant to nucleases, and are being developed for therapeutic use. Phosphorothioate ONs that target the *Bcl-2* gene (see Fig. 42.2), and the genes for Raf and PKCγ (see Fig. 42.3) are in clinical trial.

Targeting the mechanisms by which cancer cells spread in the body has the potential to be successful. Metalloproteinases are involved in both the invasiveness and metastasis of cancer (see above, pp 666–667). Agents that inhibit these enzymes (e.g. **marimastat**) are already in phase III clinical trial. Other angiogenesis inhibitors being tested clinically include an analogue of fumagillin (a fungal product) and IL-2 (which induces an anti-angiogenic protein) and a calcium-channel blocker (Baringa

1997). Another approach which has been successful in experimental animals is the use of a monoclonal antibody against an angiogenesis factor spontaneously produced by tumour cells. For a review of angiogenesis inhibitors currently under development, see Shawver et al. (1997).

Several approaches target the signal transduction mechanisms for cell division—though affecting the proliferation of normal cells may be a hazard.

One example is the development of agents which block the capacity of mutant *ras* genes to make cells malignant. The role of the Ras protein in the signal transduction for cell division has been outlined on page 668 and in Figure 42.3. In normal cells, Ras, after synthesis, moves to the cell membrane to which it becomes attached by a sort of molecular 'hook'—a farnesyl group. This group is added to the protein by the enzyme, farnesyl transferase. Compounds that inhibit this enzyme have recently been produced. They have been shown, in in vitro tests, to reverse the malignant transformation in cancer cells containing the *ras* oncogene, restoring normal growth patterns; they did not interfere with cell division in normal cells (see Travis 1993).

Some endogenous peptides are potent growth factors for small cell lung cancer cells which can themselves then produce growth-stimulating peptides. Analogues that are broad-spectrum antagonists of these growth factors for this cancer are in clinical trial.

Based on the knowledge that cancer development is associated with alterations of the cdks that promote progression through the cell cycle (Fig. 42.1), chemical inhibitors of cdks are being developed (see Meijer 1996). One such—flavopiridol—is in clinical trial.

Tyrosine kinases are critical in the proliferation pathway (Fig. 42.3). Inhibitors of these enzymes, tyrphostins, with high activity against specific tyrosine kinases are being produced and tested—so far in vitro.

Restoration of tumour suppressor gene function is under examination. More than 50% of human tumours carry a mutation of the *p53* gene (see p. 668 and Figs 42.1, 42.2 and 42.4). There is a long way to go still but preliminary studies have shown that virally mediated introduction of the wild-type (normal) *p53* gene has inhibited cancer growth in some patients. Gene therapy is discussed in Chapter 50.

The use of a retroviral vector to deliver antisense oligomers to block expression of a *ras* oncogene is being tested as a treatment of adenocarcinoma of the lung in the USA.

Agents that inhibit telomerase (see p. 666) could prove to be wide-spectrum anticancer agents, since many tumours express telomerase. This possibility is being explored.

THE TARGETING OF TOXINS AGAINST CANCER CELLS

As virtually all currently used anticancer drugs have a greater or lesser effect on normal cells, finding methods of selectively targeting cancer cells is a priority. Where tumour-specific or tumour-associated antigens can be identified, *monoclonal antibodies* against the antigens are raised (though problems arise because of the heterogeneity of antigen expression in tumour cells). These antibodies, or fragments of these antibodies, are used to direct *radioactive isotopes* or *toxic molecules* specifically to the malignant cells. Toxic molecules so used include ricin, diphtheria toxin, and *Pseudomonas aeruginosa* exotoxin A. A modification of this approach is the introduction into the body of a Fab fragment of monoclonal antibody coupled to a non-mammalian enzyme with the capacity to activate an anticancer pro-drug to a cytotoxic agent. Growth factors that preferentially bind to cancer cells can also be used to target toxins against the tumour. Clinical trials with these immunotoxins are being conducted. Photochemical activation of anticancer agents is also under examination.

Another use of monoclonal antibodies with bound toxins is to *purge* tumour cells from bone marrow taken from a patient, prior to the use of radiation and/or megadose chemotherapy regimes. Purging can also be accomplished by the use of complement (see Ch. 12, p. 200) after adding monoclonal antibodies against tumour cell antigens to the marrow in vitro. The purged marrow is then re-injected to reconstitute the bone marrow of the patient.

An unusual approach, now under test, is the use of a modified adenovirus to kill cancer cells. To replicate and lyse human cells, this virus has to enter cells while they are in the cell cycle. The modified virus expresses a protein that inactivates the *Rb* protein, one of the two main negative regulatory forces or 'superbrakes' in normal cells (see p. 664 and Figs 42.1, 42.3 and 42.4). Normal cells, which express the other superbrake—the *p53* protein—are not affected, but cancer cells that are *p53* deficient are lysed. Clinical trials are under way.

REVERSAL OF MULTIDRUG RESISTANCE

Several non-cytotoxic drugs (e.g. calcium-channel blockers) can reverse multidrug resistance. Development of related compounds could make it feasible to overcome this type of resistance. In addition, the use of antibodies, immunotoxins, antisense oligonucleotides (see above) or liposome-encapsulated agents could be useful in the elimination of cells with multidrug resistance (reviewed by Gottesman & Pastan 1993).

ENHANCEMENT OF THE HOST'S RESPONSE TO CANCER

Drugs that enhance the host's response to cancer are classified as **biological response modifiers**. Some biological response modifiers are already in use (see above). Others being investigated include various cytokines, e.g. interleukin 12.

A modification of this approach is the adoptive transfer of autologous tumour-infiltrating lymphocytes (TILs). It seems that some tumour genes that code for the antigens recognised by TILs can be characterised and cloned. Based on successful experiments in mice, it is proposed that a patient's TILs be grown up in vitro, sensitised against these antigens and then transferred to the patient.

Investigation of the efficacy of immunotherapy for tumours may be fruitful and cancer experts have been exhorted to get to grips with 'immunobabble'.

A combination of the various novel approaches to anticancer treatment cited above may be of even more potential value than their use alone. One way or another, it is likely that dramatic advances in the treatment of cancer will occur during the coming decade.

General approaches to cancer therapy

- Kill or remove malignant cells:
  - Cytotoxic drugs*
  - Surgery*
  - Irradiation*
  - Targeted cytotoxic agents (e.g. antibody-linked toxins).**
- Inactivate components of oncogene signalling pathway:
  - Inhibitors of cyclins, cdks, tyrosine kinases, Ras, etc.***
  - Antisense oligonucleotides.***
- Restore function of tumour suppressor genes:
  - Gene therapy approaches.**
- Employ tissue-specific proliferation inhibitors:
  - Oestrogens, anti-oestrogens, androgens, anti-androgens, glucocorticoids, gonadotrophin-releasing hormone analogues, octeotride.*
- Inhibit tumour growth, invasion, metastasis:
  - Inhibitors of angiogenesis**
  - Matrix metalloproteinase inhibitors.**
- Enhance host immune response
  - Cytokine-based therapies**
  - Gene therapy-based approaches.**
- Reverse drug resistance:
  - Inhibitors of multidrug resistance transporter.**

*Therapies in general use
**Therapies in development
***Potential approaches

REFERENCES AND FURTHER READING

Augustin H G 1998 Antiangiogenic tumour therapy: will it work? Trends Pharmacol Sci 19: 216–222 (*Excellent article; informative diagrams; lists endogenous regulators of angiogenesis, lists therapeutic strategies*)

Baringa M 1997 Designing therapies that target tumour blood vessels. Science 275: 482–484 (*Short coverage of new anti-angiogenesis therapies listing drugs in clinical trial*)

Barr P J, Tomei D L 1994 Apoptosis and its role in human disease. Bio/Technology 12: 487–493 (*Good coverage of the molecular mechanisms of apoptosis; lists references to numerous papers on pathophysiological disorders with disregulated apoptosis*)

Bellamy W T 1996 P-glycoproteins and multidrug resistance. Annu Rev Pharmacol Toxicol 36: 161–183 (*Detailed review*)

Brun C, Marchand S, Gilson E 1997 Proteins that bind to double-stranded regions of telomeric DNA. Trends Biochem Sci 7: 317–323 (*See particularly reference 5 in this article*)

Chabner B A, Longo D L 1996 Cancer chemotherapy and biotherapy, 2nd edn. Lippincott-Raven, Philadelphia (*Textbook with comprehensive coverage of anticancer drugs*)

Dale M M, Cunnane T C et al. 1999 The biology of cancer and anticancer drugs. In: Interactive pharmacology. Blackwell Science CD-ROM (*A simple, clear coverage with good diagrams, good animations, and MCQs*)

Fan T-P D, Jagger R, Bicknell R 1995 Controlling the vasculature: angiogenesis, anti-angiogenesis and vascular targeting of gene therapy. Trends Pharmacol Sci 16: 57–66 (*Review covering the process of angiogenesis, its role in cancer, CVS disease, and wound healing; lists angiogenesis inhibitors and discusses gene therapy*)

Finkel E 1997 Phase 1 cancer trials on mutant adenovirus near completion. Lancet 349: 547 (*Very short outline of a simple and unusual new approach to cancer therapy*)

Foye W O (ed) 1995 Cancer chemotherapeutic agents. American Chemical Society, Washington DC, p 698 (*Well-referenced textbook with emphasis on chemistry of anticancer drugs*)

Gottesman M M, Pastan I 1993 Biochemistry of multidrug resistance mediated by the multidrug transporter. Annu Rev Biochem 62: 385–427 (*Clear review*)

Grainger D J, Metcalf J C 1996 Tamoxifen: teaching an old drug new tricks. Nature Med 2: 381–385 (*The authors outline the actions and mechanisms of action of tamoxifen—anticancer, anti-osteoporotic effects*)

Greider C W, Blackburn E H 1996 Telomeres, telomerase and cancer. Scientific American (Feb): 80–85 (*Simple, clear overview with high-quality figures*)

Haber D A, Fearon E R 1998 The promise of cancer genetics. Lancet 351(SII): 1–8 (*Excellent coverage; detailed tables of mutations in proto-oncogenes and tumour-suppressor genes in human cancers*)

Harris A 1997 Antiangiogenesis for cancer therapy. Lancet 349 (suppl II): 13–15 (*Short article discussing mechanisms of tumour angiogenesis and possible clinical use of antiangiogenic drugs; one article in useful 30-page supplement on cancer with five other articles relevant for this chapter*)

Howell A, Dowsett M 1997 Recent advances in endocrine therapy of breast cancer. Br Med J 315: 863–866

Karp J E, Broder S 1995 Molecular foundations of cancer: new targets for intervention. Nature Med 1: 309–319 (*Covers tumourigenesis, and the positive and negative regulators of the cell cycle*)

Lane D 1998 The promise of molecular oncology. Lancet 351(SII): 17–20 (*Excellent*)

Lane D P 1994 p53 and human tumours. Br Med Bull 50: 582–599 (*Covers the properties, regulation of function, mutations and mechanism of action of p53 gene and the expression of p53 protein in tumours and normal tissue*)

Laurence, D R, Bennett P J, Brown M J 1997 Clinical pharmacology, 8th edn. Churchill Livingstone, Edinburgh, p 710 (*Good, well-written clinical textbook—a pleasure to read*)

Lee H-W, Blasco M A et al. 1998 Essential role of mouse telomerase in highly proliferative organs. Nature 392: 569–574

Mackensen A, Lindemann A, Mertelsman R 1997 Immunostimulatory cytokines in somatic cells and gene therapy of cancer. Cytokine and Growth Factor Rev 8: 119–128

McConkey D J, Zhivotovsky B, Orrenius S 1996 Apoptosis: molecular mechanisms and biomedical implications. Molec Aspects Med 17: 1–110 (*Monograph with chapters on the triggering, signalling and molecular regulation of apoptosis and its role in immunity, cancer and the CNS*)

Meijer L 1996 Chemical inhibitors of cyclin-dependent kinases. Trends Cell Biol 6: 393–397 (*Discusses mechanisms of action and therapeutic potential of cdk inhibitors*)

Meredith J E, Schwartz M A 1997 Integrins, adhesion and apoptosis. Trends Cell Biol 7: 146–150 (*Discusses integrin-activated survival signals and how these inhibit apoptosis*)

Orr-Weaver T L, Weinberg R A 1998 A checkpoint on the road to cancer. Nature 392: 223–224 (*Discusses the increase in mutability in the tumour cell genome*)

Rowe P M 1996 Campotothecins: new enthusiasm for an old drug. Lancet 347: 892–893 (*Short outline of mechanism of action of the campothecins*)

Rowinsky E K, Donehower R C 1995 Paclitaxel. N Engl J Med 15: 1004–1014 (*Detailed pharmacological coverage of this new anticancer agent*)

Rudin M, Thompson C B 1997 Apoptosis and disease. Annu Rev Med 48: 267–281 (*Covers regulation and clinical relevance of apoptosis*)

Schnitzer J E 1998 Vascular targeting as a strategy for cancer therapy. N Engl J Med 339: 472–473 (*Succinct article; good diagram*)

Scientific American September 1996 (*Has several papers on cancer. Those under the headings 'Fundamental Understandings', 'Improving Conventional Therapy' and 'Therapies of the Future' are relevant, simply written and very well illustrated*)

Shawver L K, Lipson K et al. 1997 Receptor tyrosine kinases as targets for inhibition of angiogenesis. Drug Discovery Today 2: 51–63

Travis J 1993 Novel anticancer agents move closer to reality. Science 260: 1877–1878

Wagner R W, Flanagan W M 1997 Antisense technology and prospects for therapy of viral infections and cancer. Mol Med Today (Jan): 31–38

Weinberg R A 1996 How cancer arises. Scientific American (Sept): 42–48 (*Simple, clear overview, listing main oncogenes, tumour suppressor genes and the cell cycle; excellent diagrams*)

43

Antibacterial drugs

A detailed classification of the bacteria of medical importance is beyond the scope of this book. However, a short list of the commoner and/or more important microorganisms which cause disease is given in Table 43.1.

Individual chemotherapeutic agents are dealt with briefly in this chapter and a general indication of their main antibacterial actions is given in Table 43.1. Some of the main diseases that may be caused by the organisms are included in the table but it should be understood that most of the organisms may, on occasion, produce other pathological conditions.

Certain principles should be borne in mind when choosing an antibiotic to treat a bacterial infection. It is important to determine the organism's susceptibility to antibacterial agents, if possible. In addition, certain host factors should be taken into account, such as previous exposure to antibiotics, age, renal and hepatic function, site of infection, concurrent administration of other drugs that might interact with the antibiotic, and whether the patient is pregnant or has a compromised immune system.

In Table 43.1, many of the organisms are classified as either Gram-positive or Gram-negative. This classification is based on whether the organisms do or do not stain with Gram's stain, but has a significance far beyond that of an empirical staining reaction. Gram-positive and Gram-negative organisms are different in several respects, not least in the structure of the cell wall, which has implications for the action of antibiotics.

The cell wall of Gram-positive organisms is a relatively simple structure, 15–50 nm thick. It consists of about 50% peptidoglycan (see p. 651 and Fig. 41.2), about 40–45% acidic polymer (which results in the cell surface being highly polar and carrying a negative charge) and about 5–10% proteins and polysaccharides. The strongly polar polymer layer influences the penetration of ionised molecules, and favours the penetration of positively charged compounds, such as **streptomycin**, into the cell.

The cell wall of Gram-negative organisms is much more complex. From the plasma membrane outwards it consists of the following:

- A periplasmic space containing enzymes and other components.

Table 43.1 General choice of antibiotics against common or important microorganisms*

Microorganism†	First choice antibiotic(s)‡	Second choice antibiotic(s)‡
Gram-positive cocci		
Staphylococcus (boils, infection of wounds, etc.)		
Non β-lactamase-producing	Penicillin G or V§	A cephalosporin, or vancomycin, or imipenem
β-lactamase-producing	A β-lactamase-resistant penicillin (e.g. flucloxacillin)	A cephalosporin, or amoxycillin + clavulanic acid, or vancomycin, or a macrolide, or a quinolone
Methicillin-resistant	Vancomycin ± gentamicin ± rifampicin	Co-trimoxazole, or ciprofloxacin, or a macrolide ± fusidic acid, or rifampicin
Streptococcus, haemolytic types (septic infections)	Penicillin G or V§ ± an aminoglycoside	A cephalosporin, or a macrolide, or vancomycin
Pneumococcus (pneumonia)	Penicillin G or V§, or ampicillin, or a macrolide	A cephalosporin
Gram-negative cocci		
Neisseria gonorrhoeae (gonorrhoea)	Amoxycillin + clavulanic acid, or ceftriaxone, or a quinolone	Spectinomycin, or cefotaxime, or a quinolone
Neisseria meningitidis (meningitis)	Penicillin G§	Chloramphenicol, or cefotaxime, or minocycline
Gram-positive rods		
Corynebacterium (diphtheria)	A macrolide	Penicillin G§
Clostridium (tetanus, gangrene)	Penicillin G§	A tetracycline, or a cephalosporin
Listeria monocytogenes (rare cause of meningitis and generalised infection in neonates)	Amoxycillin ± an aminoglycoside	Erythromycin ± an aminoglycoside
Gram-negative rods		
Enterobacteriaceae (coliform organisms)		
Escherichia coli, Enterobacter, Klebsiella		
—infections of urinary tract	An oral cephalosporin, or a quinolone	Extended-spectrum penicillin
—septicaemia	An aminoglycoside i.v., or cefuroxime	Imipenem, or a quinolone
Shigella (dysentery)	A quinolone	Ampicillin, or trimethoprim
Salmonella (typhoid, paratyphoid)	A quinolone, or ceftriaxone	Amoxycillin, or chloramphenicol, or trimethoprim
Haemophilus influenzae (infections of the respiratory tract, ear, sinuses; meningitis)	Ampicillin, or cefuroxime	Cefuroxime (not for meningitis), or chloramphenicol
Bordetella pertussis (whooping cough)	A macrolide	Ampicillin
Vibrio cholerae (cholera)	A tetracycline	A quinolone
Legionella pneumophila (pneumonia)	A macrolide ± rifampicin	
Helicobacter pylori (associated with peptic ulcer)	Metronidazole + amoxycillin + ranitidine¶ (2-week regime)	Clarithromycin + metronidazole + omeprazole¶ (1-week regime)
Pseudomonas aeruginosa		
—urinary tract infection	A quinolone	Antipseudomonal penicillins
—other infections (of burns etc.)	Antipseudomonal penicillins + tobramycin‖	Imipenem ± an aminoglycoside, or ceftazidime
Brucella (brucellosis)	Doxycycline + rifampicin	

Table 43.1 (contd)

Microorganism[†]	First choice antibiotic(s)[‡]	Second choice antibiotic(s)[‡]
Bacteroides fragilis		
—oropharyngeal infection	Penicillin G[§]	Metronidazole, or clindamycin
—gastrointestinal infection	Metronidazole, clindamycin	Imipenem
Gram-negative anaerobic rods (other than *B. fragilis*)	Penicillin G[§], or metronidazole	A cephalosporin, or clindamycin
Campylobacter (diarrhoea)	A macrolide, or a quinolone	A tetracycline, or gentamicin
Spirochaetes		
Treponema (syphilis, yaws)	Penicillin G[§]	A macrolide, or ceftriaxone
Borrelia (relapsing fever)	A tetracycline	Penicillin G[§]
Borrelia (Lyme disease)		
Leptospira (Weil's disease)	Penicillin G[§]	A tetracycline
Rickettsiae (typhus, tick-bite fever, Q fever, etc.)	A tetracycline	A quinolone
Mycobacteria (see text for details)		
Other organisms		
Mycoplasma pneumoniae	A tetracycline, or a macrolide	Ciprofloxacin
Chlamydia (trachoma, psittacosis, urogenital infections)	A tetracycline	A macrolide
Actinomyces (abscesses)	Penicillin G[§]	A tetracycline
Pneumocystis (pneumonia, especially in AIDS patients)	Co-trimoxazole (high dose)	Pentamidine, or atovaquone, or trimetrexate
Nocardia (lung disease)	Co-trimoxazole	

*This table is not meant to be a definitive guide for clinical treatment but a general indication of the main antimicrobial actions and thus of the overall usefulness of commonly used antibiotics. For a more comprehensive list, see Laurence et al. (1997). The selection of antibiotic to treat an infection will change as resistance occurs and as new agents are introduced. Susceptibility tests should be performed if possible.

[†]Only the main diseases caused by each organism are mentioned (in brackets).

[‡,±] signifies that an agent is to be used with or without another agent; if agents are to be used concomitantly, a plus sign only is used.

[§]Penicillin G = benzylpenicillin; Penicillin V = phenoxymethylpenicillin

[¶]These are anti-ulcer drugs, not antibiotics (see Ch. 21).

[||]Not in the same syringe

- A peptidoglycan layer 2 nm in thickness and comprising 5% of the cell wall mass; this is often linked to lipoprotein molecules which project outwards.
- An outer membrane consisting of a lipid bilayer similar in some respects to the plasma membrane. It contains protein molecules and on its inner aspect has lipoprotein that is linked to the peptidoglycan. Complex polysaccharides are important components on its outer surface. These are different in different strains of bacteria and are the main determinants of the antigenicity of the organism. They constitute the 'endotoxins' which, in vivo, trigger various aspects of the inflammatory reaction, activating complement, causing fever, etc. (see Ch. 12). In addition, there are proteins in the outer membrane that form transmembrane water-filled channels, termed 'porins', through which hydrophilic antibiotics can move freely.

Difficulty in penetrating this complex outer layer is probably the reason why some antibiotics are less active against Gram-negative than Gram-positive bacteria. This is the basis of the extraordinary insusceptibility to most antibiotic drugs of *Pseudomonas aeruginosa*, a pathogen which can cause life-threatening infections in neutropenic patients and patients with burns and wounds.

The lipopolysaccharide of the cell wall is also a major barrier to penetration.

Antibiotics for which penetration is a problem include **penicillin G**, **methicillin**, **the macrolides**, **rifampicin**, **fusidic acid**, **vancomycin**, **bacitracin** and **novobiocin**.

ANTIMICROBIAL AGENTS WHICH INTERFERE WITH THE SYNTHESIS OR ACTION OF FOLATE

SULPHONAMIDES

In the 1930s Domagk first demonstrated that a chemotherapeutic agent could influence the course of a bacterial infection. The drug was **prontosil**, a dye which proved to be a pro-drug, inactive in vitro and needing to be metabolised in vivo to give the active product—**sulphanilamide** (Fig. 43.1). Many sulphonamides have been developed since, and although their therapeutic importance has declined somewhat they are still useful drugs. Furthermore, chemical modification of the sulphonamide structure has given rise to several important groups of drugs, especially diuretics (thiazides; see Ch. 20), drugs for glaucoma (acetazolamide), tuberculostatic and antileprotic agents (the sulphones; see below) and oral hypoglycaemic drugs (sulphonylureas; see Ch. 22).

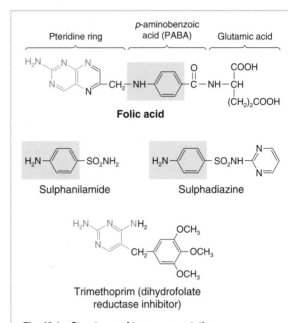

Fig. 43.1 Structures of two representative sulphonamides and trimethoprim. The structures illustrate the relationship between the sulphonamides and the PABA moiety in folic acid (light blue box), and the possible relationship between the antifolate drugs and the pteridine moiety (blue). Co-trimoxazole is a mixture of sulphamethoxazole and trimethoprim.

The clinically useful antibacterial sulphonamides are derived from sulphanilamide (Fig. 43.1), by substitution on the amide moiety (SO_2NHR). Compounds in which the amino group (NH_2) has been substituted are prodrugs that must be activated in the body, since a free amino group is necessary for antimicrobial activity.

The sulphonamides are generally used as their sodium salts, which are readily soluble in water.

Examples of sulphonamides in clinical use are:

- **sulphadiazine** (Fig. 43.1), **sulphadimidine**, **sulphamethoxazole**; short-acting, well absorbed in the gastrointestinal tract
- **sulfametopyrazine**; long-acting, well absorbed in the gastrointestinal tract
- **sulphasalazine**; poorly absorbed in the gastrointestinal tract, (see also Ch. 12, p. 237)
- **sulphamethoxazole**; given with trimethoprim, the combination constitutes **co-trimoxazole** (see below).

Mechanism of action

Sulphanilamide is a structural analogue of *p*-aminobenzoic acid (see Fig. 43.1) which is essential for the synthesis of folic acid in bacteria. As explained in Chapter 41, folate is required for the synthesis of the precursors of DNA and RNA both in bacteria and mammals, but mammals obtain their folic acid in their diet whereas bacteria need to synthesise it. Sulphonamides compete with *p*-aminobenzoic acid (PABA) for the enzyme *dihydropteroate synthetase*, and the effect of the sulphonamide may be overcome by adding excess PABA. This is why some local anaesthetics, for example **procaine** (see Ch. 40), which are PABA esters, can antagonise the antibacterial effect of these agents. The action of a sulphonamide is to inhibit growth of the bacteria, not to kill them, i.e. it is *bacteriostatic* rather than *bactericidal*. The action is negated by the presence of pus and the products of tissue breakdown since these contain thymidine and purines, which bacteria use to bypass the need for folic acid. Resistance, which is common, is plasmid-mediated (see Ch. 41) and due to the synthesis of an enzyme insensitive to the drug.

Pharmacokinetic aspects

Most sulphonamides are readily absorbed in the gastrointestinal tract and reach maximum concentrations in the plasma in 4–6 hours.

They are usually not given topically, mainly because of the risk of sensitisation and allergic reactions. An exception is **silver sulphadiazine** which is used topically in the treatment of infected burns.

The drugs pass into inflammatory exudates, and cross the placental barrier; most reach an effective concentration in the CSF, but they are no longer used to treat CNS infections.

They are metabolised mainly in the liver, the major product being an acetylated derivative which lacks antibacterial action. They are excreted in the urine.

The clinical use of sulphonamides is given on this page.

Unwanted effects

Mild to moderate side-effects are nausea and vomiting, headache and mental depression. Cyanosis due to methaemoglobinaemia may occur and is a lot less alarming than it looks. Serious adverse effects that necessitate cessation of therapy include hepatitis, hypersensitivity reactions (rashes, fever, anaphylactoid reactions), bone marrow depression and crystalluria. This last results from the precipitation of acetylated metabolites in the urine. It can be prevented by giving plenty of fluids and keeping the urine alkaline, and is less likely to occur with the more water-soluble drugs.

Clinical uses of sulphonamides

Absolute indications are very few, but sulphonamides may be used as follows:

- combined with trimethoprim (co-trimoxazole) for *Pneumocystis carinii*
- combined with pyrimethamine for drug-resistant malaria (Table 46.1), and for toxoplasmosis
- in inflammatory bowel disease and as an anti-inflammatory drug—sulphasalazine (sulphapyridine–salicylate combination) is so used
- for infected burns (silver sulphadiazine given topically)
- for some sexually transmitted infections (e.g. trachoma, chlamydia, chancroid)
- for respiratory infections; use now confined to a few special problems (e.g. infection with *Nocardia*)
- for acute urinary tract infection (now seldom used).

TRIMETHOPRIM

In structure, trimethoprim (Fig. 43.1) has some resemblance to the pteridine moiety of folate. The similarity is close enough to confuse the relevant bacterial enzyme. Trimethoprim is chemically related to the antimalarial drug, **pyrimethamine** (Fig. 46.4); both are *folate antagonists*. Bacterial dihydrofolate reductase is many times more sensitive to trimethoprim than is the equivalent enzyme in humans (Table 41.1).

Trimethoprim is active against most common bacterial pathogens, and it too is bacteriostatic. It is sometimes given as a mixture with sulphamethoxazole in a combination called **co-trimoxazole** (Fig. 43.1). Since sulphonamides affect an earlier stage in the same metabolic pathway in bacteria, i.e. folate synthesis, they can potentiate the action of trimethoprim. This is illustrated in Figure 43. 2.

Pharmacokinetic aspects

Trimethoprim is given orally, is fully absorbed in the gastrointestinal tract and widely distributed throughout the tissues and body fluids. It reaches high concentrations in the lungs and the kidneys and fairly high concentrations in the CSF. When given with sulphamethoxazole, about half of each is excreted within 24 hours. Since trimethoprim is a weak base, its elimination by the kidney increases with decreasing urinary pH.

The clinical use of trimethoprim is given on page 690.

Unwanted effects

Unwanted effects of trimethoprim include nausea, vomiting, blood disorders and skin rashes. Folate deficiency,

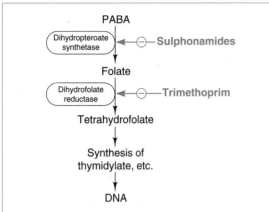

PABA

Dihydropteroate synthetase ← ⊖ — Sulphonamides

Folate

Dihydrofolate reductase ← ⊖ — Trimethoprim

Tetrahydrofolate

Synthesis of thymidylate, etc.

DNA

Fig. 43.2 The action of sulphonamides and trimethoprim on bacterial folate synthesis. See Figure 18.3 and Figure 42.11 for more detail of tetrahydrofolate synthesis, and Table 41.1 for comparisons of antifolate drugs.

with resultant megaloblastic anaemia (see Ch. 18)—a toxic effect related to the pharmacological action of trimethoprim—can be prevented by giving folinic acid. The sulphonamide moiety in co-trimoxazole can cause serious unwanted effects.

Antimicrobial agents which interfere with the synthesis or action of folate

- **Sulphonamides** are bacteriostatic; they act by interfering with folate synthesis and thus with nucleotide synthesis. Unwanted effects include crystalluria and hypersensitivities.
- **Trimethoprim** is bacteriostatic. It acts by folate antagonism.
- **Co-trimoxazole** is a mixture of trimethoprim with sulphamethoxazole, which affects bacterial nucleotide synthesis at two points.

Clinical uses of trimethoprim/co-trimoxazole

The main uses are as follows:

- for urinary tract and respiratory infections; trimethoprim, used on its own, is now usually preferred
- for infection with *Pneumocystis carinii*, which causes pneumonia in patients with AIDS, co-trimoxazole is used, in high dose.

See also Table 43.1.

BETA-LACTAM ANTIBIOTICS

PENICILLIN

In 1928, Alexander Fleming, working at St Mary's Hospital in London, observed that a culture plate on which staphylococci were being grown had become contaminated with a mould of the genus *Penicillium*, and that bacterial growth in the vicinity of the mould had been inhibited. He isolated the mould in pure culture and demonstrated that it produced an antibacterial substance which he called penicillin. This substance was subsequently extracted and its antibacterial effects analysed by Florey & Chain and their colleagues at Oxford in 1940. They showed that it had powerful chemotherapeutic properties in infected mice and that it was non-toxic. Its remarkable antibacterial effects in man were clearly demonstrated in 1941. A small amount of penicillin extracted laboriously from crude cultures in the laboratories of the Dunn School of Pathology in Oxford was tested on a policeman who had staphylococcal and streptococcal septicaemia with multiple abscesses, and osteomyelitis with discharging sinuses. He was in great pain and was desperately ill. (Sulphonamides were available but would have had no effect in the presence of pus; see p. 689.) Intravenous injections of penicillin were given every 3 hours. All the patient's urine was collected and each day the excreted penicillin was extracted and used again. After 5 days the patient's condition was vastly improved; his temperature was normal, he was eating well and there was obvious resolution of the abscesses. Furthermore, there seemed to be no toxic effects of the drug. Then the supply of penicillin ran out, his condition gradually deteriorated and he died a month later. This was the first evidence of the dramatic antibacterial effect of penicillin given *systemically* in humans. It is not generally known that *topical* penicillin had been used with success in five patients with eye infections 10 years previously by Paine—a graduate of St Mary's—who had obtained some penicillin mould from Fleming. The penicillins are extremely effective antibiotics and are very widely used.

Chemistry of penicillin

Penicillin is one of the group of β-lactam antibiotics which also includes cephalosporins, monobactams and carbapenems (Fig. 43.3). The basic nucleus of penicillin is 6-aminopenicillanic acid, which consists of a thiazolidine ring (A) linked to a β-lactam ring (B). This latter ring carries a secondary amino group. The side-chain substituents at R_1 determine the main antibacterial and

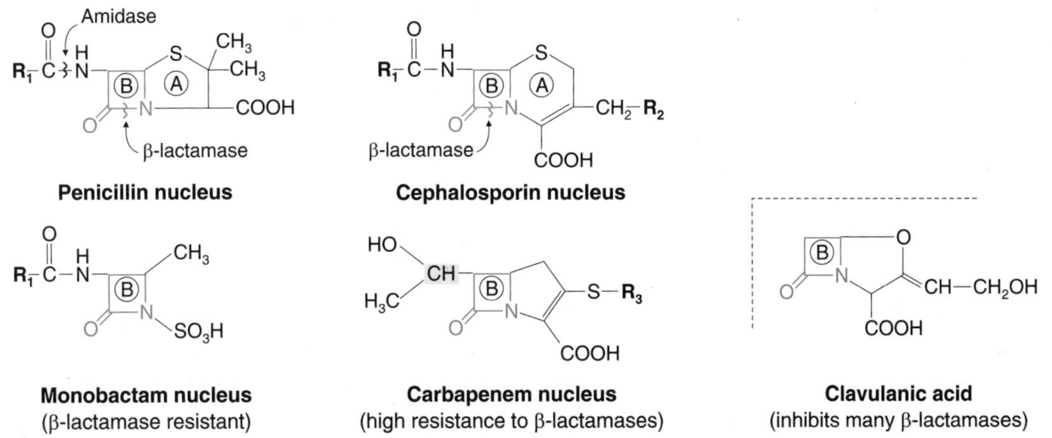

Fig. 43.3   Basic structures of four groups of β-lactam antibiotics and clavulanic acid. The structures illustrate the β-lactam ring (marked B), and the sites of action of bacterial enzymes that inactivate these antibiotics (A = thiazolidine ring). Various substituents are added at R_1, R_2, R_3, to produce agents with different properties. In carbapenems the stereochemical configuration of the part of the β-lactam ring shown shaded in light blue here is different from the corresponding part of the penicillin and cephalosporin molecules; this is probably the basis of the β-lactamase resistance of the carbapenems. The β-lactam ring of clavulanic acid is thought to bind strongly to β-lactamase, meanwhile protecting other β-lactams from the enzyme.

pharmacological characteristics of each particular penicillin (see Table 43.2).

Penicillins may be destroyed by enzymes—amidases and β-lactamases (penicillinases) (see Fig. 43.3).

Mechanisms of action

All β-lactam antibiotics interfere with the synthesis of the bacterial cell wall peptidoglycan (see Ch. 41, p. 653, Fig. 41.3). After attachment to binding sites on the bacterium (termed *penicillin-binding proteins*, of which there may be seven or more types in different organisms), they inhibit the transpeptidation enzyme that cross-links the peptide chains attached to the backbone of the peptidoglycan (see Fig. 41.3). The final bactericidal event is the inactivation of an inhibitor of the autolytic enzymes in the cell wall; this leads to lysis of the bacterium. Some organisms have defective autolytic enzymes and are inhibited but not lysed—they are referred to as 'tolerant'.

Resistance to penicillin—discussed in Chapter 41, page 660—may be due to different causes, the main ones being:

- *The production of β-lactamases*, of which there are about 50 different types. β-lactamase production is particularly important in staphylococci, though other organisms (*Neisseria gonorrhoeae*, *Haemophilus* spp., etc.) also produce these enzymes; streptococci do not. Since the introduction of penicillin, staphylococcal

resistance due to β-lactamase production has spread progressively, occurring first in staphylococcal strains in hospitals and then in strains in the community at large. In developed countries, at least 80% of staphylococci now produce β-lactamase. One solution is the concomitant use of β-lactamase inhibitors, such as **clavulanic acid** (Fig. 43.3) an inhibitor of the enzyme, which contains a β-lactam ring and is thought to bind covalently to the enzyme at or near its active site. Some enzyme molecules are irreversibly inactivated; in others, the complex is cleaved only very slowly to release the enzyme. Other β-lactamase inhibitors are **sulbactam** and **tazobactam**.

- *A reduction in the permeability of the outer membrane* and thus a decreased ability of the drug to penetrate to the target site. This occurs with Gram-negative organisms, which have an outer membrane that limits the penetration of hydrophilic antibiotics (see p. 688).
- *The occurrence of modified penicillin-binding sites.* This is particularly important in methicillin-resistant staphylococci (see pp 660–661).

Types of penicillin and their antimicrobial activity

The first penicillins were the naturally occurring benzylpenicillin and its congeners. Benzylpenicillin is active against a wide range of organisms and is the drug of first choice for many infections (see Table 43.1 and the clinical box on p. 692). Its main drawbacks are poor

Table 43.2 Penicillins

Type of penicillin	Absorption in GIT	Important properties and similar drugs
Benzylpenicillin and congeners		*Active against most Gram-positive cocci and Gram-negative bacteria. See Table 43.1. Destroyed by β-lactamases; many staphylococci now resistant*
Benzylpenicillin (penicillin G)	Poor	The treatment of choice for many infections (see Table 43.1). Given i.m. or i.v.; $t_{1/2}$ after i.m. is 30 min. Repository i.m. preparations which give more continuous, though lower, plasma concentrations are procaine penicillin and benzathine penicillin
Phenoxymethylpenicillin (penicillin V)	Good	Less potent than benzylpenicillin
β-lactamase-resistant penicillins		*Spectrum as for benzylpenicillin, but less potent. Many staphylococci now resistant*
Cloxacillin Flucloxacillin	Adequate	Given orally (except methicillin) or i.m. Cloxacillin adsorbed on food, $t_{1/2}$ 30–60 min. Excretion mostly renal, some in bile
Methicillin	Poor	
Nafcillin	Variable	Nafcillin is the most active of the β-lactamase-resistant penicillins against organisms other than benzylpenicillin-resistant *S. aureus*; reaches reasonable concentrations in the CSF. Excretion: 80% in bile, 20% in urine
Temocillin		Temocillin is effective against penicillinase-producing Gram-negative bacteria but not pseudomonads
Broad-spectrum penicillins		*Destroyed by β-lactamases produced by Staph. aureus and many Gram-negative organisms. Spectrum as for benzylpenicillin (though less potent), plus some Gram-negative bacteria*
Ampicillin	Fairly good	Given orally; food decreases absorption, $t_{1/2}$ 80 min. Excreted in bile and urine. May cause diarrhoea
Pivampicillin Bacampicillin	Good	Pro-drug releasing ampicillin in the liver. Absorption not decreased by food. Less diarrhoea than with ampicillin
Amoxycillin	Very good	Higher blood levels than ampicillin and less GIT disturbance. Can be given parenterally. $t_{1/2}$ 80 min. Available in combination with β-lactamase inhibitor, clavulanic acid
Extended-spectrum penicillins*		*Susceptible to β-lactamases. Spectrum as for broad-spectrum drugs, plus pseudomonads. Most strains of Staph. aureus are resistant*
Carbenicillin	Very poor	Also active against Proteus. Given i.v. or i.m. $t_{1/2}$ 80 min. Renal excretion
Ticarcillin	Very poor	More potent against pseudomonads. Available in combination with β-lactamase inhibitor, clavulanic acid
Azlocillin	Very poor	Very active against pseudomonads, also some strains of *Klebsiella*. Given i.v., $t_{1/2}$ 60 min. Excreted in bile and urine; clearance in bile decreased as dose increases
Piperacillin	Very poor	Has increased potency against common Gram-negative organisms

*Extended to include pseudomonads

absorption in the gastrointestinal tract (which means it must be given by injection) and its susceptibility to bacterial β-lactamases.

Various semisynthetic penicillins have been prepared by adding different side-chains to the penicillin nucleus (at R_1 in Fig. 43.3). In this way **β-lactamase-resistant penicillins** and **broad-spectrum penicillins** have been produced. More recently, **extended-spectrum penicillins** with antipseudomonal activity have been developed and have gone some way to overcoming the problem of serious infections caused by *Pseudomonas aeruginosa* (see p. 688). Details of the various types of penicillin are given in Table 43.2.

Pharmacokinetic aspects

When given orally, different penicillins are absorbed to differing degrees (see Table 43.2) depending on their stability in acid and their adsorption to food. Penicillins can be given by intramuscular or intravenous injection. Intrathecal administration is inadvisable, particularly with **benzylpenicillin**, as it can cause convulsions. The drugs are widely distributed in the body fluids, passing into joints, into pleural and pericardial cavities, into the bile, the saliva and the milk and across the placenta. Being lipid-insoluble they do not enter mammalian cells. They therefore do not cross the blood–brain barrier unless the meninges are inflamed, in which case they readily reach therapeutically effective concentrations in the CSF.

Elimination of most penicillins is mainly renal and occurs rapidly, 90% being by tubular secretion. The relatively short plasma half-life is a potential problem in the clinical use of **benzylpenicillin**, although since penicillin works by preventing cell wall synthesis in dividing organisms, intermittent rather than continuous exposure to the drug can be an advantage. Where it is not, the problem can be overcome—either by frequent dosage or by giving a slow-release preparation, such as **procaine penicillin** or **benzathine penicillin**. Tubular secretion of penicillins can be partially blocked by **probenecid**, which raises their plasma concentration and prolongs their action (see Chs 48 and 20). The fact that penicillin is excreted in the urine was made use of when the drug was first tested in the first human patient (see above).

Clinical use of the penicillins

Penicillins, often combined with other antibiotics, are crucially important in antibacterial chemotherapy. They are the drugs of choice for many infections. A list of clinical uses is given on this page. See also Table 43.1.

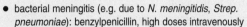

Clinical uses of the penicillins

Important uses include:

- bacterial meningitis (e.g. due to *N. meningitidis*, *Strep. pneumoniae*): benzylpenicillin, high doses intravenously
- bone and joint infections (e.g. with *Staph. aureus*): flucloxacillin
- skin and soft tissue infections (e.g. with *Strep. pyogenes* or *Staph. aureus*): benzylpenicillin, flucloxacillin; animal bites (often mixed organisms): co-amoxiclav
- pharyngitis (from *Strep. pyogenes*): phenoxymethylpenicillin orally
- otitis media (organisms commonly include *Strep. pyogenes*, *H. influenzae*): amoxicillin
- bronchitis in patients with chronic obstructive airways disease (mixed infections common): amoxicillin orally; community-acquired pneumonia, not severely ill (e.g. with *Strep. pneumoniae*): amoxycillin orally
- urinary tract infection (e.g. with *E. coli*): amoxicillin orally
- gonorrhoea: amoxicillin plus probenecid (orally) plus other antibiotics
- syphilis: procaine penicillin intramuscularly
- endocarditis (e.g. with *Strep. viridans* or *Enterococcus faecalis*): benzylpenicillin plus an aminoglycoside
- serious infections with *Pseudomonas aeruginosa*: piperacillin intravenously.

This list is not exhaustive. Treatment with penicillins is sometimes started empirically, if the likely causative organism is one thought to be susceptible to penicillin, while awaiting the results of laboratory tests to identify the organism and determine its antibiotic susceptibility.

Unwanted effects

One of the remarkable features of the penicillins is their relative freedom from direct toxic effects (other than their proconvulsant effect when given intrathecally). The main unwanted effects of the penicillins are *hypersensitivity reactions*, caused by the degradation products of penicillin which combine with host protein and become antigenic (see Ch. 49). There are cross-reactions between various types of penicillin. *Skin rashes* and *fever* are common; a delayed type of *serum sickness* occurs infrequently. Much more serious is *acute anaphylactic shock* which may, in some cases, be fatal but is fortunately very rare. Other hypersensitivity reactions seen occasionally are *vasculitis*, *interstitial nephritis* and various *haematologic disturbances*. The occurrence of these allergic reactions is unpredictable.

Injectable penicillins that contain potassium or sodium can produce electrolyte disturbances. Haemostatic defects have been reported with carbenicillin.

Penicillins, particularly the broad-spectrum type

given orally, alter the bacterial flora in the gut. This can be associated with gastrointestinal disturbances and, in some cases, with suprainfection by microorganisms not sensitive to penicillin.

CEPHALOSPORINS AND CEPHAMYCINS

Work by Abraham & Newton on a *Cephalosporium* fungus resulted in the identification of three distinct antibiotics, cephalosporins N and C, which are chemically related to penicillin, and cephalosporin P, a steroid antibiotic that resembles fusidic acid (see below). The cephamycins are β-lactam antibiotics produced by *Streptomyces* organisms and they are closely related to the cephalosporins.

Semisynthetic **broad-spectrum cephalosporins** have been produced by the addition, to the cephalosporin C nucleus, of different side-chains at R_1 and/or R_2 (see Fig. 43.3). These agents are water-soluble and relatively acid-stable. They vary in susceptibility to β-lactamases.

There are now a very large number of cephalosporins and cephamycins available for clinical use. They are usually classified arbitrarily in terms of the chronological order in which they were produced—the first generation compounds begat the second generation compounds which begat the third generation and so on. In Table 43.3 we eschew this biblical approach and classify them in terms of the method of administration, merely mentioning their genealogy in passing.

Mechanism of action

The mechanism of action of these agents is the same as that of the penicillins—interference with bacterial peptidoglycan synthesis after binding to the β-lactam-binding proteins. This is described in detail in Chapter 41 and illustrated in Figure 41.3. Resistance to this group of drugs has increased because of plasmid-encoded or chromosomal β-lactamase. Nearly all Gram-negative bacteria have a chromosomal gene coding for a β-lactamase that is more active in hydrolysing cephalosporins than penicillins; in several organisms a single-step mutation can result in high level constitutive production of this enzyme. Resistance also occurs if there is decreased penetration of the drug due to alterations to outer membrane proteins or mutations of the binding-site proteins.

The antibacterial spectrum of these agents is summarised briefly in Table 43.3.

Pharmacokinetic aspects

Some cephalosporins may be given orally (see Table 43.1) but most are given parenterally, intramuscularly (which may be painful with some agents) or intravenously. After absorption they are widely distributed in the body, passing into the pleural, pericardial and joint fluids and across the placenta. Some, such as **cefoperazone**, **cefotaxime**, **cefuroxime** and **ceftriaxone** also cross the blood–brain barrier. Excretion is mostly via the kidney, largely by tubular secretion, but 40% of ceftriaxone and 75% of cefoperazone is eliminated in the bile.

Table 43.3   Cephalosporins and cephamycins

Categories with examples	Important properties and similar drugs
Oral drugs	
Cephalexin ($t_{1/2}$ 1 h)	An example of the first-generation compounds that have reasonable activity against Gram-positive organisms and modest activity against Gram-negative organisms *Similar drugs:* Cefachlor ($t_{1/2}$ 0.8 h) is a second-generation compound with greater potency against Gram-negative organisms, but it can cause unwanted cutaneous lesions
Parenteral drugs	
Cefuroxime ($t_{1/2}$ 1.5 h)	An example of the second-generation compounds which show only moderate activity against most Gram-positive organisms but reasonable potency against Gram-negative organisms *Similar drugs:* Cephamandole, cefoxitin ($t_{1/2}$ of both approx. 1 h), good activity against Gram-negative organisms, resistant to β-lactamase from Gram-negative rods, good potency against *Bacteroides fragilis*, bowel flora
Cefotaxime ($t_{1/2}$ 1 h)	An example of the third-generation compounds which are less active against Gram-positive bacteria than those of the second generation, but more active against Gram-negative bacteria. Has some activity against pseudomonads *Similar drugs:* Ceftizoxime ($t_{1/2}$ 1.5 h); ceftriaxone ($t_{1/2}$ 8.5 h), excreted largely in the bile; cefperazone ($t_{1/2}$ 2 h), excreted mainly in the bile, can cause decrease of vitamin K-dependent clotting factors

Clinical use

Some clinical uses of the cephalosporins are given in Table 43.1 and the clinical box above.

Unwanted effects

Hypersensitivity reactions, very similar to those that occur with penicillin, may be seen. Some cross-reactions occur; about 10% of penicillin-sensitive individuals will have allergic reactions to cephalosporins. Nephrotoxicity has been reported (especially with cephradine), as has intolerance to alcohol. Diarrhoea can occur with oral cephalosporins and cefoperazone.

OTHER β-LACTAM ANTIBIOTICS

Carbapenems and monobactams

Carbapenems and monobactams (see Fig. 43.3) were developed to deal with β-lactamase-producing Gram-negative organisms resistant to broad-spectrum and extended-spectrum penicillins.

Imipenem, an example of a carbapenem, acts in the same way as the other β-lactams (see Fig. 43.3). It has a very broad spectrum of antimicrobial activity, being active against many aerobic and anaerobic Gram-positive and Gram-negative organisms, including *Listeria*, pseudo-monads and most Enterobacteriaceae. However, many of the 'methicillin-resistant' staphylococci (see p. 661) are less susceptible, and resistant strains of *P. aeruginosa* have emerged during therapy. Imipenem was originally resistant to all β-lactamases but some organisms now have chromosomal genes which code for imipenem-hydrolysing β-lactamases.

Imipenem is given intravenously. In the kidney it is partly broken down by a dehydropeptidase in the proximal tubule and is therefore given in combination with **cilastatin**, a specific inhibitor of this enzyme.

Unwanted effects are similar to those seen with other β-lactams, nausea and vomiting being the most fre-

quently seen. Neurotoxicity can occur with high plasma concentrations.

Meropenem is similar to imipenem but is not broken down by proximal tubule dehydropeptidase.

The main monobactam is **aztreonam**, a simple mono-cyclic β-lactam with a complex substituent at R_3 (see Fig. 43.3), which is resistant to most β-lactamases. This has an unusual spectrum—being active only against Gram-negative aerobic rods, including pseudomonads, *Neisseria meningitidis* and *Haemophilus influenzae*; it has no action against Gram-positive organisms or anaerobes.

It is given parenterally and has a plasma half-life of 2 hours. *Unwanted effects* are, in general, similar to those of other β-lactam antibiotics, but this agent does not necessarily cross-react immunologically with penicillin and its products, and so may not (but sometimes does) cause allergic reactions in penicillin-sensitive individuals.

ANTIMICROBIAL AGENTS AFFECTING BACTERIAL PROTEIN SYNTHESIS

TETRACYCLINES

Tetracyclines are broad-spectrum antibiotics. The group includes **tetracycline, oxytetracycline, doxycycline** and **minocycline**.

Mechanism of action
Tetracyclines act by inhibiting protein synthesis after uptake into susceptible organisms by active transport. This action is described in detail in Chapter 41 (p. 653 and Fig. 41.4). The tetracyclines are bacteriostatic, not bactericidal.

Antibacterial spectrum
The spectrum of antimicrobial activity of the tetracyclines is very wide and includes Gram-positive and Gram-negative bacteria, *Mycoplasma*, *Rickettsia*, *Chlamydia*, some spirochaetes and some protozoa (e.g. amoebae). Minocycline is also effective against *Neisseria meningitidis* and has been used to eradicate this organism from the nasopharynx of carriers; it does not penetrate the blood–brain barrier and is not used to treat meningitis.

However, many strains of organisms have become resistant to these agents and this has decreased their usefulness (see Ch. 41, p. 660). Resistance is transmitted mainly by plasmids and, since the genes controlling resistance to tetracyclines are closely associated with genes for resistance to other antibiotics, organisms may become resistant to many drugs simultaneously.

Pharmacokinetic aspects
The tetracyclines are usually given orally but can be given parenterally. The absorption of most preparations from the gut is irregular and incomplete, and is improved in the absence of food. Since tetracyclines chelate metal ions (calcium, magnesium, iron, aluminium), forming non-absorbable complexes, absorption is decreased in the presence of milk, certain antacids and iron preparations. **Minocycline** and **doxycycline** are virtually completely absorbed. The drugs have a wide distribution, entering most fluid compartments, crossing the placenta to the foetus and appearing in the milk. Minocycline is found

in high concentrations in tears and saliva. Excretion of most tetracyclines is by two routes—via the bile and via the kidney by glomerular filtration. Most tetracyclines will accumulate if renal function is impaired and will exacerbate renal failure. Doxycycline is an exception, being excreted largely into the gastrointestinal tract. Minocycline is partly metabolised.

The clinical use of the tetracyclines is given in the box on this page.

Unwanted effects
The commonest unwanted effects are gastrointestinal disturbances, due initially to direct irritation and later to modification of the gut flora. Vitamin B complex deficiency can occur as can suprainfection.

Because they chelate calcium, tetracyclines are deposited in growing bones and teeth, causing staining and sometimes dental hypoplasia and bone deformities. They should therefore not be given to children, pregnant women or nursing mothers. Another hazard in pregnant women is hepatotoxicity.

Phototoxicity (sensitisation to sunlight) has been seen, more particularly with **demeclocycline**. **Minocycline** can produce dose-related vestibular disturbances (dizziness and nausea). High doses of tetracyclines can decrease protein synthesis in host cells—an anti-anabolic effect— which could result in renal damage. Long-term therapy can cause disturbances of the bone marrow.

CHLORAMPHENICOL

Chloramphenicol was originally isolated from cultures of *Streptomyces*. The *mechanism of action* is by inhibition of protein synthesis as described in Chapter 41 (p. 653 and Fig. 41.4). Chloramphenicol binds to the 50S sub-

---

> **Clinical uses of the tetracyclines**
>
> The main uses are as follows:
>
> - They are drugs of first choice for rickettsial, mycoplasma and chlamydial infections, brucellosis, cholera, plague and Lyme disease.
> - They are drugs of second choice for infections with several different organisms (see Table 43.1).
> - They are useful in mixed infections of the respiratory tract and in acne.
>
> An unusual use of demeclocycline is for chronic hyponatraemia due to inappropriate secretion of antidiuretic hormone—the antibiotic is probably effective because it renders the renal tubule cells unresponsive to the hormone.

unit of the bacterial ribosome at the same site as do **erythromycin** and **clindamycin**. The drugs may compete and thus interfere with each other's actions if given concurrently.

Antibacterial spectrum

Chloramphenicol has a wide spectrum of antimicrobial activity, including Gram-negative and Gram-positive organisms and rickettsiae. It is bacteriostatic for most organisms but bactericidal to *H. influenzae*. As with other bacteriostatic antibiotics, it may interfere with the action of bactericidal antimicrobials if used concurrently.*

Resistance is due to the production of chloramphenicol acetyl-transferase (see p. 660) and is plasmid mediated.

Pharmacokinetic aspects

Given orally, chloramphenicol is rapidly and completely absorbed and reaches its maximum concentration in the plasma within 2 hours; it can also be given parenterally. It is widely distributed throughout the tissues and body fluids including the CSF, in which its concentration may be 60% of that in the blood. In the plasma it is 30–50% protein-bound and its half-life is approximately 2 hours. About 10% is excreted unchanged in the urine, and the remainder is inactivated in the liver.

The clinical use of chloramphenicol is given in the box on this page.

Unwanted effects

The most important unwanted effect of chloramphenicol is severe, idiosyncratic depression of the bone marrow resulting in pancytopenia (a decrease in all blood cell elements)—an effect which, though rare, can occur even with very low doses in some individuals. In a small proportion of patients (approx. 1 in 50 000), fatal aplastic anaemia may occur. Dose-related blood cell disorders occur in many individuals taking chloramphenicol for 2 weeks or more; these disappear when treatment is stopped.

Chloramphenicol should be used with great care in newborns because inadequate inactivation and excretion of the drug (see Ch. 48) can result in the 'grey baby syndrome'—vomiting, diarrhoea, flaccidity, low temperature and an ashen-grey colour—which carries a 40% mortality; if its use is essential, plasma concentrations

---

*Theoretically and in laboratory experiments, chloramphenicol interferes with the action of penicillin when given concurrently, the basis of this effect being that penicillin acts on dividing cells and chloramphenicol prevents growth and division in bacteria; however, this interference may not occur when the drugs are used clinically.

> ### Clinical uses of chloramphenicol
>
> Clinical use of chloramphenicol should be reserved for serious infections in which the benefit of the drug is greater than the risk of toxicity (see below), such as:
>
> - infections caused by *H. influenzae* resistant to other drugs
> - meningitis in patients in whom penicillin cannot be used.
>
> It is also safe and effective in:
>
> - bacterial conjunctivitis (given topically).
>
> It is effective in typhoid fever but ciprofloxacin or amoxycillin and co-trimoxazole are similarly effective and less toxic. Other possible uses are given in Table 43.1.

should be determined and the dose adjusted accordingly. Hypersensitivity reactions can occur, as can gastro-intestinal disturbances and other sequelae of alteration of the intestinal microbial flora.

AMINOGLYCOSIDES

The aminoglycosides are a group of antibiotics of complex chemical structure, resembling each other in antimicrobial activity, pharmacokinetic characteristics and toxicity. The main agents are gentamicin, **streptomycin**, **amikacin**, **tobramycin**, **netilmicin**, **neomycin** and **framycetin**.

Mechanism of action

Aminoglycosides inhibit bacterial protein synthesis (see Ch. 41, p. 653).

Their penetration through the cell membrane of the bacterium depends partly on oxygen-dependent active transport by a polyamine carrier system and they have minimal action against anaerobic organisms. Chloramphenicol blocks this transport system. The effect of the aminoglycosides is bactericidal and is enhanced by agents that interfere with cell wall synthesis.

Resistance

Resistance to aminoglycosides is becoming a problem. It occurs by several different mechanisms (see pp 660–661), the most important being inactivation by microbial enzymes of which there are nine or more. **Amikacin** was designed as a poor substrate for these enzymes; but some organisms have developed enzymes that inactivate this agent.

Resistance due to failure of penetration can be largely overcome by the concomitant use of **penicillin** and/or **vancomycin**.

Antibacterial spectrum

The aminoglycosides are effective against many aerobic Gram-negative and some Gram-positive organisms (see Table 43.1).

They are most widely used against Gram-negative enteric organisms and in sepsis. They may be given together with a penicillin in infections caused by *Streptococcus*, *Listeria* or *Pseudomonas aeruginosa* (see Table 43.1). **Gentamicin** is the aminoglycoside most commonly used, though **tobramycin** is the preferred member of this group for *P. aeruginosa* infections. **Amikacin** has the widest antimicrobial spectrum and along with **netilmicin** can be effective in infections with organisms resistant to gentamicin and tobramycin. **Neomycin** and **framycetin** are too toxic for parenteral use and are only used topically.

Pharmacokinetic aspects

The aminoglycosides are polycations and highly polar. They are not absorbed in the gastrointestinal tract, and are usually given intramuscularly or intravenously. They do not enter cells, nor do they cross the blood–brain barrier into the CNS, penetrate the vitreous humor of the eye or reach high concentrations in secretions and body fluids, though high concentrations can be attained in joint and pleural fluids. They may, however, cross the placenta. The plasma half-life is 2–3 hours. Elimination is virtually entirely by glomerular filtration in the kidney, 50–60% of a dose being excreted unchanged within 24 hours. Tissue concentrations increase during treatment (Fig. 43.4). If renal function is impaired, accumulation occurs rapidly with a resultant increase in those toxic effects (such as ototoxicity and nephrotoxicity, see below) which are dose-related.

Clinical use

Clinical uses of the aminoglycosides are given in Table 43.1.

Unwanted effects

Serious, dose-related toxic effects, with the potential for increasing with length of treatment, can occur with the aminoglycosides, the main hazards being ototoxicity and nephrotoxicity.

The *ototoxicity* involves progressive damage to and destruction of the sensory cells in the cochlea and vestibular organ of the ear. The result, usually irreversible, may be vertigo, ataxia and loss of balance in the case of vestibular damage, and auditory disturbances, including deafness, in the case of cochlear damage. Any amino-

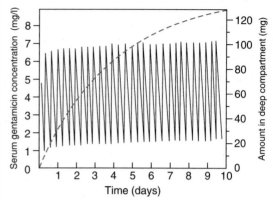

Fig. 43.4 Graph of serum and tissue concentrations of aminoglycoside antibiotics during repeated administration. The concentration in the tissues (dotted line) increases while the serum concentration (solid line) does not rise progressively. (Adapted from: Aronson J K, Reynolds D J M 1992 Br Med J 305: 1421–1424)

glycoside may produce both types of effect, but **streptomycin** and **gentamicin** are more likely to interfere with vestibular function whereas **neomycin** and **amikacin** affect mostly hearing. **Netilmicin** is less ototoxic than other aminoglycosides and is preferred when prolonged use is necessary. Ototoxicity is potentiated by the concomitant use of other ototoxic drugs (e.g. loop diuretics, p. 363).

The *nephrotoxicity* consists of damage to the kidney tubules and can be reversed if the use of the drugs is stopped. Nephrotoxicity is more likely to occur in patients with pre-existing renal disease or in conditions in which urine volume is reduced; concomitant use of other nephrotoxic agents (e.g. **cephalosporins**) increases the risk. Note that as the elimination of these drugs is almost entirely renal, their nephrotoxic action can impair their own excretion and a vicious cycle can be set up. Plasma concentrations should be monitored regularly.

A rare but serious toxic reaction is paralysis due to neuromuscular blockade, usually only seen if the agents are given concurrently with neuromuscular-blocking agents. It is due to inhibition of the calcium uptake necessary for the exocytotic release of acetylcholine (see Ch. 7).

Spectinomycin

Spectinomycin is related to the aminoglycosides in structure. Its use is confined to the treatment of gonorrhoea in patients allergic to penicillin or those whose infections are caused by penicillin-resistant gonococci.

MACROLIDES

For 40 years, **erythromycin** was the only macrolide antibiotic in general clinical use. (The term 'macrolide' relates to the structure—a many-membered lactone ring to which one or more deoxy sugars are attached.) Recently a host of new macrolide and related antibiotics have become available, the two most important of which are **clarithromycin** and **azithromycin**.

Mechanism of action

The macrolides inhibit bacterial protein synthesis by an effect on translocation (Fig. 41.4). Their action may be bactericidal or bacteriostatic, the effect depending on the concentration and on the type of microorganism. The drugs are bound to the 50S subunit of the bacterial ribosome; the binding site is the same as that of **chloramphenicol** and **clindamycin** and the three types of agent could compete, if given concurrently.

Antimicrobial spectrum

The antimicrobial spectrum of **erythromycin** is very similar to that of penicillin and it has proved to be a safe and effective alternative for penicillin-sensitive patients. Erythromycin is effective against Gram-positive bacteria and spirochaetes but not against most Gram-negative organisms, exceptions being *N. gonorrhoeae* and, to a lesser extent, *H. influenzae*. *Mycoplasma pneumoniae*, *Legionella* and some chlamydial organisms are also susceptible. See Table 43.1. *Resistance* can occur and is due to a plasmid-controlled alteration of the binding site for erythromycin on the bacterial ribosome (Fig. 41.4).

Azithromycin is less active against Gram-positive bacteria than erythromycin, is considerably more effective against *H. influenzae* and may be more active against *Legionella*. It has excellent action against *Toxoplasma gondii* (p. 737), killing the cysts.

Clarithromycin is as active, and its metabolite is twice as active, against *H. influenzae* as erythromycin; it is also effective against *Mycobacterium avium cellulare* (which can infect immunologically compromised individuals and elderly patients with chronic lung disease) and may be useful in leprosy and against *Helicobacter pylori* (see Ch. 21). Both these macrolides are effective in Lyme disease.

Pharmacokinetic aspects

The macrolides are administered orally, **azithromycin** and **clarithromycin** being more acid-stable than **erythromycin**. Erythromycin can also be given parenterally, though intravenous injections can be followed by local thrombophlebitis. They all diffuse readily into most tissues, including prostatic fluid and the placenta, but do not cross the blood–brain barrier and there is poor penetration into synovial fluid. The plasma half-life of erythromycin is about 90 minutes; that of clarithromycin is three times longer and that of azithromycin 8–16 times longer. This latter agent persists at high concentrations in the tissues (which could be significant in some infections) but its peak plasma concentration can be quite low (which needs to be taken into account in infections such as pneumococcal pneumonia which can be complicated by septicaemia). Macrolides enter and are concentrated within phagocytes—azithromycin concentrations in phagocyte lysosomes can be 40 times higher than in the blood—and they can enhance phagocyte killing of bacteria.

Erythromycin is partly inactivated in the liver; azithromycin is more resistant to inactivation and clarithromycin is converted to an active metabolite. (Effects on the P450 cytochrome system can affect the bioavailability of other drugs; see Ch. 48.) The major route of elimination is in the bile.

Clinical use

The clinical use of the macrolides is given in Table 43.1.

Unwanted effects

Gastrointestinal disturbances are common and unpleasant but not serious and occur less often with the two newer agents. With erythromycin, the following have also been reported: hypersensitivity reactions such as skin rashes and fever, transient hearing disturbances, and, rarely, with treatment longer than a fortnight, cholestatic jaundice.

Opportunistic infections of the gastrointestinal tract or vagina can occur.

LINCOSAMIDES

Clindamycin is active against Gram-positive cocci, including many penicillin-resistant staphylococci, and many anaerobic bacteria such as *Bacteroides* species.

Its *mechanism of action* involves inhibition of protein synthesis similar to that of the macrolides and chloramphenicol (Fig. 41.4).

Clindamycin can be given orally or parenterally and is widely distributed in tissues (including bone) and body fluids but does not cross the blood–brain barrier. There is active uptake into leukocytes. Its $t_{\frac{1}{2}}$ is 21 hours. Some is metabolised in the liver, and the metabolites, which are active, are excreted in the bile and the urine. *Unwanted effects* consist mainly of gastrointestinal disturbances. A potentially lethal condition, *pseudomembranous colitis*, can occur; this is an acute inflammation of the colon due to a necrotising toxin produced by a clindamycin-resistant organism, *Clostridium difficile*, which may be part of the normal faecal flora.* Vancomycin, given orally, and metronidazole (see below) are effective in the treatment of this condition.

Its *clinical use* is in infections caused by *Bacteroides* organisms and for staphylococcal infections of bones and joints. It is also used topically, as eye drops, for staphylococcal conjunctivitis.

FUSIDIC ACID

Fusidic acid is a narrow-spectrum steroid antibiotic active mainly against Gram-positive bacteria. It acts by inhibiting protein synthesis (Fig. 41.4).

Sodium fusidate is well absorbed from the gut and is distributed widely in the tissues. Some is excreted in the bile and some metabolised.

> **Antimicrobial agents affecting bacterial protein synthesis**
>
> - **Tetracyclines:** e.g. minocycline. These are orally active, bacteriostatic, broad-spectrum antibiotics. Resistance is increasing. GIT disorders are common. They chelate calcium and are deposited in growing bone. They are contraindicated in children and pregnant women.
> - **Chloramphenicol:** This is an orally active, bacteriostatic, broad-spectrum antibiotic. Serious toxic effects are possible, including bone marrow depression, grey baby syndrome. It should be reserved for life-threatening infections.
> - **Aminoglycosides:** e.g. gentamicin. These are given by injection. They are bactericidal, broad-spectrum antibiotics (but with low activity against anaerobes, streptococci and pneumococci). Resistance is increasing. The main unwanted effects are dose-related nephrotoxicity and ototoxicity. Serum levels should be monitored. (Streptomycin is an antituberculosis aminoglycoside.)
> - **Macrolides:** e.g. erythromycin. Can be given orally and parenterally. They are bactericidal/bacteriostatic. The antibacterial spectrum is the same as for penicillin. Erythromycin can cause jaundice. Newer agents are clarithromycin and azithromycin.
> - **Clindamycin:** Can be given orally and parenterally. It can cause pseudomembranous colitis.
> - **Fusidic acid:** This is a narrow-spectrum antibiotic which acts by inhibiting protein synthesis. It penetrates bone. Unwanted effects include GIT disorders.

---

*This can also occur with some penicillins and cephalosporins.

Unwanted effects such as gastrointestinal disturbances are fairly common. Skin eruptions and jaundice can occur. It is used in combination with other drugs (e.g. **flucloxacillin**) mainly for serious staphylococcal infections caused by penicillin-resistant organisms, especially osteomyelitis, since sodium fusidate is concentrated in bone. It is also used topically for staphylococcal conjunctivitis.

ANTIMICROBIAL AGENTS AFFECTING TOPOISOMERASE II

FLUOROQUINOLONES

The fluoroquinolones are synthetic antibiotics recently introduced into clinical practice. They include the broad-spectrum agents **ciprofloxacin**, **ofloxacin**, **norfloxacin**, **acrosoxacin** and **pefloxacin**, and the narrower-spectrum drugs used in urinary tract infections—**cinoxacin**, and **nalidixic acid**. (The last named was the first quinolone and is not fluorinated.) As explained on page 656, these agents inhibit topoisomerase II (a DNA gyrase), the enzyme that produces a negative supercoil in DNA, permitting transcription or replication (Fig. 43.5).

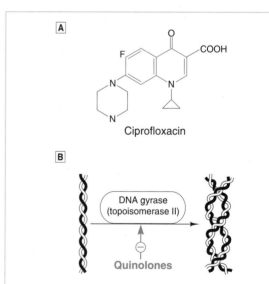

Fig. 43.5 A simplified diagram of the mechanism of action of the fluoroquinolones. [A] An example of a quinolone (the quinolone moiety is shown in blue). [B] Schematic diagram of (left) the double helix; and (right) the double helix in supercoiled form. (See also Fig. 41.6.) In essence, the DNA gyrase unwinds the RNA-induced positive supercoil (not shown) and introduces a negative supercoil.

Antibacterial spectrum and clinical use

Ciprofloxacin is the most commonly used fluoro-quinolone and will be described as the type agent. It is a broad-spectrum antibiotic, effective against both Gram-positive and Gram-negative organisms, being especially active against the latter. It has excellent activity against the Enterobacteriaceae (the enteric Gram-negative bacilli), including many organisms resistant to peni-cillins, cephalosporins and aminoglycosides, and is also effective against *H. influenzae*, penicillinase-producing *N. gonorrhoeae*, *Campylobacter* and pseudomonads. Of the Gram-positive organisms, streptococci and pneumo-cocci are only weakly inhibited and there is a high inci-dence of staphylococcal resistance. Ciprofloxacin should be avoided in methicillin-resistant staphylococcal infec-tions. Intracellular pathogens, such as *Mycobacterium tuberculosis*, *Mycoplasma*, *Chlamydia*, *Legionella* and *Brucella* species are inhibited to a variable extent and there is only low activity against anaerobic bacteria.

Clinically the fluoroquinolones are best used for infections with facultative and aerobic Gram-negative rods and cocci.* Resistant strains of *Staph. aureus* and *P. aeruginosa* have emerged.

Pharmacokinetic aspects

Given orally, the fluoroquinolones are well absorbed. The half-life of ciprofloxacin and norfloxacin is 3 hours, that of ofloxacin is 5 hours and that of perfloxacin is 10 hours. The drugs concentrate in many tissues, parti-cularly in the kidney, prostate and lung. All quinolones are concentrated in phagocytes. Most do not cross the blood–brain barrier except for pefloxacin and ofloxacin which reach, in the CSF, respectively 40% and 90% of their serum concentrations. **Aluminium** and **magnesium antacids** interfere with the absorption of the quinolones. Elimination of ciprofloxacin, norfloxacin and enofloxacin is due partly to hepatic metabolism by P450 enzymes (which they can inhibit, giving rise to interactions with other drugs; see below) and partly to renal excretion. Pefloxacin is metabolised to norfloxacin. Ofloxacin is excreted in the urine.

The clinical use of the fluoroquinolones is given on this page.

---

*When ciprofloxacin was introduced, some clinical pharmacologists and microbiologists suggested, sensibly, that to prevent emergence of resistance, it should be reserved for organisms resistant to other drugs. However, it was estimated that, in 1989, it was prescribed for 1 in 44 of Americans; so it would seem that the horse has not only left the stable but has bolted.

Unwanted effects

Unwanted effects are infrequent, usually mild and dis-appear if the agents are withdrawn. They consist mainly of gastrointestinal disorders and skin rashes. (Most antacids cannot be used to treat the gastric symptoms; see above.) Arthropathy has been reported in young indi-viduals. CNS symptoms—headache, dizziness—have occurred and, less frequently, convulsions, which have been associated with CNS pathology or concurrent use of theophylline or a non-steroidal anti-inflammatory drug. Fluoroquinolones have been reported to inhibit the binding of GABA to its receptor. Photosensitivity and hypersensitivity reactions (sometimes involving the blood cells) have been seen, as have renal disorders.

There is a clinically important interaction between **ciprofloxacin** and **theophylline** (through inhibition of P450 enzymes) which can lead to theophylline toxicity in asthmatics treated with the fluoroquinolones; theo-phylline toxicity is discussed in Chapter 19.

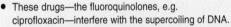

Antimicrobial agents affecting DNA topoisomerase II

- These drugs—the fluoroquinolones, e.g. ciprofloxacin—interfere with the supercoiling of DNA.
- Ciprofloxacin has a wide antibacterial spectrum, being especially active against Gram-negative enteric coliform organisms including many organisms resistant to penicillins, cephalosporins and aminoglycosides; it is also effective against *H. influenzae*, penicillinase-producing *N. gonorrhoeae*, *Campylobacter* and pseudomonads. There is a high incidence of staphylococcal resistance. It is active orally with a $t_{1/2}$ of 4.5 hours.
- Unwanted effects include GI tract upsets and hypersensitivity reactions and, rarely, CNS disturbances.
- Newer agents include ofloxacin, norfloxacin.

Clinical uses of the fluoroquinolones

The main uses are as follows:

- for complicated urinary tract infections (norfloxacin, ofloxacin)
- for *P. aeruginosa* respiratory infections in patients with cystic fibrosis
- for invasive external otitis caused by *P. aeruginosa*
- for chronic Gram-negative bacillary osteomyelitis
- for eradication of *S. typhi* in carriers
- for gonorrhoea (norfloxacin, ofloxacin)
- for bacterial prostatitis (norfloxacin)
- for cervicitis (ofloxacin).

In patients in whom penicillin cannot be used, a single dose of acrosoxacin can cure gonorrhoea.

Numerous new quinolones have been synthesised and are under test.

MISCELLANEOUS ANTIBACTERIAL AGENTS

GLYCOPEPTIDE ANTIBIOTICS

The main glycopeptide antibiotic is **vancomycin**. It is bactericidal (except against streptococci) and acts by inhibiting cell wall synthesis (see Fig. 41.3). It is effective mainly against Gram-positive bacteria, including *methicillin-resistant staphylococci*, and has been used for resistant enterococci. Resistance in these latter micro-organisms, rare during the 35 years that this agent has been used, is now emerging rapidly world-wide. It synergises with some **aminoglycoside** antibiotics against some organisms which vancomycin, on its own, does not kill.

It is not absorbed from the gut and is only given by the oral route for treatment of gastrointestinal infection with *Clostridium difficile*. For parenteral use it is given intravenously (and if infused too fast causes a histamine-induced reddening of the skin). It is widely distributed. Its plasma half-life is about 8 hours—if renal function is normal. Elimination is virtually entirely by glomerular filtration into the urine and thus it could accumulate if renal function is impaired.

The *clinical use* of vancomycin is limited mainly to pseudomembranous colitis (see under 'Clindamycin', p. 699) and the treatment of some multiresistant staphylococcal infections. It is also valuable in severe staphylococcal infections in patients allergic both to **penicillins** and **cephalosporins**, and in some forms of endocarditis.

Unwanted effects include fever, rashes and local phlebitis at the site of injection. Ototoxicity and nephrotoxicity can occur and hypersensitivity reactions are seen occasionally.

Teicoplanin, given intramuscularly or intravenously, is similar but is longer-acting.

POLYMIXIN ANTIBIOTICS

The polymixin antibiotics in use are **polymixin B** and **colistin** (polymixin E). They have cationic detergent properties and their *mechanism of action* involves interaction with the phospholipids of the cell membrane and disruption of its structure (Ch. 41, p. 656). They have a selective, rapidly bactericidal action on Gram-negative bacilli, especially pseudomonads and coliform organisms. They are not absorbed from the gastrointestinal tract.

Unwanted effects may be serious and include neurotoxicity and nephrotoxicity. Use of these drugs is limited by their toxicity and is confined largely to gut sterilisation and topical treatment of ear, eye or skin infections caused by susceptible organisms.

BACITRACIN

Bacitracin is a polypeptide antibiotic with a range of activity similar to that of penicillin, being most active against Gram-positive organisms including staphylococci producing β-lactamase. Its mechanism of action involves inhibition of cell-wall formation (see Fig. 41.3).

Bacitracin has serious toxic effects on the kidney and is therefore only used topically for infections of mouth, nose, eye and skin.

METRONIDAZOLE

Metronidazole was introduced as an antiprotozoal agent (and is dealt with in more detail on p. 735) but it is also active against anaerobic bacteria such as *Bacteroides*, clostridia and some streptococci. It is effective in the therapy of *pseudomembranous colitis*, a clostridial infection sometimes associated with antibiotic therapy (see p. 700), and is important in the treatment of serious anaerobic infections (e.g. sepsis secondary to bowel disease).

NITROFURANTOIN

Nitrofurantoin is a synthetic compound active against a range of Gram-positive and Gram-negative organisms. The development of resistance in susceptible organisms is rare and there is no cross-resistance. Its mechanism of action is not known.

It is given orally and is rapidly and totally absorbed from the gastrointestinal tract and very rapidly excreted by the kidney by both glomerular filtration and tubular secretion; thus it reaches antibacterial concentrations in the urine but not in the plasma. In renal failure, toxic blood levels ensue.

The *clinical use* of nitrofurantoin is confined to the treatment of urinary tract infections, and the drug is more active in acid urine.

Unwanted effects such as gastrointestinal disturbances are relatively common, and hypersensitivity reactions involving the skin and the bone marrow (e.g. leukopenia) can occur. Hepatotoxicity and peripheral neuropathy have been reported. (Note that nitrofurantoin interferes with the therapeutic action of some quinolones.)

- **Glycopeptide antibiotics:** e.g. vancomycin. Vancomycin is bactericidal, acting by inhibiting cell wall synthesis. It is used intravenously for multiresistant staphylococcal infections and orally for pseudomembranous colitis. Unwanted effects include ototoxicity and nephrotoxicity.
- **Polymixins:** e.g. colistin. They are bactericidal, acting by disrupting bacterial cell membranes. They are seriously neurotoxic and nephrotoxic and are only used topically.
- **Bacitracin** inhibits bacterial cell wall formation. It is used topically for superficial infections.
- **Nitrofurantoin** is orally active and is used for urinary tract infections.

ANTIMYCOBACTERIAL AGENTS

The main mycobacterial infections in man are *tuberculosis* and *leprosy*—both typically chronic infections, caused, respectively, by *Mycobacterium tuberculosis* and *Mycobacterium leprae*. A particular problem with both these conditions is that after phagocytosis, the microorganism can survive inside macrophages, unless these are 'activated' by cytokines produced by Th1 lymphocytes (see Ch. 13, pp 204–206).

DRUGS USED TO TREAT TUBERCULOSIS

Tuberculosis was for centuries a major killer disease; then 40 years or so ago, new drugs were developed and put to use and tuberculosis came to be regarded as an easily curable condition. This is so no longer—the mycobacterium which causes it has come back to haunt us: multidrug-resistant strains are now common and recent evidence suggests that strains with increased virulence have emerged (Bloom & Small 1998). An article in *Nature* (Bloom 1992) was entitled 'Tuberculosis: back to a frightening future'. The World Health Organization has declared tuberculosis to be a 'global emergency' and has estimated that in 1996 there were 8 million new cases and 3 million deaths. It has become clear that there is an ominous synergy between mycobacteria (e.g. *Mycobacterium tuberculosis*, *Mycobacterium avium*) and the AIDS virus. The disease is out of control in many parts of the world and it is now the world's leading cause of death from a single agent.

Against this background we will now consider the antituberculosis drugs. The first-line drugs are, **isoniazid**, **rifampicin**, **ethambutol** and **pyrazinamide**. Some

second-line drugs available are **capreomycin**, **cycloserine**, **streptomycin** (rarely used now in the UK), **clarithromycin** and **ciprofloxacin**; these may be used for infections with tubercle bacilli likely to be resistant to first-line drugs or when the first-line agents have to be abandoned because of unwanted reactions.

To decrease the possibility of the emergence of resistant organisms, *compound drug therapy* is employed, involving the following:

- a first phase of about 2 months consisting of three drugs used concomitantly: isoniazid, rifampicin, pyrazinamide (plus ethambutol if the organism is suspected to be resistant)
- a second, continuation phase, of 4 months, consisting of two drugs: isoniazid and rifampicin; longer-term treatment is needed in some situations, for example for patients with meningitis, bone/joint involvement, drug-resistant infection.

ISONIAZID

The antibacterial activity of isoniazid is limited to mycobacteria. It is bacteriostatic on resting organisms but can kill dividing bacteria. It passes freely into mammalian cells and is thus effective against intracellular organisms, and it is actively taken up by tubercle bacilli. The mechanism of its action is not clearly known. There is evidence that it inhibits the synthesis of mycolic acids, important constituents of the cell wall and peculiar to mycobacteria. It is also reported to combine with an enzyme that is uniquely found in isoniazid-sensitive strains of mycobacteria; this results in disorganisation of the metabolism of the cell. Resistance can occur and is due to reduced penetration of the drug. Cross-resistance with other tuberculostatic drugs does not occur.

Pharmacokinetic aspects

Isoniazid is readily absorbed from the gastrointestinal tract and is widely distributed throughout the tissues and body fluids; the concentration in the CNS is the same as that in the serum. An important point is that it penetrates well into 'caseous' tuberculous lesions (i.e. necrotic lesions, with a cheese-like consistency). Metabolism, which involves largely acetylation, depends on genetic factors that determine whether a person is a 'slow' or 'rapid' acetylator of the drug (see Chs 5 and 48).

The half-life in slow inactivators is 3 hours and in rapid inactivators, 1 hour. Isoniazid is excreted in the urine partly as unchanged drug and partly in the acetylated or otherwise inactivated form.

Unwanted effects

Unwanted effects depend on the dosage and occur in about 5% of individuals, the commonest being allergic skin eruptions. A variety of other adverse reactions have been reported, including fever, hepatotoxicity, haematological changes, arthritic symptoms and vasculitis. Liver function should be assessed before treatment is started. Adverse effects involving the central or peripheral nervous systems are largely due to a deficiency of pyridoxine (see Fig. 43.6 for explanation) and are common in malnourished patients unless prevented by administration of this substance. Pyridoxal-hydrazone formation occurs mainly in slow acetylators. Isoniazid may cause haemolytic anaemia in individuals with glucose-6-phosphate deficiency and it decreases the metabolism of the antiepileptic agents, **phenytoin**, **ethosuximide** and **carbamazepine**, resulting in an increase in the plasma concentration and toxicity of these drugs.

RIFAMPICIN (RIFAMPIN)

Rifampicin acts by binding to, and inhibiting, DNA-dependent RNA polymerase in prokaryotic but not in eukaryotic cells (Ch. 41, p. 655). It is one of the most active antituberculosis agents known. It is also active against most Gram-positive bacteria as well as many Gram-negative species. It enters phagocytic cells and can kill intracellular microorganisms including the tubercle bacillus. Resistance can develop rapidly in a one-step process and is thought to be due to chemical modification of microbial DNA-dependent RNA polymerase, resulting from a chromosomal mutation (see Ch. 41, p. 660).

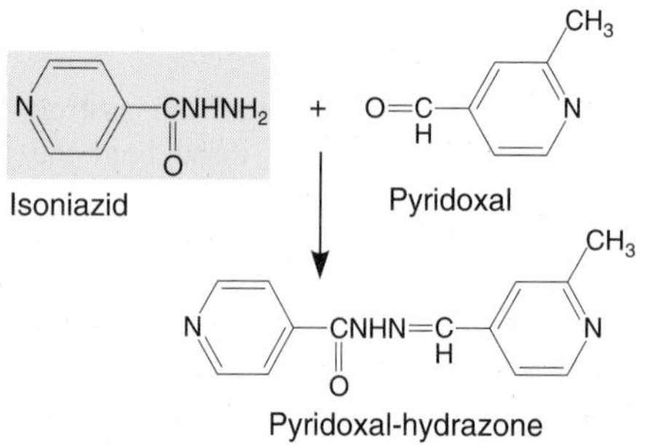

Fig. 43.6 Isoniazid, a tuberculostatic drug. In some circumstances it can cause pyridoxine deficiency by spontaneously forming a hydrazone with pyridoxal (as shown), the complex being rapidly excreted in the urine.

Pharmacokinetic aspects and unwanted effects

Rifampicin is given orally and is widely distributed in the tissues and body fluids, giving an orange tinge to saliva, sputum, tears and sweat. In the CSF it reaches 10–40% of its serum concentration. It is excreted partly in the urine and partly in the bile, some of it undergoing enterohepatic cycling. There is progressive metabolism of the drug by deacetylation during its repeated passages through the liver. The metabolite retains antibacterial activity but is less well absorbed from the gastrointestinal tract. The half-life is 1–5 hours, becoming shorter during treatment owing to induction of the hepatic microsomal enzymes.

Unwanted effects are relatively infrequent, occurring in fewer than 4% of individuals. The commonest are skin eruptions, fever and gastrointestinal disturbances. Liver damage with jaundice has been reported and has proved fatal in a very small proportion of cases. Liver function should be assessed before treatment is started. An influenza-like syndrome and a variety of symptoms of CNS disturbances have been recorded (dizziness, tiredness and confusion), as have various allergic manifestations such as urticaria and haemolysis. Rifampicin causes induction of hepatic metabolising enzymes resulting in an increase in the degradation of warfarin, glucocorticoids, narcotic analgesics, oral antidiabetic drugs, dapsone and oestrogens, the last leading to failure of oral contraceptives.

ETHAMBUTOL

Ethambutol has no effect on organisms other than mycobacteria. It is taken up by the bacteria and after a period of 24 hours it inhibits their growth. The mechanism of action is unknown. Resistance emerges rapidly if the drug is used on its own.

It is given orally and is well absorbed, reaching therapeutic plasma concentrations within 4 hours. In the blood it is taken up by erythrocytes and slowly released. It is partly metabolised and is excreted in the urine (50% of a dose as unchanged drug and 15% as metabolites). 20% appears in the faeces. The half-life is 3–4 hours. It can reach therapeutic concentrations in the CSF in tuberculous meningitis.

Unwanted effects are uncommon, the most important being optic neuritis, which is dose-related and is more likely to occur if renal function is decreased. It results in visual disturbances: initially red/green colour blindness followed by a decrease in visual acuity. Colour vision should be monitored during prolonged treatment.

Other unwanted effects are gastrointestinal disturbances, arthralgia, headache, giddiness and mental disturbances.

PYRAZINAMIDE

Pyrazinamide is inactive at neutral pH but tuberculostatic at acid pH. It is effective against the intracellular organisms in macrophages, since, after phagocytosis, the organisms are contained in phagolysosomes in which the pH is low. Resistance develops rather readily but cross-resistance with isoniazid does not occur.

The drug is well absorbed after oral administration, and is widely distributed, penetrating well into the meninges. It is excreted through the kidney, mainly by glomerular filtration.

Unwanted effects include gout, which is associated with high concentrations of plasma urates. Gastro-intestinal upsets, malaise and fever are reported. With the high doses previously used, serious hepatic damage was a possibility; this is now less likely with lower doses and shorter courses, but nevertheless, liver function should be assessed before treatment.

CAPREOMYCIN

Capreomycin is a peptide antibiotic given by intra-muscular injection. There is some cross-reaction with the aminoglycoside, **kanamycin**.

Unwanted effects are kidney damage and injury to the eighth nerve with deafness and ataxia. (The drug should not be given at the same time as streptomycin or other drugs that may damage the eighth nerve.)

CYCLOSERINE

Cycloserine is a broad-spectrum antibiotic inhibiting the growth of many bacteria including coliforms and mycobacteria. It is water-soluble and destroyed at acid pH. It is a structural analogue of D-alanine (Fig. 43.7A) and competitively inhibits cell wall synthesis by preventing the formation both of D-alanine and of the D-Ala–D-Ala dipeptide which is added to the initial tripeptide side-chain on N-acetylmuramic acid, i.e. it prevents completion of the major building block of peptidoglycan (see Figs 43.7B and 41.3). After being given orally it is rapidly absorbed and reaches peak concentrations within 4 hours. It is distributed throughout the tissues and body fluids, concentrations in the CSF being equivalent to the concentration in the blood. Most of the drug is eliminated in active form in the urine, but some (approximately 35%) is metabolised.

Unwanted effects affect mainly the central nervous system. A wide variety of disturbances may occur, ranging from headache and irritability to depression, convulsions and psychotic states.

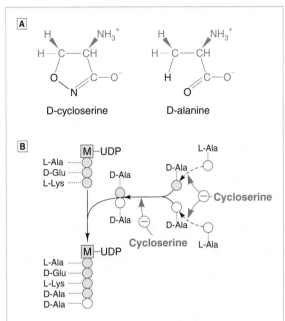

Fig. 43.7 Cycloserine. A The relationship of cycloserine to D-alanine (D-Ala). B Cycloserine inhibits an early stage of peptidoglycan synthesis; it inhibits the conversion of L-alanine (L-Ala) to D-Ala and also the conversion of two molecules of D-Ala to D-alanine-D-alanine. This is an enlarged section of Figure 41.3 and shows the peptide chain of *Staph. aureus*; N-acetylmuramic acid (M) and the four amino acids which make up the basic building block of the peptidoglycan are shown in light blue. (D-Glu = D-glutamic acid; L-Lys = L-lysine; UDP = uridine diphosphate)

Its use is limited to tuberculosis that is resistant to other drugs.

DRUGS USED TO TREAT LEPROSY

There are approximately 11 million individuals with leprosy world-wide, most being in Africa and Asia, and 600 000 new cases are detected each year. Multidrug treatment regimes initiated by WHO in 1982 are improving the outlook for this disease. Paucibacillary leprosy—leprosy with few bacilli, which is mainly *tuberculoid** in type—is treated for 6 months with **dapsone**, and **rifampicin**. Multibacillary leprosy—leprosy with numerous bacilli, which is mainly *lepromatous** in

---

*The basis of the difference appears to be that the T cells of patients with tuberculoid leprosy vigorously produce γ-interferon which enables macrophages to kill intracellular microbes, whereas in lepromatous leprosy, the immune response is dominated by interleukin-4 which blocks the action of γ-interferon. See Chapter 12.

Antituberculosis drugs

First-line drugs

- **Isoniazid** kills actively growing mycobacteria within host cells; mechanism of action unknown. Given orally it penetrates necrotic lesions, also the CSF. 'Slow acetylators' (genetically determined) respond well. It has low toxicity. Pyridoxine deficiency increases risk of neurotoxicity. No cross-resistance with other agents.
- **Rifampicin** is a potent, orally active drug, which inhibits mycobacterial RNA-polymerase. It penetrates CSF. Unwanted effects are infrequent (but serious liver damage has occurred). It induces hepatic drug-metabolising enzymes. Resistance can develop rapidly.
- **Ethambutol** inhibits growth of mycobacteria by unknown mechanism. It is given orally and can penetrate CSF. Unwanted effects are uncommon; optic neuritis can occur. Resistance can emerge rapidly.
- **Pyrazinamide** is tuberculostatic against intracellular mycobacteria by an unknown mechanism. Given orally, it penetrates CSF. Resistance can develop rapidly. Unwanted effects: increased plasma urate, liver toxicity with high doses.

Second-line drugs

- **Capreomycin** is given intramuscularly. Unwanted effects include damage to kidney and to VIIIth nerve.
- **Cycloserine** is broad spectrum. It inhibits an early stage of peptidoglycan synthesis. Given orally it penetrates the CSF. Unwanted effects affect mostly CNS.
- **Streptomycin**, an aminoglycoside antibiotic, acts by inhibiting bacterial protein synthesis. Given i.m. Unwanted effects: ototoxicity (mainly vestibular) and nephrotoxicity. Infrequently used now.

To avoid emergence of resistant organisms, compound therapy is used, e.g. three drugs initially, then two drugs later.

type—is treated for at least 2 years with **rifampicin**, **dapsone** and **clofazimine**. The effect of therapy with minocycline or the fluoroquinolones is being investigated.

DAPSONE

Dapsone (Fig. 43.8) is chemically related to the **sulphonamides** (Fig. 43.1) and, since its action is antagonised by PABA, probably acts by inhibition of folate synthesis.

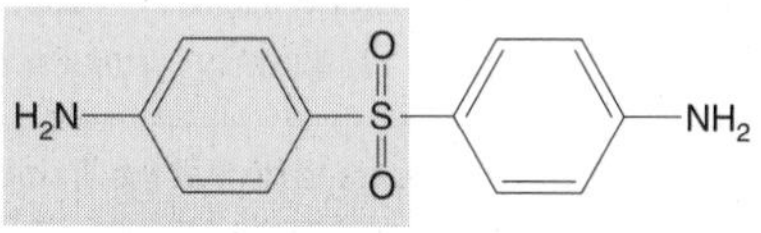

Fig. 43.8 Dapsone. The relationship with sulphanilamide (Fig. 43.1) is indicated by the light blue box.

Resistance to dapsone is increasing and treatment with combinations of drugs is now recommended.

Dapsone is given orally and is well absorbed and widely distributed through the body water and all tissues. The plasma half-life is 24–48 hours but some dapsone remains in certain tissues (liver, kidney, and, to some extent, skin and muscle) for much longer periods. There is enterohepatic recycling of the drug but some is acetylated and excreted in the urine. Dapsone is also used to treat dermatitis herpetiformis, a chronic blistering skin condition associated with coeliac disease.

Unwanted reactions occur fairly frequently and include haemolysis of red cells (usually not severe enough to lead to frank anaemia), methaemoglobinaemia, anorexia, nausea and vomiting, fever, allergic dermatitis and neuropathy. Lepra reactions (an exacerbation of lepromatous lesions) can occur and a syndrome resembling infectious mononucleosis, but which can be fatal, has occasionally been seen.

RIFAMPICIN

See page 704, under 'Drugs used to treat tuberculosis'.

CLOFAZIMINE

Clofazimine is a dye of complex structure. It has anti-inflammatory activity and is also therefore useful in patients in whom dapsone causes inflammatory side-effects. Its mechanism of action against leprosy bacilli may involve an action on DNA.

It is given orally and tends to cumulate in the body, being sequestered in the mononuclear phagocyte system. The antileprotic effect is delayed and is usually not seen for 6–7 weeks. The plasma half-life may be as long as 8 weeks.

Anti-leprosy drugs

- For tuberculoid leprosy: dapsone and rifampicin.
- For lepromatous leprosy: dapsone, rifampicin and clofazimine.
- **Dapsone** is sulphonamide-like and may inhibit folate synthesis. It is given orally. Unwanted effects are fairly frequent, a few are serious. Resistance is increasing.
- **Clofazimine** is a dye which is given orally and can cumulate by sequestering in macrophages. Action is delayed for 6–7 weeks. $t_{½}$ 8 weeks. Unwanted effects: red skin and urine, sometimes GIT disturbances.
- **Rifampicin** (see box on this page).

Unwanted effects may be related to the fact that clofazimine is a dye. Thus the skin and urine can develop a reddish colour and the lesions a blue-black discoloration. Dose-related nausea, giddiness, headache and gastrointestinal disturbances can also occur.

POSSIBLE NEW ANTIBACTERIAL DRUGS

New agents actively being sought include:

- agents to replace vancomycin for the treatment of resistant Gram-positive organisms; examples are: semisynthetic glycopeptides; the streptogramin antibiotic, quinupristin-dalfopristin; oxalidones; everninomycins (see Ford et al. 1997, Nicas et al. 1997)
- peptide antibiotics (see Hancock 1997)
- new quinolones: trovafloxacin and clinafloxacin are in Phase III trial
- new cephalosporin derivatives (e.g. cefepime, cefpirome are in development)
- new carbapenem-type compounds.

REFERENCES AND FURTHER READING

Amyes S G B, Gemmell C G (eds) 1997 Antibiotic resistance. J Med Microbiol 46: 436–470 (*Review of a symposium*)

Bloom B R 1992 Tuberculosis. Back to a frightening future. Nature 358: 538–539

Bloom B R, Small P M 1998 The evolving relation between humans and *Mycobacterium tuberculosis*. Lancet 338: 677–678 (*Editorial comment*)

Blumer J L 1997 Meropenem: evaluation of a new generation carbapenem. Int J Antimicrob Agents 8: 73–92

Brumfitt W, Hamilton-Miller J 1989 Methicillin-resistant *Staphylococcus aureus*. N Engl J Med 320: 1188–1195

Cohn D L, Bustreo F, Raviglioni M C 1997 Drug-resistant tuberculosis: review of the worldwide situation and the WHO/IUATLD global surveillance project. Clin Infect Dis 24: S121–S130

Courvalin P 1996 Evasion of antibiotic action by bacteria. J Antimicrob Chemother 37: 855–869 (*Covers recent developments in the understanding of the genetics and biochemical mechanisms of resistance*)

Donowitz G R, Mandell G L 1988 β-lactam antibiotics. N Engl J Med 318: 419–425, 490–500

Finch R 1990 The penicillins today. Br Med J 300: 1289–1290

Ford C W, Hamel J C et al. 1997 Oxalidones: new antibacterial agents. Trends Microbiol 5: 196–200 (*Promising candidates for antimicrobial action against multidrug-resistant Gram-positive bacteria*)

Gold H S, Moellering R C 1996 Antimicrobial drug resistance. N Engl J Med 335: 1445–1453 (*Excellent well-referenced review; covers mechanisms of resistance of important organisms to the main drugs; has useful table of therapeutic and preventive strategies, culled from the literature*)

Greenwood D (ed) 1995 Antimicrobial chemotherapy, 3rd edn. Oxford University Press Oxford, p 428

Hancock R E W 1997 Peptide antibiotics. Lancet 349: 418–422

Heym B, Honoré N et al. 1994 Implications of multidrug resistance for the future of short-course chemotherapy of tuberculosis: a molecular study. Lancet 344: 293–298

Hooper D C, Wolfson J S 1991 Fluoroquinolone antimicrobial agents. N Engl J Med 324: 384–394

Howie J 1986 Penicillin: 1929–1940. Br Med J 293: 158–159

Iseman M D 1993 Treatment of multidrug-resistant tuberculosis. N Engl J Med 329: 784–791

Jacoby G A, Archer G L 1991 Mechanisms of disease: new mechanisms of bacterial resistance to antimicrobial agents. N Engl J Med 324: 601–612

Jacoby G A, Medeiros A 1991 More extended-spectrum β-lactamases. Antimicrob Agents Chemother 35: 1697–1704

Just P M 1993 Overview of the fluoroquinolone antibiotics. Pharmacotherapy 13: 4S–17S

Knowles D J C 1997 New strategies for antibacterial drug design. Trends Microbiol 5: 379–383 (*Potential new approaches based on bacterial genomics*)

Laurence D R, Bennett P N, Brown M J 1997 Clinical pharmacology, 8th edn. Churchill Livingstone, Edinburgh, p 710

Lowy F D 1998 *Staphylococcus aureus* infections. N Engl J Med 339: 520–541 (*Structure of* Staph. aureus *pathogenesis of infection, resistance; extensive references; impressive diagrams*)

Moellering R C 1985 Principles of anti-infective therapy. In: Mandell G L, Douglas R G, Bennett J E (eds) Principles and practice of infectious disease. John Wiley, New York

Michel M, Gutman L 1997 Methicillin-resistant *Staphylococcus aureus* and vancomycin-resistant enterococci: therapeutic realities and possibilities. Lancet 349: 1901–1906 (*Excellent review article; good diagrams*)

Neu H C 1992 New macrolide antibiotics: azithromycin and clarithromycin. Ann Intern Med 116: 517–518

Nicas T I, Zeckel M L, Braun D K 1997 Beyond vancomycin: new therapies to meet the challenge of glycopeptide resistance. Trends Microbiol 5: 240–249

Quagliarello V J, Scheld W M 1997 Treatment of bacterial meningitis. N Engl J Med 336: 708–716

Raoult D, Drancourt M 1994 Antimicrobial therapy of rickettsial diseases. Antimicrob Agents Chemother 35: 2457–2462

Sato K, Hoshino K, Mitsuhashi S 1992 Mode of action of the new quinolones: the inhibitory action on DNA gyrase. Prog Drug Res 38: 121–132

Shimada J, Hori S 1992 Adverse effects of fluoroquinolones. Prog Drug Res 38: 133–143

Tillotson G S 1996 Quinolones: structure activity relationships and future predictions. J Med Microbiol 44: 320–324

Toshihiko U, Nakashima M 1992 Pharmacokinetic aspects of the newer quinolones. Prog Drug Res 38: 39–58

Wood M J 1991 More macrolides. Br Med J 303: 594–595

Woodford N, Johnson A P et al. 1995 Current perspectives on glycopeptide resistance. Clin Microbiol Rev 8: 585–615 (*Comprehensive review*)

44

Antiviral drugs

VIRAL INFECTION

Viruses are small infective agents consisting essentially of nucleic acid (either RNA or DNA) enclosed in a protein coat or capsid (Fig. 44.1). The coat plus the nucleic acid core is termed the nucleocapsid. Some viruses have, in addition, a lipoprotein envelope which may contain antigenic viral glycoproteins, as well as host phospho-

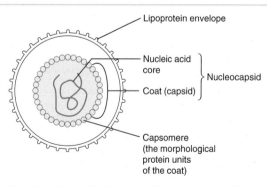

Fig. 44.1   Schematic diagram of the components of a virus particle or virion.

Lipoprotein envelope

Nucleic acid core

Coat (capsid)

Nucleocapsid

Capsomere (the morphological protein units of the coat)

lipids acquired when the virus nucleocapsid buds through the nuclear membrane or plasma membrane of the host cell. Certain viruses also contain enzymes which initiate their replication in the host cell. The whole infective particle is termed a virion. In different types of virus the genome may be double-stranded or single-stranded.

For simple descriptions of viruses see Timbury (1986), Challand & Young (1997).

EXAMPLES OF PATHOGENIC VIRUSES

Some important examples of viruses and the diseases they cause are as follows:

- *DNA viruses:* poxviruses (smallpox), herpesviruses (chickenpox, shingles, cold sores, glandular fever), adenoviruses (sore throat, conjunctivitis) and papillomaviruses (warts)
- *RNA viruses:* orthomyxoviruses (influenza), paramyxoviruses (measles, mumps), rubella virus (German measles), rhabdoviruses (rabies), picornaviruses (colds, meningitis, poliomyelitis), retroviruses (AIDS, T-cell leukaemia), arenaviruses (meningitis, Lassa fever), hepadnaviruses (serum hepatitis) and arboviruses (arthropod-borne encephalitis and various fevers, e.g. yellow fever).

Viruses are intracellular parasites with no metabolic machinery of their own. In order to replicate they have to attach to and enter a living host cell—animal, plant or bacterial—and use its metabolic processes. The binding sites on the virus are polypeptides on the envelope or capsid. The virus-specific receptors on the host cell, to which the virus attaches, are normal membrane constituents—receptors for cytokines, neurotransmitters or hormones, ion channels, integral membrane glycoproteins, etc. (Some examples of host cell receptors utilised by particular viruses are listed in Table 44.1.). The receptor/virus complex enters the cell by receptor-mediated endocytosis during which the virus coat may

Table 44.1 Some host cell structures that can function as receptors for viruses

Host cell structure	Virus
CD4 glycoprotein on helper T lymphocytes	HIV (AIDS virus)
The receptor, CCR5, for chemokines MCP-1* and RANTES†	HIV (AIDS virus)
Chemokine receptor, CXCR4, for cytokine SDF-1‡	HIV (AIDS virus)
Acetylcholine receptor on skeletal muscle	Rabies virus
Complement C3d receptor of B lymphocytes	Glandular fever virus
Interleukin-2 receptor on T lymphocytes	T cell leukaemia viruses
β-adrenoceptors	Infantile diarrhoea virus
MHC§ molecules	Adenovirus causing sore throat, conjunctivitis; T cell leukaemia viruses

*MCP-1 = **m**onocyte **c**hemoattractant **p**rotein-1
†RANTES = **r**egulated upon **a**ctivation, **n**ormal **T** cell **e**xpressed and **s**ecreted
‡SDF-1 = **s**tromal cell-**d**erived **f**actor-1
§MHC = **m**ajor **h**istocompatibility **c**omplex
For more detail on complement, interleukin-2, the CD4 glycoprotein on helper T lymphocytes, major histocompatibility complex molecules, etc., see Chapter 12. For SDF-1, see Chapter 18.

be removed. The nucleic acid of the virus then uses the cell's machinery for synthesising nucleic acid and protein and the manufacture of new virus particles.

Viral replication requires DNA or RNA synthesis, synthesis of viral proteins and glycosylation. A simplified account of viral replication is given here.

In *DNA viruses*, there is generally entry of the viral DNA into the host cell nucleus, transcription of this viral DNA into mRNA by host cell RNA polymerase followed by translation of the mRNA into virus-specific proteins. Some of these proteins are enzymes which then synthesise more viral DNA as well as proteins of the coat and envelope. After assembly of coat proteins around the viral DNA, complete virions are released by budding or after cell lysis. An example of the replication of a DNA virus is given in Figure 44.2.

In *RNA viruses*, enzymes in the virion synthesise its mRNA or the viral RNA serves as its own mRNA. This is translated into various enzymes, including RNA polymerase (which directs the synthesis of more viral RNA) and also into structural proteins of the virion. Assembly and release of virions occurs as explained above. With these viruses the host cell nucleus is usually not involved in viral replication.*

In *RNA retroviruses*, the virion contains a *reverse transcriptase* which makes a DNA copy of the viral RNA. This DNA copy is integrated into the host genome and it is then termed a 'provirus'. The provirus DNA

is transcribed into both new genomic RNA and mRNA for translation into viral proteins. The completed viruses are released by budding and many can replicate without killing the host cell. Some RNA retroviruses can transform normal cells into malignant cells. The AIDS virus is an RNA retrovirus; it is discussed in more detail below.

VIRAL PLOYS TO INVADE HOST CELLS AND EVADE HOST RESPONSES

Viruses have various invasion ploys; one such is described above—the expression of surface proteins that attach to host cell surface receptors (Table 44.1).

Viruses have also evolved mechanisms to evade the host's immune responses. The host normally deals with virus infection as follows: a virally infected cell presents, on its surface, viral peptides complexed with major histocompatibility (MHC-I) molecules; the complex is recognised by cytotoxic CD8 T cells (cytotoxic lymphocytes, CTLs)** which then kill the infected cell, probably by stimulating it to undergo apoptosis (programmed cell death; see Fig. 42.2).

Some viruses use a stealth ploy to evade this killer attack—they code for proteins that interfere with the presentation of MHC-peptide molecules. This turns off the signal that the cells are infected, enabling the viruses to remain undetected. These tactics do not, however, protect them from natural killer (NK) cells (Ch. 12,

---

*However, some RNA viruses, e.g. those causing influenza, have a requirement for active cellular transcription in the nucleus.

**MHC-I molecules are recognised by CD8 cells, MHC-II by CD4 cells (see Ch. 12 for more detail).

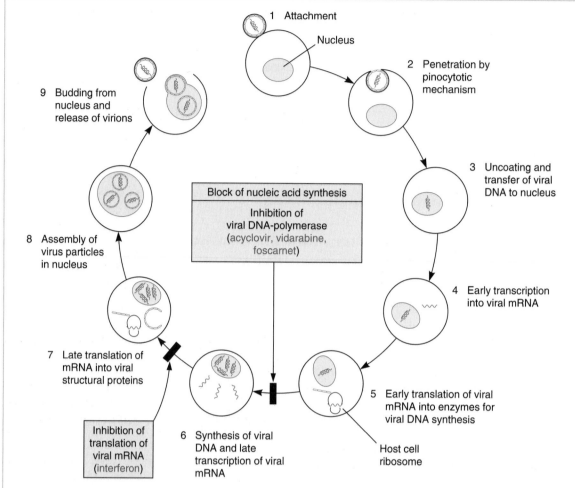

1 Attachment

Nucleus

2 Penetration by pinocytotic mechanism

9 Budding from nucleus and release of virions

3 Uncoating and transfer of viral DNA to nucleus

Block of nucleic acid synthesis

Inhibition of viral DNA-polymerase (acyclovir, vidarabine, foscarnet)

8 Assembly of virus particles in nucleus

4 Early transcription into viral mRNA

7 Late translation of mRNA into viral structural proteins

5 Early translation of viral mRNA into enzymes for viral DNA synthesis

Inhibition of translation of viral mRNA (interferon)

6 Synthesis of viral DNA and late transcription of viral mRNA

Host cell ribosome

Fig. 44.2 Schematic diagram of replication of a DNA virus (e.g. herpes simplex) in a host cell with the probable sites of action of antiviral agents. Viral components are shown in blue. In some viruses, assembly (stage 8) takes place in the host cell cytoplasm.

p. 203), which attack any cells that do not express MHC-I. This NK reaction to the absence of MHC molecules might be called the 'mother turkey' strategy (see Ch. 12, p. 203).

Some viruses, e.g. cytomegalovirus (a herpesvirus), apparently get round the mother turkey approach by adopting a 'baby turkey' ploy—they express a homologue of MHC-I (the equivalent of a baby turkey's noise) that is similar enough to the real thing to hoodwink NK cells, but not so similar that a CTL attack is triggered.

Some poxviruses after infecting a cell, express proteins that match cytokine receptors—reducing the work of synthesising the proteins by expressing only the extracellular ligand-binding domains; these pseudoreceptors, when released, bind cytokines, preventing them from

reaching their natural receptors on cells of the immune system and thus moderating the normal immune response to virus-infected cells.

Understanding of the virus–host interaction is expected to lead to new types of antiviral therapies.

THE HUMAN IMMUNODEFICIENCY VIRUS (HIV) AND AIDS

Infection with HIV* results in the acquired immune deficiency syndrome (AIDS). In 1997 it was estimated

*In fact, there are two viruses associated with AIDS—HIV-1 and HIV-2. HIV-1 cause most HIV infections world-wide; HIV-2 occurs in parts of Africa and India.

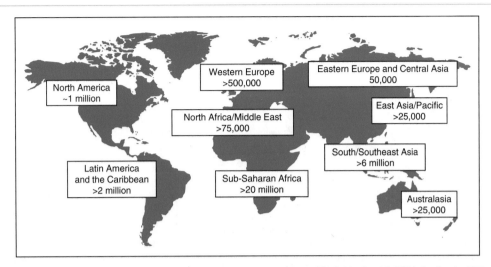

Fig. 44.3 **Figures from the United Nations AIDS programme for the number of individuals with HIV infection in 1997.** (McIlwain 1997 Nature 390: 326)

that nearly 30 million adults world-wide were infected with HIV, with the number of HIV infections increasing by five every minute. The epidemic is overwhelmingly centred on sub-Saharan Africa, where about 7% of the population is infected (see Fig. 44.3).

For a review of the pathogenesis of AIDS, see Levy (1993).

The interaction of HIV with the host's immune system is complex. Cells of the immune system have the equivalent of 'name badges' that identify them. The surface glycoprotein CD4 is the name badge of a particular group of helper T lymphocytes (see Fig. 12.3); it also occurs on macrophages and dendritic cells. HIV recognises the CD4 name badge, buttonholes the cell and infects it. Interaction of an HIV surface glycoprotein (gp 120) with CD4 is necessary but not sufficient for entry; additional interaction with a co-receptor is required for fusion of virus envelope with cell plasma membrane. Some variants of HIV are macrophage-tropic, i.e. infecting only macrophages and dendritic cells, and for these the co-receptor is a protein termed CCR5, which is the natural receptor for the β chemokines, MCP-1 and RANTES (see Ch. 12, pp. 202 and 224). Some variants are T cell-tropic and for these the co-receptor is a protein termed CXCR4.*

---

*CXCR4 is a G-protein-coupled receptor that was cloned before identification of its natural ligand—now known to be stromal cell-derived factor-1 (SDF-1).

Within the cell, HIV is integrated with the host DNA (the provirus form), undergoing transcription and generating new virions when the cell is activated. In an untreated subject, some 10^{10} new virus particles may be produced each day. Much of intracellular HIV may remain silent for a long time before being stimulated into activity when that particular T cell clone meets its intended antigen partner.

Antibodies are produced to various HIV components but it is the action of CD8 T cells (cytotoxic lymphocytes, CTLs) that initially prevents HIV spread by killing HIV-infected cells and releasing anti-HIV factors.

There is a progressive loss of CD4 cells (see Fig. 44.4); this is the defining characteristic of HIV infection. The reason for this loss is not clear; it may be due to killing by CTLs, direct virus-induced damage, etc.

Viral replication is error-prone and there are approximately 10^4–10^5 mutations per day at each site in the HIV genome, so HIV soon escapes the CTLs that recognise it initially. Although other CTLs recognise the mutated virus protein(s), further mutations in turn allow escape from these CTLs. It is suggested that wave after wave of CTLs act against new mutants as they arise, gradually diminishing the T cell repertoire, already being seriously diminished by loss of CD4 helper T cells. Eventually, the immune response fails.

There is considerable variation in the progress of the disease but the usual clinical course of HIV infection is shown in Figure 44.4. There is an initial acute flu-like

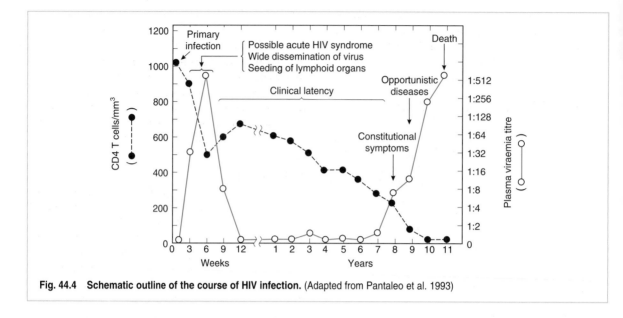

Fig. 44.4 Schematic outline of the course of HIV infection. (Adapted from Pantaleo et al. 1993)

illness associated with an increase in the number of virus particles in the blood, their widespread dissemination through the tissues and the seeding of lymphoid tissue with the virion particles. Within a few weeks the viraemia is reduced by the action of CD8 T cells specified above.

The acute illness is followed by a symptom-free period during which there is reduction in the viraemia accompanied by silent virus replication in the lymph nodes, associated with damage to lymph node architecture and the loss of CD4 lymphocytes and dendritic cells. Clinical latency (median, 10 years) comes to an end when the immune response finally fails and the signs and symptoms of AIDS appear—opportunistic infections (e.g. with *Pneumocystis carinii* or the tubercle bacillus), neurological disease (e.g. confusion, paralysis, dementia), bone marrow depression and cancers. Chronic gastrointestinal infections contribute to the severe weight loss. Cardiovascular damage and kidney damage can also occur. In an untreated patient, death usually follows within 2 years. The advent of highly active antiretroviral therapy (HAART) has changed the prognosis—in countries that can afford it. HAART is a combination of three antiviral drugs including at least one protease inhibitor (see below). There are at the time of writing 11 anti-HIV drugs available; five nucleoside reverse transcriptase inhibitors, three non-nucleoside reverse transcriptase inhibitors and four protease inhibitors. All are licensed in the USA but only eight in Europe. Most are discussed below.

With a HAART regime, HIV replication is inhibited—

its presence in the plasma being reduced to undetectable levels—and patient survival is prolonged; but the regime is complex, difficult to adhere to and may well have to be lifelong. It is also extremely expensive—which effectively prevents its use in developing countries. In any case, with the high mutation rate if the virus, resistance could be a problem in the future. HIV has certainly not yet been outsmarted.

The clinical use of currently available drugs for AIDS and HIV infection is described on page 715. It specifies the international consensus for use of anti-

Viruses

- Viruses are small infective agents consisting essentially of nucleic acid (RNA or DNA) enclosed in a protein coat.
- They are not cells and, having no metabolic machinery of their own, they are obligate intracellular parasites, i.e. they have to use the metabolic processes of the host cell which they enter and infect.
- DNA viruses usually enter the host cell nucleus and direct the generation of new viruses.
- RNA viruses direct the generation of new viruses, usually without involving the host cell nucleus (the 'flu' virus is an exception in that it does involve the host cell nucleus).
- RNA retroviruses (e.g. AIDS virus, T cell leukaemia virus) contain an enzyme, reverse transcriptase, which makes a DNA copy of the viral RNA. This DNA copy is integrated into the host cell genome and directs the generation of new virus particles.

retroviral therapy at the time of writing. The development of drugs to treat HIV infection and AIDS is progressing rapidly; possible future developments in HIV therapy are considered below (p. 717).

GENERAL ACTIONS OF ANTIVIRAL DRUGS

Because viruses share many of the metabolic processes of the host cell it is difficult to find drugs that are selective for the pathogen. However, there are some enzymes that are virus-specific and these are potential targets for drugs. Most currently available antiviral agents are only effective while the virus is replicating.

The main mechanisms of action of antiviral agents and the relevant drugs are given below.

INHIBITION OF TRANSCRIPTION OF THE VIRAL GENOME

DNA POLYMERASE INHIBITORS

Aciclovir (acyclovir)

The era of effective selective antiviral therapy began with aciclovir. This agent is a guanosine derivative (Fig. 44.5) with a high specificity for herpes simplex and varicella-zoster viruses. Herpes simplex can cause cold sores, conjunctivitis, mouth ulcers, genital infections* and, rarely but very seriously, encephalitis; in immunocompromised patients it is much more aggressive. Varicella-zoster viruses cause shingles and chickenpox. Herpes simplex is more susceptible to aciclovir than varicella-zoster. Epstein–Barr virus (a herpesvirus which causes glandular fever) is also slightly sensitive. Aciclovir has a small but reproducible effect against cytomegalovirus (CMV)—a herpesvirus which can affect the foetus with catastrophic consequences, and can cause a glandular-fever-like syndrome in adults and severe disease (e.g. retinitis, which can result in blindness) in individuals with decreased immune responses due to AIDS or the administration of immunosuppressants.

Mechanism of action

Aciclovir is converted to the monophosphate by thymidine kinase, and happily the virus-specific form of this enzyme is very much more effective in carrying out the phosphorylation than the enzyme of the host cell. It is therefore only adequately activated in infected cells, and the host cell's kinases then convert the monophosphate to the triphosphate. It is the aciclovir triphosphate that inhibits viral DNA-polymerase (Fig. 44.2), terminating the nucleotide chain. It is 30 times more potent against the herpesvirus enzyme than the host enzyme. Aciclovir triphosphate is fairly rapidly broken down within the host cells, presumably by cellular phosphatases. Resistance due to changes in the viral genes

*Venereologists (now called 'sexually transmitted disease physicians', references to Venus presumably being no longer acceptable) with a taste for cynical humour ask 'What is the difference between true love and genital herpes?', their answer being that genital herpes is for ever. (It may not be.)

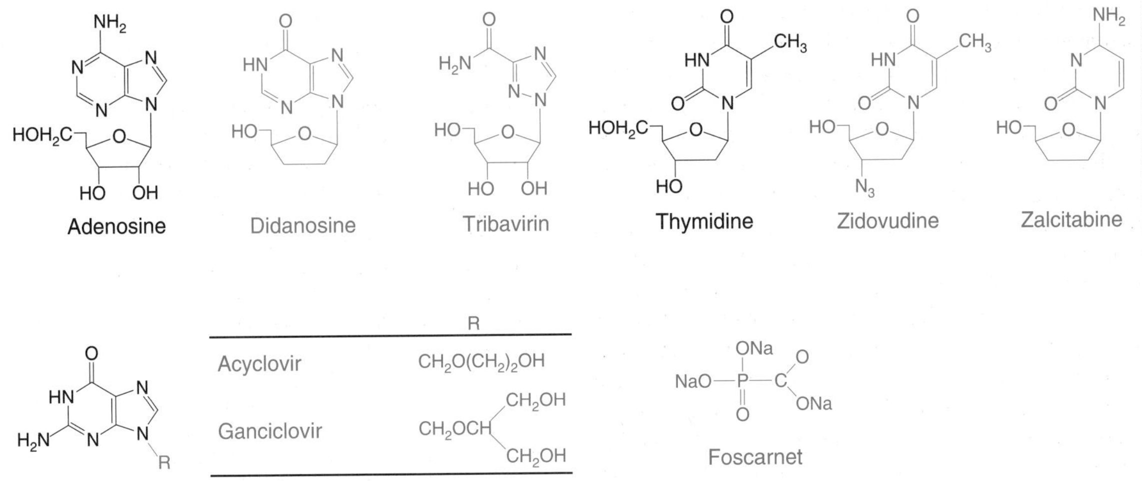

Fig. 44.5 Structures of some antiviral agents. The structures in black are found normally in vivo, those in blue are drugs.

coding for thymidine kinase or DNA polymerase has been reported and aciclovir-resistant herpes simplex virus has been the cause of pneumonia, encephalitis and mucocutaneous infections in immunocompromised patients.

Pharmacokinetic aspects

Aciclovir can be given orally, intravenously or topically. When it is given orally, only 20% of the dose is absorbed and peak plasma concentrations are reached in 1–2 hours. The drug is widely distributed, reaching concentrations in the CSF which are 50% of those in the plasma. It is excreted by the kidneys partly by glomerular filtration and partly by tubular secretion.

Unwanted effects

Unwanted effects are minimal. Local inflammation can occur during intravenous injection if there is extravasation of the solution. Renal dysfunction has been reported when aciclovir is given intravenously; slow infusion reduces the risk. Nausea and headache can occur and, rarely, encephalopathy.

Clinical use

The clinical uses of aciclovir are given on this page.

Other drugs similar to aciclovir are **valaciclovir** and **famciclovir**.

Valaciclovir is a pro-drug of aciclovir. Famciclovir is metabolised to penciclovir, the active compound, in vivo. Penciclovir has a similar action to aciclovir.

Clinical use of aciclovir

Aciclovir is used:

- to treat varicella-zoster infections (shingles), orally in immunocompetent patients, intravenously in immunocompromised patients
- to treat herpes simplex infections (genital herpes, mucocutaneous herpes and herpes encephalitis)
- to treat varicella (chickenpox) in immunocompromised patients
- prophylactically in patients who are to be treated with immunosuppressant drugs or radiotherapy and who are at risk of herpesvirus infection due to reactivation of a latent virus
- prophylactically in individuals who suffer from frequent recurrences of genital infection with herpes simplex virus.

Ganciclovir

Ganciclovir (Fig. 44.5), a synthetic nucleoside analogue, is the drug of choice for cytomegalovirus (CMV). Infection with CMV occurs particularly in immunocompro-

mised individuals; it is a frequent opportunistic infection in AIDS patients and has been a formidable obstacle to successful transplantation of organs and bone marrow (which necessitates immunosuppressive therapy).

Like aciclovir, ganciclovir has to be activated to the triphosphate and in this form it competes with guanosine triphosphate for incorporation into viral DNA. It suppresses viral DNA replication, but unlike aciclovir it does not act as a chain terminator, nor is it rapidly broken down, being shown to persist in cells infected with cytomegalovirus for 18–20 hours.

Ganciclovir is given intravenously, excreted in the urine and has a half-life of 4 hours. It has serious unwanted actions, including bone marrow depression and potential carcinogenicity and it is therefore used only for life- or sight-threatening cytomegalovirus infections in patients who are immunocompromised. Oral administration can be used for maintenance therapy in AIDS patients.

Tribavirin (ribavirin)

Tribavirin (Fig. 44.5) is a synthetic nucleoside, similar in structure to guanosine. It is thought to act either by altering virus nucleotide pools or by interfering with the synthesis of viral mRNA (Fig. 44.2). It inhibits a wide range of DNA and RNA viruses including many that affect the lower airways. In aerosol form it has been used to treat influenza and infections due to respiratory syncytial virus (an RNA paramyxovirus).

It has been shown to be effective in Lassa fever, an extremely serious arenavirus infection; given intravenously within the first 6 days of onset it has been shown to reduce to 9% a case-fatality rate previously 76%.

Foscarnet (phosphonoformate)

Foscarnet (Fig. 44.5) is a synthetic non-nucleoside analogue of pyrophosphate which inhibits viral DNA polymerase by binding directly to the pyrophosphate-binding site. It can cause serious nephrotoxicity. Given by intravenous infusion, it is a second-line drug in cytomegalovirus eye infection in immunocompromised patients.

REVERSE TRANSCRIPTASE INHIBITORS

Zidovudine (azidothymidine, AZT)

Zidovudine (Fig. 44.5) is an analogue of thymidine. In retroviruses—such as the HIV virus—it is an active inhibitor of reverse transcriptase. It is phosphorylated by cellular enzymes to the triphosphate form, in which it competes with equivalent cellular triphosphates which are essential substrates for the formation of proviral DNA by viral reverse transcriptase (viral RNA-dependent

DNA polymerase); its incorporation into the growing viral DNA strand results in chain termination. Mammalian alpha DNA polymerase is relatively resistant to the effect. However, gamma DNA polymerase in the host cell mitochondria is fairly sensitive to the compound and this may be the basis of unwanted effects. The use of zidovudine in the prevention and treatment of AIDS is outlined in the box on this page in which it features as one of the reverse transcriptase inhibitors.

Pharmacokinetic aspects
Given orally, the bioavailability of zidovudine is 60–80% and the peak plasma concentration occurs at 30 minutes. It can also be given intravenously. Its half-life is 1 hour, and the intracellular half-life of the active triphosphate is 3 hours. Zidovudine enters mammalian cells by passive diffusion and in this is unlike most other nucleosides which require active uptake. The drug passes into the CSF and brain. Most of the drug is metabolised to inactive glucuronide in the liver, only 20% of the active form being excreted in the urine.

Unwanted effects
Anaemia and neutropenia are common, particularly with long-term administration.* Other unwanted effects include gastrointestinal disturbances, paraesthesia, skin rash, insomnia, fever, headaches, abnormalities of liver function and, more particularly, myopathy. Confusion, anxiety, depression and a flu-like syndrome are also reported. The prophylactic use of the drug, short-term, in fit individuals, after specific exposure to the virus, is associated with only minor, reversible unwanted effects.

Resistance to the antiviral action of zidovudine
Because of rapid mutation the virus is a constantly moving target, thus the therapeutic response wanes with long-term use, particularly in late-stage disease. Furthermore, resistant strains can be transferred between individuals. Other factors which underlie the loss of efficacy of the drug are decreased activation of zidovudine to the triphosphate and increased virus load due to reduction in immune mechanisms.

Didanosine (dideoxyinosine, ddI)
Didanosine is a synthetic purine dideoxynucleoside analogue. It is phosphorylated in the host cell to the triphosphate, dideoxyadenosine, in which form it acts as a chain terminator and inhibitor of the viral reverse transcriptase. It is used to treat AIDS.

Pharmacokinetic aspects
Didanosine is given orally, rapidly absorbed and is actively secreted by the kidney tubules. The plasma half-life is 30 minutes but the intracellular half-life is more than 12 hours. The cerebrospinal fluid/plasma ratio is 0.2.

Unwanted effects
The main unwanted effect—occurring in > 30% of patients—is dose-related pain and sensory loss in the feet. Dose-related pancreatitis occurs in 5–10% of patients and has been fatal in a few cases. Headache and gastrointestinal disturbance are also common and insomnia, skin rashes, bone marrow depression (less marked than with AZT) and alterations of liver function have been reported.

Zalcitabine (dideoxycytidine, ddC)
Zalcitabine, a synthetic nucleoside analogue, is used in combination with zidovudine for the therapy of AIDS. It is a reverse transcriptase inhibitor and it is activated in the T cell by a different phosphorylation pathway from zidovudine. It is given orally, its plasma half-life is 20 minutes, its intracellular half-life is nearly 3 hours and its cerebrospinal fluid/plasma ratio is ~0.2.

Unwanted effects
The most important unwanted effect is a dose-related neuropathy (which can increase for several weeks after the drug has been stopped). Other unwanted effects include gastrointestinal disturbances, headache, mouth ulcers, nail changes, oedema of the lower limbs and general malaise. Skin rashes occur but may resolve spontaneously. Pancreatitis has been reported.

Treatment of HIV/AIDS

An international consensus on the use of retroviral therapy in AIDS has emerged based on the following five therapeutic principles:*

- Monitor plasma viral load and CD4 count.
- Start treatment before immunodeficiency becomes evident.
- Aim to reduce plasma viral concentration as much as possible for as long as possible.
- Use combinations of at least three drugs, e.g. two reverse transcriptase inhibitors and one protease inhibitor.
- Change to a new regime if plasma viral concentration increases.

*Modified from Montaner et al. 1997.

---

*Administration of erythropoietin and GM-CSF (see Ch. 23, p. 336) may alleviate these problems.

New **non-nucleoside reverse transcriptase inhibitors** now in use include **lamuvidine** and **stavudine**.

Non-nucleoside reverse transcriptase inhibitors under test include **nevirapine**, **delavirdine** and **loviride**. All are given orally.

INHIBITION OF POST-TRANSLATIONAL EVENTS

PROTEASE INHIBITORS

Host mRNAs code directly for functional proteins, but in HIV, the RNA is translated into biochemically inert polyproteins. A *virus-specific protease* then converts the polyprotein into various structural and functional proteins by cleavage at the appropriate positions. Since this protease does not occur in the host, it is a good target for chemotherapeutic intervention. Several protease inhibitors have now been developed, and their use, in combination with reverse transcriptase inhibitors, has transformed the therapy of AIDS. Examples of current protease inhibitors are: **saquinavir**, **ritonavir**, **indinavir**, and **nelfinavir**. The first three are licensed in Europe, all are licensed in the USA.

They are all given orally and all can cause gastro-intestinal disorders: nausea, vomiting and diarrhoea. Raised concentrations of liver enzymes in the blood are reported with ritonavir and indinavir. Ritonavir can cause paraesthesias around the mouth, and in the hands and feet, and patients on indinavir may develop kidney stones.

All inhibit the cytochrome P450 enzymes (indinavir and saquinavir to a lesser extent than ritonavir) and can interact with other drugs handled by this system, and all can increase the plasma concentration of benzo-diazepines. Preliminary evidence suggests that long-term use may lead to an unusual redistribution of cutaneous fat.

INHIBITION OF ATTACHMENT TO OR PENETRATION OF HOST CELLS

Amantadine

Amantadine* is active against influenza A virus (an RNA virus) but has no action against influenza B virus. **Rimantadine** is similar in its effects.

Mechanism of action

At two stages of viral replication within the host cell, a viral membrane protein, M_2, functions as an ion channel. The stages are: (i) the fusion of viral membrane and endosome membrane and (ii) the later stage of assembly

---

*Also used for its mildly beneficial effect in Parkinson's disease.

and release of new virions at the host cell surface. Amantadine blocks this ion channel.

Pharmacokinetic aspects and unwanted effects

Given orally, amantadine is well absorbed, reaches high levels in secretions (e.g. saliva) and most is excreted unchanged via the kidney. Aerosol administration is feasible.

Unwanted effects are relatively infrequent, occurring in 5–10% of patients, and are not serious. Dizziness, insomnia and slurred speech are the most common adverse effects.

Immunoglobulin

Pooled immunoglobulin contains antibodies against various viruses present in the population. The antibodies are directed against the virus envelope and can 'neutralise' some viruses and prevent their attachment to host cells. If used before the onset of signs and symptoms it may attenuate or prevent measles, infectious hepatitis, German measles, rabies or poliomyelitis. Hyperimmune globulin, specific against particular viruses, is used against hepatitis B, varicella-zoster and rabies.

IMMUNOMODULATORS

Interferon (IFN)

Interferons are a family of inducible proteins synthesised by mammalian cells and now produced by recombinant DNA technology. There are at least three types, α-, β-, and γ-interferon, constituting a family of hormones involved in cell growth and regulation and modulation of immune reactions. γ-interferon, termed 'immune interferon' (see Ch. 12, p. 206 and Fig. 12.3), is produced mainly by T lymphocytes as part of an immunological response to both viral and non-viral antigens, the latter including bacteria and their products, rickettsiae, protozoa, fungal polysaccharides and a range of polymeric chemicals and other cytokines. α- and β-interferons are produced by B and T lymphocytes, macrophages and fibroblasts in response to the presence of viruses and cytokines. The general actions of the interferons are described briefly in Chapter 12 (p. 225).

Mechanism of antiviral action of interferons

Interferons work by inducing, in the ribosomes of the host's cells, the production of enzymes that inhibit the translation of viral mRNA into viral proteins and thus stop the reproduction of the viruses (Fig. 44.2). Interferons bind to specific receptors on cell membranes, which may be gangliosides. They inhibit the replication of most viruses in vitro.

Pharmacokinetic aspects

Given intravenously, interferons have a half-life of 2–4 hours. With intramuscular injections, peak blood concentrations are reached in 5–8 hours. They do not cross the blood–brain barrier.

Clinical use

α-interferon is used for treatment of hepatitis B infections and AIDS-related Kaposi sarcomas, interferon α-2b for hepatitis C. There are reports that interferons can prevent re-activation of herpes simplex after trigeminal root section, and prevent spread of herpes zoster in cancer patients.

When used for antiviral chemotherapy, interferons act partly by augmenting the host's immune response (see Ch. 12).

Unwanted effects. These are common and include fever, lassitude, headache and myalgia. Repeated injections cause chronic malaise. Bone marrow depression, rashes, alopecia and disturbances in cardiovascular, thyroid and hepatic function can also occur.

POSSIBLE FUTURE DEVELOPMENTS IN ANTIVIRAL THERAPY

A variety of new approaches to antiviral therapy are being explored, particularly anti-HIV agents; some examples are given below. See also Challand & Young (1997).

Agents affecting viral attachment to host cells

This group includes drugs that interact with the sites on viruses which bind to host cells (e.g. the envelope protein, gp120, of HIV), and antagonists of the chemokine receptors that act as co-receptors for HIV. One such is AOP-RANTES, which potently inhibits infection by macrophage-tropic HIV in vitro (Simmons et al. 1997).

Agents affecting uncoating

The three-dimensional structure of the capsid of the RNA virus causing the common cold is known. Some drugs now in development can bind tightly to one of the proteins in the shell, preventing uncoating of the virion.

Agents affecting early stages of viral replication

This group includes inhibitors of integration of viral DNA into host genome, or of transcription of viral DNA.

- *Antisense oligonucleotides* (ANOs) are synthetic nucleotides of short chain length (13–20) which bind to specific portions of the viral genome by complementary base-pairing. This interferes with the function

Antiviral drugs

These act by the following mechanisms:

Inhibition of penetration of host cell
- Amantadine inhibits uncoating and is effective against influenza A virus.
- Gamma globulin 'neutralises' viruses.

Inhibition of transcription of the viral genome
DNA polymerase inhibitors:
- Aciclovir, a guanosine derivative, selectively inhibits viral DNA polymerase; effective against herpesviruses; minimal unwanted effects.
- Ganciclovir, also a guanosine derivative, is phosphorylated and then incorporated into viral DNA, suppressing its replication; used in cytomegalovirus (CMV) infection, especially CMV retinitis in AIDS patients; it can have serious unwanted effects.
- Vidarabine, an adenosine derivative, is a relatively selective inhibitor of viral DNA polymerase; effective against herpes simplex and varicella-zoster; can have serious unwanted effects.
- Tribavirin is similar to guanosine and is thought to interfere with synthesis of viral mRNA; it can inhibit many DNA and RNA viruses.
- Foscarnet inhibits viral DNA polymerase by attaching to the pyrophosphate binding site; it is fairly effective in cytomegalovirus infection.

Reverse transcriptase inhibitors (RTIs)
- Zidovudine, an analogue of thymidine, is relatively effective in HIV/AIDS. Other RTIs are zalcitabine and didanosine. They are used in combination with protease inhibitors.
- Non-nucleoside RTIs, e.g. lamuvidine and stavudine have been introduced.

Inhibition of post-translational events
- Protease inhibitors e.g. indinavir and saquinavir, inhibit cleavage of the translated inert protein into functional and structural proteins. They are used in combination with reverse transcriptase inhibitors.

Immunomodulators
- Interferons induce, in the host cells' ribosomes, enzymes which inhibit viral mRNA; they are used in hepatitis B infection and may be useful in AIDS.

of RNA by blocking RNA transport or translation. At least three antisense oligonucleotides are in phase I trial for HIV treatment (Matteucci & Wagner 1996), and an anti-cytomegalovirus ANO is in phase III clinical trial).
- *Integrase inhibitors* are being studied as potential antiviral agents.
- *Ribonucleotide reductase inhibitors.* The activity of

ribonucleotide reductase, which converts ribonucleotides to deoxyribonucleotides, is an essential step in DNA synthesis. The enzyme consists of two subunits which must form a dimer before the enzyme can act. A synthetic nonapeptide that mimics the sequence involved in the interaction between the two subunits can bind competitively to one subunit and prevents dimer formation. A shortened version of this peptide might have effective antiviral activity.

Agents affecting late stages in viral replication

A late step in viral replication is the formation of the viral envelope, which involves glycosylation; glycosylation inhibitors are being developed and tested. Cytoskeletal processes are involved in assembly and release of virus particles; agents which interfere with these processes are being sought.

In influenza virus, the action of neuraminidase is involved in the budding of new virus from infected cells. The neuraminidase inhibitor, **zanamivir**, active against both influenza A and B viruses, may have a place in therapy.

Immune-directed therapies

This group includes cytokine-based therapy, gene therapy, vaccines* and attempts to alter the balance of the host's immune responses.

- Some authorities think that an imbalance between different types of immune responses and the associated cytokines (see Ch. 12, p. 223) affects HIV replication and the progress to AIDS. Some cytokines, e.g. the primary pro-inflammatory cytokines TNF-α and IL-1 (see Ch. 12) can induce HIV expression whereas others, e.g. IL-10 and IL-16, inhibit it. CD8 T cells release soluble factors** that suppress HIV replication. Th2 cytokines (see above) inhibit the production of this factor (discussed by Fauci 1996). Various approaches to changing the balance between HIV-suppressing and HIV-inducing host responses are being considered (see Pantaleo 1997), but it is early days yet.
- Adoptive transfer of gene-modified virus-specific T lymphocytes is under test for Epstein–Barr virus infections.
- A phase I trial of gene therapy, using genes encoding two HIV proteins, is underway in Japan.
- Vaccines against the HIV coat protein gp120 are in phase I trial.

---

*Vaccines are of course already in routine use for the prevention of numerous viral infections.

**In addition to the chemokines RANTES and macrophage inhibitory protein (MIP) which compete with HIV for its co-receptors.

REFERENCES AND FURTHER READING

Bangham C R M, Phillips R E 1997 What is required of an HIV vaccine? Lancet 350: 1617–1621

Barré-Sinoussi F 1996 HIV as the cause of AIDS. Lancet 348: 31–35 (*Clear coverage of structure, genome map, genetic diversity of HIV and evolution of primate lentiviruses*)

Bonifacino J S 1996 Reversal of fortune for nascent proteins. Nature 384: 405-406. (*Gives details of viral ploys to evade immune surveillance and discusses how abnormal proteins once synthesised can be degraded*)

Cairns J S, D'Souza M P 1998 Chemokines and HIV-1 second receptors: the therapeutic connection. Nature Med 4: 563–568 (*Excellent review of therapeutic strategies that target the chemokine receptors used by HIV-1 to invade host cells*)

Challand R, Young R J 1997 Antiviral chemotherapy. Spectrum, USA, p 128 (*A monograph in the Biochemical and Medicinal Chemistry Series; emphasis on medicinal chemistry*)

Cohn J A 1997 Recent advances: HIV-1 infection. Br Med J 314: 487–491 (*Short, clear coverage of clinical course of HIV infection, laboratory tests, and the newly licensed drugs: nucleoside reverse transcriptase inhibitors (RTIs) non-nucleoside RTIs and protease inhibitors*)

D'Souza M P, Harden V A 1996 Chemokines and HIV-1 second receptors. Nature Med 2: 1293–1300 (*Very clear coverage of the relationship between HIV and β-chemokines; useful diagram*)

Fauci A S 1996 Host factors and the pathogenesis of HIV-induced disease. Nature 384: 529–534 (*Dense coverage of immune mechanisms—particularly cytokines and chemokines and their receptors—in AIDS pathogenesis*)

Flexner C 1998 HIV-protease inhibitors. N Engl J Med 338: 1281–1292 (*Excellent, comprehensive review covering mechanisms of action, clinical and pharmacokinetic properties, potential drug resistance and possible treatment failure*)

Gallo R C, Lusso P 1997 Chemokines and HIV infection. Curr Opin Infect Dis 10: 12–17 (*Clear coverage of chemokine receptors as co-receptors for HIV, and the clinical relevance for HIV infection*)

Gazzard B, Moyle G et al 1998. 1998 revision to the British HIV Association guidelines for antiretroviral treatment of HIV seropositive individuals. The Lancet 352: 314–316 (*Consensus statement from the British HIV Association*)

Hirschel B, Francioli P 1998 Progress and problems in the fight against AIDS. N Engl J Med 338: 906–908

Kärre K, Welsh R M 1997 Viral decoy vetoes killer cell. Nature 386: 446–447 (*Covers invasion ploys of HIV; very readable; useful diagram*)

Lee W M 1997 Hepatitis B virus infection. N Engl J Med 337: 1733–1745 (*Detailed review covering genome of the virus and the immunopathogenesis, clinical aspects and treatment of the infection*)

Levy J A 1993 Pathogenesis of human immunodeficiency virus infection. Microbiol Rev 57: 183–289 *(Detailed review)*

Levy J A 1996 Infection by human immunodeficiency virus: CD4 is not enough. N Engl J Med 335: 1528–1530 *(Excellent explanatory diagram of interaction of virus with CD4 and co-receptors on human cell)*

Matteucci M, Wagner R W 1996 In pursuit of antisense. Nature 384: 20–22 *(Mechanism of action of antisense oligonucleotides with emphasis on chemistry)*

Miller R H, Sarver N 1997 HIV accessory proteins as therapeutic targets. Nature Med 4: 389–394

Montaner J S G, Hogg R S, O'Shaughnessy M V 1997 Emerging international consensus for use of antiretroviral therapy. Lancet 349: 1042

Nguyen B-Y, Yarchoan R 1996 Anti-HIV drugs. In Chabner BA, Longo D L (eds) Cancer chemotherapy and biotherapy. Lippincott-Raven, Philadelphia, ch 21, 493–508 *(Structure, mechanisms of action and pharmacology of the main anti-HIV drugs—at the time)*

Pantaleo G 1997 How immune-based interventions can change HIV therapy. Nature Med 3: 483–490

Pantaleo G, Fauci A S 1996 Immunopathogenesis of HIV infection. Annu Rev Microbiol 50: 825–854 *(Detailed review of interrelation of HIV infection and immune responses; discusses how this affects the progression of the disease in different individuals: 'rapid progressors', 'typical progressors', 'long term non-progressors' and 'long-term survivors')*

Pantaleo G, Graziosi C, Fauci A S 1993 The immunopathogenesis of human immunodeficiency virus infection. N Engl J Med 328: 327–335 *(Good coverage of pathogenesis)*

Rosenberg Y J, Anreson A O, Pabst R 1998 HIV-induced decline in blood CD4/CD8 ratios: viral killing or altered lymphocyte trafficking. Immunol Today 19: 10–16

Sepkowitz K A 1998 Effect of HAART on natural history of AIDS-related opportunistic disorders. Lancet 351: 228–230

Simmons G, Clapham P R et al. 1997 Potent inhibition of HIV-1 infectivity in macrophages and lymphocytes by a novel CCR5 antagonist. Science 276: 276–279

Skehel J J 1992 Influenza virus: amantadine blocks the channel. Nature 358: 110–111

Smythe J A, Symonds G 1995 Gene therapeutic agents: the use of ribozymes, antisense, and RNA decoys for HIV-1 infection. Inflamm Res 44: 11–15

Timbury M C 1986 Notes on medical virology. Churchill Livingstone, Edinburgh

Wagner R W, Flannagan W M 1997 Antisense technology and prospects for therapy of viral infections and cancer. Mol Med Today (January): 31–38

Wain-Hobson S 1997 Down or out in blood and lymph. Nature 387: 123–124 *(Short 'News and Views' article on recent advances; very readable)*

Werther G 1998 Not all is dead in the HIV-1 graveyard. Lancet 351: 308–309 *(Short article about reservoir of latent infection)*

Wolthers K C, Schuitemake H, Miedema F 1998 Rapid CD4+ T-cell turnover in HIV-1 infection: a paradigm revisited. Immunol Today 19: 44–48

45

Antifungal drugs

FUNGAL INFECTIONS

Fungal infections are termed *mycoses* and in general can be divided into superficial infections (affecting skin, nails, scalp or mucous membranes) and systemic infections (affecting deeper tissues and organs). Many of the fungi that can cause mycoses live in association with humans as commensals or are present in the environment; but until recently, serious superficial infections were relatively uncommon and systemic infections very uncommon indeed—at least in cool and temperate climatic zones. In these zones, a fungal infection usually meant athlete's foot or oral or vaginal thrush, which caused discomfort but were hardly life-threatening. But in the last 30 years there has been a steady increase in the incidence of serious secondary systemic fungal infections. One factor has been the widespread use of broad-spectrum antibiotics, which eliminate or decrease the non-pathogenic bacterial populations that normally compete with fungi. Another has been the increase in the number of individuals with reduced immune responses due to AIDS or the action of immunosuppressant drugs or cancer chemotherapy agents; this has led to an increased prevalence of opportunistic infections, i.e. infections with fungi which are normally either innocuous or readily overcome in immunocompetent individuals.

In the UK the commonest systemic fungal disease is systemic candidiasis—an infection with a yeast-like organism. Others are cryptococcal meningitis or endocarditis, pulmonary aspergillosis, and rhinocerebral mucormycosis. Invasive pulmonary aspergillosis is now a leading cause of death in recipients of bone marrow transplants.

In other parts of the world the commonest systemic fungal infections are blastomycosis, histoplasmosis, coccidiomycosis and paracoccidiomycosis; these are often primary infections, i.e. they are not secondary to reduced immunological function or altered commensal microorganisms.

Superficial fungal infections can be classified into the *dermatomycoses* and *candidiasis*. Dermatomycoses are infections of the skin, hair and nails, caused by dermatophytes. The commonest are due to *Tinea* organisms, which cause various types of 'ringworm'. *Tinea capitis* affects the scalp, *Tinea cruris*, the groin, *Tinea pedis*, the feet (causing 'athlete's foot'), and *Tinea corporis*, the body. In superficial candidiasis, the yeast-like organism infects the mucous membranes of the mouth ('thrush') or vagina, or skin.

The drugs used in fungal infections are described briefly below and their clinical use is outlined in Table 45.1.

DRUGS USED FOR FUNGAL INFECTIONS

For detailed coverage of antifungal drugs, see Hoeprich (1995).

ANTIFUNGAL ANTIBIOTICS

Amphotericin

Amphotericin is a macrolide antibiotic of complex structure, characterised by a many-membered ring of carbon atoms.

Mechanism of action

Amphotericin binds to cell membranes (like other polyene antibiotics; see Ch. 41) and interferes with permeability and with transport functions. It forms a pore in the membrane, the hydrophilic core of the molecule creating a

Table 45.1 Outline of the uses of antifungal drugs

Disease	Drug used
Systemic infections	
Systemic candidiasis	Amphotericin ± flucytosine,* fluconazole
Cryptococcosis (meningitis)	Amphotericin ± flucytosine,* fluconazole, itraconazole
Systemic aspergillosis	Itraconazole,* amphotericin
Blastomycosis	Itraconazole,* amphotericin
Histoplasmosis	Amphotericin, itraconazole, fluconazole
Coccidiomycosis	Fluconazole, itraconazole, amphotericin
Paracoccidiomycosis	Fluconazole, itraconazole, amphotericin
Mucormycosis	Amphotericin ± flucytosine*
Disseminated sporotrichosis	Amphotericin, itraconazole
Superficial infections	
Dermatomycosis	
Tinea pedis (athlete's foot)	A topical azole, or oral itraconazole
Tinea corporis (skin ringworm)	A topical azole, oral terbinafine, oral itraconazole
Tinea cruris	
Tinea capitis	Oral itraconazole
Tinea unguium (nail infection)	Oral or topical terbinafine, topical amorolfine
Candidiasis	
Skin	A topical azole, topical nystatin
Mouth (thrush)	A topical azole or nystatin, oral fluconazole
Vagina	A topical azole, oral fluconazole
Chronic mucocutaneous candidiasis	Fluconazole, ketoconazole[†]

*Drugs of choice
[†]The potential benefits of treatment should be carefully weighed against the risk of liver damage.

transmembrane ion channel. One of the repercussions of this is a loss of intracellular K^+ ions. Amphotericin has a selective action, binding avidly to the membranes of fungi and some protozoa, less avidly to mammalian cells and not at all to bacteria. The relative specificity for fungi may be due to the drug's greater avidity for ergosterol (the fungal membrane sterol) than for cholesterol, the main sterol in the plasma membrane of animal cells. It is active against most fungi and yeasts.

Amphotericin enhances the antifungal effect of **flu-cytosine** (see below).

Pharmacokinetic aspects

Given orally, amphotericin is poorly absorbed, and it is therefore only given by this route for fungal infections of the gastrointestinal tract. For systemic infections it is complexed with sodium deoxycholate and given as a suspension by slow intravenous injection. Other preparations available for intravenous infusion include amphotericin complexed with lipids or encapsulated in liposomes. It can also be given topically.

The drug is very highly protein-bound and is found in fairly high concentrations in inflammatory exudates.

It normally crosses the blood–brain barrier poorly but penetration may be improved when the meninges are inflamed since intravenous amphotericin, used with flu-cytosine, is effective in cryptococcal meningitis. It is excreted very slowly via the kidney, traces being found in the urine for 2 months or more after administration has ceased.

Unwanted effects

The commonest and most serious unwanted effect of amphotericin is renal toxicity. Some degree of reduction of renal function occurs in more than 80% of patients receiving the drug, and, though this generally recovers after treatment is stopped, some impairment of glomerular filtration may remain. Hypokalaemia occurs in 25% of patients, requiring potassium chloride supplementation. Anaemia can also occur. Other unwanted effects include impaired hepatic function, thrombocytopenia, and anaphylactic reactions. Injection frequently results initially in chills, fever, tinnitus and headache, and about one in five patients vomit. The drug is irritant to the endothelium of the veins and local thrombophlebitis is sometimes seen after intravenous injection. Intrathecal injections can cause neurotoxicity, and topical applications a skin rash. The liposome-encapsulated and lipid-complexed preparations cause fewer adverse reactions but are considerably more expensive.

Nystatin

Nystatin is a polyene macrolide antibiotic similar in structure to amphotericin and with the same mechanism of action. There is virtually no absorption from the mucous membranes of the body or from skin and its use is limited to fungal infections of the skin and the gastrointestinal tract.

Griseofulvin

Griseofulvin is a narrow-spectrum antifungal agent isolated from cultures of *Penicillium griseofulvum*. It is fungistatic and it acts by interacting with microtubules and interfering with mitosis. It can be used to treat dermatophyte infections of skin or nails, but treatment needs to be very prolonged.

Pharmacokinetic aspects

Griseofulvin is given orally. It is poorly soluble in water and absorption varies with the type of preparation, in particular with particle size. Peak plasma concentrations are reached in about 5 hours. It is taken up selectively by newly formed skin and concentrated in the keratin.

The plasma half-life is 24 hours, but it is retained in the skin for much longer. It potently induces cytochrome P450 enzymes and causes several clinically important drug interactions.

Unwanted effects

Unwanted effects with griseofulvin use are infrequent but the drug can cause gastrointestinal upsets, headache and photosensitivity. Allergic reactions (rashes, fever) may also occur.

SYNTHETIC ANTIFUNGAL AGENTS

Flucytosine

Flucytosine (Fig. 45.1) is a synthetic antifungal agent which, given orally, is active against a limited range

Fig. 45.1 Flucytosine and 5-fluorouracil.

of systemic fungal infections, being effective mainly in those caused by yeast. If given alone, drug resistance commonly arises during treatment so it is usually combined with amphotericin for severe infections such as cryptococcal meningitis.

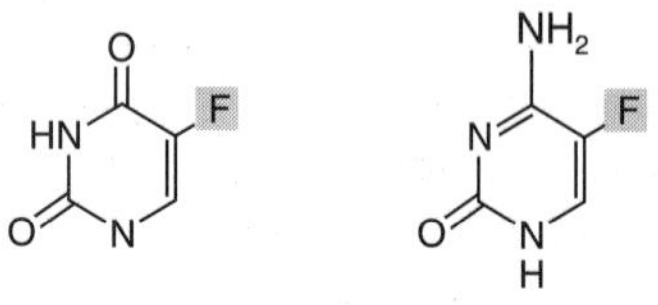

Mechanism of action

Flucytosine is converted to the antimetabolite, 5-fluorouracil (5-FU), in fungal but not human cells. 5-FU inhibits thymidylate synthetase and thus DNA synthesis (see Chs 41 and 42). Resistant mutants may emerge rapidly so this drug should not be used alone.

Pharmacokinetic aspects

Flucytosine is usually given by intravenous infusion but can also be given orally. It is widely distributed throughout the body fluids including the CSF. About 90% is excreted unchanged via the kidneys, and the plasma half-life is 3–5 hours. The dosage should be reduced if renal function is impaired.

Unwanted effects

Unwanted effects are infrequent. Gastrointestinal disturbances, anaemia, neutropenia, thrombocytopenia and alopecia have occurred, but these are usually mild and are reversed when therapy ceases. Uracil is reported to decrease the toxic effects on the bone marrow without impairing the antimycotic action. Hepatitis has been reported but is rare.

Azoles

The azoles are a group of synthetic fungistatic agents with a broad spectrum of activity. The main drugs available are **fluconazole**, **itraconazole**, **ketoconazole**, **miconazole**, **econazole**. For reviews, see Como & Dismukes (1994), Hoeprich (1995).

Mechanism of action of the azoles

The azoles inhibit the fungal P450 enzymes responsible for the synthesis of ergosterol, the main sterol in the fungal cell membrane. The resulting depletion of ergosterol alters the fluidity of the membrane and this interferes with the action of membrane-associated enzymes. The overall effect is an inhibition of replication. A further repercussion is the inhibition of the transformation of candidal yeast cells into hyphae—the invasive and pathogenic form of the parasite.

Note that the depletion of membrane ergosterol reduces the binding sites for amphotericin.

Ketoconazole

Ketoconazole was the first azole that could be given orally to treat systemic fungal infections. It is effective against several different types of fungi (see Table 45.1). It is, however, toxic (see below) and relapse is common after apparently successful treatment. It is well absorbed from the gastrointestinal tract. It is distributed widely throughout the tissues and tissue fluids but does not reach therapeutic concentrations in the CNS unless high doses are given. It is inactivated in the liver and excreted in bile and in urine. Its half-life in the plasma is 8 hours.

The main hazard of ketoconazole is liver toxicity, which is rare but can prove fatal. It may occur without overt clinical evidence and may progress after stopping the drug. Other side-effects that occur are gastrointestinal disturbances and pruritus. Inhibition of adrenocortical steroid and testosterone synthesis has been recorded with high doses, the latter resulting in gynaecomastia in some male patients. There may be adverse interactions with other drugs. Cyclosporin, terfenadine and astemizole all interfere with the metabolising enzymes, causing increased plasma concentrations of ketoconazole or the interacting drug or both. Rifampicin, H_2-receptor antagonists and antacids decrease the absorption of ketoconazole and hence decrease its plasma concentration.

Fluconazole

Fluconazole can be given orally or intravenously. It reaches high concentrations in the cerebrospinal fluid and ocular fluids and may become the drug of first choice for most types of fungal meningitis. Fungicidal concentrations are also achieved in vaginal tissue, saliva, skin and nails. It has a half-life of ~25 hours; 90% is excreted unchanged in the urine and 10% in the faeces.

Unwanted effects, which are generally mild, include nausea, headache and abdominal pain. However, exfoliative skin lesions (including, on occasion, Stevens–Johnson syndrome)* have been seen in some individuals—primarily in AIDS patients who are being treated with multiple drugs.

Hepatitis has been reported, though this is rare, and fluconazole, in the doses usually used, does not produce the inhibition of hepatic drug metabolism and of steroidogenesis which occurs with ketoconazole.

Itraconazole

Itraconazole is given orally and, after absorption (which is variable), undergoes extensive hepatic metabolism. Its half-life is ~36 hours and it is excreted in the urine. It does not penetrate the cerebrospinal fluid. Unwanted effects include gastrointestinal disturbances, headache

and dizziness. Rare unwanted effects are hepatitis, hypokalaemia and impotence. Allergic skin reactions have been reported (including Stevens–Johnson syndrome; see above). Inhibition of steroidogenesis has not been reported. Drug interactions due to inhibition of cytochrome P450 enzymes occur (similar to those described above for ketoconazole).

Miconazole

Miconazole is given orally for infections of the gastrointestinal tract. It has a short plasma half-life and needs to be given every 8 hours. It reaches therapeutic concentrations in bone, joints and lung tissue but not in the CNS, and it is inactivated in the liver. It can also be given topically. Unwanted effects are relatively infrequent, those most commonly seen being gastrointestinal disturbances, but pruritus, blood dyscrasias and hyponatraemia are also reported. There can be problems during the process of injection—the occurrence of anaphylactic reactions, dysrhythmias and fevers. The drug can have an irritant action on the venous endothelium. Because of the possibility of adverse interactions, concomitant administration with H_1-receptor antagonists, terfenadine and astemizole, should be avoided (see above, under 'Ketoconazole').

Clotrimazole, econazole, tioconazole and sulconazole

Clotrimazole, econazole, tioconazole and sulconazole are azole antifungal agents used only for topical application. Clotrimazole interferes with amino acid transport into the organism by an action on the cell membrane. It is active against a wide range of fungi, including candida organisms.

Terbinafine

Terbinafine is a highly lipophilic, keratinophilic fungicidal compound active against a wide range of skin pathogens. It acts by selectively inhibiting the enzyme, squalene epoxidase, which is involved in the synthesis of ergosterol from squalene in the fungal cell wall. The accumulation of squalene within the cell is toxic to the organism.

It is used to treat fungal infections of the nails. Given orally, it is rapidly absorbed and is taken up by skin, nails and adipose tissue. Given topically, it penetrates skin and mucous membranes. It is metabolised in the liver by the cytochrome P450 system and the metabolites are excreted in the urine. Given topically, it penetrates skin and mucous membranes.

Unwanted effects occur in about 10% of individuals and are usually mild and self-limiting. They include gastrointestinal disturbances, rashes, pruritus, headache

---

*This is a severe and usually fatal condition involving blistering of the skin, mouth, eyes and genitalia, often accompanied by fever, polyarthritis and kidney failure.

and dizziness. Joint and muscle pains have been reported and, more rarely, hepatitis.

Naftifine is similar in action to terbinafine.

Amorolfine is a morpholine derivative which interferes with fungal sterol synthesis. It is given locally as a lacquer and is reported to be effective against fungal infections of the nails.

POTENTIAL NEW ANTIFUNGAL THERAPIES

Increasing numbers of fungal strains are becoming resistant to the currently used antifungal drugs. Fortunately, drug resistance is not transferable in fungi—though this is small comfort to a patient infected with a resistant strain. An additional problem is that new strains of commensal-turned-pathogenic fungi have emerged. New and better antifungal agents are therefore being sought.

Most of the conventional antifungal drugs act on the *fungal plasma membrane*, most by interfering with ergosterol metabolism (e.g. flucytosine, azoles, terbinafine). A new azole, voriconazole, is in phase III trial; it has fungistatic action against all fungi, including resistant strains, and is fungicidal against aspergillus. A maize protein that increases fungal cell membrane permeability is also under investigation.

The targeting of other aspects of fungal structure and function is under active consideration (see Bonn 1997, 1998).

Some drugs now in clinical development—echinocandins and pradamicins—are targeted at the *fungal cell wall* which has no human homologue, and an echinocandin is in phase II trial. Two signal transduction kinases essential for fungal cell wall assembly have been identified and in vitro screens are being set up to find inhibitors of these enzymes.

Fungal protein synthesis could be another target for antifungal drug development since such synthesis requires an elongation factor that is missing from human cells.

A different approach, also being tested, is to enhance the host's ability to confront the fungal pathogen. Recombinant forms of human granulocyte-colony-stimulating factor (see Ch. 23, p. 336), for example lenograstim and molgramostim, can increase the neutrophil count in neutropenic patients with fungal infections. Early results are promising.

REFERENCES AND FURTHER READING

Bonn D 1997 New antifungals make mayhem for mycoses. Lancet 350: 870 *(Succinct summary article)*

Bonn D 1998 New strategies to combat fungal infections. Mol Med Today (February): 50

Como J A, Dismukes W E 1994 Oral azoles as systemic antifungal chemotherapy. N Engl J Med 330: 263–272 *(Comprehensive review)*

Groll A M, Piscitelli S C, Walsh T J 1998 Clinical pharmacology of systemic antifungal events: A comprehensive review of agents in clinical use, current investigational compounds and putative targets for antifungal drug developments. Adv in Pharmacol volume 44

Hartsel S, Bolard J 1996 Amphotericin B: new life for an old drug. Trends Pharmacol Sci 17: 445–449

Hoeprich P D 1995 Antifungal chemotherapy. Prog Drug Res 44: 88–127 *(Detailed coverage of main classes of drugs: chemical formulae, mode of action, pharmacokinetics, adverse effects)*

Lambert H P, O'Grady F W 1992 Antifungal agents. In: Lambert H P, O'Grady F W (eds) Antibiotic and chemotherapy. Churchill Livingstone, Edinburgh, ch 2

Polak A, Hartman P G 1991 Antifungal chemotherapy—are we winning? Prog Drug Res 37: 181–265

Ryley J F (ed) 1990 Chemotherapy of fungal diseases. Springer-Verlag, Berlin

Walsh T J 1992 Invasive fungal infections: problems and challenges for developing new antifungal compounds. In: Sutcliffe J A, Georgopapadakou N H (eds) Emerging targets in antibacterial and antifungal therapy. Chapman & Hall, New York, ch 13

Yamaguchi H, Kobayashi G S, Takahashi H 1992 (eds) Recent progress in antifungal chemotherapy. Marcel Dekker, New York

46

Antiprotozoal drugs

The main protozoa that produce disease in man are those causing malaria, amoebiasis, leishmaniasis, trypanosomiasis and trichomoniasis.

HOST–PARASITE INTERACTIONS

Mammals have developed very efficient mechanisms for dealing with invading parasites, and some of these parasites have, in turn, evolved clever tactics to evade the defensive responses of the host. One parasite ploy is to take refuge within the cells of the host where antibodies cannot reach them. Most protozoa do this, some (plasmodia species) taking up residence in red cells, some (leishmania species) infecting macrophages exclusively and some (various trypanosome species) invading many cell types. The host has, in turn, evolved strategies to deal with these intracellular parasites, namely cell-mediated immune responses involving primarily the Th1 pathway cytokines (such as IL-2, TNF-β, IFN-γ) that activate macrophages and cytotoxic CD8 T cells (Ch. 12, p. 206, Fig. 12.3). Activated macrophages kill intracellular parasites, and cytotoxic T cells collaborate with macrophages by producing macrophage-activating cytokines.

The Th1 pathway responses can be down-regulated by Th2 pathway cytokines such as TGF-β, IL-4 and IL-10 (p. 206). Some intracellular parasites have evolved mechanisms for manipulating the Th1/Th2 balance to their own advantage by stimulating production of the Th2 cytokines that down-regulate cell-mediated immune reactions. Thus, for example, the invasion of macrophages by leishmania species is associated with induction of TGF-β; and the invasion of T cells, B cells and macrophages by trypanosome species is associated with induction of IL-10.

Toxoplasma gondii, has evolved a different ploy—up-regulation of some host responses. The main, definitive host* of this protozoon is the cat, but humans can inadvertently become intermediate hosts, harbouring the asexual form of the parasite. In most individuals the disease is asymptomatic, though it can severely damage the developing foetus and can cause fatal generalised infection in AIDS patients or other immunosuppressed subjects.

In humans, *T. gondii* infects numerous cell types and has a highly virulent replicative stage; it is therefore important to the parasite that its proliferative capacity is regulated so as to ensure the survival of its host. To do this it stimulates production of IFN-γ, thus modulating the host's cell-mediated responses which then promote encystment of the parasite in the tissues.**

---

*The host that harbours the adult, sexual forms of the parasite.

**The encysted parasite is waiting patiently for its intermediate host to be eaten by its main host, a cat—a somewhat flawed stratagem when the intermediate host is a human.

Improved understanding of host–protozoon relation-ships has opened up new vistas for the development of antiprotozoan agents. The possibility of using cytokine analogues and/or antagonists to treat disease caused by protozoa is already being investigated.

MALARIA

Malaria is mosquito-borne and is one of the major killer diseases of the world, causing up to 2.7 million deaths annually and a staggering amount of chronic ill health. In some parts of Africa, 10% of the deaths of children under 5 years are due to the direct effects of malaria, and its contribution to the mortality from other diseases cannot be computed. About 50 years ago, the World Health Organization attempted to eradicate malaria using the powerful 'residual' insecticides and the highly effec-tive antimalarial drugs which had become available. By the end of the 1950s the incidence of malaria had dropped dramatically. However, during the 1970s it became clear that the attempt at eradication had failed—largely owing to the increasing resistance of the mosquito to the insec-ticides and of the parasite to the drugs—and currently malaria causes over 300 million new infections annually, many being the 'malignant' form of the infection caused by the most dangerous of the parasites, *Plasmodium falciparum*. At present about 46% of mankind lives in malarious areas (Fig. 46.1). Sporadic cases—the result of air travel—are quite common in Western Europe and the USA, where the risk of transmission is negligible, and the incidence of this travellers' malaria is rising year by year.

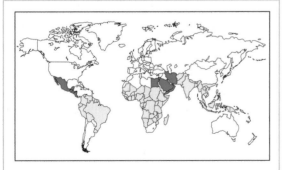

Fig. 46.1 Geographic distribution of malaria. Blue areas show regions where *P. falciparum* strains are sensitive to chloroquine; shaded areas show where they are chloroquine-resistant. (Map from Center for Disease Control and Prevention, USA; adapted from N Engl J Med 1993 329: 36).

THE LIFE CYCLE OF THE MALARIA PARASITE

The life cycle consists of a *sexual cycle*, which takes place in the female anopheline mosquito, and an *asexual cycle*, which occurs in humans (Fig. 46.2). With the bite of an infected female mosquito, *sporozoites*—usually few in number—are injected and reach the bloodstream. Within 30 minutes they disappear from the blood and enter the parenchymal cells of the liver, where, during the next 10–14 days they undergo a *pre-erythrocytic* stage of development and multiplication. At the end of this stage the parasitised liver cells rupture and a host of *merozoites* are released. These bind to and enter the red cells of the blood and form motile intracellular parasites termed *trophozoites*. The development and multiplication of the plasmodia within these cells constitutes the *erythrocytic* stage. During maturation within the red cell, the parasite remodels the host cell, inserting parasite proteins and phospholipids into the red cell membrane. The host's haemoglobin is digested and transported to the parasite's food vacuole where it provides a source of amino acids. Free haem, which would be toxic to the plasmodium, is rendered harmless by polymerisation to *haemozoin*. Some antimalarial drugs act by inhibiting the haem polymerase.

Following mitotic replication of its nucleus, the para-site in the red cell is called a *schizont*, and its rapid growth and division, *schizogony*, another phase of multiplication, results in the production of further merozoites which are released when the red cell ruptures. These merozoites then bind to and enter fresh red cells and the erythrocytic cycle starts all over again.

In certain forms of malaria, some sporozoites on entering the liver cells form *hypnozoites*, or resting forms of the parasite, which can be reactivated to continue an *exoerythrocytic cycle* of multiplication. The dormancy can last for months or years.

Malaria parasites can multiply in the body at a pheno-menal rate—a single parasite of *Plasmodium vivax* being capable of giving rise to 250 million merozoites in 14 days. To appreciate the action required of an anti-malarial drug, note that destruction of 94% of the para-sites every 48 hours will only *maintain* equilibrium and will not reduce their number or their propensity for proliferation.

Some merozoites, on entering red cells, differentiate into male and female forms of the parasite, called *gameto-cytes*. These can only complete their cycle when taken up by the mosquito, when it sucks the blood of an infected host.

The cycle in the mosquito involves fertilisation of

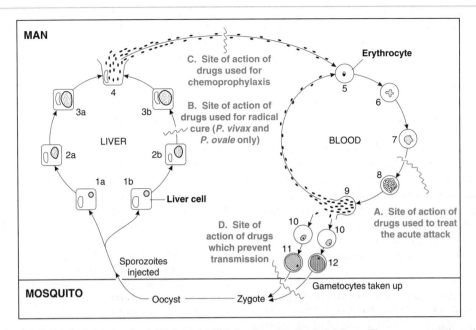

Fig. 46.2   The life cycle of the malarial parasite and the site of action of antimalarial drugs. The pre- or exoerythrocytic cycle in the liver and the erythrocytic cycle in the blood are shown: **1a** Entry of sporozoite into liver cell (the parasite is shown as a small circle containing dots and the liver cell nucleus as a white oval); **2a** and **3a** Development of the schizont in liver cell; **4** Rupture of liver cell with release of merozoites (some may enter liver cells to give resting forms of the parasite, hypnozoites); **5** Entry of a merozoite into a red cell; **6** Trophozoite in red cell; **7** and **8** Development of schizont in red cell; **9** Rupture of red cell with release of merozoites, most of which parasitise other red cells; **10, 11** and **12** Entry of some merozoites into red cells and development of male and female gametocytes; **1b** Resting form of parasite in liver (hypnozoite); **2b** and **3b** Growth and multiplication of hypnozoites. Sites of drug action: [A] Drugs used to treat the acute attack (also called 'blood schizonticidal agents' or 'drugs for suppressive or clinical cure'). [B] Drugs that affect the exoerythrocytic hypnozoites and result in radical cure of *P. vivax* and *P. ovale.* [C] Drugs that block the link between the exoerythrocytic stage and the erythrocytic stage; they are used for chemoprophylaxis (also termed 'causal prophylactics') and prevent the development of malarial attacks. [D] Drugs that prevent transmission and thus prevent increase of the human reservoir of the disease.

the female gametocyte by the male gametocyte with the formation of a zygote, which develops into an *oocyst* (sporocyst). A further stage of division and multiplication takes place leading to rupture of the sporocyst with release of sporozoites, which then migrate to the mosquito's salivary glands and enter another human host with the mosquito's bite.

The periodic episodes of fever that characterise malaria are due to the periodic synchronised rupture of red cells with release of merozoites and cell debris. The rise in temperature is associated with a rise in the concentration of tumour necrosis factor (TNF) in the plasma (see Ch. 12, p. 225).

Relapses of malaria are likely to occur with those forms of malaria that have an exoerythrocytic cycle, because the dormant hypnozoite form in the liver can

emerge after an interval of weeks or months to start the infection again.

The chief species of human malaria parasites are as follows:

- *Plasmodium falciparum*, which has an erythrocytic cycle of 48 hours in man, produces *malignant tertian malaria*—'tertian' because the fever is said to recur every third day,* 'malignant' because it is the most severe form of malaria and can be fatal. The plasmodium induces, on the infected red cell's membrane, receptors for the adhesion molecules on vascular endothelial cells (see Ch. 12, p. 203). These parasitised red

---

*The pattern is actually seldom the 'classical' 48 hours—various patterns are seen and are of no diagnostic import.

cells then stick to uninfected red cells forming clusters (rosettes). They also adhere to and pack the vessels of the microcirculation, interfering with tissue blood flow and causing organ dysfunction, for example renal failure and encephalopathy (cerebral malaria). *P. falciparum* does not have an exoerythrocytic stage, so that if the erythrocytic stage is eradicated, relapses do not occur (Fig. 46.2).

- *Plasmodium vivax* produces *benign tertian malaria*—'benign' because it is less severe than falciparum malaria and rarely fatal. Exoerythrocytic forms may persist for years and cause relapses (Fig. 46.2).
- *Plasmodium ovale*, which has a 48-hour cycle and an exoerythrocytic stage, is the cause of a rare form of malaria (see Fig. 46.2.)
- *Plasmodium malariae* has a 72-hour cycle, causes *quartan malaria* and has no exoerythrocytic cycle (Fig. 46.2).

Immunity to malaria occurs and can protect many individuals living in malarious areas. It involves mostly cell-mediated reactions (Ch. 12) the details of which are now gradually being elucidated. The immunity is lost if the individual is absent from the area for more than 6 months. There is hope that it may be possible to make vaccines for immunisation against malaria.

Malaria

- Malaria is caused by various species of plasmodia. The female anopheline mosquito injects sporozoites (the asexual form of the parasite) which can develop in the liver into:
  — schizonts (the pre-erythrocytic stage), which liberate merozoites. These infect red blood cells, forming motile trophozoites which, after development, release another batch of erythrocyte-infecting merozoites causing fever; this constitutes the erythrocytic cycle.
  — dormant hypnozoites which may liberate merozoites later (the exoerythrocytic stage).
- The main malarial parasites causing 'tertian' malaria (by definition fever 'every third day', though various patterns are seen) are:
  — *P. vivax*, which causes benign tertian malaria
  — *P. falciparum*, which causes malignant tertian malaria; unlike *P. vivax*, this plasmodium has no exoerythrocytic stage.
- Some merozoites develop into gametocytes, the sexual forms of the parasite; these, when ingested by the mosquito, give rise to further stages of the parasite's life cycle within the insect.

ANTIMALARIAL DRUGS

Antimalarial drugs are usually classified in terms of the action against the different stages of the life cycle of the parasite (Fig. 46.2).

Drugs used to treat the acute attack

Blood schizonticidal agents (Fig. 46.2, site A) are used to treat the acute attack—they are also known as drugs for suppressive or clinical cure. They act on the erythrocytic forms of the plasmodium. In infections with *P. falciparum* or *P. malariae*, which have no exoerythrocytic stage, these drugs effect a cure; with *P. vivax* or *P. ovale* the drugs suppress the actual attack but exoerythrocytic forms can cause later relapses.

This group of drugs includes quinoline–methanols (e.g. **quinine** and **mefloquine**), various 4-amino-quinolines (e.g. **chloroquine**), the phenanthrene, **halofantrine**, and agents which interfere either with the synthesis of folate (e.g. **sulphones**) or with its action (e.g. **pyrimethamine**). Combinations of these agents are frequently used. Some antibiotics, such as **tetracycline** and **doxycycline** (see Ch. 43), have proved useful when combined with the above agents. Compounds derived from qinghaosu, for example **artemether**, have also proved effective.

For a brief summary of currently recommended treatment regimes see Table 46.1. A more detailed coverage of the treatment of malaria is given by White (1996).

Drugs which effect radical cure

Tissue schizonticidal agents effect a radical cure by acting on the parasites in the liver (Fig. 46.2, site B). Only the 8-aminoquinolines (**primaquine**) have this action. These drugs also destroy gametocytes and thus reduce the spread of infection.

Drugs used for chemoprophylaxis

Drugs used for chemoprophylaxis (also known as *causal prophylactic* drugs) block the link between the exo-erythrocytic stage and the erythrocytic stage and thus prevent the development of malarial attacks. True causal prophylaxis—the prevention of infection by the killing of the sporozoites on entry into the host—is not feasible with the drugs at present in use, though it may be achieved in the future with vaccines. Prevention of the development of clinical attacks can, however, be effected by chemoprophylactic drugs that kill the parasites when they emerge from the liver after the pre-erythrocytic stage (Fig. 46.2, site C). The drugs used for this purpose are mainly those listed above: **chloroquine**, **mefloquine**,

Table 46.1 Summary of drugs used for treatment and chemoprophylaxis of malaria*

Infections	Drugs for the treatment of the clinical attack[†]	Drugs for chemoprophylaxis[‡]
All plasmodial infections except chloroquine-resistant *P. falciparum*[§]	Oral chloroquine[¶] or sulphadoxine–pyrimethamine	Oral chloroquine or proguanil

Infection with chloroquine-resistant *P. falciparum*[§]	Oral quinine[‖] plus:
	   (i) tetracycline or
	   (ii) doxycycline**
	  or
	Oral halofantrine[††]
	  or
	Oral mefloquine[‡‡]
		Oral chloroquine plus:
		   (i) proguanil or
		   (ii) doxycycline** or
		   (iii) pyrimethamine–dapsone
		  or
		Oral mefloquine[§§]

*The specific combinations of drugs used may vary in different malarious areas.
[†]See White (1996) for more detail.
[‡]See Bradley et al. (1993), Bradley & Warhurst (1995) for more detail.
[§]Chloroquine-resistant *P. falciparum* is now very widespread, and in some areas *P. vivax* has also became resistant.
[¶]If oral administration is not feasible, chloroquine can be given by infusion.
[‖]If oral administration is not feasible, quinine is given by slow intravenous infusion.
**Contraindicated in children under 12, pregnant women and nursing mothers.
[††]Can cause cardiac problems.
[‡‡]Has a fairly high incidence of adverse effects (see text for details).
[§§]Should not be used for chemoprophylaxis unless there is a high risk of chloroquine-resistant malaria.

proguanil, **pyrimethamine**, **dapsone** and **doxycycline**. They are often used in combinations.

Chemoprophylactic agents are given to individuals who intend travelling to an area where malaria is endemic. Administration should start 1 week before entering the area and should be continued throughout the stay and for at least a month afterwards. No chemoprophylactic regime is 100% effective and the choice of drug is difficult. In addition to the normal criteria used in selecting a drug, the unwanted effects of some antimalarial agents need to be borne in mind and weighed against the risk of a serious, possibly fatal, parasitaemia. A further problem is the complexity of the regimes which require different drugs to be taken at different times and the fact that different agents may be required for different travel destinations.*

For a brief summary of currently recommended regimes of chemoprophylaxis see Table 46.1. More detailed coverage is given by Bradley et al. (1993), Bradley & Warhurst (1995) and Wyler (1993).

Drugs used to prevent transmission
Some drugs (e.g. **primaquine**, **proguanil** and

pyrimethamine) have the additional action of destroying the gametocytes (Fig. 46.2, site D), preventing transmission by the mosquito and thus preventing the increase of the human reservoir of the disease—but they are rarely used for this action alone.

Antimalarial therapy and the parasite life cycle

- Drugs used to treat the acute attack of malaria (i.e. for suppressive or clinical cure) act on the parasites in the blood; they can cure infections with parasites (e.g. *P. falciparum*) which have no exoerythrocytic stage.
- Drugs used for chemoprophylaxis (causal prophylactics), i.e. to prevent malarial attacks when in a malarious area, act on merozoites emerging from liver cells.
- Drugs used for radical cure are active against parasites in the liver.
- Some drugs act on gametocytes and prevent transmission by the mosquito.

4-AMINOQUINOLINES

The main 4-aminoquinoline used clinically is **chloroquine** (Fig. 46.3). **Amodiaquine**, which has very similar action to chloroquine, was withdrawn several years ago

---

*See details of malaria chemoprophylaxis regimes for travellers in relevant copies of WHO: Weekly Epidemic Record.

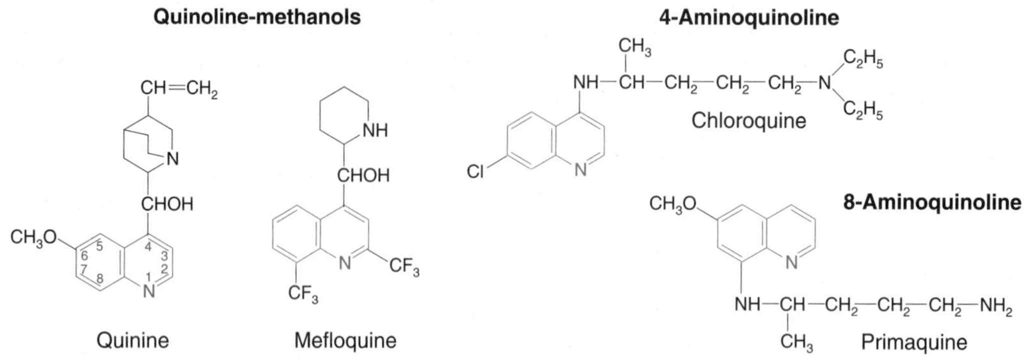

Fig. 46.3   Structures of some quinoline antimalarial drugs. The quinoline moiety is shown in blue.

because it caused agranulocytosis; but as chloroquine resistance burgeons, there is talk of resurrecting it for treatment—though not for chemoprophylaxis.

Chloroquine

Chloroquine is a very potent blood schizonticidal drug (Fig. 46.2, site A), effective against the erythrocytic forms of all four plasmodial species (if sensitive to the drug), but it does not have any effect on sporozoites, hypnozoites or gametocytes. It has a complex mechanism of action which is not fully understood. It is a weak base but its accumulation in the parasite lysosome is 1000-fold greater than is predicted on this basis. This suggests that there are additional parasite-specific drug-concentrating mechanisms; one such is now thought to be a Na^+/H^+ exchange transporter. Chloroquine inhibits digestion of haemoglobin by the parasite and thus reduces the supply of amino acids necessary for parasite viability. It also inhibits haem polymerase—the enzyme that polymerises toxic free haem to haemozoin, rendering it harmless.

Resistance

P. falciparum is now resistant to chloroquine in most parts of the world. Resistance appears to be due to increased efflux of the drug from parasitic vesicles and/or decreased uptake. There are also reports of *P. vivax* resistance to chloroquine in some areas.

Pharmacological actions

Chloroquine is a disease-modifying antirheumatoid drug (p. 238) and also has some quinidine-like actions on the heart.

Clinical use.   The clinical use of chloroquine is given in Table 46.1.

Administration and pharmacokinetic aspects

Chloroquine is given orally, is completely absorbed, is extensively distributed throughout the tissues and is concentrated in parasitised red cells. In severe falciparum malaria it may be given by frequent intramuscular or subcutaneous injection of small doses or by *slow* continuous intravenous infusion.

As explained above, chloroquine concentrates particularly in parasitised red cells. It is released slowly from the tissues and metabolised in the liver. It is excreted in the urine, 70% as unchanged drug and 30% as metabolites. Elimination is slow, the major phase having a half-life of 50 hours, and a residue persists for weeks or months.

Unwanted effects

Chloroquine has few adverse effects when given for chemoprophylaxis. With the larger doses used to treat the clinical attack of malaria, unwanted effects can occasionally occur, including nausea and vomiting, dizziness and blurring of vision, headache, and urticarial symptoms. Large doses have sometimes resulted in retinopathies. Bolus intravenous injections of chloroquine can cause hypotension and, if high doses are used, fatal dysrhythmias.

Chloroquine is considered to be safe for use by pregnant women.

QUINOLINE–METHANOLS

The two most widely used quinoline–methanols are **quinine** and **mefloquine** (Fig. 46.3).

Quinine

Quinine is an alkaloid derived from cinchona bark. It is a blood schizonticidal drug, effective against the erythrocytic forms of all four species of plasmodia (Fig. 46.2, site A), but it has no effect on exoerythrocytic forms or on the gametocytes of *P. falciparum*. Its mechanism of action is, like that of chloroquine, associated with inhibition of the parasite's haem polymerase; but quinine is not so extensively concentrated in the plasmodium as chloroquine so other mechanisms could also be involved.

With the emergence and spread of **chloroquine** resistance, quinine is now the main chemotherapeutic agent for *P. falciparum*.

Pharmacological actions

Pharmacological actions on host tissue include a depressant action on the heart, a mild oxytocic effect on the uterus in pregnancy, a slight blocking action on the neuromuscular junction and a weak antipyretic effect.

Clinical use. The clinical use of quinine is given in Table 46.1

Pharmacokinetic aspects

Quinine is usually given orally in a 7-day course, but can be given by slow intravenous infusion for severe *P. falciparum* infections and in patients who are vomiting. A loading dose may be required, but bolus intravenous administration is contraindicated because of the risk of cardiac dysrhythmias. It is well absorbed from the gastrointestinal tract and is metabolised in the liver, the metabolites being excreted in the urine within about 24 hours. The $t_{1/2}$ is 10 hours.

Unwanted effects

Given orally, quinine is bitter, so compliance is poor. It is irritant to the gastric mucosa and can cause nausea and vomiting. If the concentration in the plasma exceeds 30–60 μmol/l, 'cinchonism' is likely to occur—nausea, dizziness, tinnitus, headache and blurring of vision. Excessive plasma levels of quinine can result in hypotension, cardiac dysrhythmias and severe CNS disturbances such as delirium and coma.

Other rarer unwanted reactions that have been reported are hypoglycaemia, blood dyscrasias (especially thrombocytopenia) and hypersensitivity reactions.

Quinine can stimulate insulin release. Patients with marked falciparum parasitaemia can have low blood sugar for this reason and also because of glucose consumption by the parasite. This can cause diagnostic confusion between coma caused by cerebral malaria and hypoglycaemic coma—which responds to glucose.

'Blackwater fever', a severe and often fatal condition in which acute haemolytic anaemia is associated with renal failure, is a rare result of treating malaria with quinine or of erratic and inappropriate use of quinine for a 'fever'.

Resistance

Some degree of resistance is developing—owing to increased expression of an efflux transporter similar to the human multidrug resistance transporter, P-glycoprotein (see Ch. 42, p. 680, and Ch. 4).

Mefloquine

Mefloquine (Fig. 46.3) is a blood schizonticidal quinoline–methanol compound, active against *P. falciparum* and *P. vivax* (Fig. 46.2, site A); however, it has no effect on hepatic forms of the parasites, so treatment of *P. vivax* infections should be followed by a course of primaquine (see below) to eradicate the hypnozoites.

The *antiparasite action* is associated with inhibition of the haem polymerase; but since mefloquine, like quinine, is not as extensively concentrated in the parasite as chloroquine, other mechanisms could also be involved.

Resistance has occurred in *P. falciparum* in some areas—particularly in Southeast Asia—and is thought to be due, as with quinine, to increased expression in the parasite of an efflux transporter similar to the human multidrug resistance transporter, P-glycoprotein (see Ch. 42, p. 680, and Ch. 4).

Clinical use. The clinical use of mefloquine is given in Table 46.1.

Pharmacokinetic aspects

Mefloquine is given orally and is rapidly absorbed. It has a slow onset of action and a very long plasma half-life (up to 30 days), which may be due to enterohepatic cycling or to tissue storage.

Unwanted effects

When mefloquine is used for treatment of the acute attack, about 50% of subjects complain of gastrointestinal disturbances. Transient CNS toxicity—giddiness, confusion, dysphoria, insomnia (and sometimes psychotic symptoms and/or convulsions)—can occur and there have been a few reports of aberrant AV conduction and serious, but rare, skin diseases. Mefloquine is contraindicated in pregnant women and in women liable to become pregnant within 3 months of stopping the drug, because of its long half-life and uncertainty about its possible teratogenicity.

When used for chemoprophylaxis the unwanted actions are usually milder, but the drug should not be used in this way unless there is a high risk of acquiring chloroquine-resistant malaria.

PHENANTHRENE–METHANOLS

Halofantrine

Halofantrine is a blood schizonticidal drug. It is one of a group of compounds that were studied during the Second World War and found to have antimalarial activity but that were not developed when chloroquine was found to be successful. However, as chloroquine resistance developed, halofantrine came in from the cold. It is active against strains of *P. falciparum* that are resistant to **chloroquine**, **pyrimethamine** and **quinine**. It is effective against the erythrocytic form of *P. vivax* (Fig. 46.2, site A) but not the hypnozoites. However, it is not usually used for vivax malaria since this is generally susceptible to chloroquine. Cross-resistance between halofantrine and mefloquine in falciparum infections has been reported. Its mechanism of action is not known.

Clinical use. The clinical use of halofantrine is given in Table 46.1.

Pharmacokinetic aspects

Halofantrine is given orally. It is slowly and rather irregularly absorbed, with a peak plasma concentration approximately 4–6 hours after ingestion and a half-life of 1–2 days, though its main metabolite, which has equal potency, has a half-life of 3–5 days. Absorption is substantially increased by a fatty meal and elimination is in the faeces.

Unwanted effects

Abdominal pain, gastrointestinal disturbances, headache, a transient rise in hepatic enzymes and cough occur. Pruritus is reported but is less marked than with chloroquine. Halofantrine can produce changes in cardiac rhythm (particularly if used with other dysrhythmia-inducing drugs), and it should be used with caution in patients with a history of dysrhythmia. It has caused sudden cardiac death. Rarer reactions are haemolytic anaemia and convulsions. Because of unwanted actions halofantrine is reserved for infections caused by resistant organisms. However, decreasing sensitivity and resistance of *P. falciparum* have been reported recently.

DRUGS AFFECTING THE SYNTHESIS OR UTILISATION OF FOLATE

The folate antagonists, **pyrimethamine** and **proguanil**, inhibit the *utilisation* of folate by inhibiting dihydrofolate reductase; the **sulphonamides** and the **sulphones** inhibit the *synthesis* of folate by competing with *p*-aminobenzoic acid (see Chs 41 and 43). Combinations of folate antagonists with drugs inhibiting folate synthesis cause

sequential blockade, affecting the same pathway at different points; these combinations thus have synergistic action (see Fig. 43.2).

Pyrimethamine is a 2,4,diaminopyrimidine (see Fig. 46.4) and is similar in structure to trimethoprim (see Fig. 43.1). The structure of **proguanil** is different but it can assume a configuration similar to that of pyrimethamine (see Fig. 46.4). These compounds inhibit the formation of tetrahydrofolate with the consequences for DNA synthesis outlined in Chapter 42 (p. 675). As explained in Chapters 41 and 43, some agents (pyrimethamine, proguanil) have a greater affinity for the plasmodial enzyme than for the human enzyme. They have a slow action against the erythrocytic forms of the parasite (Fig. 46.2, site A) and proguanil is believed to have an additional effect on the initial hepatic stage (1a to 3a in Fig. 46.2) but not on the hypnozoites of *P. vivax* (Fig. 46.2, Site B). Pyrimethamine is only used in combination with either dapsone or a sulphonamide.

The main sulphonamide used in malaria treatment is **sulphadoxine** and the only sulphone used is **dapsone** (see Figs 43.8 and 46.4). Details of these drugs are given in Chapter 43. The sulphonamides and sulphones are active against the erythrocytic forms of *P. falciparum* but are less active against those of *P. vivax*; they have no activity against the sporozoite or hypnozoite forms of the plasmodia. Pyrimethamine–sulphadoxine has been extensively used for chloroquine-resistant malaria but resistance to this combination has developed in many areas.

Clinical use. The clinical use of these drugs is given in Table 46.1.

Pharmacokinetic aspects

Both pyrimethamine and proguanil are given orally and are well absorbed, though the process is slow. Pyrimethamine has a plasma half-life of 4 days and effective 'suppressive' plasma concentrations may last for 14 days; it is taken once a week. The $t_{1/2}$ of proguanil is 16 hours. It is a pro-drug, metabolised in the liver to its active form—a triazine metabolite which is excreted mainly in the urine. It must be taken daily. Details of the pharmacokinetics of dapsone are given in Chapter 43 (p. 706).

Unwanted effects

These drugs have few untoward effects if used carefully in therapeutic doses. Larger doses of the pyrimethamine–dapsone combination can cause serious reactions such as haemolytic anaemia, agranulocytosis and eosinophilic alveolitis. The pyrimethamine–sulphadoxine combination can cause serious skin reactions, blood dyscrasias and allergic alveolitis and is no longer recommended for

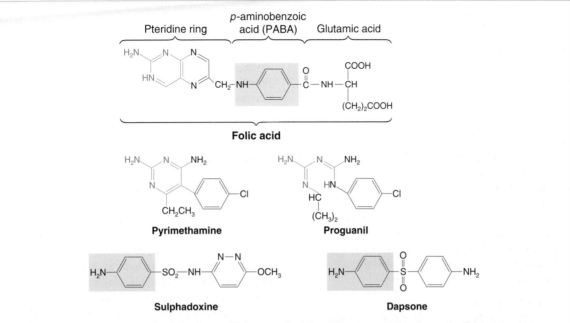

Fig. 46.4 Structures of some antimalarial drugs which act on the folic acid pathway of the plasmodia. Folate antagonists (pyrimethamine, proguanil) inhibit dihydrofolate reductase; the relationship between these drugs and the pteridine moiety is shown in blue. Sulphones (e.g. dapsone) and sulphonamides (e.g. sulphadoxine) compete with *p*-aminobenzoic acid for dihydropteroate synthetase (relationship shown in light blue). (See also Fig. 43.1.)

chemoprophylaxis. In high doses, pyrimethamine may inhibit mammalian dihydrofolate reductase and cause a megaloblastic anaemia (see Ch. 18); folic acid supplements should be given if this drug is used during pregnancy.

8-AMINOQUINOLINES

The only 8-aminoquinoline used is **primaquine** (see Fig. 46.3). The mechanism of action is not known.

Its antimalarial action is exerted against the liver hypnozoites and it is the only drug that can effect a *radical cure* of those forms of malaria in which the parasites have a dormant stage in the liver—*P. vivax* and *P. ovale*. It does not affect sporozoites and has little if any action against the erythrocytic stage of the parasite. However, it has a gametocidal action and is the most effective antimalarial drug for *preventing transmission* of the disease in all four species of plasmodia, thus reducing the human reservoir of malaria. It is almost invariably used in combination with another drug, usually **chloroquine**. Resistance to primaquine is rare, though evidence of a decreased sensitivity of some vivax strains has been reported.

Pharmacokinetic aspects
Primaquine is given orally and is well absorbed. Its metabolism is rapid and very little drug is present in the body after 10–12 hours. The $t_{1/2}$ is 3–6 hours.

Unwanted effects
Primaquine has few unwanted effects in most patients when used in normal therapeutic dosage. Dose-related gastrointestinal symptoms can occur and large doses may cause methaemoglobinaemia with cyanosis. This antimalarial drug can, however, cause haemolysis in individuals with an X-chromosome-linked genetic metabolic condition—a deficiency of glucose-6-phosphate dehydrogenase in the red cells (see p. 750). When this deficiency is present, the red cells are not able to regenerate NADPH, its concentration being reduced by the oxidant metabolic derivatives of primaquine. As a consequence, the general metabolic functions of the red cells are impaired and haemolysis occurs. Primaquine metabolites have greater haemolytic activity than the parent compound. The deficiency of the enzyme occurs in up to 15% of black males and is also fairly common in some other ethnic groups. Glucose-6-phosphate dehydrogenase activity should be estimated before giving primaquine.

Antimalarial drugs

- Chloroquine is a blood schizonticide acting by inhibiting haem polymerase—the enzyme that renders harmless the otherwise toxic free haem (derived from haemoglobin digestion); it is usually given orally ($t_{\frac{1}{2}}$ 50 h); it is concentrated in the parasite. Unwanted effects include GI tract disturbances, dizziness, urticaria; bolus i.v. injections can cause dysrhythmias.
- Quinine is a blood schizonticide; it is given orally ($t_{\frac{1}{2}}$ 10 h); it can be given by i.v. infusion if necessary. Unwanted effects include GI tract upsets, tinnitus, blurred vision and, with large doses, dysrhythmias and CNS disturbances. 'Blackwater fever' is very occasionally associated with its administration. It is usually given in combination therapy with:
  — pyrimethamine, a folate antagonist, a slow blood schizonticide, given orally ($t_{\frac{1}{2}}$ 4 days), and either
  — dapsone, a sulphone, given orally ($t_{\frac{1}{2}}$ 24–48 h), or
  — sulphadoxine, a long-acting sulphonamide ($t_{\frac{1}{2}}$ 7–9 days)
- Proguanil, a folate antagonist, is a slow blood schizonticide with some action on the primary liver forms of *P. vivax*; given orally ($t_{\frac{1}{2}}$ 16 h).
- Mefloquine is a blood schizonticidal agent active against *P. falciparum* and *P. vivax*; given orally, it acts by inhibiting the parasite's haem polymerase; onset of action is slow, and $t_{\frac{1}{2}}$ is 30 days; main unwanted effects: GIT disturbances, neurotoxicity (e.g. convulsions), psychiatric problems.
- Halofantrine is a blood schizonticidal agent active against all species of malarial parasite, including multiresistant *P. falciparum*; it is given orally, is irregularly absorbed; $t_{\frac{1}{2}}$ of parent drug is 1–2 days, of active metabolite, 3–5 days; common unwanted effects (abdominal pain, GIT disturbances, headache) are fewer than with mefloquine, but serious cardiac problems sometimes occur.
- Primaquine is effective against the liver hypnozoites, and is also active against gametocytes. Given orally its $t_{\frac{1}{2}}$ is 36 hours. Unwanted effects are mainly GI tract disturbances and, with large doses, methaemoglobinaemia. Haemolysis is produced in individuals with genetic deficiency of erythrocyte glucose-6-phosphate dehydrogenase.

Antibiotics used in malaria

Some antibiotics, for example **doxycycline** and **tetracycline**, have a place in the treatment of the acute attack of malaria and in chemoprophylaxis; see page 728 above and Table 46.1. Details of these antibiotics are given in Chapter 43 (p. 696).

QINGHAOSU (ARTEMISININ) AND RELATED COMPOUNDS

These compounds are derived from the herb, *qing hao*, a traditional Chinese remedy for malaria. The scientific name, conferred on the herb by Linnaeus, is *Artemisia*.* **Artemisinin**, a chemical extract from *Artemisia*, poorly soluble in water, is a fast-acting blood schizonticide that has been effective in treating the acute attack of both vivax and falciparum malaria (including chloroquine-resistant and cerebral malaria). **Artesunate**, a water-soluble derivative and the synthetic analogues, **artemether** and **artether**, have higher activity and are better absorbed. The compounds are concentrated in parasitised red cells. The mechanism of action is not known; it may involve damage to the parasite membrane by free radicals or covalent alkylation of proteins. These compounds do not have any effect on liver hypnozoites and are not useful for chemoprophylaxis. Artemisinin can be given orally, intramuscularly or by suppository, artemether orally or intramuscularly, artesunate intramuscularly or intravenously. They are rapidly absorbed and widely distributed, and are converted in the liver to the active metabolite, dihydroartemisinin. The half-lives are: artemisinin, about 4 hours; artesunate, 45 minutes; artemether, 4–11 hours.

There have been few *unwanted effects* so far. Transient heart block, transient decrease in blood neutrophils and brief episodes of fever have been reported.

In rodent studies, artemisinin potentiated the effects of mefloquine, primaquine, and tetracycline, was additive with chloroquine and antagonised the sulphonamides and the folate antagonists.

In randomised trials, the qinghaosu compounds have cured attacks of malaria, including cerebral malaria, more rapidly and with fewer unwanted effects than other antimalarial agents. Artemisinin and derivatives have been effective against multidrug-resistant *P. falciparum* in sub-Saharan Africa and, combined with mefloquine, against multidrug-resistant *P. falciparum* in Southeast Asia. However, the preclinical and clinical data are at present insufficient to satisfy the drug regulatory requirements in many countries. Artemether may become available fairly soon.

For a review of this topic, see Hien & White (1993).

POTENTIAL NEW ANTIMALARIAL DRUGS

Pyronaridine is a new synthetic schizonticidal agent derived from mepacrine, developed in China.

Atovaquone, a hydroxynapthoquinone that is licensed for the treatment of *Pneumocystis carinii* pneumonia (see below) is under test as an antimalarial.

---

*The herbs are noted for their extreme bitterness and their name derives from Artemisia, wife and sister of the fourth century king of Halicarnassus; her sorrow on his death led her to mix his ashes with whatever she drank to make it bitter.

PNEUMOCYSTIS PNEUMONIA AND ITS TREATMENT

First recognised in 1909, *Pneumocystis carinii* was presumed to belong to the protozoa, but recent studies have shown that it shares structural features with both protozoa and fungi, leaving its precise classification uncertain. Previously considered to be an innocuous microorganism widely distributed in the animal kingdom without causing disease, it now causes opportunistic infection in AIDS patients. Pneumocystis pneumonia is often the presenting symptom in an AIDS patient and it is a leading cause of death.

Many drugs have been used to treat *P. carinii* pneumonia. High-dose **co-trimoxazole** (Ch. 43, p. 689) is the drug of choice, with parenteral **pentamidine** (see above) as an alternative. Other treatment regimes include **trimethoprim–dapsone**, or **atovaquone** or **clindamycin–primaquine**. A combination of the folate antagonist, **trimethexate**, plus **folinic acid**, has been approved by the FDA for treatment of the pneumonia in the USA.

AMOEBIASIS AND AMOEBICIDAL DRUGS

Amoebiasis is an infection with *Entamoeba histolytica* produced by the ingestion of cysts of this organism. In the intestine the cysts develop into trophozoites which adhere to colonic epithelial cells by means of a lectin on the parasite membrane that has similarity to host adherence proteins (Ch. 12, p. 203). The trophozoite then lyses the host cell (hence *histolytica*) and invades the submucosa, where it may secrete a factor that inhibits γ-interferon-activated macrophages (p. 206) which would otherwise kill it. These processes may result in dysentery, though in many subjects a chronic intestinal infection can be present in the absence of dysentery. The parasite may invade the liver leading to the development of liver abscesses and in some subjects an amoebic granuloma (an amoeboma) develops in the intestinal wall. Some individuals are 'carriers'—they harbour the parasite without developing overt disease; but the cysts are present in their faeces and they can infect other individuals. The cysts can survive outside the body for at least a week in a moist and cool environment.

The use of drugs in treating this condition depends largely on the site and type of infection, and different drugs may be effective in acute amoebic dysentery, in chronic intestinal amoebiasis, in extra-intestinal infection and in the carrier state.

The main drugs currently used are: **metronidazole**, **tinidazole** and **diloxanide**. These agents may be used in combination.

The drugs of choice for the various forms of amoebiasis are as follows:

- for acute invasive intestinal amoebiasis resulting in acute severe amoebic dysentery: metronidazole (or tinidazole) followed by diloxanide
- for chronic intestinal amoebiasis: diloxanide
- for hepatic amoebiasis: metronidazole followed by diloxanide
- for the carrier state: diloxanide.

Metronidazole

Metronidazole kills the trophozoites of *E. histolytica* but has no effect on the cysts. It is the most effective drug available for invasive amoebiasis involving the intestine or the liver, but it is less effective against organisms in the lumen of the gut.

The action of metronidazole is thought to be through damage to the DNA of the trophozoite by toxic oxygen products generated from the drug by the parasite.

Pharmacokinetic aspects

Metronidazole is usually given orally and is rapidly and completely absorbed, giving peak plasma concentration in 1–3 hours, with a $t_{1/2}$ of about 7 hours. Rectal and intravenous preparations are also available. It is distributed rapidly throughout the tissues, reaching high concentrations in the body fluids, including the cerebrospinal fluid. Some is metabolised but most is excreted in urine.

Unwanted effects

There are few unwanted effects with therapeutic doses. It has a metallic, bitter taste in the mouth. Minor gastrointestinal disturbances have been reported as have CNS symptoms (dizziness, headache, sensory neuropathies). The drug interferes with alcohol metabolism and alcohol should be strictly avoided. Metronidazole should not be used in pregnancy.

Other similar drugs are **tinidazole** and **nimorazole**. Tinidazole is eliminated more slowly than metronidazole, having a half-life of 12–14 hours. *Unwanted effects* are similar to those seen with metronidazole.

Diloxanide

Both diloxanide itself and, more particularly, an insoluble ester, **diloxanide furoate**, are effective against the non-invasive intestinal parasite. The drugs have a direct amoebicidal action, affecting the amoebae before encystment. Diloxanide furoate is given orally, the unabsorbed moiety being the amoebicidal agent. It has no serious adverse effects.

LEISHMANIASIS AND LEISHMANICIDAL DRUGS

There are a variety of *Leishmania* organisms that cause disease, mainly in tropical and subtropical regions. The World Health Organization estimates that there are about 1 million cases world-wide, with 400 000 new cases each year. With increasing international travel, leishmaniasis is being imported into areas where it was not previously seen and opportunistic infections are now being reported (particularly in AIDS patients).

The parasite exists in two forms—a flagellated form, found in a sandfly (the insect vector) which feeds on warm-blooded animals, and a non-flagellated form, which occurs in the bitten mammalian host. In the latter, the parasite is taken up by the mononuclear phagocyte system where it remains alive and viable.

There are several clinical types of leishmaniasis—a simple skin infection which may heal spontaneously, a mucocutaneous form (in which there may be large ulcers of the mucous membranes) and a visceral form ('kala azar'). In this last, the parasite spreads through the bloodstream and causes hepatomegaly and splenomegaly, anaemia and intermittent fever.

The main drugs used in visceral leishmaniasis are pentavalent antimony compounds, **sodium stibogluconate**, and **meglumine antimoniate**, but resistance to these agents is increasing. Sodium stibogluconate is given intramuscularly or by slow intravenous injection in a 10-day course. It is rapidly eliminated in the urine—70% being excreted within 6 hours. More than one course may be required. Unwanted effects are anorexia, vomiting, bradycardia and hypotension. Coughing and substernal

pain may occur during intravenous infusion. Combination of sodium stibogluconate with γ-interferon (Ch. 12, p. 225) is being investigated.

Pentamidine isethionate (see below) can be used in antimony-resistant leishmaniasis.

Other drugs used in leishmaniasis are liposomally incorporated **amphotericin** (also used as an antifungal agent; p. 720) and **metronidazole** (see above), which is effective against cutaneous lesions.

Possible approaches to the treatment of leishmaniasis are discussed by Olliaro & Bryceson (1993).

TRYPANOSOMIASIS AND TRYPANOSOMICIDAL DRUGS

There are three main species of trypanosome that cause disease in humans—*T. gambiense* and *T. rhodesiense*, which cause sleeping sickness in Africa, and *T. cruzi*, which causes Chagas' disease in South America. In both types of disease there is an initial local lesion at the site of entry, followed by bouts of parasitaemia and fever. Damage to organs is caused by the toxins released, involving the CNS (in sleeping sickness), and the heart and sometimes liver, spleen, bone and the intestine (in Chagas' disease).

The main drugs used for African sleeping sickness are **suramin**, with **pentamidine** as an alternative, in the haemolymphatic stage of the disease and the arsenical, **melarsoprol**,* for the late stage with CNS involvement (see Wang 1995).

Drugs used in Chagas' disease include **primaquine** (see above), and **puromycin** (see Ch. 43), **nifurtimox*** and **benznidazole*** (the latter two used in the acute disease only), but there is, in essence, no really effective treatment for this condition.

Suramin

Suramin was introduced into the therapy of trypanosomiasis in 1920. It does not kill the parasites immediately but induces biochemical changes which result in the organisms being cleared from the circulation after an interval of 24 hours.

The drug binds firmly to host plasma proteins and the complex enters the trypanosome by endocytosis; it is then liberated by lysosomal proteases. It has a selective action on trypanosomal enzymes.

It is given by slow intravenous injection. The blood concentration drops rapidly during the first few hours and

---

*Not available in the UK.

then more slowly over the succeeding days. A low concentration remains for 3–4 months. It tends to accumulate in the mononuclear phagocyte system of the host and is also found in the cells of the proximal tubule in the kidney.

Unwanted effects

Suramin is relatively toxic, particularly in a malnourished patient, the main toxic effect being on the kidney. Other slowly developing adverse effects reported include optic atrophy, adrenal insufficiency, skin rashes, haemolytic anaemia and agranulocytosis. A small proportion of individuals have an immediate idiosyncratic reaction to suramin injection—nausea, vomiting, shock, seizures, and loss of consciousness.

Pentamidine isethionate

Pentamidine has a direct trypanocidal action in vitro. It is rapidly taken up in the parasites by a high-affinity energy-dependent carrier and is thought to interact with the DNA. Pentamidine is given intravenously or by deep intramuscular injection, usually daily for 10–15 days and, after absorption from the injection site, it soon leaves the circulation. It is eliminated slowly—only 50% of a dose being excreted over 5 days. Fairly high concentrations of the drug persist in the kidney, the liver and the spleen for several months. Its usefulness is limited by its unwanted effects—an immediate decrease in blood pressure, with tachycardia, breathlessness and vomiting, and later serious toxicity, such as kidney damage, hepatic impairment, blood dyscrasias and hypoglycaemia.

TRICHOMONIASIS AND TRICHOMONICIDAL DRUGS

The principal *Trichomonas* organism that produces disease in humans is *T. vaginalis*. Virulent strains cause inflammation of the vagina in females and sometimes of the urethra in males.

The main drug used in therapy is **metronidazole** (p. 735). **Tinidazole** is also effective.

TOXOPLASMOSIS AND TOXOPLASMOCIDAL DRUGS

Toxoplasma gondii is a protozoan that infects cats and other animals. Oocysts in the infected animal's faeces can infect humans, giving rise to sporozoites, then to trophozoites and finally to cysts in the tissues. In many individuals, toxoplasmosis is self-limiting or even asymptomatic, but infection with the protozoan during pregnancy can cause serious disease in the foetus. Immunocompromised individuals (e.g. AIDS patients) are also very susceptible.

The treatment of choice is **pyrimethamine–sulphadiazine** (to be avoided in pregnant patients); **trimethoprim–sulphamethoxazole** or parenteral **pentamidine** is also used and, more recently, **azithromycin** has shown promise.

NEW APPROACHES TO ANTIPROTOZOAL THERAPY

Enzyme inhibitors

Protozoan enzymes for which inhibitors are being sought include:

- *T. cruzi* protease (cruzain), which is essential for parasite replication
- *T. cruzi* trans-sialidase which promotes attachment to host cells
- cysteine proteases of *Entamoeba histolytica* and *Leishmania*
- *proteosomes* in plasmodia.

Proteosomes are large complexes containing the enzymes responsible for ubiquitin-dependent proteolysis thought to be involved in the remodelling that the plasmodium undergoes in its life cycle in the host. Small proteosome inhibitors are available and could possibly be modified so as to be parasite-selective.

Vaccines. Clinical trials of a DNA vaccine encoding a *P. falciparum* circumsporozoite protein is under way.

The *Plasmodium falciparum* genome is being sequenced. This should provide information that could eventually allow the function of various parasite proteins to be elucidated, and hopefully lead to novel antimalarial drugs.

Cytokine-based therapies

The relationship between host and parasite is determined largely by host cytokines, and as more understanding of the role of cytokines is gained, the possibility of utilising this for therapy is being studied. Agents being considered include peptide antagonists at cytokine receptors, soluble cytokine receptors, anti-cytokine antibodies, soluble cytokine receptors and mutant cytokines. IL-2 has been shown to protect monkeys against malaria.

REFERENCES AND FURTHER READING

Adams S A, Robson S C et al. 1993 Immunological similarity between the 170 kD amoebic adherence glycoprotein and human β2 integrins. Lancet 341: 17–19

Berent A R, Craig A G 1997 *Plasmodium falciparum*—sticky jams and PECAM pie. Nature Med 3: 1315–1316 (*Deals with malaria parasites and host adhesion molecules*)

Bradley D J, Warhurst D 1995 Malaria prophylaxis: guidelines for travellers. Br Med J 310: 709–714 (*Excellent review of chemoprophylaxis regimes*)

Bradley D et al. 1993 Prophylaxis against malaria for travellers from the United Kingdom. Br Med J 306: 1247–1252

Bryson H M, Goa K L 1992 Halofantrine. A review of its antimalarial activity, pharmacokinetic properties and therapeutic potential. Drugs 43: 236–258

Cox F E G 1992 Malaria: getting into the liver. Nature 359: 361–362

Croft A, Garner P 1997 Mefloquine to prevent malaria: a systematic review of trials. Br Med J 315: 1412–1416 (*Analysis of 10 trials to assess the efficacy and tolerability of mefloquine*)

Croft S L 1997 The current status of antiparasite chemotherapy. Parasitology 114: S3–S15 (*Comprehensive coverage of current drugs and outline of approaches to possible future agents*)

Foley M, Tilley L 1997 Quinoline antimalarials: mechanisms of action and resistance. Int J Parasitol 27: 231–240 (*Good, short review; useful diagrams*)

Fu S, Xiao S-H 1991 Pyronaridine: a new antimalarial drug. Parasitol Today 7: 310–313

Haldar K 1996 Sphingolipid synthesis and membrane formation by *Plasmodium*. (*Biochemical insights into effects of parasite growth within red cell; potential targets for new drugs*)

Hien T T, White N J 1993 Qinghaosu. Lancet 341: 603–608 (*Good background article on qinghaosu*)

Hudson A T 1993 Atavoquone—a novel broad-spectrum anti-infective drug. Parasitol Today 9: 66–68

Hughes W, Leoung G et al. 1993 Comparison of atovaquone (556C80) with trimethoprim–sulfamethoxazole to treat *Pneumocystis carinii* pneumonia in patients with AIDS. N Engl J Med 328: 1521–1527

Kalinna B H 1997 DNA vaccines for parasitic infections Immunobiol Cell Biol 75: 370–375

Knight R 1980 The chemotherapy of amoebiasis. J Antimicrob Chemother 6: 577–593

Krishna S 1997 Malaria. Br Med J 315: 730–732 (*Good, short review in series 'Science, medicine and the future'; useful diagram*)

Lell B, Luckner D et al. 1998 Randomised placebo-controlled study of atovaquone plus proguanil for malaria prophylaxis in children. Lancet 351: 709–713 (*States that this is highly effective and well tolerated*)

Martinez S, Marr J J 1992 Allopurinol in the treatment of American cutaneous leishmaniasis. N Engl J Med 326: 741–744

Martinez-Palomo A, Espinosa-Cantellano M 1998 Amoebiasis: new understandings and new goals. Parasitol Today 14: 1–3

Masur H 1992 Prevention and treatment of Pneumocystis pneumonia. N Engl J Med 327: 1853–1860

Mishra M, Biswas U K et al. 1992 Amphotericin versus pentamidine in antimony-unresponsive kala-azar. Lancet 340: 1256–1257

Murphy G S, Basri H et al. 1993 Vivax malaria resistant to treatment and prophylaxis with chloroquine. Lancet 341: 96–100

Nosten F, ter Kuile F O et al. 1993 Cardiac effects of antimalarial treatment with halofantrine. Lancet 341: 1054–1056

O'Brien C 1997 Beating the malaria parasite at its own game. Lancet 350: 192 (*Clear, succinct coverage of mechanisms of action and resistance of current antimalarials and potential new drugs; useful diagram*)

Olliaro P L, Bryceson A D M 1993 Practical progress and new drugs for changing patterns of leishmaniasis. Parasitol Today 9: 323–328 (*Useful coverage of antileishmaniasis drugs*)

Petri W A, Clark C G 1993 International seminar on amebiasis. Parasitol Today 9: 73–76

Radloff P D, Phillips J et al. 1996 Atovaquone and proguanil for *Plasmodium falciparum* malaria. Lancet 347: 1511–1514

Reed S G 1995 Cytokine control of the macrophage parasites *Leishmania* and *Trypanosoma cruzi*. In: Boothroyd J C, Komuniecki R (eds) Molecular approaches to parasitology. Wiley-Liss, New York, pp 443–453 (*Thought-provoking coverage of interaction between parasites and host cytokines*)

Riley E 1997 Malaria vaccines: current status and future prospects. J Pharm Pharmacol 49 (suppl 2): 21–27

Sher A 1995 Regulation of cell-mediated immunity by parasites: the ups and downs of an important host adaptation. In: Boothroyd J C, Komuniecki R (eds) Molecular approaches to parasitology. Wiley-Liss, New York, pp 431–442 (*Thought-provoking coverage of host–parasite interactions*)

Targett G A 1998 Malaria—variety is the price of life. Nature Med 4: 267–268 (*The biological roles of the surface proteins of malaria-infected red cells*)

Ter Kuile F O, Dolan G et al. 1993 Halofantrine versus mefloquine in treatment of multidrug-resistant falciparum malaria. Lancet 341: 1044–1049

Thakar C P, Kumar M, Kumar P, Mishra B N, Pandey A K 1988 Rationalisation of regimes of treatment of kala-azar with sodium stibogluconate in India: a randomised study. Br Med J 296: 1557–1560

Wang C C 1995 Molecular mechanisms and therapeutic approaches to the treatment of African trypanosomiasis. Annu Rev Pharmacol Toxicol 35: 93–127 (*Detailed review*)

Warren E, George S, et al. 1997 Advances in the treatment and prophylaxis of *Pneumocystis carinii* pneumonia. Pharmacotherapy 17: 900–916

White N J 1996 The treatment of malaria. N Engl J Med 335: 800–806 (*Excellent review of drug treatment and management of malaria*)

Winstanley P 1996 Pyronaridine: a promising drug for Africa? Lancet 347: 2–3

Wirth D F 1995 Drug resistance and transfection in *Plasmodium*. In: Boothroyd J C, Komuniecki R (eds) Molecular approaches to parasitology. Wiley-Liss, New York, pp 227–241

Wyler D J 1993 Malaria chemotherapy for the traveller. N Engl J Med 329: 31–37

47

Anthelminthic drugs

A large proportion of mankind harbours helminths (worms) of one species or another. In some cases these infections result mainly in discomfort and do not cause substantial ill health, an example being threadworms in children. Other worm infections, such as schistosomiasis (bilharzia) and hookworm disease, can produce very serious morbidity. In many countries, particularly those in tropical and subtropical regions, almost all the indigenous population is infected with hookworms and/or other helminths and the problem of the treatment of helminthiasis is, therefore, one of very great practical importance.

HELMINTH INFECTIONS

Humans are the primary (definitive) hosts for most, but not all, helminth infections; in other words, most worms reproduce sexually in the human host, producing eggs or larvae that pass out of the body and infect the secondary (intermediate) host.

There are two clinically important types of worm infections—those in which the worm lives in the host's alimentary canal, and those in which the worm lives in other tissues of the host's body.

The main examples of worms that live in the host's *alimentary canal* are:

- **Tapeworms (cestodes)**: *Taenia saginata, Taenia solium, Hymenolepis nana, Diphyllobothrium latum.* In Asia, Africa and parts of America about 82 million people harbour one or other of these tapeworm species. Only the first two are likely to be seen in the UK.

  The usual intermediate hosts of the two most common tapeworms (*T. saginata* and *T. solium)* are

cattle and pigs, respectively. Humans become infected by eating raw or undercooked meat containing the larvae, which have encysted in the animals' muscle tissue. (In some circumstances, the larval stage of *T. solium* can develop in humans, resulting in *cysticercosis*, a condition characterised by encysted larvae in the muscles and the viscera or, more seriously, in the eye or the brain.)

Hymenolepis nana can have both the adult stage (the intestinal worm) and the larval stage in the same host, which may be human or rodent, though some insects (fleas, grain beetles) can also serve as intermediate hosts. The infection is usually asymptomatic.

Diphyllobothrium latum has two sequential intermediate hosts—a freshwater crustacean and a freshwater fish. Humans become infected by eating raw or incompletely cooked fish containing the larvae. Vitamin B_{12} deficiency sometimes occurs (see Ch. 18).

- **Intestinal roundworms (nematodes)**: *Ascaris lumbricoides* (common roundworm), *Enterobius vermicularis* (threadworm), *Trichuris trichiura* (whipworm), *Strongyloides stercoralis* (threadworm in USA), *Necator americanus, Ankylostoma duodenale* (hookworms). It is estimated that 1000 million people harbour *A. lumbricoides*, 500 million *T. trichiura*, and 500 million *E. vermicularis*, while at least 800 million have hookworm infection.

The main examples of worms that live in the *tissues* of the host are:

- **Trematodes or flukes:** *Schistosoma haematobium, Schistosoma mansoni, Schistosoma japonicum.* These cause schistosomiasis (bilharzia). The adult worms of both sexes live and mate in the veins or venules of the gut wall or the bladder. The female lays eggs which pass into the bladder or gut and produce inflammation of these organs, resulting in haematuria in the former case and, occasionally, loss of blood in the faeces in the latter. The eggs hatch in water after discharge from the body and give rise to *miracidia*, which enter the secondary host—a particular species of snail. After a period of development in this host, free-swimming *cercariae* emerge. These are capable of infecting humans by penetration of the skin. About 200 million people are infected with one or other of the schistosomes.

- **Tissue roundworms:** *Trichinella spiralis, Dracunculus medinensis* (guinea-worm) and the filariae, which include *Wuchereria bancrofti, Loa loa, Onchocerca volvulus* and *Brugia malayi.*

  The adult filariae live in the lymphatics, connective tissues or mesentery of the host and produce live embryos or microfilariae, which find their way into the bloodstream. They may be ingested by mosquitoes or similar biting insects when they feed. After a period of development within this secondary host, the larvae pass to the mouthparts of the insect and are re-injected into humans. Major filarial diseases are caused by *Wuchereria* or *Brugia*, which cause obstruction of lymphatic vessels producing elephantiasis; other related diseases are onchocerciasis (in which the presence of microfilariae in the eye causes 'river-blindness') and loiasis (in which the microfilariae cause inflammation in the skin and other tissues).

  In guinea-worm infection, larvae released from crustaceans in wells and water-holes are ingested and migrate from the intestinal tract to mature and mate in the tissues; the gravid female then migrates to the subcutaneous tissues of the leg or the foot where she may protrude through an ulcer in the skin. The worm may be up to a metre in length and has to be removed surgically or by slow mechanical winding of the worm on to a stick over a period of days.*

  T. spiralis causes trichinosis; the larvae from the viviparous female worms in the intestine migrate to skeletal muscle, where they become encysted.

- **Hydatid tapeworm:** *Echinococcus* species. These are cestodes for which canines are the primary (definitive) hosts, and sheep the intermediate hosts. The primary, intestinal stage does not occur in humans, but under certain circumstances humans can function as the intermediate host, in which case the larvae develop into *hydatid cysts* within the tissues.

---

*In 1980 there were 2 million cases of guinea-worm infection world-wide. In 1986 the World Health Organization initiated a programme to eradicate this worm. The target date, set in 1990, was 1995. At that date the total number of cases had fallen by about 95%, mainly because of public health measures. However, 160 000 cases were reported that year and it has still not been completely eradicated.

Some nematodes that usually live in the gastrointestinal tract of animals may infect humans and penetrate tissues. A skin infestation, termed 'creeping eruption' or 'cutaneous larva migrans' is caused by the larvae of dog and cat hookworms. Toxocariasis or 'visceral larva migrans' is caused by larvae of cat and dog roundworms of the *Toxocara* genus.

ANTHELMINTHIC DRUGS

To be an effective anthelminthic,** a drug must be able to penetrate the cuticle of the worm or gain access to its alimentary tract.

An anthelminthic drug can act by causing paralysis of the worm, or by damaging its cuticle, leading to partial digestion or to rejection by immune mechanisms. Anthelminthic drugs can also interfere with the metabolism of the worm, and since the metabolic requirements of these parasites vary greatly from one species to another, drugs that are highly effective against one type of worm are ineffective against others. Individual drugs are described briefly below; indications for their use are given in Table 47.1. For a comprehensive coverage of antiparasitic drugs and their clinical uses, see Liu & Weller (1996).

Benzimidazoles

The benzimidazole anthelminthics include **mebendazole, thiabendazole** and **albendazole**. These compounds are broad-spectrum agents and constitute one of the main groups of anthelminthics used clinically. They bind to free β-tubulin, inhibiting its polymerisation and thus interfering with microtubule-dependent glucose uptake. They have a selective inhibitory action on helminth microtubular function, being 250–400 times more potent in helminth than in mammalian tissue. The effect takes time to develop and the worms may not be expelled for several days.

Only 10% of mebendazole is absorbed after oral administration; a fatty meal increases absorption. It is rapidly metabolised, the products being excreted in the urine and the bile within 24–48 hours. It is given as a single dose for threadworm and twice daily for 3 days for hookworm and roundworm infestations. Thiabendazole is rapidly absorbed from the gastrointestinal tract, very rapidly metabolised and excreted in the urine in conjugated form. It is given twice-daily for 3 days for guinea-

---

**Helmins, helminthos = worm, hence 'anthelminthic' or 'anthelmintic': medicine acting against parasitic worms (Concise Oxford Dictionary).

Tabel 47.1 Drugs used in helminth infections*

Helminth	Drugs used
Threadworm (pinworm)[†] (*Enterobius vermicularis*)	Mebendazole,[‡] albendazole,[‡] (piperazine, pyrantel)
Strongyloides stercoralis (called 'threadworm' in the USA)	Albendazole,[‡] thiabendazole, ivermectin[§]
Common roundworm (*Ascaris lumbricoides*)	Mebendazole,[‡] pyrantel (piperazine), levamisole[§]

Other roundworms (filariae)
    Wuchereria bancrofti, Loa loa
    Onchocerca volvulus
	
	Diethylcarbamazine, ivermectin
	Ivermectin[§]

Guinea-worm (*Dracunculus medinensis*)	Praziquantel,[‡] (mebendazole, metronidazole)[¶]
Trichiniasis (*Trichinella spiralis*)	Thiabendazole,[‡] mebendazole,[‡] (pyrantel)
Tapeworm (*Taenia saginata, Taenia solium*)	Praziquantel,[‡] niclosamide
Cysticercosis (infection with larval *T. solium*)	Praziquantel,[‡] albendazole
Hydatid disease[‖] (*Echinococcus granulosus*)	Albendazole,[‡] praziquantel
Hookworm (*Ankylostoma duodenale, Necator americanus*)	Mebendazole,[‡] albendazole,[‡] pyrantel
Whipworm (*Trichuris trichiura*)	Mebendazole,[‡] albendazole,[‡] diethylcarbamazine

Blood flukes (*Schistosoma* species)
    S. haematobium
    S. mansoni
    S. japonicum
	
	Praziquantel,[‡] metriphonate[‡§]
	Praziquantel,[‡] oxamniquine
	Praziquantel[‡]

Cutaneous larva migrans (*Ankylostoma caninum*) Visceral larva migrans (*Toxacara canis*) }	Albendazole,[‡] thiabendazole (diethylcarbamazine)

*Based largely on Liu & Weller (1996) and Croft (1997).
[†]Combination of hygienic measures with anthelminthics essential.
[‡]Indicates drug of first choice. Drugs less commonly used are given in brackets.
[§]Available in the UK on a 'named patient' basis.
[¶]See Chapter 46.
[‖]Surgery may be needed for cysts.

worm and strongyloides infestations, and for up to 5 days for trichinosis and for cutaneous larva migrans.

Unwanted effects are few with mebendazole though gastrointestinal disturbances can occasionally occur. Unwanted effects with thiabendazole are more frequent but usually transient, the commonest being gastrointestinal disturbances, though headache, dizziness and drowsiness are reported and allergic reactions (fever, rashes) can occur. More serious toxic effects (such as parenchymal liver damage) have been seen in a few cases.

Albendazole, the most recently introduced benzimidazole, is a broad-spectrum anthelminthic. Given orally it is rapidly absorbed and metabolised to the sulphoxide and sulphone which may be responsible for its anthelminthic actions. The plasma concentration of its active metabolite is 100 times greater than that of mebendazole. Unwanted effects—mainly gastrointestinal disturbances—are not common and usually do not require discontinuation of the drug.

Praziquantel

Praziquantel is a broad-spectrum anthelminthic drug (available but not marketed in the UK). It is the drug of choice for all species of schistosomes and is effective in cysticercosis, for which there was previously no effective therapy.

It acts by altering calcium homeostasis in the helminth cells. This causes contraction of the musculature and eventually results in paralysis and death of the worm. It has been suggested that praziquantel modifies the parasite so that it becomes susceptible to the host's normal immune responses (see Sher 1995).

The drug affects not only the adult schistosomes but also the immature forms and the cercariae—the form of the parasite that infects humans by penetrating the skin (see above, p. 740).

Praziquantel has no pharmacological effects in humans in therapeutic dosage. Given orally it is rapidly absorbed; much of the drug is rapidly metabolised to inactive metabolites on first passage through the liver and the metabolites are excreted in the urine. The plasma half-life of the parent compound is 60–90 minutes.

Mild *unwanted effects* occur but are usually transitory and rarely of clinical importance. They include gastro-intestinal disturbance, dizziness, aching in muscles and joints, skin eruptions and low-grade fever. Some effects are more marked in patients with a heavy worm load and may be due to products released from the dead worms.

Piperazine

Piperazine can be used to treat infections with the common roundworm (*Ascaris lumbricoides*) and the threadworm (*Enterobius vermicularis*)—which is called 'pinworm' in the USA. It reversibly inhibits neuro-muscular transmission in the worm, probably by acting like GABA, the inhibitory neurotransmitter on GABA-gated chloride channels in nematode muscle. The paralysed worms are expelled alive.

Piperazine is given orally and some but not all is absorbed. It is partly metabolised and the remainder is eliminated, unchanged, via the kidney. The drug has singularly little pharmacological action in the host.

Unwanted effects are uncommon but gastrointestinal disturbances, urticaria and bronchospasm occur occa-sionally and some patients experience dizziness, para-esthesias, vertigo, incoordination.

Used to treat roundworm, piperazine is effective in a single dose. For threadworm, a longer course (7 days) at lower dosage is necessary. This drug has been largely superseded by the benzimidazoles.

Pyrantel

Pyrantel is a derivative of tetrahydropyrimidine that is thought to act by depolarising the helminth neuro-muscular junction, causing spasm and paralysis. It also has some anticholinesterase activity. There is poor ab-sorption from the gastrointestinal tract after oral dosing—more than 50% of the drug being eliminated in the faeces.

It is generally regarded as a safe drug. Unwanted effects are mild and transitory and involve mostly gastrointestinal upsets. Dizziness and fever have been reported, but no serious effects on blood, kidney or liver. It has been largely superseded by the benzimidazoles.

Niclosamide

Niclosamide was the drug of choice for tapeworm infec-tions, but has now largely been superseded by prazi-quantel. The scolex (the head of the worm with the parts that attach to the host intestinal cells) and a proximal segment are irreversibly damaged by the drug; the worm separates from the intestinal wall and is expelled. Neither the larvae nor the ova are affected. For *T. solium* the drug is given in a single dose after a light meal, followed by a purgative 2 hours later. A purgative is necessary because the damaged tapeworm segments may release ova, which are not affected by the drug, so there is a theo-retical possibility that cysticercosis may develop. For other tapeworm infections, it is not necessary to give a purgative after administration of niclosamide. There is negligible absorption of the drug from the gastrointestinal tract.

Unwanted effects are few, infrequent and transient. Nausea and vomiting can occur.

Oxamniquine

Oxamniquine is active against *Schistosoma mansoni*, affecting both mature and immature forms. Its mecha-nism of action may involve intercalation in the DNA and its selective action may be related to the ability of the parasite to concentrate the drug. Resistance has occurred in some geographical areas. It is given orally, is well absorbed, and is metabolised in the gut wall and in the liver to inactive metabolites that are excreted in the urine. It has a short half-life of 1–2 hours and is eliminated from the plasma by 10–12 hours.

Unwanted effects of transient dizziness and headache are reported in 30–95% of patients in various studies, and gastrointestinal disturbances in 10–20% of patients. Symptoms caused by CNS stimulation may occur and include hallucinations and convulsive episodes. Allergic manifestations and other symptoms, which appear several days after treatment has stopped, may be related to the release of products from the dead fluke.

Metriphonate

Metriphonate (only available in the UK on a 'named patient' basis) is an organophosphate anticholinesterase that was originally used as an insecticide. It was subse-quently found to be effective against *Schistosoma haema-tobium* and is now one of the drugs of choice for infections with this blood fluke. It is a pro-drug, giving rise spontaneously to the active drug, **dichlorvos**, in vivo. Its action is thought to be due to an inhibitory effect on cholinesterases in the helminth, causing paralysis. The ova of the fluke are not affected. Given orally it is absorbed rapidly and the parent compound is cleared from the plasma within 8 hours. The plasma concentration of active metabolite constitutes about 1% of that of the parent compound and both are cleared from the tissues within 1–2 days.

Effects on the host enzymes occur but do not usually result in serious physiological changes. Plasma cholinesterase activity is inhibited and there is a marked decrease in red cell acetylcholinesterase activity. Recovery from these effects takes 4–15 weeks, the plasma enzyme recovering more rapidly.

Unwanted effects occur in some patients (gastrointestinal disturbances, bronchospasm, dizziness) but usually last less than a day. Foetal damage has been reported.

Diethylcarbamazine

Diethylcarbamazine is a piperazine derivative that is active in filarial infections caused by *W. bancrofti* and *L. loa*. Diethylcarbamazine rapidly removes the microfilariae from the blood circulation and has a limited effect on the adult worms in the lymphatics, but it has little action on microfilariae in vitro. It has been suggested that it modifies the parasite so that it becomes susceptible to the host's normal immune responses. It may also interfere with the parasite's arachidonate metabolism.

The drug is given orally, is absorbed and is distributed throughout the cells and tissues of the body, excepting adipose tissue. It is partly metabolised and both the parent drug and its metabolites are excreted in the urine, being cleared from the body within about 48 hours.

Unwanted effects are common but transient, subsiding within a day or so even if the drug is continued. Side-effects due to the drug itself are gastrointestinal disturbances, arthralgias, headache and a general feeling of weakness. Allergic side-effects referable to the products of the filariae are common and vary with the species of worm. In general these start during the first day's treatment and last 3–7 days; they include skin reactions, enlargement of lymph glands, dizziness, tachycardia and gastrointestinal and respiratory disturbances. When these symptoms disappear, larger doses of the drug can be given without further problem. The drug is not used in patients with onchocerciasis in whom it can have serious unwanted effects.

Levamisole

Levamisole (not marketed in the UK) is effective in infections with the common roundworm (*Ascaris lumbricoides*). It has a nicotine-like action, stimulating and subsequently blocking the neuromuscular junctions. The paralysed worms are then passed in the faeces. Ova are not killed. The drug is given orally, is rapidly absorbed and is widely distributed. It crosses the blood–brain barrier. It is metabolised in the liver to inactive metabolites, which are excreted via the kidney. Its plasma half-life is 4 hours. When single-dose therapy is used, *unwanted effects* are few and soon subside. They include gastrointestinal disturbances, dizziness and skin eruptions. High concentrations can have nicotinic actions on autonomic ganglia in the mammalian host.

Ivermectin

Ivermectin (available in the UK on a 'named patient' basis) is a semisynthetic agent derived from a group of natural substances, the avermectins, obtained from an actinomycete. It has potent anthelminthic activity against filaria in man, being the drug of choice for onchocerciasis, which causes 'river blindness'; it has also given good results in *Wuchereria bancrofti*, which causes elephantiasis. A single dose kills the immature microfilariae of *Onchocerca volvulus* but not the adult worms. Ivermectin reduces the incidence of onchocercal blindness by up to 80%. The drug also has activity against infections with some roundworms: common round worms, whipworms, threadworms—both the UK variety (*E. vermicularis*) and the US variety (*S. stercoralis*)—but not hookworms.

It is given orally and has a half-life of 11 hours.

It is thought to paralyse the worm by opening chloride channels and increasing chloride conductance (see Rohrer & Schaeffer 1995). Its binding site is different from that in mammalian species and distinct from that of all other effector molecules of the chloride channel.

Unwanted effects include skin rashes, fever, giddiness, headaches and pains in muscles, joints and lymph glands. In general, the drug is well tolerated.

REFERENCES AND FURTHER READING

Burnham G M 1997 Ivermectin where *Loa loa* is endemic. Br Med J 350: 2–3

Burnham G M 1998 Onchocerciasis. Lancet 351: 1341–1346

Cairncross S 1995 Victory over guineaworm disease: partial or Pyrrhic? Lancet 346: 1440

Cook G C 1992 Use of protozoan and anthelmintic drugs during pregnancy: side-effects and contraindications. J Infect 25: 1–9

Croft S L 1997 The current status of antiparasite chemotherapy. Parasitology 114: S3–S15 (*Comprehensive coverage of current drugs and outline of approaches to possible future agents*)

Day T A, Bennett J L, Pax R A 1992 Praziquantel: the enigmatic antiparasitic. Parasitol Today 8: 342–344

Fisher M H, Mrozik H 1992 The chemistry and pharmacology of the avermectins. Annu Rev Pharmacol Toxicol 32: 537–553

Kalinna B H 1997 DNA vaccines for parasitic infections Immunobiol Cell Biol 75: 370–375

Klein R D, Geary T G 1996 Prospects for rational approaches to anthelmintic discovery. Parasitology 113: S217–S234

Liu L X, Weller P F 1996 Antiparasitic drugs. N Engl J Med 334: 1178–1184 *(Excellent, up-to-date coverage of antiparasitic drugs and their clinical use)*

Martin R J, Robertson A P, Bjorn H 1997 Target sites of anthelminthics. Parasitology 114 (suppl): S111–S124

Moodley M, Moosa A 1989 Treatment of neurocysticercosis: is praziquantel the new hope? Lancet 1: 262–263

Rohrer S P, Schaeffer J M 1995 Ivermectin. In: Boothroyd J C, Komuniecki R (eds) Molecular approaches to parasitology. Wiley-Liss, New York, pp 93–107 *(Mechanism of action of ivermectin)*

Sher A 1995 Regulation of cell-mediated immunity by parasites: the ups and downs of an important host adaptation. In: Boothroyd J C, Komuniecki R (eds) Molecular approaches to parasitology. Wiley-Liss, New York, pp 431–442. *(Thought-provoking coverage of host–parasite interactions)*

Thompson D P, Klein R D, Geary T G 1996 Prospects for rational approaches to anthelmintic discovery. Parasitology 113: S217–234

Whitworth J 1992 Treatment of onchocerciasis with ivermectin in Sierra Leone. Parasitol Today 8: 138–140

World Health Organization 1995 WHO model prescribing information: drugs used in parasitic diseases, 2nd edn. WHO, Geneva

GENERAL TOPICS

48

Individual variation and drug interaction

Variability in the effect of a drug, given either to different individuals or to the same individual on different occasions, can be caused by differing concentrations of the drug at its site of action or by different responses to the same drug concentration. The first kind is often called *pharmacokinetic variation*, and can occur because of differences in absorption, distribution, metabolism or excretion of the drug. Variability of the second kind is called *pharmacodynamic variation*, and its possible causes are legion. In most cases, the variation is *quantitative* in the sense that the drug produces a larger or smaller effect, or acts for a longer or shorter time, while still exerting qualitatively the same effect. In other cases, the action is *qualitatively* different. Such instances are known as *idiosyncratic* reactions (the OED defines an idiosyncrasy as 'the physical constitution peculiar to an individual or class') and are often caused by genetic or immunological differences between individuals.

Effects on the absorption and elimination of drugs of factors such as bioavailability, food intake and gastric and urinary pH were discussed in Chapters 4 and 5. All of these contribute substantially to quantitative variations in drug responses. In this chapter some other important factors responsible for variation in drug response are presented under five headings:

- age
- genetic factors
- idiosyncratic reactions
- disease
- drug interactions.

> **Individual variation**
>
> - Variability is a serious problem when drugs are used clinically; if not taken into account it can result in:
>   — lack of efficacy
>   — unexpected side-effects.
> - Types of variability may be classified as:
>   — pharmacokinetic
>   — pharmacodynamic
>   — idiosyncratic.
> - The main causes of variability are:
>   — age
>   — genetic factors
>   — physiological states (e.g. pregnancy)
>   — pathological states (e.g. kidney or liver disease)
>   — drug interactions.

EFFECTS OF AGE

The main reason that age affects drug action is that drug metabolism and renal function are less efficient both in newborn babies and in old people, so that, with some exceptions, drugs tend to produce greater and more prolonged effects at the extremes of life. Other age-related factors, such as variations in pharmacodynamic sensitivity, are also important with some drugs. Physiological factors (e.g. altered cardiovascular reflexes) and pathological factors (e.g. hypothermia), which are common in elderly people, also influence drug effects. Body composition changes with age, fat contributing a greater proportion to body mass in the elderly with consequent changes in distribution volume of drugs. Elderly people consume more drugs than do younger adults, so the potential for drug interactions is also increased.

Effect of age on renal excretion of drugs
Renal function in the newborn, normalised to body surface area, measured either as glomerular filtration rate

or as maximal tubular secretory rate, is only about 20% of the adult value. Accordingly, plasma elimination half-lives ($t_{1/2}$) of various drugs that are mainly eliminated by the kidney are longer in neonates than in adults (Table 48.1). In babies born at term renal function increases to values similar to those in young adults in less than a week, and indeed continues to increase to a maximum of approximately twice the adult value at 6 months of age. The increase in renal function occurs more slowly in premature infants. Renal immaturity in premature infants can have a very large effect on drug elimination. Thus, in premature newborn babies the antibiotic **gentamicin** has a plasma half-life of 18 hours or greater, compared with 1–4 hours for adults and approximately 6 hours for babies born at term. It is therefore necessary to reduce and/or space out doses to avoid toxicity in premature babies.

From the age of about 20 years, renal function begins to decline slowly, falling by about 25% at age 50 and by 50% at age 75. This change in glomerular filtration is accompanied by a reduced rate of renal elimination of drugs, but is not reflected by an increase in plasma creatinine concentration, which typically remains within the normal adult range despite diminished renal function. This is because creatinine *synthesis* is reduced in elderly persons because of their reduced muscle mass. Failure to recognise this and reduce the dose of drugs that are eliminated by renal excretion can lead to drug toxicity. Figure 48.1 shows that the renal clearance of **digoxin** in young and old subjects is closely correlated with creatinine clearance. Consequently, chronic administra-

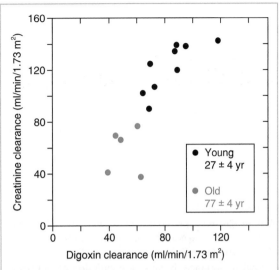

Fig. 48.1 Relationship between renal function (measured as creatinine clearance) and digoxin clearance in young and old subjects. (From: Ewy G A et al. 1969 Circulation 34: 452)

Table 48.1 Effect of age on plasma elimination half-lives (mean or range, h) of various drugs

Drug	Term neonate*	Adult	Elderly
Drugs that are mainly excreted unchanged in the urine			
Gentamicin	10	2	4
Lithium	120	24	48
Digoxin	200	40	80
Drugs that are mainly metabolised			
Diazepam	25–100	15–25	50–150
Phenytoin	10–30	10–30	10–30
Sulphamethoxypyridazine	140	60	100

*Even greater differences from mean adult values occur in premature babies.
Data from: Reidenberg 1971 Renal function and drug action. Saunders, Philadelphia; and from: Dollery 1991 Therapeutic drugs. Churchill Livingstone, Edinburgh

tion over the years of the same daily dose of digoxin to an individual as he or she ages leads to a progressive increase in plasma concentration, and is a common cause of glycoside toxicity (see Ch. 14).

Effect of age on drug metabolism

Several enzymes that are important for drug metabolism, for example hepatic microsomal oxidase, glucuronyl transferase, acetyl transferase and plasma esterases, have low activity in neonates, especially if they have been born prematurely. These enzymes take 8 weeks or longer to reach the adult level of activity. The relative lack of conjugating activity in the newborn can have serious consequences, as in *kernicterus* caused by drug displacement of bilirubin from its binding sites on albumin (see below) and in the 'grey baby' syndrome caused by the antibiotic **chloramphenicol** (see Ch. 43). This sometimes fatal condition, at first thought to be a specific biochemical sensitivity to the drug in young babies, actually results simply from accumulation of very high tissue concentrations of chloramphenicol because of slow hepatic conjugation. Chloramphenicol is no more toxic to babies than to adults provided the dose is reduced to make allowance for this. Slow conjugation is also one reason why **morphine** (which is excreted mainly as the glucuronide) is not used as an analgesic in labour, since drug transferred via the placenta has a long $t_{1/2}$ in the newborn baby, and can cause prolonged respiratory depression.

The activity of hepatic microsomal enzymes declines slowly (and very variably) with age, and the distribution volume of lipid-soluble drugs increases, because the proportion of the body that is fat increases with advancing age. The increasing $t_{1/2}$ of the anxiolytic drug, **diazepam** with advancing age (Fig. 48.2), is one consequence of this. Some other benzodiazepines and their active metabolites show even greater age-related increases in $t_{1/2}$. Since this pharmacokinetic parameter determines the time-course of drug accumulation during repeated dosing (Ch. 5) insidious effects, developing over days or weeks, can occur in elderly people and may be misattributed to age-related memory impairment rather than to drug accumulation. The effect of age is less marked for many other drugs, but even though the mean $t_{1/2}$ may not change much, there is often a striking increase in the *variability* of $t_{1/2}$ between individuals with age. This is of some clinical importance, because a population of old people will contain some individuals with grossly reduced rates of drug metabolism whereas such extremes do not occur so commonly in younger populations, and drug regulatory authorities increasingly require studies in elderly patients before granting a product licence.

Age-related variation in sensitivity to drugs

There are many instances where the same plasma concentration of a drug causes different effects in young and old subjects. Thus, anxiolytic and hypnotic drugs such as benzodiazepines (Ch. 33) produce more confusion and less sedation in elderly than in young subjects, and hypotensive drugs often cause postural hypotension in elderly patients.

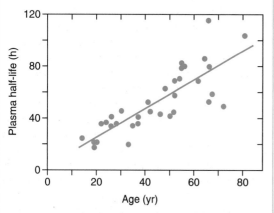

Fig. 48.2 Increasing plasma half-life for diazepam with age in 33 normal subjects. (From: Klotz U et al. 1975 J Clin Invest 55: 347)

Effects of age

- At birth and in old age, renal and hepatic function are generally impaired relative to other ages, so drug effects are prolonged and accumulation tends to occur.
- Premature infants have particularly poor renal and hepatic function in relation to drug clearance. These functions mature in the first few weeks of life.
- Renal and hepatic function decline slowly and variably after middle age, so inter-individual variation is greater in the elderly.
- Body composition changes with age, fat contributing a greater proportion to body mass in the elderly with consequent changes in distribution volume of drugs (increased for lipid-soluble drugs like diazepam, reduced for polar drugs like digoxin in old people).
- Physiological factors in the elderly (e.g. impaired cardiovascular reflexes) may qualitatively alter drug effects.
- Pathological factors that influence drug metabolism (e.g. hypothermia) are commoner in the elderly.
- Elderly people consume more drugs, so the potential for drug interactions is increased.

GENETIC FACTORS

Genetic influences on drug metabolism

Studies on identical and non-identical twins have shown that much of the individual variability in $t_{1/2}$ for various drugs is genetically determined. Thus $t_{1/2}$ values for **antipyrene**, a probe of hepatic drug oxidation, and for **coumarin** in pairs of identical twins are 6–22 times less variable than in fraternal twins. There is a continuous, roughly Gaussian, distribution of pharmacokinetic characteristics of many drugs within a population. Figure 48.3 shows the approximately Gaussian distribution of plasma concentrations achieved 3 hours after administration of a standard oral dose of **salicylate** to 100 subjects; genetic factors cause only part of this variation, the rest being due to the influence of physiological factors (e.g. gastrointestinal motility, urine flow and urinary pH) on absorption or elimination of the drug. Figure 48.3 also shows the distribution of plasma concentrations measured after an oral dose of **isoniazid**. In contrast to salicylate, the distribution is *bimodal*. The plasma concentration was < 20 µmol/l in about half the population in which the mode was approximately 9 µmol/l, whereas in the other half (plasma concentration > 20 µmol/l) the mode was approximately 30 µmol/l. The elimination of isoniazid depends mainly on acetylation, involving acetyl-CoA and an acetyltransferase enzyme (Ch. 43). The white

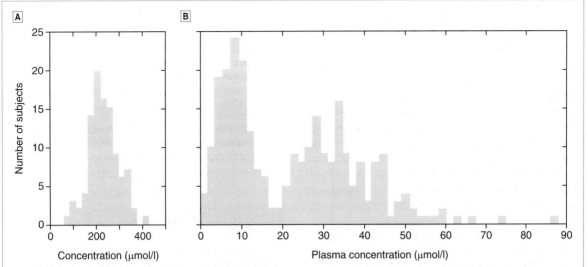

Fig. 48.3   Distribution of individual plasma concentrations for two drugs in humans. [A] Plasma salicylate concentration 3 hours after oral dosage with sodium salicylate at 0.19 mmol/kg. [B] Plasma isoniazid concentration 6 hours after oral dosage at 71 μmol/kg. Note the normally distributed values for salicylate, compared with the bimodal distribution with isoniazid. (From: (A) Evans & Clarke 1961 Brit Med Bull 17: 234–240; (B) Evans et al 1960 Brit Med J 2: 485–491)

population contains roughly equal numbers of 'fast acetylators' and 'slow acetylators', a situation described by population geneticists as a 'balanced polymorphism'. Family studies have shown that the characteristic of fast or slow acetylation is controlled by a single recessive gene associated with low hepatic acetyltransferase activity. Other ethnic groups have different proportions of fast and slow acetylators. Isoniazid causes two distinct forms of toxicity. One is peripheral neuropathy, which is produced by isoniazid itself and is commoner in slow acetylators. The other is hepatotoxicity, which has been related to conversion of the acetylated metabolite to acetylhydrazine and is commoner in fast acetylators, at least in some populations. This type of genetic variation thus produces a qualitative change in the pattern of toxicity caused by the drug in different populations. Acetyltransferase is also important in the metabolism of other drugs, including **hydralazine** (Ch. 15), **procainamide** (Ch. 14) and various sulphonamides (Ch. 43).

The list of drug-metabolising enzymes that are subject to polymorphic variation is now quite long. Drugs for which such variation is important include **phenytoin**, an anticonvulsant (Ch. 36); **debrisoquine**, a hypotensive drug that is obsolete therapeutically but useful because it is a convenient indicator for several other drugs metabolised by the same form of cytochrome P450 (Ch. 5); and **mercaptopurine**, an antitumour drug (Ch. 42).

Suxamethonium provides a well-studied example of genetic variation in the rate of drug metabolism due to a Mendelian autosomal recessive trait. This short-acting neuromuscular-blocking drug is widely used in anaesthesia and is normally rapidly hydrolysed by plasma cholinesterase (Ch. 7). About 1 in 3000 individuals fail to inactivate suxamethonium rapidly and experience prolonged neuromuscular block if treated with it; this is due to a recessive gene that gives rise to an abnormal type of plasma cholinesterase. The abnormal enzyme has a modified pattern of substrate and inhibitor specificity. It is detected by measuring the effect of the inhibitor **dibucaine**, which inhibits the abnormal enzyme less than the normal enzyme. Heterozygotes hydrolyse suxamethonium at a more or less normal rate, but their plasma cholinesterase has reduced sensitivity to dibucaine, intermediate between normals and homozygotes (Fig. 48.4). There are other, non-genetic, reasons why suxamethonium hydrolysis may be impaired in an individual patient (see p. 129), so it is important to discover whether this genetic abnormality is present in patients who experience prolonged paralysis following treatment with this drug, and to test family members who may be affected.

Sex differences in the rate and pattern of drug metabolism are important in several mammals, but not in humans.

Ethnic differences can be important. For example,

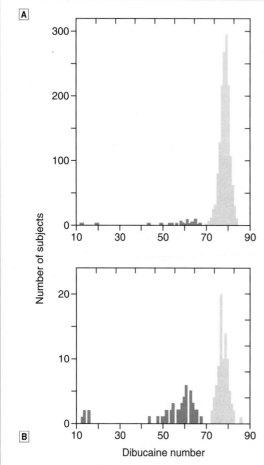

Fig. 48.4 Distribution of plasma cholinesterase phenotypes in humans. Dibucaine number is a measure of the percentage inhibition of plasma cholinesterase by 10^{-5} mol/l dibucaine. The abnormal enzyme has, in addition to low enzymic activity, a low dibucaine number. [A] Normal population. [B] Families of subjects with low or intermediate dibucaine numbers. (From: Kalow 1962 Pharmacogenetics. W. B. Saunders, Philadelphia)

Chinese subjects differ from whites in the way in which they metabolise **ethanol**, producing a higher plasma concentration of acetaldehyde which can cause flushing and palpitations (Ch. 39). Chinese subjects are considerably more sensitive to the cardiovascular effects of **propranolol** (Ch. 8) than whites, whereas black subjects are less sensitive. Despite their increased sensitivity to β-adrenoceptor antagonists, Chinese subjects metabolise propranolol consistently *faster* than whites, implying that the difference relates to pharmacodynamic differences in sensitivity at or beyond the β-adrenoceptors.

Genetic factors

- Genetic variation is an important source of pharmacokinetic variability.
- There are several examples of clear-cut genetic polymorphism, including:
  — fast/slow acetylators (hydralazine, procainamide, isoniazid)
  — plasma cholinesterase variants (suxamethonium)
  — hydroxylase polymorphism (debrisoquine).
- Several ethnic differences in drug metabolism are known (e.g. propranolol).

IDIOSYNCRATIC REACTIONS

An idiosyncratic reaction is a qualitatively abnormal, and usually harmful, drug effect that occurs in a small proportion of individuals. For example, **chloramphenicol** causes aplastic anaemia in approximately 1:50 000 patients (p. 697). In many cases, genetic anomalies are responsible, though the mechanisms are often poorly understood. *Glucose-6-phosphate dehydrogenase (G6PD) deficiency* is the basis for the most common form of genetically determined adverse reaction to drugs, a discovery that stemmed from investigation of the antimalarial drug **primaquine** (Ch. 46) which, while well tolerated in most individuals, causes haemolysis leading to severe anaemia in 5–10% of Afro-Caribbean men. This reaction, in sensitive individuals, also occurs with other drugs, including **dapsone, doxorubicin** and some sulphonamide drugs, and after eating the bean *Vicia fava* or inhaling its pollen. This underlies the condition known as 'favism' characterised in severely affected individuals by life-threatening haemolysis. This was described in antiquity in Mediterranean countries and in China. G6PD deficiency is inherited as a sex-linked recessive. The enzyme is necessary to maintain the content of reduced glutathione (GSH) in red cells, GSH being necessary to prevent haemolysis. Primaquine and related substances reduce red cell GSH harmlessly in normal cells, but enough to cause haemolysis in G6PD-deficient cells. Interestingly, heterozygote females, who show no tendency to haemolysis, have an increased resistance to malaria, providing a selective advantage that accounts for the persistence of the gene in regions where malaria is endemic.

The *hepatic porphyrias* are prototypic pharmacogenetic disorders. Although individually rare, they are clinically important. The well-intentioned use of sedative, antipsychotic or analgesic drugs in patients with undiagnosed hepatic porphyrias can be lethal, whereas with appropriate supportive management recovery from acute attacks is usually excellent. These disorders are characterised by absence of one of the enzymes required for haem synthesis, with the result that various porphyrin-containing haem precursors accumulate, giving rise to acute attacks of gastrointestinal, neurological and behavioural disturbances. Many drugs, especially but not exclusively those that induce hepatic mixed function P450 oxidase enzymes (e.g. barbiturates, **griseofulvin**, **carbamazepine**, oestrogens), can precipitate acute attacks in susceptible individuals. Porphyrins are synthesised from δ-amino laevulinic acid (ALA), formed by ALA synthase in the liver. This enzyme is induced, like various other hepatic enzymes, by drugs such as barbiturates, resulting in increased ALA production and, hence, increased porphyrin accumulation.

Various other diseases also cause genetically determined idiosyncratic reactions. These include *malignant hyperthermia* (see Ch. 7), a metabolic reaction to drugs including **suxamethonium** and various inhalational anaesthetic and antipsychotic drugs, and caused by an inherited abnormality in the Ca^{2+} release channel of the sarcoplasmic reticulum in striated muscle (and also cardiac muscle; see Ch. 14) known as the *ryanodine receptor*. The alcohol-induced flushing and nausea that occurs in a proportion of subjects treated with **chlorpropamide** (Ch. 22) is another example of an idiosyncratic reaction with autosomal dominant inheritance; its biochemical basis is unknown but may be related to the fact that, in addition to its principal action on the B-cells of the pancreatic islets (Ch. 22), chlorpropamide is also an inhibitor of aldehyde dehydrogenase.

Idiosyncratic reactions

- Harmful, sometimes fatal, reactions that occur in a small minority of individuals.
- Reactions may occur with low doses.
- Genetic factors may be responsible (e.g. primaquine sensitivity, malignant hyperthermia), though often the cause is poorly understood (e.g. bone marrow depression with chloramphenicol).

EFFECTS OF DISEASE

Detailed consideration of the many diseases that are important as a cause of individual variation is beyond the scope of this book. Disease can cause pharmacokinetic or pharmacodynamic variation. Common disorders such as impaired *renal* or *hepatic* function predispose to toxicity by causing unexpectedly intense or prolonged drug effects. Drug absorption is slowed in conditions causing *gastric stasis* (e.g. *migraine*), and may be incomplete in patients with *malabsorption* due to ileal or pancreatic disease or to oedema of the ileal mucosa caused by heart failure or nephrotic syndrome. Nephrotic syndrome (characterised by heavy proteinuria, oedema and a reduced concentration of albumin in plasma) not only alters drug absorption because of oedema of intestinal mucosa, and drug disposition by altered binding to plasma albumin, but also causes insensitivity to diuretics such as **frusemide** that act on ion transport mechanisms on the luminal surface of tubular epithelium (Ch. 20) because of binding to albumin in tubular fluid. *Hypothyroidism* is associated with increased sensitivity to several widely used drugs (e.g. **pethidine**), for reasons that are poorly understood. *Hypothermia* (to which elderly persons, in particular, are predisposed) markedly reduces the clearance of many drugs.

Other disorders, although unusual, are important because they illustrate mechanisms that may prove to be of more general applicability. Examples include:

- *Diseases that influence receptors*:
  — *myasthenia gravis*, an autoallergic disease

Variation due to disease

Pharmacokinetic alterations
- In absorption:
  — gastric stasis (e.g. migraine)
  — malabsorption (e.g. steatorrhoea from pancreatic insufficiency)
  — oedema of ileal mucosa (e.g. heart failure, nephrotic syndrome).
- In distribution:
  — altered plasma protein binding (e.g. of phenytoin in chronic renal failure)
  — impaired blood–brain barrier (e.g. to penicillin in meningitis).
- In metabolism:
  — hepatic cirrhosis and portal hypertension
  — hypothermia.
- In excretion:
  — acute and/or chronic renal failure.

Pharmacodynamic alterations
- In receptors (e.g. myasthenia gravis, nephrogenic diabetes insipidus, familial hypercholesterolaemia).
- In signal transduction (e.g. pseudohypoparathyroidism, familial precocious puberty).
- Mechanism unknown (e.g. increased sensitivity to pethidine in hypothyroidism).

characterised by antibodies to nicotinic acetylcholine receptors (Ch. 7)
— X-linked *nephrogenic diabetes insipidus*, characterised by abnormal vasopressin receptors
— *familial hypercholesterolaemia*, an inherited disease of LDL-receptors (Ch. 16).

- *Diseases that influence signal transduction mechanisms*:
  — *pseudohypoparathyroidism*, which stems from impaired coupling of receptors with adenylate cyclase
  — *familial precocious puberty*, and hyperthyroidism caused by *functioning thyroid adenomas*, which are each caused by mutations in G-protein-coupled receptors that result in the receptors remaining 'turned on' even in the absence of the hormones that are their natural agonists.

DRUG INTERACTIONS

The administration of one drug (A) can alter the action of another (B) by one of two general mechanisms:*

- modification of the pharmacological effect of B without altering its concentration in the tissue fluid (*pharmacodynamic interaction*)
- alteration of the concentration of B that reaches its site of action (*pharmacokinetic interaction*).

For such interactions to be important clinically it is necessary that the therapeutic range of drug B is narrow (i.e. that a small reduction in effect will lead to loss of efficacy and/or a small increase in effect will lead to toxicity). For pharmacokinetic interactions to be clinically important it is also necessary that the concentration–response curve of drug B is steep (so that a small change in plasma concentration leads to a substantial change in effect). For many drugs these conditions are not met: even quite large changes in plasma concentrations of relatively non-toxic drugs like **penicillin** are unlikely to give rise to clinical problems because there is usually a comfortable safety margin between plasma concentrations produced

---

*A third category of pharmaceutical interactions should be mentioned, in which drugs interact in vitro so that one or both are inactivated. No pharmacological principles are involved, just chemistry. An example is the formation of a complex between thiopentone and suxamethonium, which must not be mixed in the same syringe. Heparin is highly charged and interacts in this way with many basic drugs; it is sometimes used to keep intravenous lines or cannulae open, and can inactivate basic drugs if they are injected without first clearing the line with saline.

by usual doses and those resulting in either loss of efficacy or toxicity. Several drugs do have steep concentration–response relationships and a narrow therapeutic margin and drug interactions can cause major problems, for example with antithrombotic, antidysrhythmic and anti-epileptic drugs, lithium and several antineoplastic and immunosuppressant drugs.

Pharmacodynamic interaction

Pharmacodynamic interaction can occur in many different ways (including those discussed under 'Drug antagonism' in Ch. 1). There are many mechanisms, and some examples of practical importance are probably more useful than attempts at classification. Consider the following:

- β-adrenoceptor antagonists diminish the effectiveness of β-receptor agonists, such as **salbutamol** or **terbutaline** (Ch. 8).
- Many diuretics lower plasma potassium concentration (see Ch. 20), and thereby enhance some actions of cardiac glycosides and predispose to glycoside toxicity (Ch. 14).
- Monoamine oxidase inhibitors increase the amount of noradrenaline stored in noradrenergic nerve terminals and thereby interact dangerously with drugs, such as **ephedrine** or **tyramine**, that work by releasing stored noradrenaline. This can also occur with tyramine-rich foods—particularly fermented cheeses such as Camembert (see Ch. 35).
- **Warfarin** competes with vitamin K, preventing hepatic synthesis of various coagulation factors (see Ch. 17). If vitamin K production in the intestine is inhibited (e.g. by antibiotics), the anticoagulant action of warfarin is increased. Drugs that cause bleeding by distinct mechanisms (e.g. **aspirin**, which inhibits platelet thromboxane A_2 biosynthesis and can damage the stomach—Ch. 13) increase the risk of bleeding caused by warfarin.
- Sulphonamides prevent the synthesis of folic acid by bacteria and other microorganisms; **trimethoprim** inhibits its reduction to tetrahydrofolate. Given together the drugs have a synergistic action of value in treating *Pneumocystis carinii* (Ch. 46).
- Non-steroidal anti-inflammatory drugs (NSAIDs; Ch. 13), such as **ibuprofen** or **indomethacin**, inhibit biosynthesis of prostaglandins, including renal vasodilator/natriuretic prostaglandins (PGE_2, PGI_2). If administered to patients receiving treatment for hypertension, they cause a variable but sometimes marked increase in blood pressure, and if given to patients

being treated with diuretics for chronic heart failure can cause salt and water retention and hence cardiac decompensation.*

- H_1-receptor antagonists, such as **mepyramine**, commonly cause drowsiness as an unwanted effect. This is more troublesome if such drugs are taken with alcohol, and may lead to accidents at work or on the road.

Pharmacokinetic interaction

All of the four major processes that determine the pharmacokinetic behaviour of a drug—absorption, distribution, metabolism and excretion—can be affected by coadministration of other drugs. Such interactions have received a great deal of attention, and examples have sprouted in the literature like mushrooms. Some of the more important mechanisms are given here, with examples.

Absorption

Gastrointestinal absorption is slowed by drugs that inhibit gastric emptying, such as **atropine** or opiates, or accelerated by drugs (e.g. **metoclopramide**; see Ch. 21) which hasten gastric emptying. Alternatively, drug A may interact with drug B in the gut in such a way as to inhibit absorption of B (cf. pharmaceutical interactions; see footnote, p. 752). Thus calcium (and also iron) forms an insoluble complex with **tetracycline** and retards its absorption; **cholestyramine**, a bile acid binding resin used to treat hypercholesterolaemia (Ch. 16), binds several drugs (e.g. **warfarin**, **digoxin**) preventing their absorption if administered simultaneously. Another example is the addition of **adrenaline** to local anaesthetic injections: the resulting vasoconstriction slows the absorption of the anaesthetic, thus prolonging its local effect (Ch. 40).

Effects on drug distribution

One drug may alter the distribution of another, but such interactions are seldom clinically important. Displacement of a drug from binding sites in plasma or tissues transiently increases the concentration of *free* (unbound) drug, but this is followed by increased elimination so a new steady state results, in which *total* drug concentration in plasma is reduced but the free drug concentration is similar to that before introduction of the second 'displacing' drug. There are several direct consequences of potential clinical importance:

- Toxicity from the transient increase in concentration of free drug, before the new steady state is reached.

*The interaction with diuretics may involve a pharmacokinetic interaction in addition to the pharmacodynamic effect described here, because NSAIDs can compete with weak acids, including diuretics, for renal tubular secretion, see below.

- If dose is being adjusted according to measurements of total plasma concentration, it must be appreciated that the target therapeutic concentration range will be altered by coadministration of a displacing drug.
- When the displacing drug additionally reduces elimination of the first, so that not only is the free concentration increased acutely, but also chronically at the new steady state, severe toxicity may ensue.

Though many drugs have appreciable affinity for plasma albumin and therefore might potentially be expected to interact in these ways, there are rather few instances of clinically important interactions of this type. Protein-bound drugs that are given in large enough dosage to act as 'displacing agents' include **aspirin** and various sulphonamides, as well as **chloral hydrate** whose metabolite, trichloracetic acid, binds very strongly to plasma albumin. Displacement of *bilirubin* from albumin by such drugs in jaundiced premature neonates could have clinically disastrous consequences: bilirubin metabolism is undeveloped in the premature liver, and unbound bilirubin can cross the blood–brain barrier (which is also incompletely developed) and cause *kernicterus* (staining of the basal ganglia by bilirubin). This causes a distressing and permanent disturbance of movement known as choreoathetosis, characterised by involuntary writhing and twisting movements in the child.

Phenytoin dose is adjusted according to measurement of its concentration in plasma, and such measurements do not routinely distinguish bound from free phenytoin (that is, they reflect the total concentration of drug). Introduction of a displacing drug in an epileptic patient stabilised on phenytoin (Ch. 36) reduces the total plasma phenytoin concentration owing to increased elimination of free drug, but no loss of efficacy because the concentration of unbound (active) phenytoin at the new steady state is unaltered. If it is not appreciated that the therapeutic range of plasma concentrations has been reduced in this way, an increased dose may be prescribed resulting in toxicity.

There are several instances where drugs that alter protein binding additionally reduce elimination of the displaced drug, causing clinically important interactions. **Phenylbutazone** displaces **warfarin** from binding sites on albumin and more importantly selectively inhibits metabolism of the pharmacologically active *S* isomer (see below), prolonging prothrombin time and resulting in increased bleeding (Ch. 17). Salicylates displace **methotrexate** from binding sites on albumin and reduce its secretion into the nephron by competition with the anion secretory carrier (Ch. 5). **Quinidine** and several other

Table 48.2   Examples of drugs that induce or inhibit drug-metabolising enzymes

Drugs modifying enzyme action	Drugs whose metabolism is affected
Enzyme induction	
Phenobarbitone and other barbiturates	Warfarin
Rifampicin	Oral contraceptives
Griseofulvin	Corticosteroids
Phenytoin	Cyclosporin
Ethanol	(as well as drugs listed in left-hand column)
Carbamazepine	
Enzyme inhibition	
Disulfiram	Warfarin
Allopurinol	Mercaptopurine, azathioprine
Ecothiopate and other anticholinesterases	Suxamethonium, procaine, propanidid
Chloramphenicol	Phenytoin
Corticosteroids	Various drugs, e.g. tricyclic antidepressants, cyclophosphamide
Cimetidine	Many drugs, e.g. amiodarone, phenytoin, pethidine
MAO inhibitors	Pethidine
Erythromycin	Cyclosporin, theophylline
Ciprofloxacin	Theophylline

antidysrhythmic drugs including **verapamil** and **amiodarone** (Ch. 14) displace **digoxin** from tissue-binding sites while simultaneously reducing its renal excretion, and can consequently cause severe dysrhythmias due to digoxin toxicity.

Effects on drug metabolism

Some examples of drugs that inhibit or induce drug metabolism are shown in Table 48.2. Enzyme induction (e.g. by barbiturates, ethanol or **rifampicin**; see Ch. 5) is an important cause of drug interaction. Over 200 drugs cause enzyme induction and thereby decrease the pharmacological activity of a range of other drugs. Since the inducing agent is normally itself a substrate for the induced enzymes, the process can result in slowly developing tolerance, although this pharmacokinetic kind of tolerance is generally less important clinically than tolerance that results from pharmacodynamic adaptations (e.g. to opioid analgesics; Ch. 37), and the lethal dose of inducing drugs such as the barbiturates is only moderately increased in chronic users.

Many clinically important drug interactions result from enzyme induction, a few of which are listed in Table 48.2. Figure 48.5 shows how the antibiotic **rifampicin**, given for 3 days, reduces the effectiveness of **warfarin** as an anticoagulant. Conversely, enzyme induction can increase toxicity of a second drug whose toxic effects are mediated via a metabolite. **Paracetamol** toxicity is a case in point (see Fig. 49.1): it is due to *N*-acetyl-*p*-benzoquinone imine, which is formed by cytochrome P450. Consequently the risk of serious hepatic injury following paracetamol overdose is increased in patients whose cytochrome P450 system has been induced, for example by chronic use of alcohol. It is likely that part of the variability in rates of drug metabolism between individuals results from varying exposure to environmental contaminants, some of which are strong enzyme inducers.

Enzyme induction can be exploited therapeutically, by administering **phenobarbitone** to premature babies to induce glucuronyl transferase, thereby increasing bilirubin conjugation and reducing the risk of kernicterus (see above).

Enzyme inhibition, particularly of the P450 system, is caused by many drugs. This can slow the metabolism, and hence increase the action, of other drugs metabolised by the enzyme. Such effects can be clinically important: an example of topical interest is the interaction between the non-sedating antihistamine **terfenadine** and the imidazole antifungal drugs such as **ketoconazole** and other drugs that inhibit the CYP3A subfamily of P450 enzymes, mentioned in Chapter 5. This can result in prolongation of the Q–T interval* on the electrocardiogram and a form

---

*The Q–T interval (see Fig. 14.1) normally varies physiologically with the heart rate; this is corrected for by calculating a corrected Q–T interval ('Q–Tc') by dividing by the square root of the R–R interval.

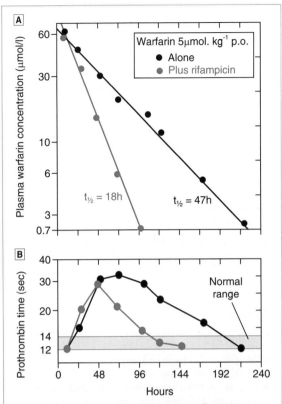

Fig. 48.5 Effect of rifampicin on the metabolism and anticoagulant action of warfarin. [A] Plasma concentration of warfarin (log scale) as a function of time following a single oral dose. After the subject was given rifampicin (600 mg daily for a few days), the plasma half-life of warfarin decreased from the normal value of 47 hours (black curve) to 18 hours (blue curve). [B] The effect of a single dose of warfarin on prothrombin time under normal conditions (black curve) and after rifampicin administration (blue curve). (Redrawn from: O'Reilly 1974 Ann Intern Med 81: 337)

Table 48.3 Stereoselective and non-stereoselective inhibition of warfarin metabolism

Stereoselective inhibition of clearance of *S* isomer
Phenylbutazone
Metronidazole
Sulphinpyrazone
Trimethoprim–sulphamethoxazole
Disulfiram

Stereoselective inhibition of clearance of *R* isomer
Cimetidine*
Omeprazole*

Non-stereoselective inhibition of clearance of *R* and *S* isomers
Amiodarone

*Minor effect only on prothrombin time
From: Hirsh 1991 N Engl J Med 324: 1865–1875

of ventricular tachycardia in susceptible individuals. *Grapefruit juice* contains a psoralen that inhibits CYP3A and reduces the metabolism of terfenadine and other drugs, including cyclosporin and several calcium channel antagonists. To make life even more difficult, several inhibitors of drug metabolism influence the metabolism of different stereoisomers selectively. Examples of drugs that inhibit the metabolism of the active *S* and less active *R* isomers of warfarin in this way are shown in Table 48.3.

The therapeutic effects of some drugs are a direct consequence of enzyme inhibition (e.g. the xanthine oxidase inhibitor, **allopurinol**, used to prevent gout;

Ch. 13). Xanthine oxidase metabolises several cytotoxic and immunosuppressant drugs, including **mercapto-purine** (the active metabolite of **azathioprine**), whose action is thus potentiated and prolonged by allopurinol. **Disulfiram**, an inhibitor of aldehyde dehydrogenase used to produce an aversive reaction to ethanol (see Ch. 39), also inhibits metabolism of other drugs, including **warfarin** which it potentiates. **Metronidazole**, an antimicrobial used to treat anaerobic bacterial infections and several protozoal diseases (Chs 43 and 46) also inhibits this enzyme, and patients prescribed it are advised to avoid alcohol for this reason.

In other instances, inhibition of drug metabolism is less expected since enzyme inhibition is not the main mechanism of action of the offending agents. Thus **steroids** and **cimetidine** enhance the actions of a range of drugs including some antidepressant and cytotoxic drugs. The only rule for prescribers is: if in doubt about the existence of a possible interaction, look it up (e.g. in the British National Formulary, which has an invaluable appendix on drug interactions indicating which are of known clinical importance).

Haemodynamic effects

Variations in hepatic blood flow influence the rate of inactivation of drugs that are subject to extensive pre-systemic hepatic metabolism (e.g. **lignocaine** or **propranolol**). A reduced cardiac output reduces hepatic blood flow, so negative inotropes (e.g. propranolol) reduce the rate of metabolism of lignocaine by this mechanism.

Effects on drug excretion

The main mechanisms by which one drug can affect the rate of renal excretion of another are:

- by altering protein binding, and hence filtration
- by inhibiting tubular secretion
- by altering urine flow and/or urine pH.

Inhibition of tubular secretion. **Probenecid** (Ch. 20) was developed expressly to inhibit **penicillin** secretion and thus prolong its action. It also inhibits the excretion of other drugs, including **azidothymidine** (AZT; see

Ch. 44). Other drugs have an incidental probenecid-like effect which can enhance the actions of substances that rely on tubular secretion for their elimination. Table 48.4 gives some examples. Since diuretics act from within the tubular lumen, drugs that inhibit their secretion into the tubular fluid, such as NSAIDs, can *reduce* their effect.

Alteration of urine flow and pH. Not surprisingly, diuretics tend to increase the urinary excretion of other drugs, but this is seldom clinically important. Conversely, loop and thiazide diuretics indirectly increase the proximal tubular reabsorption of Li^+ (which is handled in a similar way as Na^+) and this can cause Li^+ toxicity in patients treated with **lithium carbonate** for mood disorders (Ch. 35). The effect of urinary pH on the excretion of weak acids and bases is put to use in the treatment of poisoning (see Ch. 5), but is not a cause of accidental interactions.

Table 48.4 Examples of drugs that inhibit renal tubular secretion

Drugs causing inhibition	Drugs whose $t_{1/2}$ may be affected
Probenecid Sulphinpyrazone Phenylbutazone Sulphonamides Aspirin Thiazide diuretics Indomethacin	Penicillin Azidothymidine Indomethacin
Verapamil Amiodarone Quinidine	Digoxin
Diuretics	Lithium
Indomethacin	Frusemide
Aspirin NSAIDs	Methotrexate

Drug interactions

- They are many and varied; the rule is: if in doubt, look it up.
- Interactions may be pharmacodynamic or pharmacokinetic in origin.
- Pharmacodynamic interactions are often predictable from the actions of the interacting drugs.
- Pharmacokinetic interactions can involve:
  — effects on drug absorption
  — effects on distribution (e.g. competition for protein binding)
  — effects on hepatic metabolism (induction or inhibition)
  — effects on renal excretion.

REFERENCES AND FURTHER READING

Carmichael D J S 1992 Handling of drugs in kidney disease. In: Cameron S, Davison A M, Grünfeld J-P, Kerr D, Ritz E Oxford textbook of clinical nephrology. Oxford University Press, Oxford, pp 175–196 (*Discusses the influence on pharmacokinetics of renal failure and nephrotic syndrome, and outlines a practical approach to prescribing in such patients*)

Price-Evans D A 1993 Genetic factors in drug therapy, clinical and molecular pharmacogenetics. Cambridge University Press, Cambridge (*Scholarly tour de force. Also a surprisingly good read!*)

Rane A 1985 Drug metabolism and disposition in neonates and infancy. In: Wilkinson G R, Rawlins D M (eds) Drug metabolism and disposition. MTP Press, Lancaster

Ritter J M, Lewis L D, Mant T G K 1995 A textbook of clinical pharmacology, 3rd edn. Edward Arnold, London (*The chapters on drugs in pregnancy, at extremes of age and drug interactions provide an introduction*)

Rowland M, Tozer T N 1995 Clinical pharmacokinetics, concepts and applications. Williams & Wilkins, Baltimore, pp 203–312 (*Section IV, 'Individualization', provides more advanced treatment*)

Zhou H H, Koshakji R P, Silberstein D J, Wilkinson G R, Wood A J 1989 Altered sensitivity to and clearance of propranolol in men of Chinese descent as compared with American whites. N Engl J Med 320: 565–570 (*Chinese have greater sensitivity to propranolol than whites, despite metabolising propranolol more rapidly than whites. See also editorial comment: Kalow W 1989 Race and therapeutic drug response. N Engl J Med 320: 588–590*)

49

Harmful effects of drugs

In this chapter we discuss:

- types of adverse drug reactions
- toxicity testing in animals
- general mechanisms of toxin-induced cell damage and death
- mutagenesis and carcinogenesis
- teratogenesis
- allergic reactions to drugs.

TYPES OF ADVERSE DRUG REACTION

All drugs can produce harmful as well as beneficial effects. These are either: (a) related or (b) unrelated to the principal pharmacological action of the drug. Many adverse effects in the first category are predictable, at least if the main action of the drug is well understood, and are sometimes referred to as 'Type A' adverse reactions (Rawlins & Thompson 1985). Adverse effects unrelated to the main pharmacological effect are often also predictable when the drug is taken in excessive dose (e.g. **paracetamol** hepatotoxicity, **aspirin**-induced tinnitus, aminoglycoside ototoxicity), during pregnancy (e.g. **thalidomide** teratogenicity), or in disease (e.g. **primaquine** haemolysis in patients with G6PD deficiency). Sometimes a predictable subsidiary pharmacological

effect can have serious implications for rare susceptible individuals, especially if drug metabolism is altered by concomitant drug or food intake: in this regard there is current concern over effects of drugs on the electrocardiographic Q–T interval (see Chs 5 and 48). In addition rare unpredictable adverse effects can occur, for example: aplastic anaemia (**chloramphenicol**); anaphylaxis (**penicillin**); oculomucocutaneous syndrome (**practolol**). These *idiosyncratic* reactions are termed 'Type B' in the Rawlins & Thompson classification. They are usually severe—otherwise they would go unrecognised—and their existence is important in establishing the safety of medicines. If the incidence of an adverse reaction is 1 in 6000 patients exposed, approximately 18 000 patients would have to be exposed to the drug for three events to occur and approximately double that number for three events to be detected and their possible relationship to the drug recognised and reported, even if there were no background incidence of the event in question. Thus such reactions cannot be excluded by early-phase clinical trials (which usually expose only 1–2000 individuals to the drug), and the association may only come to light after many years of use. A recently recognised example is the association between severe primary pulmonary hypertension and several anorectic drugs, including **fenfluramine** and **dexfenfluramine** that have been used for many years. Valvular heart disease has also been linked to the use of these drugs. This supports prudence on the part of doctors in prescribing newly introduced drugs and indicates a need for continued monitoring by regulatory authorities after drugs have been licensed and marketed. Different countries have responded to this need in different ways, and harmonising the procedures of the different agencies involved is a major international challenge, currently being addressed through a body known as the International Conference on Harmonisation (ICH).

Many important unwanted effects related to the principal pharmacological actions of drugs have been discussed in previous chapters. For example, postural hypotension occurs with α_1-adrenoceptor antagonists, bleeding with anticoagulants and cardiac dysrhythmias with glycosides. In many instances, this type of unwanted effect is reversible, and the problem can often be dealt with by reducing the dose. Such effects are sometimes serious (e.g. intracerebral bleeding due to anticoagulants, hypoglycaemic coma from **insulin**) and occasionally they are not easily reversible, for example in the case of tardive dyskinesia produced by antipsychotic drugs (see Ch. 34) or the syndromes of drug dependence produced by opiate analgesics, alcohol or nicotine (see Ch. 39).

The second category of adverse reactions (i.e. those that arise by a biochemical mechanism unrelated to the main pharmacological effect of the drug) is often mediated by a chemically reactive metabolite rather than the parent drug. Toxicity may be direct or immunological in nature. Examples include liver or kidney damage, bone marrow suppression, carcinogenesis and disordered foetal development. Such effects (which are by no means confined to drugs, being liable to occur with any kind of chemical) fall conventionally into the area of toxicology rather than pharmacology.

Clinically important adverse drug reactions are diverse. Any organ system can be the principal target, or several systems can be involved simultaneously. Examples of this diversity are shown in Table 49.1. Anticipating, avoiding, recognising and responding to adverse drug reactions are among the most important parts of clinical practice. A full account of this area of therapeutics is beyond the scope of the present work.

Table 49.1 Examples of the diversity of organ systems involved in adverse drug reactions classified as to whether or not these are known to be related to the principal pharmacological action of the drug

Organ	Drug/clinical situation	Adverse effect	Related*	Unrelated†	Unknown	See Chapter
Heart	β-adrenoceptor antagonists	Heart failure	+			8, 14
	Doxorubicin	Heart failure		+		42
	Digoxin	Dysrhythmia	+			14
Brain	L-dopa, bromocriptine	Hallucinations	+, +			34
	Ethanol (alcohol withdrawal)	Hallucinations		+		39
	Muscarinic receptor antagonists	Memory impairment	+			31
	Chlorpromazine	Malignant neuroleptic syndrome			+	34
Sensory						
Eye	Ethambutol, chloroquine	Blindness (maculopathy)		+, +		43, 46
Ear	Aminoglycoside antibiotics	Deafness (sensorineural)		+		43
Taste	Captopril	Distortion		+		15
Touch/pain	Vincristine	Pain and numbness	+			42
Locomotor	β-adrenoceptor antagonists	Fatigue	+			8
	Fibrates (myositis)	Myalgia		+		16
	Diuretics	Gout		+		20
	Prednisolone	Osteoporosis		+		24
	Phenytoin	Osteomalacia		+		36
Gastrointestinal						
Stomach	NSAIDs	Peptic ulcer	+			13
Pancreas	Asparaginase	Pancreatitis		+		42
Colon	Clindamycin, amoxycillin (pseudomembranous colitis)	Diarrhoea	+			43
Liver	Phenytoin	Hepatitis		+		36
Gall bladder	Octreotide	Gallstones			+	24

Table 49.1 (cont'd)

Organ	Drug/clinical situation	Adverse effect	Mechanism			See Chapter
			Related*	Unrelated†	Unknown	
Lung	β-adrenoceptor antagonists, NSAID	Worsening of asthma	+, +			8, 13
	Amiodarone	Interstitial fibrosis		+		14
Kidney	ACEI	Acute renal failure	+			15
	NSAID	Acute renal failure	+			13
	Aminoglycoside antibiotics	Acute renal failure		+		43
	Analgesic abuse	Chronic renal failure			+	37
	Methysergide (retroperitoneal fibrosis)	Chronic renal failure		+		9
	Penicillamine, captopril	Nephrotic syndrome	+, +			13, 15
Genitourinary tract	Cyclophosphamide (haemorrhagic cystitis)	Haematuria	+			42
	Thiazide diuretics	Erectile impotence		+		15, 20
Endocrine/ metabolism	Thiazide diuretics	Hyperglycaemia		+		15, 20
	Sulphonylureas	Hypoglycaemia	+			22
	Amiodarone	Thyroid dysfunction		+		14
	Dopamine antagonists, e.g. chlorpromazine, haloperidol, metoclopramide	Gynaecomastia/galactorrhoea	+			34, 21
Blood—haemopoietic						
Red cells	Methyldopa	Haemolytic anaemia		+		15
White cells	Carbimazole	Neutropenia		+		25
Platelets	Quinine	Thrombocytopenia		+		46
All lineages	Chloramphenicol	Aplastic anaemia		+		43
Coagulation	Stilboestrol	Thrombosis		+		26
	Heparin, Warfarin	Haemorrhage	+, +			17
Skin	Penicillins, many others	Minor measles-like ('morbilliform') rash		+		43
	Allopurinol, sulphonamides	Generalised potentially fatal erythema multiforme (Stevens–Johnson syndrome)	+, +			13, 43
Multisystem Joints/muscles/ kidneys/brain	Hydralazine	Drug-induced lupus syndrome		+		15
Foetal development	Etretinate	Teratogenesis		+		49
	Phenytoin			+		36
Carcinogenesis	Immunosuppressant and cytotoxic drugs	Cancer	+			41

* Probably related to principal pharmacological action of drug
† Probably unrelated to principal pharmacological action of drug

DRUG TOXICITY

TOXICITY TESTING AND SCOPE OF THE CHAPTER

Toxicity testing in animals is carried out on new drugs to identify potential hazards before administering them to man. It involves the use of a wide range of tests in different species, with long-term administration of the drug, regular monitoring for physiological or biochemical abnormalities, and a detailed post-mortem examination at the end of the trial to detect any gross or histological abnormalities. Such studies are performed with doses well above the expected therapeutic range, and determine which tissues or organs are likely 'targets' of toxic effects of the drug. Recovery studies are performed to assess whether toxic effects are reversible, and particular attention paid to irreversible changes such as carcinogenesis or neurodegeneration. The basic premise is that toxic effects caused by a drug are similar in man and other animals. This is inherently reasonable in view of the similarities between higher organisms at the cellular and molecular levels. There are nevertheless wide inter-species variations, so that toxicity testing in animals is not always a reliable guide. Toxic effects can range from negligible to so severe as to preclude further development of the compound. Intermediate levels of toxicity are more acceptable in drugs intended for the more severe illnesses (for example AIDS or cancers) and decisions on whether or not to continue development are often difficult. If development does proceed, safety monitoring can be concentrated on the system 'flagged' as a potential target of toxicity by the animal studies.* *Safety* of a drug (as opposed to toxicity) can *only* be established during use in humans.

GENERAL MECHANISMS OF TOXIN-INDUCED CELL DAMAGE AND DEATH

Although cell injury can be produced directly by some drugs, in most cases it is caused by reactive substances

---

*The value of toxicity testing is illustrated by experience with **triparanol**, a cholesterol-lowering drug marketed in the USA in 1959. 3 years later a team from the FDA, acting on a tip-off, paid the manufacturer a surprise visit which revealed falsification of toxicology data demonstrating cataracts in rats and dogs. The drug was withdrawn, but some patients who had been taking it for a year or more also developed cataracts. Regulatory authorities now require that toxicity testing is performed under a tightly defined code of practice ('Good laboratory practice') which incorporates many safeguards to minimise the risk of error or fraud.

> **Types of drug toxicity**
>
> - Toxic effects of drugs can be:
>   — related to the principal pharmacological action, e.g. bleeding with anticoagulants
>   — unrelated to the principal pharmacological action, e.g. liver damage with paracetamol.
> - Some adverse reactions that occur with ordinary therapeutic dosage are unpredictable, serious and uncommon (e.g. agranulocytosis with carbimazole). Such idiosyncratic reactions are almost inevitably only detected after widespread use of a new drug.
> - Adverse effects unrelated to the main action of a drug are often caused by reactive metabolites and/or immunological reactions.

formed during metabolism. Toxic metabolites can form covalent bonds with target molecules, or alter the target molecule by non-covalent interactions (Table 49.2). Some metabolites do both. The liver is of paramount importance in drug metabolism (Ch. 5), and hepatocytes are exposed to high concentrations of nascent metabolites as these are formed by cytochrome P450-dependent drug oxidation. Drugs and their polar metabolites are concentrated in renal tubular fluid as water is reabsorbed from the nephron, so renal tubules are exposed to higher concentrations than are other tissues. Furthermore, renal vascular mechanisms are critical to the maintenance of glomerular filtration, and are vulnerable to drugs that interfere with the control of afferent and efferent arteriolar contractility. It is therefore not surprising that the occurrence of hepatic and/or renal damage is a common reason for abandoning a potential new drug during toxicity testing.

Non-covalent interactions

Reactive metabolites of drugs can be involved in several related, potentially cytotoxic, non-covalent interactions including:

- lipid peroxidation
- generation of toxic oxygen radicals
- reactions causing depletion of glutathione (GSH)
- modification of sulphydryl groups.

Some of these effects are also produced by covalent reactions.

Lipid peroxidation of polyunsaturated lipids can be initiated either by reactive metabolites or by reactive oxygen species generated by such metabolites (see below). Lipid peroxyradicals (ROO$^\bullet$) can produce lipid hydroperoxides (ROOH), which produce further lipid

Table 49.2 Drugs whose reactive metabolites interact with target molecules causing potential cell damage and/or death*

Covalent interactions		Non-covalent interactions	
Drug	Dealt with in Chapter	Drug	Dealt with in Chapter
Paracetamol	13	Paracetamol	13
Hydrocortisone	24	Adriamycin	42
Stilboestrol	26	Bleomycin	42
Isoniazid	43	Nitrofurantoin	43
Iproniazid	35	Menadione	17
Paraoxon	7	Halothane[†]	32

* In many cases, though covalent binding can be demostrated, the exact mechanism of cell damage/death is not clear.
† See also below, under 'Allergic reactions to drugs'.
From: Nelson S D, Pearson P G 1990 Annu Rev Pharmacol Toxicol 30: 169

peroxyradicals. This chain reaction—a peroxidative cascade—may eventually affect much of the membrane lipid. Cell damage and eventually cell death can result from alteration of membrane permeability or from reactions of the products of lipid peroxidation with proteins. However, lipid peroxides and peroxyradicals are usually dealt with effectively, for example by glutathione peroxidase and vitamin E, and lipid peroxidation may not, in itself, be sufficient as a cause of cell death.

Generation of toxic oxygen radicals by reactive metabolites involves reduction of molecular oxygen to superoxide anion (O_2^-) followed by enzymic conversion to H_2O_2 or to reactive species such as the hydroperoxy $(HOO^\bullet)$ and hydroxyl $(OH^\bullet)$ radicals or singlet oxygen. These are cytotoxic, both directly and through lipid peroxidation (see above).

Reactions causing depletion of glutathione result in 'oxidative stress', which is a disturbance in the pro-oxidant/antioxidant balance in cells in favour of the pro-oxidant state. It can be caused by accumulation of the normal oxidative products of cell metabolism, or by the action of toxic chemicals. The glutathione (GSH) redox cycle is a protective system that minimises cell damage from oxidative stress. GSH is normally maintained in a redox couple with its disulphide, GSSG. Oxidising species convert GSH to GSSG, GSH being regenerated by NADPH-dependent GSSG-reductase. Oxidative stress depletes cellular GSH, and when it falls to about 20–30% of normal cellular defence against toxic compounds is impaired and cell death can result.

Modification of sulphydryl (SH) groups can be produced either by oxidising species that alter SH groups reversibly or by covalent interaction. Free SH groups have a critical role in the catalytic activity of many enzymes, and modification of such SH groups results in inactivation. Important targets for SH-group modification by reactive metabolites include the cytoskeletal protein actin, glutathione reductase (see above) and Ca^{2+}-transporting ATPases in the plasma membrane and endoplasmic reticulum. These maintain cytoplasmic Ca^{2+} concentration at approximately 0.1 µmol/l, in the face of an external Ca^{2+} concentration of more than 1 mmol/l. A sustained rise in cell calcium occurs with inactivation of these enzymes (or with increased membrane permeability; see above), and compromises cell viability. Lethal processes leading to cell death after acute calcium overload include activation of degradative enzymes (neutral proteases, phospholipases, endonucleases) and protein kinases, mitochondrial damage and cytoskeletal alterations (e.g. modification of association between actin and actin-binding proteins). Altered cell signalling leading to programmed cell death ('apoptosis'; see Ch. 42, p. 665) is increasingly recognised to be of paramount importance, especially in chronic toxicity.

Covalent interactions

Targets for covalent interactions include DNA, proteins/peptides, lipids and carbohydrates. Covalent bonding to DNA is a basic mechanism of action of mutagenic chemicals; this is dealt with below. Several non-mutagenic chemicals also form covalent bonds with macromolecules, but the relationship between this and cell damage is not clear. Some drugs with metabolites that form covalent bonds are listed in Table 49.2. For example, the cholinesterase inhibitor, **paraoxon**, binds acetylcholinesterase at the neuromuscular junction and causes necrosis of skeletal muscle. One toxin from a toadstool, *Amanita phalloides*, binds actin and another binds to RNA-polymerase, interfering with actin depolymerisation and protein synthesis respectively.

General mechanisms of cell damage and cell death

- Drug-induced cell damage/death is usually due to reactive metabolites of the drug, involving non-covalent and/or covalent interactions with target molecules (Table 49.2). Cell death is often 'self-inflicted', via triggering of apoptosis rather than caused by acute necrosis.
- Non-covalent interactions include:
  — lipid peroxidation; peroxyradicals produce hydroperoxides that produce further peroxyradicals and so on
  — generation of cytotoxic oxygen radicals
  — reactions causing depletion of GSH, resulting in 'oxidative stress'
  — modification of SH groups on key enzymes (e.g. Ca^{2+}-ATPases, GSSG reductase) and structural proteins.
- Covalent interactions, e.g. adduct formation between NAPBQI and cellular macromolecules (Fig. 49.1). Covalent binding to protein can produce an immunogen; binding to DNA can cause carcinogenesis and teratogenesis.

HEPATOTOXICITY

Many therapeutic drugs cause liver damage, manifested clinically as hepatitis, or (in less severe cases) only as laboratory abnormalities (e.g. increased plasma aspartate transaminase activity). **Paracetamol, isoniazid, iproniazid** and **halothane** cause cell necrosis by the mechanisms of cell damage outlined above. Genetic differences in drug metabolism (see Ch. 5) have been implicated in some instances (e.g. **isoniazid, phenytoin**). Mild drug-induced abnormalities of liver function are not uncommon but the mechanism of liver injury is often uncertain (e.g. HMG-CoA reductase inhibitors; Ch. 16). It is not always necessary to discontinue a drug when such mild laboratory abnormalities occur, but the occurrence of irreversible liver disease (cirrhosis) as a result of long-term low-dose **methotrexate** treatment (Ch. 13) for psoriasis argues for caution. Hepatotoxicity of a different kind, namely reversible *obstructive* jaundice, occurs with **chlorpromazine** (Ch. 34) and androgens (Ch. 26).

Hepatotoxicity caused by toxic doses of **paracetamol** is clinically important (paracetamol was the fourth most

common cause of death following self-poisoning in the UK in 1989). An outline of the initial reactions in which this drug is involved is given in Chapter 13, page 236 and Figure 13.1. Because the body's handling of this drug exemplifies many of the general mechanisms of cell damage outlined above, the story is taken up again here. With toxic doses of paracetamol, the enzymes catalysing the normal conjugation reactions are saturated (see Ch. 13), and mixed-function oxidases convert the drug to the reactive metabolite *N-acetyl-p-benzoquinone imine* (NAPBQI). As explained in Chapters 5 and 48, paracetamol toxicity is increased in patients in whom P450 enzymes have been induced, for instance by chronic excessive consumption of alcohol. NAPBQI initiates several of the covalent and non-covalent interactions described above and illustrated in Figure 49.1. Oxidative stress due to GSH depletion is important in leading to cell death, although the precise mechanism is not yet clear. Synthesis of new GSH depends on the availability of cysteine, but the supply of this can be limiting. **Acetylcysteine** or methionine can, within limits, increase GSH synthesis and reduce mortality in patients with severe paracetamol poisoning.

Liver damage can also be produced by immunological mechanisms (see below), which have been particularly implicated in **halothane** hepatitis (see Ch. 32).

Hepatotoxicity

- Hepatocytes are exposed to reactive metabolites of drugs as these are formed by P450 enzymes.
- Liver damage can be produced by general mechanisms of cell injury; paracetamol exemplifies many of these (see Fig. 49.1).
- Some drugs (e.g. chlorpromazine) can cause reversible cholestatic jaundice.
- Immunological mechanisms are sometimes implicated (e.g. halothane).

NEPHROTOXICITY

Drug-induced nephrotoxicity is a common clinical problem. Indeed, non-steroidal anti-inflammatory drugs (NSAIDs; Table 49.3) and angiotensin-converting enzyme inhibitors (ACEI) are currently among the commonest causes of acute renal failure. This is usually a result of their principal pharmacological actions in patients whose underlying disease results in renal haemodynamics (blood flow and glomerular filtration) that are dependent on vasodilator prostaglandin biosynthesis

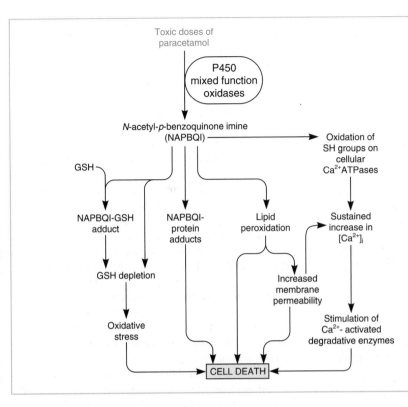

Fig. 49.1 Potential mechanisms of liver cell death resulting from the metabolism of paracetamol to N-acetyl-p-benzoquinone imine (NAPBQI). (GSH = glutathione) (Based on data from: Boobis A R et al. 1989, and Nelson S D, Pearson P G 1990 Annu Rev Pharmacol Toxicol 30: 169) See also Figure 13.1.

Table 49.3   Adverse effects of non-steroidal anti-inflammatory drugs on the kidney

Due to principal pharmacological action (i.e. inhibition of prostaglandin biosynthesis)
Acute ischaemic renal failure
Sodium retention (leading to or exacerbating hypertension and/or heart failure)
Water retention
Hyporeninaemic hypoaldosteronism (leading to hyperkalaemia)

Allergic-type interstitial nephritis (unrelated to principal pharmacological action)
Renal failure
Proteinuria

Analgesic nephropathy (unknown whether or not related to principal pharmacological action)
Papillary necrosis
Chronic renal failure

Adapted from: Murray & Brater 1993

(NSAIDs) or on angiotensin-II-mediated efferent arteriolar vasoconstriction (ACEI). *Acute renal impairment* occurs on starting the drug and is reversible if it is discontinued promptly. NSAIDs and ACEI are discussed further in Chapters 13 and 15 respectively. By reducing prostacyclin production NSAIDs can indirectly depress renin and aldosterone secretion thus predisposing to hyperkalaemia, especially if the glomerular filtration rate is also reduced. ACEI also reduce aldosterone secretion and have a similar effect.

In addition to these effects related to their main pharmacological action, NSAIDs can also cause an *allergic-type interstitial nephritis*. This is rare but severe and usually occurs several months to 1 year after starting treatment. It manifests clinically as acute renal failure often accompanied by proteinuria, or sometimes by frank nephrotic syndrome (heavy proteinuria, hypoalbuminuria and oedema). **Fenoprofen** is particularly liable to cause this type of renal damage, possibly because its metabolites bind irreversibly to albumin.

Analgesic nephropathy is a third kind of renal damage in which NSAIDs are implicated. This consists of *renal papillary necrosis* leading to chronic interstitial nephritis and severe and irreversible *chronic renal failure*. It is associated with prolonged and massive overuse of analgesics. **Phenacetin** has particularly been incriminated, but **paracetamol** and NSAIDs have not been exonerated. The role of **caffeine** (often included with analgesics and NSAIDs in combined preparations) is uncertain but could be important. It is possible that such analgesic-associated nephropathy is causally related to inhibition of renal prostaglandin synthesis, but its pathogenesis is not understood.

Captopril in higher doses than are currently recommended can cause heavy proteinuria (Ch. 15). This is due to glomerular injury and is also caused by other drugs that contain a sulphydryl group (e.g. **penicillamine**), and it is believed that it is this chemical feature rather than ACE inhibition per se that is responsible for this adverse effect.

Cyclosporin, used to prevent transplant rejection (see Ch. 13), causes renal damage via a change in renal vascular dynamics—a persistent increase in renal vascular resistance with a marked decline in glomerular filtration rate, and systemic hypertension. It alters renal prostaglandin biosynthesis.

Many drugs that cause hepatotoxicity can also cause toxic damage to the kidney, most commonly by producing necrosis of renal tubular cells. The mechanisms involved are generally similar to those described above under 'General mechanisms of cell death'.

Nephrotoxicity

- The kidney is exposed to high concentrations of drugs and drug metabolites as the urine is concentrated.
- Renal damage can be produced by general mechanisms of cell injury, which can cause papillary and/or tubular necrosis.
- Reduction in compensatory vasodilator prostaglandins can result in increased renal vascular resistance and decreased renal function.

MUTAGENESIS AND CARCINOGENICITY

Mutation is a change in the genotype of a cell, which is passed on when the cell divides. Chemical agents cause mutation by covalent modification of DNA. Certain kinds of mutation result in carcinogenesis, because the affected DNA sequence codes for a protein that is involved in growth regulation. It usually requires more than one mutation in a cell to initiate the changes that result in malignancy, mutations in proto-oncogenes (which regulate cell growth) and tumour suppressor genes (which code for products that inhibit the transcription of oncogenes) being particularly implicated (see Ch. 42). Some oncogenes code for modified growth factors or growth-factor receptors, or for elements of the intracellular transduction mechanism by which growth factors regulate cell proliferation (see p. 668). Growth factors are polypeptide mediators that stimulate cell division; examples are *epidermal growth factor* (EGF) and *platelet-derived growth factor* (PDGF). The receptors for these growth factors regulate a number of cellular processes through tyrosine phosphorylation (see Fig. 2.17). Though there are many details to be filled in, the complex connection between exposure to a mutagenic chemical and the development of a cancer is beginning to be understood.

Biochemical mechanisms of mutagenesis

Most chemical carcinogens act by modifying bases in DNA, particularly guanine, the O_6 and N_7 positions of which readily combine covalently with reactive metabolites of chemical carcinogens (Fig. 42.7). Substitution at the O_6 position is the more likely to produce a permanent mutagenic effect, since N_7 substitutions are usually quickly repaired.

The accessibility of bases in DNA to chemical attack is greatest when DNA is in the process of replication (i.e. during cell division). The likelihood of genetic damage by many mutagens is therefore related to the frequency of cell division. The developing foetus is particularly susceptible, and mutagens are also potentially teratogenic (see later section). This is also important in relation to mutagenesis of *germ cells*, particularly in the female, because in humans the production of primary oocytes occurs by a rapid succession of mitotic divisions very early in embryogenesis. Each of these primary oocytes then undergoes only two further divisions much later in life at the time of ovulation. It is thus during early pregnancy that germ cells of the developing female embryo are most likely to undergo mutagenesis, the mutations being transmitted to progeny conceived many years after exposure to the mutagen. In the male, germ cell divisions occur throughout life, and sensitivity to mutagens is continuously present.

The importance of drugs, in comparison to other chemicals such as pollutants and food additives, as a causative factor in mutagenesis has not been established, and such epidemiological evidence as exists suggests that they are uncommon (but not unimportant) causes of foetal malformations and cancers.

Mutagenesis and carcinogenicity

- Mutagenesis involves alteration of the genotype of a cell by modification of DNA.
- Carcinogenesis involves alteration of proto-oncogenes or tumour suppressor genes by mutation; more than one mutation is usually required.
- Chemical carcinogens commonly act by binding to O_6 of guanine during cell division.
- Germ cells in the female embryo undergo several rapid divisions and are therefore very vulnerable to mutagens during early development, but the effects will not be manifest till the next generation. Later in development (from infancy till reproductive adult life) female gametes are relatively resistant to mutagenesis, but if mutations do occur they can be transferred to progeny years afterwards.
- In the male, germ cell division occurs throughout life and sensitivity to mutagens is continuously present.
- Drugs are relatively uncommon (but not unimportant) causes of birth defects and cancers.

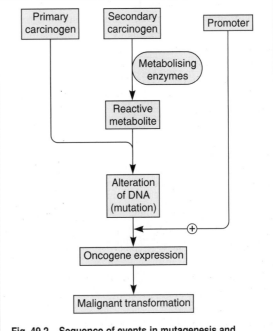

Fig. 49.2 Sequence of events in mutagenesis and carcinogenesis.

CARCINOGENESIS

Alteration of DNA is the first step in the complex, multi-stage process of carcinogenesis (see Ch. 42). Carcinogens are chemical substances that cause cancer, and can interact directly with DNA or act at a later stage to increase the likelihood that mutation will result in the production of a tumour (Fig. 49.2). Carcinogens (see Weisburger & Williams 1984) are divided into:

- *Genotoxic carcinogens* (i.e. mutagens, as discussed above). These are also termed 'initiators' and can be further divided into:
  — Primary carcinogens, which act on DNA directly
  — Secondary carcinogens, which must be converted to a reactive metabolite before they affect DNA. Most important carcinogens fall into this category.
- *Epigenetic carcinogens* (i.e. agents that do not themselves cause genetic damage, but increase the likelihood that such damage will cause cancer). There are several different types of epigenetic carcinogen, the most important being:
  — Promoters. These are not carcinogenic by themselves, but increase the likelihood of tumour development from genetically damaged cells; they can thus produce cancers when given *after* a genotoxic agent. Examples include phorbol esters, bile acids and (in large doses) saccharin. *Cigarette smoke* not

only contains carcinogenic aromatic hydrocarbons, but also has promoter activity.
  — Co-carcinogens. These substances are not carcinogenic by themselves but enhance the effect of genotoxic agents when given simultaneously; examples include phorbol esters and various aromatic and aliphatic hydrocarbons. Note that some chemicals have both genotoxic and promoter/co-carcinogenic activity. *Urban polluted air* contains substances that have carcinogenic, co-carcinogenic and promoter actions.
  — Hormones. Some tumours are hormone-dependent (see Ch. 42), the most important examples being oestrogen-dependent breast cancers and androgen-dependent prostatic cancers. Endometrial hyperplasia induced by prolonged oestrogen treatment increases the risk of uterine carcinoma unless countered by cyclical progestogen administration. This is probably due to a change in the DNA which is given expression when the cells proliferate. Hormone replacement therapy with oestrogen for postmenopausal women with an intact uterus is therefore accompanied by cyclical treatment with a progestogen (Ch. 26).

Measurement of mutagenicity and carcinogenicity

Much effort has gone into developing tests for detecting mutagenicity and carcinogenicity which can be broadly divided into:

- *In vitro tests for mutagenicity.* These rapid tests are suitable for screening large numbers of compounds, but they can give positive results on compounds that are not subsequently shown to be carcinogenic in tests on whole animals, and can miss known carcinogens.
- *Whole animal tests for carcinogenicity.* Such tests are expensive and time-consuming, but are usually required by drug regulatory authorities before a new drug is licensed for use in humans. The main limitation of this kind of study is that there are important species differences, mainly to do with the metabolism of the foreign compound and the formation of reactive products.
- *Whole animal tests for teratogenesis (reproductive-toxicity testing).* Tests on pregnant animals are required for drugs that are to be used by women of reproductive potential especially (obviously) if they are to be used during pregnancy. Similar limitations of such tests apply as with carcinogenicity testing.

In vitro tests for genotoxic carcinogens

Bacteria have great advantages as a test system for measuring mutagenicity because of their high replication rate. The most widely used assays are variations on the *Ames test*, which measures the rate of back-mutation (i.e. reversion from mutant to wild-type form) in a culture of *Salmonella typhimurium*. The normal, wild-type strain can grow in a medium containing no added amino acids, because it can synthesise all the amino acids it needs from simple carbon and nitrogen sources. The test makes use of the fact that a mutant form of the organism cannot make histidine in this way and therefore only grows on a medium containing this amino acid. The test involves growing the mutant form on a medium containing a small amount of histidine, the drug to be tested being added to the culture. After several divisions, the histidine becomes depleted, and the only cells that continue dividing are those that have back-mutated to the wild-type. A count of colonies following subculture on plates deficient in histidine gives a measure of the mutation rate.

Primary carcinogens cause mutation by a direct action on bacterial DNA but most carcinogens have to be converted to an active metabolite (see above). Therefore it is necessary to include, in the culture, enzymes that catalyse the necessary conversion. An extract of liver from a rat treated with **phenobarbital** to induce liver enzymes is usually employed. There are many variations based on the same principle.

Other short-term in vitro tests for genotoxic chemicals include measurements of mutagenesis in mouse lymphoma cells, and assays for chromosome aberrations and sister chromatid exchanges in Chinese hamster ovary ('CHO') cells. However, all the in vitro tests give some false positives and some false negatives.

In vivo tests for carcinogenicity

In vivo tests for carcinogenicity entail detection of tumours in groups of test animals. Carcinogenicity tests are inevitably slow, since there is usually a latency of months or years before tumours develop. Furthermore, tumours can develop spontaneously in control animals, and the results often provide only equivocal evidence of carcinogenicity of the test drug, making it difficult for industry and regulatory authorities to decide on further development and possible licensing of a product. None of the tests so far described can reliably detect *epigenetic carcinogens*. To do this it is necessary to measure the effect of the test substance on tumour production with a threshold dose of a genotoxic agent. Such tests are being evaluated.

Few therapeutic drugs are known to increase the risk of cancer, the most important groups being drugs that act on DNA, i.e. cytotoxic and immunosuppressant drugs, and sex hormones, e.g. oestrogen which increases

---

Carcinogens

- Carcinogens can be:
  - *Genotoxic*, i.e. causing mutations directly (primary carcinogens) or after conversion to reactive metabolites (secondary carcinogens)
  - *Epigenetic*, i.e. increasing the possibility that a mutagen will cause cancer, though not themselves mutagenic. Epigenetic carcinogens include 'promoters' which increase cancer rate if given after the mutagen, and 'co-carcinogens' which increase the rate if given with it. Phorbol esters have both actions.
- New drugs are tested for mutagenicity and carcinogenicity.
- The main test for mutagenicity measures back-mutation, in histidine-free medium, of a mutant *Salmonella typhimurium* (which, unlike the wild type, cannot grow without histidine) in the presence of:
  - the chemical to be tested
  - a liver microsomal enzyme preparation for generating reactive metabolites. Colony growth indicates that mutagenesis has occurred. Some false positives and false negatives occur.
- Carcinogenicity testing involves chronic dosing of groups of animals. It is expensive and time-consuming.
- There is no really suitable test for epigenetic carcinogens.

the occurrence of endometrial cancer and possibly also cancer of other sex hormone-responsive organs. **Pyrimethamine** (Ch. 46) is mutagenic in high concentrations, and carcinogenicity testing in strain A mice (but not other strains or species) was positive for a threefold increase in lung tumours. **Methoxsalen** (a psoralen used together with ultraviolet light (PUVA) in special centres for treatment of the skin disease, psoriasis) is both mutagenic and carcinogenic in animal models, and may increase the incidence of skin cancer in humans.

Registration of pharmaceuticals requires a comprehensive assessment of their genotoxic potential. Since no single test is adequate, the usual approach recommended by the ICH (ESRA Rapporteur 4: 5–7 1997) is to carry out a battery of in vitro and in vivo tests for genotoxicity. The following battery is often used:

- a test for gene mutation in bacteria
- an in vitro test with cytogenetic evaluation of chromosomal damage
- an in vivo test for chromosomal damage using rodent haemopoietic cells

- reproductive toxicity testing (see below)
- carcinogenicity testing.

TERATOGENESIS AND DRUG-INDUCED FOETAL DAMAGE

The term 'teratogenesis' is used to signify the production of gross structural malformations during foetal development, to distinguish it from other kinds of drug-induced foetal damage such as *growth retardation*, *dysplasia* (e.g. iodide-associated goitre) or asymmetric limb reduction due to vasoconstriction caused by **cocaine** (see Ch. 39) in an otherwise normally developing limb. A list of drugs that can affect foetal development adversely is given in Table 49.4.

It has been known that external agents can affect foetal development since about 1920, when it was discovered that X-irradiation during pregnancy could cause foetal malformation or death. Nearly 20 years later the importance of *rubella* infection was recognised, but it was not until 1960 that drugs were implicated as causative

Table 49.4   Drugs reported to have adverse effects on human foetal development

Agent	Effect	Teratogenicity*	See Chapter
Thalidomide	Phocomelia, heart defects, gut atresia, etc.	K	49
Penicillamine	Loose skin, etc.	K	13
Warfarin	Saddle nose, retarded growth, defects of limbs, eyes, CNS	K	17
Corticosteroids	Cleft palate and congenital cataract—rare		24
Androgens	Masculinisation in female		26
Oestrogens	Testicular atrophy in male		26
Stilboestrol	Vaginal adenosis in female foetus, also vaginal or cervical cancer 20+ years later		26
Anticonvulsants			
Phenytoin	Cleft lip/palate, microcephaly, mental retardation	K	36
Valproate	Neural tube defects, e.g. spina bifida	K	36
Carbamazepine	Retardation of foetal head growth	S	36
Cytotoxic drugs (esp. folate antagonists)	Hydrocephalus, cleft palate, neural tube defects, etc.	K	42
Aminoglycosides	8th cranial nerve damage		43
Tetracycline	Staining of bones and teeth, thin tooth enamel, impaired bone growth	S	43
Ethanol	Foetal alcohol syndrome	K	39
Retinoids	Hydrocephalus, etc.	K	49
Angiotensin-converting enzyme inhibitors	Oligohydramnios, renal failure		15

* K = known teratogen (in experimental animals and/or humans); S = suspected teratogen (in experimental animals and/or humans)
Adapted from: Juchau 1989 Annu Rev Pharmacol Toxicol 29: 165

agents in teratogenesis: the shocking experience with **thalidomide** led to a widespread reappraisal of many other drugs in clinical use, and to the setting up of drug regulatory bodies in many countries. The majority of birth defects (about 70%) occur with no recognisable causative factor. Drug or chemical exposure during pregnancy are believed to account for only about 1% of all foetal malformations. While this percentage may appear small, the total numbers are substantial and result in appalling suffering as well as major social and economic effects on families and the community.

Mechanism of teratogenesis

The timing of the teratogenic insult in relation to the stage of foetal development is critical in determining the type and extent of damage produced. Mammalian foetal development passes through three phases (Table 49.5):

- blastocyst formation
- organogenesis
- histogenesis and maturation of function.

Cell division is the main process occurring during *blastocyst formation*. During this phase, drugs can cause death of the embryo by inhibiting cell division, but provided the embryo survives, its subsequent development does not generally seem to be compromised, although there is evidence that **ethanol** may affect development at this very early stage (see Ch. 39).

It is during *organogenesis*, which occurs during days 17–60 in the first trimester of pregnancy, that drugs can cause gross malformations. The structural organisation of the embryo occurs in a well-defined sequence: eye and brain, skeleton and limbs, heart and major vessels, palate, genitourinary system. The type of malformation produced thus depends on the time of exposure to the teratogen.

The cellular mechanisms by which teratogenic substances produce their effects are not at all well understood.

There is a considerable overlap between mutagenicity and teratogenicity. In one large survey, among 78 compounds, 34 were both teratogenic and mutagenic, 19 were negative in both tests and 25 (among them **thalidomide**) were positive in one but not the other. It therefore seems that damage to DNA is important, but, as with carcinogenesis, it is certainly not the only factor. The control of morphogenesis is poorly understood; vitamin A derivatives (retinoids) are involved and are potent teratogens. Known teratogens also include a number of drugs (e.g. **methotrexate** and **phenytoin**) that do not react directly with DNA, but inhibit its synthesis by their effects on folate metabolism. Administration of **folate** during pregnancy *reduces* the frequency of both spontaneous and drug-induced malformations, especially neural tube defects.

In the final stage of *histogenesis and functional maturation*, the foetus is dependent on an adequate supply of nutrients, and development is regulated by a variety of hormones. Gross structural malformations do not arise from exposure to mutagens at this stage, but drugs that interfere with the supply of nutrients or with the hormonal milieu may have deleterious effects on growth and development. Exposure of a female foetus to androgens at this stage can cause masculinisation. **Stilboestrol** was commonly given to pregnant women with a history of recurrent miscarriage during the 1950s (for unsound reasons) and causes dysplasia of the vagina of the infant and an increased incidence of carcinoma of the vagina in the teens and twenties.

Testing for teratogenicity

The **thalidomide** disaster dramatically brought home the need for routine teratogenicity studies on potential new therapeutic drugs. Assessment of teratogenicity in humans is a particularly difficult problem, for various reasons. One is that the 'spontaneous' malformation rate is high (3–10% depending on the definition of a

Table 49.5 The nature of drug effects on foetal development			
Stage	Gestation period in humans	Main cellular processes	Affected by
Blastocyst formation	0–16 days	Cell division	Cytotoxic drugs
Organogenesis	17–60 days approx.	Division	
		Migration	Teratogens
		Differentiation	
		Death	
Histogenesis and functional maturation	60 days to term	As above	Miscellaneous drugs, e.g. alcohol, nicotine, antithyroid drugs, steroids

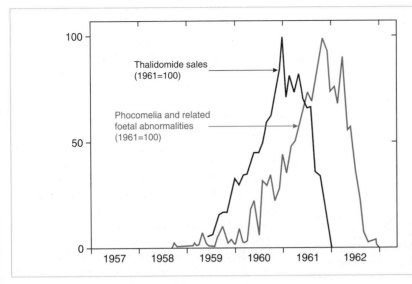

Fig. 49.3   Incidence of major foetal abnormalities in Western Europe following the introduction and withdrawal of thalidomide.

significant malformation) and highly variable between different regions, age groups and social classes. Large-scale studies are required, which take many years and much money to perform, and usually give suggestive, rather than conclusive, results.

In vitro methods, based on the culture of cells, organs or whole embryos, have not so far been developed to a level where they satisfactorily predict teratogenesis in vivo, and most regulatory authorities require terato-genicity testing in one rodent (usually rat or mouse) and one non-rodent (usually rabbit) species. Pregnant females are dosed at various levels during the critical period of organogenesis, and the foetuses are examined for struc-tural abnormalities. However, poor cross-species corre-lation means that tests of this kind are not reliably predictive in humans, and it is usually recommended that new drugs are not used in pregnancy unless it is essential.

Some definite and probable human teratogens

Though many drugs have been found to be teratogenic in varying degrees in experimental animals, relatively few are known to be teratogenic in humans (see Table 49.4). Some of the more important are discussed below.

Thalidomide

Thalidomide is virtually unique in producing, at thera-peutic dosage, virtually 100% malformed infants when taken in the first 3–6 weeks of gestation. It was intro-duced in 1957 as a hypnotic and sedative with the special feature that it was extremely safe in overdosage, and it was even recommended specifically for use in pregnancy

(with the advertising slogan 'the safe hypnotic'). As was then normal, it had been subjected only to acute toxicity testing, and not to chronic toxicity* or teratogenicity testing. Thalidomide was marketed energetically and successfully, and the first suspicion of its teratogenicity arose early in 1961 with reports of a sudden increase in the incidence of *phocomelia* ('seal limbs'; an absence of development of the long bones of the arms and legs) which had hitherto been virtually unknown. At this time approximately 1 000 000 tablets were being sold daily in West Germany. Reports of phocomelia came simultane-ously from Hamburg and Sydney, and the connection with thalidomide was made. The drug was withdrawn late in 1961, by which time an estimated 10 000 malformed babies had been born (Fig. 49.3). In spite of intensive study, its mechanism of action remains poorly under-stood. Study of the many cases of thalidomide terato-genesis in humans showed very clearly the correlation between the time of exposure and the type of malfunction produced (Table 49.6).

---

*A severe peripheral neuropathy, leading to irreversible paralysis and sensory loss, was reported within a year of the drug's introduction and subsequently confirmed in many reports. The drug company responsible was less than punctilious in acting on these reports (see Sjostrom H, Nilsson R 1972 Thalidomide and the power of the drug companies. Penguin Books, London), which were soon eclipsed by the discovery of teratogenic effects, but the neurotoxic effect was severe enough in its own right to have necessitated withdrawal of the drug from general use, although even today thalidomide still has a few highly specialised applications under tightly controlled and restricted conditions.

Table 49.6	Thalidomide teratogenesis
Day of gestation	Type of deformity
21–22	Malformation of ears
	Cranial nerve defects
24–27	Phocomelia of arms
28–29	Phocomelia of arms and legs
30–36	Malformation of hands
	Anorectal stenosis

Cytotoxic drugs

Many alkylating agents (e.g. **chlorambucil** and **cyclophosphamide**) and antimetabolites (e.g. **azathioprine** and **mercaptopurine**) can cause malformations when used in early pregnancy, but more often lead to abortion (see Ch. 42). Folate antagonists (e.g. **methotrexate**) produce a much higher incidence of major malformations, evident in both live-born and still-born foetuses.

Retinoids

Etretinate, a retinoid (i.e. vitamin A derivative) with marked effects on epidermal differentiation, is a known teratogen and causes a high proportion of serious abnormalities (notably skeletal deformities) in exposed foetuses. It is used by dermatologists to treat severe psoriasis and other skin diseases. It accumulates in subcutaneous fat and in consequence is eliminated extremely slowly, detectable amounts persisting for many months after chronic dosing is discontinued. Because of this, women should avoid pregnancy for at least 2 years after treatment. **Acitretin** is an active metabolite of etretinate. It is equally teratogenic, but tissue accumulation is less pronounced and elimination may therefore be more rapid.

Heavy metals

Lead, *cadmium* and *mercury* all cause fetal malformations in humans. The main evidence comes from Minamata disease, named after the locality in Japan where an epidemic occurred when the local population ate fish contaminated with methylmercury that had been used as an agricultural fungicide. In the developing foetus, this impaired brain development resulting in cerebral palsy and mental retardation, often with microcephaly. Mercury, like other heavy metals, inactivates many enzymes by forming covalent bonds with sulphydryl and other groups, and this is presumed to be responsible for these developmental abnormalities.

Anti-epileptic drugs

Congenital malformations are increased two- to threefold in babies of epileptic mothers. Interestingly, all existing anti-epileptic drugs have been implicated including **phenytoin** (particularly cleft lip/palate), **valproate** (neural tube defects) and **carbamazepine** (spina bifida and hypospadias—a malformation of the male urethra) as well as newer agents.

Warfarin

Administration of warfarin (see Ch. 17) in the first trimester is associated with nasal hypoplasia and various central nervous system abnormalities, affecting roughly 25% of babies. In the last trimester it must not be used because of the risk of intracranial haemorrhage in the baby during delivery.

Anti-emetics

Anti-emetics have been widely used in treating morning sickness in early pregnancy, and some are teratogenic in animals. Results of surveys in humans are inconclusive, providing no clear evidence of teratogenicity. Nevertheless, it is prudent to avoid the use of these drugs in pregnant patients if possible.

Teratogenesis and drug-induced foetal damage

- Teratogenesis means production of gross structural malformations of the foetus, e.g. the absence of limbs after thalidomide. Less comprehensive damage can be produced by many other drugs (see Table 49.4). <1% of congenital foetal defects are attributed to drugs given to the mother.
- Gross malformations can be produced only if teratogens act during organogenesis. This occurs during the first 3 months of pregnancy but after blastocyst formation. Drug-induced foetal damage is rare during blastocyst formation (exception: foetal alcohol syndrome) and after the first 3 months.
- The mechanisms of action of teratogens are not clearly understood, though DNA damage is a factor in many cases.
- New drugs are tested in pregnant females of one rodent and one non-rodent (e.g. rabbit) species.

ALLERGIC REACTIONS TO DRUGS

Allergic reactions of various kinds are a very common form of adverse response to drugs. Most drugs, being low-molecular-weight substances, are not immunogenic in themselves. A drug or its metabolites can, however, interact with protein to form a stable conjugate that can function as an *immunogen* (see Ch. 12). In some instances, the immunological basis for such responses has been well worked out, but very often it is inferred from the clinical characteristics of the reaction, and direct evidence of an immunological mechanism is lacking. The main criteria that are suggestive of an immune response are:

- The reaction has a time-course different from that of the pharmacodynamic effect, i.e. it is either delayed in onset, occurring a few days after administration of the drug, or occurs only with repeated exposure to the drug.
- Sensitisation and/or the subsequent allergic reaction may occur with doses that are too small to elicit pharmacodynamic effects.
- The reaction conforms to one of the clinical syndromes associated with allergy—types I, II, III and IV of the Gell & Coombs classification (Ch. 12, p. 209, and below)—and is unrelated to the pharmacodynamic effect of the drug.

The overall incidence of allergic drug reactions is variously reported as being between 2 and 25%. The great majority are relatively harmless skin eruptions. Serious reactions (e.g. *anaphylaxis*, *haemolysis* and *bone marrow depression*) which can be fatal, are rare. Penicillins, which are the commonest cause of drug-induced anaphylaxis, produce this response in an estimated 1 in 50 000 patients exposed.

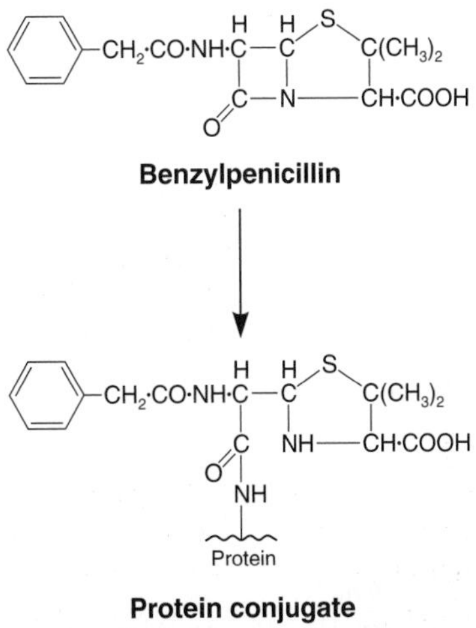

Immunological mechanisms

The formation of an immunogenic conjugate between a small molecule and an endogenous protein requires covalent bonding. In most cases, reactive metabolites, rather than the drug itself, are responsible. Such reactive metabolites can be produced during drug oxidation or by photo-activation in the skin. They may also be produced by the action of toxic oxygen metabolites generated by activated leukocytes. Rarely (e.g. in *drug-induced lupus erythematosus*) the reactive moiety interacts with nuclear components (DNA, histone) rather than proteins to form an immunogen (see below). The mechanism for covalent coupling of **benzylpenicillin** to protein is shown in Figure 49.4. Metabolites of penicillin such as *benzylpenicillenic acid* also couple to proteins, forming immunogens. Conjugation with a macromolecule is usually essential, although penicillin is an exception, because it can form sufficiently large polymers in solution to elicit an anaphylactic reaction in a sensitised individual, even without conjugation to protein.

Clinical types of allergic response to drugs

In the Gell & Coombs classification of hypersensitivity reactions (Ch. 12), types I, II and III are antibody-

Fig. 49.4 Mechanism of formation of protein conjugate by penicillin.

mediated and type IV is cell-mediated. Unwanted reactions to drugs involve both antibody- and cell-mediated reactions. The more important clinical manifestations of hypersensitivity include: anaphylactic shock, haematological reactions, allergic liver damage and other hypersensitivity reactions.

Anaphylactic shock

Anaphylactic shock—a type I hypersensitivity response—is a sudden and life-threatening reaction that results from the release of *histamine* and *other mediators* (Ch. 12). The main features include urticarial rash, swelling of soft tissues, bronchoconstriction and hypotension.

Penicillins are the drugs most likely to cause anaphylactic reactions, and account for about 75% of anaphylactic deaths, reflecting the frequency with which they are used in clinical practice. Other drugs that can cause anaphylaxis include: various enzymes, for example **streptokinase** (Ch. 17), **asparaginase** (Ch. 42); hormones, for example ACTH (Ch. 24), insulin (Ch. 22); **heparin** (Ch. 17); dextrans; radiological contrast agents; vaccines; and other serological products. Anaphylaxis with local anaesthetics (Ch. 40) and the surface antiseptic, chlorhexidine, and with many other drugs has been reported but is uncommon. Anaphylaxis is treated by injection of **adrenaline** (which is life-saving in this circumstance), corticosteroids and antihistamines.

It is feasible to carry out a skin test for the presence of anaphylactic hypersensitivity, by injecting a minute dose of the drug intradermally. This is sometimes done if a patient reports that he or she is allergic to a particular drug. However, the test is not completely reliable, and false negative results are not uncommon. Furthermore, the test dose itself may elicit a severe reaction. The use of *penicilloylpolylysine* as a skin test reagent for penicillin allergy is an improvement over the use of penicillin itself, because it bypasses the need for conjugation of the test substance, thereby reducing the likelihood of a false negative. Other specialised tests are available to detect the presence of specific IgE in the plasma, or to measure histamine release from the patient's basophils, but these are not used routinely.

Other drug-induced type I hypersensitivity reactions include *bronchospasm* (see Ch. 19) and *urticaria*.

Haematological reactions

Drug-induced haematological reactions can be produced by type II, III or IV hypersensitivity (see p. 209). Type II reactions can affect any or all of the formed elements of the blood, which may be destroyed by effects either on the circulating blood cells themselves or on their progenitors in the bone marrow. They involve antibody binding to a drug–macromolecule complex on the cell surface membrane. The antigen–antibody reaction activates complement leading to lysis (Fig. 12.1) or provokes attack by killer lymphocytes or phagocytic leukocytes. *Haemolytic anaemia* has been most commonly reported with sulphonamides and related drugs (Ch. 43) and with the antihypertensive drug, **methyldopa** (see Ch. 8). With methyldopa, significant haemolysis occurs in less than 1% of patients, but the appearance of antibodies directed against the surface of red cells is detectable in 15% by the Coombs' test. The antibodies are directed against Rh antigens, but it is not known how methyldopa produces this effect. *Drug-induced agranulocytosis* (complete absence of circulating neutrophils) is usually delayed 2–12 weeks after beginning drug treatment but may then be sudden in onset. It often presents with mouth ulcers, a severe sore throat or other infection. Serum from the patient lyses leukocytes from other individuals, and circulating antileukocyte antibodies can usually be detected immunologically. The main groups of drugs associated with agranulocytosis are NSAIDs (especially **phenylbutazone**; Ch. 13), **carbimazole** (Ch. 25) and **clozapine** (Ch. 34). Sulphonamides and related drugs (e.g. thiazides and sulphonylureas) are uncommon but well-documented causes of agranulocytosis. This is a rare, but highly dangerous condition, because recovery when the drug is stopped is often absent or incomplete and the marked reduction of blood granulocytes makes the patient extremely vulnerable to bacterial infections. This type

of antibody-mediated leukocyte destruction must be distinguished from the direct effect of cytotoxic drugs (see Ch. 42), most of which cause granulocytopenia. With these latter drugs, however, the effect is rapid in onset, predictably related to dose and reversible. *Thrombocytopenia* (reduction in platelet numbers) can be caused by type II reactions to **quinine** (Ch. 46), **heparin** (Ch. 17) and thiazide diuretics (Ch. 20). Some drugs (notably **chloramphenicol**) can suppress all three haemopoietic cell lineages giving rise to *aplastic anaemia* (anaemia with associated agranulocytosis and thrombocytopenia).

The distinction between type III and type IV hypersensitivity reactions in the causation of haematological reactions is not clear cut, and it is likely that either or both mechanisms are often involved.

Allergic liver damage

Most drug-induced liver damage is due to the direct toxic effects of drugs or their metabolites as described above. However, hypersensitivity reactions are sometimes involved, a particular example being **halothane**-induced hepatic necrosis (see Ch. 32). *Trifluoracetylchloride*, a reactive metabolite of halothane, couples to a macromolecule to form an immunogen. Most patients with halothane-induced liver damage have antibodies that react with halothane–carrier conjugates. There is evidence from rabbit experiments that the halothane–protein antigens can be expressed on the surface of the liver cells. Destruction of the cells occurs by type II hypersensitivity reactions involving killer T cells. If antigen–antibody complexes are released by damaged cells, type III reactions can contribute.

Enflurane may also cause antibody-mediated liver damage, and apparent cross-sensitisation with halothane is reported.

Other hypersensitivity reactions

The clinical manifestations of type IV hypersensitivity reactions are diverse, ranging from minor skin rashes to generalised autoimmune disease. Fever may accompany these reactions. Skin rashes can be antibody-mediated, but are usually cell-mediated. They range from mild eruptions to fatal exfoliation. In some cases the lesions are photosensitive, probably because of degradation of the drug to reactive substances in the presence of UV light.

Some drugs (notably **hydralazine** and **procainamide**) can produce an autoimmune syndrome resembling *systemic lupus erythematosus* (SLE). This is a multisystem disorder in which there is immunological damage to many organs and tissues (including joints, skin, lung, CNS and kidney) caused particularly, but not exclusively, by type III hypersensitivity reactions. The prodigious array of antibodies directed against 'self' components has been termed 'an autoimmune thunder-storm'. The antibodies react with determinants shared by many molecules, for example the phosphodiester backbone of DNA, RNA and phospholipids. In drug-induced SLE, the immunogen may result from the reactive drug moiety interacting with nuclear material, and in the effector phase, joint and pulmonary damage is common. The condition usually resolves when treatment with the offending drug is stopped.

Allergic reactions to drugs

- Drugs or their reactive metabolites can bind covalently to tissue proteins to form immunogens. Penicillin (which can also be immunogenic by forming polymers) is an important example.
- Drug-induced allergic (hypersensitivity) reactions may be antibody-mediated (types I, II, III) or cell-mediated (type IV). Important clinical manifestations include:
  — *Anaphylactic shock* (type I). This is life-threatening, by obstructing respiration. Many drugs can cause the condition; most deaths are due to penicillin.
  — *Haematological reactions* (type II, III or IV). These, along with examples of causative drugs, are: haemolytic anaemia (sulphonamides and methyldopa), agranulocytosis, which can be irreversible (sulphonamides, chloramphenicol and carbimazole) and thrombocytopenia (quinine, heparin and thiazide diuretics).
  — *Allergic liver damage* (type II, III). The reactive metabolite of halothane couples to liver proteins to form an immunogen.
  — *Skin rashes* (type I, IV). These occur with many drugs, are usually type IV and usually mild, though some can be life-threatening.
  — *Drug-induced systemic lupus erythematosus* (mainly type II). This involves antibodies to nuclear material.

REFERENCES AND FURTHER READING

Alison M R, Sarraf C E 1995 Apoptosis: regulation and relevance to toxicology. Hum Exp Toxicol 14: 234–247 (Review)

Anonymous 1997 Drug-induced agranulocytosis. Drug Ther Bull 35: 49–52 (*Considers which drugs are most commonly involved, how to minimise risk and how to manage*)

Boobis A R, Fawthrop D J, Davies D S 1989 Mechanisms of cell death. Trends Pharmacol Sci 10: 275–280 (*Oxidising species convert GSH to GSSG. GSH is usually regenerated by NADPH-dependent GSSG-reductase; but when the rate of GSH oxidation to GSSG exceeds the capacity of this enzyme, GSSG is removed from the cell by active transport*)

Briggs G G, Freeman R K, Sumner J Y 1994 Drugs in pregnancy and lactation, 4th edn. Williams & Wilkins, Baltimore (*Invaluable reference guide to foetal and neonatal risk for clinicians caring for pregnant women*)

Brimblecombe R W, Dayan A D 1993 Preclinical toxicity testing. In: Burley D M, Clarke J M, Lasagna L (eds) Pharmaceutical medicine, 2nd edn. Edward Arnold, London. pp 12–32 (*Scholarly review*)

De Weck A L 1983 Immunopathological mechanisms and clinical aspects of allergic reactions to drugs. In: De Weck A L, Bundgaard H (eds) Allergic responses to drugs. Handbook of experimental pharmacology. Springer-Verlag, Berlin, vol 63, pp 75–135

Farrar H C, Blumer J L 1991 Fetal effects of maternal drug exposure. Annu Rev Pharmacol 31: 525–547 (*Reviews teratology, foetal drug effects, teratogenesis and foetal pharmacology*)

Hanson J W, Streissguth A P, Smith D W 1978 The effects of moderate alcohol consumption during pregnancy on fetal growth and morphogenesis. J Paediatr 92: 457–460

Hay A 1988 How to identify a carcinogen. Nature 332: 782–783

Hinson J A, Roberts D W 1992 Role of covalent and noncovalent interactions in cell toxicity: effects on proteins. Annu Rev Pharmacol Toxicol 32: 471–510

Huff J, Haseman J, Rall D 1991 Scientific concepts, value, and significance of chemical carcinogenesis studies. Annu Rev Pharmacol Toxicol 31: 621–652

Jones J K, Idänpään-Heikkilä J E 1993 Adverse reactions, postmarketing surveillance and pharmacoepidemiology. In: Burley D M, Clarke J M, Lasagna L (eds) Pharmaceutical medicine, 2nd edn. Edward Arnold, London, pp 145–180

Kenna J G, Knight T L, van Pelt F N A M 1993 Immunity of halothane metabolite-modified proteins in halothane hepatitis. Ann NY Acad Sci 685: 646–661

Lutz W K, Maier P 1988 Genotoxic and epigenetic chemical carcinogens: one process, different mechanisms. Trends Pharmacol Sci 9: 322–326

Moss A J 1993 Measurement of the QT interval and the risk of QTc prolongation: a review. Am J Cardiol 72: 23B–25B

Murray M D, Brater D C 1993 Renal toxicity of the nonsteroidal anti-inflammatory drugs. Annu Rev Pharmacol Toxicol 33: 435–465

Nicotera P, Bellomo G, Orrenius S 1992 Calcium-mediated mechanisms in chemically-induced cell death. Annu Rev Pharmacol Toxicol 32: 449–470 (*Discusses the role of calcium in the early development of cell damage*)

Pohl L R, Satoh H, Christ D D, Kenna J G 1988 The immunologic and metabolic basis of drug hypersensitivities. Annu Rev Pharmacol 28: 367–387

Pumford N R, Halmes N C 1997 Protein targets of xenobiotic reactive intermediates. Annu Rev Pharmacol Toxicol 37: 91–117 (*Intrinsic versus idiosyncratic toxicity*)

Rawlins M D, Thomson J W 1985 Mechanisms of adverse drug reactions. In: Davies D M (ed) Textbook of adverse drug reactions, 3rd edn. Oxford University Press, Oxford, pp 12–38 *(Type A/type B classification)*

Scales M D C 1993 Toxicity testing. In: Griffin J P, O'Grady J, Wells F O (eds) The textbook of pharmaceutical medicine. Queen's University Press, Belfast, pp 53–79 *(Thoughtful review)*

Timbrell J A 1982 Principles of biochemical toxicology. Taylor & Francis, London

Uetrecht J 1989 Mechanism of hypersensitivity reactions: proposed involvement of reactive metabolites generated by activated leucocytes. Trends Pharmacol Sci 10: 463–467

Venitt S 1981 Microbial tests in carcinogenesis studies. In: Gorrod J W 1981 Testing for toxicity. Taylor & Francis, London *(Describes some of the many variants of the Ames test)*

Weinberg R A 1984 Cellular oncogenes. Trends Biochem Sci 9: 131–133

Weisburger J H, Williams G M 1984 New, efficient approaches to tests for carcinogenicity of chemicals based on their mechanisms of action. In: Zbinden G et al. (eds) Current problems in drug toxicology. Libbey, Paris *(Scheme of classification of carcinogens)*

50

Gene therapy

The history of therapeutics has been punctuated by monumental innovations (e.g. surgery, immunisation, antibiotics) that are conceptually simple but have changed the world. Gene therapy, the genetic modification of cells to prevent, alleviate or cure disease, has certainly not done that—yet; indeed, at the time of writing no gene therapy product has been licensed for general use. The concept of introducing nucleic acid into cells of the body in order to treat or prevent disease is, however, so appealing that vast resources (both public and private) have been committed to its development. There are several reasons for this appeal. First, the approach offers the potential for radical cure of single gene diseases such as cystic fibrosis and the haemoglobinopathies, which are collectively responsible for much misery throughout the world. Second, many much commoner conditions, including malignant, neurodegenerative and infectious diseases, have a large genetic component. Conventional treatment of such disorders is, as readers of this book will appreciate, woefully inadequate, so a completely new approach has enormous attraction. Finally, an ability to control gene expression could revolutionise the management of diseases in which there is no genetic component at all.*

---

*If a lamb can be grown from the nucleus of a cell from the udder of an adult sheep, it does not take an H G Wells to imagine what this could mean for amputees or other victims of trauma, although it must be admitted with the present state of the art such applications still appear far-fetched.

The gene for vascular endothelial growth factor is being used to stimulate the growth of new blood vessels around blockages in atherosclerotic arteries, and preliminary results have been encouraging. More mundanely, if a deficient protein (such as factor VIII, insulin or erythropoietin) could be synthesised in vivo, this would have great practical advantages over recurrent injections of purified or synthetic protein in diseases such as haemophilia (Ch. 17), diabetes (Ch. 22) or chronic renal failure (Ch. 18).

Using modern techniques it is possible to identify and clone genes, alter DNA or RNA in the laboratory and produce large amounts of this modified, recombinant, nucleic acid. Such recombinant nucleic acid, coding for a gene that it is hoped will have therapeutic effect, can be introduced into host chromosomes via plasmids and transposons (see Ch. 43). The gurus are emphatic that 'the conceptual part of the gene therapy revolution has indeed occurred …'—so where are the therapies? The devil, of course, is in the detail: in this case the details of pharmacokinetics (gene delivery to appropriate target cells), pharmacodynamics (*controlled* expression of the gene in question), safety, clinical efficacy and long-term practicability. These problems are formidable: an analogy is to put oneself in the shoes of a barber-surgeon cutting for stone on Samuel Pepys. Such a practitioner would surely have imagined the *concept* of abdominal surgery (to relieve obstruction from a strangulated hernia or tumour for instance), but realisation of the dream would needs await discoveries in the fields of anaesthesia and aseptic technique in the 19th and 20th centuries.

In the case of gene therapy, perhaps the most fundamental hurdle is the delivery problem; here modern virology offers more than a whiff of the possibilities of gene delivery for therapeutic use, and other techniques are also available that can introduce functional nucleic acids into mammalian cells (see below). It is this sense of the possible in the setting, on the one hand, of a concept so simple that any broadsheet reader can apprehend it and, on the other, great prizes (humanitarian, scientific and commercial) that has led inevitably to great expectations and, perhaps equally inevitably, to frustration at the lack of practical progress. Here we concentrate on principles that have emerged thus far in the confident beliefs:

- that nucleic acid based therapies will be developed that are safe and effective
- that this will radically change medicine; but that
- the full impact of these changes will not be realised for many years.

At present there is a broad consensus that attempts at gene therapy should focus exclusively on somatic cells and a moratorium has been agreed on therapies intended to alter the DNA of germ cells and hence influence the next generation.

Definition and potential uses

- Gene therapy is the genetic modification of cells to prevent, alleviate or cure disease; current efforts are directed to somatic and not to germ cells.
- Potential applications:
  — radical cure of single gene diseases (e.g. cystic fibrosis, haemoglobinopathies)
  — amelioration of diseases with or without a genetic component, including many malignant, neurodegenerative and infectious diseases.

TECHNICAL ASPECTS

GENE DELIVERY

The transfer of recombinant nucleic acid into target cells—the 'drug distribution' problem—is critical to the success of gene therapy. Nucleic acid must pass from the extracellular space across the plasma and nuclear membranes, and be incorporated into the chromosomes. Since DNA is highly negatively charged and single genes have molecular weights around 10^4 times greater than conventional drugs, the problem is of a different order from the equivalent stage of routine drug development. Various approaches have been developed, most of which involve inserting the therapeutic gene into a drug delivery system called a '*vector*', often in the form of a *suitably modified virus* (see below).

There are two main strategies for delivering genes into patients: *in vivo* and *ex vivo*. The in vivo strategy is to inject a suspension of a vector containing the therapeutic gene directly into the patient—either intravenously, in which case some form of targeting of the vector to the organ or tissue on which it is intended to act is highly desirable—or into a tissue on which it is hoped that it will act (e.g. directly into a malignant tumour). The ex vivo strategy is to remove cells from the patient (e.g. stem cells from marrow or circulating blood, or myoblasts from a biopsy of striated muscle) treat them with the vector, and inject the genetically altered cells back into the patient.

An ideal vector would be safe, highly efficient (i.e. insert the therapeutic gene into a large fraction of target cells), and selective in that it would lead to expression of the therapeutic protein in the target cells but not to the expression of viral proteins. It would cause *persistent* expression, avoiding the need for repeated treatment provided the cell into which it is inserted is itself long-lived. This is a problem with a therapeutic target such as the airway epithelium. This malfunctions in the autosomal recessive disorder cystic fibrosis owing to deficiency of a membrane chloride ion transporter known as the cystic fibrosis transport regulator (CFTR). Epithelial cells in the airways are continuously dying off and being replaced, so even if the *CFTR* gene were stably transfected into the epithelium, there would still be a need for periodic retreatment unless the gene can be inserted into the progenitor ('stem') cells. Similar problems are to be anticipated in other cells that turn over continuously such as gastrointestinal epithelium and skin. (Repeat administration of therapeutic drugs is, of course, usually needed, but in the case of macromolecules and viruses causes problems associated with immune responses.)

Viral vectors. Viruses take over the metabolic machinery of the cells they invade, and some are expert at fusing with their nucleic acid. Most strategies for gene delivery utilise these properties. While producing a tantalising glimpse of the possible,* there remain substantial practical problems with this approach, partly at least because as viruses have evolved the means to invade human cells, so humans have evolved enzymes and immune responses that thwart them. The field is currently seething with activity.

Retroviral vectors have the attraction that, if introduced into stem cells, their effects are persistent because they become incorporated into and replicate with host DNA and so are passed down to each daughter during cell

---

*Rather like a would-be abdominal surgeon in the 17th century contemplating the use of general anaesthesia when his only experience of it was intoxication with alcoholic beverages.

division. Against this, since they are inserted randomly into the chromosome, they may cause damage (see below). Furthermore, since they are relatively promiscuous as regards the cells they infect they could produce undesired effects, including effects on germ cells, if administered in vivo. They are therefore currently used for ex vivo attempts at therapy. The life cycle of naturally occurring retroviruses are exploited to create vectors for use in gene therapy (see Fig. 50.1). For the future, it is hoped that it will be possible to alter the retroviral envelope to increase specificity, so that the vector could be administered systemically but would home in only on the desired target cell population. An example of this approach is the substitution of the envelope protein of a non-pathogenic vector (e.g. mouse leukaemia virus, which is not pathogenic for humans and has been evaluated as a potential

retrovirus vector for use in humans) with the envelope protein of human vesicular stomatitis virus, in order specifically to target epithelial cells. Most retrovirus vectors are unable to penetrate the nuclear envelope, and therefore only infect dividing cells since the nuclear membrane dissolves during cell division. Consequently, they do not infect non-dividing cells such as adult neurons.

Adenovirus vectors are popular because of their perceived safety and because of the high transgene expression that can be achieved. They transfer genes to the nucleus of the host cell, but (unlike retroviruses) these are not inserted into the host genome and so do not produce effects that outlast repeated cell divisions. Adenovirus vectors have been used to attempt in vivo gene therapy. The lack of insertion into host chromosomes obviates

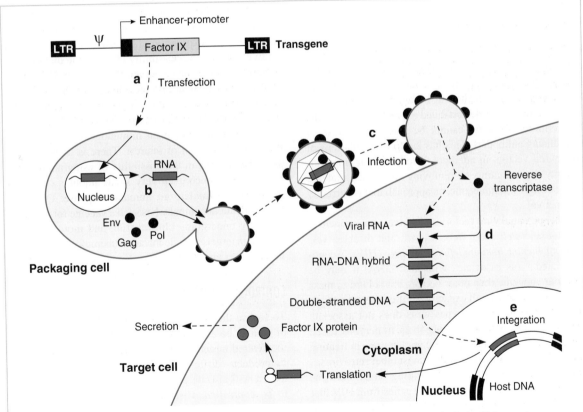

Figure 50.1 Strategy for making retroviral vectors. The transgene (the example shows the gene for factor IX) in a vector backbone is introduced (a) into a packaging cell, where it is integrated into a chromosome in the nucleus and (b) transcribed to make vector mRNA which is packaged into the retroviral vector and shed from the packaging cell. It then infects the target cell (c). Virally encoded reverse transcriptase (d) converts vector RNA into an RNA–DNA hybrid, and then into double-stranded DNA which is integrated (e) into the genome of the target cell which can then transcribe and translate it to make factor IX protein. (From: Verma I M, Somia N 1997 Nature 389: 239–242)

the risk of disturbing the function of vital cellular genes and the theoretical risk of carcinogenicity that this imparts (see below), but at the cost of producing only a temporary effect. Adenovirus vectors are genetically modified by making deletions in the viral genome, thereby making the virus unable to replicate and cause widespread infection in the host while at the same time creating space in the viral genome for the therapeutic transgene to be inserted. One of the first adenoviral vectors lacked part of a growth-controlling region called E_1. This defective virus is grown in a cell line that substitutes for the missing E_1 function. Recombinant virus is produced by infecting complementing cells with a plasmid generated from the cloned DNA of therapeutic interest plus an expression cassette and portions of adenoviral DNA. Recombination between this and the 'backbone' of the E_1-deficient adenoviral genome results in a virus encoding the desired transgene. This approach led to seemingly spectacular results, demonstrating gene transfer to cell lines and animal models of disease, but has been disappointing (especially for cystic fibrosis) in humans. The main problem has been that low doses (administered by aerosol to patients with this disease) have produced only very low efficiency transfer, whereas higher doses have resulted in inflammation and a host immune response, and short-lived expression of the gene. Furthermore, treatment cannot be repeated because of neutralising antibodies. This has led to manipulations of adenoviral vectors in attempts to reduce their immunogenicity, by mutating or removing the genes that are most strongly immunogenic, an approach that is currently very active.

Other potential viral vectors under investigation include *adeno-associated virus*, *herpes virus*, and disabled versions of *human immunodeficiency virus* (*HIV*). Adeno-associated virus associates with host DNA; it may be less immunogenic than other vectors but is hard to mass produce and has a small capacity, so it cannot be used to carry large transgenes. Herpes virus does not associate with host DNA but is very long-lived in nervous tissue and could therefore have specific applications in treating neurological disease. HIV, unlike most other retroviruses (see above), can infect non-dividing cells such as neurons. It is possible to remove the genes from HIV that permit its replication and substitute marker genes that are expressed following injection into rat brain, and it is hoped that therapeutic genes could be inserted similarly. Alternatively, it may prove possible to transfer those genes that permit HIV to penetrate the nuclear envelope to other non-pathogenic retroviruses.

Non-viral vectors include a variant of liposomes

(Ch. 4). Plasmids (diameter up to approximately $2\,\mu m$) are too big to package in regular liposomes (diameter 0.025–$0.1\,\mu m$), but larger particles can be made using positively charged lipids ('*lipoplexes*') which interact with negative charges on cell membranes and negatively charged DNA, improving delivery into the cell nucleus and incorporation into the chromosome. Such particles have been used to deliver the genes for HLA-B7, interleukin-2 and CFTR. They are much less efficient than viruses and attempts are currently under way to improve this by incorporating various viral signal proteins (membrane fusion proteins, for example) in their outer coat. Meanwhile, direct injection into solid tumours (e.g. melanoma, breast, kidney and colon cancers) can achieve high local concentrations within the tumour.

Biologically erodable microspheres made from polyanhydride copolymers of fumaric and sebacic acids (see Ch. 4) can be loaded with plasmid DNA. A plasmid with bacterial β-galactosidase activity formulated in this way and given by mouth to rats can result in systemic absorption and expression of the bacterial enzyme in the rat liver, raising the possibility of oral gene therapy!

Surprisingly, it has emerged that plasmid DNA itself ('*naked DNA*') can access the nucleus and be expressed, albeit much less efficiently than when it is packaged in a vector.* Such DNA carries no risk of viral replication and is not necessarily itself immunogenic,** but cannot be targeted to a cell of interest. There is currently considerable interest in the possibility of using naked DNA for *vaccines*, since even very small amounts of foreign protein can stimulate an immune response. One large pharmaceutical company has such a vaccine for influenza currently undergoing clinical trial, and more ambitious long-term targets include malaria, tuberculosis, chlamydia, helicobacter and hepatitis.

CONTROLLING GENE EXPRESSION

To realise the full potential of gene therapy, it will not, of course, be enough to transfer the gene selectively to the desired target cells and keep it there still expressing its product—difficult though these goals are. For many uses it will also be essential for the activity of the gene to be *controlled*. Historically it was the realisation of

---

*The discovery came from its use—injected into striated muscle—as a 'negative' control that turned out positive.

**This is a theoretical concern, since antibodies directed against DNA are characteristic of several autoimmune diseases including systemic lupus erythematosus.

Gene delivery and expression

- Gene delivery is one of the main hurdles to making gene therapy practicable.
- Recombinant genes are transferred via a plasmid to a vector, often a suitably modified virus.
- There are two main strategies for delivering genes into patients:
  — *in vivo* injection of the vector containing the therapeutic gene directly into the patient (e.g. into a malignant tumour)
  — *ex vivo* treatment of cells from the patient (e.g. stem cells from marrow or circulating blood, or myoblasts from a biopsy of striated muscle) followed by reinjection into the patient.
- An ideal vector would be safe, efficient (i.e. insert the gene into a large fraction of target cells), selective (i.e. lead to expression of the therapeutic protein but not of viral proteins) and would cause persistent expression of the therapeutic gene.
- Viral vectors include:
  — *Retroviruses*, which infect many different types of dividing cells and become incorporated randomly into host DNA.
  — *Adenoviruses*, genetically modified by deletions in the genome that make them unable to replicate and create space for the therapeutic transgene. They transfer genes to the nucleus but not to the genome of the host cell. Problems with current adenovirus vectors include a strong immune response, inflammation and short-lived expression. Treatment cannot be repeated because of neutralising antibodies.
  — *Adeno-associated virus*, which associates with host DNA, is non-immunogenic but is hard to mass produce and has a small capacity.
  — *Herpes virus*, which does not associate with host DNA but is very long-lived in nervous tissue and could therefore have specific applications in treating neurological disease.
  — Disabled versions of *human immunodeficiency virus* (*HIV*) which, unlike most other retroviruses infects non-dividing cells including neurons.
- Non-viral vectors include:
  — A variant of liposomes (Ch. 4), made using positively charged lipids and called '*lipoplexes*'.
  — *Biologically erodable microspheres* (see Ch. 4) hold out a possibility of orally active gene therapy.
  — Plasmid DNA itself ('*naked DNA*'), can access the nucleus and be expressed, albeit much less efficiently than when it is packaged in a vector. It is being used to develop new vaccines.
- Once transferred, it will be essential, for many uses, for the activity of the therapeutic gene to be *controlled*. One promising approach to this is to use a tetracycline-inducible expression system.

how difficult this was going to be that diverted attention from the haemoglobinopathies (which were the first projected targets of gene therapy). Correction of these disorders demands an appropriate *balance* of alpha and beta globin chain synthesis in addition to synthesis of wild type rather than mutant polypeptide. For this and for many other potential applications more or less precisely controlled gene expression will be essential. It has not yet proved possible to control transgenes in human recipients, but there are potential ways of achieving this. One hinges on the use of a tetracycline-inducible expression system. This was first applied in cultured cells but has recently been extended to the mouse in vivo. Myoblasts were engineered for doxycyclin-inducible and skeletal-muscle-specific expression of *erythropoietin* by using two retroviral vectors. After intramuscular injection of these cells, the transgene became detectable in skeletal muscle of the recipient, and it proved possible to switch erythropoietin production (and consequently the haematocrit) in the mouse on or off by treatment with doxycyclin over a period of several months (Fig. 50.2). To carry this strategy further, it will be necessary to discover ways whereby *physiological* stimuli can control expression of the therapeutic gene. This will clearly be a great deal more difficult for situations where very rapid responses (e.g. to changing blood glucose in a diabetic) are needed.

SAFETY

In addition to safety concerns specific to any particular therapy (e.g. polycythaemia, thrombosis and hypertension from overexpression of erythropoietin; see above and Fig. 50.2), a number of concerns relate generally to the use of viral vectors. These are selected to be non-pathogenic for humans, or modified to render them non-pathogenic, but there is a concern that such agents could acquire virulence during use. Viral proteins may be expressed that are immunogenic and can elicit an inflammatory response, which is harmful in some situations (e.g. in the airways in patients with cystic fibrosis). Viruses such as retroviruses that insert randomly into host DNA could damage the genome and interfere with the protective mechanisms that normally regulate the cell cycle (see Ch. 42). Consequently, if they happen to disrupt an essential function this could, at least theoretically, increase the risk of malignancy. The limited clinical experience to date has generally been reassuring, and has not so far provided evidence of general problems.

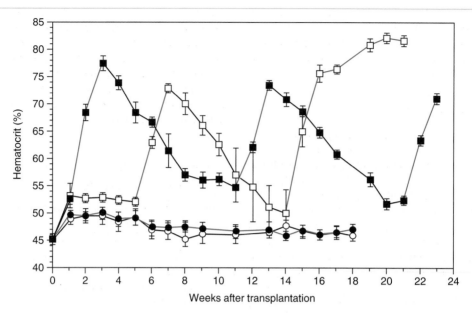

Figure 50.2 **Control of erythropoietin secretion by doxycycline in mice transplanted with myoblasts containing an erythropoietin transgene with (squares) or without (circles) a second transgene that confers doxycyclin-inducibility.** Intermittent administration of doxycycline via drinking water turned on the secretion of erythropoietin in the animals that had received the doxycycline-inducibility gene, and hence increased haematocrit, over a 5-month period. (From: Bohl D, Naffakh N, Heard J M 1997 Nature Med 3: 299–305)

Safety

- There are safety concerns specific to any particular therapy (e.g. polycythaemia from overexpression of erythropoietin), and additional general concerns relating, for example, to vectors.
- Viral vectors:
  — might acquire virulence during use
  — viral proteins may be immunogenic
  — can elicit an inflammatory response
  — could damage the host genome and interfere with the cell cycle; this could, at least theoretically, increase the risk of malignancy.
- The limited clinical experience to date has generally been reassuring, and has not so far provided evidence of insurmountable general problems.

THERAPEUTIC ASPECTS

SINGLE GENE DEFECTS

Single gene disorders are individually relatively uncommon. As mentioned above, the haemoglobinopathies were the first projected targets of gene therapy (in the 1980s), but early attempts were put on 'hold' because of the problem posed by the need to control precisely the expression of the genes encoding the different polypeptide chains of the haemoglobin molecule. The focus shifted to a rare genetic disorder called *adenine deaminase deficiency* which results in severe combined immunodeficiency. This led to the first *therapeutic* gene transfer protocol to be approved by the National Institutes of Health. It was hoped that expression of the gene for the deficient enzyme in any amount would be therapeutically beneficial in this disorder, and in one patient there is anecdotal evidence of at least partial success, although interpretation is clouded by the ongoing therapeutic use of infusions of the deficient enzyme. Tight regulation of therapeutic protein biosynthesis may not be essential in some other disorders (e.g. cystic fibrosis and the haemophilias). Attempts at gene therapy for these and for other single gene disorders continue: protocols that have been approved for clinical trials by the recombinant DNA advisory committee include alpha$_1$-antitrypsin deficiency (which causes chronic lung disease), chronic granulomatous disease (an X-linked disease in which neutrophils malfunction), familial hypercholesterolaemia (see Ch. 16), Duchenne muscular dystrophy (another X-linked disease, in which affected boys become progressively disabled) and various lysosomal storage disorders including Gaucher's disease and Hunter's syndrome (in which abnormal lipids or mucopolysaccharides accumulate in various organs).

GENE THERAPY FOR CANCER

Approximately half of all current clinical gene therapy research is on cancer. The first gene transfer experiment to be approved by the National Institutes of Health was a non-therapeutic protocol in the late 1980s designed to introduce a marker gene (conferring resistance to an analogue of neomycin) into a class of lymphocytes that infiltrate various tumours ('tumour infiltrating lymphocytes'). Gene transfer was performed ex vivo, and the cells reinjected into the patient in order to track their subsequent redistribution. This strategy has been useful in tracking other cells and hence identifying the cause of relapse following bone marrow transplantation for various leukaemias. Various therapeutic approaches are under investigation: there is excellent evidence from animal models for the potential usefulness of several of these, but experience with conventional antineoplastic drugs (Ch. 42) cautions against extrapolation to the clinical situation. Promising approaches include restoring protective mechanisms such as p53; inactivating oncogene expression (e.g. by a retroviral vector bearing a construct that produces an antisense transcript RNA to the K-*ras* oncogene; see below); delivering a gene (e.g. that encoding thymidilate kinase, *tK*) to malignant cells thus rendering them sensitive to drugs, such as ganciclovir, that are activated by tK; delivery of proteins to healthy host cells in order to protect them (e.g. addition of the multidrug resistance channel—see Ch. 42—to bone marrow cells ex vivo thereby rendering them resistant to drugs used in chemotherapy and protecting the patient from the neutropenia and thrombocytopenia that is otherwise predictably caused by such treatment); tagging cancer cells with genes (e.g. for antigens such as HLA-B7 or cytokines such as granulocyte-macrophage colony-stimulating factor—GMCSF—and interleukin-2) that when expressed render malignant cells more visible to the immune system of the host and trigger a vigorous defensive response. Gap junctions between malignant cells may help to propagate the desired effect from cells that have taken up the therapeutic gene to neighbouring cells. Among studies using these approaches are ongoing clinical trials in head and neck cancer involving injection into the tumour of recombinant adenoviral vectors containing the human p53 gene, and trials in glioblastoma (a brain tumour that

affects 4000–5000 people in the UK each year) involving herpes virus vectors carrying a gene to activate a prodrug. The most clinically advanced program for glioblastoma currently is a phase III trial using a retroviral vector encoding the herpes simplex virus *tK* gene, which is administered into the tumour at the time of surgery and may render the tumour susceptible to drugs such as ganciclovir—see above.

> **Gene therapy for cancer**
>
> Promising approaches include:
>
> - restoring protective mechanisms such as p53
> - inactivating oncogene expression
> - delivering a gene to malignant cells thus rendering them sensitive to drugs
> - delivery of a gene to healthy host cells to protect them from chemotherapy
> - tagging cancer cells with genes that make them immunogenic.

GENE THERAPY AND INFECTIOUS DISEASE

In addition to the approaches to vaccine development using naked DNA mentioned above, there is considerable interest in the potential of gene therapy for HIV infection and AIDS. Currently, approximately 10% of all clinical gene therapy research is focused on this area. The objectives are to stop HIV replicating in infected cells and to prevent it from spreading to uninfected cells, ideally by rendering stem cells (which differentiate into immune cells) resistant to HIV before they mature. Various strategies are under investigation including the use of genes that code for variants of HIV-directed proteins that serve as blocking agents (so-called 'dominant-negative' mutations, e.g. *REV* which began clinical testing in 1995), RNA decoys and soluble forms of CD4 (the cellular receptor whereby HIV gains access to lymphocytes; Ch. 44) that will bind, and hopefully inactivate, HIV extracellularly.

OTHER GENE-BASED APPROACHES

So far, we have largely been considering the addition of whole genes, but there are other, related nucleic acid-based therapeutic strategies. One is to attempt to *correct* a gene that has been altered by mutation; this has the enormous theoretical advantage that the corrected gene would remain under physiological control, avoiding the problems discussed above in the section on controlling gene expression. This approach is in its infancy and is beyond the range of this textbook.

Other therapeutic approaches that are in effect gene therapies are conventionally excluded from this terminology. These include organ transplantation to correct a gene deficiency (e.g. liver transplantation to correct LDL receptor deficiency in homozygous familial hypercholesterolaemia; Ch. 16) or the use of conventional drugs to alter gene expression (e.g. the use of hydroxyurea to increase the expression of γ-chain globin and hence increase foetal haemoglobin and ameliorate the severity of sickle cell anaemia).

Another method, known as the 'antisense oligonucleotide' approach—which we describe briefly here—has enormous theoretical appeal. This consists of the use of short (15–25) sequences of nucleotide bases (oligonucleotides) that are complementary to part of a gene or gene product that it is desired to inhibit. These snippets of genetic material can be designed to influence the expression of a gene either by forming a triplex (three-stranded helix) with a regulatory component of chromosomal DNA, or by complexing a region of messenger RNA. Oligonucleotides can cross plasma and nuclear membranes by endocytosis as well as by direct diffusion, despite their molecular size and charge. However, there are abundant enzymes that cleave foreign DNA in plasma and in cell cytoplasm so methylphosphorate analogues have been synthesised in which a methyl group substitutes for an oxygen atom in the nucleotide backbone. Another approach is the use of phosphothiorate analogues in which a negatively charged sulphur atom substitutes for an oxygen (so called 'S-oligomers'). This increases water solubility as well as conferring resistance to enzymic degradation. The oligomer needs to be at least 15 bases long to confer specificity and tight binding. Following parenteral administration, such oligomers distribute widely (although not to the central nervous system) and work in part by interfering with the transcription of mRNA and in part by stimulating its breakdown by ribonuclease H which cleaves the bound mRNA. This approach is being investigated in clinical studies in patients with viral disease (including HIV infection) and malignancy (including the use of *BCL-2* antisense therapy administered subcutaneously in patients with non-Hodgkin lymphoma).

Other gene-based approaches

- Correction of a gene that has been altered by mutation would be ideal. This is in its infancy.
- '*Antisense oligonucleotides*' are short (15–25) sequences of nucleotide bases (oligonucleotides) that are complementary to part of a gene or gene product that it is desired to inhibit. They influence the expression of a gene either by forming a triplex (three-stranded helix) with a regulatory component of chromosomal DNA, or by complexing a region of messenger RNA.
- Oligonucleotides can cross plasma and nuclear membranes, but there are abundant enzymes that cleave foreign DNA so water-soluble methylphosphorate or phosphothiorate analogues that are resistant to enzymic degradation are used.
- This approach is being used in clinical trials in HIV infection and malignancy.

REFERENCES AND FURTHER READING

The 'Scientific American' published an issue devoted to gene therapy in June 1997 which is an excellent introduction, including articles by T Friedmann (on 'overcoming the obstacles to gene therapy'), P L Felgner (on non-viral strategies for gene therapy), R M Blaese (on gene therapy for cancer) and by D Y Ho and R M Sapolsky (on gene therapy for the nervous system).

Askari F K, McDonnell W M 1996 Antisense-oligonucleotide therapy. N Engl J Med 334: 316–318

Blau H M, Springer M L 1995 Gene therapy—a novel form of drug delivery. N Engl J Med 333: 1204–1207 (*Succinct molecular pharmacological view*)

Blau H M, Springer M L 1995 Muscle-mediated gene therapy. N Engl J Med 333: 1554–1556

Brenner M K 1996 Gene transfer to hematopoietic cells. N Engl J Med 335: 337–339 (*Pluripotent stem cells could provide stable populations of genetically altered cells within each haematopoietic lineage*)

Channon K M, George S E 1997 Improved adenoviral vectors: cautious optimism for gene therapy. Q J Med 90: 105–109 (*'Second generation' adenoviral vectors with the potential for long-term transgene expression with little or no chronic inflammatory response*)

Docherty K 1997 Gene therapy for diabetes mellitus. Clin Sci 92: 321–330 (*Reviews experimental approaches to engineering glucose-responsive B cell and non-B cell lines, and in vivo transfer of the insulin gene in animals*)

Friedmann T 1996 Human gene therapy—an immature genie, but certainly out of the bottle. Nature Med 2: 144–147 (*Commentary on the mood swings of the gene therapy community by a founding father*)

Leiden J M 1995 Gene therapy—promise, pitfalls and prognosis. N Engl J Med 333: 871–872 (*Editorial discussing two negative trials in the same issue, one on adenoviral vector mediated gene transfer in cystic fibrosis, pp 823–831, and the other, pp 832–838, on myoblast transfer in the treatment of*

Duchenne muscular dystrophy)

Matteucci M D, Wagner R W 1996 In pursuit of antisense. Nature 384 (suppl): 20–22 *(First generation antisense oligodeoxynucleotides (ODNs) are undergoing clinical trial in HIV and CMV infections, various malignancies and to prevent restenosis after balloon angioplasty; also discusses second and third generation phosphothiorate and other modifications of ODNs)*

Verma I M, Somia N 1997 Gene therapy—promises, problems and prospects. Nature 389: 239–242 *(The authors, from the Salk Institute, describe the principle of putting corrective genetic material into cells to alleviate disease, the practical obstacles to this, and the hopes that better delivery systems will overcome these.*

Weichselbaum R R, Kufe D 1997 Gene therapy of cancer. Lancet 349 (suppl II): 10–12 *(Discusses vectors, selective transgene expression and transduction, therapeutic genes, immunogene therapy, gene replacement, transfer of resistance to cytotoxic therapy and clinical trials)*

Wilson J M 1996 Adenoviruses as gene-delivery vehicles. N Engl J Med 334: 1185–1187 *(Briefly reviews the development of adenovirus as vector for the CFTR gene which is defective in patients with cystic fibrosis, and the problems that result from immune responses to such vectors)*

Appendix
Some important pharmacological agents

Students may feel overwhelmed by the number of drugs described in pharmacology textbooks. We would emphasise that it is more important to understand general pharmacological principles and to appreciate the pharmacology of the main *classes* of drugs than to attempt to memorise details of individual agents. Specific drugs are best learned about when they are encountered in the setting of general topics such as chemical transmission, in practical classes or (for therapeutic drugs) near the patient's bedside. The following list identifies examples of some of the more important pharmacological agents. It is *not* intended as a starting point to learning pharmacology, and we would caution against the approach of attempting to memorise lists of names and properties. The examples we provide here are divided into agents of primary and secondary importance. In some geographic areas one or another class of drug will have more or less importance (e.g. anthelminthics are very important in regions where schistosomiasis is common, less so in the UK), so these categories are meant only as a broad guide. The list includes not only drugs used therapeutically but also endogenous mediators/transmitters and certain important drugs used as experimental tools; these are shown in italics. A working knowledge of drugs in the 'primary importance' category, including effects and mode of action, and (for those used therapeutically) pharmacokinetic properties, side effects, toxicity and main uses should be built up gradually as they are encountered during training. For drugs in the second category, an awareness of the mechanism of action is usually sufficient, and also, where appropriate, an understanding of how they differ from those in the primary category.

The choice and prioritisation of drugs in clinical use is inevitably somewhat arbitrary, and local variations will be encountered (e.g. as to which ACEI or NSAID is stocked in the hospital pharmacy). If the student or doctor comes to these (e.g. when changing to a job in a new hospital) with a sound appreciation of *general* principles of pharmacology and of the specifics of the *classes* of the agents involved, he or she will readily be able to look up and understand the information needed about the specific agent favoured locally to use it sensibly. (Learning how to cope with change is one of the main educational objectives defined in the General Medical Council's recommendations on undergraduate medical training – 'Tomorrow's doctors'—and this is one example of its importance.)

The drugs are grouped broadly as in the chapters of the text, and may appear more than once in the lists.

Primary	Secondary
1. Pharmacological agents and cholinergic transmission	
Agonists	
acetylcholine	carbachol
suxamethonium (succinylcholine)	*nicotine*
	pilocarpine
Antagonists	
atropine	tropicamide
	pirenzepine
tubocurarine	atracurium
	α-bungarotoxin
	vecuronium
hexamethonium	trimetaphan
anticholinesterases and ( ) related drugs	
Neostigmine	edrophonium
	dyflos
	(pralidoxime—cholinesterase reactivator)

Primary	Secondary

2. Pharmacological agents and noradrenergic transmission

Agonists

adrenaline (epinephrine)	clonidine
noradrenaline (norepinephrine)	phenylephrine
isoprenaline (isoproterenol)	
salbutamol	

Antagonists

propranolol	atenolol
prazosin	metoprolol

Drugs affecting noradrenergic neurons

guanethidine	*tyramine*
	amphetamine
methyldopa	*cocaine*
	reserpine
	α-methyltyrosine
	imipramine
	phenelzine

3. Other peripheral mediators (5-HT, purines, peptides and nitric oxide) and agents related to them

Drugs acting on 5-HT receptors

5-hydroxytryptamine (5-HT, serotonin)	ergotamine
ondansetron	
methysergide	
sumatriptan	

Drugs acting on purinoceptors

adenosine	theophylline
ATP	
ADP	

Renin-angiotensin system

angiotensin	
captopril	
losartan	

Various peptides

bradykinin	*atrial natriuretic peptide (ANP)*
endothelin	calcitonin
oxytocin	*calcitonin gene-related peptide (CGRP)*
vasopressin	*cholecystokinin*
	neuropeptide Y (NPY)
	octreotide
	substance P
	vasoactive intestinal polypeptide (VIP)

Nitric oxide

nitric oxide (NO)
L-N^G-monomethyl arginine (LNMMA)

$L\text{-}N^G\text{-monomethyl arginine (LNMMA)}$

4. Local hormones, inflammation and allergy (including anti-inflammatory and immunosuppressant drugs)

Eicosanoids — **Leukotriene antagonists and 5-lipoxygenase inhibitors:**

		montelukast
prostaglandins		zileutin
thromboxanes	*eicosanoids*	
prostacyclin		
leukotrienes		

Cyclo-oxygenase inhibitors (NSAIDs)

aspirin
ibuprofen
indomethacin

Histamine and antihistamines

histamine	
mepyramine	terfenadine
	fexofenadine
ranitidine	cimetidine

Drugs used in gout

allopurinol	colchicine
	probenecid
	sulphinpyrazone

Immunosuppressant drugs

azathioprine	tacrolimus
cyclosporin	
methotrexate	
prednisolone	

Other disease modifying antirheumatic drugs:

auranofin
hydroxychloroquine
penicillamine
sulphasalazine

Other mediators

cytokines (e.g. interleukins)
platelet activating factor (PAF)
interferon beta

Primary	Secondary	Primary	Secondary

5. Drugs affecting the cardiovascular system

Anti-dysrhythmic drugs (Vaughan-Williams classification)

Class I: lignocaine	flecainide
Class II: atenolol	metoprolol
Class III: amiodarone	sotalol
Class IV: verapamil	
Unclassified: adenosine	
digoxin	

Anti-anginal drugs
Nitrates:
glyceryl trinitrate
isosorbide mononitrate

β-blockers: atenolol	metoprolol
Ca²⁺ antagonists:	
amlodipine	
nifedipine	diltiazem

Anti-hypertensive drugs
Thiazide diuretics:

bendrofluazide	hydrochlorothiazide

β-adrenocetor antagonists:
atenolol
ACEI and angiotensin II
(AT1 receptor) antagonists:

captopril	lisinopril
enalapril	trandolapril
losartan	irbesartan

Ca²⁺ antagonists:
amlodipine
nifedipine
α₁-adrenoceptor antagonists:

doxazosin	prazosin
	terazocin

Other vasodilators:

lisinopril	hydralazine
	minoxidil
	nitroprusside

Centally-acting drugs:

	methydopa
	moxonidine

Drugs used in heart failure and shock

Diuretics: frusemide	bendrofluazide
amiloride	
ACE inhibitors: captopril	
enalapril	
Cardiac glycosides: digoxin	
Drugs acting on catecholamine	
receptors:	dobutamine
	dopamine

Drugs used to prevent atherosclerosis

Statins: simvastatin	pravastatin
Fibrates: bezafibrate	gemfibrozil
Resins: cholestyramine	colestipol

6. Drugs used in haemostasis and thrombosis

Oral anticoagulants and antagonists
warfarin
vitamin K

Heparin and ( ) antagonists

heparin	(protamine)
low molecular weight heparins	
(eg tinzaparin)	

Antiplatelet drugs:

aspirin	dipyridamole
	prostacyclin
	ticlopidine

Fibrinolytic drugs and ( ) inhibitors
of fibrinolysis:

streptokinase	(tranexamic acid)
tissue plasminogen activator	

7. Drugs affecting the respiratory system

β₂ adrenoceptor agonists:

salbutamol	salmeterol
	terbutaline

Inhaled glucocorticoids:
beclomethasone
Inhaled muscarinic antagonists:
ipratropium
Xanthine alkaloids:
theophylline

Other inhaled drugs used
for asthma prophyaxis:

	cromoglycate

Leukotriene antagonists and
5-lipoxygenase inhibitors:

	montelukast
	zileutin

Antitussive drugs:

	codeine

8. Drugs affecting the kidney

Thiazide diuretics:

bendrofluazide	hydrochlorothiazide

Loop diuretics:

frusemide	bumetanide

K⁺-sparing diuretics:

spironolactone	triamterene
amiloride	

Osmotic diuretics:	mannitol
Carbonic anhydrase inhibitors:	acetazolamide
Vasopressin (V₂) agonist:	desmopressin

Primary	Secondary

9. Drugs affecting the gastrointestinal system

Ulcer-healing drugs:
H$_2$-receptor antagonists:

ranitidine	cimetidine

Proton pump inhibitors:

omeprazole	lansoprazole

Antibiotics for *Helicobacter pylori*
See section 30

Prostaglandin analogues:	misoprostol

Aluminium complexes:	sucralfate

Laxatives:
lactulose
senna

Antiemetics:
domperidone
metoclopramide
ondansetron

Emetics:

	ipecacuanha

Antidiarrheal drugs:

codeine	loperamide

**Drugs for inflammatory
  bowel disease**
sulphasalazine

Antispasmodics:	hyoscine
	cyclizine

10. Drugs affecting the endocrine pancreas

Hormones:

insulin	*amylin*
glucagon	*somatostatin*

Sulphonylureas:

tolbutamide	glibenclamide
	gliburide

Biguanides:
metformin

α-glucosidase inhibitors:	acarbose

Thiazolidinediones:	troglitazone

11. Thyroid hormones and anti-thyroid drugs

Hormones and precursors:

thyroxine	liothyronine
	iodine/iodide

Antithyroid drugs:

carbimazole	propylthiouracil
	radioiodine (^{131}I)

12. Obesity

	leptin
	neuropeptide Y

13. Anterior pituitary and adrenal glands

Glucocorticoids:
prednisolone
hydrocortisone
dexamethasone
Mineralocorticoids:
fludrocortisone

Pituitary hormones:	corticotrophin (ACTH)
	growth hormone
	somatostatin
	octreotide

14. Sex hormones and related drugs

Oestrogens:
oestradiol
Anti-oestrogens:

tamoxifen	clomiphene

Progestogens:

progesterone	norethisterone

Anti-progestogens:
mifepristone
Androgens:
testosterone
Anti-androgens:

cyproterone	finasteride

**Gonadotropin releasing hormone
  analogues:**

	buserelin

15. Drugs acting on the uterus

ergometrine
oxytocin
dinoprostone (PGE$_2$)

Primary	Secondary

16. Drugs and bone

parathyroid hormone (PTH)   calcitonin
vitamin D   calcium salts
oestrogen
etidronate

17. Haemopoietic system

Haematinic drugs:
ferrous sulphate
folic acid
vitamin B_{12}

Hormones and growth factors: erythropoietin
granulocyte colony-
   stimulating factor
   (GCSF)
granulocyte – macrophage
   colony-stimulating
   factor (GMCSF)
thrombopoietin

18. Chemical mediators in the central nervous system

Neurotransmitters and ( ) related drugs
  (see also lists 1- 3):
glutamate

NMDA   (ketamine – NMDA
   channel blocker)
(dizocilpine – NMDA
   channel blocker)

kainic acid
glycine   *(strychnine – glycine*
   antagonist)
GABA   *(baclofen – GABA_B -*
   receptor agonist)
(bicuculline – GABA_A-
   receptor antagonist)

Amines
noradrenaline
dopamine
5-HT
acetylcholine
histamine   melatonin

19. Neurodegenerative diseases

Parkinson's disease:
levodopa   selegiline
carbidopa   benztropine
bromocriptine amantadine
   apomorphine
   MPTP

Amyotrophic lateral sclerosis   riluzole

Alzheimer's disease: donepezil

20. General anaesthetics

Inhalational:
halothane   ether
enflurane
isoflurane
nitrous oxide

Intravenous:
propofol   etomidate
   ketamine
   thiopentone

21. Anxiolytic, hypnotic and related drugs

Benzodiazepines and ( ) antagonists
temazepam   nitrazepam
diazepam   lorazepam
   (flumazenil)

Barbiturates: amylobarbitone

Other: buspirone ($5HT_{1A}$
   receptor agonist)

22. Antipsychotic drugs

Classical:
chlorpromazine   fluphenazine
haloperidol   thioridazine

Atypical:
clozapine   risperidone
olanzapine   sulpiride

Primary	Secondary	Primary	Secondary

23. Drugs used in affective disorders

Tricyclic antidepressants:

amitriptyline — imipramine
mianserin

SSRIs:

fluoxetine — fluvoxamine
sertraline

MAOIs:

moclobemide — phenelzine
tranylcypromine

Atypical antidepressants:

— mianserin
maprotiline

Antimanic drugs ("mood stabilizers")

lithium — carbamazepine

24. Anti-epileptic drugs and centrally-acting muscle relaxants

phenytoin — phenobarbitone
carbamazepine — diazepam
valproate — clonazepam
ethosuximide
vigabatrin
gabapentin
baclofen

25. Analgesics and related substances

Opioids and ( ) antagonists:

morphine — fentanyl
codeine — methadone
pentazocine — diamorphine
(naloxone) — pethidine

Mild analgesics (see also under list 4):

aspirin
paracetamol

Other analgesic drugs:

— tramadol
carbamazepine
amitriptyline

Other compounds involved in nociception:

enkephalins and endorphins — *dynorphin*
substance P
capsaicin

26. Central nervous system stimulants and psychotomimetics

amphetamine — methylphenidate
cocaine — *MDMA ("ecstasy")*
caffeine — *LSD*
phencyclidine
strychnine
bicuculline
leptazol

27. Drug dependence and drug abuse

opiates (morphine, diamorphine) — Δ^9-tetrahydrocannabinol (THC)
nicotine
ethanol — *anandamide*
cocaine — solvents
benzodiazepines
amphetamine

28. Local anaesthetics and other drugs that affect Na$^+$ or K$^+$ channels

Local anaesthetics:

lignocaine — amethocaine
tetracaine

Selective Na$^+$-channel antagonists:

— *tetrodotoxin (TTX)*

K$^+$-channel antagonists

— *tetraethylammonium (TEA)*
4-aminopyridine
sulphonylureas (see list 10)

K$^+$-channel activators:

— *cromakalim*

29. Cancer chemotherapy

Alkylating agents and related compounds:

cyclophosphamide — lomustine
cisplatin

Antimetabolites:

cytarabine — fluorouracil
methotrexate — mercaptopurine

Cytotoxic antibiotics:

doxorubicin

Plant derivatives:

vincristine — etoposide
paclitaxel

Hormones and related drugs:

prednisolone
tamoxifen

Primary	Secondary

30. Anti-bacterial agents

Bacterial cell wall inhibitors:

benzylpenicillin	piperacillin
flucloxacillin	cefadroxil
amoxycillin	cefotaxime
vancomycin	ceftriaxone

Topoisomerase inhibitors:
ciprofloxacin

Folate inhibitors:

trimethoprim	sulphonamides

Bacterial protein synthesis inhibitors:

gentamicin	amikacin
tetracycline	
chloramphenicol	
erythromycin	clarithromycin

Anti-anaerobic drugs:
metronidazole

Antimycobacterial agents

isoniazid	ethambutol
rifampicin	streptomycin
pyrazinamide	dapsone

31. Antiviral agents

DNA polymerase inhibitors:

acyclovir	foscarnet
	ganciclovir
	tribavirin

Reverse transcriptase inhibitors:

zidovudine	didanosine
	zalcitabine

Protease inhibitors:
saquinavir

Immunomodulators: interferons

32. Antifungal drugs

Polyene antibiotics:

amphotericin	nystatin

Azoles:

fluconazole	miconazole

Antimetabolites: flucytosine

Others: terbinafine

33. Anitprotozoal drugs

Antimalarials:

chloroquine	pyrimethamine plus sulphadoxine
quinine	artemesenin
primaquine	

For *Pneumocystis pneumoniae*:
co-trimoxazole (high dose)

Amoebicidal drugs:
metronidazole

Leishmanicidal drugs: antimonials (eg stibogluconate)
pentamidine

Trypanosomicidal drugs: suramin
pentamidine

Toxoplasmocidal drugs: pyrimethamine-sulphadiazine

34. Anthelminthic drugs

Broad spectrum:	mebendazole
Round worm, threadworm:	piperazine
Schistosomes:	praziquantel
River blindness:	ivermectin

This Appendix is adapted from the Appendix in Dale M M, Dickenson A H, Haylett D G 1996 Companion to Pharmacology, 2nd edn. Churchill Livingstone, Edinburgh, with permission.

Index

Humoral factors/control
  coronary flow, 258
  immune response, *see* Antibodies
Huntington's disease, 512
Hydatid disease (echinococcosis), 740
  therapy, 741
Hydralazine
  in heart failure, 296
  in hypertension, 290
Hydrazide, *see* Isoniazid
Hydrocarbons, aromatic, receptor for, 83
Hydrochlorothiazide, 363, 364
  development, 359
  dose–response curves, 362
Hydrocortisone (cortisol), 416
  in depression, levels, 552
  use, 417
    in asthma, 347
Hydrolytic reactions, 81–2
Hydromorphone, 599
Hydroxocobalamin, 333, 334
  use, 335
25-Hydroxycholecalciferol (calcifediol),
    structure/synthesis, 456, 458
6-Hydroxydopamine, 156, 157
  amphetamine and effects of, 607
5-Hydroxyindoleacetic acid (5-HIAA), 165, 490
  in carcinoid syndrome, 173
  depression and, 552
Hydroxylation, ring, of tricylic antidepressants,
    558
3-Hydroxy-3-methylglutaryl-coenzyme A, *see*
    HMG-CoA; HMG-CoA reductase
    inhibitors
Hydroxyprogesterone/hydroxyprogesterone
    hexanoate, 442
11-β-Hydroxysteroid dehydrogenase, 425–6
5-Hydroxytryptamine (serotonin), 164–74, 490–2
  anxiety and, 537
  biosynthesis/degradation, 165, 490
  clinical conditions involving, 171–4
  in CNS, *see* Central nervous system
  depression and, 551, 552
  distribution, 164–5
  effects/actions/role, 165–6
  in neurotransmission, 104, 105
  nociception and, 488, 585
  schizophrenia and, 541–2
  uptake inhibitors, *see* 5-Hydroxytryptamine
    (re)uptake inhibitors
5-Hydroxytryptamine receptor(s) (in general/
    unspecified), 167–8, 491
  antagonists
    as anti-emetics, 378–9, 673, 681
    as antipsychotics, 542
    H₁-receptor antagonist as, 241
  classification/subtypes, 167–8, *see also*
      specific subtypes below
  in CNS, 491
  drugs (in general) acting on, 169
  LSD action, 490, 541, 612
5-Hydroxytryptamine receptor type-1, 167, 168,
    491
  in CNS, 491
  ergot alkaloids as antagonists and partial
      agonists of, 170
  type-1A, 167, 168, 491
  type-1A agonists, 167
    as anxiolytics, 492, 529, 537
    unwanted effects, 537
  type-1A antagonists, 167, 537
  type-1B, 167, 491
    agonists/antagonists, 167

type-1C, *see* 5-Hydroxytryptamine receptor
    type-2
type-1D, 167, 168, 491
  agonists, 167
  agonists, in migraine, 169, 172
  antagonists, 167
  partial agonist, 172
5-Hydroxytryptamine receptor type-2 (5HT₂),
    167, 168, 491
  antagonists (non-selective/unspecified), 169
    in carcinoid syndrome, 173–4
  antidepressant actions, 555, 556
  in CNS, 491
  type-2A, 167, 168
    agonists/antagonists, 167
    antagonists, vasodilator effects, 166
  type-2B, 167
    agonists/antagonists, 167
  type-2C (old classification=5HT₁C), 167
    agonists/antagonists, 167
5-Hydroxytryptamine receptor type-3 (5-HT₃),
    167, 168, 491
  agonists, 167
  antagonists, 167
    as anti-emetics, 169, 378–9
    as anxiolytics, 492, 538
  in CNS, 491
  vomiting and, 378
5-Hydroxytryptamine receptor type-4 (5-HT₄),
    167
  agonists, 167
    as prokinetics, 169
  antagonists, 167
5-Hydroxytryptamine receptor type-5 (5-HT₅),
    167
5-Hydroxytryptamine receptor type-6 (5-HT₆),
    167
5-Hydroxytryptamine receptor type-7 (5-HT₇),
    167
  agonists/antagonists, 167
5-Hydroxytryptamine/noradrenaline uptake
    inhibitors as anxiolytics, 538
5-Hydroxytryptamine (re)uptake inhibitors
  in obesity, 407
  selective (SSRIs), 553, 554, 558, 558–9
    as anxiolytics, 538
    pharmacokinetics, 559
    unwanted effects, 554, 559
  tricyclic antidepressants as, 556, 557, 558
5-Hydroxytryptophan metabolism, 165, 490
Hydroxyurea, 679–80
25-Hydroxyvitamin D₃, *see* Calcifediol
Hymenolepsis nana, 739
Hyoscine (scopolamine), 119–20, 122
  effects, 121, 122
    anti-emetic, 378
    on learning/memory, 494
    unwanted, 378
Hyperactivity disorder, 609
Hyperaldosteronism, primary/secondary (Conn's
    syndrome), 418
Hyperalgesia, 581, 581–2
Hyperbola, rectangular, occupancy–drug
    concentration relationship producing, 6
Hypercalcaemia, 460
  management, 362, 462
Hypercholesterolaemia, 307
  endothelial NOS synthase and, 195
  familial, 752
    homozygous, 306
Hyperglycaemia
  β-blocker effects, 154–5
  in diabetes, 391

rebound, with insulin, 394
  glucocorticoid-induced, 423
Hyperkalaemia with ACE inhibitors, 292
Hyperlipidaemia/hyperlipoproteinaemia, *see*
    Dyslipidaemia
Hyperphosphataemia, 460
Hyperpolarisation in heart, 262
Hyperpyrexia/hyperthermia
  malignant, 129–30, 523, 751
  with salicylates, 235
Hyper-reactivity/hyper-responsiveness,
    bronchial, in asthma, 340–1
Hypersensitivity (allergic) reactions, 209–10,
    770–3, *see also* Allergy
  to antipsychotics, 547
  to penicillin, 693, 771
  type I (anaphylactic/immediate), 209, 771–2
    adrenoceptor agonists with, 152
  type II (cytotoxic antibody-dependent), 209,
    772
  type III (immune complex-mediated), 209,
    772
  type IV (delayed-type/cell-mediated), 209–10,
    772
Hypertension (intracranial), osmotic diuretics in,
    366
Hypertension (vascular), 293–5, *see also*
    Eclampsia
  causes
    antidepressants, 561
    oral contraceptives, 448
  diabetes and co-existing, 392
  drugs treating, *see* Antihypertensives
  portal, 287
Hyperthermia, *see* Hyperpyrexia
Hyperthyroidism (thyrotoxicosis), 431
  drugs used in, 155, 432–4, 434
  oral anticoagulant potentiation in, 317
  signal transduction affected in, 752
Hypertonicity in renal medulla, 357
Hypertrophic pyloric stenosis, 193, 196
Hyperuricaemia, *see* Gout
Hypnotics, *see* Anxiolytic agents
Hypnozoites, plasmodial, 726, 727
  drugs acting against, 733
Hypoaldosteronism, 320
Hypocalcaemia, 460
Hypoglycaemia
  with β-blockers, 155
  with insulin, 394
  with sulphonylureas, 396
Hypoglycaemic agents, oral, 359, 393, 394–7
  development, 359
  structure, 396
Hypokalaemia with loop diuretics, 363
Hypokinesia in Parkinson's disease, 508
  levodopa effects, 510–11
Hypoparathyroidism, 461
Hypoperfusion, *see* Shock
Hypophosphataemia, 460
Hypotension, 297–9
  levodopa causing, 511
  loop diuretics causing, 363
  MAO inhibitors causing, 561
  morphine-like drugs causing, 596
  NO in
    donor of, in treatment, 195, 196
    role, 192
  post-exercise, ganglion blocking drugs
      causing, 124
  postural/orthostatic
    antipsychotics causing, 547
    ganglion blocking drugs causing, 124